Vascular and Endovascular Surgical Techniques

Fourth edition

Vascular and Endovascular Surgical Techniques

Fourth edition

Edited by

Roger M Greenhalgh MA, MD, MChir, FRCS

Associate Editors

Jean-Pierre Becquemin MD
Alun Davies DM, FRCS
Peter Gaines MRCP, FRCR
Peter Harris MD, FRCS
Krassi Ivancev MD, PhD
Adam Mitchell MB BS, FRCAS, FRCR
Dieter Raithel MD, PhD

W.B. SAUNDERS

London • Edinburgh • New York • Philadelphia • St Louis • Sydney • Toronto 2001

WB SAUNDERS
An imprint of Harcourt Publishers Limited

This book is printed on acid-free paper

Fourth edition published 2001

ISBN 0 7020 2643 3

British Library Cataloguing in Publication Data
A catalogue record for this book is available from the British Library

Library of Congress Cataloging in Publication Data
A catalog record for this book is available from the Library of Congress

Note
Medical knowledge is constantly changing. As new information becomes available, changes in treatment, procedures, equipment and the use of drugs become necessary. The editors, contributors and the publishers have taken care to ensure that the information given in this text is accurate and up to date. However, readers are strongly advised to confirm that the information, especially with regard to drug usage, complies with the latest legislation and standards of practice.

Existing UK nomenclature is changing to the system of Recommended International Nonproprietary Names (rINNs). Until the UK names are no longer in use, these more familiar names are used in this book in preference to rINNs, details of which may be obtained from the British National Formulary.

Commissioning Editor: Sue Hodgson
Project Development Manager: Paul Fam
Project Manager: Jane Duncan
Project Controller: Nora Naughton
Designer: Andy Chapman
Cover illustration: Lynne Larson, MA, CMI

Typeset by Phoenix Photosetting, Chatham, Kent
Printed and bound in Great Britain at The Bath Press, Bath

The Publisher's policy to use paper manufactured from sustainable forests

Contents

Section 9: OPEN VISCERAL AND RENAL ARTERIAL TECHNIQUES

Section 10: ENDOVASCULAR RENAL ARTERIAL TECHNIQUES

Section 11: OPEN TECHNIQUES FOR AORTIC ANEURYSM

Section 12: OPEN ABDOMINAL AORTIC PROCEDURES

Section 13: TECHNIQUES FOR MANAGEMENT OF PROSTHETIC GRAFT INFECTION

Section 14: EXTRA-ANATOMIC OPEN VASCULAR TECHNIQUES

Section 15: ENDOVASCULAR STENT-GRAFT TECHNIQUES FOR ABDOMINAL AORTIC ANEURYSM

A: Investigations

B: Highlights of commercially available stent-graft systems

C: Special difficulties

Section 16: UPPER LIMB OPEN VASCULAR TECHNIQUES

Section 17: UPPER LIMB ENDOVASCULAR TECHNIQUES

Section 18: LOWER LIMB OPEN VASCULAR TECHNIQUES

Section 19: LOWER LIMB ENDOVASCULAR TECHNIQUES

Section 20: AMPUTATIONS

Contributors

Andros G, MD
Section of Vascular Surgery
Hospital of the Good Samaritan
Los Angeles
California, USA

Ascer E, MD
Vascular Surgery
Maimonides Medical Center
Brooklyn
New York, USA

Baird RN, ChM, FRCS
Consultant Surgeon
Bristol Royal Infirmary
Bristol, UK

Bansal V
Division of Vascular Surgery
The Union Memorial Hospital
Baltimore, Maryland, USA

Barbar SA, MB BS, FCPS(Radiology), FPCR
Specialist Registrar
Royal Free Hospital
London, UK

Barros D'Sa AAB, OBE, MD, FRCS, FRCSEd
Hon Professor of Vascular Surgery
The Queen's University of Belfast
Consultant Vascular Surgeon
Royal Victoria Hospital
Belfast, N Ireland, UK

Bates MC, MD, FACC
Senior Scientist,
Cardiovascular Research Camcare
Health Education
and Research Institute;
Clinical Professor in Medicine,
Robert C Byrd Health Sciences Centre;
Director Circulatory Dynamics
Laboratory, CAMC, Charleston, WV;
Clinical Professor in Medicine, Marshal
University, Huntington, WV, USA

Becquemin J-P, MD
Department of Vascular Surgery
Henri Mondor Hospital
AP/HP Paris
University Paris XII
Creteil, France

Beebe HG, MD
Clinical Professor of Surgery
University of Michigan Medical School
Director, Jobst Vascular Center
Toledo, Ohio, USA

Bell PRF, MB, ChB, FRCS (Eng), FRCS (Glasgow), MD
Professor of Surgery
Faculty of Medicine & Biological Sciences,
Robert Kilpatrick Building
Leicester Royal Infirmary
Leicester, UK

Benedetti-Valentini F, MD
Professor of Vascular Surgery
Chairman 2nd Department of Vascular Surgery
Policlinico Umberto 1
"La Sapienza" University of Rome
Rome, Italy

Bensaïd Y
Clinique Chirurgicale D
CHU Avicenne
Rabat, Morocco

Bergan JJ, MD, FACS
Medical Director
Vein Institute of La Jolla
La Jolla, California
USA

Bergentz SE, MD
Department of Surgery
Lund University
Malmo General Hospital
Malmo, Sweden

Biasi GM, MD, FACS
Department of Vascular Surgery
Bassini Teaching Hospital
University of Milan
Cinisello Balsamo
Milan, Italy

Bleyn J, MD
Antwerp Blood Vessel Centre
Cogels-Osy
Berchem
Antwerp, Belgium

Bolia A, MBCh(Glasgow), DMRD, FRCR
Consultant Vascular Radiologist
University Hospitals of Leicester NHS Trust
Leicester Royal Infirmary
Leicester, UK

Bonvini S
Vascular Surgery Clinic
Padua University
Padua, Italy

Browse NL, MD, PRCS
Department of Surgery
St Thomas' Hospital
London, UK

Buckenham TM, MB, ChB, FRACR, FRCR
Professor, Department of Medical Radiology
The University of Edinburgh
The Royal Infirmary of Edinburgh
Edinburgh, UK

Burnand KG, MS, FRCS
Professor of Surgery
Guy's, King's & St Thomas's School of Medicine
St Thomas' Campus
London, UK

Cao PG, MD
Head, Division of Vascular Surgery
Policlinico Monteluce
Perugia, Italy

Chabert V
Service de Radiologie
CHU Rangueil
Toulouse
France

Chang BB, MD
Assistant Professor of Surgery
Institute for Vascular Health and Disease
Albany Medical College
New York
USA

Chuter TAM, MD
Associate Professor of Surgery in Residence
Division of Vascular Surgery
UCSF
San Francisco
California, USA

Clayton G, MRCS
Clinical Fellow
Department of Vascular Surgery
Imperial College School of Medicine
Charing Cross Hospital
London, UK

Cleveland TJ, FRCS, FRCR
Consultant Vascular Radiologist
Sheffield Vascular Institute
Northern General Hospital
Sheffield, UK

Cockett FB, MS, FRCS
Consulting Surgeon
St Thomas' Hospital
London, UK

Colonna M, MD
Department of Vascular Surgery
University Hospital of Rome
Cattedra de Chirurgie Vascolare
Dell'Universita di Roma
"La Sapienza"
Policlinico Umberto 1
Rome, Italy

Concina P
Service de Radiologie
CHU Rangueil
Toulouse
France

Coppi G, MD
Head, Division of Vascular Surgery
S Agostino General Hospital
Modena, Italy

Courbier R
Cardiovascular Surgery Division
Hôpital St Joseph
Marseille
France

Criado FJ, MD
Director, Center for Vascular Intervention
Union Memorial Hospital/MedStar Health
Baltimore, Maryland
USA

D'Addato M, MD
Chairman, Department of Vascular Surgery
Policlinico S Orsola
University of Bologna
Bologna, Italy

Darling RC III, MD
Head, Associate Professor of Vascular Surgery
Institute for Vascular Health and Disease
Albany Medical College
New York, USA

Davies AMA, DM, FRCS
Reader in Surgery
Charing Cross Hospital
London, UK

DeBakey ME, MD
Department of Surgery &
DeBakey Heart Center
Baylor College of Medicine
Houston
Texas, USA

Deriu G
Professor of Vascular Surgery
Vascular Surgery Clinic
Padua University
Padua, Italy

De Vries AC
St Antonius Hospital
Nieuwegein
The Netherlands

Diethrich EB
Medical Director
Arizona Heart Institute
Phoenix
Arizona, USA

Do-Dai-Do, MD, PD
Division of Angiology
University of Berne
Inselspital
Switzerland

Donayre C, MD
Department of Surgery
Harbor – UCLA Medical Center
University of California
Torrance
California, USA

Dulawa LB, MD
Vascular Laboratory
Saint Joseph Medical Center
Burbank
California, USA

Ehrenfeld WK, MD
Professor of Surgery
University of California at San Francisco
San Francisco
California, USA

Edwards RD, MRCP, FRCR
Consultant Interventional Radiologist
Gartnavel General Hospital
North Glasgow University Hospitals NHS Trust
Glasgow UK

Eikelboom BC, MD, PhD
Professor and Chief of Vascular Surgery
Division of Vascular Surgery
Department of Surgery G.04.232
University Hospital Utrecht
Utrecht
The Netherlands

Ellis H, CBE, DM, MCh, FRCS
Professor of Surgery
Division of Anatomy and Cell Biology
UMDS Guy's Hospital Campus
London, UK

Fadda GF, MD
Department of Vascular Surgery
University Hospital of Rome
Cattedra de Chirurgia Vascolare
Dell'Universita di Roma
"La Sapienza"
Policlinico Umberto 1
Rome
Italy

Faraglia V, MD
Dipartimento di Urologia
U Bracci
Universita degli Studi di Roma
"La Sapienza", Policlinico Umberto 1
Rome, Italy

Fiorani P, MD
Professor of Vascular Surgery
University Hospital of Rome
Cattedra de Chirurgia Vascolare
Dell'Universita di Roma
"La Sapienza"
Policlinico Umberto 1
Rome, Italy

Frigatti F
Vascular Surgery Clinic
Padua University
Padua, Italy

Gaines PA, MRCP, FRCR
Consultant Vascular Radiologist
Sheffield Vascular Institute
Northern General Hospital
Sheffield, UK

Gale SS, MD
Attending Vascular Surgeon
Jobst Vascular Center
Toledo, Ohio, USA

Gordon RL, MD
Division of Vascular Surgery
UCSF
San Francisco
California, USA

Greenfield LJ, MD
Chairman, Department of Surgery
University of Michigan Health System
Section of Vascular Surgery TC2210
Ann Arbor
Michigan, USA

Greenhalgh RM, MA, MD, MChir, FRCS
Professor of Surgery and Chairman
Department of Surgery
Charing Cross and Westminster Medical School
London, UK

Grego F
Vascular Surgery Clinic
Padua University
Padua, Italy

Griffin MB, DIC, MSc
Senior Ultrasonographer
Irvine Laboratory for Cardiovascular Investigation and Research
Department of Vascular Surgery
Imperial College School of Medicine
St Mary's Hospital
London, UK

Gupta SK, MD
Section Chief
Department of Surgery
Guthrie Clinic
Sayre, Pennsylvania, USA

Harris PL, MD, FRCS
Consultant in Vascular Surgery
Broadgreen Hospital
Liverpool, UK

Harris RW, MD
Vascular Surgeon
Vascular Laboratory
St Joseph Medical Center
Burbank
California, USA

Hartley DE, MD
Centre for Health Services Research
Department of Public Health
Clifton Street Building
University of Western Australia
Nedlands
Western Australia

Henry M, MD
Interventional Cardiologist
Co-Director, Polyclinique d'Essey
Essey-les-Nancy, France

Hollier LH, MD, FACS, FACC
Professor and Chairman
Department of Surgery
Mount Sinai School of Medicine
New York, USA

Horsch S, MD
Professor of Surgery
Academic Teaching Hospital Cologne-Porz; Chief, Vascular Surgical and Surgical Clinic
Krankenhaus Porz am Rhein
Cologne, Germany

Ivancev K, MD, PhD
Department of Diagnostic Radiology
Malmo University Hospital
Lund University
Malmo, Sweden

Jackson MJ, FRACS
Regional Vascular Unit
St Mary's Hospital
London, UK

Jackson JE, MRCP, FRCR
Department of Diagnostic Radiology
Hammersmith Hospital
London, UK

Jamieson C, MS, FRCS
Consulting Surgeon
St Thomas' Hospital London, UK;
Honorary Consultant Surgeon
Hammersmith Hospital and Royal Postgraduate Medical School
London, UK

Jausseran JM
Service de Chirurgie Cardio-Vasculaire
Hôpital Saint-Joseph
Marseille
France

Joffre F
Service de Radiologie
CHU Rangueil
Toulouse, France

Jicha DL, MD
Department of Surgery
University of California at San Francisco
San Francisco
California, USA

Katzen BT, MD
Medical Director
Miami Vascular Institute
Baptist Hospital
Miami
Florida, USA

Kessel DO, MD, MRCP, FRCP
Department of Radiology
St James's University Hospital
The Leeds Teaching Hospitals
Leeds, UK

Kieffer E, MD
Professor of Vascular Surgery
Service de Chirurgie Vasculaire
Groupe Hospitalier
Pitié Salpetriere
Paris, France

Kolvenbach R, PhD
Professor of Surgery
Department of Vascular Surgery
Augusta Hospital
Düsseldorf
Germany

Kopchok GE, MD
Department of Surgery
Harbor – UCLA Medical Center
University of California
Torrance, California , USA

Koul B, MD, PhD
Chief Surgeon
Cardiothoracic Surgery
Lund University Hospital
Lund
Sweden

Kretschmer G, MD
University Clinics of Surgery
University of Vienna
Vienna, Austria

Lane RJ, MS, FRCS, FRCSE, DDU, FRACS
Visiting Vascular Surgeon
The Royal North Shore Hospital
St Leonards
New South Wales, Australia

Lawrence-Brown MMD, FRACS
Consultant Vascular Surgeon
Mount Medical Centre
West Perth, Australia

Leather RP, MS FRCS, FRCSE, DDU, FRACS
Professor of Surgery
Albany Medical College
Albany, New York, USA

Lennox AF, MB BS, MSc, FRACS
Vascular Fellow
Royal Prince Alfred Hospital
Department of Surgery
University of Sydney
Camperdown
Sydney, Australia

Lepidi S
Vascular Surgery Clinic
Padua University
Padua, Italy

Lindh M
Department of Diagnostic Radiology
Malmo University Hospital
Lund University
Malmo, Sweden

McCollum CN, MD, FRCS
Professor of Surgery
University of Manchester
South Manchester University Hospital
Research and Teaching Building
West Didsbury,
Manchester, UK

Mahler F, MD
Professor of Internal Medicine
Division of Angiology
Inselspital,
Berne, Switzerland

Mannick JA, MD
Professor of Surgery
Harvard Medical School;
Department of Surgery
Brigham & Women's Hospital
Harvard Medical School
Boston
Massachussets, USA

Mansfield AO, ChM, FRCS
Professor of Surgery
St Mary's Hospital
London, UK

Massabuau P
Service de Radiologie
CHU Rangueil
Toulouse, France

May J
Endovascular Research Unit
Department of Surgery
Blackburn Building D06
University of Sydney
Sydney, Australia

Messina L, MD
Division of Vascular Surgery
UCSF
San Francisco
California, USA

Meites G
Service de Radiologie
CHU Rangueil
Toulouse, France

[†]Miller JH, MB BS, FRCS, FACS
[deceased]

Mingazzini P, MD
Associate Professor
Dipartimento di Medicina Sperimentale e Patologia
Universita "La Sapienza"
Rome, Italy

Moll FL, MD
Department of Surgery
St Antonius Hospital
Nieuwegein
The Netherlands

Moss JG, FRCS (Ed), FRCR
Consultant Interventional Radiologist
Gartnavel General Hospital
North Glasgow University Hospitals
NHS Trust
Glasgow, UK

Myhre HO, MD, PhD
Professor and Chairman
Department of Surgery
Trondheim University Clinic
Trondheim, Norway

Nachbur B, MD
Professor of Surgery Emeritus
University of Berne
Berne, Switzerland

Natali J
Membre des Academies Nationales de Chirurgie et de Medecine
Paris, France

Nicholson TA, BSc, MB ChB(Hons), MSc, FRCR
Consultant Cardiovascular Radiologist
Department of Radiology
Hull Royal Infirmary
Hull, UK

Nicolaides AN, MS, FRCS, FRCSE
Professor of Vascular Surgery
Irvine Laboratory for Cardiovascular Investigation and Research
Department of Vascular Surgery
Imperial College School of Medicine
St Mary's Hospital
London, UK

Niederle B, MD
University Clinics of Surgery
University of Vienna
Vienna, Austria

Oblath RW, MD
St Joseph Medical Center
Burbank
California
USA

Otal P
Service de Radiologie
CHU Rangueil
Toulouse
France

Parodi JC, MD
Director, Instituto Cardiovascular de Buenos Aires
Blanco Encalada
Buenos Aires
Argentina

Parvin S, MD, FRCS
Consultant Vascular Surgeon
Royal Bournemouth Hospital
Bournemouth, UK

Patel SC, MS
Division of Vascular Surgery
The Union Memorial Hospital
Baltimore,
Maryland
USA

Perry MO, MD
Professor Emeritus
Department of Vascular Surgery
University of Texas Southwestern Medical School
Dallas,
Texas, USA

Petitjean C
Clinique Alleray-Labrouste
Paris
France

Picchi G, MD
Chief, Section of Vascular Surgery
2nd Surgical Clinic
University of Padua
Padua
Italy

Platts AD, MD
Consultant Radiologist
Royal Free Hospital
London, UK

Proctor MC, MS
Department of Surgery
University of Michigan Medical School
Ann Arbor
Michigan, USA

Ragazzi R
Vascular Surgery Clinic
Padua University
Padua
Italy

Raithel D, MD, PhD
Professor of Surgery
Chief, Section of Vascular Surgery
Klinikum Sud Nurnberg
Vasculare und Endovasculare Chirurgie
Nurnberg, Germany

Ramos TK, MD
Department of Surgery
Creighton University
Omaha, USA

Reilly LM, MD
Division of Vascular Surgery
UCSF
San Francisco
California, USA

Reilly MK, PhD, MD
Department of Surgery
Division of Vascular Surgery
Texas Technical University
Health Sciences Center
School of Medicine
Lubbock, Texas, USA

Rich NM, MD, FACS
Chairman, Department of Surgery
F Edward Hebert School of Medicine
Uniformed Services University of the Health Sciences
Betheseda, Maryland, USA

Rizzo L, MD
I Cattedra di Chirurgia Vascolare
Dell'Universita di Roma
"La Sapienza"
Policlinico Umberto I
Rome, Italy

Robbs JV, ChM (CT), FRCSEd
Head of Department of Surgery
University of Natal Medical School
Durban, South Africa

Robertson I, MD
St James's University Hospital
The Leeds Teaching Hospitals
Leeds, UK

Robinson K, MS, FRCS
Consulting Surgeon
Chelsea & Westminster
Queen Mary Hospital
London, UK

Rose SS, FRCS
Consulting Surgeon
University Hospital of South Manchester
Manchester UK

Rossi P, MD
Professor of Radiology
"La Sapienza" University of Rome
Policlinico Umberto 1
Rome, Italy

Rousseau H
Professor of Radiology
Service de Radiologie
CHU Rangueil
Toulouse
France

Royle JP, MB BS, FRCS(Ed), FRCS, FRACS, FACS
Associate Professor of Surgery
University of Melbourne
Victoria,
Australia

Ruberti U, MD
Professor and Chief
Institute of General and Cardiovascular Surgery
University of Milan
Milan
Italy

Saether OD, MD
Department of Surgery
Trondheim University Clinic
Trondheim,
Norway

Sandmann W, MD
Professor of Surgery
Chief, Vascular Surgery
Heinrich-Heine University
Düsseldorf
Germany

Schneider E, MD
Division of Angiology
Department of Internal Medicine
University of Zurich
Zurich, Switzerland

Schneider PA, MD
Saint Joseph Medical Center
Burbank
California
USA

Scott J
Department of Radiology
St James's University Hospital
The Leeds Teaching Hospitals
Leeds, UK

Semmens JB, PhD
Director, Centre for Health Services Research
Department of Public Health
Clifton Street Building
University of Western Australia
Nedlands
Western Australia

Shah DM, MD
Director, Vascular Institute
Albany Medical College
Albany
New York, USA

Smedile G-L
Department of Vascular Surgery
Henri Mondor Hospital
AP/HP Paris
University Paris XII
Creteil
France

Soula P
Service de Radiologie
CHU Rangueil
Toulouse
France

Speziale F, MD
Department of Vascular Surgery
University Hospital of Rome
Cattedra de Chirurgia Vascolare
"La Sapienza"
Policlinico Umberto 1
Rome
Italy

Stancanelli V, MD
Head, Division of Vascular Sugery
S Maria delle Croci General Hospital
Ravenna
Italy

Stansby G, MChir, FRCS
Professor of Vascular Surgery
Northern Vascular Unit
Freeman Hospital
High Heaton
Newcastle-under-Lyme
UK

Stoney RJ, MD
Professor of Surgery
Department of Surgery
University of California at San Francisco
San Francisco
California, USA

Taurino M, MD
Department of Vascular Surgery
University of Rome
"La Sapienza"
Policlinico Umberto 1
Rome,
Italy

Taylor PR, MA, FRCS
Consultant Vascular Surgeon
Guy's Hospital Medical School
London, UK

Tealdi DG, MD
Associate Professor of Vascular Surgery
University of Milan
Milan, Italy

Teijink JAW
Department of Surgery
St Antonius Hospital
Nieuwegein
The Netherlands

Theorides T, MD
Department of Surgery
Section of Vascular Surgery
Utrecht University Hospital
Utrecht
The Netherlands

Thompson JE, MD, FACS
Attending Surgeon
Baylor University Medical Center
Dallas,
Texas, USA

Thompson JF, MS, FRCS(Ed), FRCP
Consultant Surgeon
Directorate of Surgery
Royal Devon and Exeter NHS Trust
Exeter, UK

van der Heijden FHWM, MD
Department of Surgery
Onze Lieve Vrouve
Gasthurs, Amsterdam
The Netherlands

van Reedt Dortland RWH, MD
Department of Surgery
Section of Vascular Surgery
Utrecht University Hospital
Utrecht
The Netherlands

Van Urk H, MD, PhD, FRCS(Ed)
Professor of Surgery
Department of Vascular Surgery
University Hospital Dykzigt
Rotterdam, The Netherlands

Vasquez O, BA
Division of Vascular Surgery
UCSF
San Francisco
California, USA

Veith FJ, MD
Professor of Surgery
Division of Vascular Surgery
Albert Einstein College of Medicine and Montefiore Medical Center
Bronx,
New York, USA

Wagner O, MD
Professor of Surgery
Krankenshaus der Barmherzigen Bruder
Chirurgische Abeteilung
Vienna, Austria

Watkinson A, MD, MB BS, FRCS, FRCR
Consultant Radiologist
Royal Free Hospital NHS Trust
London, UK

Weiyun Yu
Endovascular Research Unit
Department of Surgery
Blackburn Building D06
University of Sydney
Sydney, Australia

Wengerter KR, MD
Albert Einstein College of Medicine and
Montefiore Medical Center
Bronx, New York, USA

White GH
Endovascular Research Unit
Department of Surgery
Blackburn Building D06
University of Sydney
Sydney
Australia

White RA, MD
Chief Vascular Surgery
Associate Chairman
Department of Surgery
Harbor – UCLA Medical Center
University of California
Torrance
California, USA

Whitaker SC, MRCP, FRCR
Consultant Radiologist
Imaging Centre
Diagnostic Imaging Directorate
Queen's Medical Centre
University Hospital,
Nottingham UK

Whittemore AD, MD
Associate Professor
Harvard Medical School;
Surgeon
Brigham and Women's Hospital
Boston
Massachusetts, USA

Wolfe JHN, MS, FRCS
Consultant Vascular Surgeon and
Honorary Senior Lecturer
St Mary's Hospital Medical School;
Consultant Vascular Surgeon and
Honorary Senior Lecturer
Royal Postgraduate Medical School
Hammersmith Hospital
London, UK

Wunderlich M, MD RG
Department of Surgery
General Hospital
Hollabrunn
Austria

Yao JST, MD, PhD
Professor of Surgery
Northwestern University Medical
School
Department of Surgery
Wesley
Chicago
USA

Zarka ZA, MD MSc
Research Fellow
Irvine Laboratory for Cardiovascular
Investigation and Research
Department of Vascular Surgery
Imperial College School of Medicine
St Mary's Hospital
London, UK

Preface

Since the last edition there has been revolution after revolution. The first was the explosion of endovascular techniques which have provided an alternative to tried and trusted methods. At present there is insufficient evidence in terms of durability for us to be certain whether the endovascular methods are superior in the long term – but even if they are equivalent, the patient preference with smaller incisions and less pain, will drive us to favour the endovascular approach.

The second revolution is the thirst for evidence and proof that the interventions we perform are of definite benefit. It is chilling to learn that there is a 1% rupture rate per year following endovascular aneurysm repair according to EUROSTAR data. That same figure of 1% rupture rate per year was recorded in the UK small aneurysm trial in the surveillance arm where no surgery had been performed for aortas of an equivalent size. Therefore at this time we must stiffen our sinews and demand evidence for every intervention. Where there is no evidence or insufficient evidence more and more clinicians are looking for it.

The next welcome development has been more evolution than revolution. The collaboration which now exists in some parts of Europe in particular between vascular radiologists and vascular surgeons is highly commendable and certainly appreciated by patients. There is inevitably a turf war but it is certainly better for a patient if a vascular radiologist and a vascular surgeon discuss the complete range of managements and come to a rational decision based on current best evidence. The combination of skills is vital.

Finally, there is an escalation of technology to communicate continuing medical education. We now have PowerPoint presentations at meetings and cine and movie within PowerPoint presentations. CD-Rom has become a regular feature. This throws into question the value of an atlas such as this. The associate editors and I have approached this edition with that in view. Out has gone every chapter in which there is not an up-to-date message. In have come new endovascular and vascular chapters. We have retained some classics. Our view is that an atlas like this now has to compete not only with other atlases but also with other modalities which communicate continuing medical education. Nevertheless we feel that this atlas will find its place alongside the operating rooms in many of the leading vascular centres around the world. Surgeons in training will find it very helpful to look at the stages of procedures shown here. It has been an enormous pleasure to bring it together.

I am grateful to the publishing team at Harcourt, and Rosie Naylor, for help in preparation of this edition. Without them we would not have been able to produce the book on time.

R M Greenhalgh
March 2001

Planning the intervention

Roger M Greenhalgh

Introduction

Before a procedure is chosen, the vascular surgeon must always consider if the patient really requires an operative procedure at all. It is absolutely essential to be certain that the odds are very good that any operative procedure is likely to produce the desired effect. It takes much less time to learn a technique than to learn the indications for the application of the technique and when it is better not to intervene at all.

At first consultation, the patient and the referring doctor expect to learn the intentions of the vascular specialist. In order to give a sensible opinion, it is necessary to achieve accurate diagnosis at the first consultation which is achievable these days by improved non-invasive vascular imaging. Second, if an operation or operative technique is contemplated, it is important to know if the patient is fit for the procedure.

First consultation assessment

There is no substitute for a very careful history. It is vital to understand the patient's complaints and how these affect the quality of life relative to age and occupation. Patients with arterial disease are usually smokers over many years and may have concomitant arterial disease elsewhere. In the history it is important to establish if concomitant arterial disease is symptomatic and if the patient suffers from diabetes or hypertension.

The cardiac status is particularly important if a patient requires a general anaesthetic and operative procedure. More than half of patients with peripheral arterial disease have resting electrocardiographic changes indicating ischaemic heart disease and a greater number have abnormalities on the ECG after a period of exercise. At least 10% of patients with peripheral arterial disease are diabetic and more than 30% are likely to be hypertensive. It is important that hypertension is controlled from the point of view of reducing risk of stroke. In addition, the use of β-blocker drugs can exacerbate intermittent claudication and there are usually better alternative ways of controlling hypertension.

Complete physical examination is essential, recognizing the generality of arterial disease and the importance of the heart and chest in terms of mortality risk at operative procedures. Careful examination of a patient with an abdominal aortic aneurysm is vital and it should be noted if any pulsating and expansile swelling is tender. Peripheral pulses are graded normal 2, reduced 1 and absent 0. Patients with venous disease and venous ulceration must always be examined in the standing position in a good light. There it can be noted if there are obviously clinically incompetent long or short saphenous veins or obvious perforating veins on the medial or lateral aspects of the leg relating to any ankle ulcers.

1

Vascular imaging is now possible at first consultation. Ideally, colour coded duplex scanning is available close to the consultation area for patient convenience. Where necessary the arterial tree can be scanned from the diaphragm downwards including the iliac, femoral popliteal and proximal tibial vessels. From the history and physical examination, the clinician can indicate to the vascular technologist the expected diagnosis and appropriate imaging can be performed. The images are transferred ideally to a simple chart as shown. For suspected renal or visceral artery stenoses, images of these vessels can also be performed with the appropriate duplex probe.

Illustration 1 which shows a colour duplex scan of aorta, visceral, renal and peripheral arteries is an example of disease demonstrated at first consultation in a patient presenting with symptoms of peripheral arterial disease. The patient complained of bilateral buttock claudication and right calf claudication and the image shows

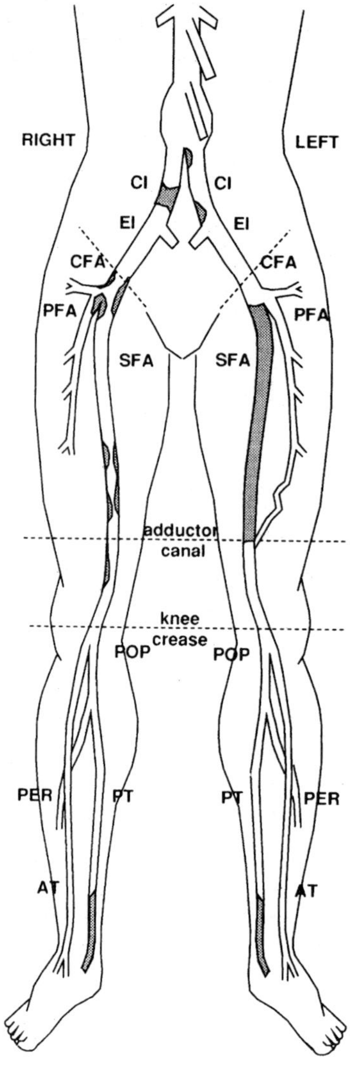

1

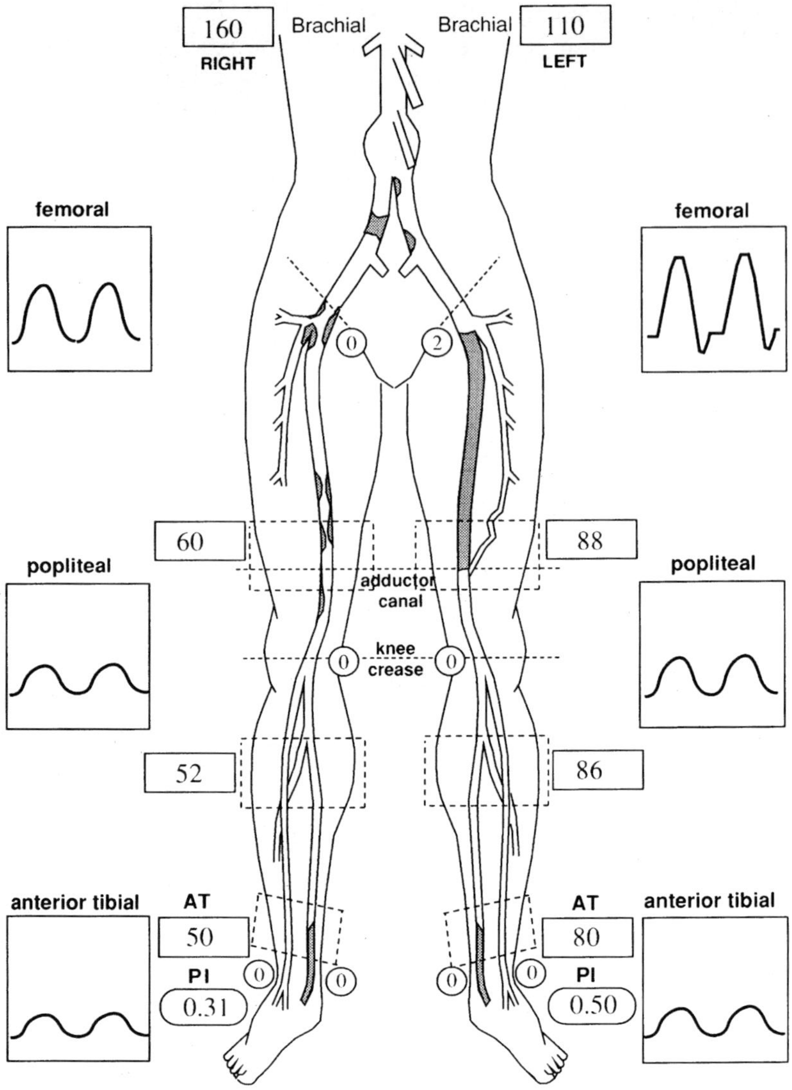

2

a 75% stenosis of the right common iliac and a 50% stenosis of the left common iliac artery with disease in more peripheral vessels, including a long occlusion of the left superficial femoral artery with already well developed collateral circulation. There is also evidence of early aortic dilatations, a small abdominal aortic aneurysm, which must be taken into account.

2

Illustration 2 shows palpable pulses, Doppler segmental pressures and velocity profiles of aorta, visceral, renal and peripheral arteries. Alongside the peripheral arterial image (1), it is useful to have segmental pressure readings and an opportunity to recall the pulse findings. The normal pulse is shown as 2, reduced pulse as 1 and absent pulse as 0. Pulses are felt at the femoral, popliteal posterior tibial and dorsalis pedis positions. On the chart are also indicated segmental pressure findings in the thighs, calves and ankles and waveforms of the velocity profiles are indicated. This provides additional numerical data relating to the severity of the disease whereas the Doppler imaging merely shows distribution of disease. It is still useful to express ankle pressures as a proportion of the right brachial pressure (pressure index, PI) and these are indicated on the chart also. For patients with a pressure index of >0.9, it is appropriate and more sensitive to use the 1 minute exercise test (Laing and Greenhalgh, 1980). After walking on a treadmill for 1 minute at 4 kilometres per hour on a 10 degrees slope, a fall of Doppler pressure of >30 mm of mercury indicates abnormality. This implies that somewhere between the ankle and infrarenal aorta, there is significant disease contributing to this fall of pressure with exercise. For patients with suspicious symptoms, normal pressures at rest and normal exercise tests, it is highly unlikely that they have significant arterial disease and the clinician should consider very carefully any possible alternative diagnosis, such as sciatica. Today such definitive assessments are at first consultation alongside the clinician. In Illustration 2 the right femoral pulse velocity waveform is monophasic or 'damped' which relates to the common iliac occlusion above and absent femoral pulse. The pressure readings in the right leg, 60, 52 and 50 mmHg respectively, are consistent with the scan finding or relatively little disease below the right groin. On the left, the femoral pulse velocity waveform is triphasic and normal and coincides with a normal feeling pulse.

3

For patients with asymptomatic carotid arterial disease, transient ischaemic attack, transient stroke, established stroke, progressing stroke or crescendo transient ischaemic attacks, it is appropriate to perform duplex scanning of the carotid and vertebral arteries at once. Also for patients with peripheral arterial disease, the carotid arteries are scanned for presence of asymptomatic arterial disease. It is now well within the compass of vascular technologists to scan accurately the carotid bifurcation, assess disease in the proximal common carotids and even using the appropriate probes, proximal subclavian and innominate vessels. The direction of blood flow in vertebral arteries is well within the compass of the investigation these days and retrograde flow in a vertebral in association with an occluded first part of the subclavian is picked up reliably at once. Transcranial Doppler can give further information about the middle cerebral artery, the whole of the circle of Willis, basilar artery and distal vertebral vessels but this is seldom required at first consultation.

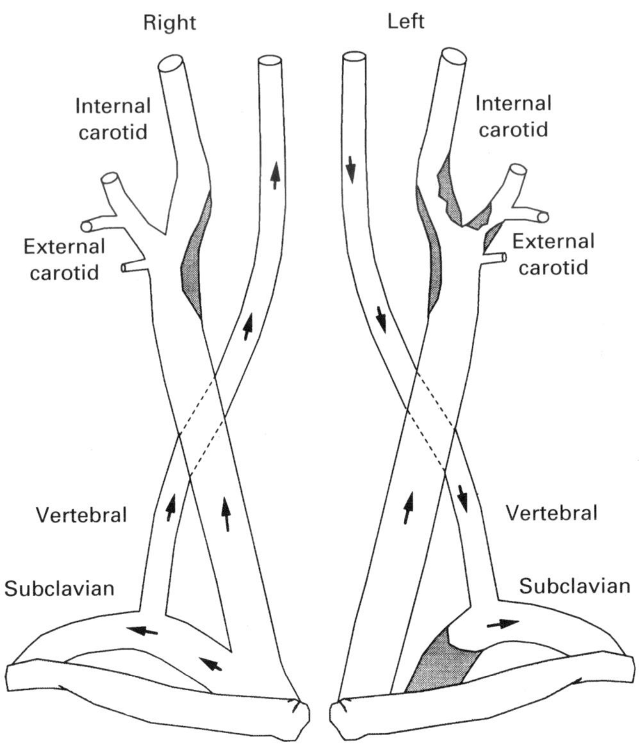

3

4

Approximately 10% of patients with intermittent claudication or symptomatic carotid artery disease have an abdominal aortic aneurysm by ultrasound (external diameter of >3 cm), (MacSweeney *et al.*, 1993). The abdominal aorta is scanned with simple B mode ultrasound at first consultation. The colour duplex scan can be used for this but a simpler B mode ultrasound scan is perfectly satisfactory. In this illustration an abdominal aortic aneurysm has been discovered at first consultation.

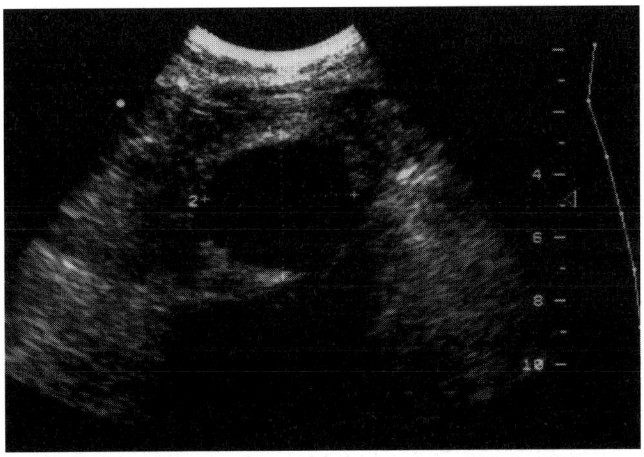

4

5

For patients with arterial disease, the Harp-Nasor classification of category and severity at first consultation is a useful summary. This can then be upgraded on future occasions. This classification stresses that for any patient with arterial disease there is likely to be concomitant disease elsewhere. The categories of disease are Heart, Aneurysm, caRotid and Peripheral (HARP). Within a category of disease are various severities Normal Asymptomatic Symptomatic Operation Recurrence. In the associated chart, it can be seen how the classification is used and encourages the clinician to think about arterial disease elsewhere and to note from time to time if there is progression of arterial disease in a particular category or whether another part of the body has become affected.

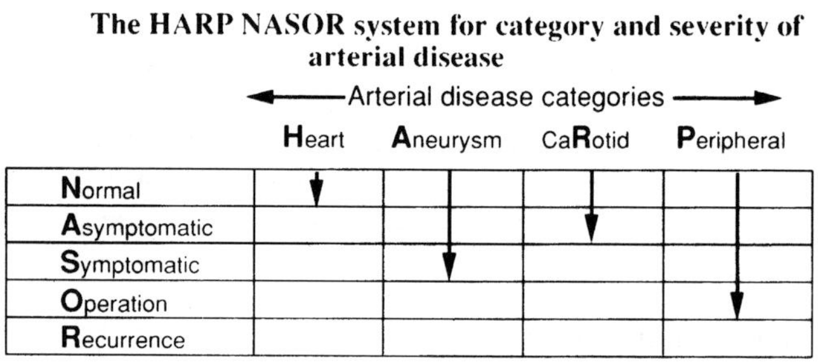

5

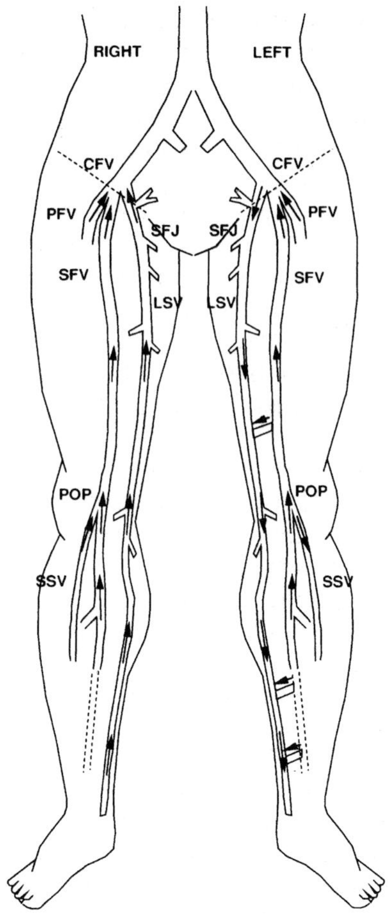

6

6

Venous scanning has become as sophisticated as arterial scanning and this chart shows the type of information which can now be available at first consultation. Colour duplex scan can follow the direction of flow and whether the deep veins are competent, incompetent or obstructed. It is possible to see with the colour code system, exactly where the blood passes through the deep fascia into the superficial system. Perforating veins can be marked accurately and sites of incompetence into the long and short venous system can be pin-pointed. This is particularly helpful for patients with venous ulceration or complex venous problems, such as complex recurrent varicose veins. The venous scans are most revealing and on many occasions, for patients who have had years and years of venous ulceration and previous surgery, it has been possible to remedy problems such as an incompetent vein coming from a medial or lateral aspect of a common femoral vein. The high pressure-blood can be traced on many occasions to immediately above where ankle ulceration of long-standing exists. With this careful pin-pointing of the underlying problem, it is possible to reduce the size of operation incisions to an absolute minimum and patients can be admitted on the same day as operations, sometimes discharged as day cases or at most kept overnight for 24 hours. Healing of most venous ulceration is the four-layer bandage technique used at the Riverside Venous Ulcer project (Moffatt *et al.*, 1992) and is achieved without hospital admission.

Contrast imaging of veins and arteries

Venography is required less and less these days and for patients with suspected venous thrombosis, colour duplex scan is ideal. The calf vein and pelvic veins can be scanned in rapid time. This is also a vital investigation for patients with suspected thromboembolism. In planning deep venous surgery, ascending and descending venography is still advocated by many and will be discussed in the appropriate chapter later in this Atlas. Arteriography and CT scanning can be performed as an outpatient procedure these days. Indications for arteriography vary somewhat in different parts of the world and some are moving towards avoiding arteriography for symptomatic carotid disease and relying entirely upon duplex scanning. Personally I am still persuaded that an arch flush angiogram with 5 French gauge catheter releasing a small amount of contrast from the arch of the aorta and using digital subtraction angiography produces excellent confirmatory visualization of the major vessels and intracranial views. It may be that we are close to abandoning some of these techniques for regular use but for the present, the majority of surgeons use contrast studies before planning surgery. There is no indication for translumber aortography today. Gone are the days when a patient needed to be admitted to hospital for a general anaesthetic and a needle was driven through the back for this outmoded procedure. Often the patient was not fit for the investigation but would have been fit to have limb and life saving procedures. It is remarkable that this procedure is still being practised.

Arteriography for aortic aneurysm is somewhat controversial, particularly as CT scans show such fine detail and can show exactly the upper and lower extremities and sometimes details of renal and visceral vessels. The intravenous digital subtraction angiogram is helpful, particularly for looking at the vessels off the aorta, enabling operation planning. Magnetic resonance imaging for all at affordable costs is awaited.

Decision of procedure for the patient and referring doctor

At first consultation it has been seen that a very precise diagnosis is possible. It should be communicated at once to the patient and the referring doctor. All of the benefit of this superb first consultation diagnosis is that the various options for management can be discussed. Endovascular procedures should always be preferred and applied where possible. These enable the patient to be admitted to hospital for the shortest possible period of time. They are cost-effective and are considered for lesser degrees of arterial disease for which a formal bypass would not be appropriate. If the only option is a full bypass, this should be considered against the patient's symptoms and the hospital stay expected and the age and condition of the patient. For an elective procedure, the patient should be asked to stop smoking before the elective procedure is undertaken. If the patient is at risk of stroke or bursting of aneurysm or has severe ischaemic rest pain, then of course the operation should go ahead nevertheless and the patient advised not to smoke. If the patient has mild intermittent claudication for example and an endovascular procedure or say femoropopliteal bypass is contemplated, then it is known that recurrence is more likely if the patient smokes (Wiseman *et al.*, 1990). Consequently, it is reasonable to expect the patient to stop smoking before the procedure is offered.

It is one of the great advances of vascular surgery in the last 5 years that instant diagnosis and imaging at the first consultation has become possible with the opportunity to discuss all options with a patient from the start.

Acknowledgement
Illustrations by Rachel Cuming.

References

Laing SP, Greenhalgh RM (1980). Standard exercise test to assess peripheral arterial disease. *Br Med J* **280**: 13.

MacSweeney STR, O'Meara M, Alexander C *et al.* (1993). High prevalence of unsuspected abdominal aortic aneurysm in patients with confirmed symptomatic peripheral or cerebral arterial disease. *Br J Surg* **80**: 582.

Moffatt CJ, Franks PJ, Oldroyd M *et al.* (1992). Community clinics for leg ulcers and impact on healing. *Br Med J* **305**: 1389.

Wiseman S, Kenchington G, Dain R *et al.* (1989). Influence of smoking and plasma factors on patency of femoropopliteal vein grafts. *Br Med J* **299**: 643.

Wiseman S, Powell JT, Greenhalgh RM *et al.* (1990). The influence of smoking and plasma factors on prosthetic graft patency. *Eur J Vasc Surg* **4**: 57.

Techniques of anastomosis

Roger M Greenhalgh

Introduction

The various techniques of anastomosis, or joining of blood vessels, fall into two main types: end-to-end anastomosis and end-to-side anastomosis. Various graft materials are preferred for bypass in different parts of the body and these are described in detail in subsequent chapters. For replacement of large vessels such as the aorta, Dacron has become the material of choice. Essentially, Dacron prostheses are of two main types, woven and knitted. The woven variety has the advantages that it does not require any preclotting of the Dacron and it does not leak blood. Its disadvantage is that it is rather stiff and when cut it frays. It is advisable to cut woven Dacron with an electric diathermy needle so that the ends are sealed, but this can be quite a tricky procedure compared with the precise cutting of a knitted Dacron graft which can be performed with scissors. The great advantage of knitted Dacron is that it can be shaped exactly as required but must be preclotted. Preclotting can be achieved by taking approximately 100 ml of blood from a nearby vein such as the vena cava and syringing it down through the graft so that the blood pours through the holes. The blood is then caught in a dish and syringed through the graft again and again with some pressure until the interstices become blocked by the clotting blood. The blood is then squeezed out of the Dacron which should be leak-proof and it is ready for anastomosis. To dispense with or minimize preclotting, collagen impregnation and albumen coating of Dacron has been introduced. An externally supported Dacron graft has gained much favour and may prove ideal in sites where it is important that the graft should not be squashed, such as for axillofemoral bypass.

Dacron is perhaps the material of choice for the replacement or bypass of arteries ranging in size from the aorta to the common femoral artery. Expanded polytetrafluoroethylene (ePTFE) is mainly used in long straight tubes for the replacement of smaller arteries than is deal for Dacron. However, a bifurcated graft of PTFE is now available to replace or bypass the aortic bifurcation; it does not require preclotting and is easy to work. Patients who are expected to have a PTFE graft should begin aspirin and dipyridamole 48 h before surgery to minimize postoperative graft thrombosis. It is an excellent graft material for femorofemoral crossover, axillobifemoral bypass and bypass of the femoral artery in the thigh.

Human umbilical vein does not require preclotting and remains an alternative to autologous vein for bypass from the groin to below the knee. It is also advisable to give aspirin and dipyridamole 48 h before the insertion of this graft as this is thought to reduce the risk of graft thrombosis.

Antibiotics and suture materials

When a prosthetic graft material is to be used it is advisable to commence prophylactic antibiotics either the day before surgery or at the time of the premedication 1 h before the operation. Some surgeons prefer to begin a day early, but virtually all would agree that it is essential to have satisfactory antibiotic levels in the blood at the time the graft material is implanted. The most threatening organism is *Staphylococcus aureus* and flucloxacillin is effective against this, but if this is used on its own there is a small risk of infection of the graft from Gram-negative organisms and it is, therefore, wise to combine ampicillin with flucloxacillin. Some prefer to use a cephalosporin prophylactic antibiotic which has anti-staphylococcal ability as well as providing cover for the Gram-negative organisms.

Fashions have changed for the choice of suture for vascular anastomosis. Only recently silk was in common usage but it is now used very rarely. It fragments after some time, but those who use it maintain that the strength of the anastomosis is in the healing of the graft to the vessel. Mersilene handles like silk; it is a braided material made of Dacron and so, in many respects, is ideal for anastomosing a Dacron graft to a large vessel. It has the advantages that is does not slip and it is easy to use. Polypropylene is a slippery monofilament suture which is without doubt the most commonly used suture material for vascular anastomoses. Using a double-ended atraumatic needle of polypropylene, great flexibility of anastomotic technique is achieved. A disadvantage of this material, however, is that when it is tied it slips and it is wise to place up to six knots to guarantee a secure anastomosis. The slippery quality of polypropylene can, however, be used to advantage; sutures can be left long and the graft slid down along their length before tying.

Lighting and magnification

It is essential to perform any anastomosis in good light. Not every operating room has an excellent lighting system and the best can be adjusted by the surgeon himself. The types which have sterile handles are the easiest to use, and at least two and preferably four lights, which can all be adjusted by the surgeon, are ideal. Few vascular surgeons have this facility. The absolute minimum is two good lights, but, all too frequently, it is not possible for the surgeon to adjust them himself. In such instances an alternative is for the surgeon to wear a fibre optic headlight. The best variety have a sterile adjuster so that once again the surgeon can direct the light exactly where it is required.

It takes time to adjust to any form of magnification but × 2.5 magnification with a simple loupe is easy to use. The focal length is usually about 50 cm but this can be varied according to the particular circumstances. For anastomoses to vessels of 2 or 3 mm diameter such as tibial vessels, this degree of magnification is essential. For smaller vessels of 1–2 mm diameter an operating microscope is required and a triploscope is ideal. This has a split beam, enabling the surgeon and assistant and a television camera to view the same work through one prism. Microvascular anastomoses require special training in a laboratory and should not be attempted in theatre by the novice surgeon.

All vascular anastomoses are either end-to-end or end-to-side. The different techniques described here are variations of end-to-end and end-to-side techniques. *It is a vital principle of all anastomoses, whether end-to-end or end-to-side, that the edges should always be everted. In this way the intima of the artery and lining of the graft material are brought into apposition.*

Techniques

End-to-end anastomosis of a graft to a large vessel

1

For an end-to-end anastomosis of large vessels (such as the aorta) it is convenient to use a polypropylene suture and place the first four or five sutures before pulling down the graft. This facilitates careful placement of the sutures in the back row. It is much easier to do this rather than to place anchoring stitches which make the subsequent adjacent suturing more difficult. It is important to take a deep bite of the posterior wall in the artery and pull it up into a ridge. It is not necessary to cut the vessel right across. Rather it can be cut approximately halfway to two-thirds across and opened like the leaves of a book. The posterior sutures are then placed long as shown.

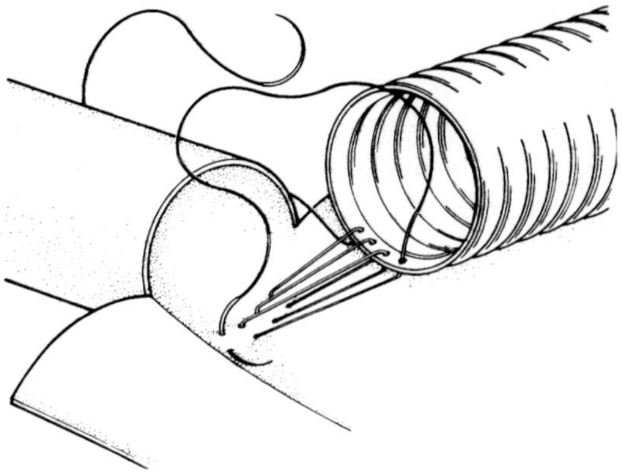

1

2

After the graft is pulled down the suturing is continued to the mid-point, the polypropylene sutures being pulled tight in opposite directions as suturing proceeds to avoid slippage. Slippage will lead to leakage around the back of the anastomosis which is difficult to correct subsequently.

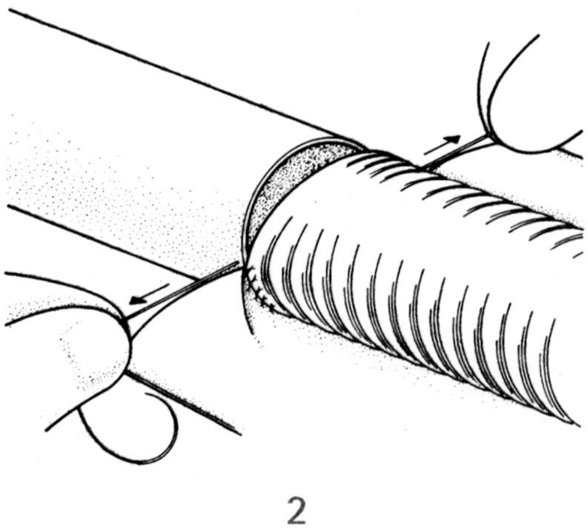

2

3, 4

The suturing is continued over and over until the sutures meet. Frequently, it does not matter if the needle passes from the Dacron to the artery or from the artery to the Dacron. Whichever is the more comfortable should be performed. However, if it is anticipated that passing the needle from aorta to Dacron will dissect atheroma it is then essential to pass the needle in the conventional method from Dacron to aorta at all times.

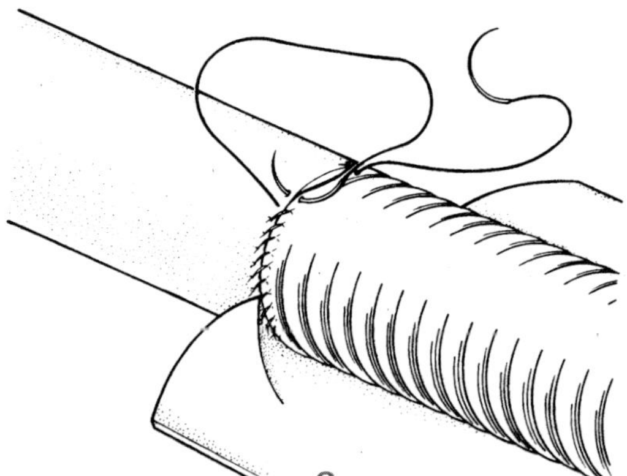

3

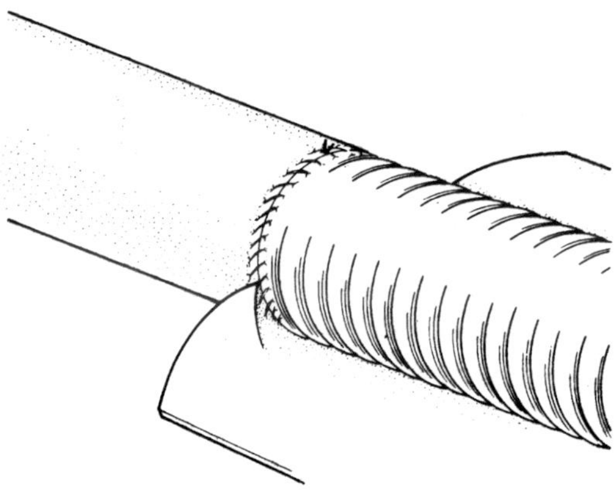

4

End-to-end anastomoses of smaller vessels

5

Wherever smaller vessels are to be anastomosed end-to-end, the vessel should be cut obliquely as shown. This will increase the length of the suture line thus reducing tension and will minimize the risk of stenosis.

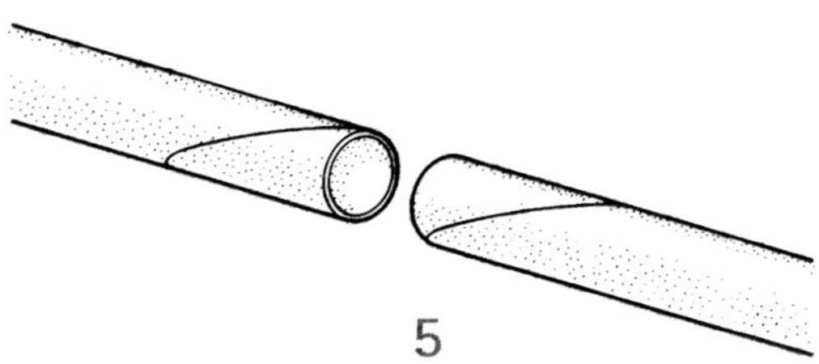

5

6

Two double-ended polypropylene sutures are passed through the opposing cut ends of the vessels.

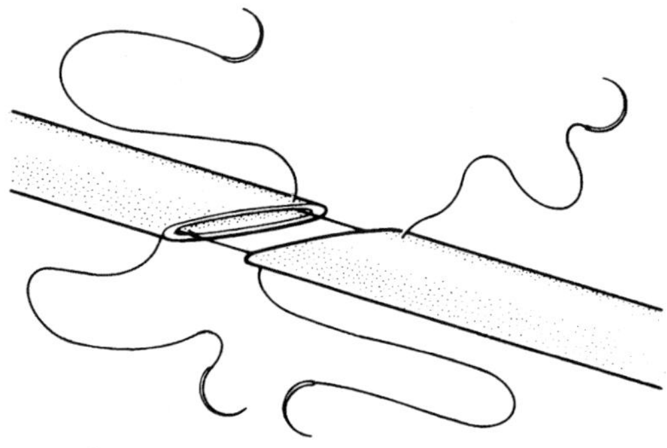

6

7, 8

One end is tied and the other is held with rubber-shod mosquito forceps. One end of the tied suture is used to sew over and over towards the other comer, while the other is held as a stay suture with rubber-shod mosquito forceps. On completion of one side, the vessel is rotated as shown.

The other side is sewn over and over between the held suture ends. At the end of the procedure the polypropylene sutures are cut long to avoid slippage.

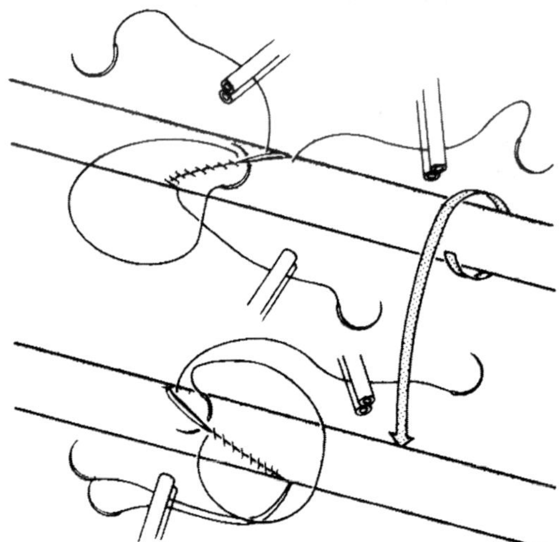

7, 8

End-to-side anastomosis

9

This illustration shows a conventional method of anastomosis of a Dacron limb to the side of the common femoral artery. The arteriotomy is cut to match the length of the obliquely cut Dacron tube and sutures are passed

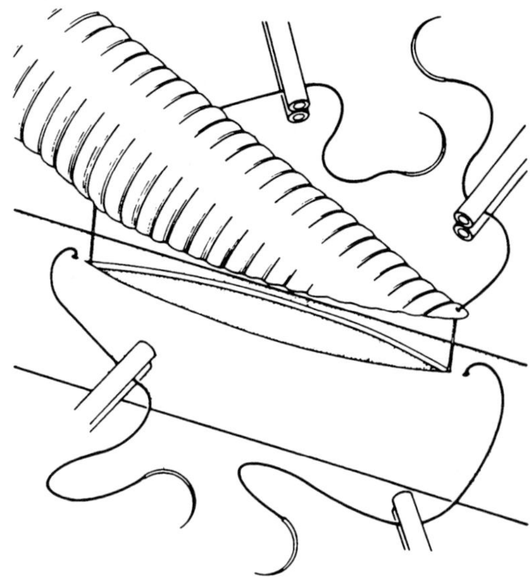

9

through each apex and tied and held with rubber mosquito forceps.

10

Suturing progresses forwards from the heel and backwards from the toe. Again, most surgeons sew from Dacron to artery to avoid freeing atheroma from the artery wall, but in some instances this is not essential. The disadvantage of this technique is that the toe end can pull away from the apex and once the sutures are pulled down it is difficult to place the adjacent sutures, particularly at the heel end. This technique is perfectly satisfactory when performed on the common femoral artery but when the Dacron is angled into the origin of the profunda artery this recipient vessel can be very thin and the Dacron frequently pulls away from the apex causing tearing of the vessel.

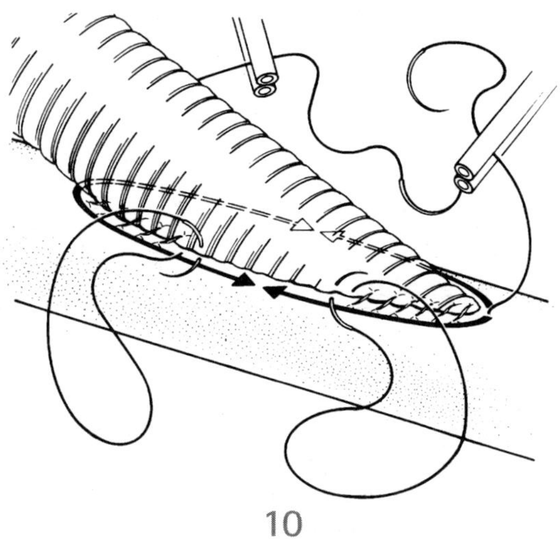

10

Alternative end-to-side method with eccentric stitch

11

Illustration 11 shows autologous reverse vein with carefully placed dots along its length so that twisting is avoided when it is tunnelled. In this illustration the first double-ended suture is placed at the heel of the anastomosis as before but the second is placed eccentrically rather than at the apex. The suturing progresses as before, forwards from the heel suture and backwards from the eccentric stitch. The other eccentric stitch is continued forwards around the toe of the graft to meet the other suture. This minimizes the risk of the graft tearing from the apex.

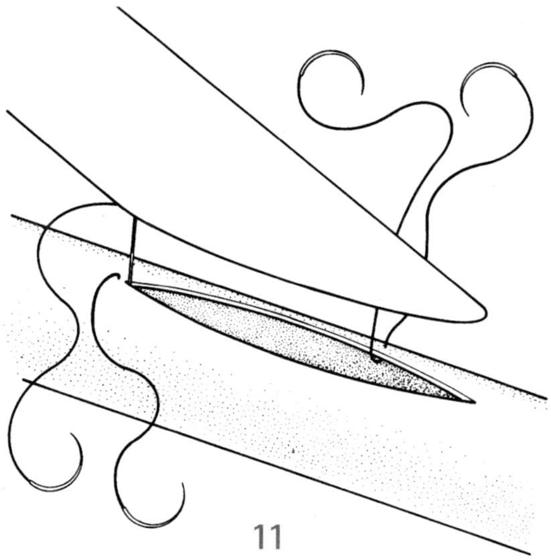

11

Alternative end-to-side anastomoses using a loose stitch at the heel end

12, 13

This method is commonly used for anatomosing the end of ePTFE to the side of the popliteal artery. It is very convenient, especially for the more experienced vascular surgeon, to place the sutures at the heel end of the graft and leave them long as shown. When the first suture is pulled down and tied as described above, it can be quite difficult to place sutures on either side. This method shown here makes the rest of the anastomosis very easy. It is essential that the sutures be placed without any crossing and it is also vital to use polypropylene because of its slippery quality.

The rest of the anastomosis is either with one double-ended polypropylene suture carried around the toe of the anastomosis to meet the other suture or else a second double-ended suture can be adopted and tied in the

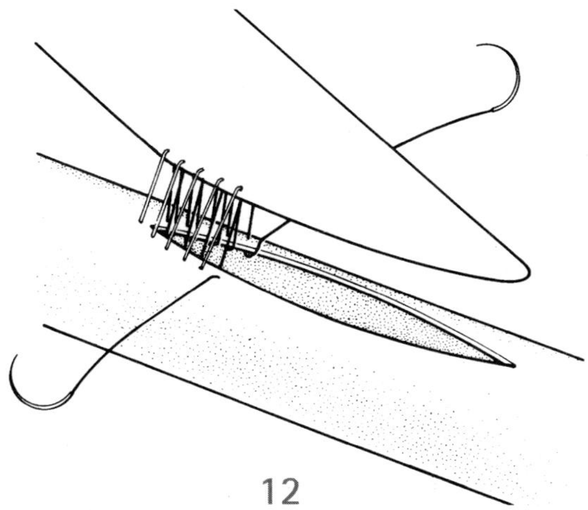

12

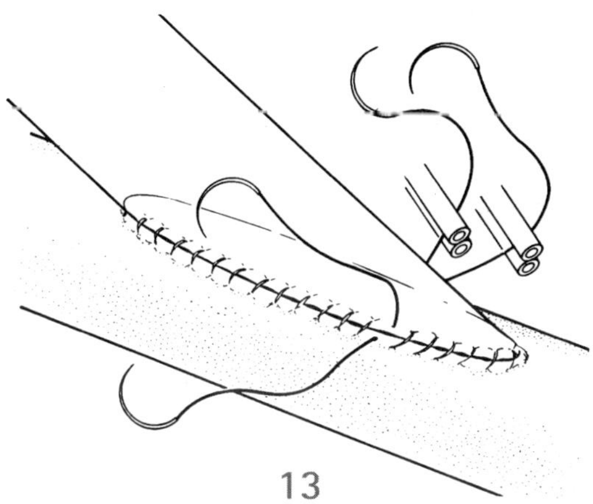

13

eccentric position as shown. With practice a single double-ended polypropylene suture is the fastest way of anastomosis and is technically satisfactory.

14

In illustration 12 a long suture is sewn over and over so that on one side the sewing is from graft to artery and from the other side it is from artery to graft. Some surgeons prefer to avoid this and instead insert the first suture as a mattress stitch so that it then becomes possible to complete the anastomosis by sewing with both needles from graft to artery. This is more like the conventional approach and will pin the atheroma to the artery wall. However, the disadvantage is that it leads to many 'backhand' sutures and this prolongs the anastomosis. If the surgeon is prepared to turn so that he always sews 'forehand' and does not mind whether he sews from graft to artery or artery to graft the whole procedure can be completed much more easily, but this is not possible if there is any risk of dissecting the diseased artery wall.

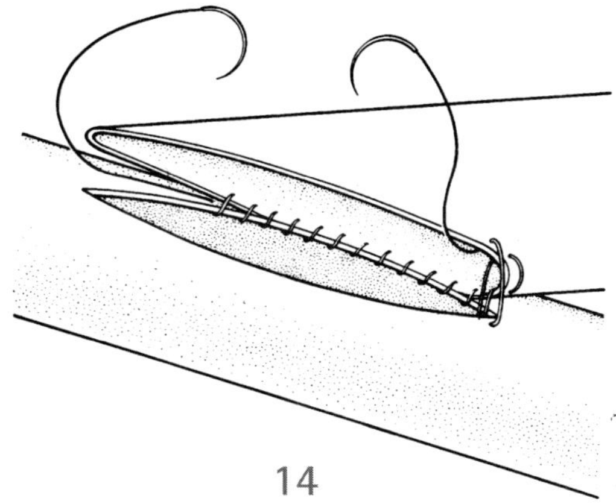

14

End-to-side anastomoses in a small vessel using interrupted sutures

15

The example shown is the umbilical vein with its Dacron sheath being anastomosed to a small vessel. The heel of the graft is sewn in the usual way. It is essential to pick up the whole thickness of the graft material including the intima and the Dacron mesh with each stitch. For the toe end of the graft it may be preferable to use interrupted stitches so that they can be placed accurately before being tied. It is a very useful technique and provides an alternative method of ensuring accurate placement of the sutures in this vital part of the anastomosis.

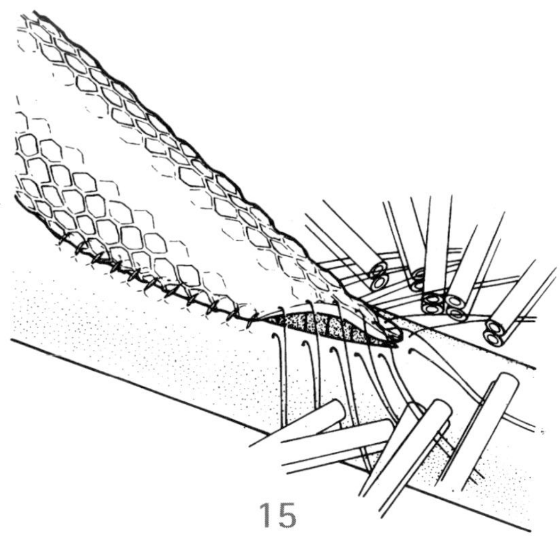

15

16, 17

On completion of the anastomosis the interrupted sutures are tied, held long and then cut one by one.

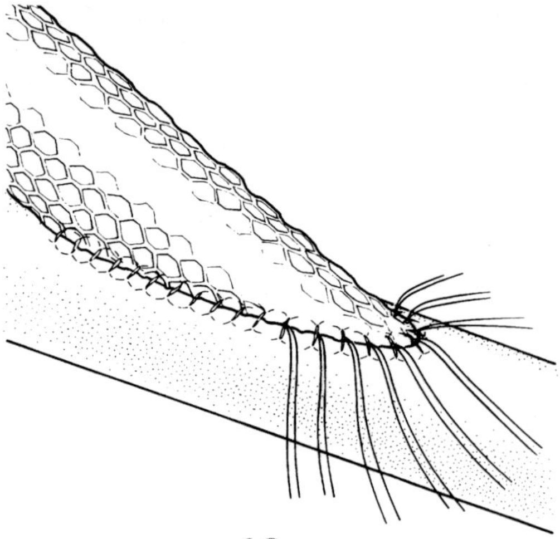

16

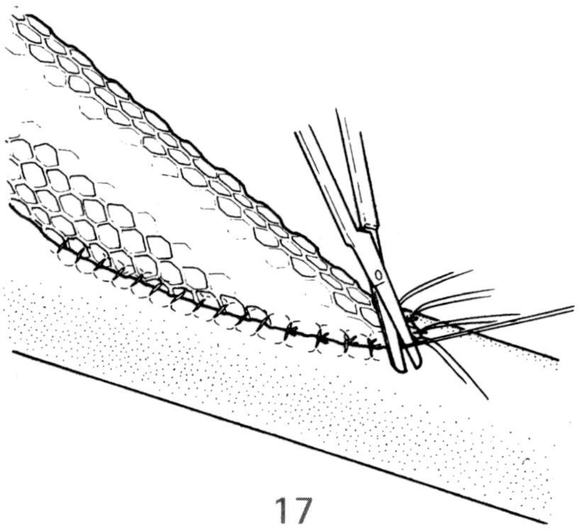

17

Confirming patency

Patency must be assessed before the wound is closed. Each surgeon has his own method of doing this and the subject cannot be dealt with in any detail here. The most conventional test, however, is to perform an on-table operative arteriogram. This will demonstrate the anatomy of the anastomoses and if nothing else it is a very useful teaching manoeuvre. Many anastomoses which were thought to be satisfactory are discovered by this method to be unsatisfactory. Such quality control leads to improved surgery.

The electromagnetic flow probe provides physiological data and is very much quicker than the operative arteriogram. The flow probe is placed around the graft and the volume flow per minute is measured. Additionally, a waveform of the flow is printed out for a permanent record.

Another method of checking an anastomosis is by direct pressure readings above the inflow and below the outflow. The needle can be connected to a thin polythene catheter which the anaesthetist attaches to a three-way tap to which the radial line is attached for monitoring. This technique is in its infancy and is probably best used in conjunction with flow readings.

Duplex scanning is now used in the operating room. A sterile Doppler probe may be used to image the vessel and assess the velocity of the blood flow in it.

Digital subraction angiography is also of tremendous value. It enables operative arteriography to be performed much more easily and can play back the result in order to minimize the problem of the timing of taking the film.

Wound closure

Clearly, meticulous aseptic technique is vital whenever prosthetic material is introduced into the body because if any infection is present the graft will be rejected. Wound infection can be minimized by closing the wound very carefully in several layers and it can be helpful to mop the wound edges with an aqueous solution of chlorhexidine. Before the final placement of the skin sutures a spray of povidone-iodine is given. Groin wounds are the most difficult and a subcuticular polypropylene suture fixed in place with beads is an ideal method of closure. This suture is removed after 7 days and leaves a good cosmetic result.

Acknowledgement

Illustrations by A George.

Intraoperative proof of patency

Bert C Eikelboom, Alexander C De Vries

Introduction

Technical errors during vascular reconstructive surgery should be detected intraoperatively because they are partly responsible for the failure of these procedures. Graft failure of up to 18% within 1 month of femorocrural bypass surgery, and complications like stroke and restenosis after carotid endarterectomy, are to some degree caused by technical inaccuracies such as intimal flaps, anastomotic and endarterectomy suture line strictures, and intraluminal thrombi.

Intraoperative detection of these imperfections will enhance quality and patency in vascular surgery. The two most common and readily available techniques – angiography and Doppler flow assessment – will be described in detail. Other techniques, such as vascular endoscopy, outflow resistance measurement, as well as the more sophisticated forms of ultrasound assessment (e.g. spectral analysis and duplex scanning), will be discussed briefly.

Angiography

Intraoperative angiography is considered to be the best form of intraoperative assessment, especially in lower limb bypass surgery. In general, we prefer to use Doppler ultrasound, as described in the next section, because we find it a less time-consuming screening technique before angiography. We perform prebypass intraoperative angiography if more information is required regarding the outflow tract.

Modern X-ray facilities in the operating room include fluoroscopy, a reference monitor, immediate replay, subtraction and roadmapping. A free-standing radiolucent operating table facilitates the investigation.

1, 2, 3

The foot lies at an angle of 45 degrees and the plate is placed flat on the table so that the angiogram is effectively shot obliquely through the leg. Depending on the type of bypass surgery, slightly different access routes are used. For the most common – angiography of autologous reversed saphenous vein bypass – we prefer to perform the proximal anastomosis first, allowing arterial blood pressure to straighten the graft and thus avoid kinking and rotation. In this way graft inflow can also be checked. After completion of the distal anastomosis, angiography is performed as shown, via a proximal side branch of the vein in the functioning graft.

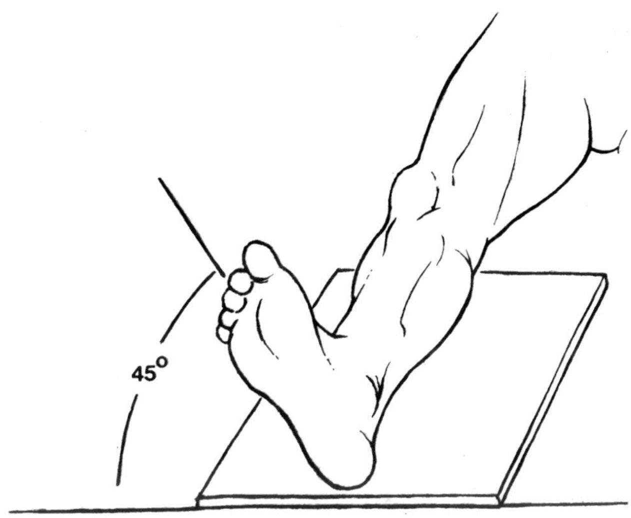

1

4

Alternatively, a vein bypass can be punctured using a standard infusion needle system (venflon 1.4 mm od) as advocated for synthetic graft assessment. *In situ* bypass can be assessed in exactly the same way as reverse vein, but Doppler techniques are our preferred procedures.

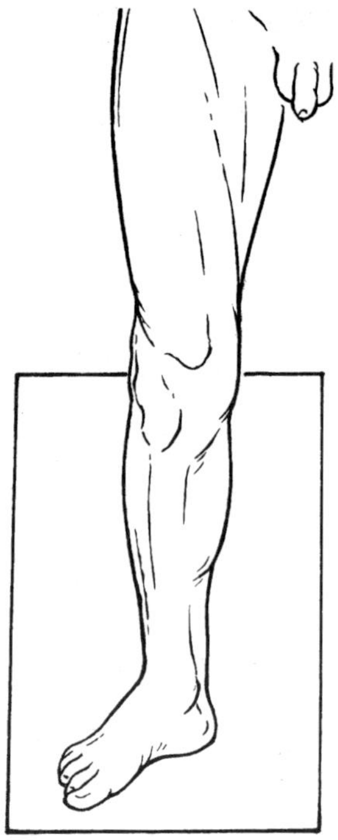

2

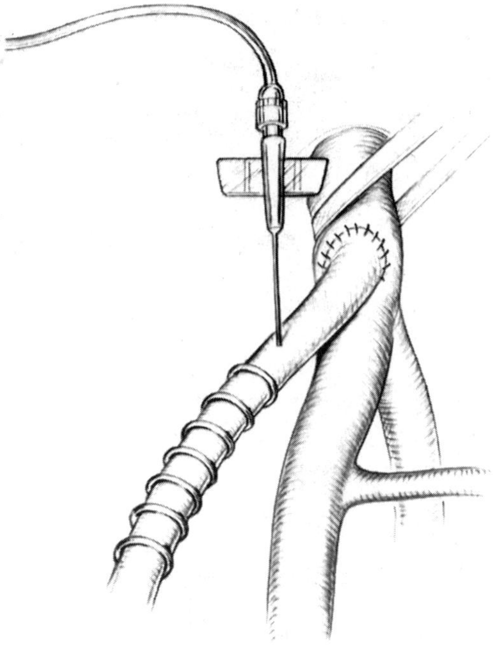

4

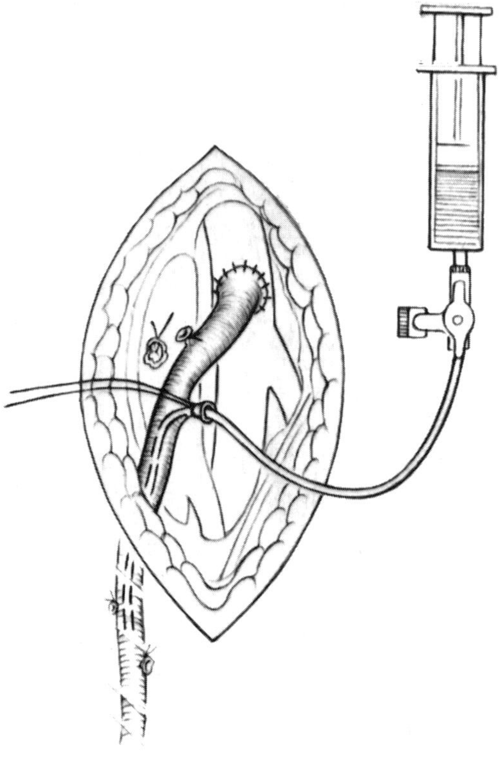

3

Even in experienced hands, erroneous anastomosis to the venous system is possible on occasions and a distal bypass outflow angiogram will alert the surgeon to this mistake. Sometimes, the distal anastomosis is performed first to allow better exposure. The angiogram is then performed before the upper anastomosis is completed.

Following distal outflow angiography, flushing with heparinized saline is advised. If necessary, additional X-rays are performed of the foot region or the graft itself.

5

In the previous illustration an externally supported polytetrafluoroethylene (PTFE) bypass is cannulated with a simple butterfly needle. Alternatively, as is shown here, at the end of both anastomoses a bypass (vein or prosthesis) can be occluded and a distal silastic catheter can be passed towards the lower anastomosis to allow good contrast delineation of the critical run-off area.

Doppler flow assessment

6

The Doppler system is a valuable tool for screening technical difficulties during vascular reconstructive surgery. We use this system in the most simple form, which comprises sterilizable probes connected to the basic apparatus which remains outside the operative field. Only audible processing is used. The apparatus remains on standby during all vascular surgery. It is less time-consuming and there are no disadvantages. It is used before or in some instances instead of angiography.

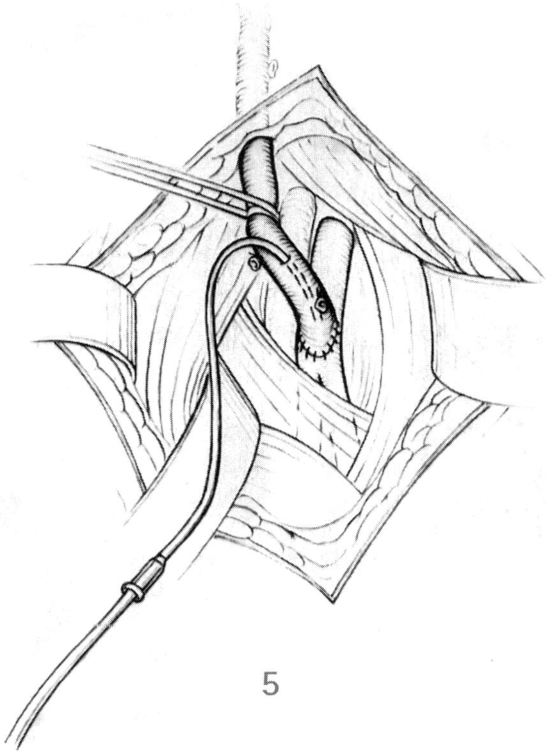

5

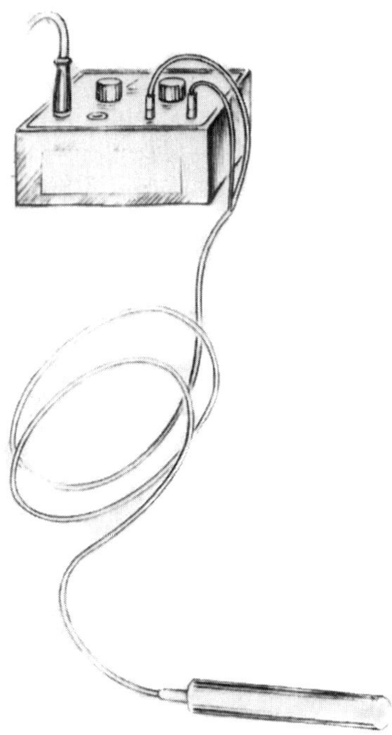

6

7

During surgery the functioning graft or reconstructed area is checked. The probe is placed near to the vessel to be assessed, preferably at an angle of 60 degrees.

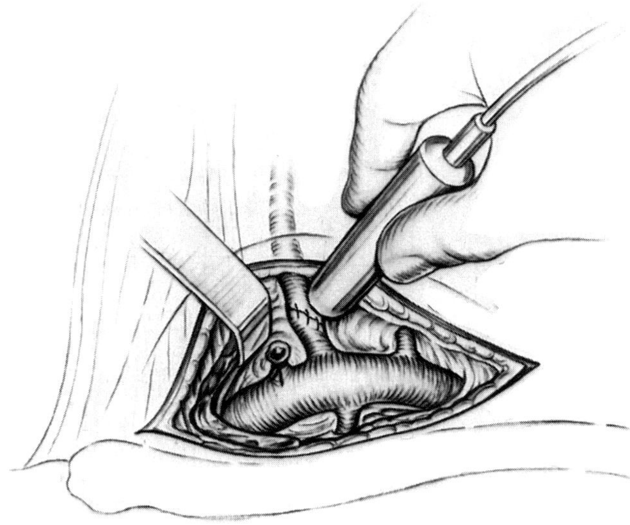

7

Conduction of ultrasound is easily achieved by placing both the probe and the vessel under heparin saline solution in a vertebral-truncus thyrocervical transposition, as shown. In this way audible signals are processed. These sounds are easily recognized, even by untrained ears. A 'good' signal is characterized by an uninterrupted flow with three components, i.e. a triphasic pattern. A 'poor' signal consists of so-called 'damped' signals of short systolic peaks of low frequency with intermissions without any recognizable flow. The haemodynamic equivalent of this is a stepwise, slow flow through the assessed vessel. The traces are shown from a directional Doppler trace but the ear can tell the difference. Stenoses are recognized by frequency shifts, while at the site of anastomoses some turbulence must be accepted. For *in situ* bypass surgery, it can be used to locate side branches as previously described (Greenhalgh *et al.*, 1985).

Miscellaneous techniques

Spectrum analysis of directional Doppler ultrasound

Doppler-derived signals can be interpreted more accurately by means of computer processing, i.e. spectral analysis. The spectrum is then visualized and can be further analysed by means of indexes. These analyses require meticulously obtained samples and are therefore not always ideal for intraoperative use. Moreover, the indexes obtained are not easily interpreted.

Duplex scanning

Duplex scanning combines Doppler with B-mode ultrasound. This image allows visualization of reconstructed areas (Flanigan, 1985). The apparatus is expensive and requires its operators to be highly trained. The scan heads used are large in comparison to the operative site to be analysed. They are not sterilized but covered by plastic bags. The instrument itself needs constant operation and adjustment, which means that a technician and a skilled surgeon skilled in the use of ultrasound are required in the operating theatre. On the other hand, it offers all ultrasound possibilities, which makes this system the most versatile for the trained operator. When this system is operational, it offers the best information possible, especially for carotid surgery.

Angioscopy

Angioscopy has become increasingly accepted as an adjunct to *in situ* bypass grafting. It helps to identify valves, which can be destroyed under direct vision, and it helps to occlude side-branches either externally through small incisions or from within the lumen using coils. The value of these techniques has not yet fully been established. Other applications include technical control after bypass, endarterectomy or thrombectomy.

Outflow resistance measurement

This technique offers outflow resistance measurements (Ascer and Veith, 1985). The value of this parameter is limited and the system is not yet commercially available.

Flow measurement

Electromagnetic flow measurement has been largely abandoned owing to technical problems (difficult probe fit) and because results have been of limited value. In the future, it will probably be replaced by Doppler-derived volume flow measurement which offers greater technical simplicity.

Summary

Doppler ultrasound, where simple audible processing is satisfactory for intraoperative use, offers a valuable tool in vascular reconstructive surgery. It is less time-consuming and requires little experience. It is advocated for screening and technical inaccuracies. We prefer its use before angiography, especially in peripheral bypass surgery. Of the other techniques mentioned, duplex scanning is the most promising. It offers all ultrasound-derived possibilities, including true visualization. However, its complexity makes its use in intraoperative application limited as yet.

Acknowledgement

Illustrations by R N Lane.

References

Ascer E, Veith FJ (1985). Outflow resistance measurements in infrainguinal bypass operations by injecting saline and measuring the integral of pressure. In *Diagnostic Techniques and Assessment Procedures in Vascular Surgery.* Greenhalgh RM ed. London/Orlando: Grune and Stratton.

Flanigan DP (1985). Peroperative Doppler testing and imaging in patients with lower limb ischaemia. In *Diagnostic Techniques and Assessment Procedures in Vascular Surgery.* Greenhalgh RM ed. London/Orlando: Grune and Stratton.

Greenhalgh RM, Heather BP, Green IL, McCollum CN (1985). Intra-operative detection of arteriovenous fistulae after *in situ* vein bypass. In *Diagnostic Techniques and Assessment Procedures in Vascular Surgery.* Greenhalgh RM ed. London/Orlando: Grune and Stratton.

Leoprecht H, Weber H, Monnig J (1985) Vascular endoscopy. In *Diagnostic Techniques and Assessment Procedures in Vascular Surgery.* Greenhalgh RM ed. London/Orlando: Grune and Stratton.

Direct reconstruction of intrathoracic great vessels

E Kieffer, C Petitjean,
Y Bensaïd, J Natali

Introduction

Direct surgical management of intrathoracic great vessel disease was used exclusively in the first years following the pioneering work of Bahnson *et al.* (1959) and Davis *et al.* (1956). Reconstruction of the innominate artery, left common carotid artery or multiple lesions was performed through a median sternotomy, and a posterolateral thoracotomy was used for left subclavian artery procedures. However, owing to the magnitude of these operations in poor-risk patients, operative mortality remained high (Crawford *et al.*, 1969), leading to a progressive decrease in indications for intrathoracic procedures and the introduction of extrathoracic reconstructions. By far the most popular of these has been the carotid-subclavian bypass (Dietrich *et al.*, 1967), but other operations have been developed including direct reimplantation of subclavian artery into the common carotid artery (Edwards and Wright, 1972) and various types of crossover cervical bypasses (Finkelstein *et al.*, 1972; Sethi *et al.*, 1975; Manart and Kempczinski, 1980).

The cervical procedures facilitate surgical management of most isolated lesions of the intrathoracic great vessels. Their low operative risk and clinical effectiveness certainly make their use valid and logical in the management of isolated subclavian or common carotid lesions, particularly left subclavian artery lesions, which are the most commonly found and whose direct surgical management is possible only through left thoracotomy. However, it is our opinion that most cases of innominate artery and multiple lesions are best treated using direct reconstruction through a median sternotomy.

The purpose of this chapter is to describe the most commonly performed procedures in our 10-year experience including 142 patients treated by direct intrathoracic procedures.

Patterns of intrathoracic arterial lesions

A knowledge of arterial pathology is important as it governs the type of reconstructive procedure to be used.

Most occlusive lesions are atherosclerotic in origin. They are usually very localized, although sometimes multiple.

Atherosclerotic involvement of the aortic arch, leading to ostial stenosis, is the most frequently encountered lesion. Each of the three intrathoracic great vessels – the innominate artery, the left common carotid artery and the left subclavian artery – may be involved. Different combinations of these lesions are possible, but when all three are involved it is called the 'aortic arch syndrome'. Lesions of the middle part of the innominate artery or the left subclavian artery, not involving the aortic origin of these vessels, are much rarer, as are localized lesions of the bifurcation of the innominate artery, extending in various degrees to the right subclavian artery and/or to the right common carotid artery.

Ulcerated atherosclerotic lesions, especially in the innominate artery, may lead to embolization in the brain, eye or upper extremity. Haemodynamic consequences are to be expected only in the presence of tightly stenosing and/or completely occluding lesions, especially when multiple. Innominate artery and left subclavian artery occlusions are usually segmental, sparing the bifurcation of the artery or remaining proximal to the origin of the left vertebral artery. In such cases some form of reversed flow in the vertebral artery and right common carotid artery is present. Occlusion of the left common carotid artery always extends at least up to the carotid bifurcation. The presence of a significant stenotic lesion, at this level usually leads to an extensive occlusion including the whole length of the internal carotid artery, sparing the external carotid artery, whose distal part is revascularized by numerous collateral branches coming from the ipsilateral subclavian artery and contralateral external carotid artery. In the presence of a normal carotid bifurcation, left common carotid artery occlusion is usually only segmental, with the internal carotid artery remaining patent, often with a reversed flow to the external carotid artery.

Takayasu's arteritis is usually localized to the middle or distal part of the common carotid and/or subclavian arteries (Kieffer and Natali, 1983). Involvement of the intrathoracic great vessels is less frequent but, when present, it is commonly associated with severe involvement of the aortic arch, leading to a complete form of 'aortoarteritis'.

Traumatic lesions are uncommon. They may be observed following penetrating or blunt deceleration injuries. The latter usually results in avulsion of the artery at its origin on the aortic arch (Kieffer *et al.*, 1977) but rupture of the middle part of the intrathoracic segment is possible. Acute lesions leading to emergency operations are beyond the scope of this chapter. Chronic sequelae include occlusions, false aneurysms and arteriovenous fistulae.

Congential lesions of the intrathoracic great vessels may be associated with the left or right aortic arch. A retro-oesophageal subclavian artery is present in 0.5% of the normal population but surgery is only indicated in the occasional symptomatic case. Isolation of the innominate or left subclavian artery is much less common. These abnormalities are usually found in association with intracardiac and/or aortic congenital lesions but may be completely isolated.

Although anatomically frequent, especially in the innominate artery, kinking is usually not haemodynamically significant and should lead to surgery only on very rare occasions. Spontaneous aneurysms are atherosclerotic or luetic in origin but remain much rarer than occlusive lesions.

Special preoperative preparation

The intrathoracic nature of the procedure obviously necessitates a precise assessment of the patient's cardiopulmonary status and medical treatment of all treatable abnormalities whenever possible. Pulmonary function should be assessed precisely. Preoperative pulmonary physiotherapy is often indicated in this middle-aged smoking population. Cardiac abnormalities should be looked for carefully through history and a standard ECG. Coronary angiography and cardiac catheterization should have broad indications even in the presence of stable angina, since coronary artery bypass, if indicated, should be performed in the same operative session. Arterial hypertension should be treated preoperatively in order to allow for safe lateral clamping of the aorta and prevent cardiac and cerebral complications. A computed tomography (CT) scan should be obtained in the presence of any permanent neurological symptoms.

Although non-invasive ultrasonic techniques are of great value and should be obtained routinely, angiography is necessary for a precise assessment of the cerebral circulation. Arch aortography should visualize not only the intrathoracic vessels but also the carotid bifurcations and vertebral arteries. Distal arteries may be difficult to visualize in the presence of multiple extensive occlusions. In rare cases we used to begin the operation with surgical exploration of one or both of the carotid bifurcations. More recently, most of these problems have been overcome using non-invasive techniques and intra-arterial digitalized subtraction angiography.

Special intraoperative monitoring for these procedures

Much of this is as described in the first chapter: 'Planning the intervention'. Blood pressure is recorded through an intra-arterial line placed either in the radial artery opposite the artery to be revascularized or in either of the femoral arteries in the presence of multiple lesions. Cardiac function assessment by a Swan-Ganz catheter should be routinely used since intraoperative lowering of the blood pressure using halothane or preferably sodium nitroprusside or trinitrin is often necessary to allow for precise and safe lateral clamping of the aorta. Multiple venous lines are also used, avoiding the cervical and left brachial regions because the left innominate vein may have to be transected in order to obtain adequate access to the lesions.

We use no special intraoperative cerebral monitoring such as EEG or pressure measurements. The only routine cerebral protective measures taken are: 1) systemic heparinization during arterial clamping (0.5 mg/kg, with neutralization by protamine sulphate at the end of the procedure); 2) avoidance of hypotension during arterial clamping and of hypertension in the postoperative period; and 3) sequential declamping of the arteries, beginning with the non-cerebral arteries (external carotid artery or distal subclavian artery). In the presence of multiple proximal lesions, revascularization should begin with the most stenotic lesion(s). Similarly, tandem intrathoracic and cervical lesions should be treated sequentially, beginning with the more proximal one.

The use of cardiopulmonary bypass may be necessary in a few selected situations, the most frequent of these being simultaneous coronary revascularization. Circulatory arrest using deep hypothermia has been used in a few cases to perform transaortic endarterectomy of multiple proximal lesions of the great vessels (Thevenet *et al.*, 1968). However, although this technique seems logical and appealing, reasonable clinical and angiographic indications remain rare and the whole procedure may seem unnecessarily complicated.

Shunting devices such as Gott (Murray *et al.*, 1971) or Javid shunts inserted into the ascending aorta have no routine indication but may be used in very selected cases in order to avoid a prosthetic bypass if endarterectomy or reimplantation necessitates simultaneous clamping of both the innominate artery and left common carotid artery.

The operations

Incisions and approaches to the great vessels

Anterolateral thoracotomy through the second or third intercostal space has been advised by some surgeons (Crawford *et al.*, 1969). However, this approach only allows for the proximal implantation of a bypass. In addition, tunnelling through the thoracic inlet seems to be a rather blind procedure, carrying the risk of venous trauma. We have used this approach only for very selected indications for subclavian artery reconstruction such as failure or infection of a cervical procedure or associated extensive lesions of the contralateral subclavian artery and common carotid arteries, precluding their use as an inflow source (Kieffer and Natali, 1983).

Left posterolateral thoracotomy through the fourth intercostal space is unique in providing direct access to the whole length of the intrathoracic portion of the left subclavian artery. However, it has several drawbacks that explain its declining use in recent years: distal exposure is limited to the origin of the vertebral artery; associated surgery is not possible: above all respiratory complications are more frequent than with a median sternotomy. Except for aneurysmal lesions, this route involves an unduly extensive technique for isolated lesions of the left subclavian artery, since they may be managed easily through a much simpler cervical approach.

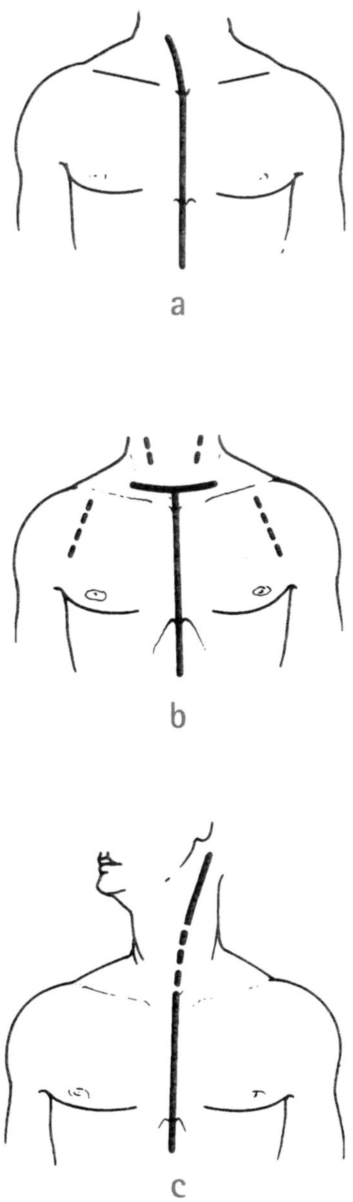

1

1a, b, c

The standard approach is through a median sternotomy. Aside from its simplicity, well-known advantages of this route include 1) low rate of respiratory complications (as evidenced by cardiac surgery in the aged patient); 2) possibility of extension to all supra-aortic vessels, either intrathoracic (except perhaps the origin of the left subclavian artery) or cervical, as well as to the abdomen (sternolaparotomy); and 3) possibility of associated cardiac surgery.

One or more complementary cervical incisions are usually necessary, according to the vessel(s) to be revascularized. The innominate and left common carotid arteries are approached by a short presternomastoid incision at the base of the neck, permitting a very easy direct approach (**1a**). The proximal subclavian arteries are approached through the same incision, which is sufficient to give access to the subclavian artery medial to the internal jugular vein and to permit its dissection up to the scalenus muscles, beyond the origin of the vertebral artery. On the left side, the proximal subclavian artery is reputedly difficult if not impossible to approach through sternotomy. In fact this is possible after section of the vertebral vein and thoracic duct, although this does not allow for safe clamping of the aortic arch at the origin of the artery.

The approach to the distal subclavian artery necessitates a complementary supraclavicular incision on either side (**1b**), with section of the sternomastoid and scalenus muscles and reclination of the phrenic nerve. The entire aortic arch and its proximal branches may be approached through a low horizontal cervicotomy without sectioning of the sternomastoid muscles, provided the approach to the subclavian arteries does not have to go beyond the scalenus muscles (**1b**). The carotid bifurcation is approached by presternomastoid incision either by extending the sternotomy, especially if the neck is short, or by a separate approach (**1c**). The axillary arteries are easily reached by deltopectoral incisions (**1b**). The transection or removal of the clavicle does not offer any additional advantage. Multiple great vessel lesions can be approached by combining these cervical incisions, particularly if the low horizontal cervicotomy is completed by one or more separate distal approaches to the carotid and/or axillary arteries. For all distal revascularizations (axillary artery or carotid bifurcation), complementary cervicotomies are done at the beginning of the operation in order to confirm the possibility of revascularization suggested by angiography.

2

To approach the arterial axis on either side, it is necessary to transect the subhyoid muscles and the thymic remnants. The left innominate vein hides the aortic arch and the proximal part of the great vessels. It does not have to be isolated for distal revascularization (axillary artery and carotid bifurcation). When revascularizing a proximal artery it is usually sufficient to mobilize the vein by complete dissection and division of its lower (thymic) and upper (thyroid) branches. Detachment of the jugular–subclavian venous confluence from the posterior part of the sternal manubrium is useful to allow for a broad sternal opening without undue tension on the vein. However, it may be divided without hesitation, especially if a wide approach to the aortic arch is required and surgery on the proximal left subclavian artery in anticipated. Transection of the left innominate vein usually has no long-lasting effect except for a transient oedema of the left upper extremity, possibly followed by the development of prethoracic collateral circulation. The latter may be an uncosmetic sequela in young female patients. We do not usually reconstruct the vein at the end of the operation, although this presents no particular difficulty.

At the end of the procedure, the thymic remnants and subhyoid muscles are sutured in front of the intrathoracic portion of the reconstruction. If entered, the pericardium is left partially opened. Closure is made according to routine techniques, following pericardial, mediastinal and cervical drainage.

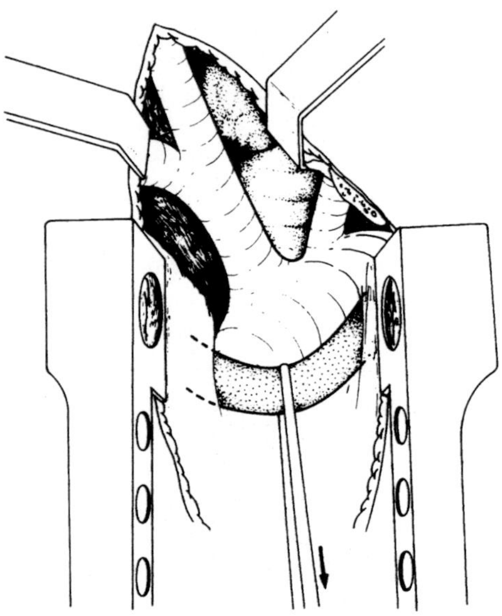

2

Innominate artery reconstruction

Among isolated lesions of the intrathoracic great vessels, those involving the innominate artery present the most logical indications for direct intrathoracic surgery (Kieffer, 1975). In our opinion, cervical bypasses are justified only in very occasional poor-risk patients. Crossover subclavian–subclavian or axilloaxillary bypasses using the left subclavian artery as an inflow source should be avoided since the artery is the most likely to be or become diseased.

Two reconstructive techniques will be described in detail: endarterectomy and bypass.

Innominate endarterectomy

This technique is applicable only in selected cases of atherosclerotic occlusive disease. Exposure of the entire length of the innominate artery, proximal parts of the left common carotid artery, right common carotid artery and right subclavian artery, as well as the upper aspect of the aortic arch is necessary (see Illustrations 1a, 2). The left innominate vein is retracted towards the lower part of the incision. The pericardium is usually not opened.

3

The first step is to make sure that wide lateral clamping of the aortic arch is possible safely. The following two conditions must be fulfilled (Kieffer, 1975).

First, sufficient space must be present in the upper aspect of the aortic arch between the origins of the innominate artery and the left common carotid artery. Inadvertent partial clamping of the left common carotid artery may be complicated by left cerebral embolism due to trauma of an associated non-significant lesion frequently involving the proximal part of the artery. Simultaneous complete clamping of both vessels, such as may be necessary in the presence of a common trunk between the innominate artery and the left common carotid artery, will usually be followed by cerebral

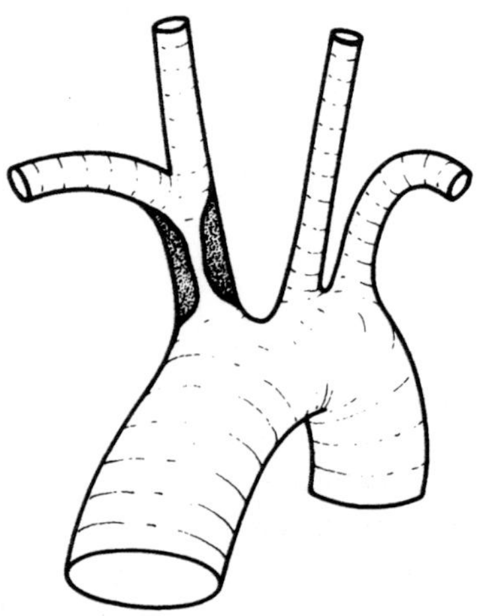

3

ischaemia of variable magnitude. In most of these cases aortoinnominate bypass seems preferable. However, endarterectomy remains possible if a shunting device is inserted between the ascending aorta and one of the common carotid arteries.

Second, involvement of the upper aspect of the aortic arch by the pathological process must be minimal if endarterectomy is to be performed with complete security. In our opinion, extensive indications for conventional endarterectomy (Carlson *et al.*, 1977) carry the risk of intra- or postoperative haemorrhage or dissection and for this reason should be discouraged. If endarterectomy must be performed despite the risks, cardiopulmonary bypass with deep hypothermia and circulatory arrest should be used in order to perform a transaortic operation (Thevenet *et al.*, 1968), but this somewhat complex technique seems unwarranted for an isolated innominate artery lesion.

4

When the two above-mentioned conditions are fulfilled, one may proceed to innominate endarterectomy. Under controlled hypotension and with the patient systemically heparinized the aortic arch is widely clamped around the origin of the innominate artery using a specially designed J clamp.

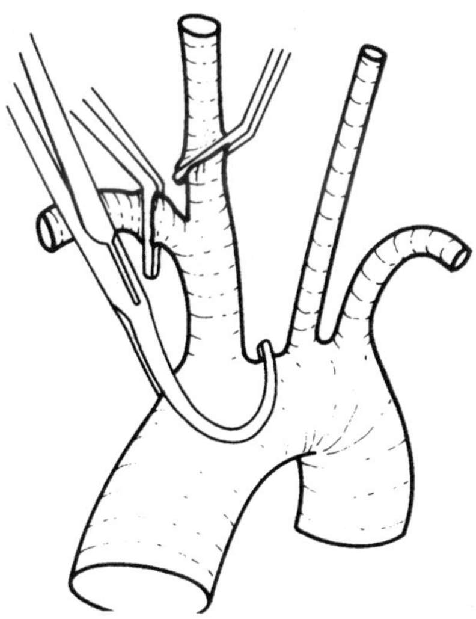

4

5

The right common carotid artery and right subclavian artery are then clamped separately using right-angle clamps, whatever the distal extension of the innominate artery lesion may be. A longitudinal arteriotomy of the innominate artery is made, extending proximally to the aorta in order to obtain adequate visualization of the origin of the innominate artery and aortic lumen.

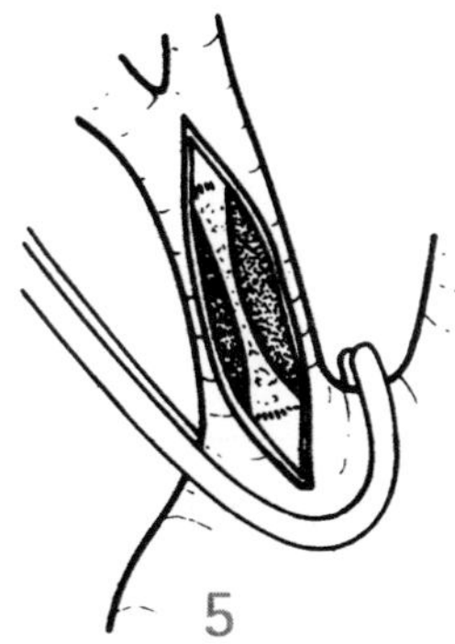

5

6, 7, 8

Using an adequate spatula, endarterectomy is begun at the middle part of the innominate artery. The plane of cleavage should not be too external, especially in the proximal part of the artery, if the hazards of aortic

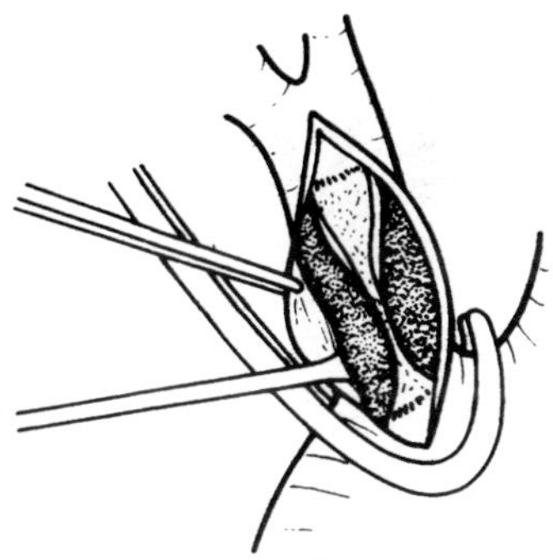

6

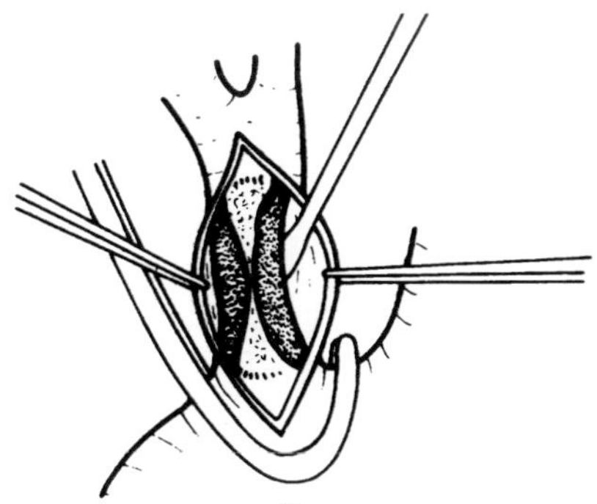

7

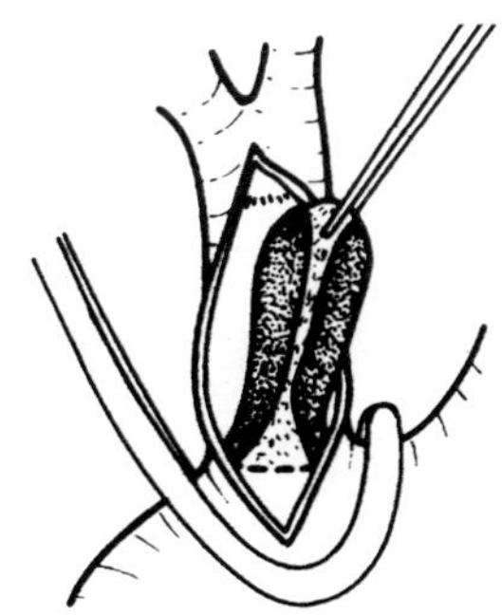

8

dissection, rupture or secondary dilatation of the artery are to be avoided.

The distal limit of the endarterectomy is usually very clear and no intimal fixation is necessary in these circumstances.

9

However, when the distal intima remains thick and easy to mobilize, one should not hesitate to tack it with a few 6/0 monofilament sutures. The proximal intima must usually be transected with scissors at the origin of the vessel, and its posterior aspect tacked using one or two 5/0 monofilament sutures.

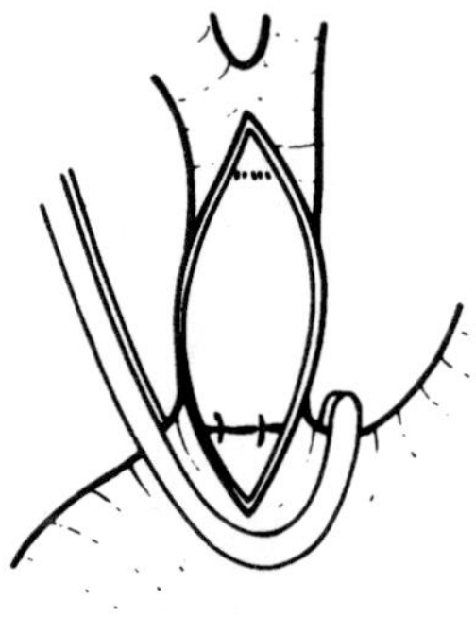

9

10a, b

Closure of the arteriotomy is usually performed using a 5/0 monofilament continuous suture (10a). Patch angioplasty (10b) is used in rare cases such as in a small innominate artery or when post-stenotic dilatation would result in relative stenosis of the proximal part of the artery. We prefer to use a knitted Dacron velour patch since a vein patch may lead to late dilatation.

a

b

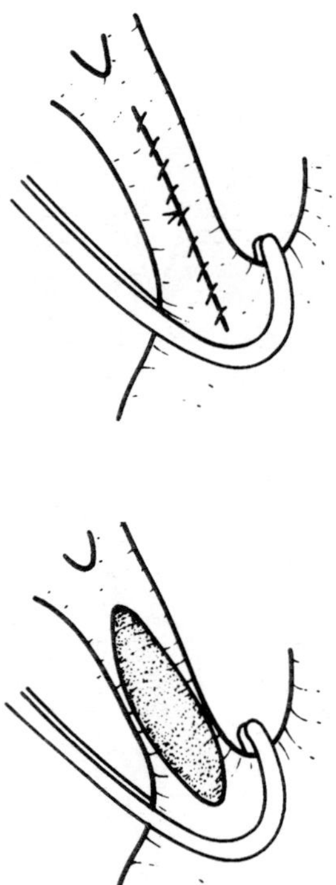

10

11, 12

Whichever form of closure is used, declamping is done sequentially, first towards the right subclavian artery and then towards the right common carotid artery.

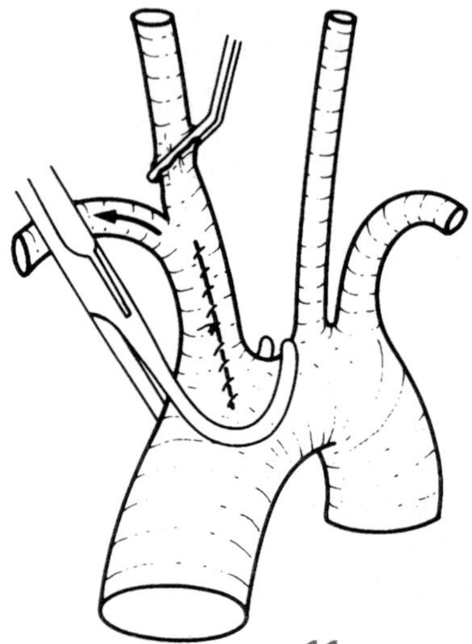

11

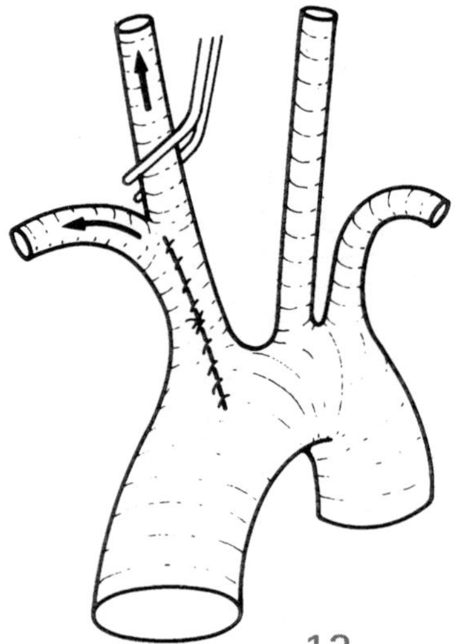

12

13

Distal extension of the lesion may necessitate associated endarterectomy of the right subclaviar artery and/or right common carotid artery. However, this extended procedure should not be performed in the presence of subclavian artery lesions extending distal to the origin of

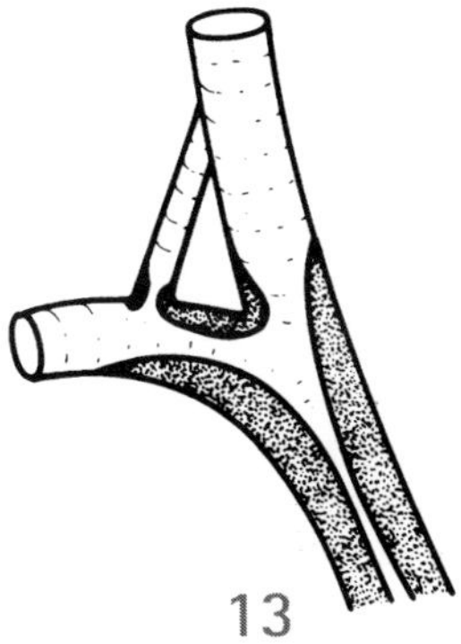
13

the vertebral artery. Separate clamping of right common carotid artery, distal right subclavian artery and vertebral artery is applied distally and the innominate arteriotomy is extended up to the level of the right vertebral artery. In most cases lesions stop proximal to the vertebral artery and endarterectomy of the proximal subclavian artery is performed easily under direct vision.

14, 15

Associated stenosis of the vertebral artery may be treated by trans-subclavian endarterectomy. On rare occasions tacking the distal intima of the subclavian artery may be indicated. The right common carotid artery is completely transected 1 or 2cm above its origin and endarterectomy of the proximal part of the artery is done using an eversion technique. In the presence of extensive lesions of the right common carotid artery and carotid bifurcation, a conventional endarterectomy of the birfurcation is performed. The middle and distal parts of the right common carotid artery are then endarterectomized using an eversion technique through the distal arteriotomy.

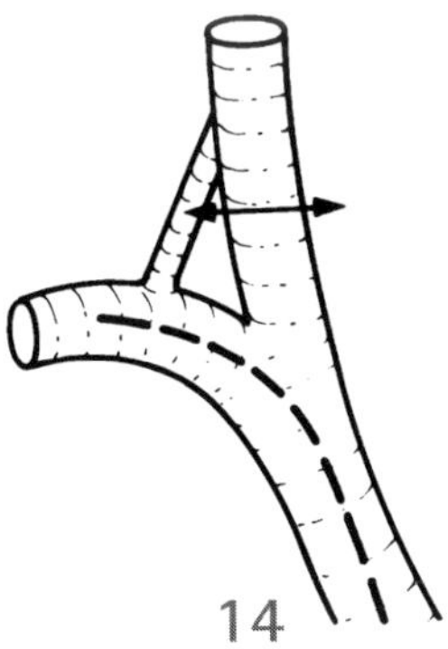
14

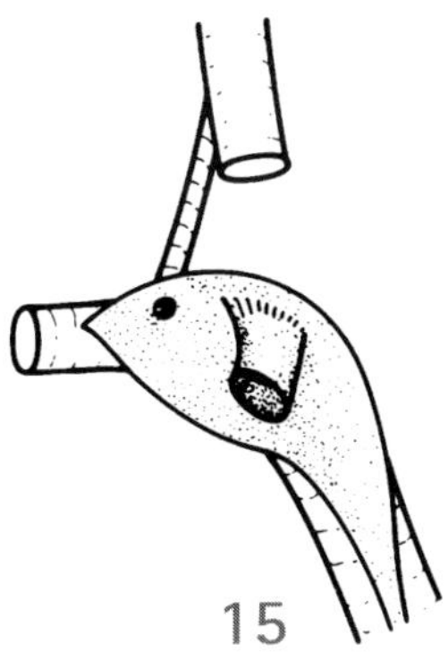
15

16

The two segments of the right common carotid artery are then anastomosed using a 5/0 monofilament continuous suture and the longitudinal innominate-subclavian arteriotomy is closed using either a continuous suture (as shown) or a Dacron patch angioplasty.

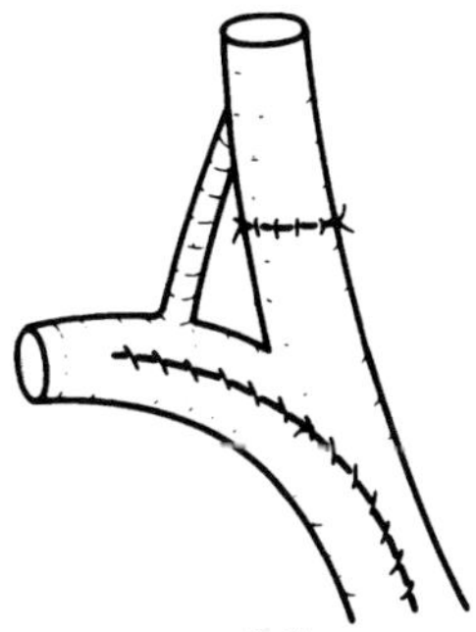
16

Aortoinnominate artery bypass

17

The incision used is shown in illustration **1b**. This technique has much broader indications than endarterectomy, since it is nearly always possible. Once the innominate artery and its bifurcation have been freed,

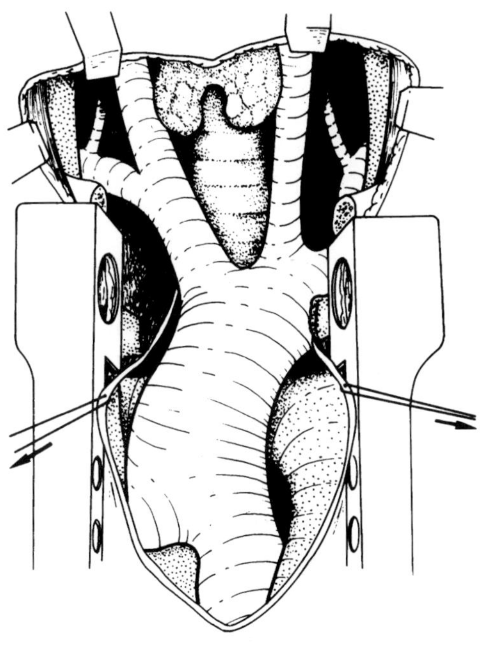
17

the upper part of the pericardium is opened longitudinally and its edges suspended from those of the sternal incision in order to expose the ascending aorta. Palpation of the latter will rarely lead to the unexpected discovery of extensive and/or heavily calcified lesions which preclude use of the procedure. In such exceptional cases, an alternative technique would be to extend the incision to the upper part of the abdomen and to use the supracoeliac aorta as an inflow source (Kieffer and Natali, 1983). Although complete transection may be necessary, extensive dissection usually facilitates the appropriate mobilization of the left innominate vein.

18

A knitted Dacron prosthetic graft of suitable size (8, 10, or sometimes 12 mm) is preclotted. When the chosen calibre is 10 mm or more, a tube graft is used. If the calibre is less than 10 mm, we prefer to use a bifurcated graft, only one of its branches and the adjacent part of its body being used. This permits the performance of a wide proximal anastomosis using large bites without any risk of inadvertent anastomotic stenosis.

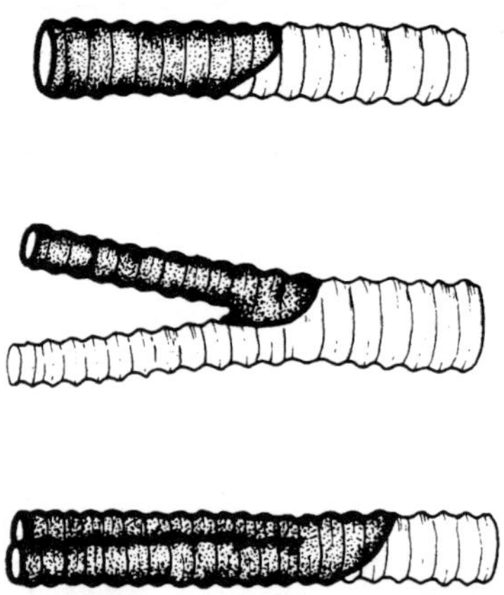

18

19

Palpation of the ascending aorta is performed very carefully in order to avoid either incomplete clamping with its associated risk of uncontrolled haemorrhage or a complete but traumatic clamping with the risk of fracture and/or dissection of the aorta. Heparin is not yet administered. The middle part of the right anterolateral aspect of the ascending aorta is widely clamped using a J clamp. Lowering the blood pressure to around 100 mmHg has the distinct advantages of avoiding aortic clamp trauma and allowing precise placement of the clamp. Indeed, the anterior aspect of the aorta should be avoided since placement of a graft in this position carries the risk of postoperative compression by the sternum. A 2–3 cm longitudinal aortotomy is performed. If the ascending

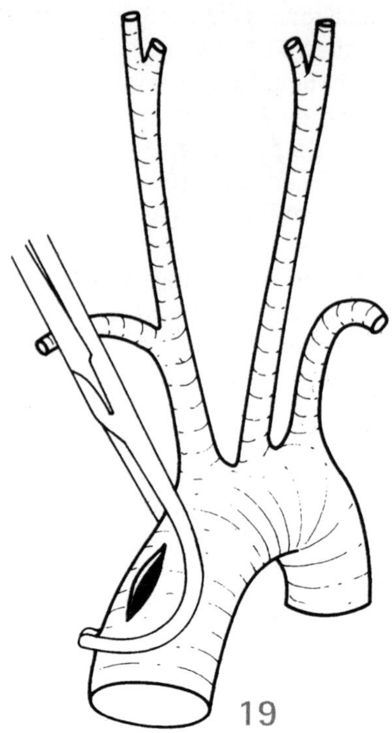

19

aorta is too thick and rigid a quadrangular or oval-shaped segment has to be excised in order to avoid proximal anastomotic stenosis.

20

The graft is bevelled and anastomosed to the aorta using a 3/0 or 4/0 monofilament continuous suture taking large bites through the aortic wall. After slow removal of

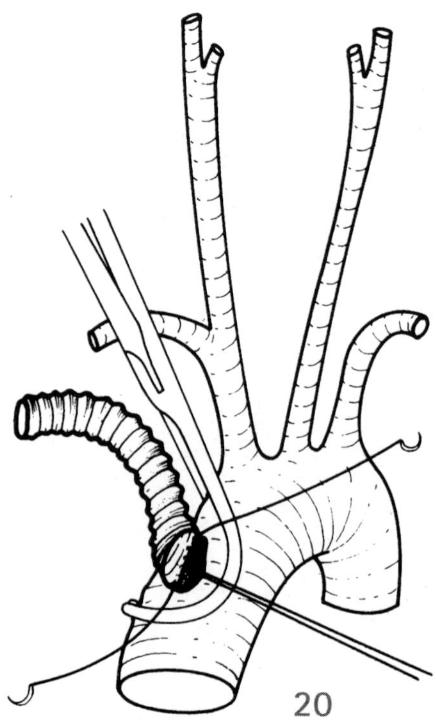

20

the clamp, the anastomosis is gently compressed in order to avoid any aortic wall haematoma. The anastomosis is then checked and should any complementary suture be necessary, this is made after reclamping the aorta. Preclotting of the graft is completed as necessary. The precise length necessary to reach the distal innominate artery is calculated with pressure in the graft. The graft is then reclamped close to its origin and any intraluminal clots are carefully removed by aspiration and lavage with non-heparinized saline solution. Any thrombus left on the wall of the graft might cause cerebral embolism when the bypass is made functional.

21, 22

Heparin is then administered systemically and the blood pressure is allowed to return to normal levels. The origin of the innominate artery and both its branches are clamped using a straight aortic clamp and two right-angle clamps respectively. If its bifurcation appears normal, the distal part of the innominate artery is completely transected and anastomosed to the graft in an end-to-end fashion using 4/0 or 5/0 monofilament continuous suture.

In the presence of associated lesions of one or both of the distal branches of the innominate artery, blind distal endarterectomy should be avoided and modifications of the distal anastomosis become necessary.

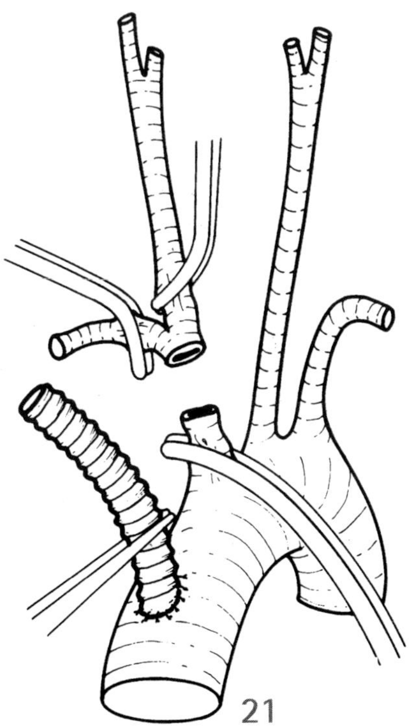

21

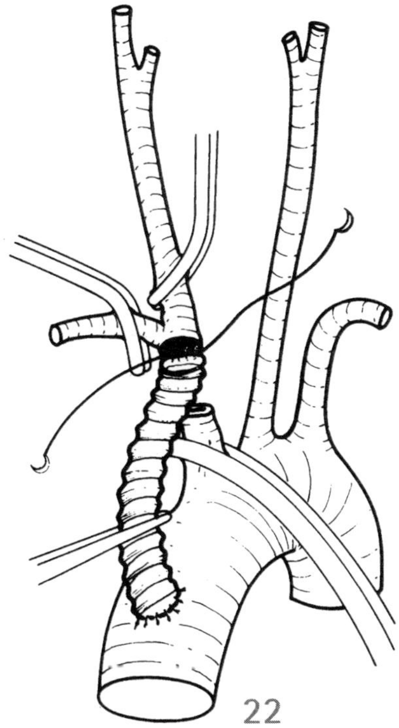

22

23, 24

When one of the branches is stenosed by a smooth localized plaque, a longitudinal incision is made and the graft may be anastomosed in a spatulated end-to-end fashion.

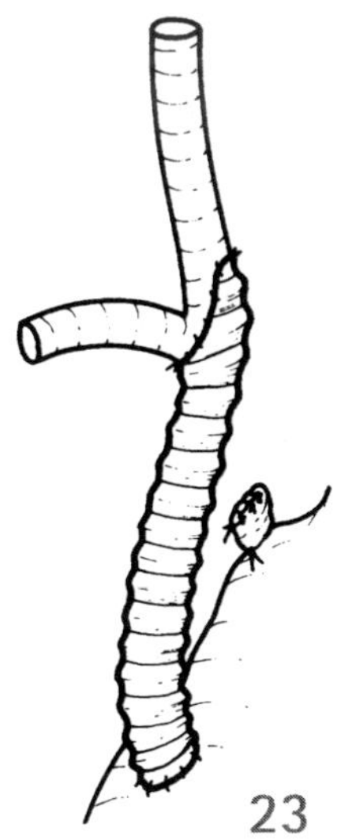

23

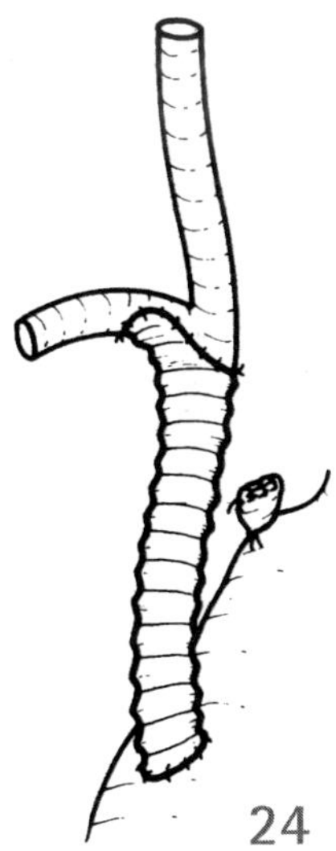

24

25, 26

Otherwise, we prefer to transect the two branches distal to the stenotic lesion (Edwards and Wright, 1972) and perform a short sequential bypass.

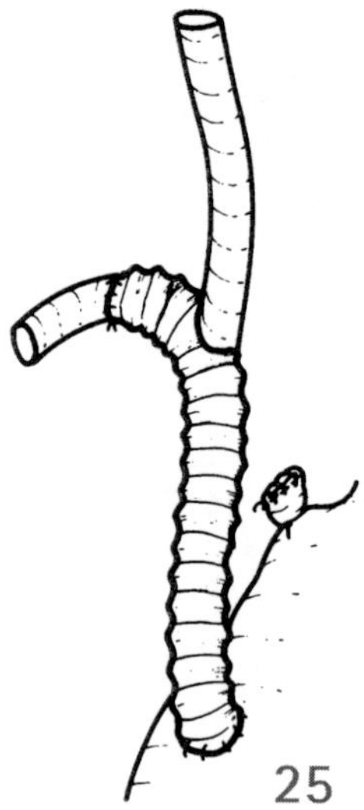

25

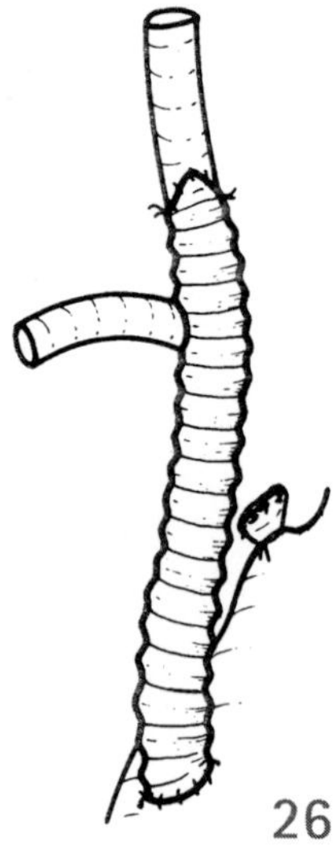

26

27, 28

With both methods declamping is done in the usual manner.

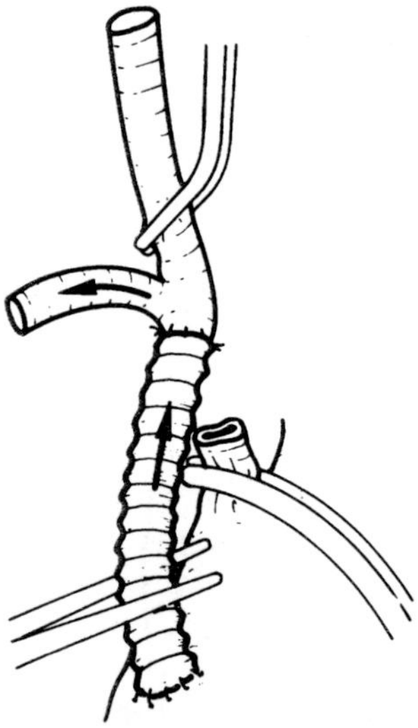

27

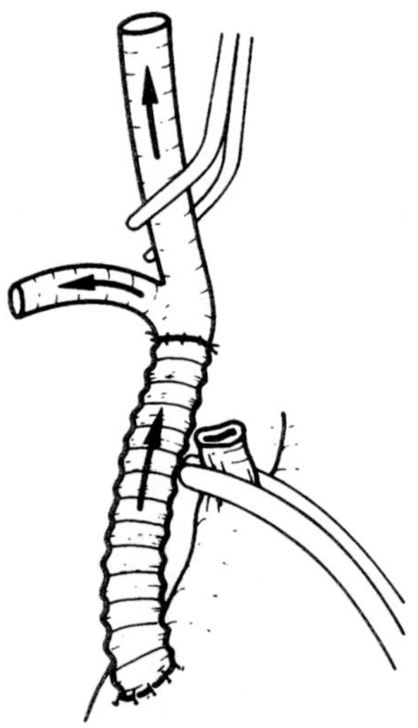

28

29, 30

The proximal stump of the innominate artery is then closed using a continuous over-and-over 2/0 braided Dacron or 3/0 monofilament suture, the choice depending on the presence of heavily calcified lesions in the proximal part of the artery.

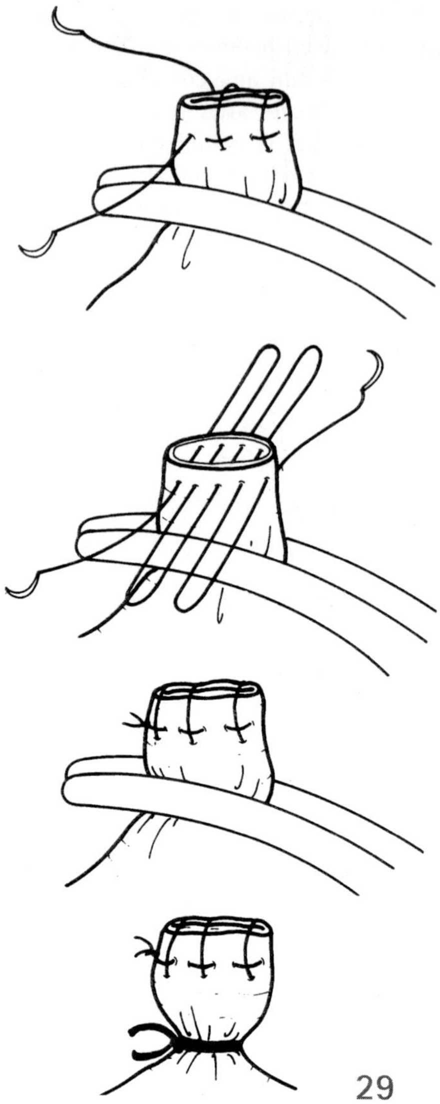

29

Alternative techniques

These are used on rare occasions. Resection and grafting may be done in the presence of aneurysmal or traumatic lesions without involvement of the origin of the artery or in the rare case of intraoperative failure of endarterectomy.

Resection followed by end-to-end anastomosis is the logical technique for managing the very rare cases of kinking in which surgical correction is necessary.

Isolated patch angioplasty may be applicable in a few selected cases of proximal non-ulcerated atherosclerotic lesion, when endarterectomy seems impractical.

Left common carotid artery reconstruction

In many cases an isolated lesion of the left common carotid artery is a good indication for extrathoracic reconstruction using a subclavian–carotid bypass (Dietrich *et al.*, 1967). This is particularly true in poor-risk patients, where the cervical procedure is simpler and much safer. However, the left subclavian artery may

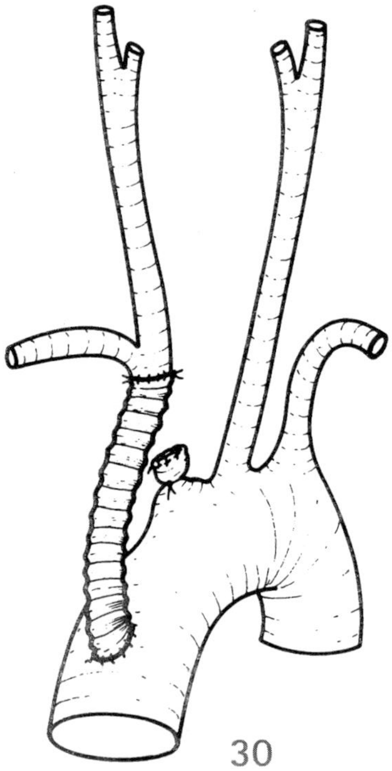

30

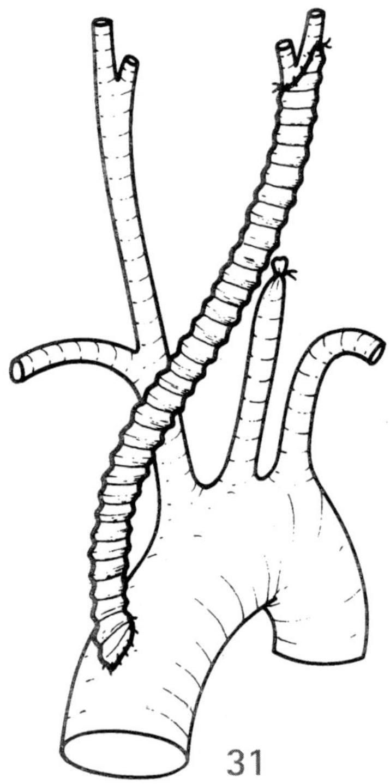

31

already be diseased at the time of initial evaluation or may become diseased afterwards. Conversely, its use as an inflow source seems to be unwarranted in younger patients, leading to consideration of intrathoracic reconstruction.

Endarterectomy is usually impractical because of the difficulty or impossibility of clamping the aortic arch between the innominate artery and the left subclavian artery. Reimplantation into a neighbouring artery is sometimes performed in order to avoid the placement of a prosthetic graft. However, reimplantation into the intrathoracic part of the left subclavian artery is illogical for reasons already mentioned and in any case can be performed through a simpler cervical approach. Reimplantation into the innominate artery is more attractive but necessitates simultaneous clamping of both arteries.

31

Aortocarotid bypass thus appears to be the logical procedure in these cases. A 6-, 7- or 8-mm knitted Dacron graft is selected, using part of a bifurcated graft. Alternatively, a saphenous vein graft may be used in young patients with small arteries, as may be encountered in Takayasu's arteritis (Kieffer and Natali, 1983). The technical steps of the procedure are the same as in the previously described aortoinnominate bypass. The length of the graft must be evaluated after temporary closure of the sternal retractor, in order to avoid overestimation with its attendant hazard of kinking. Although the distal anastomosis may be intrathoracic, in most cases it has to be performed to the carotid bifurcation.

Left subclavian artery reconstruction

Isolated lesions of the left subclavian artery are almost always an indication for a cervical approach using either carotid-subclavian bypass (Dietrich *et al.*, 1967) or, preferably, direct reimplantation of the left subclavian artery into the left common carotid artery (Edwards and Wright, 1972). A direct approach using a posterolateral thoracotomy is rarely indicated except for aneurysm or trauma. However, to avoid a crossover cervical bypass in good-risk patients, atherosclerotic occlusive disease may be best treated through a thoracic incision when the left common carotid artery appears impractical as a source of inflow. Endarterectomy of aortosubclavian bypass may be used. Anatomical indications and technical steps are similar to those described for management of innominate artery lesions.

Management of multiple occlusive lesions

General principles

Whatever their aetiology, multiple lesions constitute a logical indication for intrathoracic procedures (Kieffer, 1975; Thevenet, 1979; Crawford *et al.*, 1983). A one-stage complete revascularization, including the left subclavian artery, if diseased, is always preferable, since secondary reconstruction of the initially untreated lesion would prove difficult or even necessitate a left thoracotomy.

Multiple revascularizations are usually performed using the bypass principle, according to the following guidelines:

1. Multiple grafts are possible only if the ascending aorta is not too short, too small and/or too thick. This technique is particularly suitable if vein grafts are being used. Multiple prosthetic grafts are more likely to cause compression of the veins and airway in the thoracic inlet, especially in young female patients, and should be avoided.
2. Bifurcated grafts are simpler, but even when small sizes are used (16/8 or preferably 14/7) and the length of the body graft is tailored to be as short as possible, they may be a major cause of compression in the thoracic inlet, leading to serious complications such as venous and tracheoesophageal compression and, at a later stage, stenosis or even occlusion of one or more of the grafts.
3. Sequential grafts are to be preferred in most cases. One large prosthetic tube graft (10–12 mm) is selected to revascularize the largest vessel, usually the innominate artery. The proximal anastomosis is performed first and the graft is sequentially anastomosed to the arteries to be reconstructed, either directly or using an intermediate smaller tube graft (6–8 mm).

Application of these principles to the many possible anatomical combinations is determined mainly by the surgeon's imagination and ingenuity.

References

Bahnson H T, Spencer F C, Quattlebaum K (1959). Surgical treatment of occlusive disease of the carotid artery. *Ann Surg* **149**: 711.

Carlson R E, Ehrenfeld W K, Stoney R J, Wylie E J (1977). Innominate artery endarterectomy. *Arch Surg* **112**: 1389.

Crawford E S, DeBakey M E, Morris G C Jr, Howell J F (1969). Surgical treatment of occlusion of the innominate, common carotid, and subclavian arteries. *Surgery* **65**: 17.

Crawford E S, Stowe C L, Powers R W Jr (1983). Occlusion of the innominate, common carotid, and subclavian arteries: Long-term results of surgical treatment. *Surgery* **94**: 781.

Davis J B, Grove W J, Julian O C (1956). Thrombotic occlusion of the branches of the aortic arch. *Ann Surg* **144**: 124.

Dietrich E B, Garrett H E, Ameriso J *et al.* (1967). Occlusive disease of the common carotid and subclavian arteries treated by carotid subclavian bypass. *Am J Surg* **111**: 800.

Edwards W H, Wright R S (1972). Current concepts in the management of arteriosclerotic lesions of the subclavian and vertebral arteries. *Ann Surg* **175**: 975.

Ehrenfeld W K, Wilbur B G, Olcott C N, Stoney R J (1979). Autogenous tissue reconstruction in the management of infected prosthetic grafts. *Surgery* **85**: 81.

Finkelstein N M, Byer A, Bush B F (1972). Subclavian-subclavian bypass for the subclavian steal syndrome. *Surgery* **71**: 142.

Kieffer E (1975). Stenoses et occlusions atheromateuses du tronc arteriel brachiocephalique. *J Chirurg* **110**: 493.

Kieffer E, Natali J (1982). Ascending aorto-abdominal aorta by-pass. Technical considerations, indications and report of 15 cases. In *Extra-anatomic and Secondary Arterial Reconstruction*. **Greenhalgh R M** ed. London: Pitman, pp. 313–333.

Kieffer E, Natali J (1983). Supra-aortic trunk lesions in Takayasu' arteritis. In *Cerebrovascular Insufficiency*. **Bergan J J, Yao J S T** eds. New York: Grune and Stratton, pp. 395–415.

Kieffer E, Tricot J F, Cousin M T *et al.* (1977). Desinsertions traumatiques du tronc arterial brachiocéphalique. *Ann Chirurg Thorac Cardiovasc* **16**: 323.

Manart F D, Kempczinski R F (1980). The carotid-carotid bypass graft. *Arch Surg* **115**: 669.

Murray G F, Brawley R K, Gott V L (1971). Reconstruction of the innominate artery by means of a temporary heparin-coated shunt bypass. *J Thorac Cardiovasc Surg* **62**: 34.

Ochsner J L, Mills N L (1979). Profound hypothermia and circulatory arrest in control and repair of infected aortic prosthesis. *J Cardiovasc Surg* **20**: 1.

Selle J G, Cook J W, Elliott C M *et al.* (1982). Simultaneous revascularization for complex brachiocephalic and coronary artery diseases. *Surgery* **90**: 97.

Sethi G K, Scott S M, Takaro T (1975). Extrathoracic bypass for stenosis of innominate artery. *J Thorac Cardiovasc Surg* **69**: 213.

Stolf N A G, Bittencourt D, Verginelli G, Zerbini E J (1983). Surgical treatment of ruptured aneurysms of the innominate artery. *Am J Thorac Surg* **35**: 394.

Thevenet A (1979). Surgical management of atheroma of the aortic dome and origin of supra aortic trunks. *World J Surg* **3**: 187.

Thevenet A, Chaptal P A, Negre E (1968). L'arrêt circulatoire en hyppothermie profonde dans la chirurgie des branches de la crosse de l'aorte. *Ann Chirurg Thorac Cardiovasc* **7**: 69.

Carotid endarterectomy

Jesse E Thompson

Introduction

Carotid endarterectomy is the procedure most frequently employed in the operative treatment of cerebral ischaemic syndromes due to atherosclerotic disease. Clinical considerations determine the indications and contraindications for operation. These are listed in detail in Table 1. The principal indication is transient cerebral ischaemia since strokes can be prevented and troublesome episodes of ischaemia are largely abolished. Indication for operation is also based on a critical evaluation of operative risk, since a high proportion of these patients have hypertension and generalized atherosclerosis, especially coronary disease.

Table 1. Indications for carotid endarterectomy in cerebrovascular insufficiency

Indications
1. Transient cerebral ischaemia
2. Stable strokes (selected)
3. Asymptomatic stenoses (selected)
4. Chronic cerebral ischaemia (selected)
Contraindications
1. Acute profound strokes
2. Progressing strokes
3. Severe intracranial disease
4. Other severe generalized disorders (e.g. cancer)

Table 2 summarizes the appropriate timing of operations for the various clinical categories. There is considerable difference of opinion regarding operation for acute carotid thrombosis following arteriography or endarterectomy. If an operation can be performed immediately (1–2 h), it is probably a justifiable and worthwhile procedure. Controversy has also developed over the advisability of performing emergency endarterectomy on patients with unstable or fluctuating deficits and with crescendo transient ischaemic attacks. Management of these patients is fraught with difficulty. Although computed tomography and magnetic resonance imaging scans are helpful, in the absence of totally reliable methods for distinguishing between cerebral infarction and reversible ischaemia without infarction, the results of therapy, whether surgical or medical, are unpredictable. In general, if the deficit is mild and the lesion severe, emergency operation is justified. Patients with significant bilateral lesions should have bilateral endarterectomies, but in separate stages at least 1–2 weeks apart or even longer.

Table 2. Timing of carotid endarterectomy for cerebrovascular insufficiency

Elective operation
1. Stable stroke, recent or old
2. Transient cerebral ischaemia
3. Asymptomatic stenosis
4. Chronic cerebral ischaemia (rare)
Delayed operation (days to weeks)
1. Mild stroke
2. Fluctuating stroke
Emergency operation (rarely necessary)
1. Frank stroke –disappearance of bruit –slowly worsening –fluctuating, unstable
2. Transient cerebral ischaemia –severe stenosis, especially if bilateral –disappearance of bruit –crescendo transient ischaemic attacks
3. Carotid thrombosis immediately following arteriography or endarterectomy.

Technique of carotid endarterectomy

Technical considerations are of the utmost importance in carotid endarterectomy, since the limits of tolerance to temporary occlusion of the blood supply to the brain may be quite narrow. Safety factors must be employed which will eliminate in most instances the occurrence or aggravation of neurological deficits. Any method of carotid endarterectomy should carry low mortality, few complications, satisfactory immediate and long-term anatomical results, and good functional results relative to cerebrovascular insufficiency. The technique to be described has evolved over a period of 36 years and has proved safe and reliable. It involves the routine use of a temporary inlying bypass shunt.

1

Operation is performed under light general anaesthesia. The head is turned away from the side to be operated upon and placed on a rubber ring. The shoulders are elevated slightly using a folded sheet but there should be no undue extension of the neck. An oblique incision is made along the anterior border of the sternocleidomastoid muscle, curving medialward at its lower end, centered over the bifurcation of the common carotid artery, and curved slightly inferior to the lobe of the ear at the upper end.

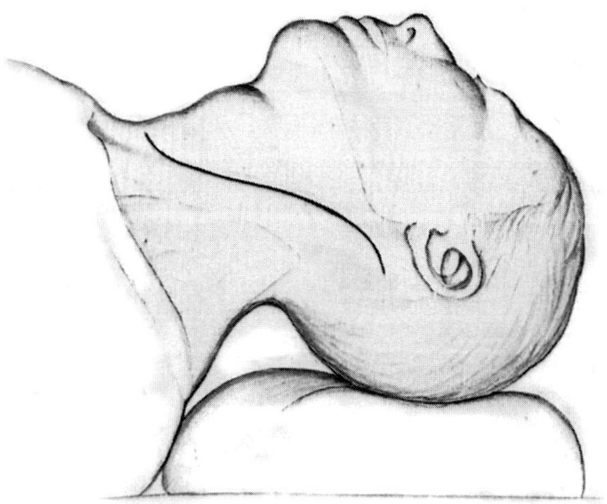

1

2

Adequate exposure of the common carotid and of the internal and external carotid divisions is essential. The carotid sinus area is infiltrated with 1% lidocaine to prevent hypotension and bradycardia. The artery is freed completely including division of the carotid sinus plexus if necessary.

One must avoid injury to the mandibular branch of the facial nerve and the vagus, hypoglossal and superior laryngeal nerves. A small branch of the external carotid artery, supplying the sternocleidomastoid muscle, usually passes over the hypoglossal nerve holding it down as a sling. This small artery should be ligated and divided to free the hypoglossal nerve off the external and internal carotid divisions. Though rarely necessary, the superior thyroid artery may be ligated and divided to facilitate dissection and exposure. An umbilical tape is first placed around the external carotid artery. Umbilical tapes are then placed around the common and internal carotid arteries and segments of No. 16 French rubber catheters are threaded over the tapes to act as tourniquets.

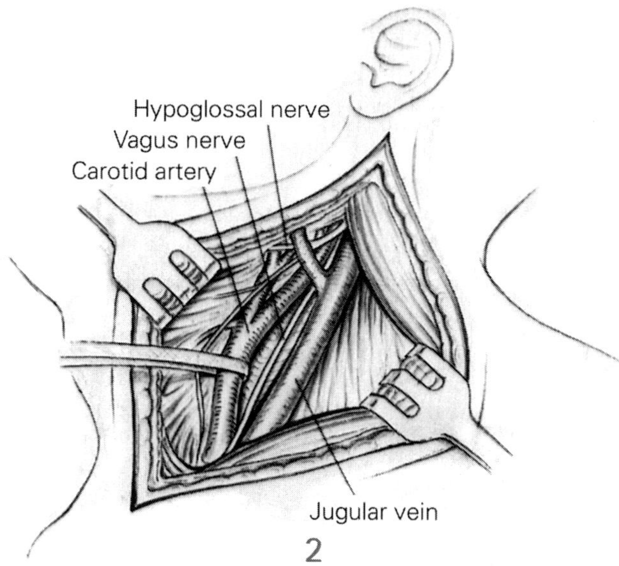

2

3

The occluding plaque is usually located at the bifurcation of the common carotid and extends only a short distance into the internal carotid. The distal internal carotid is ordinarily soft and thin-walled and is freed up for at least 1 cm beyond the palpable distal end of the plaque. Utmost gentleness is used throughout manipulation and the artery is simply palpated, never squeezed, since

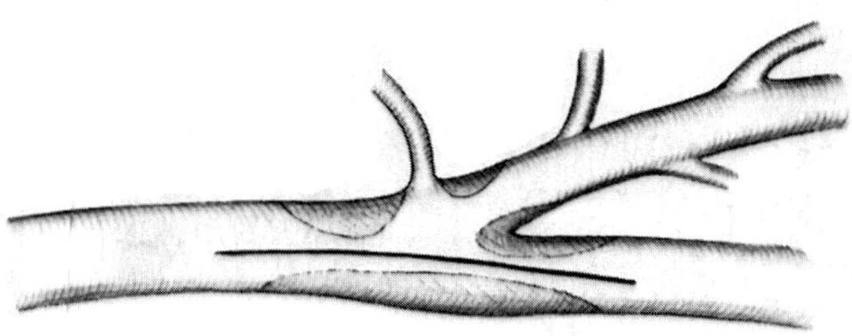

3

platelets, thrombi or atherosclerotic debris may break off and embolize intracranially.

When satisfactory exposure is obtained, systemic herarinization is affected with 3500–5000 units of heparin. The external carotid is occluded with a bulldog clamp and heparinized locally with 10 ml of a solution containing 100 units of heparin per ml. The common carotid is then clamped proximally with an angled vascular clamp. The distal internal carotid is occluded with a soft bulldog clamp and a linear arteriotomy is made from the common carotid into the internal carotid beyond the distal extent of the plaque. It is important that the internal carotid be opened beyond the plaque and that the entire extent of plaque be visualized in order to facilitate the succeeding steps of the operation.

4

A plastic catheter shunt is then inserted into the distal internal carotid and the artery allowed to backflow.

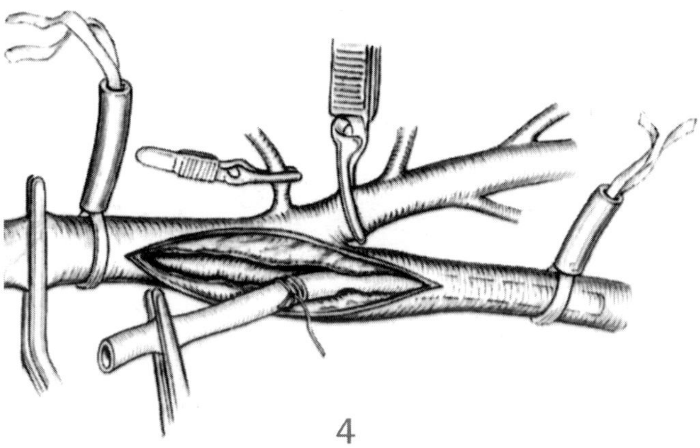

4

5

The proximal end of the plastic shunt is then placed into the common carotid lumen and the umbilical tapes with rubber tourniquets are made snug.

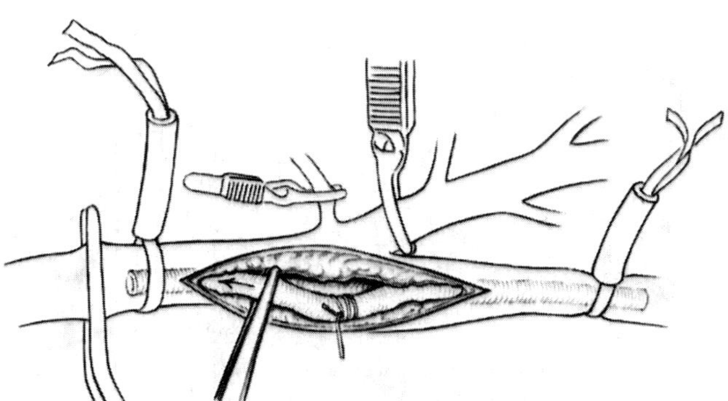

5

6

Cerebral blood flow is thus restored through the shunt. This step of the operation requires 45–90s.

The average size shunt which fits the distal internal carotid is a No. 10 French plastic catheter about 9 cm in length. A No. 8 or No. 12 catheter may be used as a shunt if the artery is smaller or larger than usual. The internal diameter of the No. 10 catheter used is 2.5 mm. With normal levels of blood pressure this shunt carries approximately 125 ml of blood per min. Experience has shown that this is an adequate flow during the period required for endarterectomy.

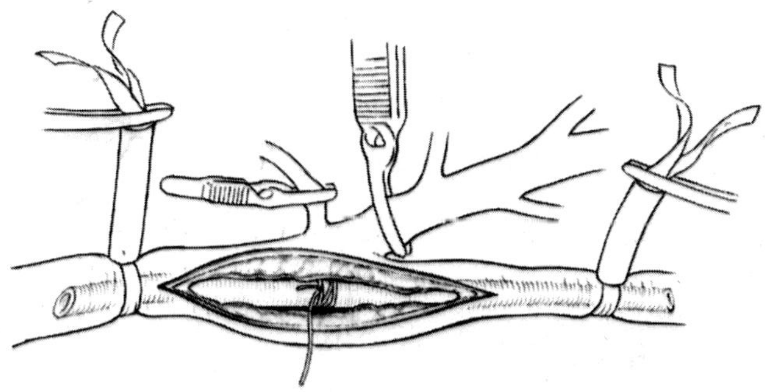

6

7

With the intraluminal shunt in place one may endarterectomize the vessel without undue haste. The appropriate plane is entered with a fine pointed clamp or other dissector and the plaque dissected from the common carotid, the bifurcation, first portion of the external carotid and that portion of the internal carotid containing the plaque.

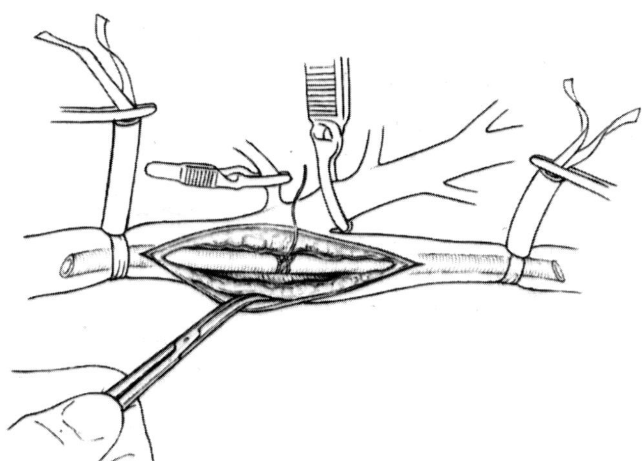

7

8

The distal end of the plaque in the internal carotid usually feathers off quite smoothly leaving only thin intima above, which should not be disturbed. Small bits of debris may be lifted out with forceps or flushed out with saline. It is of the utmost importance that the distant extent of the endarterectomy be visualized so that no large pieces of intima be left to dissect distalward and produce a postoperative occlusion.

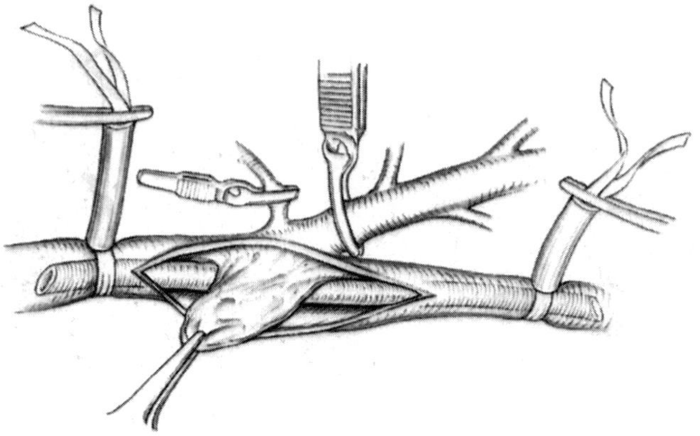

8

9

Occasionally, it is advisable to secure the distal intima with a few interrupted stitches to prevent dissection. Some 6/0 polyester sutures serve well to tack down the intima as well as to close the arteriotomy. It is also important to endarterectomize carefully the origin of the external carotid, since this artery is an important source of blood supply to the brain.

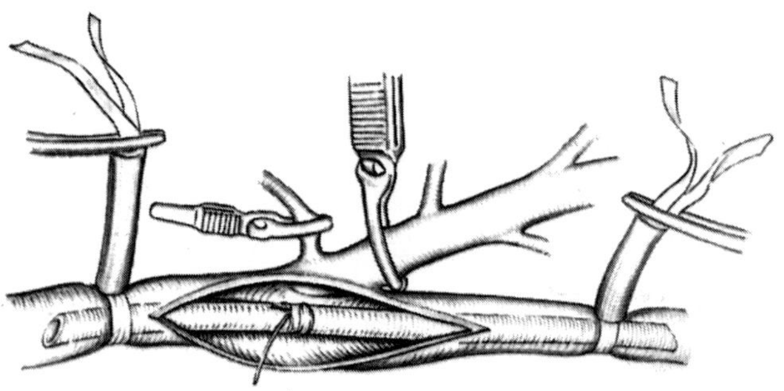

9

10

The arteriotomy is then closed with running sutures of 6/0 polyester beginning at each end. Immediately prior to placing the final three or four sutures the common carotid and internal carotid are clamped and the shunt removed. The vessels are then flushed. The final sutures are quickly placed and tied. At this point the internal carotid is allowed to backflow and is then reclamped.

Clamps are removed from the external carotid and common carotid arteries and flow restored into the external carotid allowing any debris or air to be flushed into it rather than into the internal carotid. The clamp is then removed from the internal carotid and flow restored to the brain. The occlusion time during this final step is 1–2 min. The heparin is then reversed with protamine, if necessary.

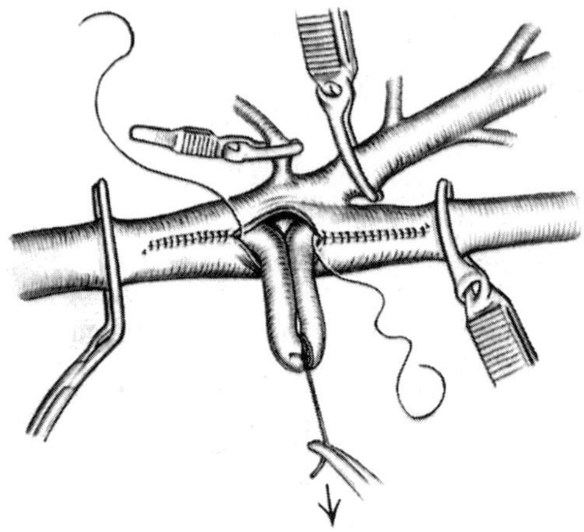

10

11, 12

One may vary the technique of arteriotomy closure by using a thin-blade, partially occluding clamp to include the unfinished portion of the suture line after the shunt is removed. In this way cerebral blood flow is quickly established and the suture line is then completed.

If one is concerned about completeness of endarterectomy or the quality of pulsation in the internal carotid following restoration of flow, arteriograms may be performed on the operating table. Some surgeons perform

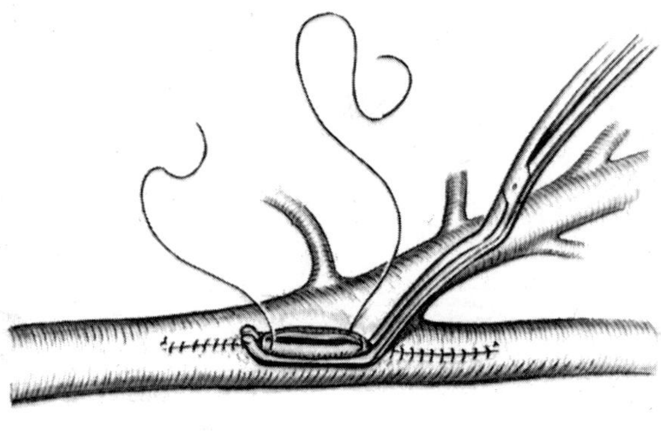

11

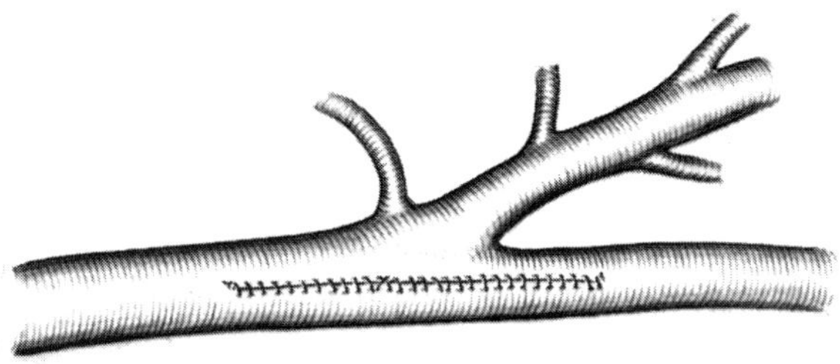

12

this step routinely, but the author has not found its routine use necessary. A sterile Doppler probe to check the signals in the internal carotid is useful at this point.

It is rarely necessary to use a patch graft for closure of the arteriotomy, but if the artery is quite small, a patch graft of autologous vein or prosthetic material may be used. The wound in the neck is then closed anatomically in two layers with interrupted sutures of fine cotton. A small rubber drain is brought out of the lower end of the wound and is removed 24h postoperatively. Bilateral operations when necessary are done in separate stages about 1 week apart to avoid complications of laryngeal oedema, transient hypoglossal paresis, and cerebral oedema.

It is important that adequate levels of blood pressure be maintained during the operation and in the immediate postoperative period. The most satisfactory way to achieve this is to administer 500–1000 ml of lactated Ringer's solution during the operation and postoperatively. Vasopressors are occasionally necessary even when adequate fluids have been given. Routine postoperative heparinization is not used. Aspirin is administered postoperatively.

The technique may vary depending upon variation in pathology. If the plaque is a long one and extends quite far distally, a longer arteriotomy is necessary as is a longer shunt. At times it is prudent to close the distal portion of the arteriotomy and move the shunt proximalward before completing the endarterectomy at the common carotid bifurcation. Occasionally, one finds a plaque in the common carotid 1 cm or so proximal to the bifurcation. In this case, the arteriotomy may be extended proximally, as it is important to remove this plaque as well.

Rarely does one encounter patients with bilaterally occluded internal carotid arteries which cannot be opened by operation. Under these circumstances it is important that patency of the external carotid arteries be maintained, and endarterectomy of the orifices of these arteries may be necessary to improve collateral cerebral blood flow. The shunt technique is easily adapted to endarterectomy of the external carotid arteries.

The technique as described depicts carotid endarterectomy with the aid of a temporary inlying shunt, which is the most reliable method for cerebral support. Some surgeons use the shunt routinely in all partially occlusive lesions, some use it selectively based on an assessment of cerebral collateral circulation, while a few rarely if ever use it. Those who advocate selective shunting rely on one of several criteria of inadequacy of cerebral collateral circulation. Some test the patient under local anaesthesia and use a shunt if temporary clamping cannot be tolerated. Others, using general anaesthesia, insert a shunt if internal carotid artery stump pressure is below 50–55 mmHg or if EEG changes occur upon carotid clamping. In the hands of experienced operators, comparable results may be obtained using selective shunting.

Acknowledgements

Thanks to Little, Brown for permission to reproduce Illustrations 1, 2, 4, 5, 6, 7, and 9 from Thompson (1984), and JB Lippincott for permission to reproduce Illustrations, 3, 8, 10, 11 and 12 from Thompson (1988).

Illustrations by RN Lane.

References

Thompson JE (1984). Carotid endarterectomy with shunt. In *Mastery of Surgery*. Nyhus LM, Baker RJ eds. Boston: Little, Brown.

Thompson JE (1988). Thrombo-obliterative disease of the vessels of the aortic arch. In *Hardy's Textbook of Surgery*, 2nd edn. **Hardy JD** ed. Philadelphia: JB Lippincott.

Thompson JE (1993). Standard carotid endarterectomy. In *Surgery for Stroke*. **Greenhalgh R, Hollier LH** eds. London: WB Saunders Co., pp. 149–156.

Selective shunting during carotid endarterectomy

Roger M Greenhalgh

Introduction

The previous chapter by J E Thompson fully discusses indications and his personal incision and mandatory shunting technique for carotid endarterectomy. Here, a curved incision is described which is preferred by some surgeons for cosmetic reasons; arguably this approach allows equivalent access to the carotid artery. The use of an intraluminal shunt for every procedure is not my practice because its very use carries a morbidity from dislodging artereal debris which can embolize to the brain.

The operation

Position of patient and anaesthesia

1

The skin is prepared and the towels are placed so that the whole neck area and the earlobe can be seen. The intended skin incision is marked in ink with cross-stripping marks to show the correct apposition points for the eventual skin closure. It is convenient to secure the towels and maintain sterility by using a plastic drape after the skin has been marked. The skin incision is placed as shown in relation to the anterior border of the sternomastoid muscle. Many surgeons prefer a longitudinal incision down the anterior border of the sternomastoid but this is less cosmetic and does not provide better exposure. The skin crease incision is preferable and care should be taken to ensure that it is at least two fingers' breadth away from the angle of the jaw for fear of damage to the cervical branch of the facial nerve. The great auricular and other cutaneous nerves are shown and these must be avoided as the incision is deepened through the platysma muscle to locate the anterior border of the sternomastoid. This is the vital landmark to find, because the rest of the dissection is continued along the plane of the anterior border of this important muscle.

2

The carotid sheath is approached by dividing and transfixing the common facial vein. A simple ligature for this

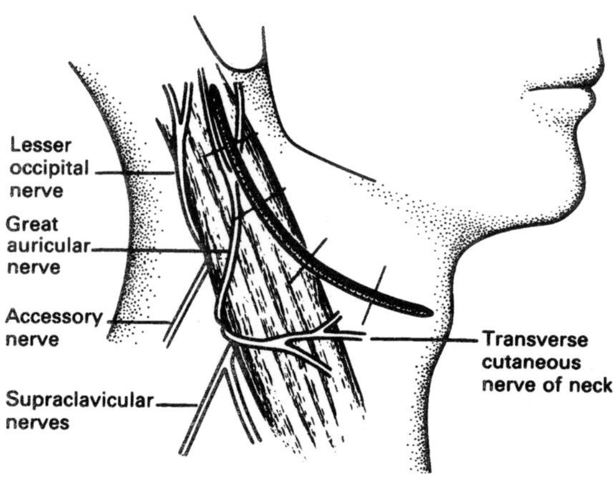

1

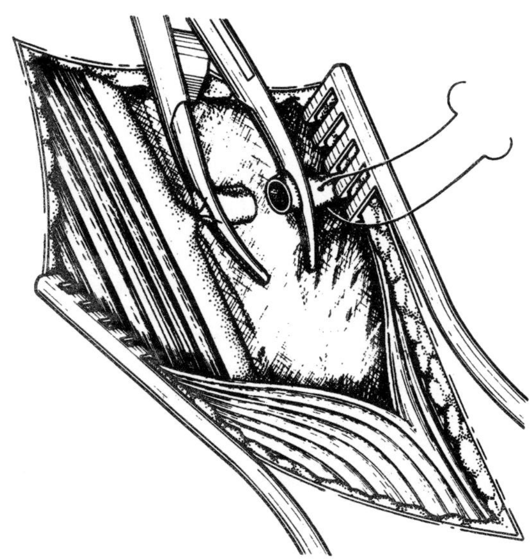

2

vein is frequently inadequate as tremendous pressures are achieved during extubation and when coughing occurs. The dissection then continues as described in the previous chapter.

Selective intraluminal shunting

3, 4

The subsequent figures concentrate on the carotid vessel itself. The patient is given 5000 units of heparin intravenously and after 3 min a clamp is placed across the external carotid artery. A needle attached to a monitoring line is placed in the external carotid artery as this avoids risk of embolization to the brain. Pressure in this artery is measured using the monitoring equipment. When the pressure is displayed on the monitoring system the common carotid is cross-clamped using a very soft clamp such as the Fogarty clamp with Silastic implants. This provides a 'back pressure' or 'stump pressure' reading.

At this stage the internal carotid artery is behaving as a side arm to the circle of Willis and this pressure is an estimate of the pressure in that circle. Those surgeons who, like the author, take notice of this reading will, in practice, find that one of two things happens the moment the common carotid artery is clamped: either the pressure falls slightly but stays at around 90 mmHg mean pressure with a pulsatile waveform, or the pressure suddenly falls and the waveform goes flat. As soon as the pressure falls to below 50 mmHg the author waits no longer but inserts an intraluminal shunt. If the pressure is above 50 mmHg and the waveform is pulsatile, no shunting is performed. Others use different methods for deciding whether to use a shunt, such as monitoring with the electroencephalogram.

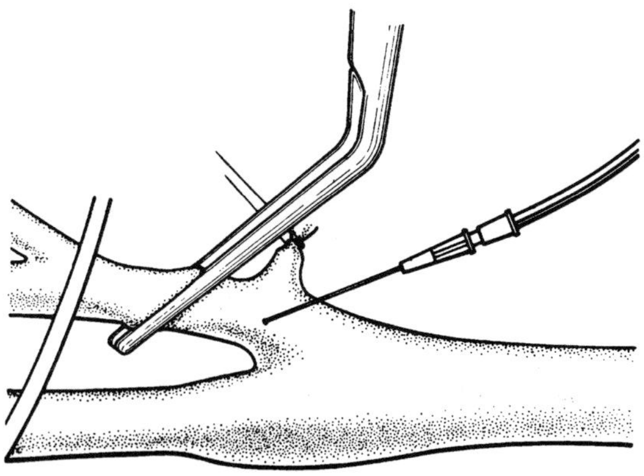

3

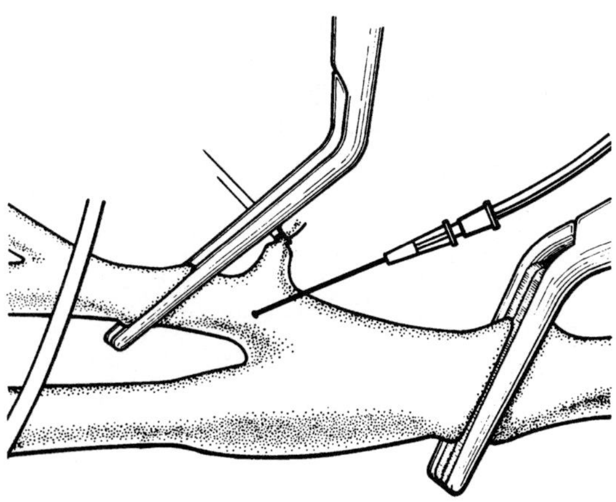

4

Shunting technique

5

When it is decided that an intraluminal shunt should be used, the author's preference is for the Javid shunt. This is a plastic shunt which fits comfortably into the common carotid below and the internal carotid above. Special ring clamps can be used to hold it in place as shown. As soon as the use of an intraluminal shunt for cerebral protection is indicated, an artery clip is placed across the Javid shunt, the larger end of the shunt is introduced into the common carotid artery below the atheroma and the ring clamp is made secure.

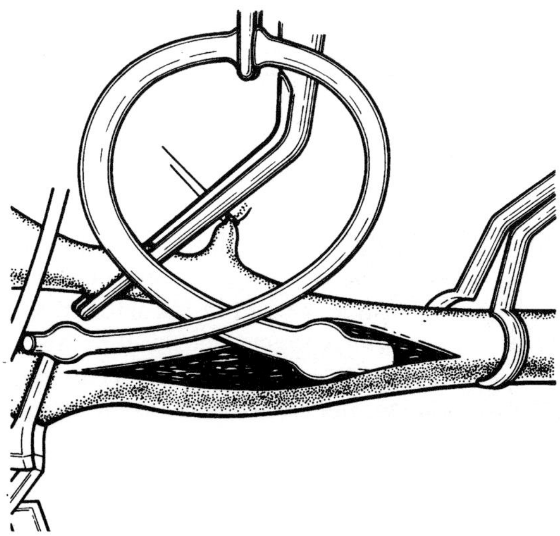

5

6

The artery clip is then momentarily removed to allow forward squirt to occur onto a swab. This clears both the shunt and the common carotid artery of any debris, minimizing the risk of embolization to the brain, and indicates that a good flow can be delivered to the brain.

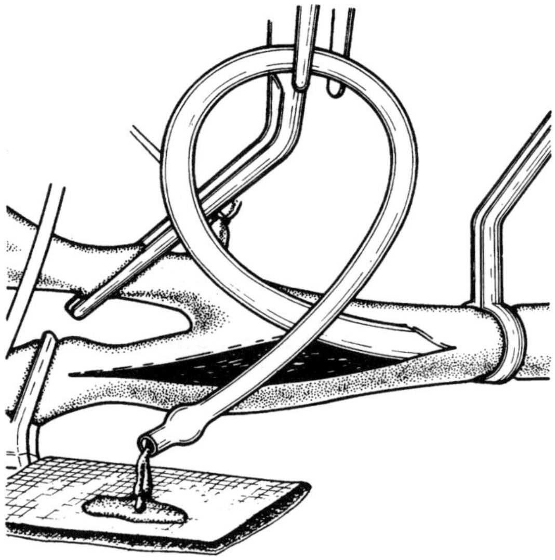

6

7

The artery clip is replaced on the Javid shunt and the bulldog clamp is removed from the internal carotid artery, allowing backbleeding to occur, which removes any debris from this vessel. The shunt is then gently manipulated into the internal carotid artery well above the diseased bifurcation.

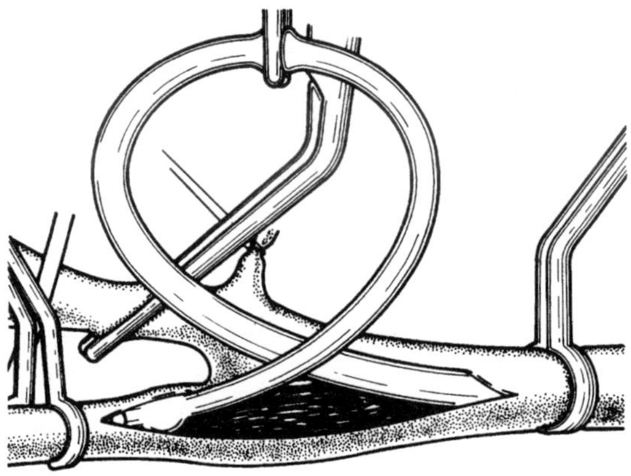

7

8

The smaller ring clamp is now secured and the artery clip is taken off the shunt. This allows blood flow to pass through the shunt from the common carotid to the internal carotid artery so that endarterectomy can be performed without any hurry.

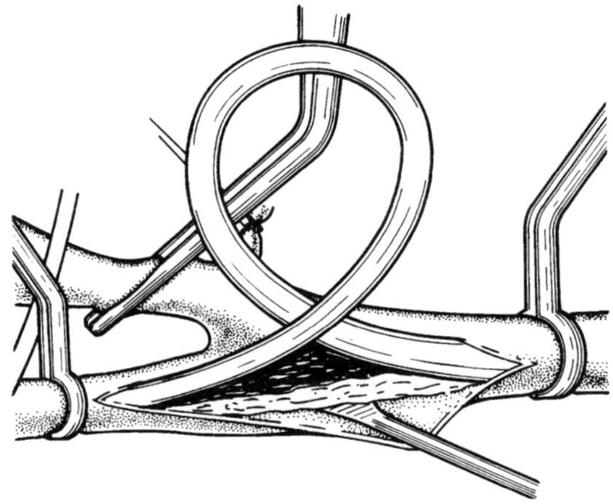

8

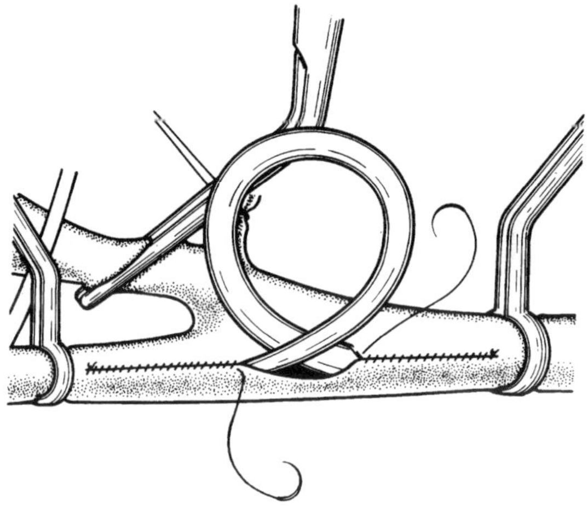

9

9

Suturing is performed as before. The shunt is no hindrance; in fact, it acts as a stent and can be a very useful aid to performing a good suture line. When no more suturing can be performed, the shunt is once again clamped with an artery clip and the ring clamps are removed; the former arterial clamps are then replaced and the shunt is removed. The arteriotomy is closed, the sutures tied and the unclamping procedure is exactly as described previously.

Acknowledgement
Illustrations by A George.

Approach to the internal carotid artery at the skull base

Wilhelm Sandmann

Introduction

In contrast to the rather uniform and frequent appearance of atherosclerosis at the carotid bifurcation, the lesions of the internal carotid artery at the skull base show a much more variable morphology and remain a challenge even for the experienced vascular surgeon. In our experience, with 60 reconstructions over 10 years, stenotic lesions have outweighed aneurysms by 2 : 1. Fibromuscular dysplasia appeared in 31%, chronic trauma in 26% atherosclerosis in 21%, spontaneous dissection in 10% and other diseases in 12%. Embolism from local thrombus formation was the major cause of preoperative transitory ischaemic attacks or strokes. Therefore, the distal segment of the internal carotid artery is not only difficult to approach for anatomical reasons but delicate to repair. Manipulation at the diseased vessel wall before clamping inevitably causes cerebral embolism. Sometimes the reconstruction has to be performed with a weakened arterial wall. Although indications for reconstruction of the internal carotid artery at the skull base are rather rare and amount to only 0.5% of all carotid operations at our institution, the approach to the skull base and technical details for reconstruction are described in this chapter.

Like other reconstruction in areas difficult to approach, surgery at the skull base requires excellent diagnostic work-up. Large skull-base aneurysms can be palpated through the nasopharynx and may be measured by computed tomography scanning of the neck. Doppler studies are helpful to detect flow-restricting lesions, but neither extra- or transcranial Doppler examination nor angiography can predict if longer time periods of clamping will be tolerated. The majority of these patients are much younger than the typical atherosclerotic patient. Therefore, collateral flow is not restricted by generalized occlusive disease and the risk of clamping ischaemia is very low. At least in our experience, recurrent or new postoperative deficits could not be attributed to temporary interruption of cerebral blood flow.

Superselective catheterization using conventional techniques or intra-arterial digital subtraction angiography in at least two planes is mandatory to determine the aetiology, anatomical extension and emboligenic potential of the disease and to visualize intracranial circulation.

Applied surgical anatomy

The extracranial portion of the internal carotid artery can be divided into three segments. The first extends from the bifurcation, where the hypoglossal nerve crosses the internal carotid artery at the level of the third vertebra. At the beginning of the second segment the hypoglossal nerve joins the sheath of the vagus nerve. At this level the architecture of the arterial wall changes from the elastic to the muscular type. Spontaneous dissections usually originate from this transition zone. The second segment reaches up to the body of C2, which is about the tip of the styloid process, where the superior laryngeal nerve leaves the vagus nerve in a dorsomedial direction. The internal jugular vein and the vagus nerve accompany the internal carotid artery within the same sheath. At the bifurcation the position of nerve and vein is lateral and not very close to the internal carotid artery, whereas at the skull base both are in a more dorsal position and the vein becomes rather close to the artery. The third segment extends from the tip of the styloid process to the carotid canal, which is entered obliquely. The view into the canal is hampered both caudally and laterally by a squamous portion of the temporal bone, which is located between the styloid process and the petrotympanica fissure below the acoustic canal.

1

The patient is placed in a supine position on the operating table with the head slightly elevated and turned

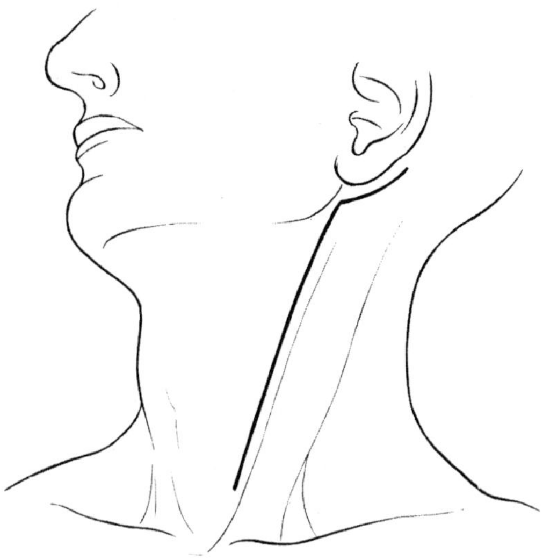

1

towards the opposite side. The skin is incised vertically along the anterior border of the sternocleidomastoid muscle just behind the ear lobe.

2

After transection of the platysma, the posterior facial vein and the posterior belly of the digastric muscle can be seen in front of the carotid artery.

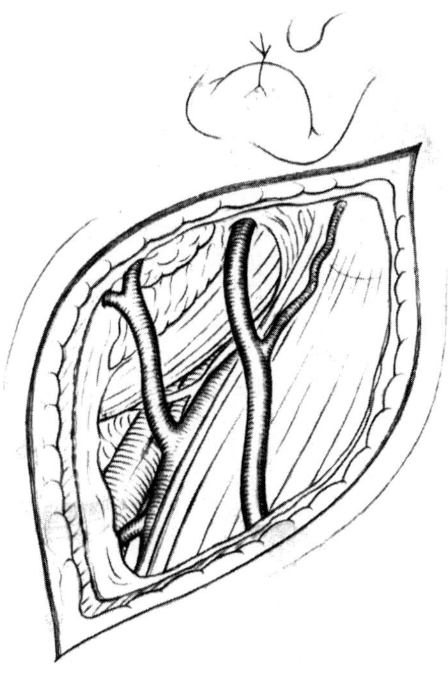

2

3

The internal carotid artery is exposed stepwise. The descendens hypoglossi is seen passing down from the hypoglossal nerve and may be divided if it helps the exposure. Any vessels lying in front of the hypoglossal nerve are divided.

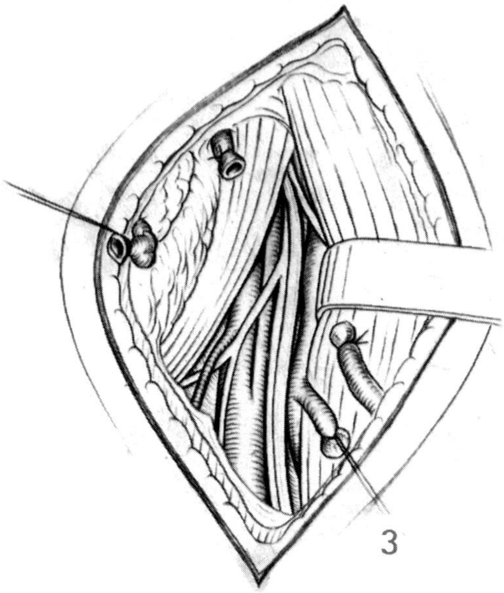

3

4

The digastric muscle is divided using electrocautery. The occipital artery or a major branch, usually located behind the digastric muscle, is ligated to avoid postoperative bleeding. Most of the skull-base arterial lesions begin at about this level.

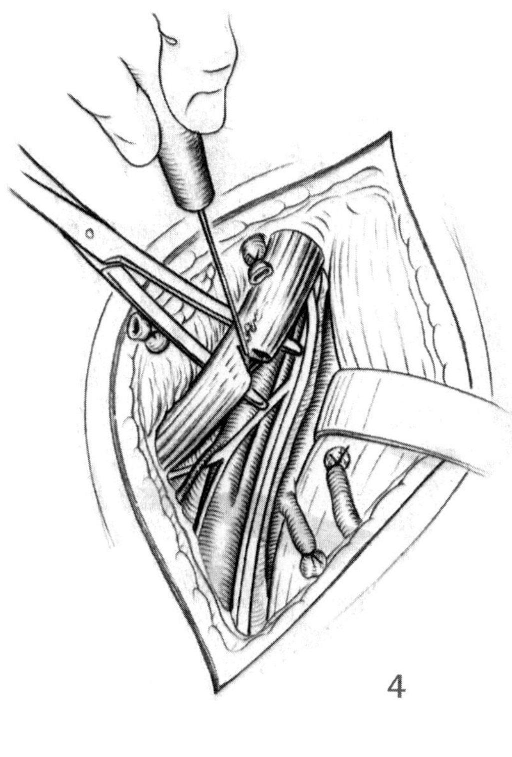

4

5

Before exposure of the diseased segment, the patient is fully heparinized and the internal carotid artery is clamped near the bifurcation. A long but shallow retractor is placed against the styloid process, which usually breaks at its base. The retractor is pulled towards the skull base and a second retractor is placed more laterally, so that a tunnel is created around the diseased internal carotid artery. The glossopharyngeal nerve and the rami pharyngei are identified and mobilized using a silicon vessel loop.

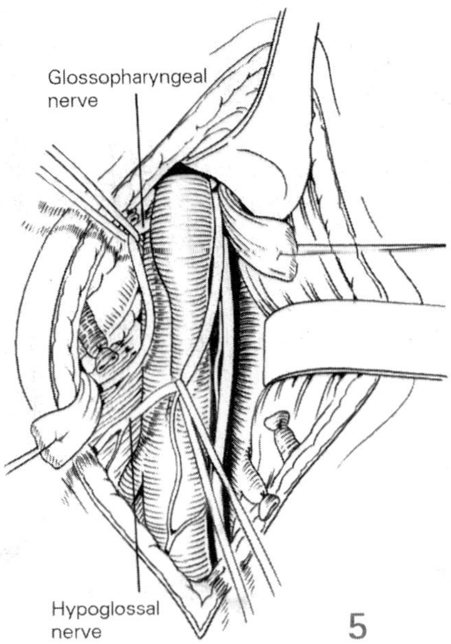

5

6

At this point the internal carotid artery is cross-clamped below the lesion and divided.

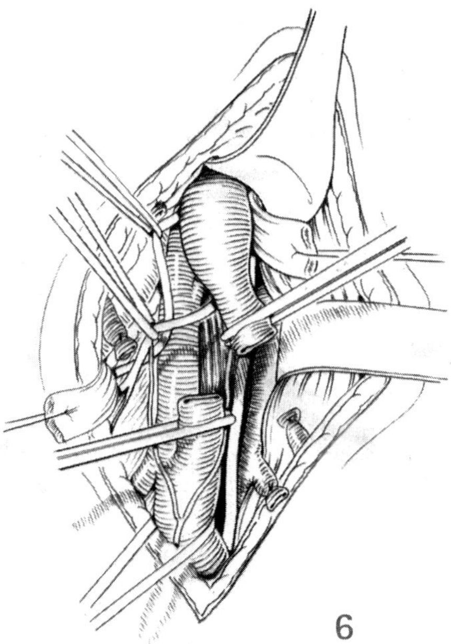

6

7

A suitable segment of harvested saphenous vein is pulled over a 3F balloon catheter. The internal carotid artery is opened and backbleeding is controlled by the balloon catheter.

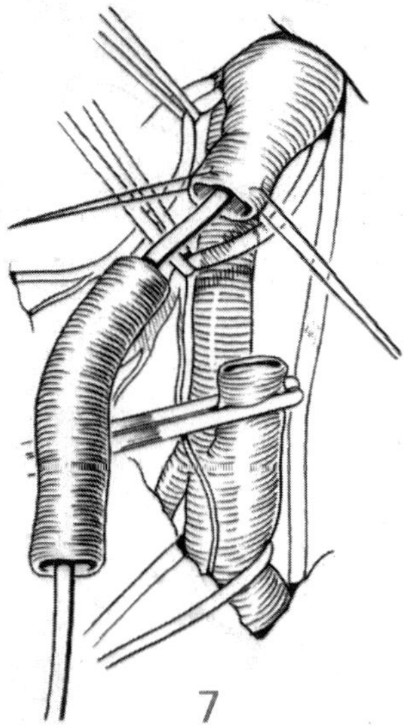

7

8

In patients with aneurysms, the aneurysmal sac is partially resected and the graft is anastomosed from the inside (the graft inclusion technique) with absorbable suture material using interrupted sutures to avoid stenosis of the anastomosis.

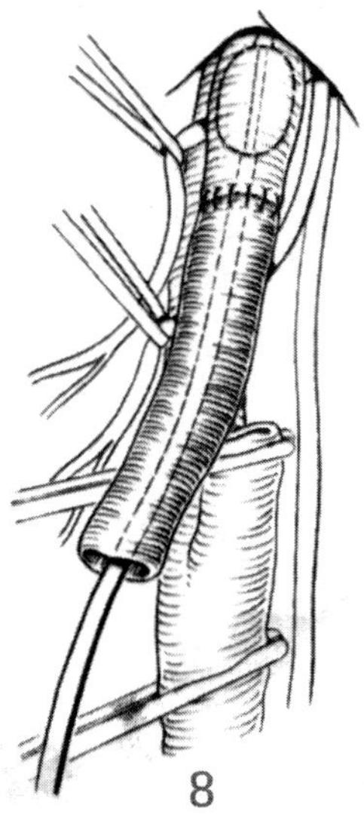

8

9

After the distal anastomosis has been performed, the vein graft is pulled through beneath the glossopharyngeal and hypoglossal nerves.

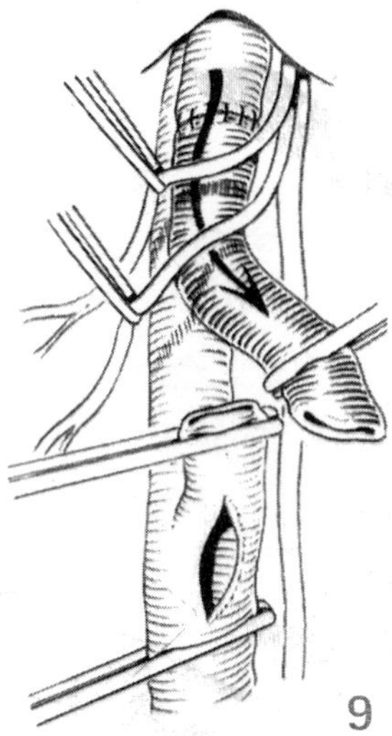

9

10, 11

The common and external carotid arteries are cross-clamped and the common carotid artery is incised. The stump of the internal carotid artery is oversewn and the

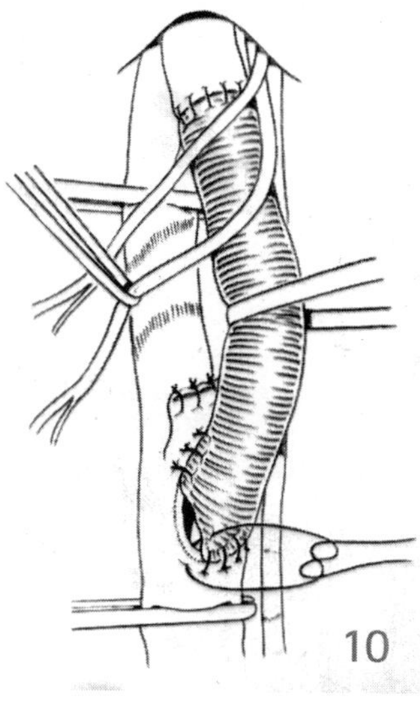

10

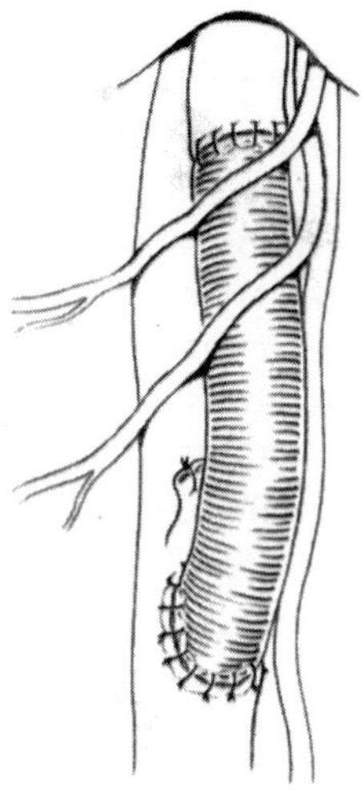

11

graft is anastomosed further proximally. The graft has to be anastomosed with a certain tension, because the neck is overextended and turned through almost 90 degrees. Before the proximal anastomosis is performed, the optimal length of the graft is determined by turning the head into the normal position.

After the anastomosis, arteriography is performed on the operating table because on occasion a very distal anastomosis cannot otherwise be checked. During cross-clamping, the patient is ventilated with 100% oxygen and anaesthesia is maintained by intravenous methods.

In patients with lesions extending just to the entrance of the carotid canal the lateral wall can be removed using a chisel. It is possible to perform the distal anastomosis 1 cm within the carotid canal. However, at this point, the operation becomes complicated and the surgeon needs to have had great experience of such reconstructions. Early proximal clamping during the dissection avoids embolization. The interrupted suture technique using monofilamentous absorbable suture material avoids stenosis of the anastomosis at the skull base. A shunt cannot be used in extremely high lesions, though through-graft balloon catheter blockage is very helpful. Although the author prefers operative angiography, electromagnetic flow measurement is an alternative to detect critical stenoses or distal occlusions during the procedure. Heparinization is necessary throughout clamping to avoid distal thrombosis. Graft length must be checked in the normal head position at the end of the procedure to ensure that kinking and twisting will not occur.

Excision of carotid body chemodectoma

Averil O Mansfield

Introduction

1

Paraganglia are widely disseminated organs with sensory and perhaps local neurosecretory function. Those APUD cells with an affinity for chrome salts are known as chromaffin paraganglia and their tumours are phaeochromocytomas. Those without chrome salt affinity are the non-chromaffin paraganglia; their most common tumour affects the carotid body. The most common sites of non-chromaffin paraganglion tumours are illustrated. In the author's experience the second most common paraganglioma in the neck is of vagal origin. On angiography this is seen as a vascular tumour which does not splay the internal and external carotids apart. When vocal cord paralysis also exists the preoperative diagnosis is complete.

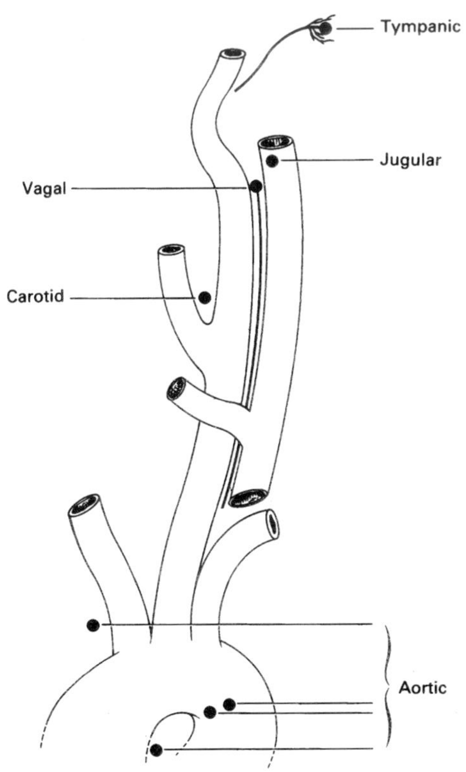

1

Histological distinction between benign and malignant tumours is not possible and only the development of metastases can determine malignancy. This is fortunately uncommon.

There has been much discussion about whether it is necessary to remove these usually benign tumours, but in the author's experience the tumour can be removed safely with little or no risk of recurrence and it is usually easier to deal with this tumour while it is small, rather than to wait until it is an advanced tumour involving local cranial nerves.

Investigations

The important and diagnostic investigation is the angiogram. Normally, this consists of a selective carotid injection and views in two planes. Intravenous digital subtraction angiography, where available, avoids the risk of a carotid injection and when doubt exists about the presence of a tumour this technique is a valuable first investigation and may be all that is required.

Duplex Doppler scanning may also be a useful non-invasive test.

The cranial nerves must be examined with care and indirect laryngoscopy must be a routine preliminary examination. The oropharynx should be inspected.

Carotid body tumours are rarely secretory but the routine examination for vanillylmandelic acid should prevent unexpected problems.

Large and particularly vascular tumours should be considered for preoperative embolization to reduce the technical problems in excising them. However, the evidence that this helps is anecdotal and the procedure carries some risk.

Position of patient

The patient is placed supine with the head of the table slightly elevated. A pad is placed longitudinally between the scapulae (a litre bag of intravenous fluid is suitable). The head, supported in a head ring, is extended and turned towards the opposite side. A bladder catheter may be inserted if a large tumour is to be removed.

Preoperative preparation

The usual preparations for major vascular surgery are undertaken and the blood pressure should be maintained at normal levels. Although hypotensive anaesthesia is an attractive theoretical prospect, it may increase the risk of stroke occurring during carotid manipulation. In addition to normal diathermy, the provision of a bipolar coagulator is valuable. A nerve stimulator may sometimes be helpful.

It is often helpful to palpate the oropharynx before starting the operation to assess the size of the tumour.

Nasal intubation in a high tumour may increase access.

The operation

Incision

2

The incision can be made exactly as in the previous chapter but the author prefers to make it along the anterior border of the sternomastoid muscle from the mastoid process to the lower part of the neck. The exact position depends on the level of the tumour.

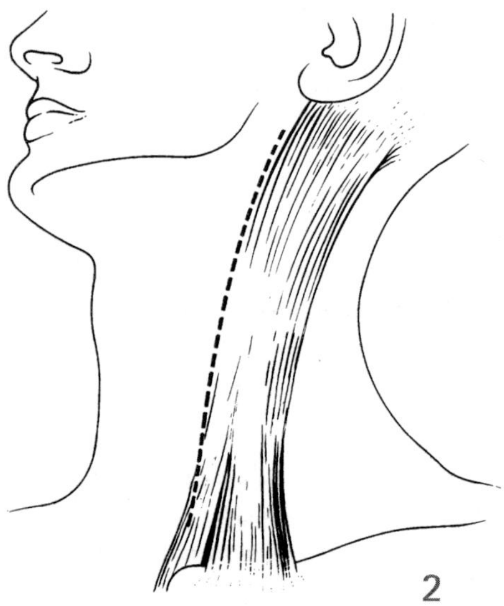

2

3

If the upper part of the tumour extends well above the angle of the mandible, the upper part of the incision may usefully be extended around the ear and anterior to the external auditory meatus, as in the routine approach to the parotid gland.

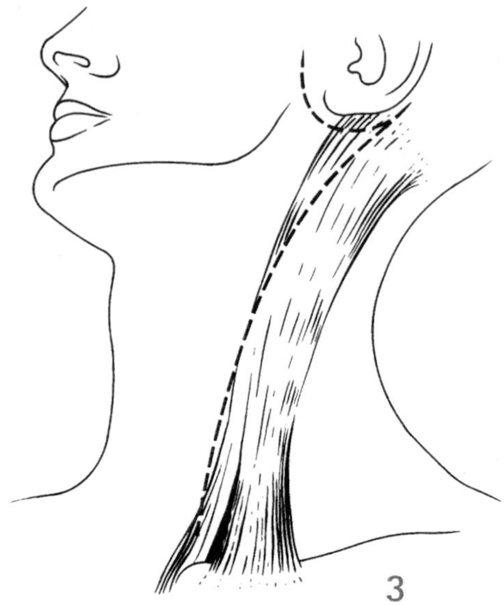

3

4

Cutaneous nerves cross the incision and are divided but the great auricular nerve is preserved.

The platysma is divided and the anterior border of the sternomastoid is exposed. Exposure is developed from the mastoid process to the lower limit of the wound by 'walking over' the muscle until the internal jugular vein comes into view. The muscle can then be mobilized and retracted with a self-retaining Travers retractor.

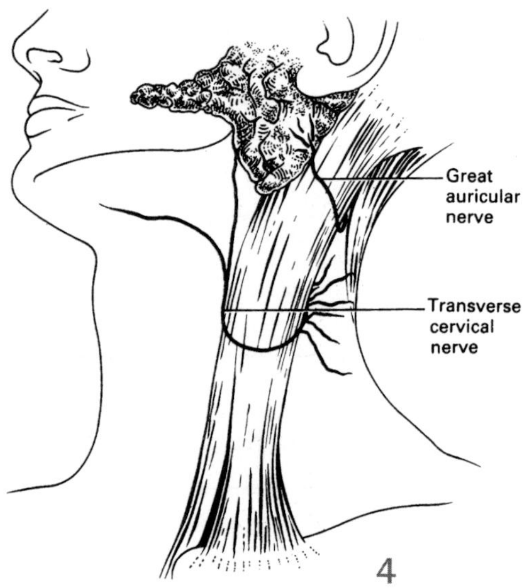

4

Internal jugular vein

5

The internal jugular vein is now dissected from the artery throughout its visible course, taking care not to injure the adjacent vagus nerve in the groove between artery and vein. The common facial vein and any other anterior tributaries are ligated and divided. The Travers retractor with its rounded 'teeth' can safely be used to retract the vein.

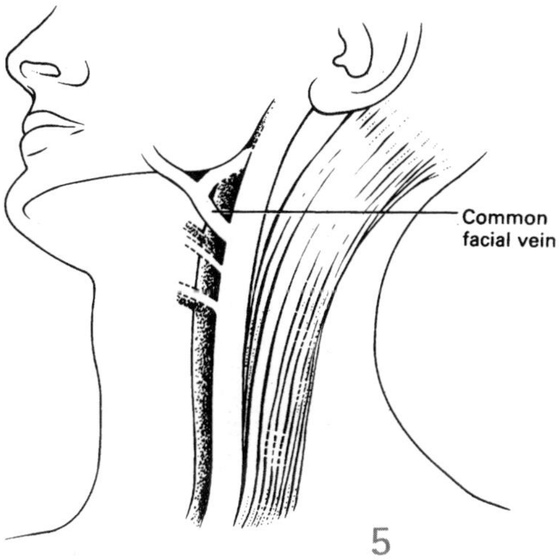

5

6

The vagus nerve is carefully identified throughout its course in the neck. The hypoglossal nerve can usually be identified and preserved but sometimes its course is within the tumour and it can only be dissected out at a later stage. The ansa cervicalis is usually visible and, if possible, is preserved.

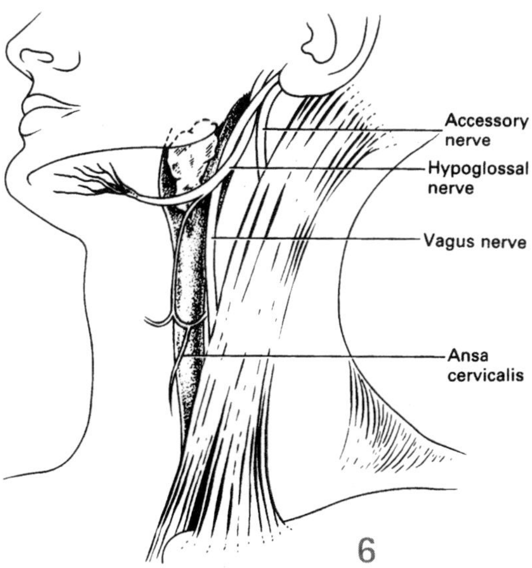

6

7

Carotid arteries

In the common form of chemodectoma, the carotid body tumour, the tumour begins at the level of the carotid bifurcation and the internal and external carotids are splayed apart by it. In the simplest form the carotid vessels are clearly identifiable throughout, but in more complex tumours the arteries may be embedded in and surrounded by the tumour.

The internal and external carotids will come closer together again above the tumour and it is important to identify the internal carotid at that level, i.e. beyond that upper limits of the tumour, before commencing the dissection, in order to ensure its safety.

From then on the operation consists of the safe and meticulous dissection of the carotid vessels from the tumour. As most of the blood supply is derived from the external carotid the dissection is begun with that vessel.

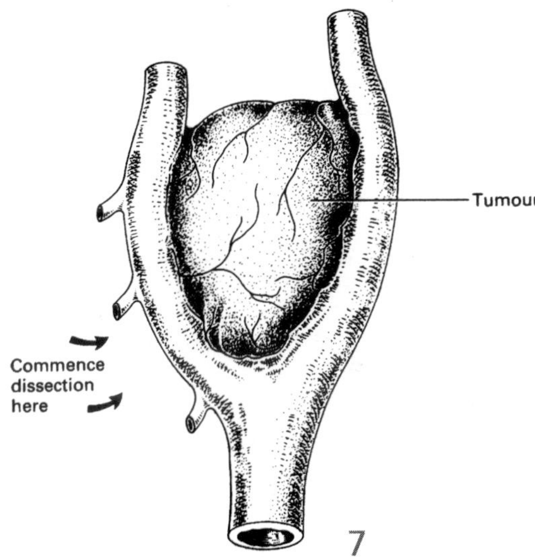

7

The upper end of the dissection

When the carotid body tumour is confined to within the bifurcation which is at or below the angle of the mandible there is no need for this upper part of the operation. However, in the high and extensive tumours this is the most important and the most difficult part of the operation and these routine steps undertaken before exposure of the tumour will facilitate the excision.

8

First the facial nerve is identified by following up the sternomastoid until the posterior belly of the digastic is displayed and then dissection is carried out in the angle above this and between the posterior belly of the

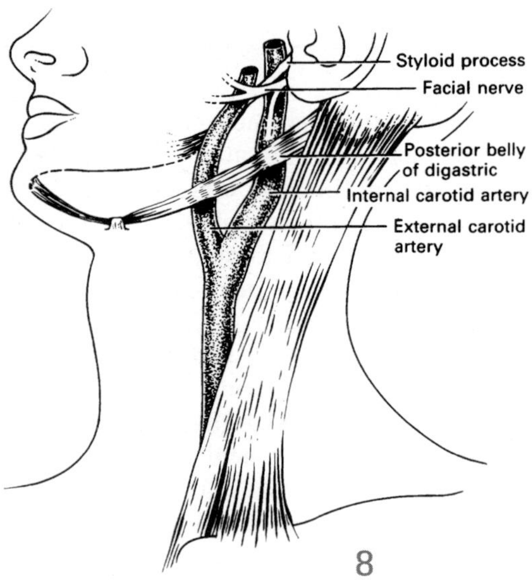

8

digastric and the mastoid process. There is usually no difficulty in recognizing the facial nerve but if any doubt exists the nerve stimulator can be valuable. The reason for displaying the facial nerve is simply to ensure its safety during the remainder of the dissection.

9

The posterior belly of the digastric can then be divided along with the stylohyoid. The occipital artery may have to be divided because it runs backwards along the inferior edge of the stylohyoid. The transverse process of the atlas can be palpated. It must remembered that deep to these muscles are the accessory nerve, the internal jugular vein and the carotid arteries. The styloid process is palpated in the depths between the mastoid process and the mandible. The styloid can then, if necessary, be fractured, allowing the space to open up further. Using this approach the author has never found it necessary to employ the alternative methods of anterior dislocation of the temporomandibular joint or osteotomy of the ramus of the mandible.

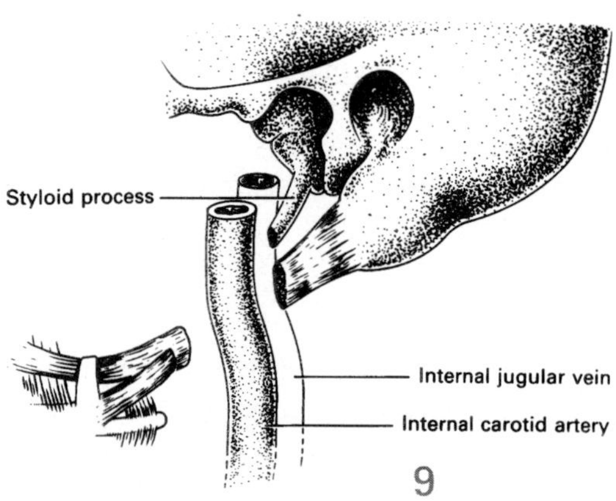

9

The dissection

10

Beginning with the external carotid side of the tumour, the plane between the tumour and vessel wall is identified and developed. The so-called white line of Gordon-Taylor in the adventitia can often be identified (as illustrated), but in other cases, when the tumour is particularly vascular, this is not apparent. Numerous small vessels will course between the vessel and the tumour and the diathermy is invaluable. The bipolar coagulator is very helpful for the numerous tiny vessels encountered. Larger feeding vessels are ligated and divided. Each such division renders the tumour less vascular but the vessels cannot be sought for and ligation must wait until the tumour is peeled off the carotid and they are exposed in the course of the dissection.

If the tumour completely surrounds the vessels it is usually necessary to divide the tumour in order to reach the correct plane of dissection. Again, any such dissection is best carried out on the external carotid side of the lesion. The dissection will then proceed over the external carotid to its anterior surface and similarly to its posterior surface. It is very important to avoid twisting the tumour, and hence the vessels, as this may result in cessation of flow up the internal carotid.

The lumen is most easily entered during the final stages of separation from the vessels in the 'crutch' between internal and external carotids. This is because the exact configuration of the vessels is unknown and because traction may be exerted on the tumour at this stage.

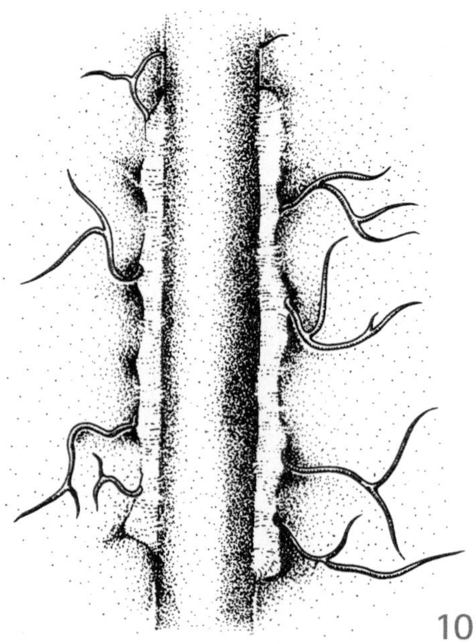

10

11

When the posterior surface of the tumour is being separated from the deep tissues it is very important to avoid injury to the glossopharyngeal nerve, which is in an immediate posterior relation in most moderate-sized tumours. It is not easy to identify and must be assumed to be in danger.

When the tumour has finally been separated from the vessels it will appear smaller and firmer. Most of the bleeding ceases at this stage although an occasional vessel in the tumour bed is diathermied using bipolar coagulation, ensuring first that the cranial nerves are not close by. The author employs suction drainage routinely.

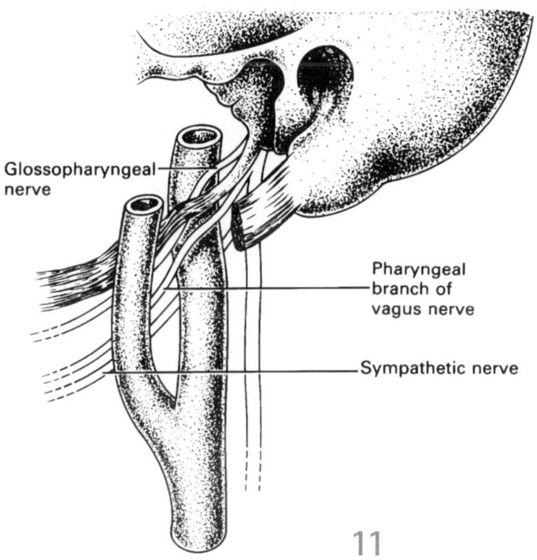

11

Shunt

A shunt, such as the Javid or Brenner shunt, should be available, so that if unexpected carotid injury occurs it can be inserted when prolonged clamping is envisaged.

12

Use of the shunt in order to reduce blood loss has also been advocated, although the author has no experience of this method. The shunt is inserted from the common carotid to the internal carotid, cutting off the orifice of the external carotid and hence the supply to the tumour. Consequently, the tumour is less vascular and the vessels safer.

Ligation of the external carotid to aid haemostasis has been suggested. However, the ligation would have to be at the origin of the external carotid and if this can be dissected out the operation is half completed; little would seem to be gained from ligation at that stage.

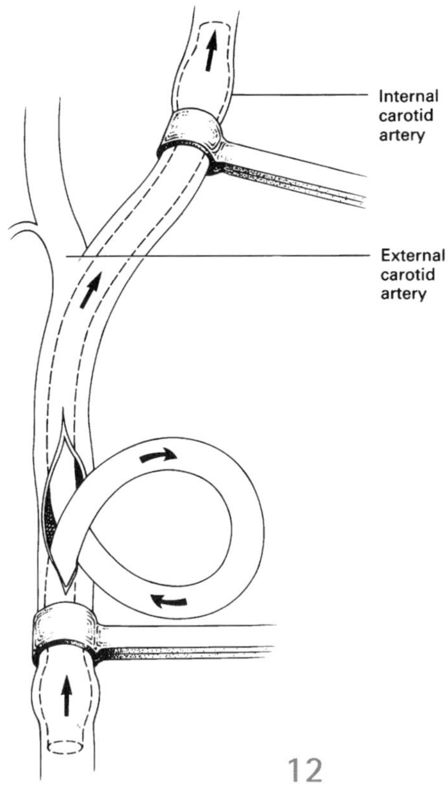

12

Complications

Stroke

Stroke is potentially the most worrying risk of the operation, but the author has had no experience of this. Reports would suggest two possible causes: injury to the internal carotid, and thrombosis as the result of stasis, which may be caused by twisting the vessels or by a haematoma in the vessel wall. In the older age group there is always the possibility of atheroma at the bifurcation and its embolization as the result of manipulation.

Cranial nerve injury

Three cranial nerves are anatomically closely related. Preoperative examination is essential as they may already be affected by tumour. The vagus nerve, except in chemodectomas arising from the vagus, can usually be easily identified and preserved. The hypoglossal is always seen crossing or entering the tumour and should be preserved, provided this does not prejudice the safety or completeness of the excision. The glossopharyngeal is the most difficult to identify and its injury can have serious effects on swallowing.

Arterial injury

If the vessel wall is entered accidentally it can usually be repaired with a 6/0 polypropylene suture. Arterial clamps must always be available. Invasion of the arterial wall by the tumour is rare, but when encountered it will require resection of the artery and vein graft replacement.

Haemorrhage

This can be steady and prolonged but rarely becomes a problem under the conditions of wide exposure, as advocated. Haemorrhage is only a serious problem when the tumour is an unexpected finding at attempted biopsy of a lump in the neck.

Haematoma

As there is a large dead space, suction drainage is necessary.

Conclusion

Carotid body tumours are slow growing and usually benign. They can be bilateral and may be associated with other tumours of APUD cells. Small tumours are easily removed, provided a preoperative diagnosis is made by angiography so that adequate wide exposure can be made. The necessary instruments for arterial repair should always be available but will rarely be required. A carotid shunt should also be available but the author has rarely used one and its use should not be regarded as routine.

Careful identification and preservation of the cranial nerves is a necesary part of the operation, but occasionally one or more of these nerves will already be involved in the tumour and have to be sacrificed.

Acknowledgement

Illustrations by D Konyn.

The technique of carotid stenting

PA Gaines

Introduction

Over the last decade the endovascular treatment of carotid occlusive disease has undergone major changes. The first description was of intraoperative simple balloon angioplasty following which percutaneous access was employed usually from the groin. Patrice Bergeron, a French surgeon, championed the use of direct carotid puncture using modified short sheaths, wires and balloon shafts. Following the involvement of American cardiologists the practice is now primarily based upon guiding catheters or long sheaths, and very low profile systems particularly 0.014 wires, 3F balloons and stents with crossing profiles approaching 5F. More recently there has been particular focus upon mechanical cerebral protection systems. This chapter deals with the basic technique of carotid stent placement for occlusive disease. Cerebral protection systems are dealt with elsewhere.

Patient selection

Local issues will determine whether asymptomatic as well as symptomatic patients are treated. Since there is only one large randomized trial that shows equivalence of outcome between surgery and endovascular techniques (CAVATAS) in those patients with symptomatic high-grade stenoses it is our practice to focus primarily on this group of patients. However, it would also seem reasonable to treat those patients who are thought to be at high risk from surgical intervention and for whom there are some outcome data from stenting that suggest that it may be a safer alternative (e.g. surgical restenosis, radiotherapy neck, high lesions). In addition there is current interest in managing those patients with asymptomatic high-grade carotid disease who require coronary bypass grafts. Those with arteritis and fibromuscular hyperplasia are potentially other rare groups that benefit from endovascular techniques elsewhere in the arterial system and may therefore be suitable for endovascular carotid intervention.

We do not treat those patients' common carotid origin of disease because of the potential for dislodging emboli whilst placing the long sheath. Very tortuous brachiocephalic or common carotid arteries make easy safe placement of the sheath difficult and again these are probably best managed surgically. Some units would also prefer to treat those patients with marked tonsillar loops surgically so that the loop can be resected. Visible fresh thrombus and total occlusions remain absolute contraindications.

Patient preparation

Patients should be reviewed in clinic so that complications can be discussed and other forms of treatment (surgery or simple medical therapy) can be given fair representation. Only then, after time for consideration, can informed consent be obtained.

Patients will already have best medical therapy. In particular this includes smoking cessation, management of hypertension, diabetes and hyperlipidaemias, and antiplatelet therapy. Most units use aspirin 75–150 mg per day, and in addition clopidogrel is added for the periprocedural period. There is no evidence base for this practice in the carotid system. However, until that evidence is available, we are beholden to do whatever we can to reduce embolization and acute clot formation and, based on the coronary work with the thienopyridine derivatives, the addition of clopidogrel makes sense. Clopidogrel should be started at least 3 days prior to the procedure and continued for 2 weeks. Alternatively some units give clopidogrel 300 mg immediately in the morning, undertake the procedure in the afternoon, and continue clopidogrel 75 mg/day for 2 weeks.

Technique

Initial arterial access is usually via the groin. Occasionally the carotids may be approached from the arms or via direct carotid puncture (see above).

Heparin (5000 international units) is given immediately after arterial access. This will provide a kaolin-cephalin clotting time of more than twice normal for 45 minutes which will cover the majority of procedures. If extra heparin is given as boluses the activated prothrombin time should be prolonged to at least 200 milliseconds.

Selective catheterization of the common carotid artery is performed. Usually this can be done using a simple shaped catheter e.g. Headhunter, but occasionally a sidewinder is required.

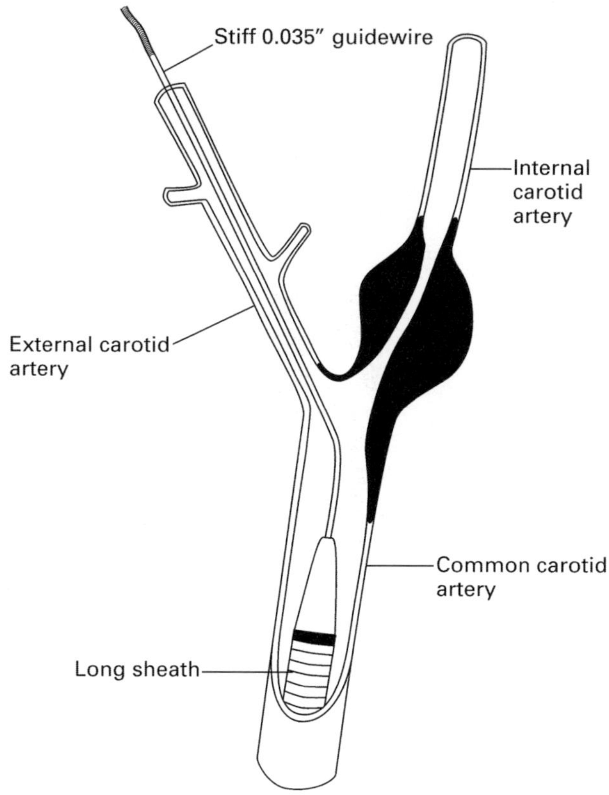

1

1

It is now necessary to place a stiff 0.035 guidewire into the external carotid artery so that a long sheath or guide catheter can be placed into the common carotid artery (1). It is important not to cross the internal-carotid stenosis with the stiff 0.035 wire. This unit prefers the Arrow 7F sheath but the Cook carotid sheath is also excellent. Guide-catheters have the disadvantage of not having a central catheter which therefore leaves the potential for the blunt end to pick up atheroma in the common carotid artery and embolize it distally. The central catheter of the sheath and 0.035 wire are then removed and atropine introduced into the common carotid artery. This is to block the baroreceptors and so inhibit any stimulation during balloon inflation. A pressurized bag of heparinized saline is attached to the side-arm of the sheath to allow continuous perfusion.

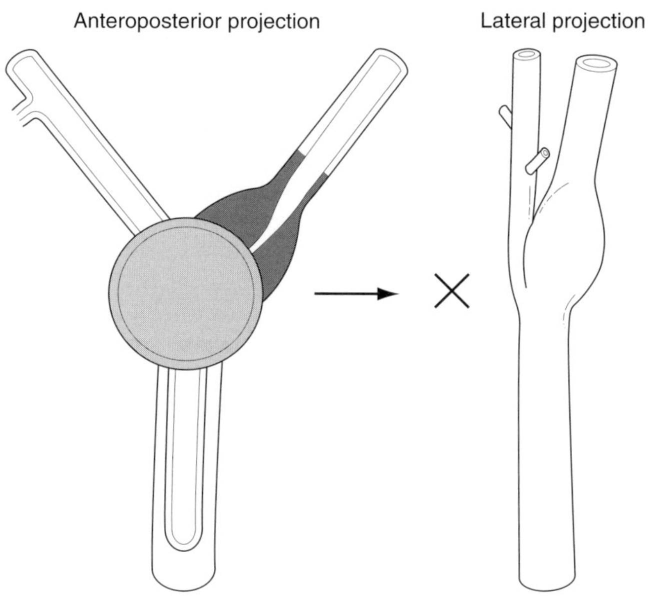

2

2

It is now necessary to size the internal carotid artery and common carotid artery to use the correct diameter stents, cerebral protection devices and post-deployment balloons (2). This can be performed in two ways. The guide-catheter or sheath can be used as the reference diameter. Alternatively, and the system we prefer, is to place a large coin of known diameter over the carotid bifurcation in the anteroposterior projection. The tube is then swung round 90 degrees so that the bifurcation is imaged in the lateral projection and the view is centred half way between the carotid bifurcation and the coin. There are now no magnification or parallax errors and an arteriogram is performed. The coin can reliably be used as the reference object to measure the vessels.

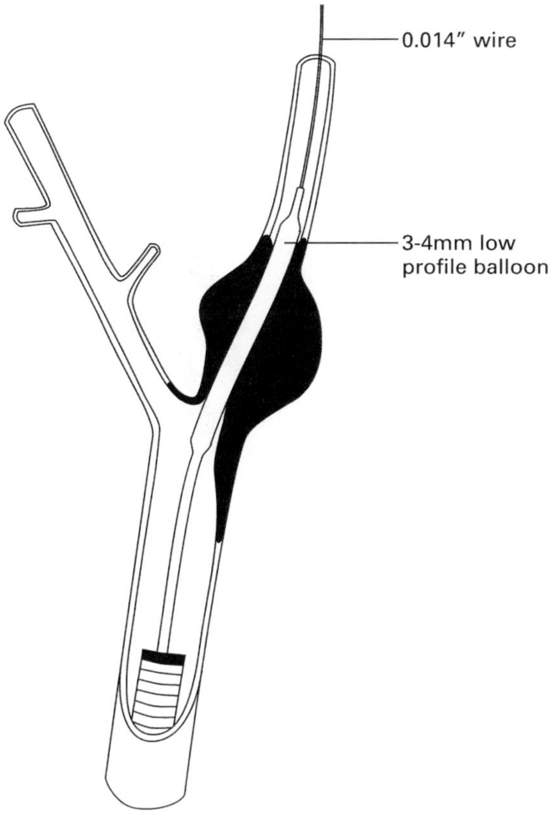

3

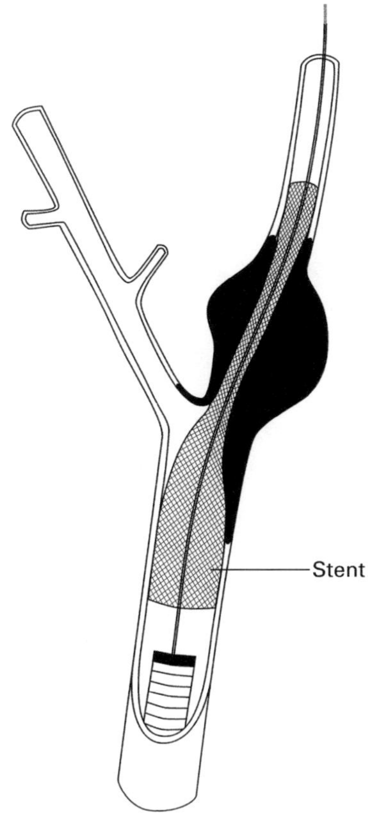

4

3

An 0.014 wire is now used to cross the internal carotid artery lesion and the tip left below the base of skull (3). Above this level the vessels are very prone to spasm. Because the current stent delivery systems are too large to cross a high-grade carotid stenosis without 'dottering' the lesion it is necessary to balloon dilate the stenosis to 3 or 4 mm depending upon the stent. The 0.014 wire facilitates the use of 3F shaft balloons and this should reduce embolization compared with the larger shaft sizes. Throughout the procedure inflation times are kept short (approximately 15 seconds) to reduce cerebral ischaemia times.

4

The stent is deployed across the lesion (4). Complete coverage should be encouraged which means that in the majority of occasions, with current stent technology, the external carotid artery is covered. This very rarely causes any problems. Many retrieval systems benefit for a little wait before they are retrieved through the stent to allow full deployment.

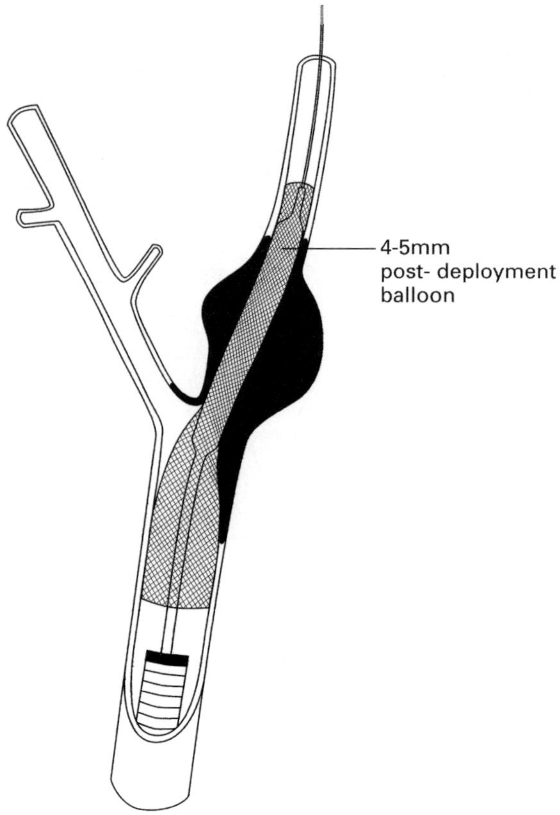

5

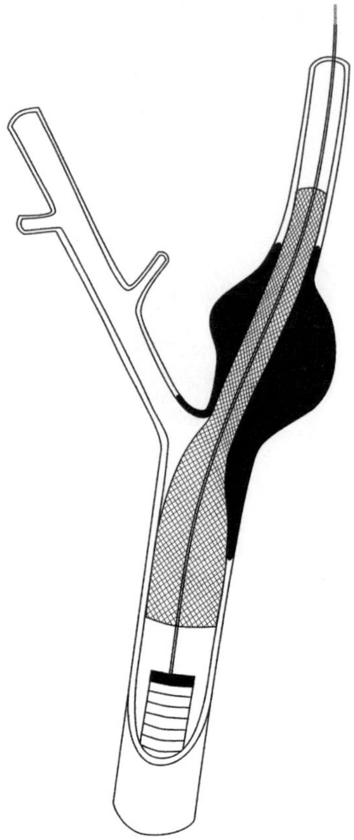

6

5

It is necessary to fully expand the self-expanding stents by post-deployment balloon dilatation (5). The size of balloon can be gauged from the initial sizing obtained at step 5. It is probably preferable not to oversize the balloons and to try to keep the balloon within the boundary of the stent whilst dilating. The Wallstent has a tendency to curl in at the top end and it is our practice to gently hand-inflate a balloon to ensure apposition of the top of the stent to the arterial wall.

6

The final result is confirmed by a completion arteriogram (6).

Protected carotid angioplasty and stenting with the PercuSurge GuardWire system

Michel Henry

Description of the system

1, 2, 3

The PercuSurge GuardWire™ system (1) (PercuSurge Inc ... Sunnyvale, CA USA) consists of three main components.

1. The GuardWire temporary occlusion catheter is a 0.014 or 0.018 inch angioplasty wire constructed of a hollow nitinol hypotube. Incorporated into the distal wire segment is an inflatable elastomeric balloon capable of occluding vessel outslow. A marker shows the location of the balloon. The diameter of the balloon (5 or 6 mm) is chosen depending on the diameter of the artery. The terminal part of the wire is floppy, shapable to cross the lesion, much like coronary wires and is 3.5 cm long. The wire is available in two lengths (190 and 300 cm) allowing a 'monorail' or 'over the wire' technique for balloon dilatation and stenting (1 and 2).
2. The proximal end of the hypotube wire incorporates a Microseal™ allowing inflation and deflation of the distal occlusion balloon utilizing a Microseal adapter.

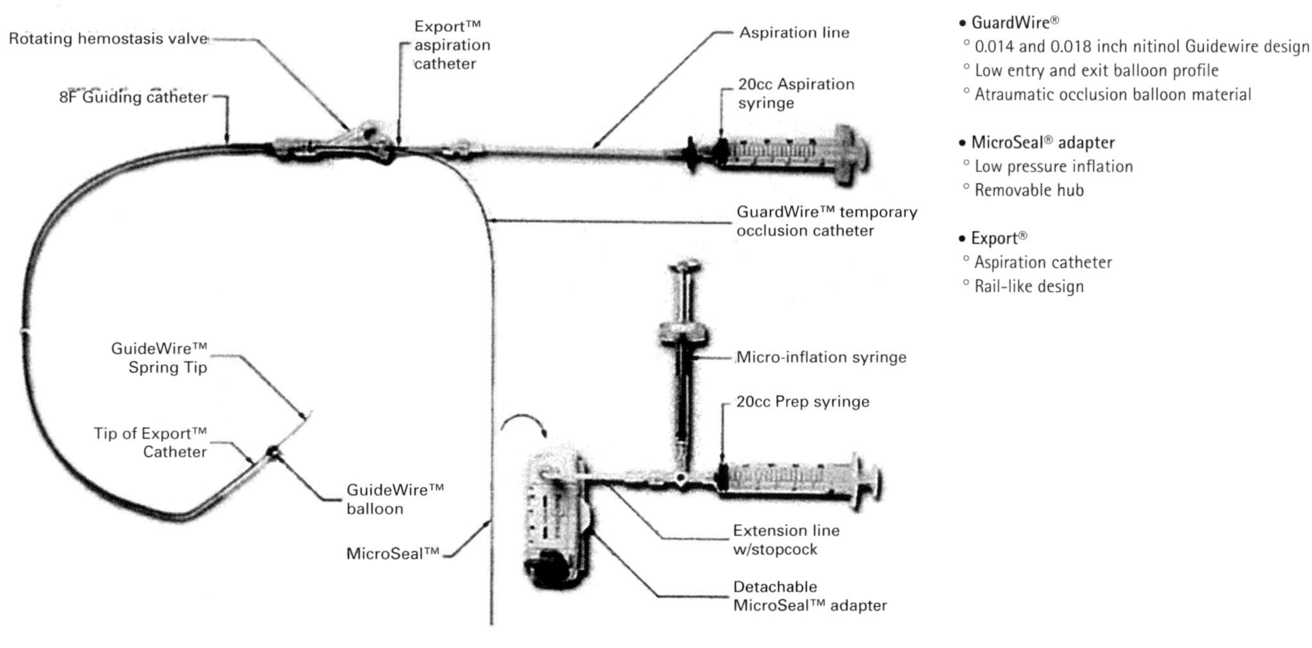

1

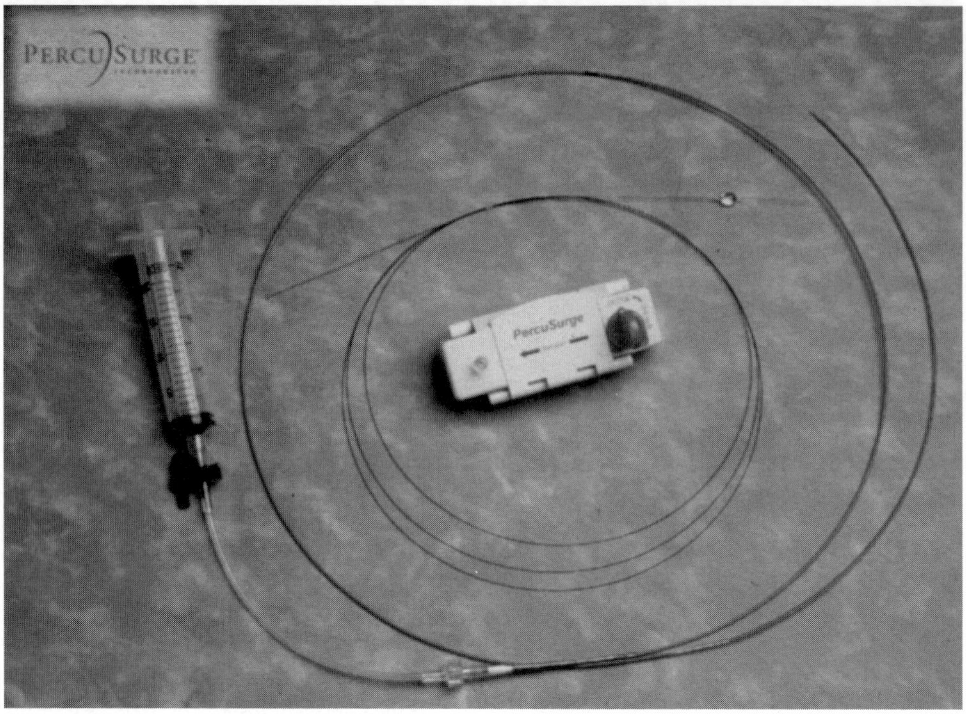

GuardWire temporary occlusion and aspiration system

2

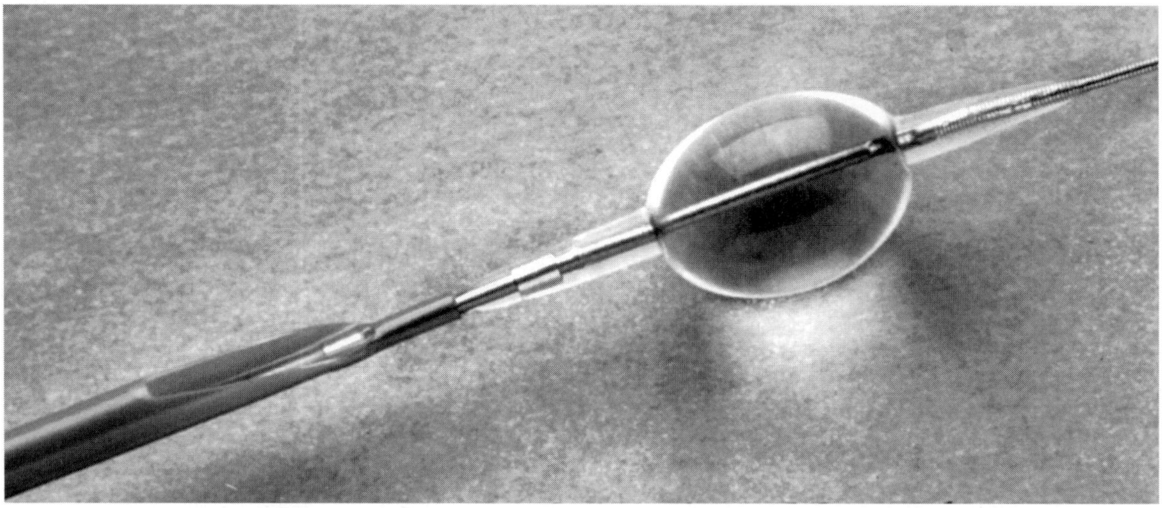

Export aspiration catheter mounted on GuardWire temporary occlusion catheter

3

The Microseal keeps the elastomeric balloon inflated while allowing catheter exchange at the proximal end similar to commonly used guidewires (2).

3. The Export™ aspiration catheter is placed over the shaft of the GuardWire to aspirate the debris generated by the procedure.

Angioplasty and stenting procedure

General technique

An 8 or 9F guiding catheter is initially placed into the common carotid artery using the femoral approach. The Guardwire is then slowly advanced through the guiding catheter. The lesion is crossed and the marker of the balloon is placed 2 or 3 cm beyond the lesion.

The Microseal adapter is attached and the occlusion balloon slowly inflated with a fixed volume of dilute contrast deriving vessel outflow, thus, blood flow is oriented towards the external carotid artery. On detaching the Microseal adapter the occlusion remains inflated. At this point, angioplasty and stenting are performed. Any debris generated is then removed from the internal carotid artery using the following two steps.

1. The aspiration catheter is advanced over the wire into the vessel. A 20-cc syringe is connected to the proximal extremity of this catheter to retrieve particulate debris, at the level of the treated area and close to the protection balloon. The aspirated blood is subsequently sent to a laboratory for analysis.

2. The aspiration catheter is then removed. Lavage cleaning of the treated area may be performed using saline injections through the guiding catheter or the aspiration catheter The injection is performed with an injection pump at a rate of 2 ml per second for 10 seconds. If the occlusion is tolerated a second saline injection may be performed; it is particularly desirable to advance the guiding catheter or the aspiration catheter to the level of the stent, close to the protection balloon. This cleaning encourages the particles towards the external carotid artery.

Balloon occlusion techniques

Two different techniques of emboli removal are possible. In the first method, the occlusion balloon may remain inflated during both stages of the procedure, i.e. pre-dilatation of the stenosis and stent implantation. In this case aspiration and flushing are performed only once after stent dilatation.

The second technique consists of deflating the occlusion balloon to restore the cerebral flow between the two stages. Aspiration and flushing must be performed both after pre-dilatation and after stent dilatation. The choice of technique depends on tolerance of the occlusion, the cerebral vascularization, state of the contralateral artery, duration of the procedure, and the technical problems encountered.

It is noteworthy that with either technique the different steps of the procedure should be performed under cerebral protection (lesion dilatation, stent implantation, and stent dilatation), to avoid cerebral embolism.

4a–f

The distal balloon occlusion technique.

1. The Guardwire is passed across the lesion into the distal internal carotid artery via the guide catheter (**4a**).
2. The distal balloon is inflated to the predetermined volume (**4b**).
3. After the lesion is dilated, the stent is delivered across the lesion; any emboli are contained by the occluding balloon (**4c**).

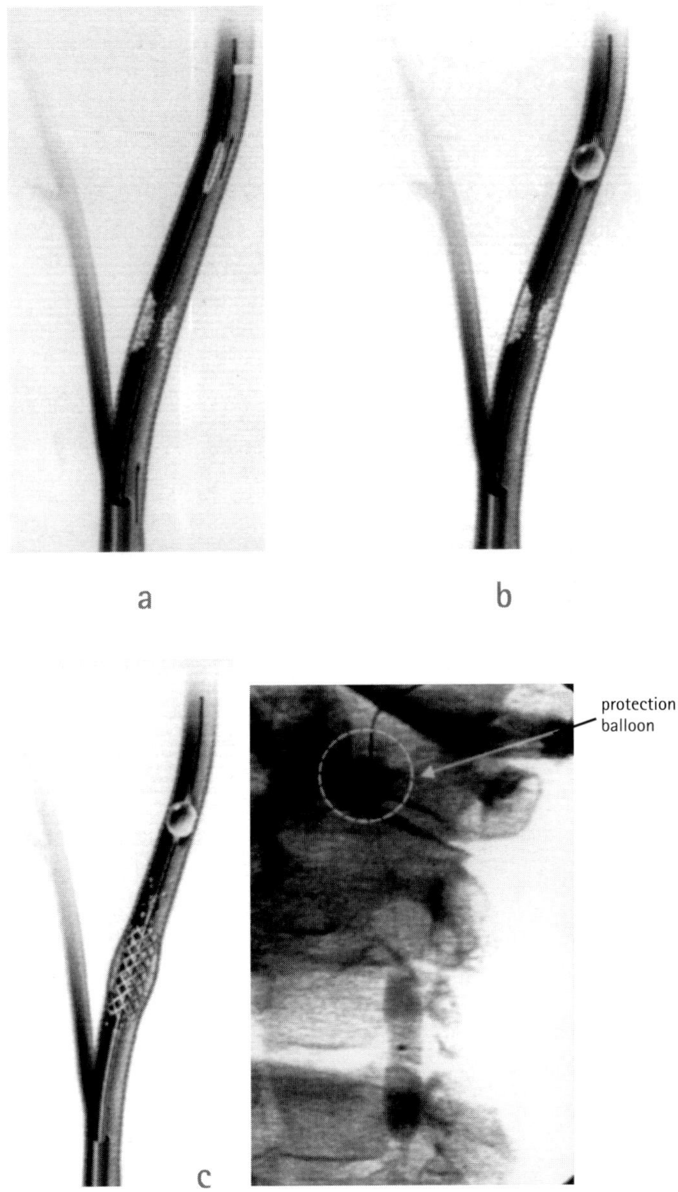

4

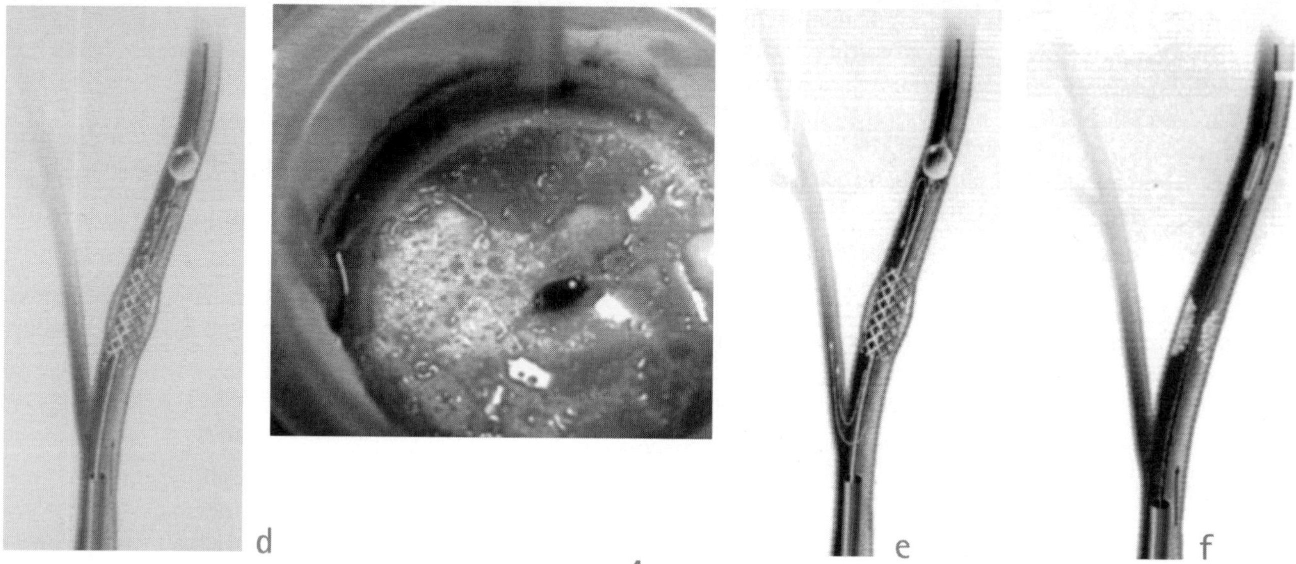

4

4. The aspiration catheter is introduced, to remove emboli and thrombi (**4d**).
5. Lavage cleaning of the dilated area (**4e**).
6. Deflation of occlusion balloon, final result (**4f**).

The MedNova NeuroShield cerebral protection system

P A Gaines

Introduction

Carotid stenting is currently undergoing rapid evolution and much attention is focussed upon strategies to reduce peri-procedural stroke. The presumed mechanism of this is cerebral embolization based upon the occasional angiographic demonstration of intracerebral emboli, transcranial Doppler data and benchtop modelling. So-called 'cerebral protection' systems are being developed which stop the flow of emboli to the brain. Three current concepts are being pursued; balloon occlusion of the internal carotid artery filters and flow reversal. The MedNova NeuroShield is a filter system that now has a CE (European Community approval) mark and is available as an adjunct to carotid stenting.

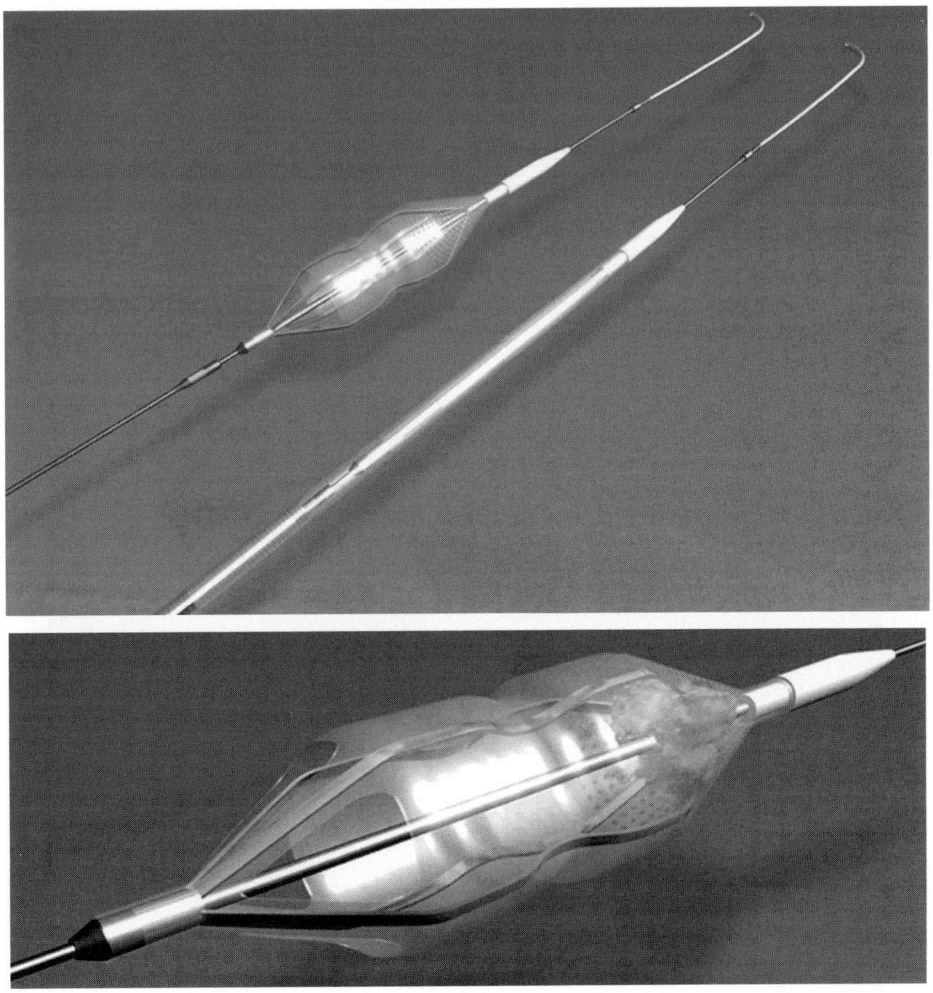

a

b

1

Description of the device

1a, b

The filter is made of a polyurethane membrane supported by gold-coated nitinol struts. The proximal entry ports are large and the distal pores 150 microns (μ) in diameter. The design of the filter provides good apposition against the vessel wall and is available in sizes to fit arteries of 3.5–6.2 mm diameter. The filter is mounted upon a 0.014 nitinol wire, which upon delivery of the NeuroShield, acts as the guidewire over which subsequent manipulations are performed. The filter has a degree of longitudinal and rotational movement upon the wire which allows for some degree of wire movement without disturbing the position of the filter. Before treatment the filter is ensheathed in an outer delivery catheter with a crossing profile of around 4F. At the tip of the system is a floppy shapeable torqueable wire which is used to cross the lesion.

2

The filter is released into position by simply pulling back the outer sheath

3

To retrieve the filter at the end of the procedure a sheath with an expandable pod at the tip is advanced to the filter (see later). The expandable pod ensures that the filter is completely covered without extrusion of debris.

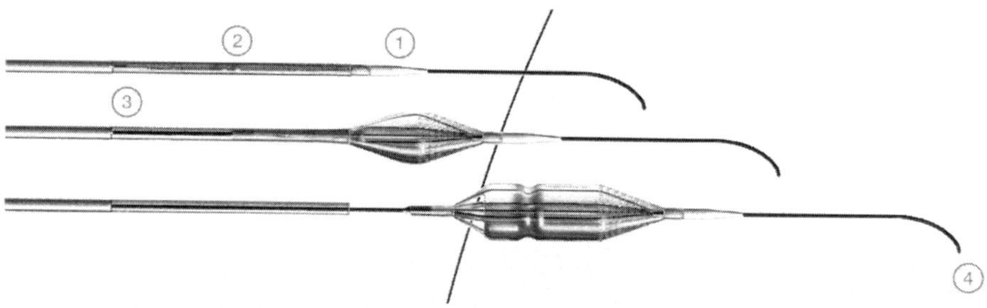

2

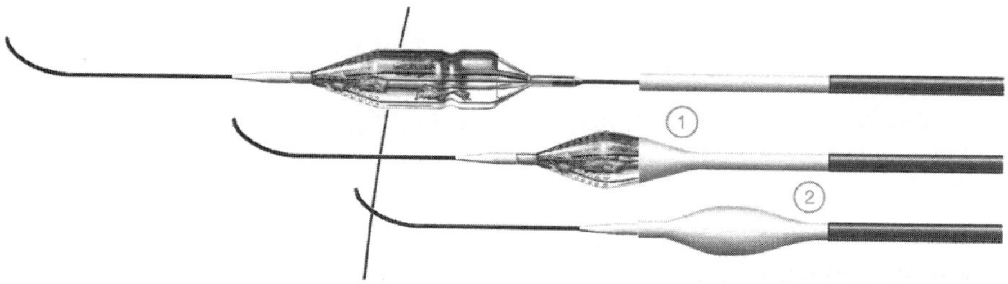

3

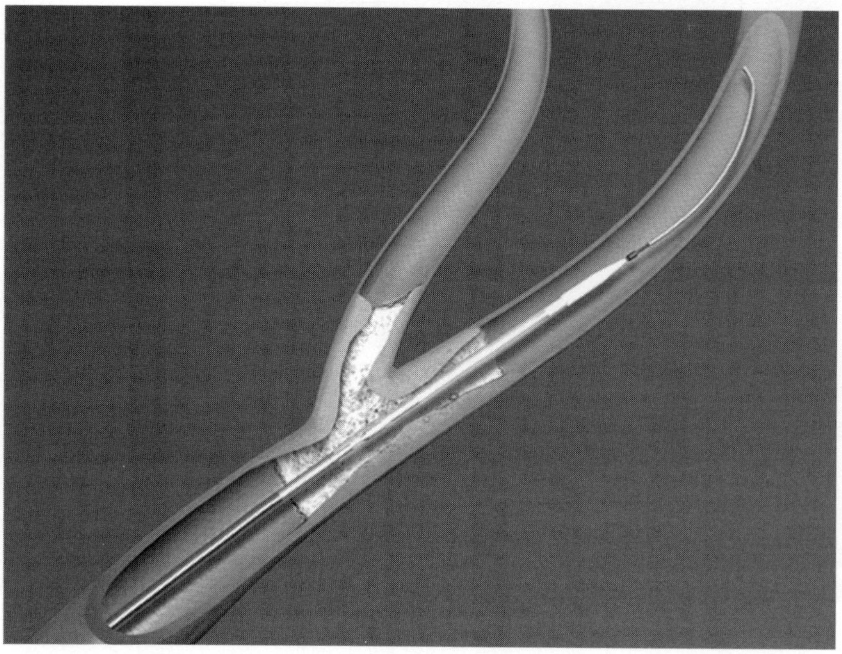

4

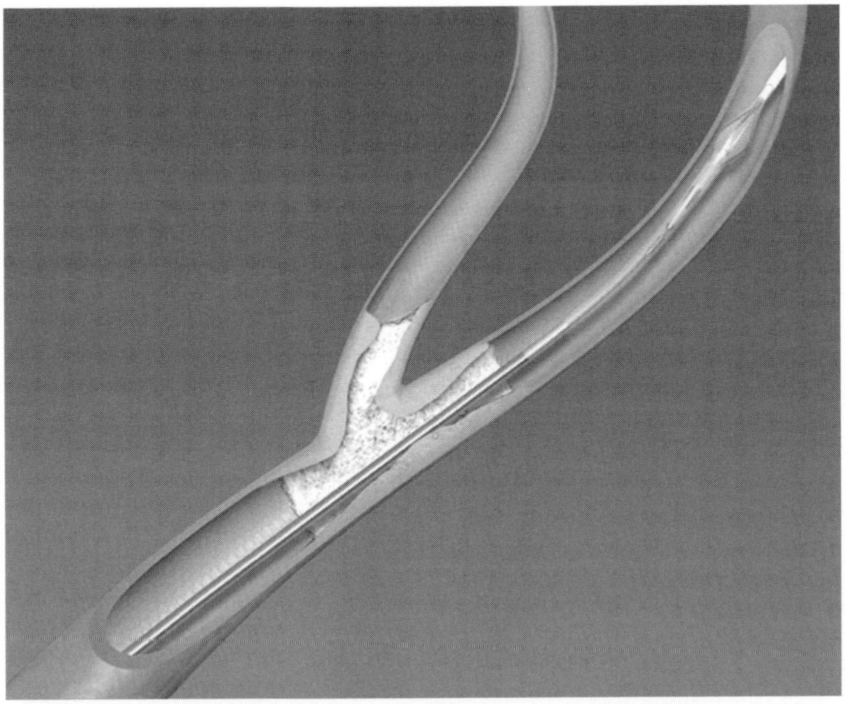

a

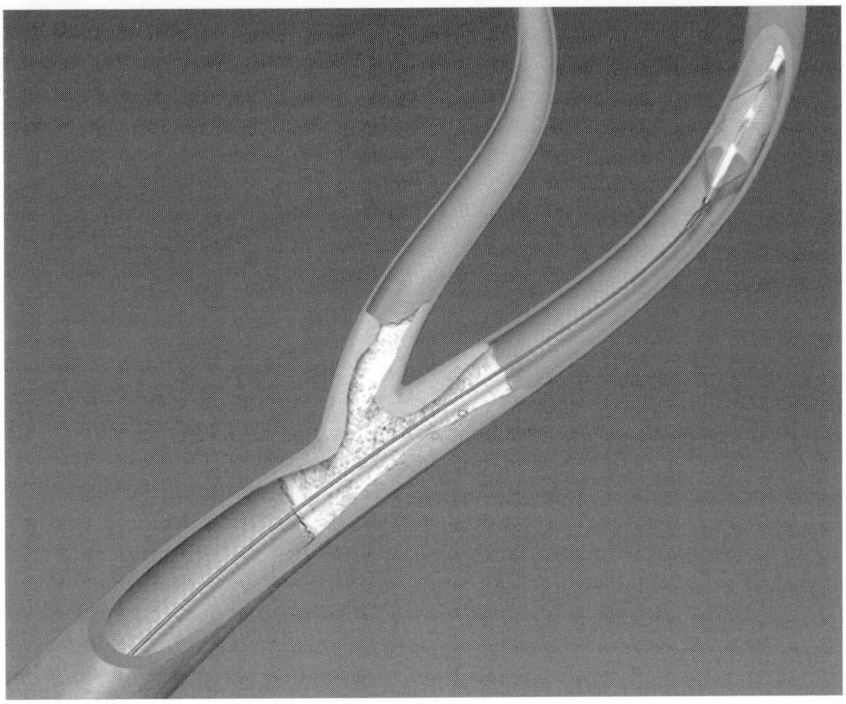

b

5

Description of use

4

Once the long sheath or guide-catheter is securely placed in the common carotid artery the enclosed filter is passed through the sheath and carefully advanced across the stenosis.

5a, b

When the device is at the appropriate deployment area the filter is deployed by retracting and removing the outer catheter.

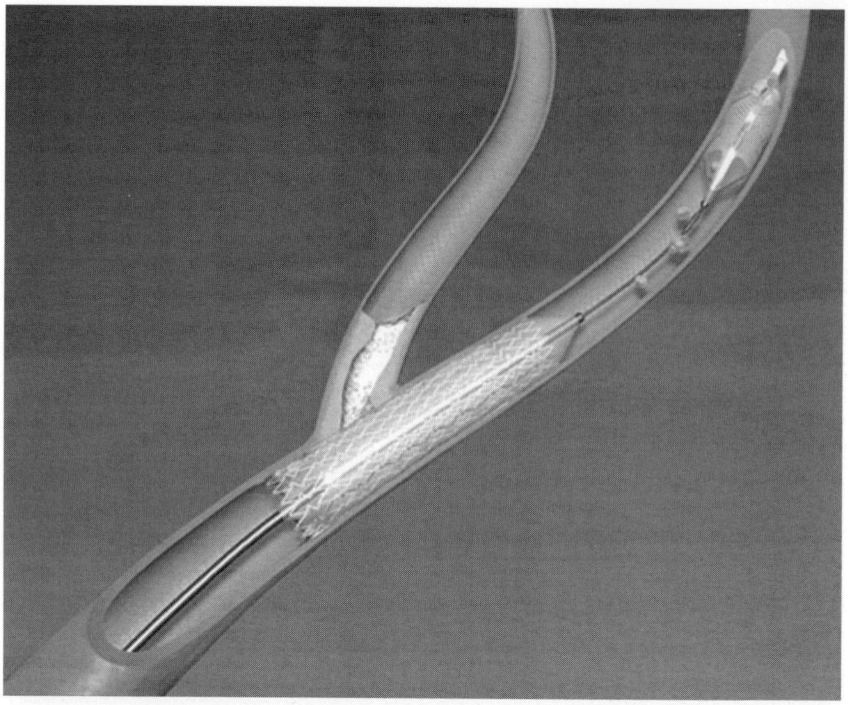

6

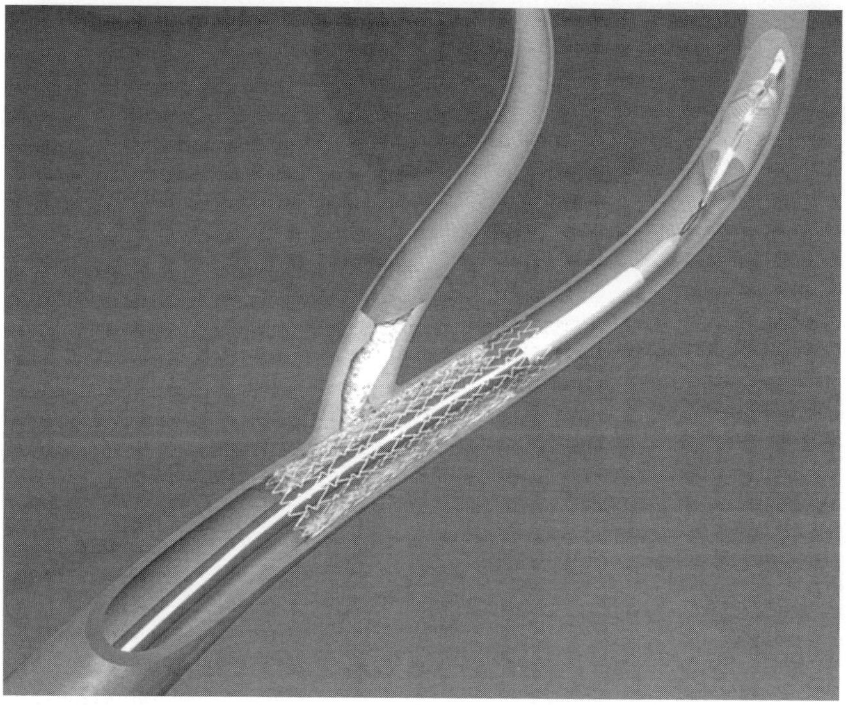

7

6

The 0.014-inch wire can now be used as the guidewire over which angioplasty and stent placement is performed. Any debris is collected within the filter.

7

To remove the device and contents of the filter at the end of the procedure the retrieval pod and centring catheter are advanced over the wire, through the stent, up to the filter.

8a, b

The centring catheter is removed and the filter withdrawn into the pod. The whole device is then removed.

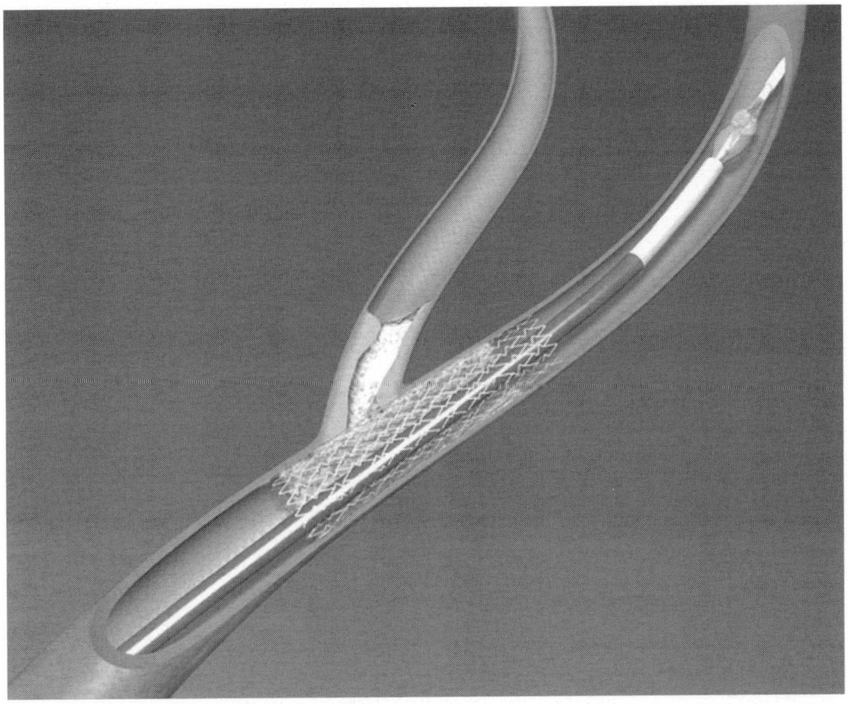

a

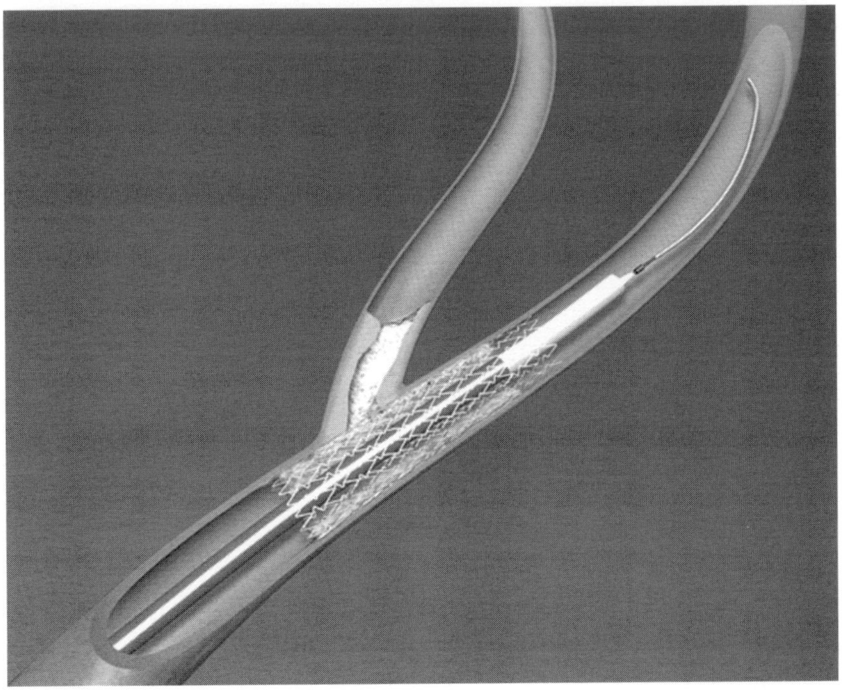

b

8

Angioplasty and stent with reversal of internal carotid flow as a cerebral protection device

Juan Carlos Parodi, Mark Cline Bates

Introduction

As technology improves and experience accumulates the endovascular treatment of extracranial cerebrovascular disease is gaining popularity and supporters. The widespread application of these techniques has been limited by a significant incidence of perioperative neurological complications ranging between 5.2 and 9.3% including a stopped trial due to an unacceptably high rate of neurological complications. The gold standard to which carotid artery angioplasty and stenting (CAS) will be compared are the results of conventional carotid endarterectomy for symptomatic patients (NASCET perioperative total neurological event rate of 5.8%) and for asymptomatic patients (ACAS perioperative total neurological event rate of 2.65%).

Despite improvements in perioperative stroke rates reported in many series of CAS in recent years, it is obvious that for CAS to become an acceptable alternative to conventional surgery for carotid occlusive disease, significant improvements have to be made to reduce procedure-related neuroembolism and its associated neurologic sequelae.

We have learned in recent years that the perioperative use of anti-platelet drugs (ticlopidine, acetyl salicylic acid (ASA), clopidogrel, anti-glycoprotein IIb/IIIa, etc); the use of coronary type hydrophilic guidewires as well as coronary balloons for pre-dilatation when needed; and stent placement in all cases regardless of angioplasty results, are strategies that have been shown to reduce thromboembolic events.

In recent years, cerebral protection devices have been designed in an attempt to reduce even further the chances of neuroembolism. Several concepts have been introduced including:

1. cerebral protection with balloon occlusion of the internal carotid artery (i.e. Percusurge®);
2. cerebral protection with balloon occlusion of the common carotid artery (Kachel's technique);

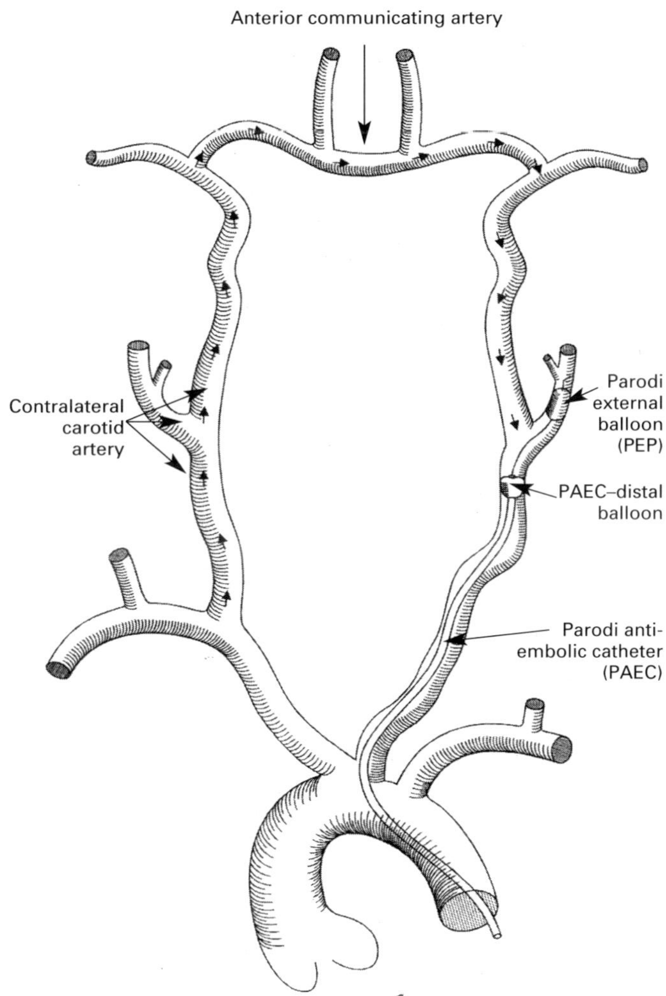

1

3. cerebral protection using filter type devices placed in the internal carotid artery (i.e. Angioguard™);
4. cerebral protection by inversion of internal carotid artery blood flow achieved by balloon occlusion of the common carotid artery and external carotid artery (Parodi device); and
5. combinations of these techniques.

1

We have designed our own Parodi anti-embolism system based on a new concept that ensures cerebral protection by producing retrograde internal carotid artery flow at the time of lesion crossing, angioplasty and stent deployment achieved by balloon occlusion of the common carotid artery and external carotid artery. Internal carotid artery flow reversal is achieved by a carotid to femoral arteriovenous shunt connecting the guiding catheter to a femoral vein introducer. This shunt can be supplemented by aspiration through the guiding catheter especially when the stent deployment device is introduced (1).

The operation

2, 3

The patient generally receives minimal preoperative sedation and on arrival in the angiographic suite the head and neck are secured with a harness to minimize movement during digital subtraction angiography and/or road mapping. The femoral artery and vein are then accessed using a modified Seldinger technique and local anaesthesia percutaneously. Specifically, an 11 Fr sheath is placed in the right common femoral artery and 6–10 Fr sheath in the ipsilateral common

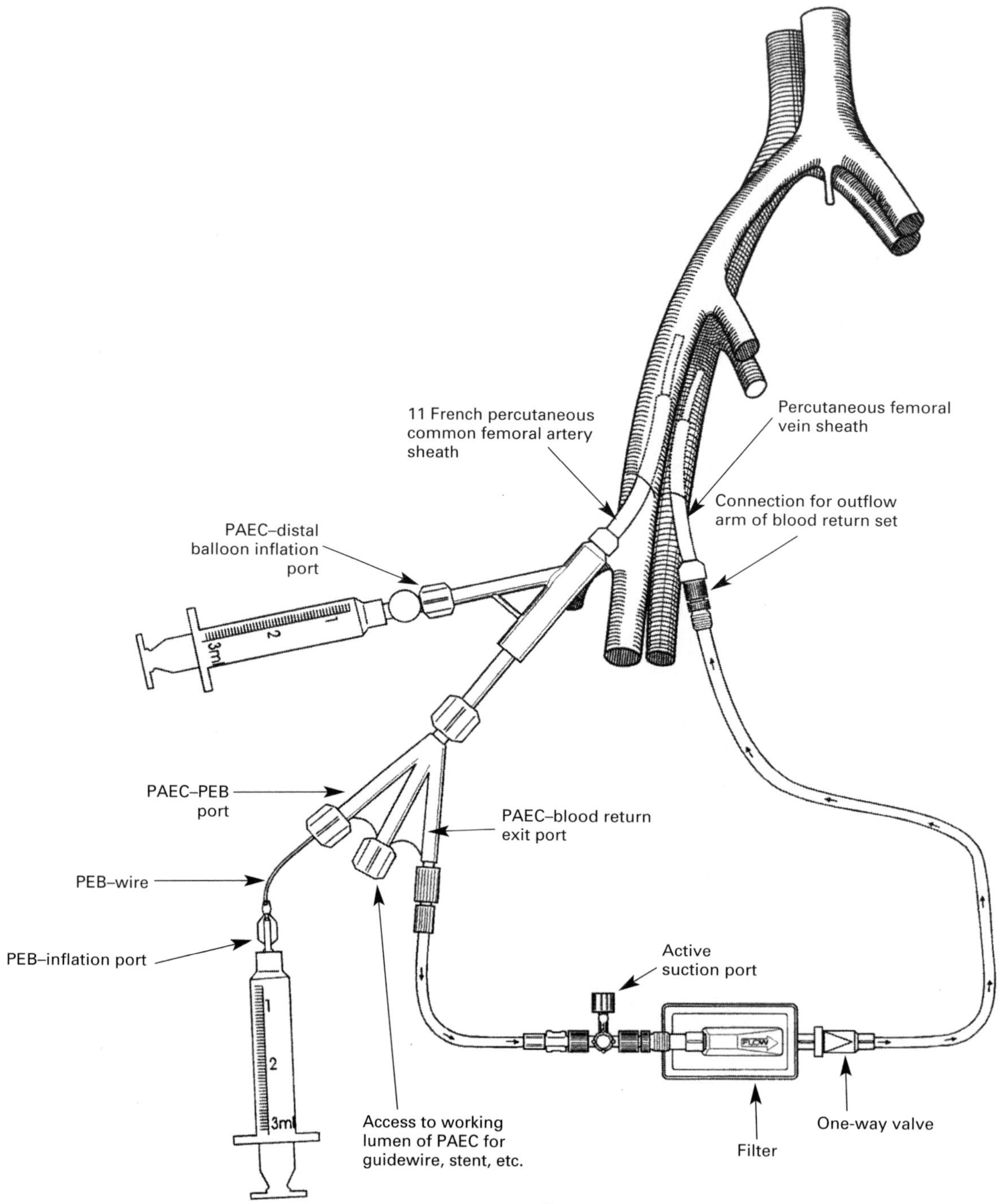

2

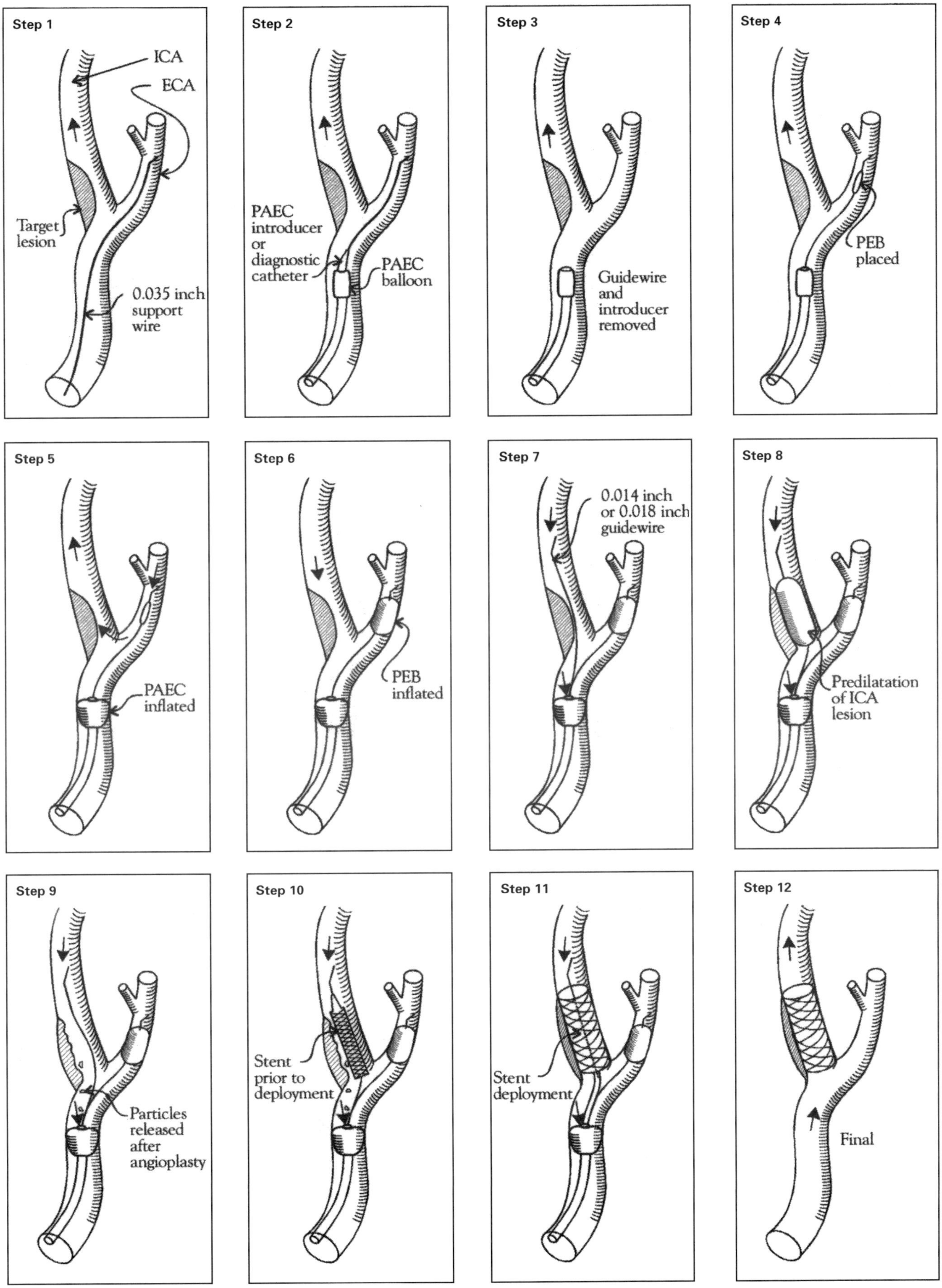
Step 1
ICA
ECA
Target lesion
0.035 inch support wire
Step 2
PAEC introducer or diagnostic catheter
PAEC balloon
Step 3
Guidewire and introducer removed
Step 4
PEB placed
Step 5
PAEC inflated
Step 6
PEB inflated
Step 7
0.014 inch or 0.018 inch guidewire
Step 8
Predilatation of ICA lesion
Step 9
Particles released after angioplasty
Step 10
Stent prior to deployment
Step 11
Stent deployment
Step 12
Final

3

femoral vein. There are those who would suggest utilization of the contralateral venous system to move the shunt out of the field into the contralateral location; however, this has not been a practical concern in our experience. After femoral access is accomplished, a diagnostic catheter is navigated into the common carotid artery using standard angiographic technique. Meticulous haemodynamic monitoring during catheter manipulation is undertaken in the hopes of avoiding hydraulic injury to intima or complex plaque theoretically reducing the risk of embolization or stroke during angiography. The steps and or details of carotid stent placement under flow reversal protection are detailed in 3. Specifically:

Step 1: Via diagnostic catheter, a 35 thousandths support guidewire is stationed in the external carotid artery.

Step 2: Over the guidewire then, the Parodi anti-embolism catheter (PAEC) is navigated into the common carotid artery below the bifurcation. Please note that the PAEC can also be introduced over a shaped diagnostic catheter depending on the preferred technique of the individual operator.

Step 3: The introducer catheter and 35 thousandths inch guidewire are then extricated leaving the PAEC in position in the common carotid artery.

Step 4: Under fluoroscopic guidance, the Parodi external balloon on a wire is then advanced into or steered into the external carotid artery where it is positioned at the base of the common carotid artery hopefully also occluding the superior thyroid artery.

Step 5: The common carotid artery PAEC balloon with its unique funnel shape is inflated in the common carotid artery. Please note that most patients, will at this point, have flow from the external to the internal carotid artery and this is supported not only in early clinical experience with the Parodi anti-embolism system, but also with the animal studies predating the human experience by 2–3 years.

Step 6: The Parodi external balloon (PEB) is inflated and at this time, the arterial venous shunt system can be connected. (See 2 for a description of the arterial venous shunt and connections.) The venous exit port on the proximal portion of the PAEC is connected to the afferent arm of the arterovenous fistula or shunt and at the same time, the distal portion of the shunt is connected to the venous system. The shunt should be cleared and there is also a port for active flow reversal. The active flow reversal port can be used for pulling back blood and this active flow reversal may be beneficial during times when a high burden of soft material or embolic disease is expected.

Step 7: The internal carotid artery lesion is crossed with a soft-tipped 0.014 or 0.018″ wire depending on the operator preference.

Step 8: Over the wire then the internal carotid artery lesion is dilated with a balloon-dilating catheter.

Step 9: The balloon is removed and particles that are illustrated in this diagram flow naturally with retrograde flow into the arteriovenous shunt system away from the patient's intracranial system.

Step 10: The stent is then positioned in the internal carotid artery. The radio-opaque markers on the PEB system make positioning the stent very simple without contrast injection. However, at this point, if it is felt that contrast is necessary to define the lesion prior to stent placement, this can simply be done by injecting a small amount of contrast into the vessel.

Step 11: Following stent placement and post-dilatation the delivery system is removed. This is all done during active flow reversal protection.

Step 12: The PAEC balloon is deflated while active suction is being applied through the active suction port with a 20-cc syringe. This helps retrieve any theoretical border particles that were not captured during stenting with active PAEC flow reversal. The catheter is then removed and completion angiograms are performed.

Complications

Early experience with the Parodi anti-embolism system has been very encouraging with minimal complications. There is a concern during active flow reversal (suction) that rapid withdrawal of a large volume of blood (20 cc) over a short period of time could produce syncopal or very transient change in level of consciousness. This may or may not have untoward clinical sequelae. However, in response to those findings, we have suggested using 10-cc withdrawal during active flow reversal manoeuvres. The current first generation delivery design requires a 10–11 Fr arterial sheath and access complications are also a concern. For that reason, minimizing sheath size is a priority on second- and third-generation system iterations. There were theoretical concerns about the external carotid artery balloon being jailed by a stent across the bifurcation. This problem will be resolved with second-generation PEB designs, but in the meantime, we have suggested utilization of the Wall stent and attempts at avoiding sharp edged nitinol stent devices. Finally, patients with extracranial cerebrovascular disease frequently have many co-morbid conditions that place them at risk for complications with any invasive procedure. The known complications and difficulty with carotid stenting including severe vessel tortuosity, access of the carotid artery, bradycardia during balloon inflation, etc, are obviously still a concern with the Parodi anti-embolism system. It is hope that the risk of embolic complication will be minimized by protection of the brain from embolization during all manoeuvres affecting the target lesion including crossing with the wire, balloon angioplasty, stent placement, etc.

Technical modifications in the repair of thoracoabdominal aortic aneurysms

Larry H Hollier

Introduction

Thoracoabdominal aortic aneurysms represent extensive deterioration of the aortic wall in patients who generally are elderly and often plagued with other degenerative diseases, especially hypertension and coronary artery disease. Failure to repair these aneurysms results in a 5-year survival rate of less than 20% (Bickerstaff *et al.*, 1982).

The advent of computerized tomography has aided greatly in the detection and delineation of the extent of thoracoabdominal aortic aneurysms. Additionally, simple suprarenal extension of abdominal aortic aneurysms are also being found with increasing frequency. In general, however, these latter aneurysms can be readily repaired by an abdominal approach and are not truly thoracoabdominal aneurysms. For purposes of this chapter, we limit the term thoracoabdominal aneurysm exclusively to mean aneurysms involving the origin of *all* the major visceral arteries. Clearly, these aneurysms require extensive technical reconstruction with revascularization of coeliac, superior mesenteric and both renal arteries, as well as the spinal cord and the lower extremities.

1a, b, c, d

Using this criterion to delineate thoracoabdominal aneurysms, we find four clinical presentations: type I, which is essentially a thoracic aneurysm that extends inferiorly to the extent that it involves the visceral vessels; type II, the classic, diffuse thoracoabdominal aneurysm with extensive involvement of the aorta both above and below the visceral arteries; type III, with aneurysmal changes starting below the middle of the thoracic aorta; type IV, aneurysmal changes that start at the level of the diaphragm and involve the visceral vessels and infrarenal aorta.

The patterns are easily differentiated by computerized tomography, with type III aneurysms being identified most commonly in our experience. Although the type II thoracoabdominal aneurysm is best treated by the classic technique described by Crawford (1974), the other anatomical configurations may allow for modifications in surgical approach so that operative time can be reduced and visceral revascularization can be facilitated. These technical modifications were actually suggested in Crawford's early publication (Crawford, 1974, Crawford *et al.*, 1978), but their utility has not been appreciated by most surgeons.

Techniques

2a, b

For all cases of thoracoabdominal aneurysm repair, the patient is placed in a semilateral position, with the buttocks resting flat on the operating table, but with the chest and shoulders rotated approximately 45 degrees anteriorly. The left arm is placed on an arm-rest rotated above and anterior to the patient's head.

The chest, abdomen and groins are scrubbed with povidone-iodine solution, then covered with sterile drapes and an adhesive plastic skin barrier. The incision extends upward from the pubis to the umbilicus, then obliquely to the left up across the costal margin and through the appropriate intercostal space. If the aneurysm involves the abdominal aorta and the origin of the visceral vessels but terminates in normal or near-normal aorta near the diaphragm (type IV), the thoracic portion of the incision is usually placed through the 9th or 10th intercostal space. If the mid- or upper thoracic aorta is involved with contiguous aneurysmal change (type I or II), the 4th or 5th intercostal space is incised.

Exposure of the infradiaphragmatic aortic may be accomplished either extraperitoneally or transperitoneally. However, if endarterectomy of the right renal, coeliac or superior mesenteric artery is required, the transperitoneal approach allows more thorough inspection of the distal vessel beyond the site of endarterectomy. Except for type I thoracoabdominal aneurysms, it

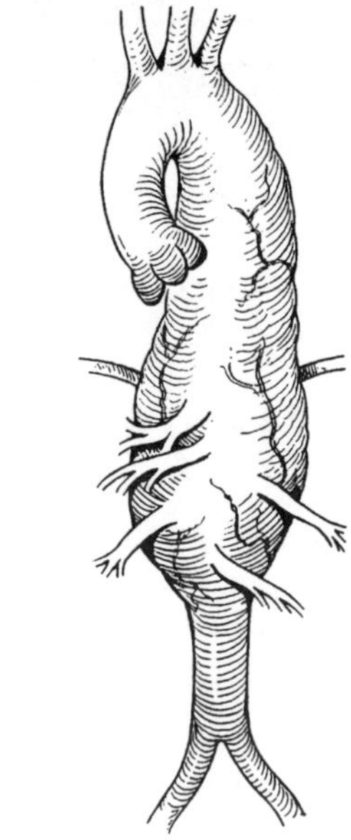

Type I

1a

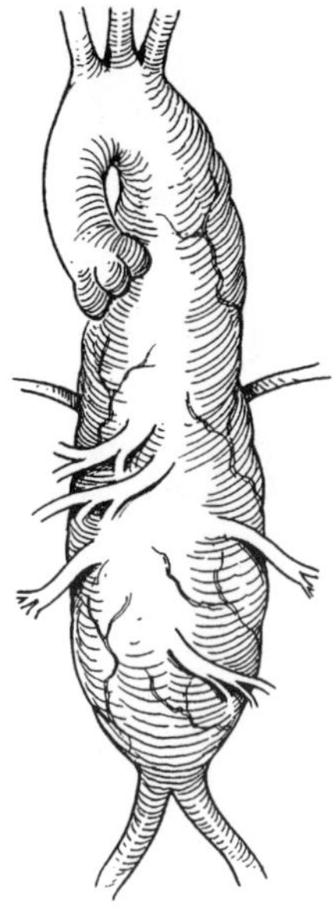

Type II

1b

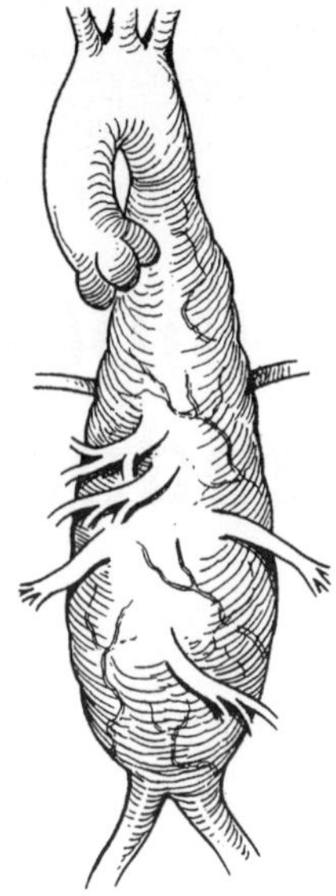

Type III

1c

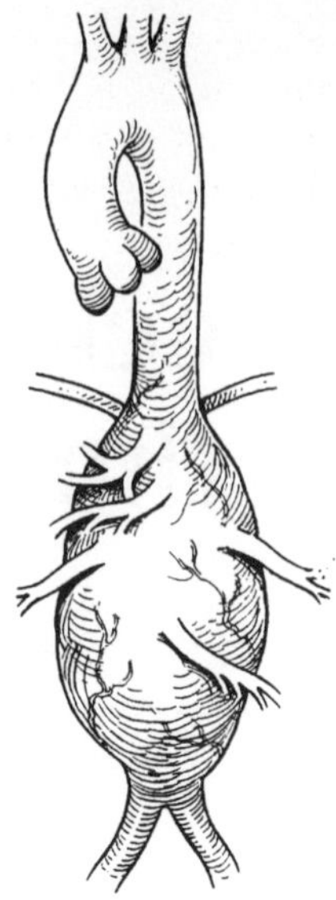

Type IV

1d

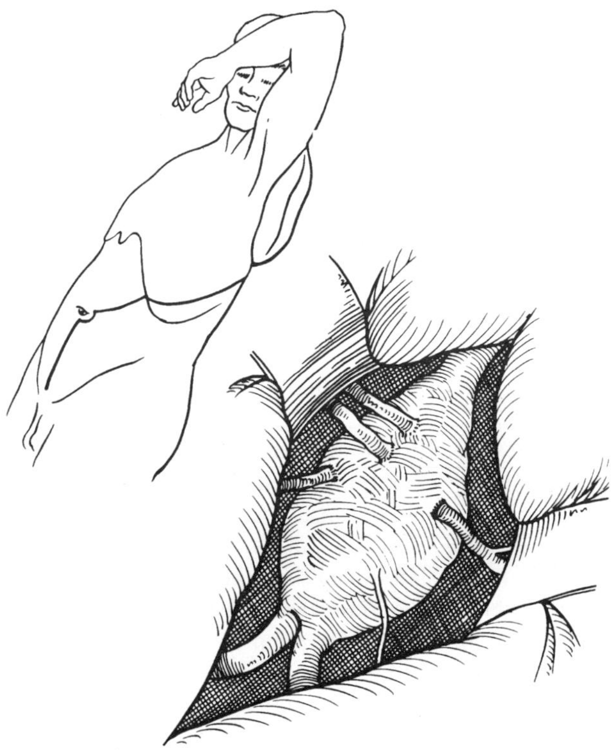

2a

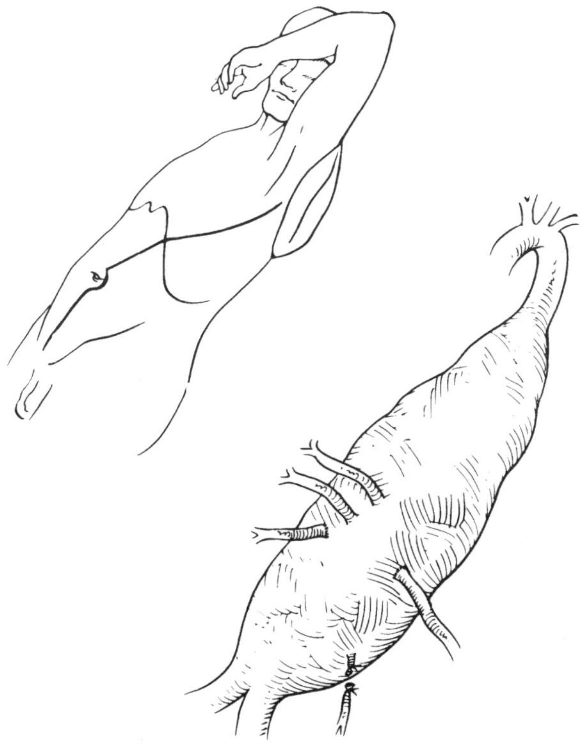

2b

is easier to reflect the left kidney along with spleen, pancreas and left colon, to expose the entire course of the aorta.

To complete exposure of the thoracoabdominal aorta, the diaphragm is divided in a circumferential rather than radial fashion, since this allows function of the left hemidiaphragm to be preserved. We place alternating green and black marking sutures in the edges of the diaphragm as it is cut so that precise approximation can be achieved at the time of closure.

Prior to manipulation of the renal vessels, mannitol 25 g and lasix 10 mg are given intravenously. This places the kidneys in a diuretic state, thereby lessening the risk of acute tubular necrosis from renal ischaemia. Systemic heparin is not given, but the visceral vessels are irrigated with heparinized saline after opening the aorta later in the operation.

After exposure to the thoracoabdominal aorta, the extent of aneurysmal change in relation to the visceral vessels is assessed. As the greatest risk in thoracoabdominal aneurysm repair is myocardial infarction related to increased left ventricular afterload and subendocardial ischaemia, every effort should be made to minimize clamping time. Some surgeons have suggested the use of femorofemoral bypass or heparincoated shunts to reduce ventricular strain, but additional complications have been noted as a direct result of these techniques. In our experience, intravenous nitroprusside has been a safe and useful means of pharmacologically off-loading the left ventricle and it avoids the problems of shunts and extracorporeal circulation. Despite vasodilatation techniques, however, prolonged cross-clamping of the thoracic aorta should be avoided, not only because of the cardiac risk, but also to lessen the risk of paraplegia.

Diffuse thoracoabdominal aneurysm

3

When widespread aneurysmal changes are noted throughout the aorta, we perform graft replacement in the manner popularized by Crawford. The entire aneurysm is exposed, proximal and distal occluding clamps are placed, and a vertical arteriotomy is made through the lateral wall along the entire length of the aneurysm. If the left kidney is left in place, the left renal vein is mobilized so that the graft may be passed beneath it without difficulty. After opening the aneurysm, a catheter is placed in the left renal artery and the kidney is perfused with iced heparinized saline to irrigate and cool it during ischaemia.

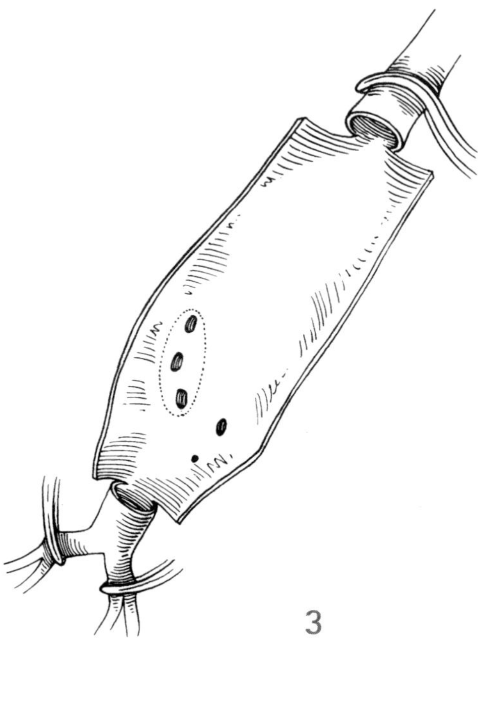

3

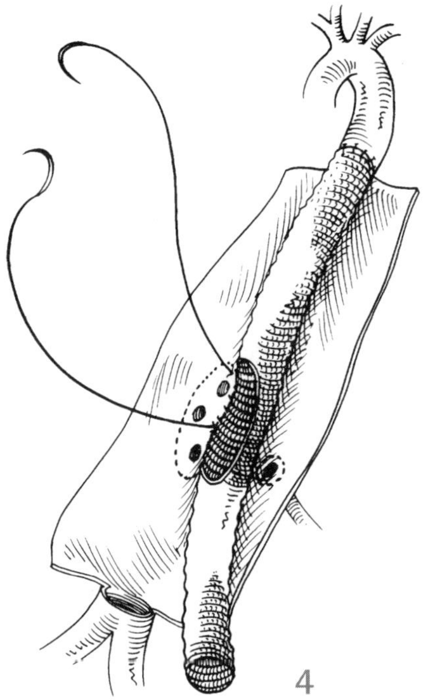

4

4

A low porosity woven graft is then sutured, end-to-end, to the partially transected proximal thoracic aorta using 0-polypropylene suture on a V-7 needle. Felt pledgets are commonly used to reinforce the anastomotic line. After the proximal anastomosis has been completed, any patent intercostal arteries are reimplanted into the graft after excising an elliptical section of the graft posteriorly. It is often possible to re-anastomose two or three pairs of intercostal arteries in one such anastomosis. Occasionally, a proximal intercostal artery can be revascularized by tailoring the proximal anastomosis obliquely to include these vessels. After intercostals have been reimplanted, the clamp is removed distally and flow is restored to the intercostal arteries. A button of graft is then excised opposite the orifices of the coeliac, superior mesenteric and right renal arteries. The graft is then sutured side-to-side to the aorta with 0-polypropylene suture, encompassing the origins of all three vessels as a single anastomosis.

5

Flow is then restored to these vessels. The total occlusion time thus far is usually no more than 30 min. Because flow through these vessels is generally more than

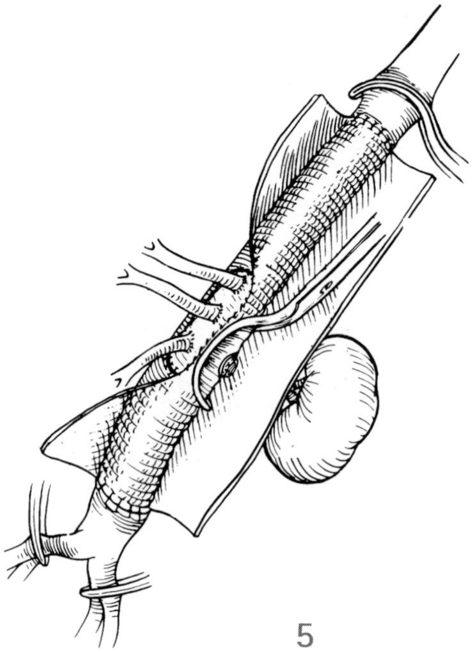

5

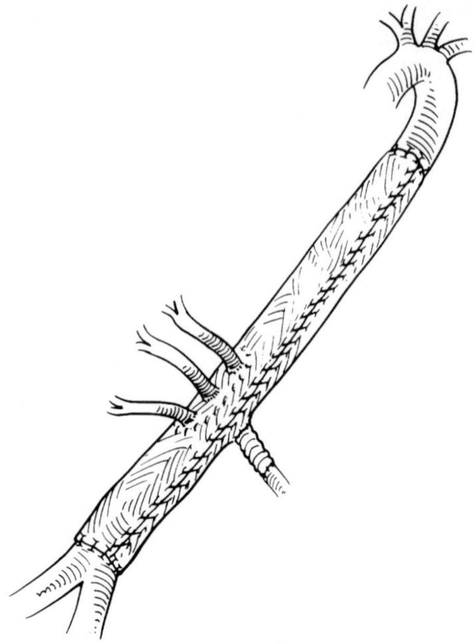

6

2000 ml per min, its early restoration provides excellent off-loading of the left ventricle. The distal anastomosis to the aortic bifurcation is then performed and flow is cautiously restored to the lower extremities. If significant iliac disease is present, a woven bifurcation graft may be used instead of the straight graft.

After lower extremity flow has been restored, the left renal artery may be implanted into the graft directly.

6

If stenosis of the left renal artery is noted, we use a short-segment (6 or 8 mm) Dacron graft to revascularize the left kidney. After completion of all anastomoses, the sac of the aneurysm is closed tightly around the graft for added haemostasis.

Vessels are examined for adequacy of pulses, and flows are measured in the revascularized arteries. The abdominal viscera are then restored to their normal anatomical position and the diaphragm is closed with interrupted horizontal mattress sutures of 2/0 braided Dacron. Two chest tubes are placed through separate stab incisions to drain the left chest, and the chest and abdominal incisions are closed in layers in standard fashion.

Low thoracoabdominal aneurysm

With increasing frequency, we see patients who have thoracoabdominal aneurysms which involve the entire abdominal aorta, including the site of origin of the visceral vessels, but in whom the aorta is relatively normal from the diaphragm upwards. In this situation we find that slight technical modifications can significantly reduce the time of increased afterload on the left ventricle.

7

A low thoracoabdominal approach is utilized (see Illustration 2a), and the aorta is dissected as previously described, although only the lower third of the thoracic aorta need be exposed in these cases. Because of the proximity of normal aorta to the visceral vessels, clamp time can be minimized by including a tongue of aorta bearing the orifices of these vessels in an oblique proximal anastomosis.

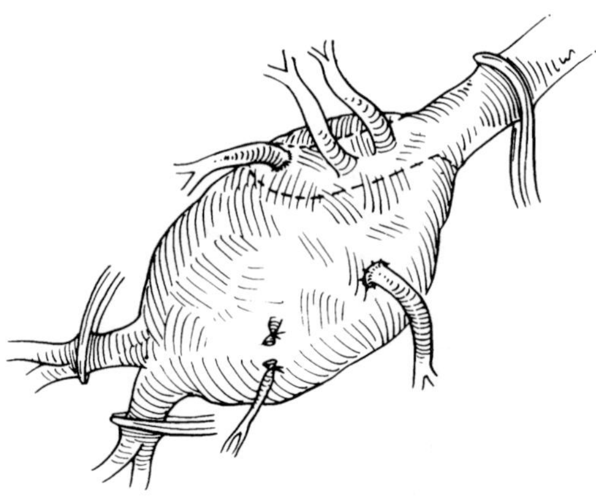

7

8

The woven low-porosity Dacron graft is trimmed as shown and an anastomosis is fashioned to provide revascularization of the coeliac, superior mesenteric and right renal arteries in conjunction with the proximal anastomosis. The proximal clamp can then be repositioned on to the graft below the right renal artery and visceral flow can be restored. Total occlusion time to this stage of the procedure is usually 15 min.

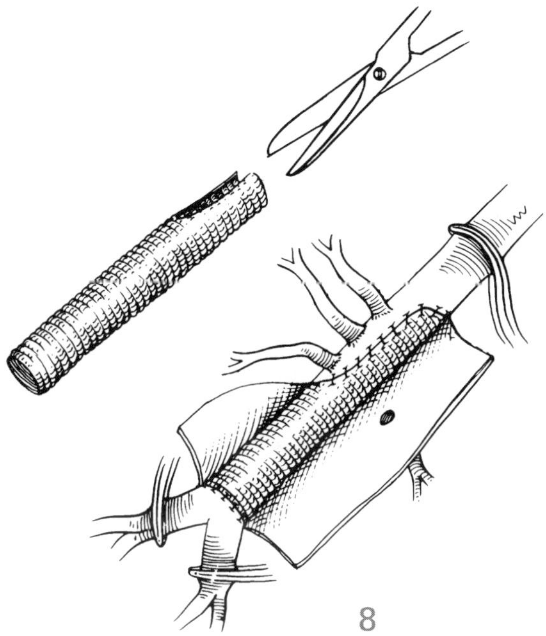

8

9

The distal anastomosis and left renal revascularization are then performed as previously described, and the sac of the aneurysm is closed over the graft with a running suture of 3/0 polypropylene.

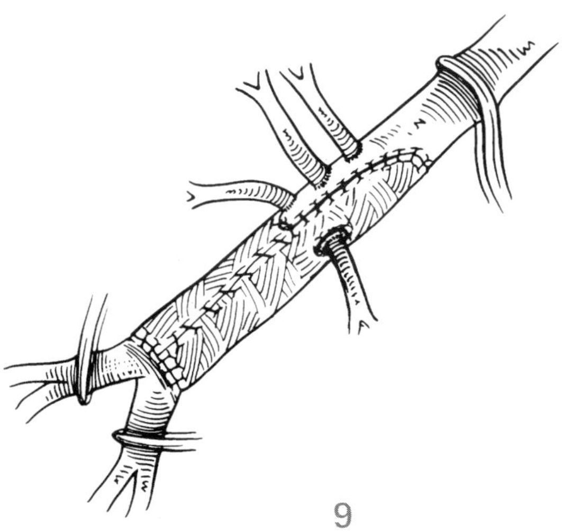

9

10, 11, 12

Thoracic aneurysm with abdominal extension

Some patients have thoracoabdominal aneurysms that are primarily thoracic aneurysms (type 1), but the aneurysmal changes extend down below the diaphragm and involve the aorta at the site of origin of the visceral vessels. In such cases, operative time may be reduced by incorporating the visceral revascularization with the distal anastomosis. Total aortic occlusion time in these cases is generally no more than 30 min.

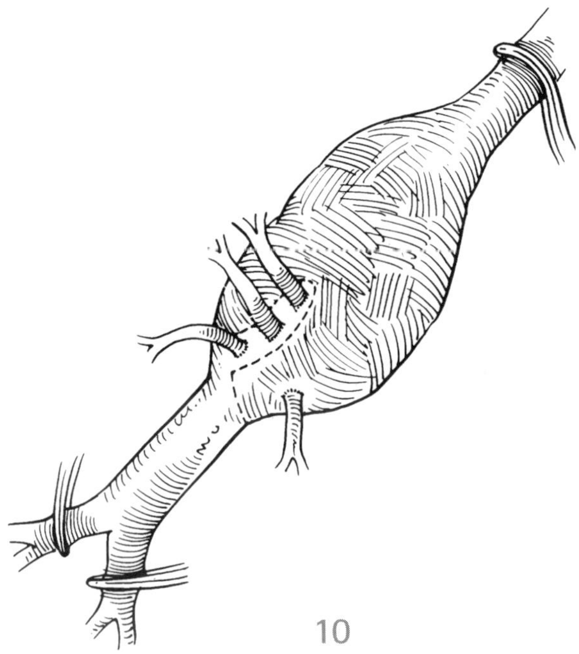

10

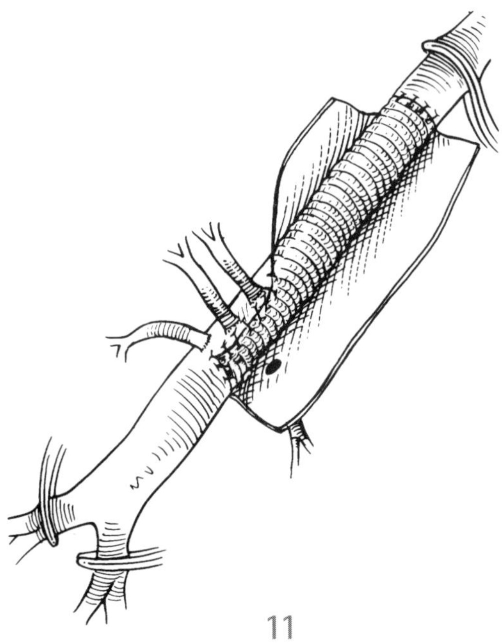

11

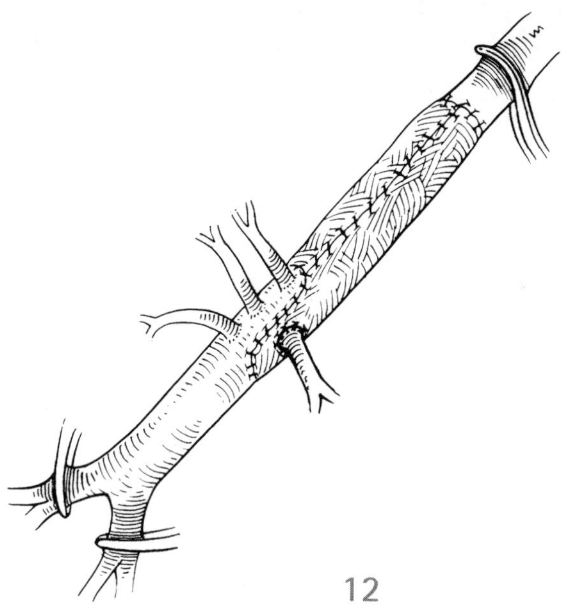

12

In all variations of revascularization procedures described here, the visceral and spinal artery anastomoses are performed in a side-to-side fashion; that is, the aortic wall is not incised in 'button' fashion around the orifices, but the reimplantations are done by suturing into the inside of the intact aortic wall. This is most clearly shown in Illustration **4**.

Prevention of paraplegia

Despite the use of evoked potential monitoring, heparin-bonded shunts, femorofemoral or atriofemoral bypass, or routine intercostal reimplantation, paraplegia still occurs. Obviously, when technically feasible, use of shunts or bypass can reduce the risk of paraplegia if clamp time is expected to be prolonged, but they are often ineffective, especially in type II aneurysms.

Recent experimental and clinical experience with spinal fluid drainage has suggested that this technique may improve spinal cord perfusion and may increase the safe clamp time. This may allow a longer safe interval in which to reimplant the intercostal arteries to revascularize the spinal cord.

After endotracheal anaesthesia is instituted, the patient is placed on his right side and an 18 gauge spinal needle is introduced intrathecally between the 4th and 5th lumbar vertebrae and a silastic catheter is introduced. A total of 10–15 dl of spinal fluid is taken and the needle is withdrawn, leaving the intrathecal catheter in place; the catheter is then connected to a pressure transducer for continuous monitoring. If the spinal fluid pressure rises during the case, additional spinal fluid is withdrawn to keep the spinal pressure below 10 mmHg.

It is important to remember that spinal fluid drainage alone does not prevent paraplegia and is not a substitute for intercostal artery reimplantation which is mandatory in some patients. Additionally, it seems unlikely that it will reduce the incidence of paraplegia that sometimes occurs several days after otherwise successful repair of thoracoabdominal aneurysms.

Complications and results

Use of the techniques mentioned above has resulted in expeditious repair of thoracoabdominal aneurysms with acceptable morbidity and mortality. We have now operated on over 200 patients who underwent repair of non-dissecting thoracoabdominal aneurysms. Long-term dialysis was needed in less than 3% of patients. The most common complicated encounters were pulmonary (20%), particularly the need for prolonged ventilation.

A total of 97% of patients survived sufficiently long to determine neurological function. Overall, paraplegia or paraparesis occurred in 4% of those patients who had type I and type II thoracoabdominal aneurysms. The incidence of spinal cord injury was 6.6%. Spinal drainage was not used in any patient early in the series. Since routine spinal fluid drainage was instituted, we have not yet seen paraplegia occur when intercostal arteries have been reimplanted.

Continuing experience and the relaxation of surgical indications will undoubtedly increase the mortality and morbidity of any series. Nonetheless, careful preoperative evaluation and preparation, careful and expeditious surgical technique, and meticulous attention to postoperative management, will improve salvage in patients with thoracoabdominal aortic aneurysms.

References

Bickerstaff L K, Pairolero P C, Hollier L H *et al.* (1982). Thoracic aortic aneurysms: A population-based study. *Surgery* **92**: 1103.

Crawford E S (1974). Thoracoabdominal and abdominal aortic aneurysms involving renal, superior mesenteric, and celiac arteries. *Annl Surg* **179**: 763.

Crawford E S, Snyder D M, Cho G C *et al.* (1978). Progress in treatment of thoracoabdominal and abdominal aortic aneurysms involving celiac, superior mesenteric and renal arteries. *Annl Surg* **188**: 404.

Hollier L H (1987). Protecting the brain and spinal cord. *J Vasc Surg* **5**: 524.

Hollier L H, Symmonds J B, Pairolero P C *et al.* (1988). Thoracoabdominal aortic aneurysm repair: Analysis of postoperative morbidity. *Arch Surg* **123**: 871.

Hollier L H, Money S R, Naslund T C *et al.* (1992). Risk of spinal cord dysfunction in patients undergoing thoracoabdominal aortic replacement. *Am J Surg* **164**: 210.

McCullogh J L, Hollier L H, Nugent M (1988). Paraplegia after thoracic aortic occlusion. Influence of cerebrospinal fluid drainage. *J Vasc Surg* **7**: 153.

Endovascular thoracoabdominal aneurysm repair

Timothy A M Chuter, Roy L Gordon, Linda M Reilly, Oscar Vasquez, Louis Messina

Introduction

Endovascular thoracoabdominal aortic aneurysm repair appears to be technically feasible (Chuter *et al.*, 2001). The potential advantages are enormous, given the poor life-expectancy of patients with untreated thoracoabdominal aortic aneurysm (Crawford and DeNatale, 1986) and the high mortality and morbidity rates of open repair (Svensson *et al.* 1993).

Preoperative imaging

Computed tomography and calibrated catheter angiography are used to assess the feasibility of endovascular repair and make the measurements necessary for stent-graft sizing. Specific exclusion criteria include:

1. Aneurysm or untreatable stenosis of the coeliac artery, superior mesenteric artery, or renal arteries.
2. Multiple renal arteries.
3. Coeliac artery length <2 cm.
4. Artery of Adamkiewicz in the area to be repaired, especially in thoracoabdominal aortic aneurysms types II or III.

Device description

The components are:

1. The primary stent-graft. This component has one orifice proximally and five orifices distally; one for each stent-graft extension.
2. The lower body extension. This component (or collection of components) is essentially a system for abdominal aortic aneurysm repair. Its configuration depends on the state of the infrarenal aorta. Extensive infrarenal involvement necessitates a bifurcated lower body extension for bilateral iliac implantation.
3. Visceral extensions. These simple tubular stent-grafts bridge the gap between the side branches of the primary stent-graft and the branches of the visceral aorta.

Device fabrication

The primary stent-graft

The primary stent-graft is sewn together from several tubular pieces of standard vascular graft material using CV-6 Goretex suture (WL Gore, Inc., Flagstaff, AZ). The trunk and the anterior visceral branches are of woven polyester (Cooley Verisoft, Meadox Medicals, Inc,, Oakland, NJ). The renal branches are of Goretex extended polytetrafluroethylene (ePTFE) (WL Gore, Inc., Flagstaff, AZ).

The diameters depend on the diameters of the corresponding arteries. The trunk is oversized 4–6 mm relative to the proximal aortic implantation site. The stent-graft side branches have approximately the same diameters as the aortic branches. The distal lumen is 20 mm in diameter.

The trunk of the primary component has two stents. An uncovered, barbed (Zenith) Gianturco Z-stent is attached to the proximal end of the trunk for anchoring. An unbarbed Gianturco tracheobronchial Z-stent is sutured within the trunk for sealing. This Z-stent is packaged in pairs with a nominal diameter of 35 mm, although the actual resting diameter is more than 50 mm once the nylon connecting sutures have been removed.

Each side-branch has a small biliary Z-stent sutured to its outer surface as a radio-opaque marker of the underlying graft. Other radio-opaque markers are sutured to the anterior surface of the trunk and to the end of each side branch. These guide axial orientation and longitudinal position.

The length of the primary stent-graft varies according to the extent of descending thoracic aortic involvement. It has to be long enough for: 2.5 cm overlap with healthy proximal aorta, 2 cm overlap between side branches and visceral extensions, 1–2 cm gap between the distal end of each side branch and the corresponding aortic branch orifice.

The lower body extension

The lower body extension is made from a Zenith Trifab abdominal aortic aneurysms repair system (Cook, Inc., Bloomington, IN). The only modification is replacement of the proximal sealing stent with the proximal attachment stent. The trunk of this system has a 24-mm diameter.

Visceral extensions

Several manufacturers produce suitable visceral extensions. To work well this component needs flexibility, full stent support and a flexible low-profile delivery system. We use the PTFE-covered Smart Stent (Cordis, Corp., Miami, FL) because it does not shorten, takes bends easily, and has stents both inside and out. The outer stents generate high friction where they meet arteries or other stent-graft components. One alternative is the Wallgraft, which has the advantage that it is available in the USA (for tracheobronchial use). Unfortunately, the Wallgraft, like the Wallstent, shortens as it expands.

Operation

Interventional suite versus operating room

We prefer to perform this procedure in the interventional suite. Even the best mobile C-arms overheat during magnified fluoroscopy in the full lateral position. The resulting image degradation complicates the procedure considerably. Endovascular repair of a thoracoabdominal aortic aneurysms requires imaging from the neck to the groin with frequent changes in the position and orientation of the field. A floating table and power-driven C-arm speed up these field changes significantly.

Position on the operating table

Our imaging table dictates patient position. Only with the patient in the supine position can we obtain the necessary anteroposterior and lateral views. In the usual left-side-up decubitus position, one or both of these views are obscured by the steel bars which run down the sides of the table.

General points

All patients receive general endotracheal anaesthesia. Cerebrospinal fluid drains are inserted by lumbar puncture. If evoked potentials change during the operation, we drain spinal fluid and support the blood pressure pharmacologically to improve spinal perfusion. Heparin is given to maintain an activated clotting time twice control. In addition, we irrigate all indwelling sheaths with heparinized saline.

Arterial access

1

The main body and the distal extension are inserted through the surgically exposed femoral arteries. We prefer oblique incisions over the usual longitudinal incisions. The main body of the stent-graft requires a 20 French sheath. The distal extension is inserted through 18 and 14 French sheaths.

The visceral extensions are inserted through the surgically exposed brachial artery; right or left, depending on arch anatomy. In theory, right-sided access carries a greater risk of stroke, but it sometimes provides a less tortuous route to the descending thoracic aorta. A 12 French sheath is inserted from the brachial artery to the proximal descending thoracic aorta (1). This helps guide the delivery systems through the aortic arch and minimizes the risk of stroke. Illustration 1 shows the main body of the stent-graft with its coeliac (1), superior mesenteric (2) and left renal (3) branches. The brachial sheath (4) traverses the aortic arch.

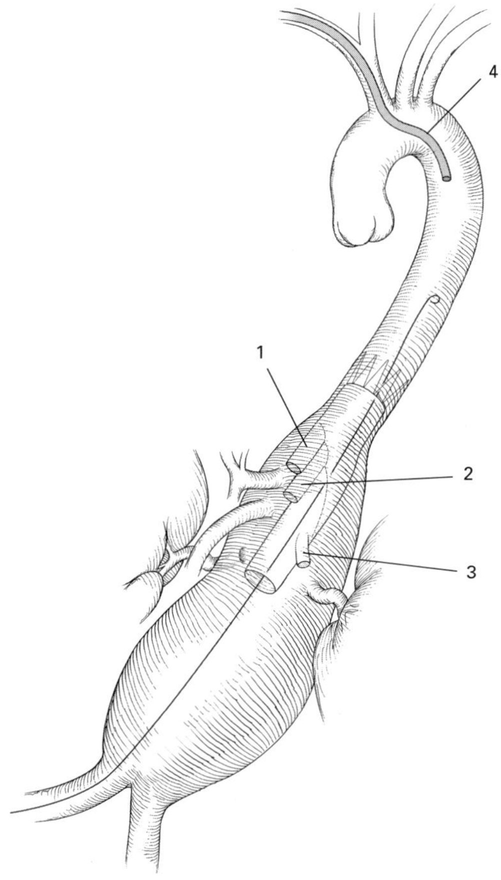

1

Main body of the stent-graft

We advance the stent-graft to the desired level and rotate it, together with the sheath, until the coeliac and superior mesenteric artery side branches lie anteriorly. A transbrachial catheter is used for angiographic localization of the renal arteries. The goal is to position the distal ends of the prosthetic renal side branches 1–2 cm above the corresponding renal artery orifices. The self-expanding stent-graft deploys spontaneously as the sheath is withdrawn (1).

Visceral extensions

2, 3, 4, 5, 6, 7

We catheterize each side branch of the main body from the brachial access site. The catheter exits the main body of the stent-graft and is directed into the corresponding branch artery through a 'road map' of the area (2). The coeliac branch of the main body is catheterized (arrow) from the arm. Another small bolus of contrast confirms catheter position. The choice of catheter and guidewire depends on the anatomy. A long multi-purpose A end hole catheter with a Roadrunner hydrophilic guidewire (both from Cook, Inc., Bloomington, IN) is a good combination to try first.

To provide the delivery system with more support, we change the Roadrunner guidewire for a stiff (Amplatz, Cook or Medtronic) guidewire with a small-radius J tip.

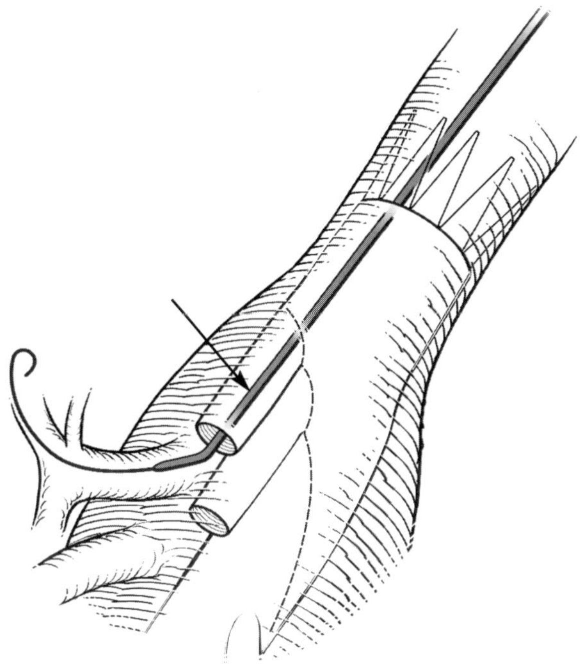

2

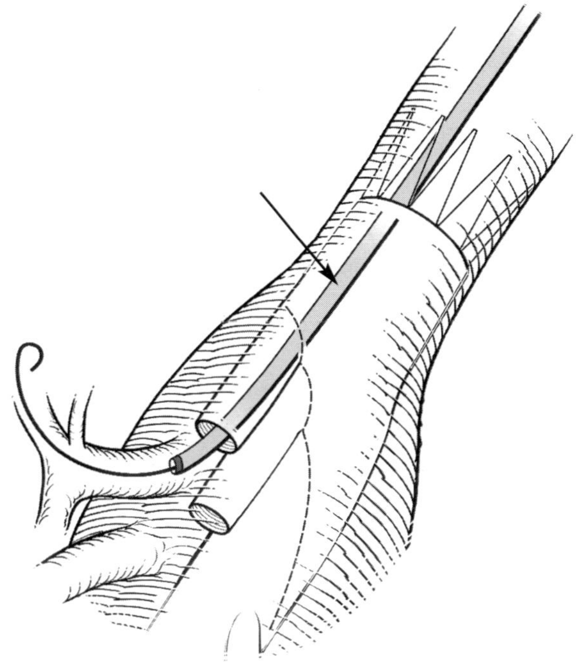

3

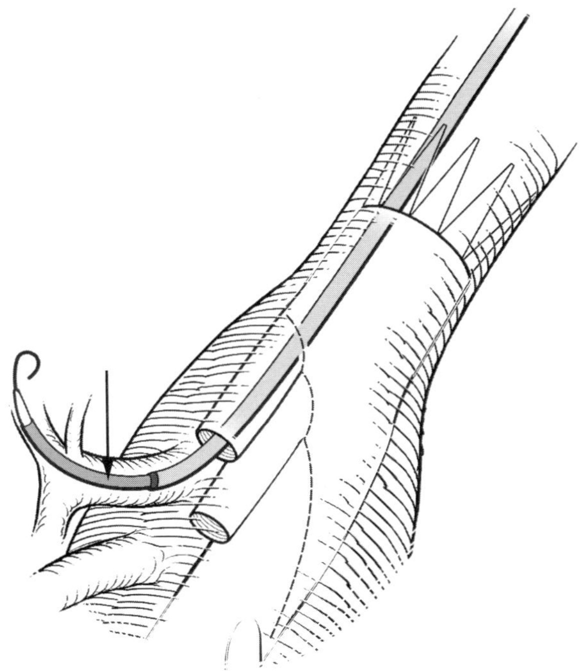

4

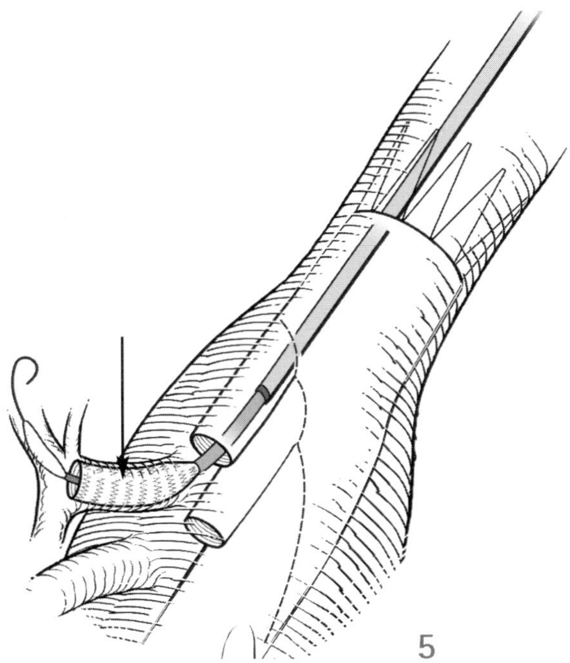

5

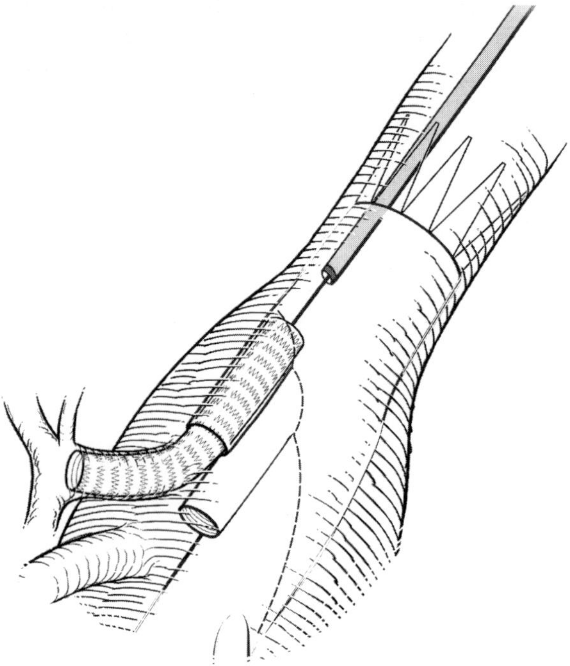

6

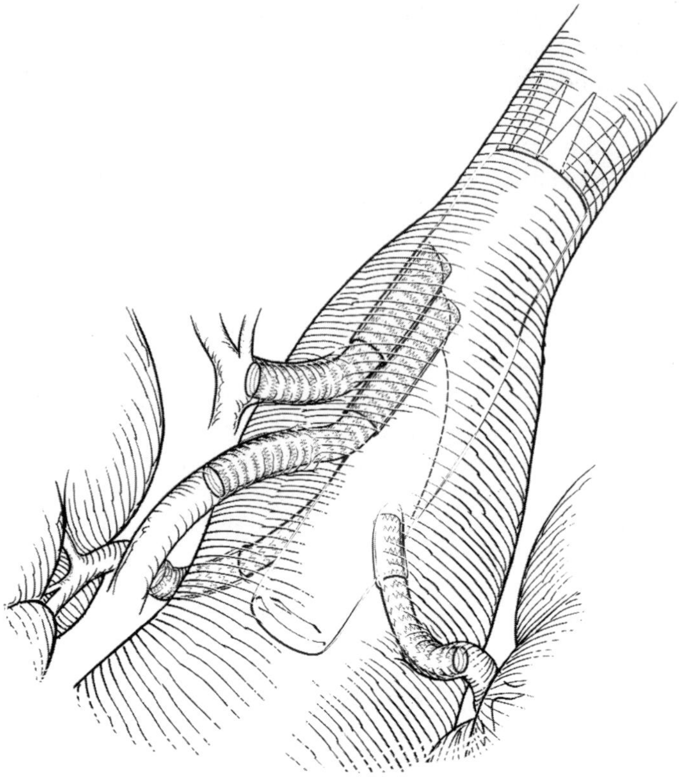

7

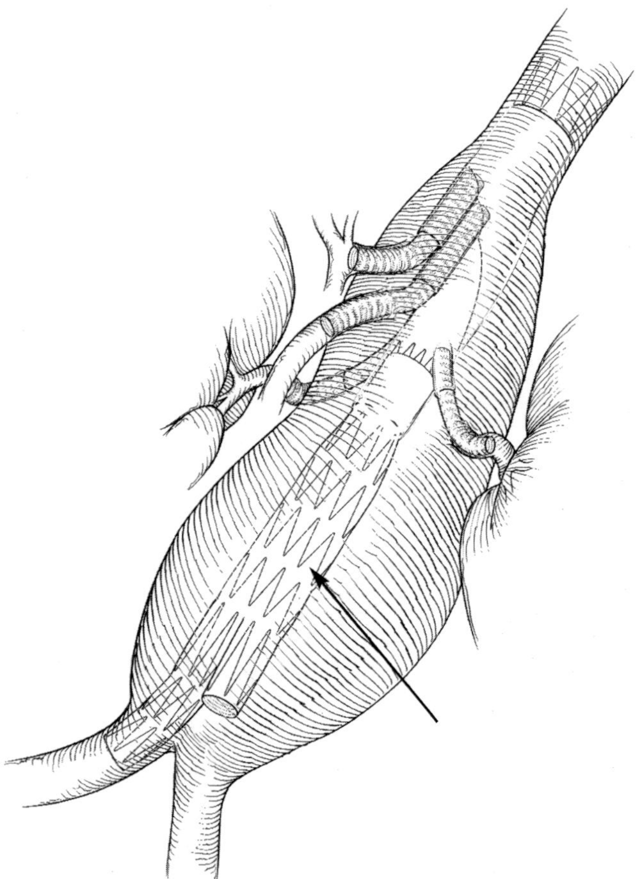

8

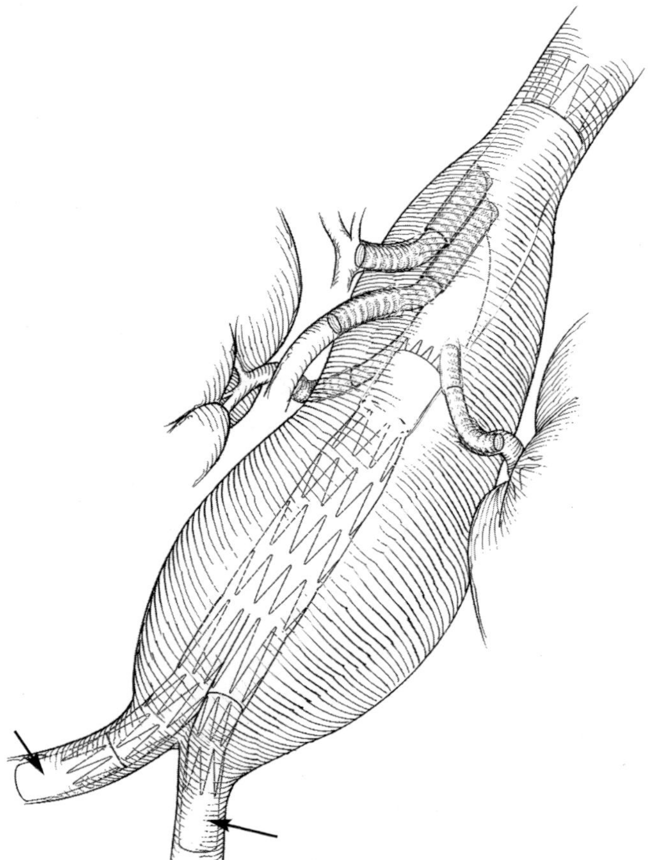

9

Having replaced its dilator, we watch the tip of the wire, while advancing a guiding catheter (arrow, 3) from the arm, though the main body of the stent-graft, and into the side branch. (3). This sheath provides a means of angiography and allows atraumatic passage of the delivery system (arrow, 4) for the visceral extension from the brachial access site into the branch artery (4). The visceral extension (arrow, 5) is deployed so that there is at least 2 cm of overlap with both the branch artery and the main body of the stent-graft (5, 6). If this is not feasible using one extension, we add another, starting distally. Another injection of contrast through the brachial sheath confirms stent-graft position, patency and seal before removing the guidewire.

We repeat his sequence until both renal arteries, the superior mesenteric artery, and the coeliac artery have all been grafted (7).

Distal extension

8, 9

Insertion of the distal extension is very like endovascular abdominal aortic aneurysm repair using a Zenith system, except for differences in delivery of the main component (trunk), which we have to insert through an 18 French homemade delivery system having removed the proximal stent. The system is a fully stented, three-component, bifurcated stent-graft. Having deployed the trunk (arrow, 8), we extend both limbs of this component into the iliac arteries (9). Once the distal extension is in place, the entire stent-graft combination has one inflow from the thoracic aorta and six outflows into the coeliac, superior mesenteric, renal, and iliac arteries (9).

Conclusion

If, as experience with endovascular thoracoabdominal aortic aneurysm repair grows, we find no serious, specific, unavoidable complications, the potential advantages are very great. One concern is the risk of paraplegia. An endovascular stent-graft covers more of the non-dilated thoracic aorta than a sutured graft and endovascular technique does not afford the opportunity for intercostal artery reimplantation. On the other hand, endovascular repair avoids some of the factors, such as aortic cross-clamp and haemodynamic instability, that contribute to the risk of paraplegia in the open operation (Svensson *et al.* 1993).

References

Chuter TAM, Gordon RL, Reilly LM *et al.* (2001). An endovascular system for thoracoabdominal aortic aneurysm repair. *J Endovasc Ther* **8**:25–33.

Crawford ES, DeNatale RW (1986). Thoracoabdominal aortic aneurysm: observations regarding the natural course of the disease. *J Vasc Surg* **3**:578.

Svensson LG, Crawford ES, Hess KR *et al.* (1993). Experience with 1509 patients undergoing thoracoabdominal aortic operations. *J Vasc Surg* **17**:357–370.

Endoluminal treatment of aortic traumatic rupture with stent-graft

H Rousseau, P Soula, P Otal, V Chabert, P Massabuau, G Meites, P Concina, F Joffre

Introduction

Acute rupture of the thoracic aorta due to blunt chest trauma is a life-threatening injury accounting for up to 18% of deaths in motor vehicle accidents. The site of aortic rupture is the isthmus in 84–90% of cases. The natural history of the patient with aortic transection is self-selective and death follows a bimodal distribution with the majority dying at the scene while approximately 15–20% of the victims reach the hospital alive owing to the preserved continuity of adventitia and mediastinal structures surrounding the injured aorta. Of those potentially curable patients the overall mortality is estimated to be 32% with one-third dying before surgical repair is attempted. Since Parmley's report in 1958 on the natural history of the injury, many aspects of aortic transection have changed which alter survival rates, through the creation of heparin-less partial bypass techniques and, more recently, through the development of endovascular intervention.

The configuration and type of pathology of the traumatic pseudoaneurysms of the thoracic aorta present specific technical difficulties. If aneurysms of the descending thoracic aorta offer a configuration that is easily amenable to an endovascular repair with few technical difficulties, in contrast, aneurysms extending proximally to the subclavian artery such as traumatic pseudoaneurysms represent a real challenge.

1

Precise sizing is critical to those endovascular procedures. In our institution we use data from digital subtraction angiograms with calibrated catheter and spiral computed tomography (CT) with three-dimensional reconstructions. We find that the multiple angle of views provided by three-dimensional reconstructions offer a unique way to thoroughly evaluate neck length, topography of aneurysm in relation to branch vessels and aortic diameters. Illustration 1 shows schemes of pre-stent grafting measurement points. The diameters of pseudoaneurysm, pseudocoarctation, native aortic lumens, proximal neck, distal neck, left subclavian arterial ostium were measured. We feel that in the near future spiral CT might be the only imaging study needed prior to stent-gaft therapy. However, due to a lack of strong scientific data confirming this premise, we keep performing pre-procedure angiograms with a calibrated catheter as a

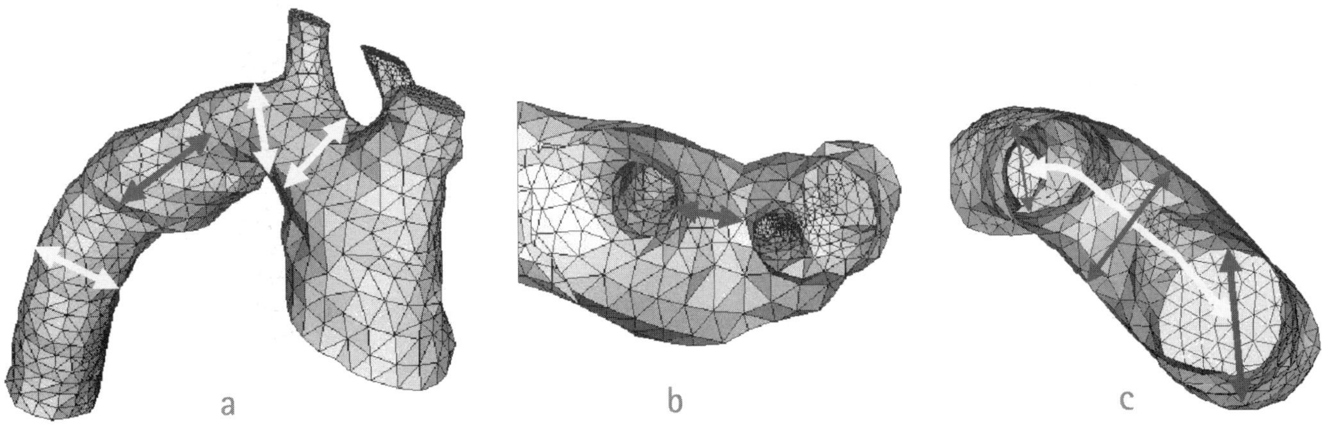

1

complementary investigation. Moreover, digital subtraction angiography provides a better evaluation of iliac arteries which is mandatory prior to introducing the large delivery systems of the currently used stent-grafts. The graft diameters are oversized by 10% to achieve a tight friction seal and the length is at least 4 cm greater than the lesion.

Three type of straight stent-grafts are commercially available: Excluder (WL Gore and associates), Talent (Medtronic) and AneuRx (Medtronic), whose diameters range from 24 to 44 mm and lengths from 80 to 100 mm. The only device with a 15-mm bare stent at the proximal end is the Talent device. Radio-opaque markers at both ends of the polytetrafluoroethylene or polyester outer covering allow a more precise placement. Introduction calibre ranges from 22 to 25 French.

Technique

The team of cardiovascular surgeons and interventional radiologists performs the endovascular procedure with the patient under general anaesthesia, with endobronchial intubation and mechanical ventilation. The procedure is conducted in a sterile radiological vascular interventional suite. The patient is positioned in dorsal decubitus and the operative field is prepared and draped for thoracotomy in case the endovascular device cannot be deployed or a major complication occurs. Cardiopulmonary bypass equipment should be readily available, if such a complication does occur.

Additional brachial arterial accesses are gained to allow: 1) easy completion of control angiograms during procedure; 2) straightforward marking off of the left subclavian artery ostium just before stent-graft deployment; and in some cases 3) direct invasive arterial pressure monitoring.

The common femoral artery is surgically exposed, following intravenous administration of 5000 international units of heparin and a standard 18 G arterial needle is used to puncture the anterior wall of the artery directly, a 5 Fr vascular sheath is placed, and a 0.0035 inch diameter soft guidewire is advanced gently through the lesion up to the ascending aorta. The vascular sheath is withdrawn over an exchange-length stiff wire (Back-up Meier, Boston Scientific Vascular, Watertown, MA). A transverse arteriotomy is performed and the 22–25 French delivery device is introduced over the guidewire. An angiography of the thoracic aorta is performed, via the right brachial approach, in the left anterior oblique projection. The purpose of this angiogram is to ensure that the patient and image intensifier are positioned optimally to monitor accurate placement of the stent-graft. Alternatively angiography can be performed by a contralateral femoral approach, the catheter remaining in place during the stent-graft insertion.

Under fluoroscopic and transoesophageal echocardiographic (TOE) guidance the delivery system is advanced until the sheath is correctly positioned with the first leading platinum marker on the compressed stent-graft at approximately 2 cm proximally to the pre-established level. Prior to release, nifedipine is administered intravenously to decrease the mean arterial blood pressure to a range of 50–70 mmHg and to decrease downstream migration of the stent-graft.

2

Under fluoroscopic guidance the delivery system is advanced until the sheath is correctly positioned with the first leading platinum marker on the compressed stent-graft at approximately 2 cm proximally to the pre-established level. For the Talent device the outer sheath is then slowly withdrawn up to the first ring of non-covered stent graft. An angiography is then performed to confirm the position of the stent-graft. The device is withdrawn approximately 2 cm to the pre-established level, and the outer sheath is then rapidly withdrawn completely to fully deploy the implant, while the pushing mandrel is maintained in fixed position. Left brachial arterial access allows straightforward marking off of the left subclavian artery ostium just before stent-graft deployment and direct invasive arterial pressure monitoring.

The latex balloon is positioned in the first leading lumen of the stent-graft and is inflated to fully anchor the neck of the stent into the non-aneurysmal wall of the aorta. If a perigraft leak exists owing to poor sealing and apposition of the stent-graft to the aortic wall, thereafter the prosthesis can be modelled with large angioplasty valvuloplasty balloons. Completion angiography and TOE should demonstrate exclusion of the false aneurysm. Finally the introducer delivery system is removed and the arteriotomy is repaired.

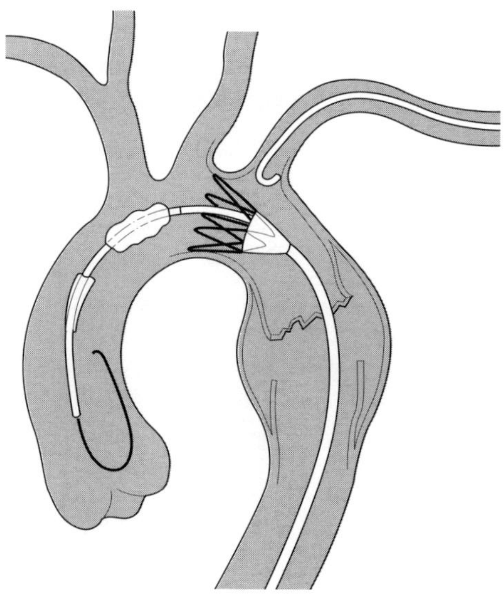

2

Patients are extubated immediately after the procedure and are usually monitored in the intensive care unit for the first 24 hours after the procedure. On the next day patients are transferred to a regular nursing unit and they are discharged from the hospital 5 days later. Anticoagulation is maintained for 48 hours and then followed by aspirin (250 mg per day). Prior to discharge, all the patients undergo a follow-up chest X-ray and contrast-enhanced spiral CT examination to evaluate the shape and position of the stent-graft, the absence of perigraft leak. A repeat CT is performed at 6 months and yearly thereafter.

Alternative access methods are required if the patient has extensive iliofemoral occlusive disease or small arteries: 1) retroperitoneal access to the distal aorta or common iliac artery; 2) access into existing aortobifemoral bypass graft; and 3) access into a newly placed surgical aortofemoral or aortic tube graft. In rare difficult cases, a right brachial artery approach allows a 2.60 m long 0.035 inch stiff guidewire to be tethered between the two vascular accesses assuring a rigid axis and smooth tracking of the device.

As for abdominal aortic aneurysm repairs, the proximal neck of the thoracic aorta needs to be at least 1.5 cm in order to perform a safe deployment of the prosthesis and avoid impingement of the subclavian artery proximally. In several selected cases, a pre- or post-deployment subclavian carotid bypass can be performed, in order to exclude the pseudoaneurysm and maintain upper limb perfusion. In our experience, in several cases we deployed the stent-graft with the first proximal non-covered end upon the left subclavian artery ostium due to the close proximity of the pseudoaneurysmal sac. As long as only the bare portion of the stent-graft covered the ostium of the left subclavian artery, this artery remained patent. In one patient we had to cover the left subclavian artery ostium by the polyester tube to exclude the pseudoaneurysm and the patency of the left subclavian artery was obtained by placing two Palmaz stents. Finally, one Talent stent-graft was customized to include a 17 × 21 mm proximal indentation in the covered portion, centred on the external curvature connecting bar, in order to avoid covering the left subclavian artery ostium with the polyester tube. This modification was dictated by the particular configuration of the aortic rupture, with an almost non-existent neck between the left subclavian artery ostium and the upper limit of the pseudoaneurysmal neck.

This approach may be a viable therapeutic option for acute traumatic rupture of the aorta, but appropriately controlled prospective studies including cost-benefits are needed before we can recommend its widespread use.

Less invasive combined surgical and endovascular stent-graft treatment for descending thoracic aortic aneurysms: surgical technical aspects

Bansi Koul, Krassi Ivancev

Introduction

Open surgical resection, with or without cardiopulmonary bypass, is the standard recommended treatment for the descending thoracic aortic aneurysms. However, open surgical resection involves a long posterolateral thoracotomy, which is time-consuming, painful and associated with impaired early postoperative lung function. Quality of the aorta in patients with descending thoracic aortic aneurysms is usually poor and the aorta is invariably lined with loose thrombi. If cardiopulmonary bypass, with or without deep hypothermic circulatory arrest, is needed for the surgical excision of the descending thoracic aortic aneurysms, the descending thoracic aorta may therefore not be suitable site for direct arterial cannulation and not also for retrograde perfusion from the femoral arteries. Moreover, through a posterolateral thoracotomy, it may not be possible to provide retrograde brain perfusion during hypothermic circulatory arrest. It may be difficult to get suitable access to the ascending aorta and the caval veins, normally employed for cardiopulmonary bypass, through a posterolateral thoracotomy incision.

A mid-line sternotomy, which is routinely performed for most of the open-heart surgery today, is less painful and patients can be mobilized faster and earlier postoperatively. A mid-line sternotomy provides adequate access to the caval veins and the ascending aorta for cardiopulmonary bypass. Early postoperative pulmonary damage is less and the incision is well suited for retrograde brain perfusion. A mid-line sternotomy, however, provides poor exposure of the descending thoracic aorta and is not recommended for the resection of descending thoracic aortic aneurysms. Supradiaphragmatic descending thoracic aorta may, on the other hand, be approached though this incision but the access is restricted and therefore amenable for minor surgical procedures only.

Percutaneous transluminally placed endovascular stent-grafts have been shown to be a feasible alternative treatment in patients with descending thoracic aortic aneurysms, and especially those at poor surgical risk (Dake *et al.* (1998); Greenberg *et al.*, 2000). The intermediate and long-term post-operative results of the procedure, however, are awaited (Resch *et al.*, 2001). One of the major limitations of endovascular stent-graft treatment, however, rests with the morphology of the proximal and distal neck of the descending thoracic aortic aneurysms (diameter, length and the tissue quality). Percutaneous transluminal aneurysm exclusion technique by endovascular stent-grafts is, on the other hand, a less invasive operation than the open surgical resection of the aneurysm.

Combining endovascular stent-grafting with open surgical modification of the aneurysm neck morphology through a mid-line sternotomy may therefore serve following goals in the treatment of descending thoracic aortic aneurysms;

1. The combined procedure is less invasive and less time consuming
2. Patients who are anatomically unsuitable may be rendered suitable for endovascular stent-grafting by addition of a less invasive open surgical procedure through a mid-line sternotomy
3. Cardiopulmonary bypass, if needed, can be performed with standard cannulation technique with satisfactory extracorporeal blood flows. Additional deep hypothermic circulatory arrest, if needed, can be complemented with retrograde brain perfusion, increasing the safety margins of the procedure

4. The combined procedure permits performance of endovascular stent-grafting simultaneously with one or many of the following complementary cardiac procedures, namely; coronary artery bypass grafting, repair of ascending aortic and aortic arch aneurysms, repair of aortic valve insufficiency etc making the entire procedure safer, less morbid and cost-effective
5. The combined procedure has the potential of combining the documented reliability of the open surgery with the least invasiveness of the endovascular stent-grafting and thereby making the treatment of descending thoracic aortic aneurysms reliable, safer, less invasive and thereby more economical.

These less invasive combined procedures may, in selected cases, be planned in stages to make the treatment less complicated. In the following sketches we have outlined the surgical technical aspects of some of the combined procedures that we have performed in the past few years.

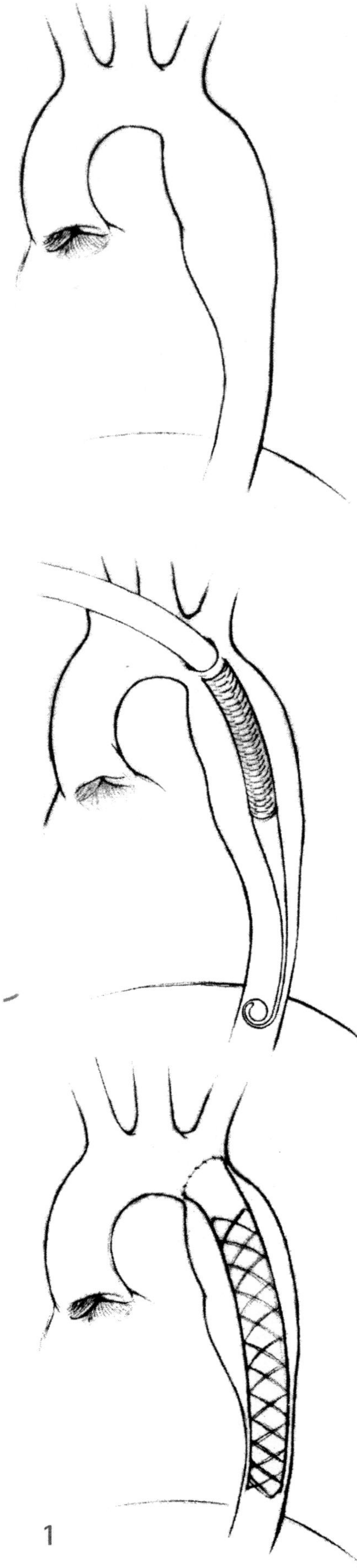

a b 1 c

1a, b, c

A descending thoracic aortic aneurysm with short dilated proximal neck is not suitable for isolated endovascular stent-grafting (**1a**). The distal neck of the aneurysm is suitable for endovascular stent-grafting. The ascending aorta and the arch of aorta are normal.

Under cardiopulmonary bypass and deep hypothermic circulatory arrest, the delivery system with an endovascular stent-graft is negotiated into the descending thoracic aorta through an aortic arch incision in an antegrade fashion (**1b**). A mid-line sternotomy has been employed for the combined open and endovascular procedure. This approach permits retrograde brain perfusion during the period of hypothermic circulatory arrest.

The endovascular stent-graft is deployed with good distal fixation of the stent-graft. The proximal unstented part of the stent-graft is surgically sutured to the aortic wall distal to the origin of the left subclavian artery incorporating the anterior half of the stent-graft in the suture line of the aortotomy.

2a, b

An isolated descending thoracic aortic aneurysm with short and wide proximal neck has been rendered suitable for endovascular stent-grafting by banding of the proximal descending thoracic aorta (**2a**). A teflon band has been sutured in place through a mid-line sternotomy and the endovascular stent-graft delivered through the groin in a retrograde fashion.

An endovascular stent-graft has been deployed and the teflon-band can be further tightened, if needed.

The distal end of the stent-graft is optimally placed without any external band (**2b**).

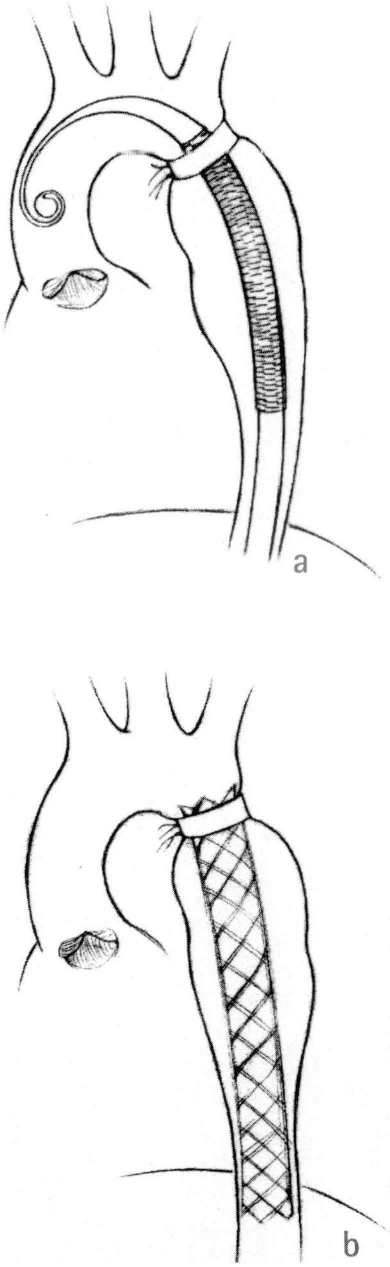

2

3

Banding of the proximal and distal neck of a wide descending thoracic aortic aneurysm achieved through a mid-line sternotomy is shown in **3**. The stent-graft has been subsequently deployed through the groin incision in a retrograde fashion.

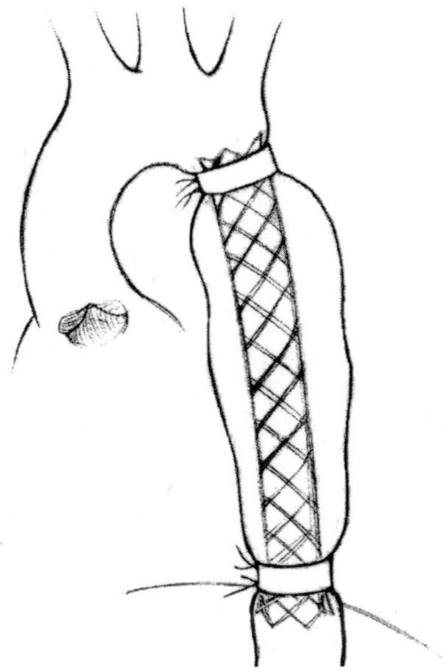

3

4a, b, c, d

A stented elephant-trunk graft is shown in **4a**. About 7.5–10 cm of the vascular graft has been covered by stainless steel Z-stents. The stented elephant-trunk graft will be left hanging in the proximal aneurysmatic descending thoracic aorta for subsequent extension with another stent-graft to exclude the descending thoracic aortic aneurysm.

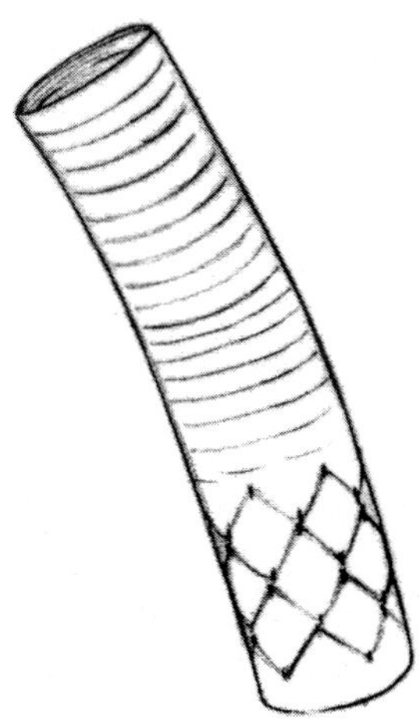

4a

The non-stented portion of the vascular graft has been inverted into the stented elephant-trunk graft and has been thereafter sutured to the aortic wall, distal to the origin of the left subclavian artery (**4b**). Note that the ascending aorta, the aortic arch and the proximal descending thoracic aorta are all aneurysmatic. The dilated sinotubular junction in the ascending aorta has resulted in aortic valve incompetence.

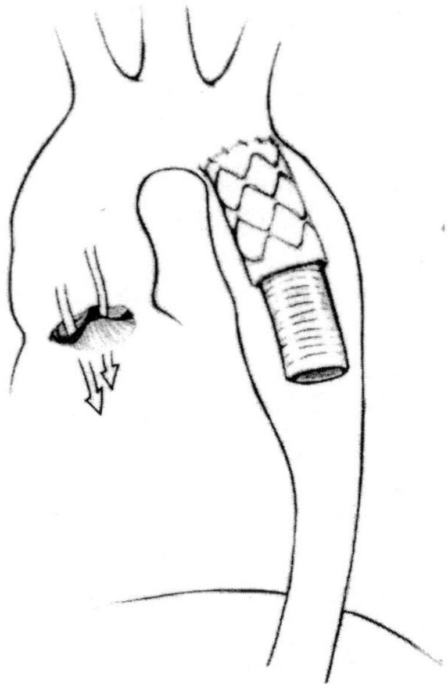

4b

The ascending aorta and the aortic arch have been excised leaving a common cuff of aorta at the base of the neck vessels (**4c**). The proximal unstented part of the elephant-trunk graft has been everted and used for reconstruction of the arch, neck vessels and the ascending aorta. The aortic valves can be made competent by remodelling of the sinotubular junction or of the entire aortic root.

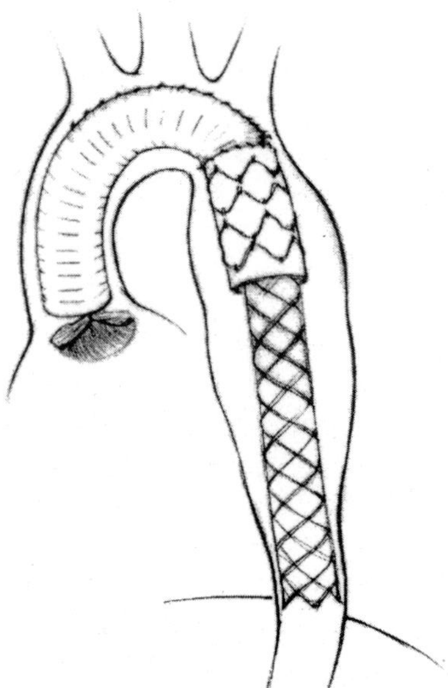

4c

In the second stage (usually after 6–12 weeks) the stented elephant-trunk graft is extended distally to exclude the descending thoracic aortic aneurysm (**4d**). A new stent-graft has been deployed in the descending thoracic aorta through a groin incision in a retrograde fashion. The proximal end of the descending thoracic stent-graft has been telescoped in the stented elephant-trunk graft. The stented elephant-trunk cannot prolapse into the aortic arch during the procedure and permits easy and controlled deployment of the thoracic stent-graft.

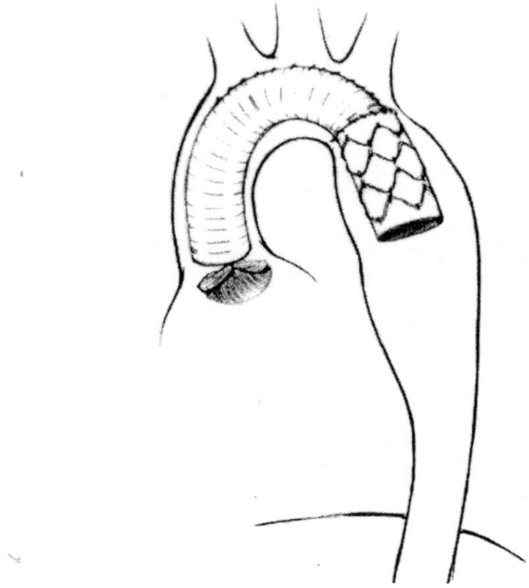

4d

References

Dake MD, Miller DC, Mitchell RS *et al.* (1998). The 'first generation' of endovascular stent-grafts for patients with aneurysms of the descending thoracic aorta. *J Thorac Cardiovasc Surg* 116:689–703; discussion 703–704.

Greenberg R, Resch T, Nyman U *et al.* (2000). Endovascular repair of descending thoracic aortic aneurysms: an early experience with intermediate-term follow-up. *J Vasc Surg* 31:147–156.

Resch T, Koul B, Dias NV *et al.* (2001). Changes in aneurysm morphology and stent-graft configuration after endovascular repair of descending thoracic aortic aneurysms *J Thorac Cardiovasc Surg* (in press).

Transperitoneal approaches to the abdominal aorta and its branches

Tammy K Ramos, Ronald J Stoney

Introduction

In 1951 Charles Dubost performed the first abdominal aortic aneurysm repair using a left subthoracic retroperitoneal approach (Dubost *et al.*, 1952). Since that time, multiple approaches to the abdominal aorta and its branches have been described and compared. Although there are many differences among the various approaches, they differ primarily by location of the incision (abdominal vs flank), anatomic route to the aorta (transperitoneal vs extraperitoneal) and the number of body cavities involved abdominal vs thoracoabdominal). The controversy over which approach is superior has been focused on perioperative morbidity. During the past decade, the left flank-extraperitoneal approach has been revitalized. Several studies Johnson *et al.*, 1986; Peck *et al.*, 1986; Sicard *et al.*, 1987; Leather *et al.*, 1989; Gregory *et al.*, 1989) have suggested that it is less morbid than the traditional midline-transperitoneal approach. The only prospective study (Cabria *et al.*, 1990) did not substantiate these findings. Although perioperative morbidity is a major consideration when selecting an approach to the abdominal aorta and its branches, the overriding consideration should be which approach provides the required exposure to perform the optimal repair of the aortic disease.

Adequate exposure of any arterial bed is determined by the distribution and extent of pathology in the artery wall, the surgical objective, and the anticipated reconstructive technique. Atherosclerosis is the most common disease involving the abdominal aorta and its branches and it may result in obstruction to blood flow, thromboembolism, and aneurysmal degeneration. Therefore, the therapeutic objectives of treatment are reperfusion of distal arterial beds, removal or exclusion of embolic sources, and replacement of unstable arterial walls. These objectives can be accomplished by two fundamental reconstructive techniques: endarterectomy and grafting (replacement; bypass – with or – without exclusion). Endarterectomy and replacement grafting require unrestricted exposure of the aorta and its branches. Bypass grafting can usually be accomplished with limited exposure of the inflow and outflow vessels.

After the necessary exposure is determined, then the best approach to achieve it can be selected. This chapter will present our methods for achieving and maintaining optimal exposure of the abdominal aorta and its branches. Our current practice is to employ a full-length midline abdominal incision and one of three transperitoneal approaches, the infracolic approach, the transcrural approach, or the medial visceral rotation approach.

Optimal exposure of the abdominal aorta and its branches requires that the area of interest be brought into view and that unobstructed access to the area be maintained throughout the reconstruction. The retroperitoneal location of the aorta, its fixation to the spine by the diaphram, its proximity to major venous structures and its coverage by abdominal viscera present a challenge for exposing this area. The superficial wound margins must be widely *retracted* throughout the procedure; the soft tissue and viscera must be mobilized, displaced and *retained* for long periods of time. The use of self-retaining retractors has helped to overcome the challenge of aortic exposure. We use the Omni-Tract vascular retractor system (Omni-Tract Surgical, A Division of Minnesota Scientific, Inc., St Paul, Minnesota), which is a table-mounted, self-retaining mechanical retractor that provides extended exposure or simultaneous multi-site exposure for an indefinite period of time.

Infracolic approach

The abdominal cavity is entered through a full-length midline incision extending from the xiphoid process to the symphysis pubis. After exploration, the Omni-Tract vascular retractor system is assembled. When this incision is used, the primary joint of the wishbone frame should be positioned so that it sets one hand-breadth cephalad to the incision and one hand-breadth above the lower sternum. The wound edges are retracted laterally from the mid-portion of the incision using the Mayo swivel retractors. Special care is always taken to protect the soft tissue and viscera by using moistened sponges beneath the retractor blades. The stomach is decompressed with a nasogastric tube. The transverse colon and omentum are wrapped in a moist sponge and reflected cephalad over the wound edges where they are retained with splanchnic retractors. The small bowel is placed in an intestinal bag and displaced to the right.

1

These manoeuvres bring the midline retroperitoneum into view. The infrarenal aorta is exposed by incising the posterior peritoneum just to the right of the midline from the aortic bifurcation to the base of the transverse colon mesentery. Proximally the periaortic tissue is divided and the left renal vein is identified and circumferentially mobilized.

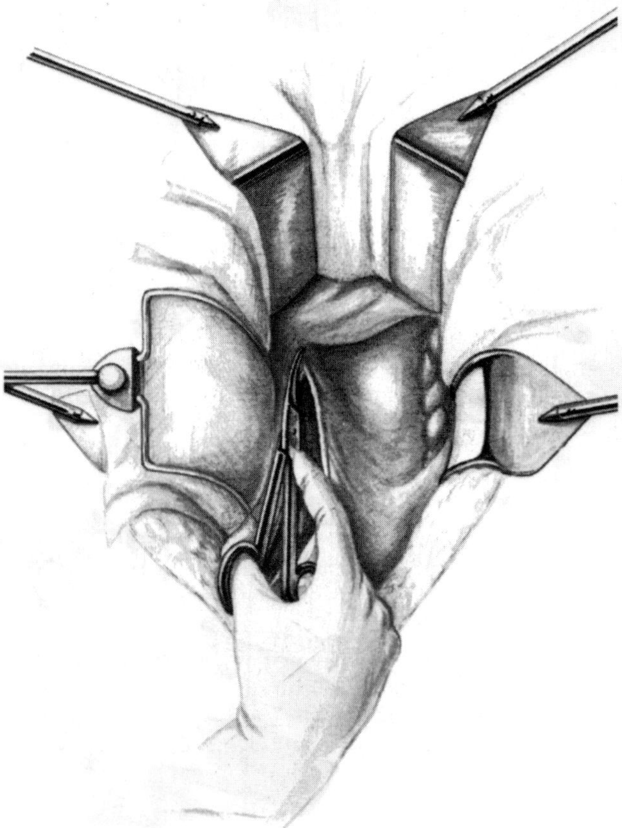

1

2

Visualization of the juxtarenal aorta is facilitated by displacing the left renal vein cephalad using the renal vein retractor. Now mobilization of the proximal infrarenal aorta can be safely accomplished by dissecting in the plane of Leriche.

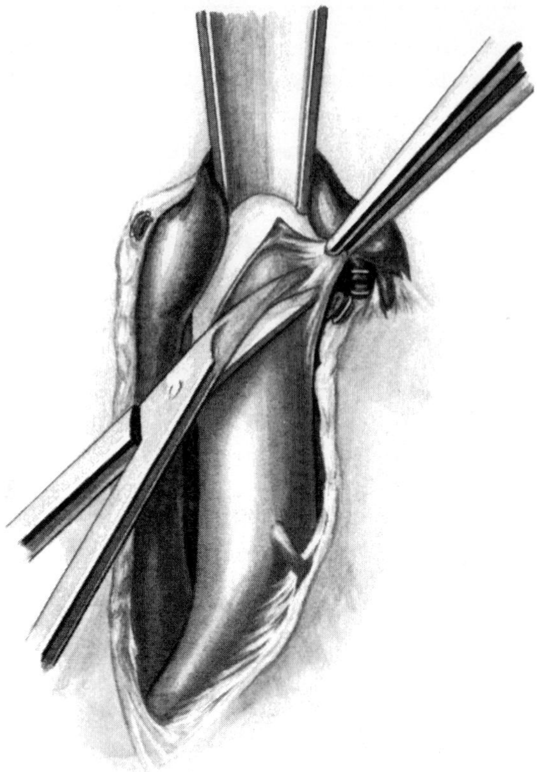

2

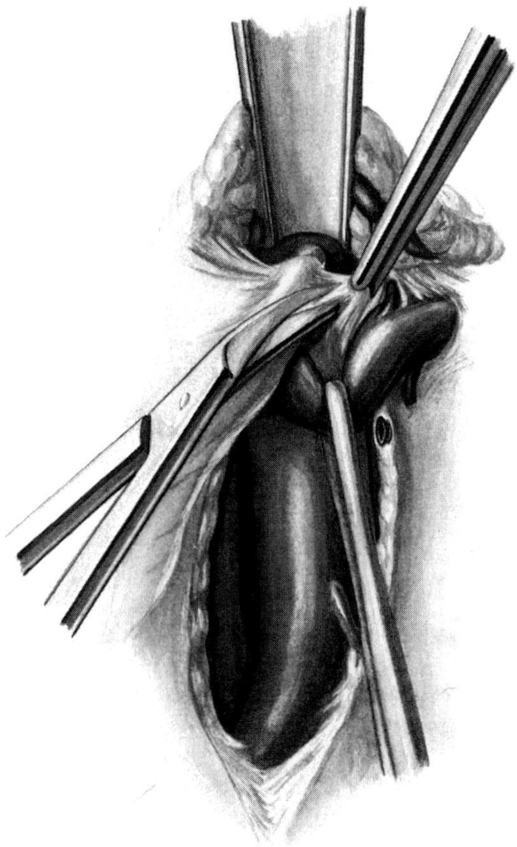

3

3

Exposure of the pararenal aorta requires that the left renal vein be circumferentially dissected to its junction with the inferior vena cava. Approximately 2 cm of the inferior vena cava is freed adjacent to this junction to ensure adequate mobility. Flexible tubing placed around the left renal vein serves as an atraumatic mobile retractor. The autonomic ganglian tissue is dissected from the anterior surface of the aorta until the origin of the superior mesenteric artery is identified. This may require cephalad, then caudad retraction of the left renal vein. The renal vein retractor is then placed to retain the left renal vein and pancreas cephalad and the splanchnic retractors are repositioned deeper in the wound so that the dissected periarterial tissue is pulled laterally away from the aorta.

4

Division of the musculotendinous crura of the diaphragm opens up the confined space cephalad to the renal arteries and greatly facilitates mobilization of the suprarenal aorta and renal arteries.

The entire infrarenal aorta and the inferior mesenteric artery can be exposed by carrying the dissection caudally along the anterior surface of the aorta. When exposing the common iliac arteries, the incision in the posterior peritoneum must be extended distally over the right common iliac artery. This avoids the autonomic nerves crossing over the left common iliac artery.

Transcrural approach

5

The abdominal cavity is entered through an upper midline abdominal incision extending from above the xiphoid to below the umbilicus. The self-retaining retractor system is assembled and the wound edges are retracted laterally as described above. Resection of the xiphoid process facilitates upper abdominal exposure. The left triangular ligament is divided, the left lobe of the liver is folded on itself and retained to the right using the malleable slotted swivel blade. The lessor sac is entered through a vertical incision in the gastrohepatic ligament and the oesophagus and stomach are displaced to the left and held with a splanchnic retractor. The midline posterior peritoneum is incised. The muscle fibres of the diaphragm are separated, uncovering the median arcuate

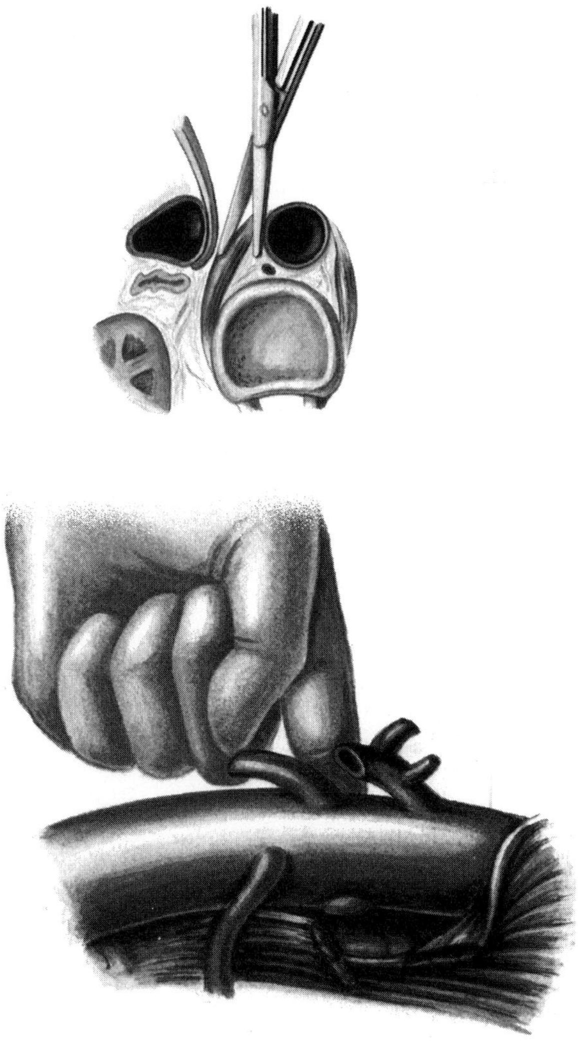

4

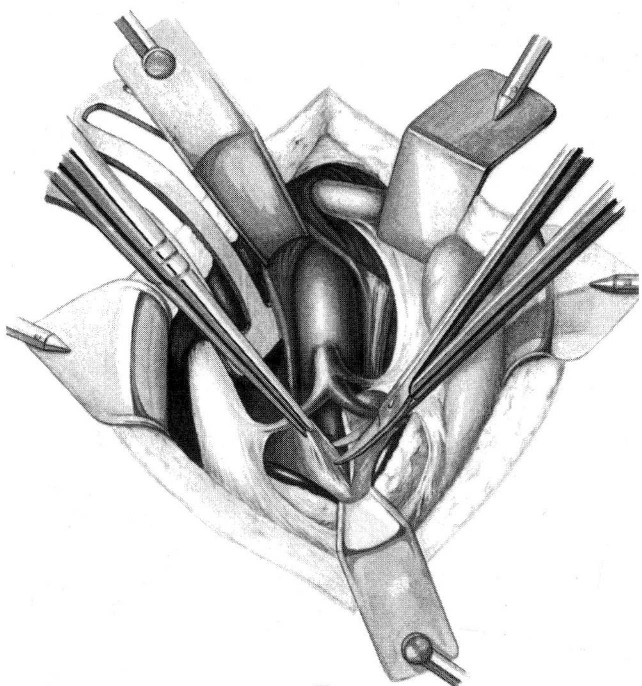

5

ligament lying immediately cephalad to the origin of the coeliac axis. Division of the median arcuate ligament exposes the distal thoracic and supracoeliac abdominal aorta. Dissection of the autonomic ganglion tissue along the left anteriolateral surface of the aorta allows the coeliac axis and the paramesenteric aorta to be mobilized. The crura of the diaphragm and freed periaortic tissue can now be displaced away from the sides of the aorta using the renal vein retractors. Dissection in the plane of Leriche is carried caudally to mobilize the proximal superior mesenteric artery behind the pancreas.

6

The spleen and pancreas are protected with moistened sponges and retained with spleachnic retractors. The remainder of the anteriorly mobilized viscera is retained to the right by repositioning the retractor. In addition, to ensure adequate perfusion of the displaced viscera, the retractors are periodically released and repositioned. The peritoneum is reflected from the left crus of the diaphragm. The triangular ligament is incised and the left lobe of the liver is folded on itself and held to the right by repositioning the more cephalad splanchnic retractor. The aorta is now clearly in view, crossed only by the left renal vein, the autonomic ganglia tissue and the muscle of the left crus of the diaphragm.

Exposure of the upper abdominal aorta also requires circumferential dissection of the left renal vein to its entry into the inferior vena cava. Flexible tubing placed around the left renal vein allows it to be widely retracted. Caudal retraction of the left renal vein exposes the origin of the renal arteries. The left renal artery can easily be freed from its origin to the renal hilum. Right lateral retraction of the inferior vena cava brings the proximal 2–3 cm of the right renal artery into view. The dense autonomic ganglia on the left anteriolateral surface of the aorta is resected and the musculotendinous left crus of the diaphragm is divided to mobilize the supracoeliac aorta and to expose the major visceral branches. Transection of the median arcuate ligament and separation of the muscle fibres of the diaphragm exposes the distal thoracic aorta within the mediastinum. The crura

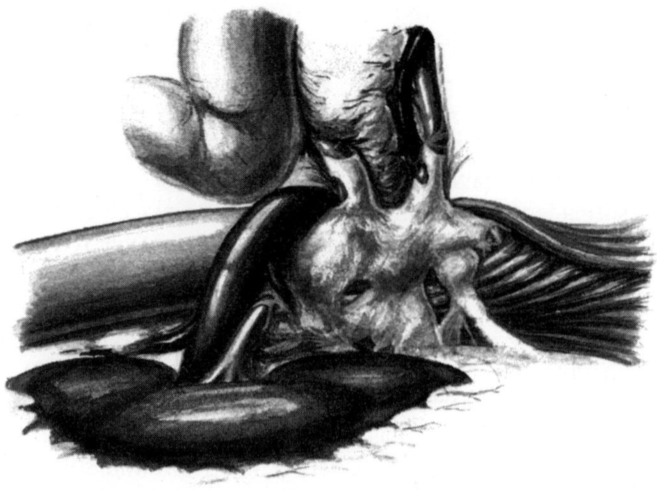

6

of the diaphragm and freed periarterial tissue can now be displaced using the renal vein retractors as described with the transcrural approach.

Mobilization of the lower abdominal aorta proceeds by incising the loose areaolar tissue along its left lateral surface. Reflection of this tissue to the right reveals the origin of the inferior mesenteric artery with the course of this vessel now vertical as a result of the colon displacement. In addition to the aortic bifurcation and the common iliac arteries, the entire length of the left internal and external iliac arteries are easily accessible for mobilization.

Summary

Table 1 summarizes the three approaches described above. The infracolic approach is simple. In most cases, it provides adequate exposure of the diseased para- and infrarenal abdominal aorta. Access to the upper abdominal aorta is limited with the infracolic approach; therefore, in some cases of pararenal aneurysmal disease, the exposure is inadequate. When the proximal extent of the aneurysm is juxtaposed to the origin of the superior mesenteric artery, some prefer to combine the infracolic

Table 1 Comparison of approaches to the abdominal wall aorta and its branches

Approach	Exposure	Limitations	Advantages	Disadvantages
Infracolic	Para- and infrarenal aorta and branches	Supracoeliac and paravisceral aorta and branches	Simple, Often adequate	Restricted
Transcrural	Supracoeliac and proximal paravisceral aorta and branches	Para- and infrarenal aorta and branches	Direct, Effective control	Restricted, Limited options
Medial visceral rotation	Entire abdominal aorta and branches	Right paramesenteric aorta, Right renal hilum, Right iliac artery bifurcation	Unrestricted, Maximum options	Complex, Indirect

approach with the transcrural approach to achieve safe proximal aortic control. However, this provides discontinuous aortic exposure separated by the transverse colon and pancreas, which prevent both segments of the aorta from being viewed simultaneously. The medial visceral rotation approach may be a superior option in this situation since it provides continuous exposure of the upper abdominal aorta.

The transcrural approach provides very limited access to the upper abdominal aorta and its branches. However, it is a direct approach to the supracoeliac aorta that provides rapid and effective proximal aortic control for the treatment of more distal aortic disease or for the treatment of visceral occlusive disease with aortovisceral bypass.

Although the medial visceral rotation approach to the aorta is indirect and more complex to establish than the above two approaches, it provides unrestricted, continuous exposure of the distal thoracic aorta and the entire abdominal aorta and its branches. Virtually all aortic disease can be treated when it is exposed using the medial visceral rotation approach. This approach maximizes the reconstructive options available to the surgeon and allows for flexibility in handling unanticipated problems.

Acknowledgements

This paper was supported in part by the Pacific Vascular Research Foundation, San Francisco, California.

Illustrations by Eileen S Natuzzi MS, MD.

References

Cabria RP, Brewster DC, Abbott WM *et al.* (1990). Transperitoneal versus retroperitoneal approach for aortic reconstruction: A randomized prospective study. *J Vasc Surg* **11**: 314.

Dubost C, Allary M, Oeconomos N (1952). Resection of an aneurysm of the abdominal aorta: Reestablishment of the continuity by a preserved human arterial graft, with results after five months. *Arch Surg* **64**: 405.

Gregory RT, Wheeler JR, Snyder SO *et al.* (1989). Retroperitoneal approach to aortic surgery. *J Cardiovasc Surg* **30**: 185.

Johnson JN, McLoughlin GA, Wake PN, Helsby CR (1986). Comparison of extraperitoneal and transperitoneal methods of aorto-iliac reconstruction. *J Cardiovasc Surg* **27**: 561.

Leather RP, Shah DM, Kaufman JL *et al.* (1989). Comparative analysis of retro-peritoneal and transperitoneal aortic replacement for aneurysm. *Surg Gynecol Obstet* **168**: 387.

Peck JJ, McReynolds DG, Baker DH, Eastman AB (1986). Extraperitoneal approach for aortoiliac reconstruction of the abdominal aorta. *Am J Surg* **151**: 620.

Sicard GA, Freeman MG, Vander Woude JC, Anderson CB (1987). Comparison between the transabdominal and retro-peritoneal approach for reconstruction of the infrarenal aorta. *J Vasc Surg* **5**: 19.

Subcostal rooftop incision and retroperitoneal exposure of the type IV thoracoabdominal aneurysm

Mark J Jackson, John H N Wolfe

Introduction

Surgical access to the upper abdominal aorta and renal arteries remains awkward. Thoracoabdominal aneurysms are classically repaired via a thoracoabdominal incision. However, this carries with it considerable morbidity. Perioperatively there are more respiratory complications and in the long-term there are consequences of diaphragmatic injury and intercostal pain. For the predominantly intra-abdominal (Type IV) aneurysms we have employed a completely abdominal approach.

This transabdominal, retroperitoneal approach is suitable for elective operations and affords good access to the entire abdominal aorta and both renal arteries and allows clamping of the distal thoracic aorta. Although the retroperitoneal exposure of the aorta was used for the first repair of an abdominal aortic aneurysm by Dubost and has been championed more recently by others, it has not been widely accepted. The disadvantage of the standard retroperitoneal approach is the poor exposure of the pararenal and suprarenal aorta.

Although a number of surgeons have championed the cause of the entirely retroperitoneal approach we are of the opinion that ready observation of the vascularity of the gut and viscera is an advantage for more complex aneurysms.

Operative technique

We describe the technique of transabdominal retroperitoneal exposure for Type IV thoracoabdominal aneurysms and juxtarenal aneurysms.

Incision

1

The incision is a high chevron or 'rooftop' abdominal incision with a left-sided subcostal extension. The rectus sheath and muscles are fully transected bilaterally, the peritoneal cavity is entered and falciform ligament divided. Any adhesions are divided and a general laparotomy carried out.

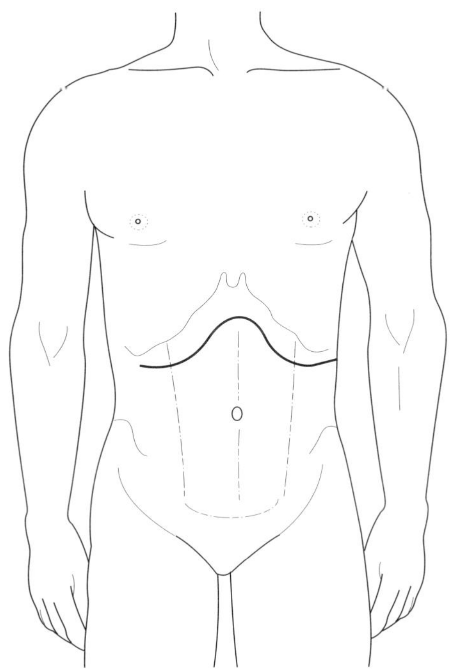

1

The small bowel is swung to the right side (extra-abdominally). Although it is preferable to pack the gut within the abdominal cavity, this is not usually possible with the extensive exposure required. The sigmoid colon is retracted medially to expose the posterior peritoneum.

Mobilization of colon from left paracolic gutter

2

Incision of the posterior parietal peritoneum of the left paracolic gutter is commenced inferiorly. The plane that

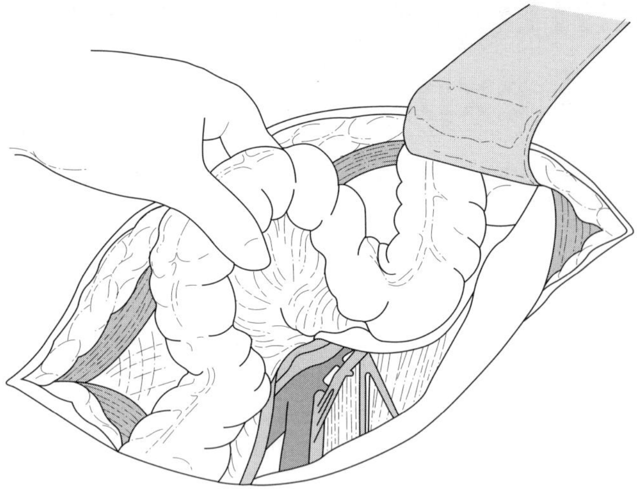

2

is dissected is posterior to gonadal vessels, left ureter, kidney and Gerota's fascia. Care is taken to leave the psoas fascia intact with the ilioinguinal, iliohypogastric and genitofemoral nerves beneath it. The lumbar branch of the left suprarenal vein is divided to allow the left kidney to be mobilized completely and rotated medially.

Retroperitoneal exposure of abdominal aorta

3

The aorta is exposed inferiorly on its left lateral aspect leaving lumbar vessels and sympathetic chain intact posterolaterally and midline visceral and renal branch origins to the patient's right. An important trick is to mobilize medially (behind the kidney and pancreas) to the level of the diaphragm before starting to swing the lateral attachments toward the midline. In this way the spleen is impacted against the surrounding tissues rather than the attachments being put under tension, risking a capsular tear.

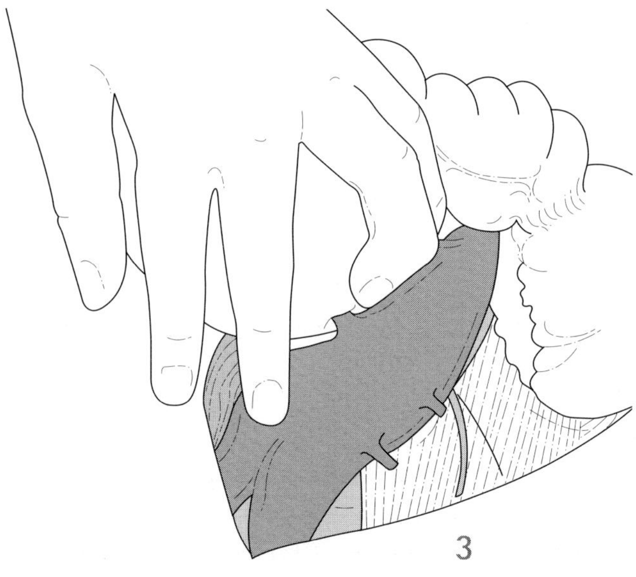

3

Complete left-sided medial visceral rotation

4

Once the tunnel along the psoas has been achieved by separating the loose areolar tissue (behind Gerota's fascia, the spleen, pancreas, left kidney, splenic flexure and stomach) these organs are dissected *en-bloc* to the patient's right. Toward the end of this part of the dissection the left renal artery should be identified but not dissected. The left ureter is identified, preserved and the mesentery retracted to expose both common iliac arteries. If there are associated iliac artery aneurysms it may be necessary to expose the distal right common iliac artery directly through the posterior peritoneum.

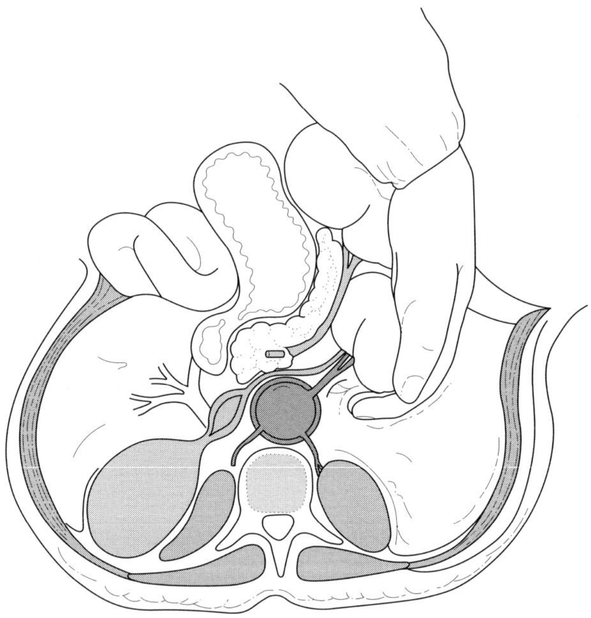

4

Exposure of the aneurysm

5

The length of the aneurysm is exposed. The viscera (in particular the left kidney and pancreas) are not directly visible through the fascia lying posterior to them. The origins of the left renal, superior mesenteric and coeliac vessels (and of lesser importance, the inferior mesenteric) can be located by palpation but should not be dissected. Careful attention is given to adequately wrapping the viscera in moist abdominal packs, especially the spleen's exposed diaphragmatic surface. An appropriate self-retaining retraction system is employed at this stage.

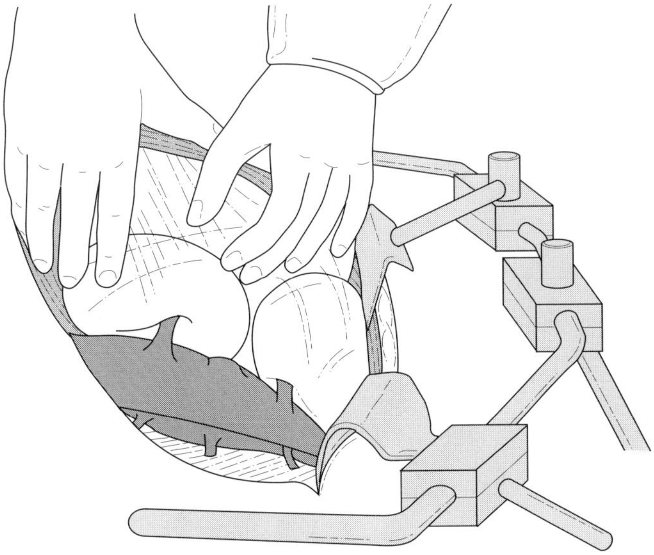

5

Incision of the left crus of the diaphragm

6

The crura are exposed which entails division of the left inferior phrenic artery. The lowermost fibres of the left crus are dissected off the aneurysm neck and divided superiorly under direct vision to expose the normal calibre lower thoracic aorta. Care is taken not to breach the costophrenic recess of the pleural cavity. Several centimetres of lower thoracic aorta can be exposed. The lower thoracic aorta must be dissected out almost circumferentially but a nylon tape should not be used. This is unnecessary and increases the risk of damaging an important lower thoracic spinal artery.

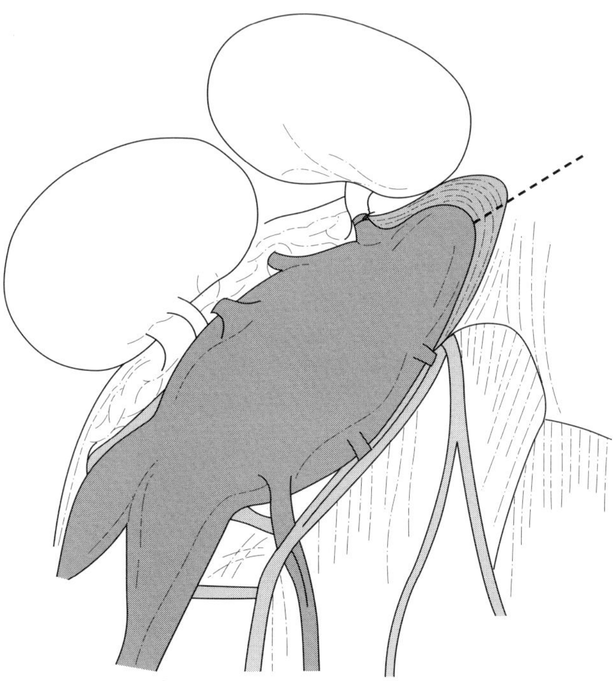

6

Supracoeliac clamp within thorax

7

It is preferable to place a straight or slightly curved aortic clamp and this can usually be accomplished in an anteroposterior fashion. This can be applied well up in the thorax via this approach depending on the length of the incision in the left crus and diaphragm.

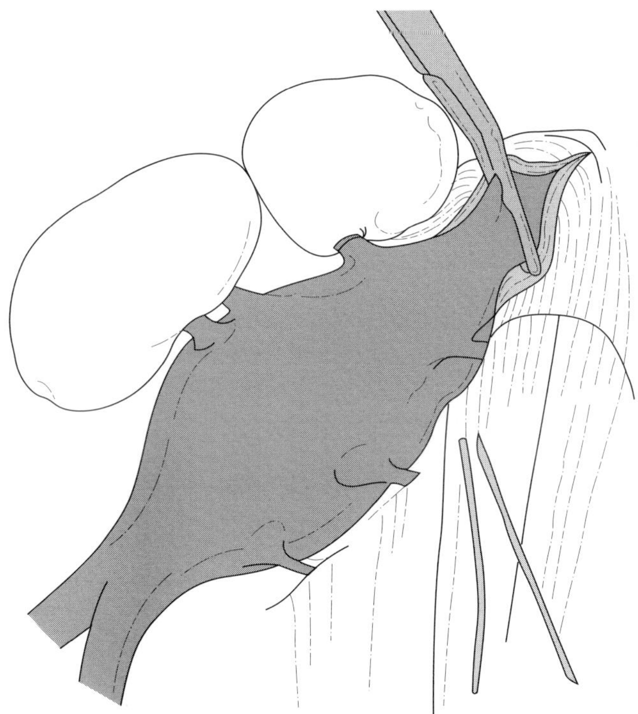

7

Aneurysm retaining-sutures Oblique visceral vessel patch

8

The aneurysm is opened widely on its anterolateral aspect. Great care is taken with the position of the incision at the level of the renal arteries particularly if there is a waist in the aneurysm at this point. If the incision is too anterior the left renal artery will be transected. Lumbar, median sacral, and inferior mesenteric ostia are oversewn. Retaining sutures are placed on the edge of the sac and the anatomy is confirmed. Care is taken to

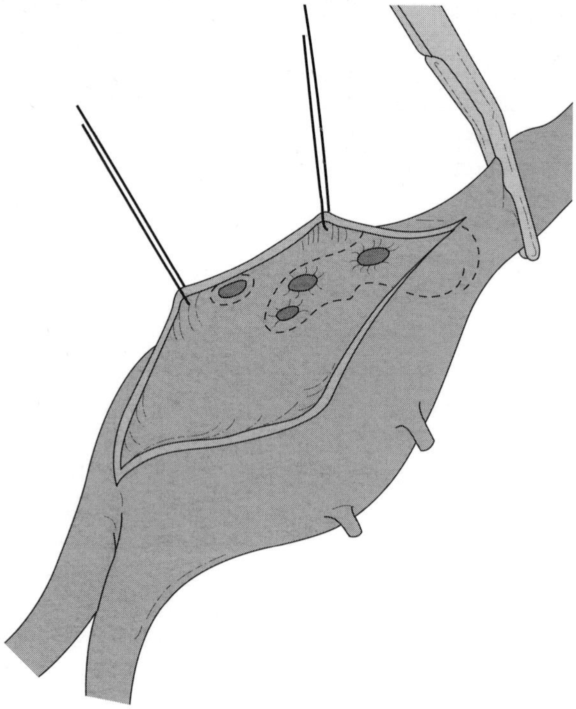

8

positively identify all four major visceral branches and ensure back bleeding. Gentle pressure on the viscera over the origins of these vessels can control retrograde bleeding in most cases without the need for temporary occlusion catheters. We believe that the occlusion balloon can damage the artery and that the static blood in the vessel is liable to thrombose. In some cases all four vessels can be incorporated within the same oblique patch but usually the left renal artery is anastomosed separately.

Left renal implantation

9

The graft may be fenestrated to allow a side-to-side anastomosis with the left renal artery. Care must be taken to cut the hole in the graft towards the left so that the artery does not kink when the viscera are returned to the abdominal cavity. Sometimes flow in the other arteries can be restored while anastomosing the left renal artery but, more usually, there is insufficient space and only after completion of this anastomosis can the clamp be positioned on the infrarenal graft to allow re-perfusion of the visceral circulation. Once the visceral patches are complete, tension should be taken off the bowel mesentery to improve blood flow and reduce the risk of damage to small mesenteric vessels. This also avoids tension on the graft suture-line. Following this revascularization the sac should be carefully scrutinized for back bleeding from the lumbar arteries. These may not bleed until the circulation has been re-established.

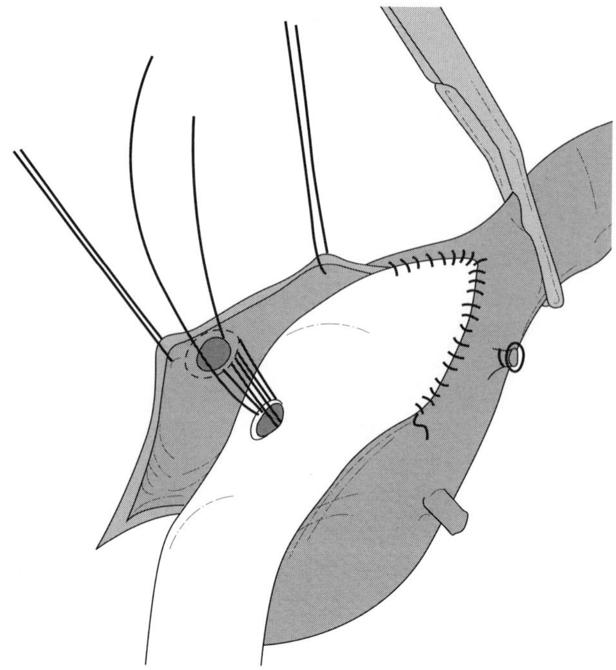

9

Completed graft

10

The distal anastomosis is completed in the routine manner as a tube or bi-iliac anastomoses. In the latter case the left limb should be plumbed initially as is expedites the re-perfusion of at least one lower limb and pelvis and avoids the need for repeated movement of retractors and visceral abdominal and pelvic contents. The free margin of the aneurysm sac wall should be sutured with a continuous suture to control troublesome bleeding that frequently occurs after unclamping.

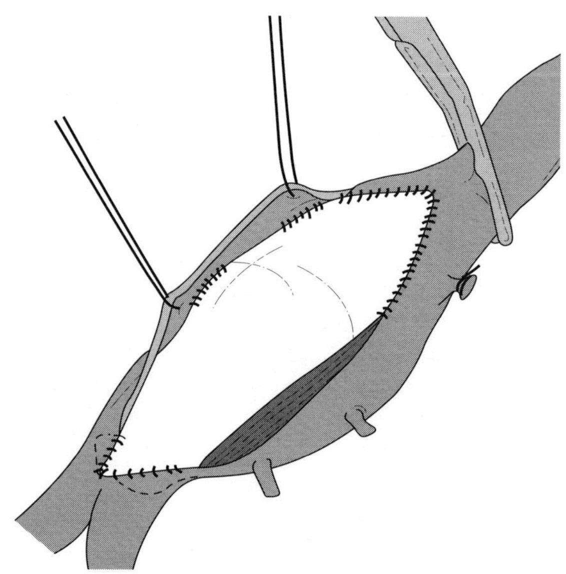

10

Extraperitoneal approach to the renal and suprarenal aorta

Charles N McCollum

Introduction

The standard transperitoneal approach to the infrarenal aorta has been almost universally adopted over nearly four decades. There is no doubt that this approach through either a midline or preferably transverse incision, provides the widest exposure of the infrarenal aorta and is relatively easy to perform in an abdomen clear of adhesions. However, the earliest aneurysm repairs were performed by Dubost in 1952 using an extraperitoneal approach which was popularized by Robb (1963). Several studies suggested less physiological stress, reduced blood loss and a shorter period of postoperative ileus when an extraperitoneal approach is used (Cambria *et al.*, 1990; Darling *et al.*, 1992; Nevelsteen *et al.*, 1988). Having used both approaches, I prefer a transverse subumbilical incision and transperitoneal approach for the infrarenal aorta as exposure is clearly better. The exception being when previous surgery suggests multiple adhesions or where there is a right-sided colostomy or ileostomy.

Suprerenal aneurysms have traditionally been exposed using a thoracoabdominal incision. Although providing excellent access, division of the costal margin, circumferential incision in the diaphragm and collapse of the left lung combine to greatly increase morbidity and mortality. Many surgeons approaching the suprarenal aorta, even as far as the lower thoracic aorta, are now using an abdominal approach. This can be via midline, bilateral subcostal (roof-top) or transverse incision with mobilization of the left-sided abdominal viscera ('medial rotation') and a retroperitoneal approach to the aorta. Providing adequate fixed retraction is available, this same segment of aorta can be exposed with less trauma to the patient through an oblique left-sided incision and extraperitoneal approach. It has been suggested that this gives poor access to the right renal artery, but I have not found that this is a problem. However, exposure of the right iliac bifurcation and external iliac artery cannot be achieved; a separate right groin incision exposing the common femoral artery would then be required.

Indications

This extraperitoneal approach is ideal for peri-renal and suprarenal aneurysm giving exposure up to approximately 10cm above the diaphragmatic hiatus. Other indications include:

1. patients exposed previously to multiple laparotomies, particularly if these have resulted in right-sided stomas;
2. patients requiring aortobifemoral reconstruction for occlusive disease;
3. infrarenal aortic aneurysm repair where there is a horseshoe kidney.

I have also used this approach for unusual arterial disease such as Takyasau's arteritis involving the origin of the visceral vessels. Finally, we are starting to use this approach to secure the distal end of an endovascular stent-graft inserted for a thoracic aneurysm where the aneurysm extends down to and involves the origin of the visceral vessels such that distal fixation cannot be achieved by endovascular technique alone.

Preoperative preparation

Essentially this is the same for any other major aortic procedure. Preoperative admission to the high dependency unit to place central and arterial lines allows intravenous fluid administration to maintain full hydration while the patient is being starved. Repeated fluid challenges are given to identify the filling pressures that each individual patient requires to optimize cardiac performance. It is more convenient for the arterial line to be placed in the right wrist as the left arm will be positioned in a sling and will not be easily accessible for the anaesthetist during the procedure. Mannitol is administered prior to suprarenal aortic clamping in an effort (unproven) to reduce the ischaemia-reperfusion injury and maintain renal function on declamping.

The operation

General anaesthesia is essential with an epidural catheter for the administration of bupivacaine and diamorphine for analgesia, both during and following surgery. In patients with a preoperative haemoglobin higher than 130g/litre, acute normovolaemic haemodilution is performed to reduce preoperative haemoglobin to approximately 105–110g/litre. This fresh autologous blood is reserved for re-infusion on wound closure at the end of the procedure. Intraoperative cell salvage is used during surgery thereby avoiding homologous blood in the majority of patients, even those undergoing surgery for thoracoabdominal aneurysms.

1

The patient is placed supine on the operating table with the buttocks flat but the left shoulder raised on a bean bag to an angle of approximately 40 degrees. The left arm is suspended in a padded sling from the underside of the frame used for a Rochard retractor. This retractor frame should be positioned so that the horizontal bar is approximately 20–30 cm above the patient's mouth giving adequate access for the surgical assistants and placing the Rochard frame an appropriate distance above the incision. Although several incisions have been advocated for extraperitoneal aortic surgery, an almost transverse oblique incision overlying the costal margin from the tenth rib and extending across the midline below the umbilicus works well. Exposure is better if the skin is incised across the costal margin and access is poor unless the incision extends at least 5–10 cm from the right of the midline. If there is any risk that the thoracic cavity may need to be opened then this incision should cross the costal margin over the ninth or even eighth intercostal space. This is a simple muscle-cutting incision which is deepened through the muscles, including the rectus, down to the transversus fascia. This fascia is then carefully incised to expose the peritoneum towards the lateral end of the incision. The extraperitoneal plane is quite easily developed laterally and inferiorly but is thin and adherent superiorly behind the rectus sheath. Great care is needed to gently strip the peritoneum from the posterior aspect of the rectus sheath and from the inferior aspect of the costal margin onto the diaphragm. Where an infrarenal procedure is planned, particularly aortobifemoral reconstruction for occlusive disease, then it may not be necessary to strip the peritoneum from the undersurface of the diaphragm. However, where the aorta must be exposed at the level of the renal arteries or above, access is poor if the peritoneum is not stripped fully from the diaphragm and the entire abdominal contents,

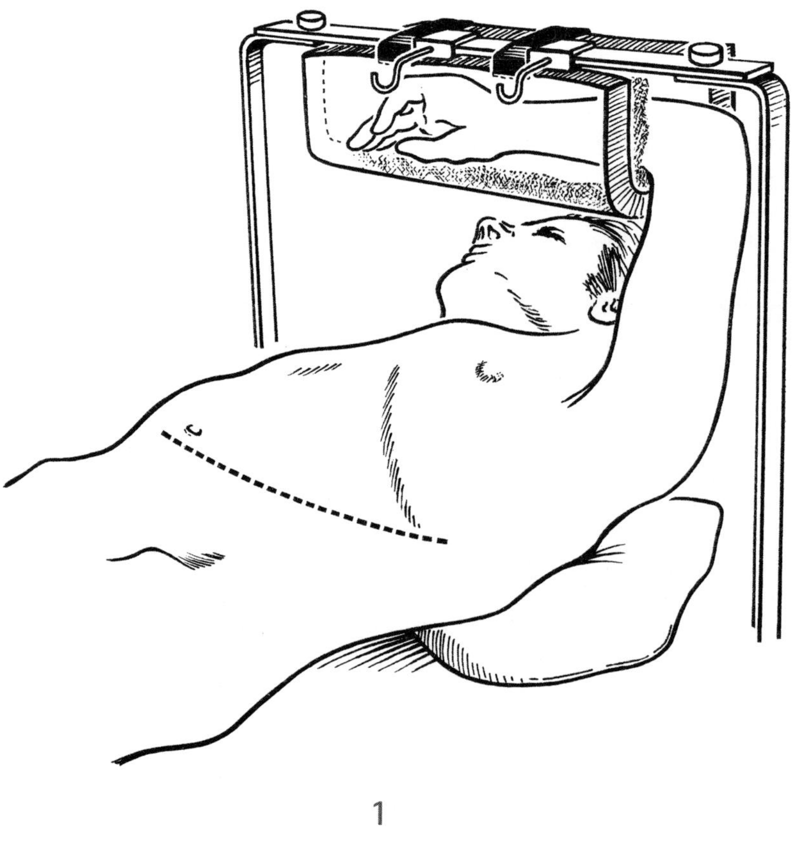

1

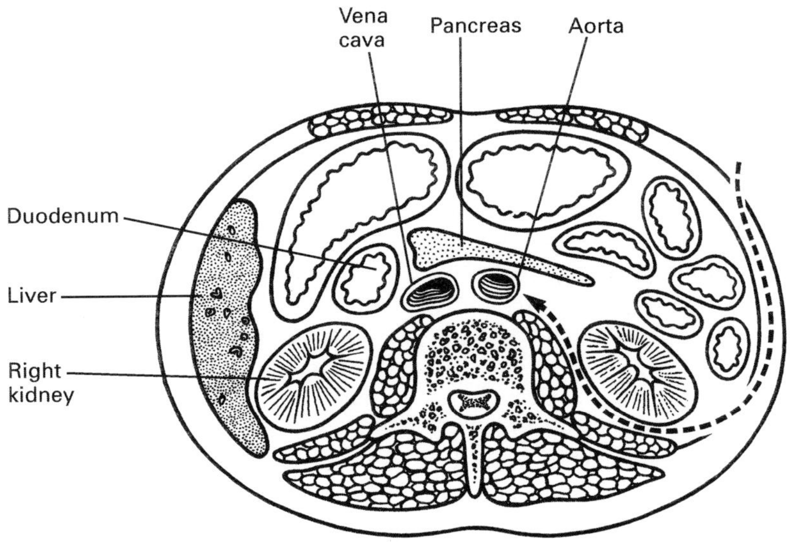

2

including the spleen, mobilized into the right abdomen.

Surgeons not familiar with this approach will usually become disheartened during the early part of this exposure as it involves careful dissection to avoid multiple tears in the peritoneum and as exposure to the aorta appears difficult initially.

2

Access to the infrarenal aorta at the level of the inferior mesenteric artery can be achieved without mobilizing the left kidney. Under these circumstances, the peritoneum is merely stripped starting in the left iliac fossa and moving up the left flank and across from the left iliac artery to the aortic bifurcation. However, exposure of the perirenal or suprarenal aorta is best achieved with full mobilization of the abdominal viscera, including the left kidney and spleen. As the peritoneum is stripped medially, it is important that the left ureter and gonadal vessels are lifted forward and remain adherent to the peritoneum. Once the spleen has been mobilized, it should be protected by a large, warm abdominal swab and held to the right with an appropriate wide-bladed retractor.

3

Following the initial mobilization of the peritoneum, a medium or large Rochard retractor blade may be inserted into the upper lateral aspect of the wound and fixed to the Rochard frame applying firm upward retraction.

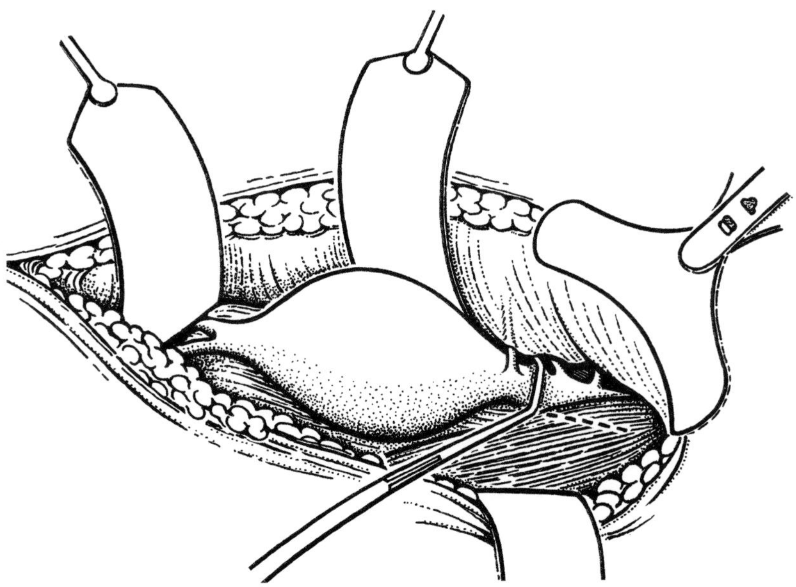

3

Without this retraction, access above the coeliac access is difficult if not dangerous. Exposure of the aorta starts from the external iliac artery on the left which is easily exposed as the retroperitoneal space is opened. The plane adjacent to the artery is developed up the common iliac artery and then the posterolateral aspect of the aorta. There is a surprising amount of tissue that initially appears adherent to the lateral aspect of the aorta but this plane immediately adjacent to the aortic wall is easily developed forward to the anterior aspect of an aortic aneurysm following ligation of the inferior mesenteric artery.

This posterolateral approach to the aorta is essential to stay behind the left renal artery. It is difficult to see or even feel this artery and the connecting vein from the renal vein to the hemiazygous vein is a helpful marker. This vein almost invariably lies close to the left aortic wall just below the left renal artery and must be divided between ligatures in order to expose the peri-renal aorta. Keeping posteriorly on the left lateral aspect of the aorta also allows better access to the lumbar arteries which frequently need to be divided before the suprarenal aorta can be clamped.

Where the aorta can be clamped just above the renals, the aorta only needs to be exposed up to the level of the coeliac axis. This exposure will involve separating the left crus of the diaphragm from the aorta, a manoeuvre relatively easily performed by blunt dissection. Once the operating surgeon is confident that the aorta can be safely clamped should bleeding occur, further exposure of the suprarenal aorta should be completed only after the retroperitoneum has been dissected away from the aortic aneurysm with the right side of the aorta visible below the renal arteries. At this stage, an apparently difficult exposure suddenly becomes very much easier. Exposure of the peri-renal aorta is then completed by gently identifying the lumbar arteries and dividing these between metallic clips. If aortic clamping just below the superior mesenteric artery is planned, it is helpful to divide the lumbars from just above the superior mesenteric artery to just below the renal arteries. A space is easily developed across the anterior aorta just below the superior mesenteric artery so that an aortic Satinsky clamp may be applied after the anaesthetist has administered heparin and mannitol.

4

Exposure of the aorta up to and above the coeliac axis initially involves separating the diaphragmatic cruri and then dividing the fibres of the left crus using scissors. There is an excellent plane around the aorta at this level and gentle digital dilatation of the diaphragmatic hiatus allows surprisingly good exposure of the distal thoracic aorta for up to 10cm. Any thoracic or lumbar branches may be divided between metallic clips so that the aorta can be mobilized circumferentially. An appropriate angled Satinsky clamp may then be applied after the anaesthetist has administered heparin and mannitol. The iliac arteries would have been exposed previously and angled Debakey clamps may now be applied anywhere throughout the left iliac system, but on the right, clamping beyond the common iliac artery is not possible.

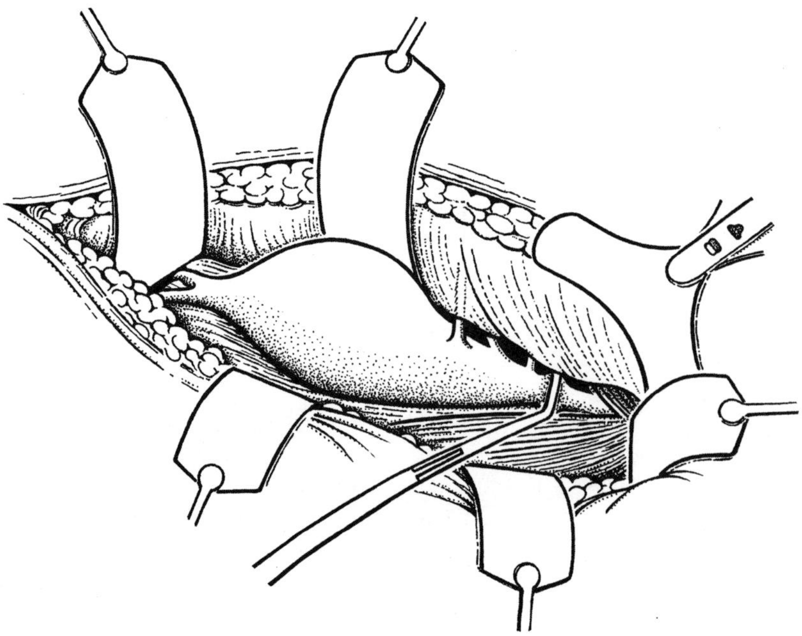

4

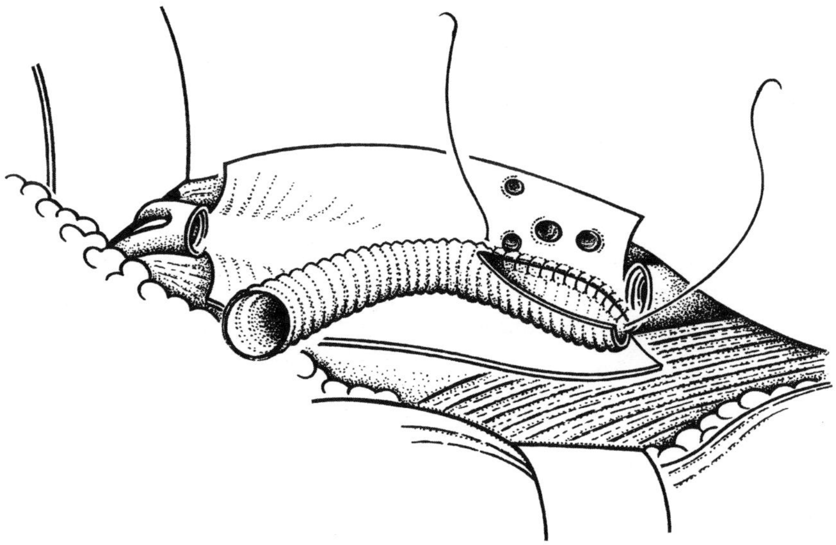

5

5

The aorta is not opened until the lateral and anterior aspects of the aneurysm are fully exposed and the origins of the coeliac axis, superior mesenteric and left renal artery identified. These origins do not need to be exposed and needless dissection only risks injury. A bold incision is made on the lateral aspect of the infrarenal aorta rapidly opening the entire sac but curving the incision carefully behind the origin of the left renal artery. Lumbar arteries may then be sutured from the inside using 2/0 Vicryl or Dexon. It is helpful to proceed rapidly at this stage as there is minimal back bleeding from the visceral vessels initially and the application of clamps or insertion of occluding balloons should not be required. The top end of an appropriate collagen or albumen-sealed Dacron graft may then be tailored to fit the aorta proximally with an oblique opening to incorporate the orifices of the coeliac axis, superior mesenteric and right renal arteries. This suture line may progress rapidly with large bites in the aorta using 3/0 or even 2/0 Prolene if the aorta is severely disease. I start by parachuting the graft down to the posterior aortic wall proximally and proceed with an oblique suture line to the right wall of the aorta behind the visceral arteries. The distal end of this oblique anastomosis is then taken around the inferior margin of the right renal artery and extended anterior to the left margin of the superior mesenteric artery. It is then easier to complete the anastomosis using the upper needle to suture the tailored Dacron tube around the proximal aorta and then obliquely along the aortic wall to the left of the visceral vessels completing the anastomosis anteriorly. The lumen is then carefully flushed to remove all debris and a clamp applied to the Dacron graft immediately distally, allowing reperfusion of the visceral vessels. The anaesthetist should be given 3–5 minutes warning so that the circulating volume and filling pressure may be increased prior to reperfusion as the blood pressure would otherwise fall. Where the proximal anastomosis is infrarenal, great care should be taken to avoid injuring the left renal artery while suturing to the anterior aortic wall. Surgeons unfamiliar with this approach may forget that the left renal artery cannot be seen but is now wrapped across the front of the aorta just above the level of an infrarenal anastomosis. This renal artery is easily lacerated by the suture needle leading to unexpected and difficult to control bleeding when the suprarenal clamp is removed.

The distal end of the Dacron may then be cut to length. For a tube graft, an end-to-end anastomosis to the aortic bifurcation using 3/0 Prolene can be completed rapidly as access is excellent. Where a bifurcated graft is required, the easiest anastomosis, usually to the left iliac system, should be performed first using 4/0 Prolene to ensure rapid reperfusion of the pelvis and lower limbs.

6

Having established perfusion to the legs, a small Satinsky clamp may then be applied to the antero-left aspect of the Dacron graft in a suitable location to re-implant the origin of the left renal artery. It should not be necessary to use an interposition graft which is prone to kinking as the left kidney is returned to its renal bed. It is convenient to cut a slightly larger hole in the Dacron than required so that the anastomosis can be rapidly performed using 3/0 rather than 4/0 Prolene.

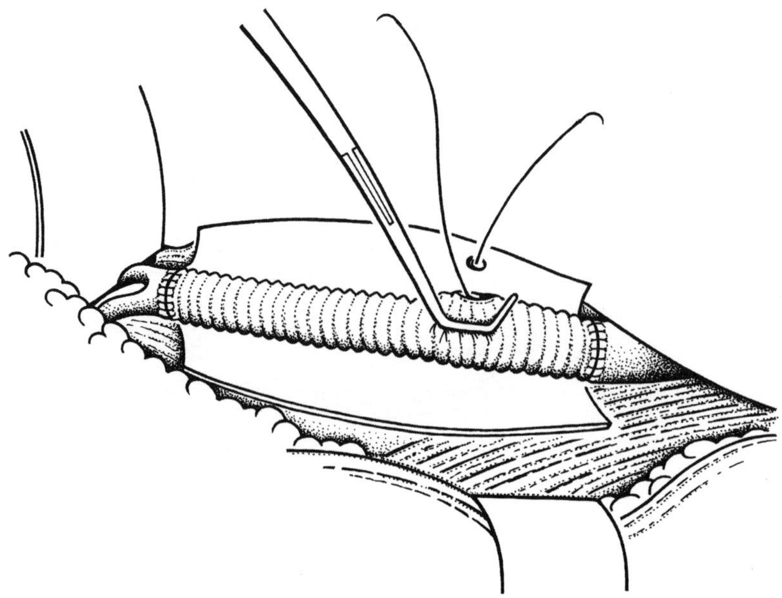

6

Closure

Having carefully ensured that there is no bleeding from the lumen of the aneurysm or from any of the anastomoses, the aneurysm sac should be trimmed and closed firmly around the Dacron graft down to the aortic bifurcation using 3/0 Prolene. The aim is to achieve secure closure with a snug fit around the visceral vessels wherever possible. The left retroperitoneal space should then be washed with warm saline and carefully inspected for blood streaming into the saline as a sign of bleeding. Packing the upper retroperitoneal space early in the procedure with a large and hot abdominal swab usually secures excellent haemostasis. An appropriate vacuum drain can be placed through the left iliac fossa extending up to just below the diaphragm and behind the spleen. Mass closure of the muscles are performed using No 1 Prolene or nylon, taking large bites less than one centimetre apart. Cosmetic closure of the skin is achieved using subcutaneous Prolene.

Postoperative care and complications

Anaesthesia may usually be reversed immediately following surgery as pain is well controlled by epidural analgesia. Postoperative ventilation is rarely required as pulmonary complications are infrequent. A positive fluid balance is beneficial presumably due to retroperitoneal and visceral oedema. Preoperative optimization on the Intensive Treatment Unit or High Dependency Unit assists by identifying the filling pressures necessary to achieve optimal cardiac function. These filling pressures are initially achieved by reinfusing blood taken during acute normovolaemic haemodilution and then maintained with clear fluids. Homologous blood transfusion should rarely be needed but should be given if the haemoglobin falls below 80g/litre during surgery or 90g/litre postoperatively following the re-infusion of all available autologous blood.

As paralytic ileus is unusual following an extraperitoneal approach, the nasogastric tube may usually be removed the next morning. With good epidural analgesia, most patients can be mobilized from the first postoperative day when the drain can also be removed. Patients undergoing an extraperitoneal approach, even to the suprarenal aorta, are usually ready to go home by the sixth to seventh postoperative day.

Acknowledgement

Illustrations by R Keith Harrison.

References

Cambria RP, Brewster DC, Abbott WM *et al.* (1990). Transperitoneal versus retroperitoneal approach for aortic reconstruction: A randomised prospective study. *J Vasc Surg* **11**: 314–325.

Darling RC, Shah DM, McClellan WR *et al.* (1992). Decreased morbidity associated with retroperitoneal exclusion treatment for abdominal aortic aneurysm. *J Cardiovasc Surg* **33**: 65–69.

Dubost C, Allary M, Oeconemos N (1952). Resection of an aneurysm of the abdominal aorta. *Arch Surg* **64**: 405–408.

Nevelsteen A, Smet G, Weymans M *et al.* (1989). Transabdominal or retroperitoneal approach to the aorto-iliac tract: A pulmonary function study. *Eur J Vasc Surg* **69**: 795–806.

Rob C (1963). Extraperitoneal approach to the abdominal aorta. *Surgery* **53**: 87–89.

Surgical techniques for visceral artery revascularization

William K Ehrenfeld, Douglas L Jicha, Ronald J Stoney

Introduction

Atherosclerotic visceral artery lesions may cause acute or chronic visceral ischaemia. The chronic form is also known as 'abdominal angina' (Dunphy, 1936; Mikkelsen, 1957). Acute occlusion of one or more visceral arteries due to thrombosis of an atherosclerotic artery or embolus from a proximal source may lead to bowel infarction. Bowel infarction is a surgical emergency requiring immediate removal of the affected bowel and possibly the offending clot or the atherosclerotic lesion. This is rarely technically feasible. Chronic mesenteric insufficiency with abdominal angina is a relatively rare condition. Extensive collateral vessels readily develop between the visceral aortic branches – coeliac axis, superior mesenteric artery, inferior mesenteric artery – and the hypogastric (internal iliac) arteries. These collateral pathways may be so efficient that very rarely gradual occlusion of all major aortic branches may actually occur without bowel infarction. Usually, involvement of two or more visceral branches cause symptoms. The main collateral circuits are: 1) the gastroduodenal and pancreaticoduodenal arteries between the coeliac axis and the superior mesenteric artery; 2) the middle and left colic arteries between the superior mesenteric artery and the inferior mesenteric artery ('meandering mesenteric artery', the arc of Riolan); and finally 3) the sigmoid and haemorrhoidal vessels between the inferior mesenteric artery and the internal iliac arteries. Although at least two of the three major visceral arteries are severely narrowed or occluded in 85% of patients with abdominal angina, the symptoms are related more to the inadequacy of the collateral blood flow than to the actual number of obstructed primary arteries (Wylie *et al.*, 1980). Occlusion of the coeliac axis along with poor collateralization may occasionally cause bowel or organ ischaemia. Chronic occlusion of either the superior mesenteric artery or inferior mesenteric artery only does not usually cause ischaemia.

The syndrome most typical of chronic intestinal ischaemia afflicts women between the ages of 50 and 70 years and includes: 1) epigastric postprandial cramping pain; 2) weight loss due to pain and/or fear of eating; 3) bowel motility disturbances (nausea, vomiting, diarrhoea and/or constipation) caused by bowel ischaemia. Malabsorption is seldom present, and there are no specific diagnostic laboratory tests. Evidence of atherosclerotic disease in other peripheral arteries is found in approximately 33% of the affected patients and an epigastric bruit is heard in 70%. The definitive diagnosis depends upon abdominal arteriography using both the anteroposterior projection, which best delineates collateral formation, and lateral or oblique projections, which best illustrate the degree of vessel obstruction. The stenotic lesions are usually seen at or near the vessel origins.

Unusual causes of visceral artery stenosis are fibromuscular dysplasia and median arcuate ligament compression of the coeliac axis and occasionally includes the superior mesenteric artery. Cases of compression of these vessels by the coeliac ganglionic nerve fibres have been reported. These cases are often atypical and are the subject of continuing surgical controversy.

During the past 25 years numerous methods for visceral artery revascularization have been evaluated including retrograde synthetic or autogenous grafts, transvisceral artery thromboendarterectomy and reimplantation. Two basic procedures are now preferred: transaortic thromboendarterectomy and antegrade synthetic graft bypass grafting.

Operative indications and preoperative preparations

Revascularization is indicated in patients with characteristic symptoms and significant stenosis of one or more visceral branches as seen by arteriography. The objectives are to relieve pain and prevent bowel infarction. Prophylactic visceral revascularization may also be indicated in coexisting aortoiliac and aortorenal vascular procedures (Stoney *et al.*, 1977). Intra-abdominal disease of non-vascular origin must be thoroughly excluded before operation. Intravenous hyperalimentation may be required in the catabolic patient with profound weight loss to restore an anabolic state. When prosthetic grafts are used, antibiotics are given intraoperatively and during the next 48 hours.

Antegrade prosthetic grafting

Atherosclerotic visceral artery lesions, in conjunction with lesions in the renal arteries, may be part of an unusually extensive atherosclerotic process of the abdominal aortic wall, which can make grafting at this level technically difficult. Antegrade prosthetic visceral bypass reconstructions may be desirable as the grafts will originate from the usually undiseased distal thoracic aorta. Antegrade graft placement is haemodynamically superior to retrograde placement which may predispose to early graft thrombosis. The antegrade route is shorter and usually requires shorter grafts. Retrograde bypass is particularly awkward for revascularization of the superior mesenteric artery since this artery arises from the aorta at an acute angle and is quite mobile, predisposing to kink and occlusion. Arterial autografts are ideal for revascularization procedures involving the renal arteries (Ehrenfeld *et al.*, 1982). However, in visceral artery revascularization, synthetic grafts are preferred since the most common autografts, the hypogastric (internal iliac) arteries, constitute part of the visceral collateral system. The hypogastric artery autograft is generally too short for antegrade revascularization of the superior mesenteric artery. Venous autografts are not used, since it is thought that they frequently cause dilatation, stenosis and late occlusion (Stanley *et al.*, 1973). Flanged knitted Dacron prostheses (5 or 6 mm) are preferred for single vessel bypass, and bifurcated grafts (10 × 5 mm or 12 × 6 mm) are used when both the coeliac axis and the superior mesenteric artery are revascularized. Visceral erosion by these grafts has not occurred in our series. Revascularization of both the coeliac axis and the superior mesenteric artery is preferred when indicated and feasible, since they supply 90% of splanchnic blood flow. This procedure is commonly used in patients with operative risk factors that preclude thoracoabdominal exposure. Despite temporary aortic occlusion of 20–30 min, the results with this procedure are excellent, with a long-term graft patency and durable relief of abdominal angina in over 90% of patients.

Operative technique

An upper midline incision extending from the xiphoid to the umbilicus is used. The coeliac artery and the supracoeliac aorta are reached by first dividing the gastrohepatic ligament. After division of the triangular ligament, the left lobe of the liver is retracted to the right and the oesophagus and the stomach to the left in order to expose the posterior fibres of the diaphragm.

1a–d

Illustration **1a** shows the anterior approach to the coeliac artery and supracoeliac aorta. The inset depicts a typical coeliac atherosclerotic lesion with contiguous aortic involvement. Isolated coeliac disease is a more common cause of symptoms than isolated superior mesenteric artery disease. The arcuate ligament and diaphragmatic crura are divided in the midline to expose the distal thoracic aorta (**1b**). The coeliac ganglionic fibres are dissected and resected from around the artery. The aorta is temporarily occluded at a level 5 cm proximal to the coeliac axis origin and also distal to the origin of the coeliac axis, after intravenous administration of 2000–4000 international units of heparin. An elliptical disc of the aortic wall is cut out from the anterior surface of the aorta (**1c**). A 6-mm flanged Dacron graft (made from 12 × 6 mm bifurcation graft) is anastomosed to the aortotomy site with a running 4/0 synthetic suture. Thereafter, the aortic clamps are released and a vascular clamp is applied on the proximal portion of the graft. The graft is then anastomosed end-to-end to the undiseased distal artery (**1d**).

2a–c

If bypass to both the coeliac and the superior mesenteric artery is planned, the superior mesenteric artery is also exposed by further dissection and resection of the cocliac nerve fibres overlying the aorta. This manoeuvre frees the body of the pancreas which can then be elevated from the aorta with ease and retracted caudally, thus exposing the first 4–5 cm of the superior mesenteric artery. An elliptical aortotomy is made on the right anterolateral aspect of the aorta (**2a**). With this technique, the two graft limbs will line up parallel to the coeliac axis and the superior mesenteric artery, respectively, without kinking and buckling of the graft. A flanged tubular bifurcation graft (12 × 6 mm) is anastomosed between aortic clamps to the aorta using a 4/0 suture. The body of the graft is then clamped and aortic flow is restored. Thereafter the coeliac axis is clamped, transected and the proximal end is oversewn. An end-to-end anastomosis is performed between the graft limb and the distal, nondiseased coeliac artery using either interrupted or running 5/0 sutures. The clamp is then shifted to the right superior mesenteric artery limb and the same procedure is used for the superior mesenteric artery (**2b**). The right (superior mesenteric artery) limb of the bifurcated graft lies behind the pancreas to parallel the course of the superior mesenteric artery (**2c**). The full length of the retropancreatic course of the superior mesenteric artery limb is visualized in (**2c**) by the artist's cutaway of a section of pancreas. The adequacy of the reconstruction may be assessed by electromagnetic flow probe measurement. Alternatively, intraoperative ultrasound B-mode imaging with Doppler flow velocity measurement can be

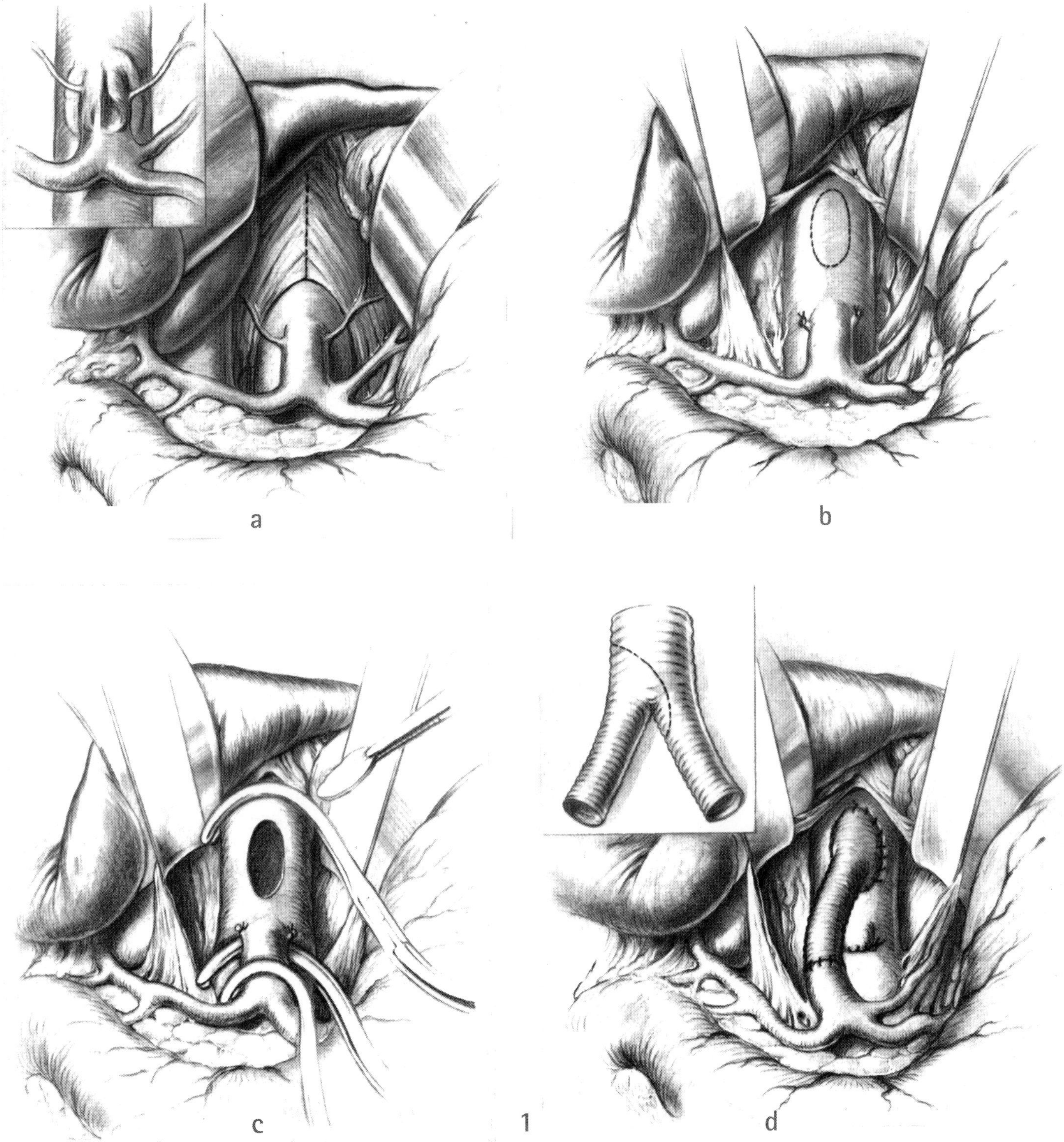

a b c d

1

used. Postoperative arteriography is also performed to verify the operative result.

Transaortic endarterectomy

The atherosclerotic lesion in the coeliac axis is invariably limited to the very proximal portion of this short artery. Even when this vessel is occluded by atherosclerosis, the distal half of the artery maintains its patency as a result of collateral flow through its three terminal branches. Superior mesenteric artery occlusion is generally more extended. When the orifice is occluded the clot usually progresses to the first major distal branch, 5–8 cm from the origin. The short lesion in coeliac stenosis or occlusion is easily removed by a simple transaortic endarterectomy. The longer lesion in superior mesenteric artery

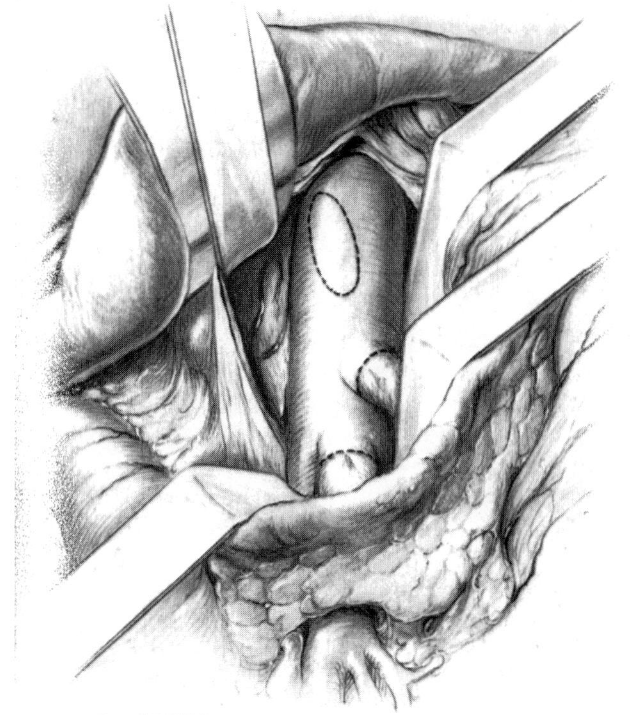

a

2

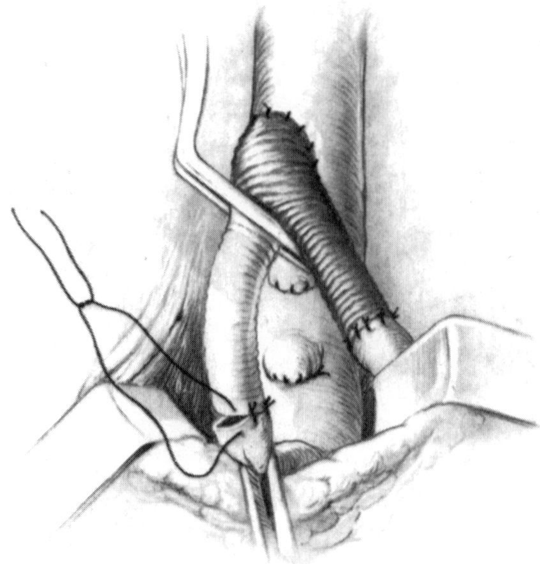

b

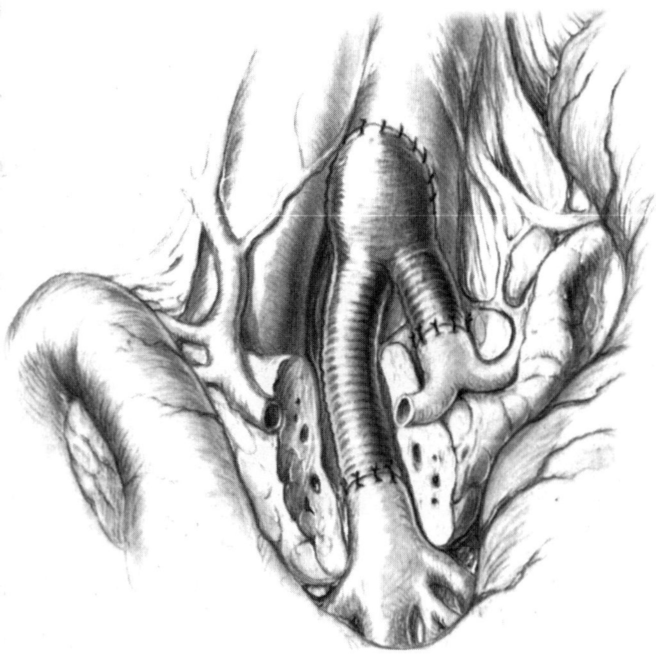

c

occlusion may require an additional angioplasty. Transarterial endarterectomy through the diseased vessel only is no longer used because of the difficulty in removing the aortic intimal lesion surrounding the visceral artery orifice. The ventral course of the visceral arteries and the position of the superior mesenteric artery under the pancreas make access for endarterectomy of these arteries extremely difficult with the conventional transperitoneal approach. It is technically feasible, but exposure is not optimal. This problem has been solved by the use of the thoracoabdominal retroperitoneal approach which provides complete exposure of the aorta and its visceral and renal branches from the distal thoracic aorta to the aortic bifurcation (Stoney *et al.*, 1977). This approach is particularly advantageous in the presence of coexistent distal aortic or aortorenal atherosclerotic disease requiring additional surgical repair. Recently, we have used a new exposure that eliminates the need for thoracotomy by performing left median visceral rotation.

Operative technique

With the patient in the supine position, a midline incision is made extending from above the xiphoid to the pubis. Using a self-retaining retractor (Omni-Tract, Minnesota Scientific Co., Minnesota) to obtain 'handless exposure', the small intestine is placed in a 'bowel bag' to the right. Mobilization of the descending colon is begun laterally and the plane is developed cephalad with incision of the splenorenal ligament. Combined blunt and sharp dissection are then employed to rotate the spleen, pancreas and left colon to the right. The left kidney, adrenal gland, ureter and gonadal vein are left in place. The left renal vein is fully mobilized to the inferior vena cava allowing for retraction or, if necessary, division. Following division and reflection of the dense autonomic ganglia on the left anterior surface of the aorta, the left diaphragmatic crura is incised longitudinally. The aorta is then circumferentially mobilized together with the superior mesenteric artery, coeliac axis and renal arteries when necessary (Sauer and Stoney, 1989).

3a, b, c

After application of proximal and distal aortic clamps as well as individual clamps on the visceral and renal arteries, excellent exposure of the coeliac and the superior mesenteric artery orifices is provided by a 'trap door' aortotomy in the anterolateral aortic wall. The dissected renal vein is retracted caudally.

If the aortic atheroma is confined to the anterior aorta, the endarterectomy is limited to the undersurface of the 'trap door' as shown here. When advanced atheromatous disease involves the whole circumference of the aorta, a sleeve endarterectomy is performed. The aortic intima is transected to the cleavage plane in the outer media and the aortic endarterectomy is carried out.

3d, e, f

Removal of the intimal lesions of the visceral artery orifices are then performed individually. Gentle traction is applied to the freed aortic intimal core while the media of the visceral artery is pushed away by a blunt dissection instrument (**3d**). In the coeliac axis, the short intimal core separates easily at the end-point under direct vision. Similarly, when the superior mesenteric artery orifice is not occluded, the atheroma is separated and the end-point is visualized using the extraction endarterectomy technique. If the lesion occludes the superior mesenteric artery, organized thrombus propagates to the first re-entry collateral (usually the left colic branch). The separation or end-point may not be visible from the aortic orifice. The aortotomy is closed and aortic blood flow is restored prior to clamping the superior mesenteric artery

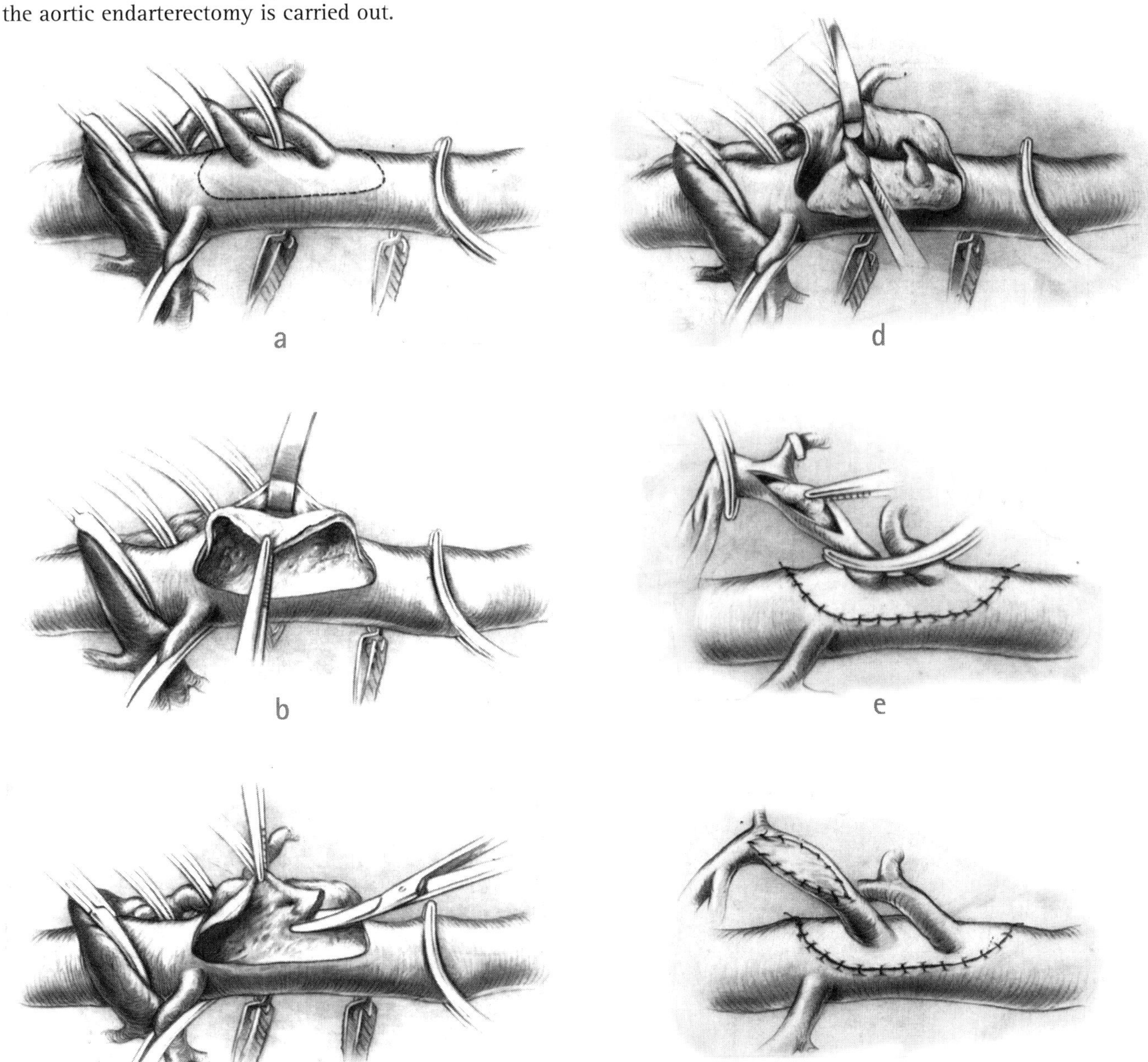

3

at its origin. A longitudinal superior mesenteric artery arteriotomy is made to a point beyond the occlusion. The specimen is removed, visualizing the smooth transition to normal intima (3e), and the arteriotomy is closed with a vein patch to prevent narrowing (3f). When indications for concomitant renal artery revascularization are present, the longitudinal aortotomy is extended to the infrarenal level to facilitate a contiguous transaortic bilateral renal endarterectomy.

As with the bypass grafting procedures, the adequacy of the endarterectomy is checked by electromagnetic flow probe measurement or ultrasound B-mode imaging with Doppler flow measurement. Intraoperative arteriography is rarely performed.

Transaortic visceral endarterectomy is suitable for most patients and can be extended for simultaneous correction of coexisting renal artery lesions or aortic atherosclerotic ('coral reef') lesions. Left medial visceral rotation allows excellent exposure of the entire abdominal aorta and its four major branches for the employment of this technique. Further, the transabdominal approach allows treatment of occlusive lesions causing acute visceral ischaemia and bowel infarction which require thrombectomy, visceral reconstruction and appropriate bowel resection. Synthetic grafts are usually avoided when gross contamination is present.

Postoperative care, complications and results

Intravenous infusion and nasogastric suction are maintained until the return of normal bowel movements. Prolonged supracoeliac occlusion of the aorta may cause acute tubular necrosis (rare), and urinary output should therefore be monitored and kept at a high level. Traumatic pancreatitis may occur from excessive manipulation of the pancreas during its dissection and retraction (rare). In over 250 cases requiring supracoeliac clamping other than for pararenal or thoracoabdominal aneurysmal disease, there have been no instances of paraplegia. Bowel infarction may occur due to graft occlusion or damage of pre-existing collaterals during the revascularization procedure, although this has not been experienced in this series.

Eighty-eight patients with primary chronic visceral ischaemia were treated at the University of California, San Francisco between 1959 and 1993. Follow-up is available for 97.3% of them. Treatment of primary chronic visceral ischaemia included transaortic endarterectomy in 51 patients and antegrade aortovisceral bypass in 26 patients. A durable relief of symptoms was obtained with both procedures and which was nearly identical at 1- and 5-year follow-up (Cunningham *et al.*, 1991). Recurrent symptoms of chronic visceral ischaemia developed in eight patients (10%). Five patients were cured after successful repeated revascularization. Antegrade visceral bypass and transaortic endarterectomies provide durable relief of chronic visceral ischaemia and protect patients from progression to acute visceral gangrene.

References

Cunningham CG, Rapp J, Reilly I *et al.* (1991). Chronic intestinal ischemia: Three decades of surgical progress. *Annl Surg* **214**: 276.

Dunphy J E (1936). Abdominal pain of vascular origin. *Am J Med Sci* **192**: 102.

Ehrenfeld WK, Stoney RJ, Wylie EJ (1982). Autogenous arterial grafts. In *Biologic and Synthetic Vascular Prostheses.* **Stanley JC** ed. New York: Grune and Stratton.

Mikkelson WP (1957). Intestinal angina: Its surgical significance. *Am J Surg* **94**: 262.

Rapp JH, Reilly LM, Qvarfordt PG *et al.* (1985). Durability of endarterectomy and antegrade grafts in the treatment of chronic visceral ischemia. *J Vasc Surg* **3**: 799.

Sauer L, Stoney, RJ (1989). Transabdominal exposure of the pararenal and suprarenal aorta by medial visceral rotation. *Semin Vasc Surg* **2**: 209.

Stanley JO, Ernst CB, Fry WJ (1973). Fate of 100 aortorenal vein grafts: Characteristics of late graft expansion, aneurysmal dilatation, and stenosis. *Surgery* **74**: 931.

Stoney RJ, Wylie EJ (1976). Surgery of the celiac and mesenteric arteries. In *Vascular Surgery: Principles and Techniques*, 2nd edn. **Haimovici H** ed. New York: McGraw-Hill.

Stoney RJ, Ehrenfeld WK, Wylie EJ (1977). Revascularization methods in chronic visceral ischemia caused by atherosclerosis. *Annl Surg* **186**: 468.

Wylie EJ, Stoney RJ, Ehrenfeld WK (1980). *Manual of Vascular Surgery*, Vol. 1. New York: Springer-Verlag.

Surgical techniques for renal artery revascularization

Douglas L Jicha,
William K Ehrenfeld, Ronald J Stoney

Introduction

Since Goldblatt *et al.* (1934) discovered the impact of renal artery stenosis on hypertension, extensive surgical experience with renal artery lesions has been acquired. Currently, renovascular hypertension is the most common indication for renal artery surgery, although prevention of renal failure and restoration of renal function have become increasingly important goals in recent years. This has been possible due to improved surgical and anaesthetic techniques, as well as precise intraoperative haemodynamic monitoring and perioperative critical care.

Occlusive lesions of the renal artery are predominantly due to atherosclerosis and fibromuscular dysplasia. A variety of historic operative techniques have been used for atherosclerotic lesions with varying results including nephrectomy, arterial reimplantation and transrenal artery thromboendarterectomy with and without patching. We have evaluated and subsequently abandoned these methods because of disappointing early and late failure rates, and currently employ transaortic endarterectomy and aortorenal bypass exclusively to treat hypertension and renal dysfunction due to renovascular disease. Fibromuscular dysplastic renal artery disease involves the middle and distal thirds of the renal artery and causes renovascular hypertension most commonly in young female patients. The use of *in situ* and *ex vivo* aortorenal bypass, depending on the extent of distal involvement, has proven effective and durable. This chapter will describe the common lesions and our preferred methods of revascularization.

1a, b, c, d, e

Following administration of intravenous heparin and mannitol which ensure anticoagulation and a diuresis, the aorta is occluded proximal to the superior mesenteric artery and distal to the renal arteries. Proximal clamping below the superior mesenteric artery is possible in cases where the inferior border of the superior mesenteric artery is greater than 2 cm cephalad to the renal ostia. Individual clamps are used to control back bleeding from the renal arteries, the superior mesenteric artery and the pararenal lumbar arteries. A longitudinal aortotomy of approximately 6–8 cm in length is created on the anterior surface of the aorta and extended proximally, between the renal arteries, and then is curved to the left of the superior mesenteric artery (**1a**).

The endarterectomy is fashioned to remove a sleeve of the pararenal aorta with bilateral opposed or multiple orificial lesions extending into the proximal renal arteries. The endarterectomy is begun in the aortic component of the plaque and follows a plane in the outer portion of the media of the diseased artery. After the aortic atherosclerotic core is freed, the distal end is transected at a point of minimal intimal thickening. When the cylinder of the entire aortic intima is separated just below the superior mesenteric artery, the proximal intimal sleeve is transected. The entire aortic plaque has been dissected before the renal orifice lesions are separated (**1b**).

Removal of the renal artery orifice disease is performed individually. Gentle traction is applied to the freed aortic intimal core while the media of the renal artery is pushed away with a Halle dissector (**1c**). This manoeuvre facilitates prolapse of the renal artery into the aortic lumen. The intimal core separates at the well-defined atherosclerotic end-point under direct vision (**1d**). The battery powered Auto Sector (Omni-Tract Surgical) (**1e**) facilitates these manoeuvres and is preferred since it shortens the endarterectomy and the renal ischaemia. After removal of any residual intimal fragments, the renal arteries are back bled, irrigated with 4 degrees C Ringer's lactate and the aortotomy is closed with a continuous 4–0 suture.

Failure to complete the removal of atheroma by transaortic endarterectomy occurs in less than 1% of patients. If an end-point problem is suspected, following restoration of aortic flow, the renal artery is clamped proximally and distally. The residual atheroma is removed through a transverse arteriotomy under direct

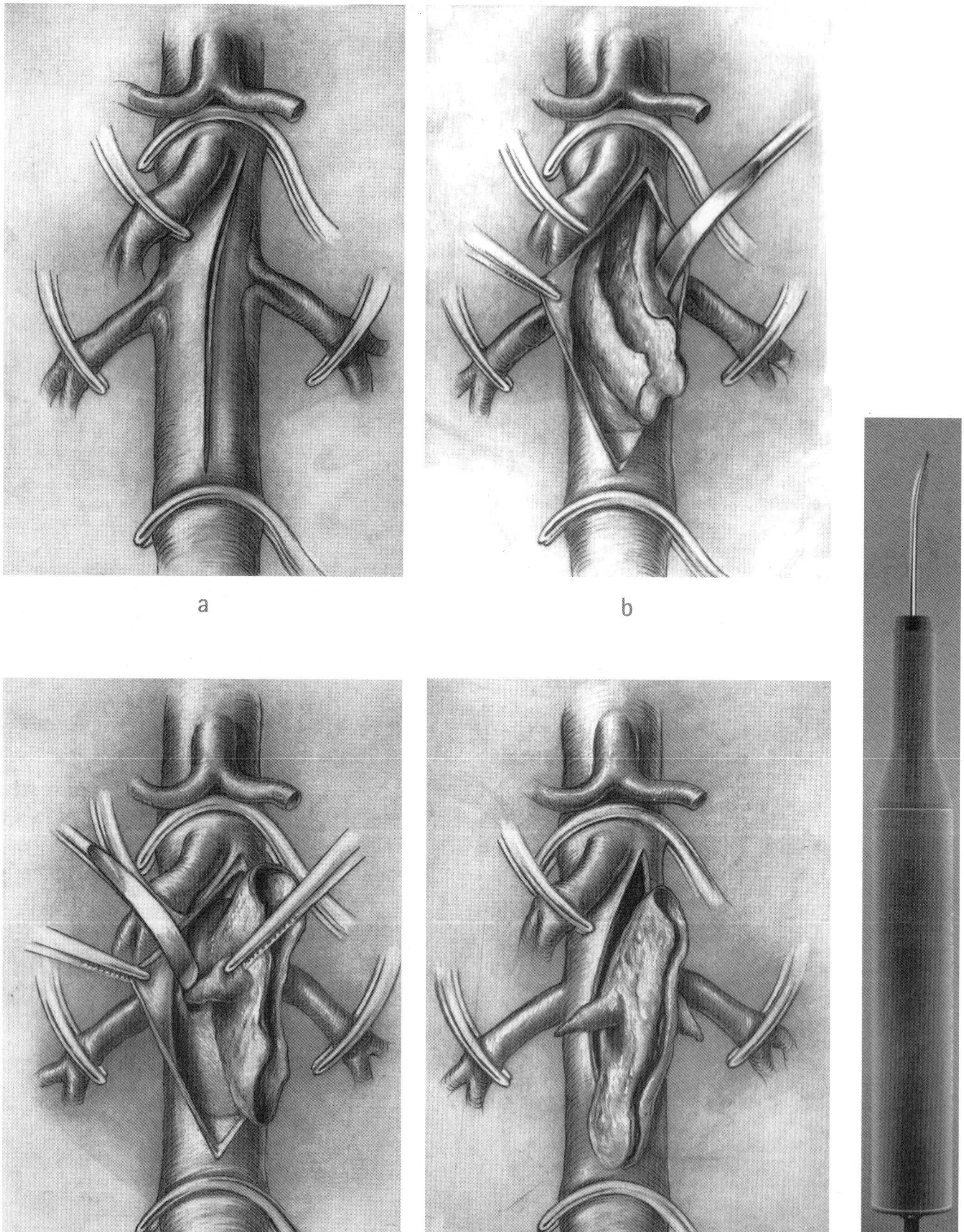

1

vision and a stable end-point is verified. The arteriotomy is closed with interrupted sutures to prevent narrowing.

With experience, renal ischaemia time rarely exceeds 20–30 min. In kidneys with renal dysfunction (creatinine 2.0 or greater), warm ischaemia tolerance is reduced when compared with normally functioning kidneys. To minimize ischaemic damage, we instill 4 degrees C Ringer's lactate solution periodically into the renal arteries during the ischaemic period to produce renal cooling.

Intraoperative evaluation of the results of transaortic endarterectomy is best performed with Doppler ultrasound (B-mode imaging with Doppler flow velocity measurements). This allows visual and haemodynamic confirmation of a satisfactory technical result prior to wound closure.

Pararenal atherosclerotic disease

Transaortic renal endarterectomy

Atherosclerotic renal artery stenosis or occlusion typically involves the pararenal aorta and renal ostia, producing variable degrees of aortic and renal artery narrowing. Typically, disease extends 1–2 cm into the renal artery and has a well-demarcated, palpable end-point. The typical location of the pararenal atherosclerotic lesions makes aortorenal bypass potentially a less suitable option because:

1. A calcified atherosclerotic aorta poses technical problems at the proximal graft anastomosis.
2. Progressive aortic atherosclerosis predisposes the proximal graft anastomosis to late stenosis or occlusion.
3. Approximately 60% of patients require a second graft to relieve bilateral renal ischaemia.

Transaortic endarterectomy is particularly suitable for repair of pararenal atherosclerosis since the aortic component is completely removed with the orificial extension through the open aorta (Wylie, 1975).

Operative technique

A midline incision is made from the xyphoid to the pubis and the pararenal aorta is exposed using an infracolic posterior peritoneal approach. Using a self-retaining retractor (Omni-Tact, Minnesota Scientific Co., Minnesota) to obtain 'handless exposure', the pararenal aorta and renal arteries are exposed and circumferentially mobilized.

Combined aortorenal atherosclerosis

When transaortic endarterectomy is combined with aortic grafting, as described above, we use the transected aorta for endarterectomy to avoid intersection of suture lines of a longitudinal aortotomy and the end-to-end graft anastomosis. This allows complete revascularization of bilateral single or multiple renal arteries, and aortic continuity is established with prosthetic graft anastomosed to the infrarenal aortic cuff. It can be performed with renal ischaemic times that are comparable with the longitudinal aortotomy approach (Stoney *et al.*, 1989).

Operative technique

Exposure of the pararenal aorta is obtained via a midline incision in the same manner as described with transaortic renal endarterectomy. After identical mobilization of the pararenal aorta, the renal arteries and the superior mesenteric artery, all branches are controlled to allow concurrent disease to be repaired. A self-retaining retractor (Omni-Tract) facilitates this exposure.

2a, b, c

After complete mobilization, heparin is administered and the aorta and its branches are controlled as described. Transaortic endarterectomy is facilitated by elevating the pararenal aorta to allow inspection of the lumen directly (2a). The dissection plane is established between the aortic atheroma and the outer media (2b). This plane is developed circumferentially (2c). Longitudinal division of the plaque is sometimes helpful. This allows each renal endarterectomy to proceed without the contralateral renal atheroma tethering the specimen in the aortic lumen.

2d, e

The endarterectomy plane is extended cephalad by traction on the mobilized atheromata through the end of the aorta. Further traction on the aortic specimen and the renal artery clamp facilitates prolapse of the renal artery. A well defined end-point is obtained with continued traction and gentle pushing of the residual artery away from the lesion (2d). After both renal endarterectomies are completed, the plaque is transected at a level just distal to the superior mesenteric artery orifice and the specimen is removed (2e).

The renal arteries are irrigated with heparinized saline and the aortic graft is then attached end-to-end to the aortic stump using continuous braided Dacron suture. Renal perfusion is restored by repositioning the proximal clamp on the graft prior to distal anastomosis to minimize renal ischaemia. Intraoperative duplex scanning is used to assess the technical adequacy of the renal endarterectomy.

Pararenal aneurysmal disease

Repair of these lesions may be complicated by difficult exposure and associated atherosclerosis that impairs renal blood flow causing hypertension and renal impairment. While simultaneous correction of these coexisting lesions can be formidable, acceptable morbidity and

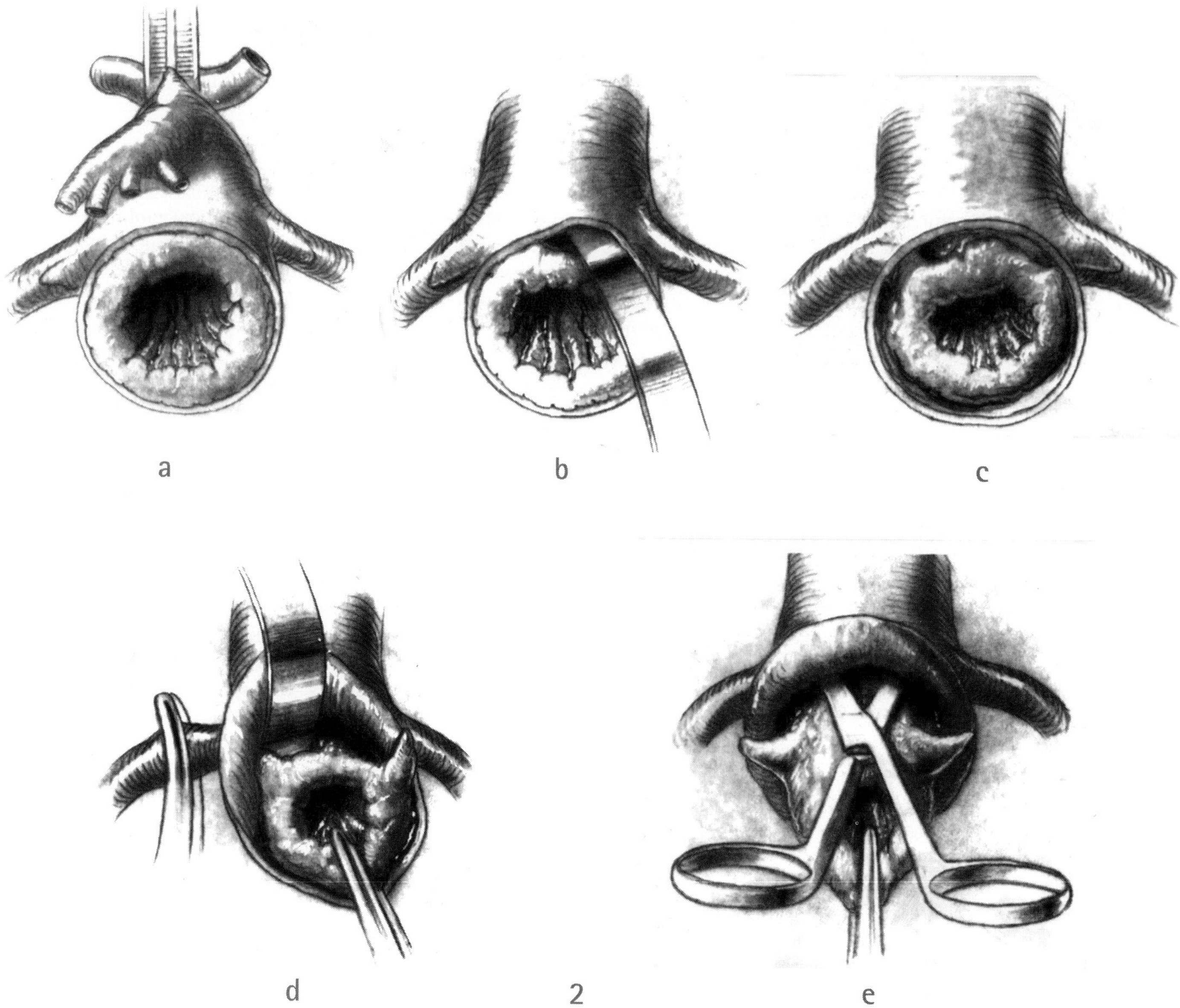

2

mortality and a durable result can be obtained with careful attention to the pattern of disease requiring operation, the technical details of the revascularization method and the perioperative care of these patients who frequently have serious comorbid disease. The surgical objective of all aortic aneurysm disease is inclusion grafting which relieves the threat of rupture. In addition, renal revascularization is accomplished by bypass or reimplantation of the renal artery to preserve or improve renal perfusion.

Operative technique

A full-length midline incision (xyphoid to pubis) is used to expose the aorta. While an infracolic posterior peritoneal approach may suffice, medial visceral rotation is often advantageous and requires mobilization of the descending colon beginning laterally. This plane is developed cephalad with incision of the splenorenal ligament. Combined blunt and sharp dissection are then employed to rotate the spleen, pancreas and left colon to the right. The left kidney, adrenal gland, ureter and gonadal vein are left in place. The left renal vein is mobilized to the inferior vena cava for retraction or, if necessary, division. Following division and reflection of the dense autonomic ganglia on the left anterior surface of the aorta, the left diaphragmatic crura is incised longitudinally. The aorta is then circumferentially mobilized. The pararenal aorta and as much of the superior mesenteric artery and coeliac axis are exposed and circumferentially mobilized as necessary (Sauer and Stoney, 1989).

3a, b

Several configurations of pararenal aortic aneurysmal disease exist. When pararenal aneurysmal disease

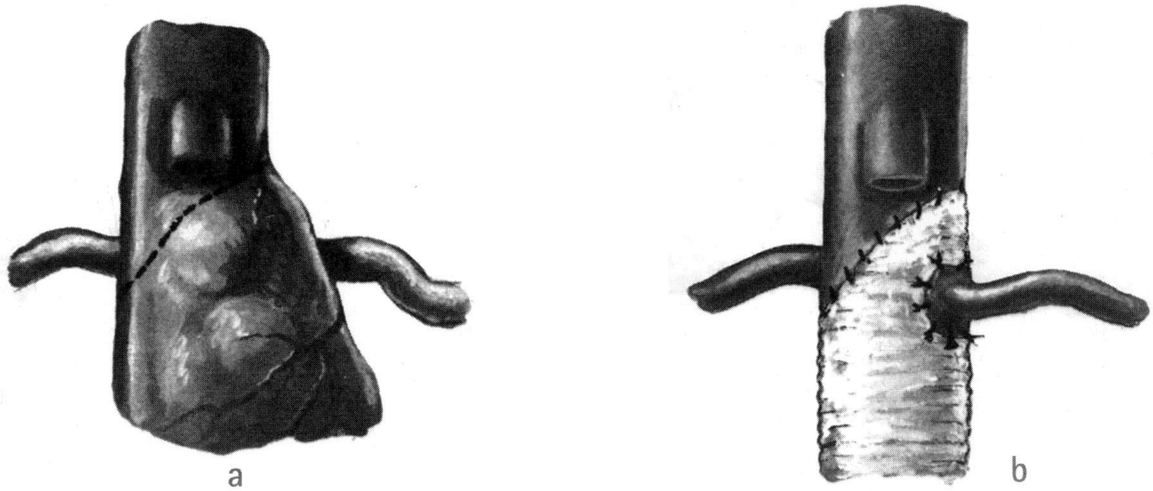

3

extends cephalad to a level beyond only one orifice (**3a**), a bevelled aortic transection may be performed. A bevelled graft is then attached end-to-end to the pararenal aorta. Reimplantation of the left renal artery, on a Carrel patch, to the side of the graft is easily performed (**3b**). This technique allows access to the right renal artery orifice as well as the superior mesenteric artery for transaortic visceral endarterectomy if indicated.

3c, d

Pararenal aortic aneurysmal disease extending above both renal artery orifices can be further complicated by extension of aneurysmal disease into the orifice of the renal arteries (**3c**). In these cases, replacement with a 5- or 6-mm Dacron graft from the aortic graft to the renal artery beyond the diseased segment is preferable. End-to-end anastomosis between the renal artery and the prosthetic graft is preferred. Careful sizing of the graft is necessary to assure a gradual curve to the graft and avoid kinking (**3d**). Intraoperative duplex is used to ensure the accuracy of the procedure.

With more complex reconstructions, special concerns must be addressed in order to minimize renal ischaemia to reduce subsequent deterioration of renal function. In patients with impaired renal function or those requiring

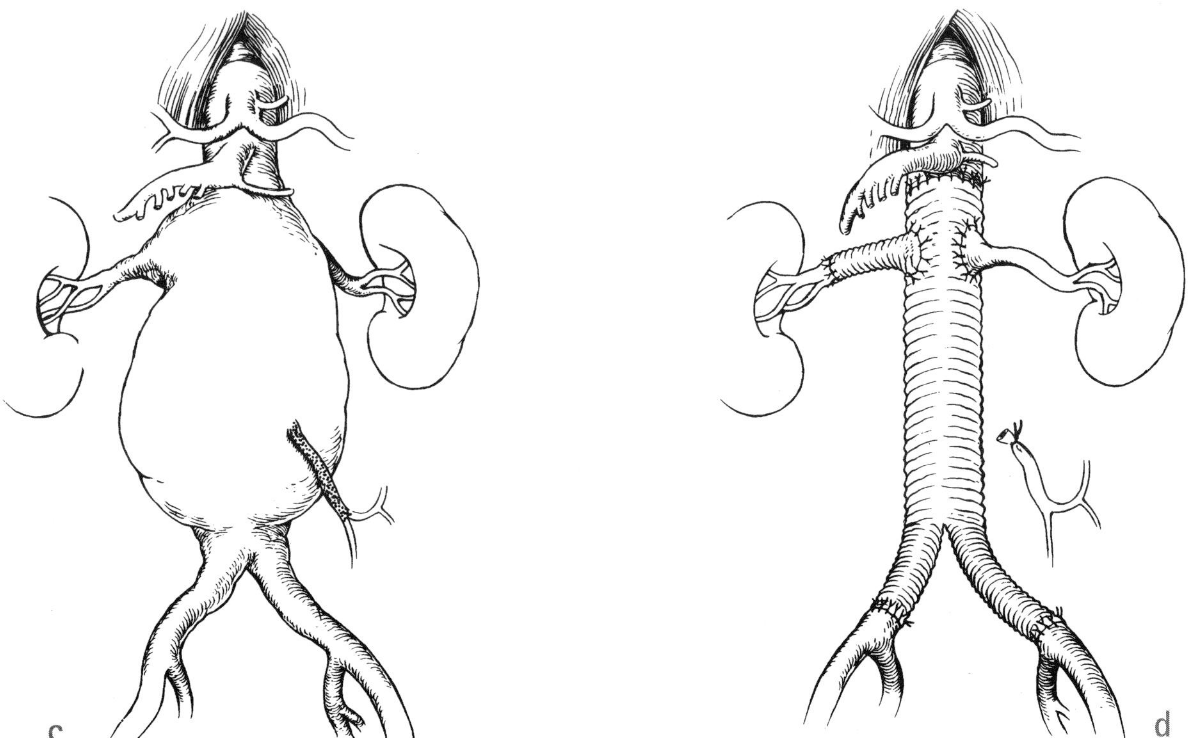

3

complex reconstructions necessitating longer ischaemic periods, renal hypothermia is maintained by placing a balloon catheter in the renal artery and infusing 4 degrees C Ringer's lactate solution. Mean renal ischaemia times with pararenal or suprarenal inclusion grafting are approximately 40 minutes, when two anastomoses are required.

Non-atherosclerotic renal artery revascularization

Non-atherosclerotic disease of the renal artery encompasses a variety of lesions including fibromuscular dysplasia, congenital bands, strictures, aneurysms and spontaneous or traumatic dissection of the renal artery. Fibromuscular dysplasia, a disease primarily of young women in otherwise good health, predominates. The distribution of these lesions is in the middle and distal third of the renal artery. Restoring normal renal perfusion and relieving or controlling hypertension are achieved using aortorenal grafting. The predominance of young patients demands durable surgical methods that allow patients to live a normal lifespan free of hypertension and the threat of a late failure of the revascularization method. We developed the concept of arterial autograft to replace diseased arterial segments and have used this preferentially for renal fibromuscular dysplasia since 1965 (Wylie, 1965).

All lesions which involve the main renal artery or the proximal renal artery branches can be repaired *in situ* using straight or bifurcated internal iliac autografts. Complex distal renal artery branch lesions or reoperative problems are performed *ex vivo* with hypothermic perfusion preservation and multibranched internal iliac autografts. These strategies achieve durable long-term results with cure of hypertension and renal salvage (Kent *et al.*, 1987). In a recent review of 71 patients at University of California, San Francisco with 1–19 year follow-up, branched internal iliac autografts allowed salvage of all but two of 78 kidneys with complex renal vascular disease. Further, hypertension was cured or improved in 97% of patients. *In situ* and *ex vivo* repair with iliac artery autograft provides a durable repair of complex distal non-atherosclerotic renal artery lesions.

Operative technique

Arterial autograft procurement

Arterial autografts are procured during the transabdominal exposure of the renal artery disease. *In situ* or *ex vivo* techniques are used depending on whether the repair is limited to the primary bifurcation branches (*in situ*) or is necessary in the more distal renal artery complex (*ex vivo*). The internal iliac artery is particularly suitable because its size closely approximates that of the renal artery in adults and children and its branches allow for branched reconstructions. Further, arterial autografts placed in children will grow with the patient. Finally, removal of the internal iliac artery does not require donor site repair because of abundant pelvic collateral circulation.

4a

The donor artery is exposed by an incision of the posterior peritoneum overlying the common iliac bifurcation. The entire internal iliac artery with the requisite number of branches is circumferentially mobilized, excised and stored temporarily in heparinized saline solution (**4a**). A larger diameter arterial autograft may be obtained from the common iliac and its two bifurcation branches. Dacron reconstruction of the donor site is required to preserve blood flow to the extremity.

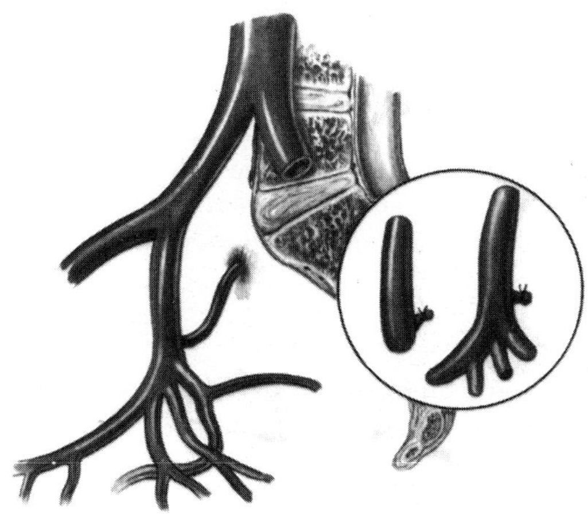

4a

4b, c, d, e

In situ *repair*

A full length midline or transverse incision allows the initial harvest of the autograft vessel from the pelvis. A self-retaining retractor (Omni-Tract) assists in exposure of the juxtarenal aorta and the renal artery with its hilar branching via the posterior infracolic approach. Mobilization of the inferior vena cava with lumbar vein ligation facilitates retrocaval autograft tunnelling for right side graft placement (**4b**). After heparin anticoagulation, the infrarenal aorta is segmentally occluded.

With rotation of the clamps to further expose the lateral aorta, a disc of aorta is excised with an ostial punch on the posterolateral aorta and an end-to-side anastomosis is created using interrupted 5–0 sutures (**4c**). Clamps are then removed from the aorta and the autograft is clamped. The native renal artery is then clamped beyond

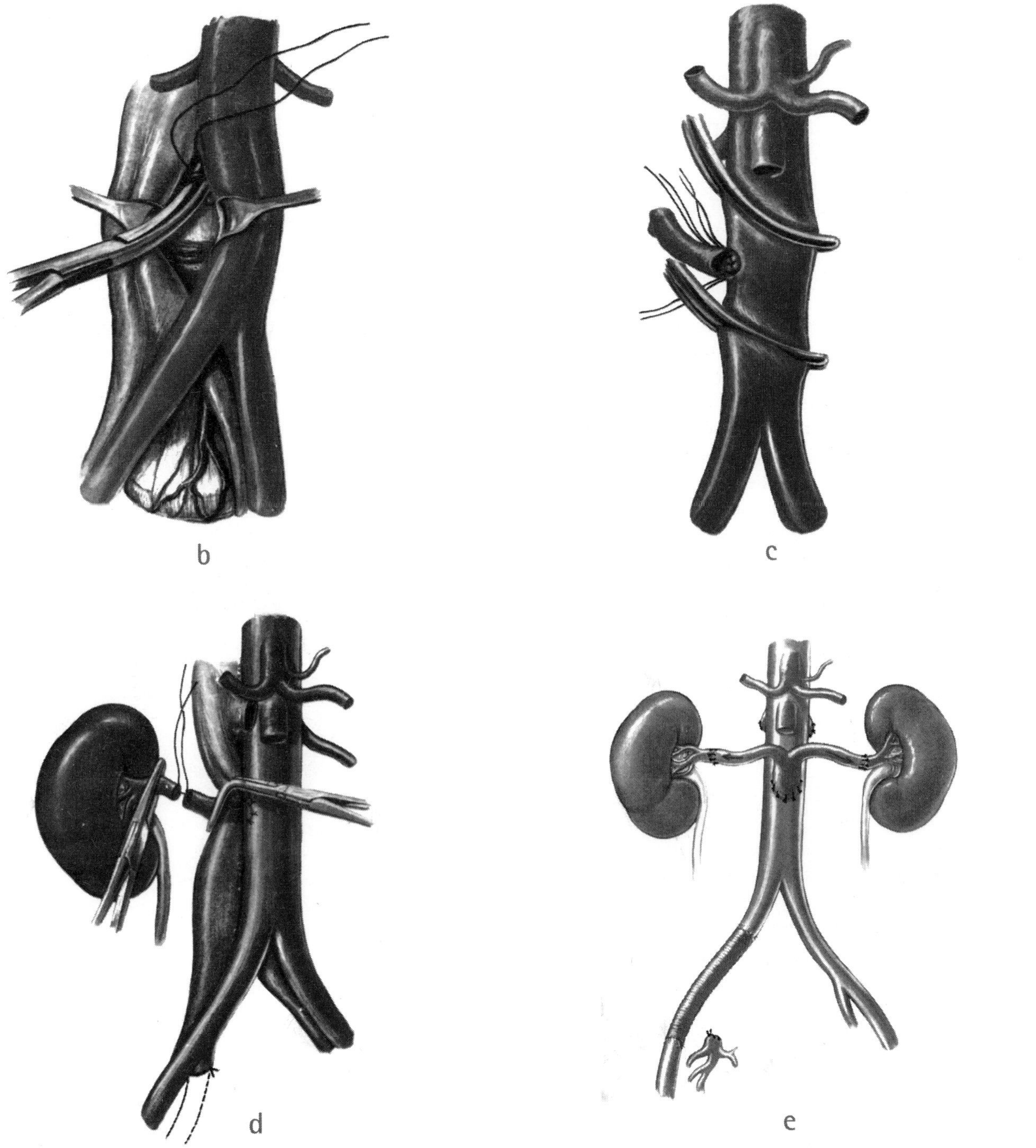

4

the disease and divided. Primary end-to-end anastomosis of the native renal artery to the autograft is performed with interrupted 6–0 sutures (**4d**). An unbranched autograft reconstruction is shown but, *in situ* procedures using the bifurcated iliac autograft are used when indicated. After perfusion is reestablished, the diseased native renal artery is excised for pathologic examination and the proximal renal artery is oversewn. Duplex scanning is used routinely to assess the technical adequacy of the repair.

Bilateral renal artery repair employing *in situ* techniques is also technically feasible either with single autograft or one bifurcated autograft as shown with common, internal and external iliac artery in (**4e**). The end-to-side common iliac artery to aortic anastomosis is generally positioned so that the longer external iliac artery is used to repair the right renal artery.

Ex vivo *repair*

Ex vivo repair is employed when renal artery disease is considered unreconstructable by *in situ* techniques. *Ex vivo* repair allows precise dissection because of improved exposure with continuous hypothermic perfusion providing optimal renal preservation. Technical problems or anastomotic leaks during the autograft reconstruction can easily be identified and repaired during perfusion rather than after reimplantation.

5a

A long midline or transverse abdominal incision is made and a self-retaining retractor (Omni-Tract) set up is used to approach the iliac donor site, the renal vasculature, the ureter and the kidney. Using right or left medial visceral rotation, the lateral peritoneal attachments of the colon, on the side of anticipated repair, are freed to expose the retroperitoneum and retract the viscera. Gerota's fascia is incised, the kidney mobilized and the renal vasculature is identified. The renal artery and vein are circumferentially mobilized to the aorta and the inferior vena cava. The ureter is mobilized, with its surrounding fat, to the pelvic brim. After mobilization, the proximal renal artery and the paracaval renal vein are divided. The kidney is elevated to the abdominal wall and flushed with 4 degrees C Ringer's lactate solution to clear the venous effluent. The renal artery is cannulated (**5a**) and the kidney is perfused at 60–75 mmHg to maintain a surface temperature of approximately 10 degrees C.

5b, c, d

During the perfusion, dissection proceeds to identify the diseased renal artery branches. Individual renal arteries are ligated and divided beyond the disease and end-to-end anastomosis of an iliac autograft branch is performed (**5b**). At each branch anastomosis is completed, perfusion is switched to the iliac artery autograft (**5c**), thereby minimizing the non perfused period to the segment of kidney supplied by the branch being repaired. Following reconstruction, the kidney is reimplanted by reanastomosing the renal vein (end-to-end) and attaching the end of the autograft to the side of the aorta (**5d**).

Sequential release of the renal vein and renal artery clamps results in prompt return of colour to the kidney and subsequent firmness of the kidney. Duplex scanning is employed intraoperatively to assess the repair prior to retroperitoneal and wound closure.

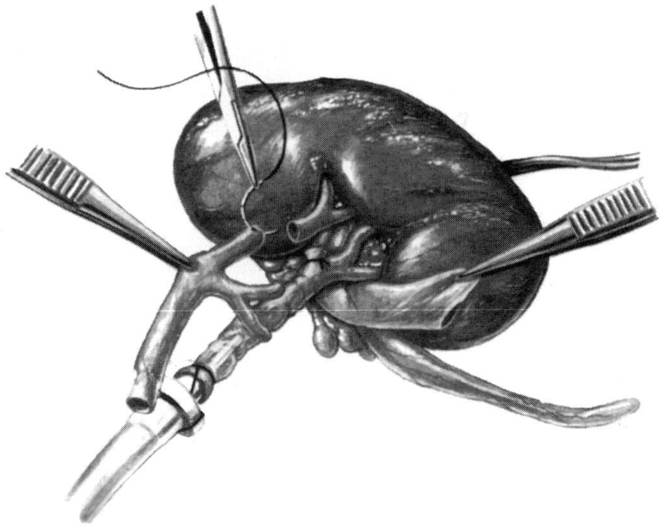

b

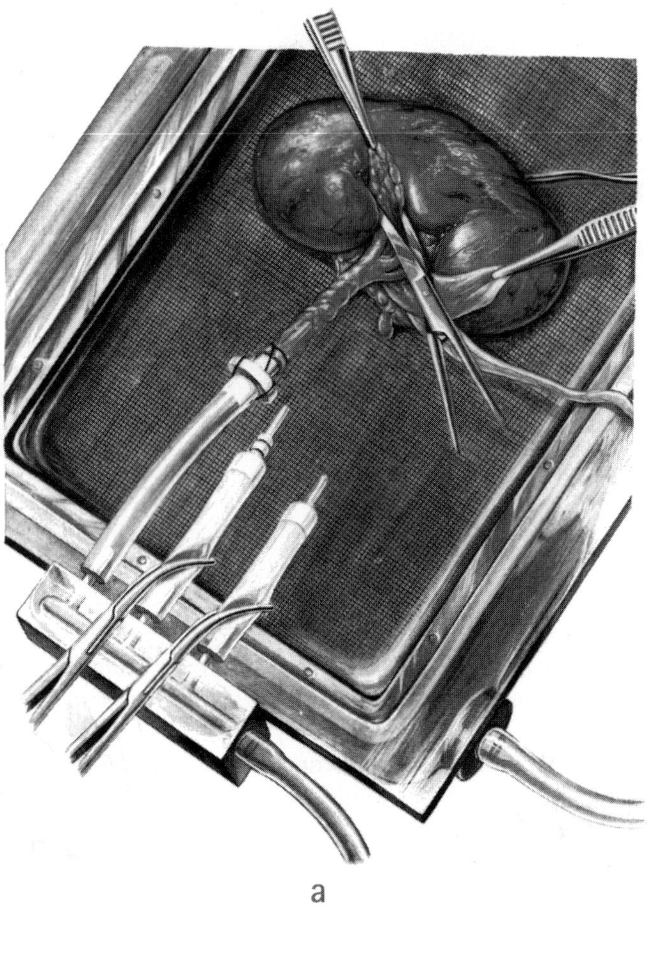

a

5

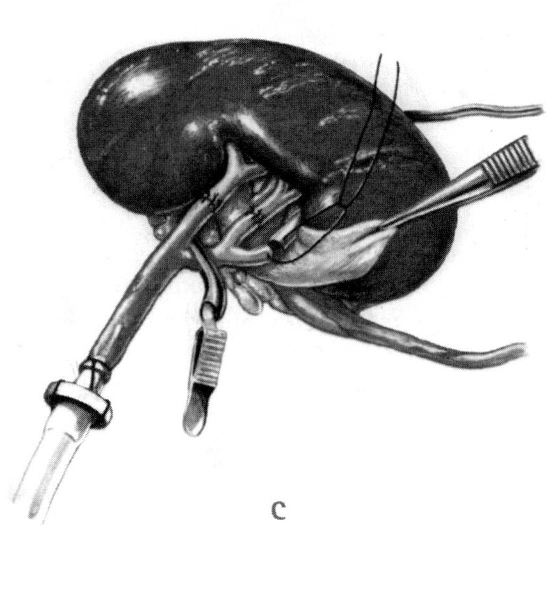

c

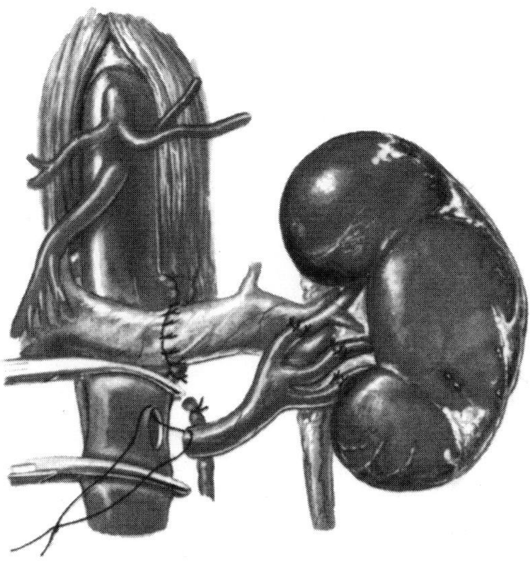

5d

Conclusion

The principal diseases of the renal vasculature are athero sclerosis and fibromuscular dysplasia. Their different patterns of distribution necessitate a variety of revascularization techniques to solve problems which they create in renal blood flow. This chapter has attempted to describe those pioneered and used at the University of California, San Francisco during the last four decades.

References

Goldblatt H, Lynch J, Hanzel RF *et al.* (1934). Studies on experimental hypertension. I. The production of persistent elevation of systolic blood pressure by means of renal ischemis. *J Exp Med* **59**: 347.

Kent KC, Salvatierra O, Reilly LM *et al.* (1987). Evolving strategies for the repair of complex renovascular lesions. *Ann Surg* **206**: 272.

Qvarfordt PG, Stoney RJ, Reilly LM *et al.* (1986). Management of pararenal aneurysms of the abdominal aorta. *J Vasc Surg* **3**: 84.

Sauer L, Stoney RJ (1989). Transabdominal exposure of the pararenal and suprarenal aorta by medial visceral rotation. *Semin Vasc Surg* **2**: 209.

Stoney RJ, Effeney DJ (1992). *Wylie's Atlas of Vascular Surgery. Thoracoabdominal Aorta and Its Branches.* Philadelphia: J B Lippincott Co.

Stoney RJ, Messina LM, Goldstone J, Reilly LM (1989). Renal endarterectomy through the transected aorta: A new technique for combined aortorenal atherosclerosis. A preliminary report. *J Vasc Surg* **9**: 224.

Wylie EJ (1965). Vascular replacement with arterial autografts. *Surgery* **57**: 14.

Wylie EJ (1975). Endarterectomy and autogenous arterial grafts in the surgical treatment of stenosing lesions of the renal artery. *Urol Clin North Am* **2**: 351.

Intervention for non-atherosclerotic renal artery stenosis

Jonathan G Moss, Richard D Edwards

Introduction

Ia, b, c

Non-atherosclerotic renal artery stenosis is far less prevalent than atherosclerotic renal artery stenosis. In some ways this is unfortunate as the technical and clinical results of endovascular intervention in this condition are far superior to those seen in atherosclerotic renal artery stenosis. Over a decade ago Tegtmeyer published 10-year cumulative patency rates of 87% following angioplasty for fibromuscular disease with cure rates for hypertension approaching 50% (1a–c). Although fibromuscular disease is the predominant non-atherosclerotic pathological process, other more esoteric entities such as Takayasu's arteritis, neurofibromatosis and middle aortic syndrome should be considered. The patient population also differs from the atherosclerotic group with children and young female adults predominantly affected. Hypertension is the presenting clinical scenario and impaired renal function is exceptional. Illustration 1 shows the situation in a 23-year-old female with hypertension. Focal right renal artery stenosis probably of the intimal variety is seen in (1a). Following a 5 mm percutaneous transluminal angioplasty (1b) there is an excellent morphological result. An angiogram at 6 months shows no evidence of restenosis (1c) and the patient remains off hypertensive medication 3 years later.

Fibromuscular dysplasia and its subgroups is a disease, which affects either the main renal artery (mid to distal) or its branches. Thirty-nine percent of main renal artery lesions extend into the first order branches and in 6% there is isolated branch vessel involvement. Aberrant arteries when present are frequently (44%) involved. Involvement of the renal artery ostium is almost unheard of and problems such as elastic recoil and dissection so commonly seen in atherosclerotic renal artery stenosis are rare. Particular and unique problems do exist, however, and include branch lesions, resistant stenoses, aneurysms and arterial spasm.

Recent advances in this area are few and focus on small platform devices permitting safer and more effective endovascular management.

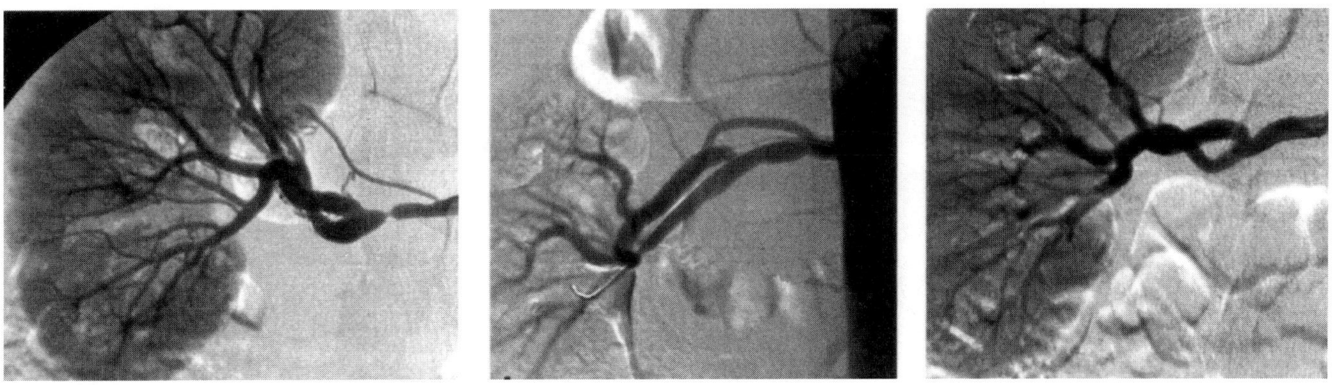

a b c

1

Non-branch lesions

These are relatively simple lesions to deal with. The normal access site is the femoral artery and having performed a flush abdominal aortogram the renal artery is selected using either a reverse curve catheter (our preference is the Sos Omni, Angiodynamics, USA) or a femorovisceral configuration. Before the stenosis is crossed 3000–5000 international units of heparin should be administered and once the renal artery has been catheterized a vasodilator is given through the catheter. The choice of vasodilator is not important, glycerol trinitrate is a reasonable choice and should be given in 150 μg aliquots up to a maximum of 500 μg. A calcium channel blocker such as verapamil 10–20 mg can be administered sublingually in addition but is not the author's, routine practice. Spasm is an issue in renal arteries and all attempts should be made to prevent it. The guidewire is the major culprit and manipulations should be gentle and minimal. The tip of the guidewire must be kept in the fluoroscopic field at all times to avoid injury to the small arterioles and prevent perforation. We prefer the TAD 11 wire (Boston Scientific, Boston, USA), which is a tapered wire with a 0.018 atraumatic tip but a relatively stiff 0.035 main shaft which provides ample support for the balloon. The wire can be pre-shaped if desired to tailor fit the anatomy. It is not unusual with the medial fibroplasia type of fibromuscular dysplasia to encounter multiple 'baffles' within the diseased section, which can impede passage of the guidewire. If difficulty is encountered crossing the lesion then a hydrophilic guidewire such as the Terumo (Terumo, Japan) is usually successful. It is best to exchange the hydrophilic wire for the TAD II once across the stenosis as it provides far more support and is less likely to become displaced during catheter exchanges. Having crossed the lesion an appropriate sized balloon is placed and inflated. The balloon should be no longer than 2 cm with a short tip and a short blunt taper to minimize trauma to the normal artery. High inflation pressures are frequently required (especially in the arteritides) and it is sensible to use an inflation device. Inflation pressures as high as 30 atmospheres may be required to fully efface the lesion. If the lesion is resistant to dilatation then it is worth pre-dilating with an undersized balloon e.g. 3 mm, which can tolerate higher pressures than, say a 6 mm balloon.

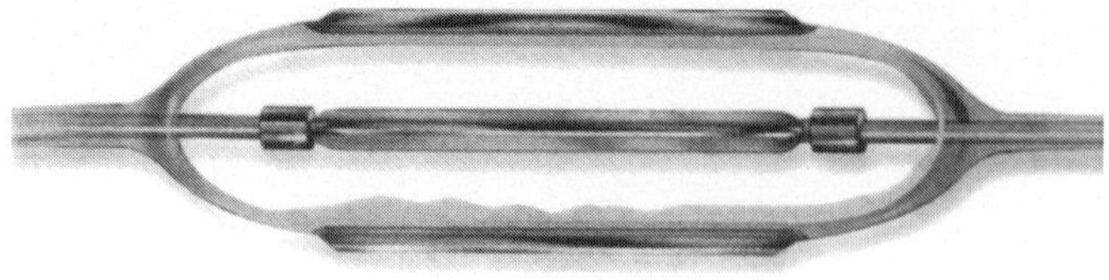

2

2, 3

More recently cutting angioplasty balloons have become available which are useful if conventional high-pressure balloons fail. Three blades, attached to the balloon surface at 120-degree intervals (2), cut the stenosis as the balloon inflates. The blades are protected by the wrap of the balloon material, permitting atraumatic passage across the stenosis. As the balloon is inflated the exposed blades relieve the 'hoop stress' by making three small controlled incisions. The expanded balloon then flattens or dilates the cut area with the minimal amount of trauma. Photomicrographs of an artery are shown (3)

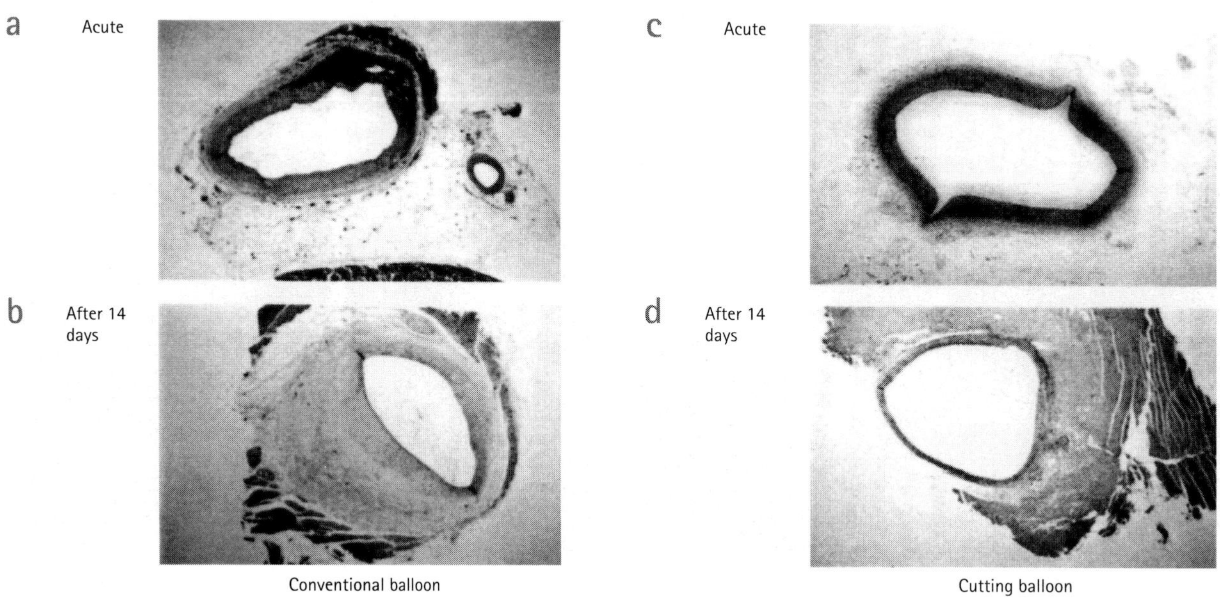

3

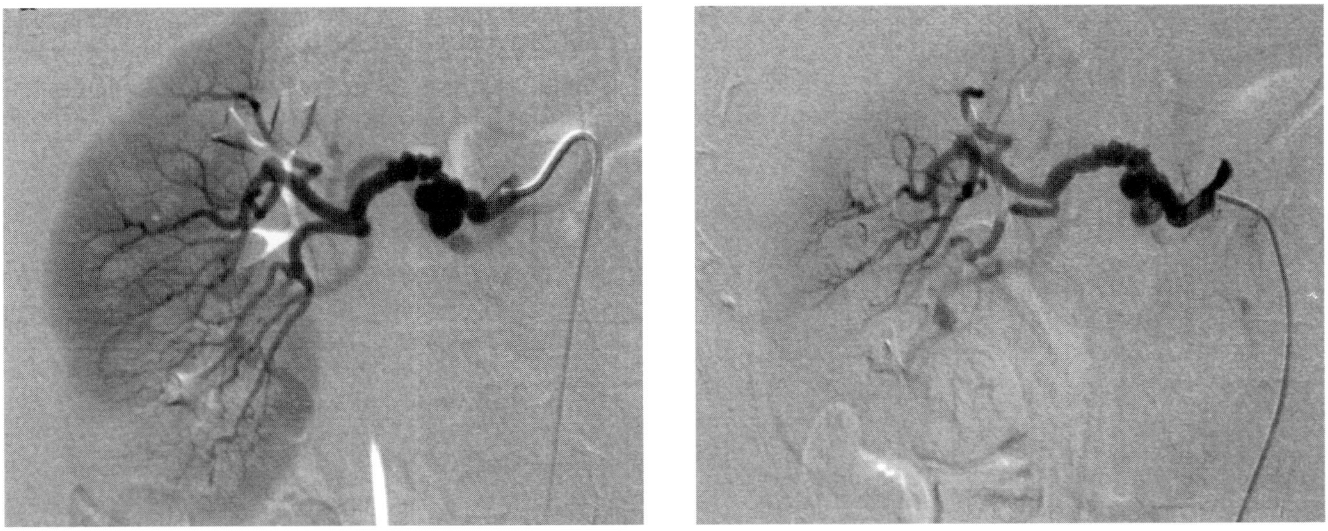

a b
4

before and 14 days after balloon angioplasty with a conventional (a, b) and cutting balloon (c, d). Less intimal and medial damage is present with the cutting balloon. The largest diameter currently available is only 4 mm but this is sufficient to precut the lesion, allowing the introduction of an appropriate sized conventional balloon. It is important to remember that these balloons are only licensed for use in the coronary arteries at present and their use in the renal arteries is 'off label'.

4, 5

It may be difficult to demonstrate angiographic improvement following angioplasty in patients who have the classical 'string-of-beads' appearance i.e. where a series of web-like stenoses coexist with focal aneurysmal dilatations (**4a, b**). This patient had severe hypertension (**4a**). Little angiographic improvement is seen following angioplasty (**b**) but the pressure gradient across the diseased segment dropped from 44 to 5 mm Hg. In this situation, measurement of the pressure gradient across the lesion is useful in assessing the response to angioplasty. A 4 F end-hole catheter or open-ended guidewire should be used for pressure measurement to minimize the reduction in luminal diameter.

Stents are very rarely required in non-atherosclerotic renal artery stenosis and the authors have only used one where a spontaneous medial dissection in the right renal artery complicated a case of fibromuscular dysplasia (**5a**). An iliorenal saphenous vein graft, performed 10 months previously had thrombosed (arrowhead). Following placement of a Palmaz PS 20 stent (arrow) (**5b**) the dissection was effaced. A follow-up angiogram at 24 months showed continued patency (**5c**).

Branch lesions

These lesions are more problematic to treat but again offer a good therapeutic outcome if successful. Four factors should be taken into account;

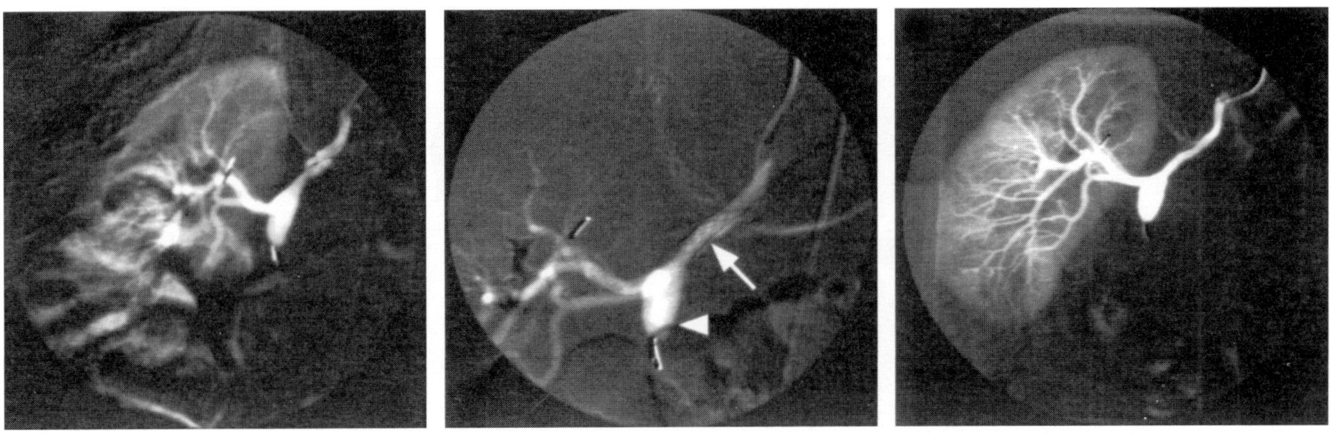

a b c
5

1. the calibre of the artery (which is typically 2–3 mm);
2. the susceptibility of small arteries to spasm;
3. the diameter of the main vessel proximal to a bifurcation if a 'kissing balloon' technique is to be used;
4. the lack of support the small platform balloons and wires offer.

It is best to use small platform balloon systems when dilating branch renal arteries. These tend to invoke less spasm and are less traumatic when crossing a tight lesion. A conventional 5 F shafted balloon may 'Dotter' the lesion when advanced across a branch stenosis risking dissection or other damage. In contrast the small platform balloons are on a 3.5–3.9 F shaft and much less likely to 'Dotter'.

6a, b

It is sensible to use a guiding catheter for three reasons:

1. it provides support for the balloon;
2. it allows two balloons to be passed for the 'kissing technique';
3. it permits the injection of contrast to aid accurate crossing and dilatation of the lesions (**6a, b**).

Traditionally a guiding catheter requires to be placed through a sheath, however the latest guide-sheaths (Cordis, Miami, USA and Guidant, USA) are supplied with integral dilators which obviate the need for a sheath and help minimize the size of the access site puncture. It should be remembered that a 7 F guiding catheter makes the same size hole in an artery as a 5 F sheath. The size of the guiding catheter will depend on how many balloons are to be inserted and whether they are of conventional construction, rapid exchange or 'balloon on a wire' configuration. A single balloon will fit through a 6–7 F guiding catheter and two balloons require a 7–8 F guiding catheter. A Tuohy-Borst adaptor will be required and if two balloons are to be inserted this will need to have two side arms rather than one.

Guiding catheters come in a variety of shapes and usually the renal double curve is the most appropriate for a femoral approach. A multipurpose shape is best for an arm approach and the guiding catheter need to be 90 cm in length with a long balloon system (usually 120 cm). It is a matter of judgment whether to choose an arm or femoral approach. At least 80–90% of renal artery stenosis can be tackled successfully from a femoral approach, which has a reduced complication rate, compared with any of the arm access sites.

It is best to begin by placing the guiding catheter at the ostium of the renal artery and then crossing the lesion with a small platform 0.014–0.018 wire (Guidant USA), contrast can be injected to aid passage of the wire. Some workers use roadmapping but the authors find respiratory movement usually degrades the image unacceptably. If a bifurcation lesion is present a second wire is then placed in the other branch and appropriate sized balloons (typically 3 mm) placed in 'kissing' fashion. It is vital at this stage to remember that both balloons will occupy the vessel proximal to the bifurcation and this vessel must be capable of tolerating this magnitude of dilatation. For example two 'kissing' 3 mm balloons require a 6 mm pre-bifurcation artery (**6a, b**). If this is not possible then only one balloon should be inflated at once. The balloons are then withdrawn across the lesion leaving the wires in place. A completion angiogram is performed through the guiding catheter.

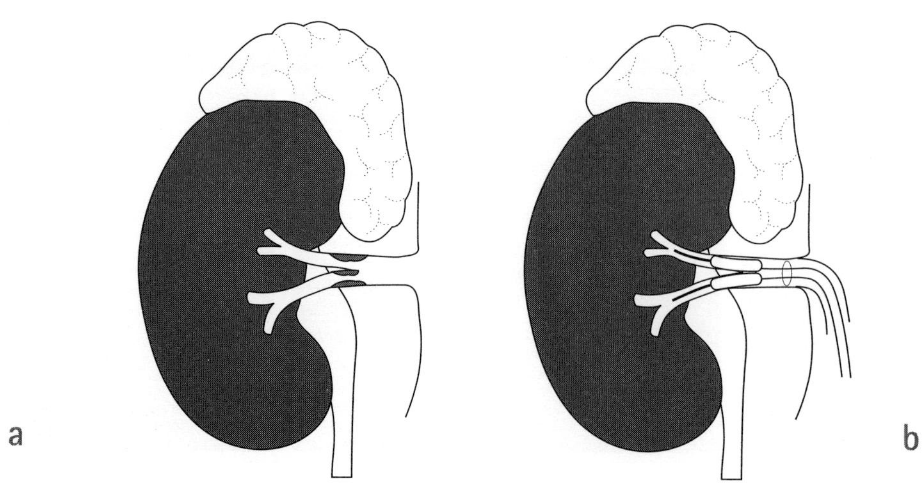

6

7

Recently rapid exchange balloon systems have become available for renal angioplasty. Once the domain of the cardiologist they offer the advantage of rapidly exchanging the balloon catheter and obviate the need for long exchange length wires (**7**).

An alternative to the conventional balloon or rapid exchange system is the 'balloon-on-a-wire' (TEG wire Boston Scientific, USA). Originally developed by Tegtmeyer it consists of a balloon mounted on an 0.035 guidewire through which the balloon is inflated. Beyond the balloon is a 2 cm 0.014–0.018 atraumatic platinum wire tip. These devices are very torqueable and do not require any wire balloon exchanges. However, the deflated balloon usually has to be left across the lesion for the post percutaneous transluminal angioplasty angiographic film and may degrade the image.

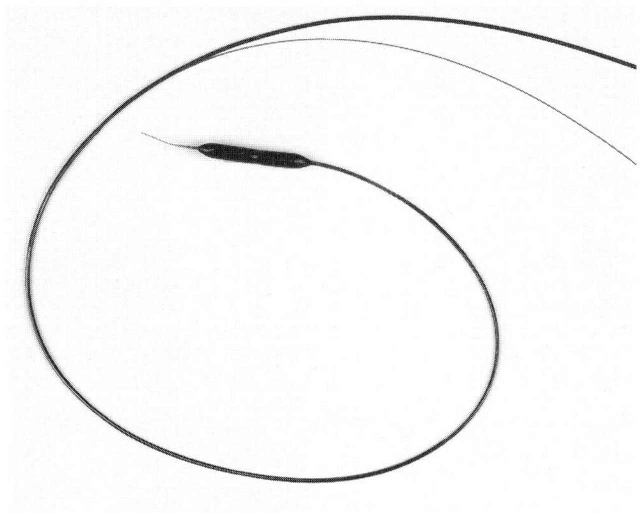

7

Ostial atherosclerotic disease

K Ivancev, M Lindh

Introduction

Ostial renal stenosis may be associated with uncontrolled hypertension and/or impaired renal function. When such a condition is suspected, non-invasive imaging, including renal captopril scintigraphy or Doppler ultrasound and magnetic resonance angiography is helpful to select the candidates for further invasive treatment (Soulez *et al.*, 2000). Open surgical renal artery reconstruction is today used mostly as an adjunctive procedure with aortic reconstructions (Darling *et al.*, 1999). Percutaneous transluminal renal angioplasty and percutaneous transluminal stent placement have been shown to be equally efficaceous, particularly for control of renal hypertension, as open surgery, without the high rate of morbidity and mortality associated with the latter (Weibull *et al.*, 1993; Xue, *et al.*, 1999). Ostial lesions are, by definition, lesions situated within 5 mm from the origin of the renal artery, and are often caused by atherosclerotic plaques in the aortic wall. Because of this, they respond poorly to percutaneous transluminal renal angioplasty and therefore often require placement of stents (van de Ven *et al.*, 1999; Rodriguez-Lopez *et al.*, 1999). Primary stenting of ostial renal artery stenosis has contributed to improved long-term blood pressure control (Rocha-Singh *et al.*, 1999; Rees, 1999) and it is now waiting for a close comparison, preferably as a randomized study comparing percutaneous transluminal stent placement with medical treatment only.

The following is a description of a technique applied for endovascular stenting of ostial renal artery stenosis.

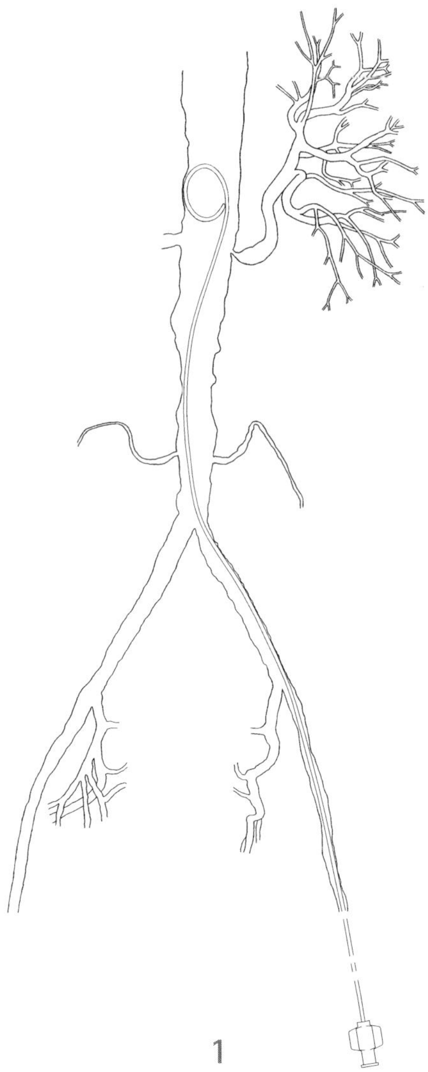

1

1

Based on pre-intervention, non-invasive imaging study, the ipsilateral common femoral artery is punctured and used as an access site. An ipsilateral site access considerably facilitates placement of subsequent devices into the stenotic main renal artery. Angiography is performed, either with iodinated contrast medium or, in case of impaired renal function, with carbon dioxide (CO_2). Once the lesion is visualized a calibrated measurement is made of the diameter of the normal renal artery, i.e. the segment distal to the post-stenotic dilatation.

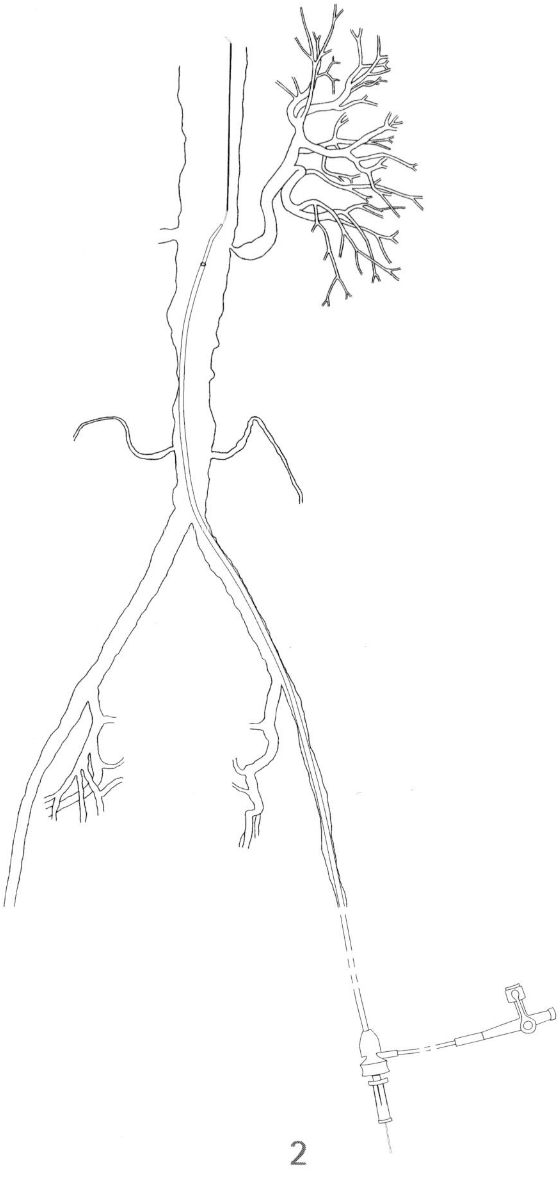

2

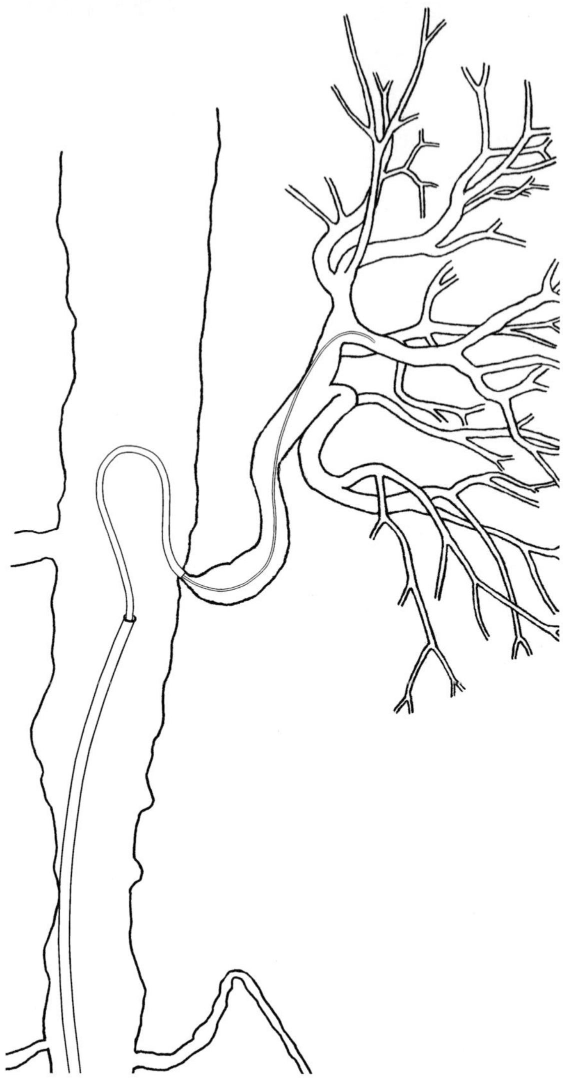

3

2

A 6F braided introducer, preferably with a curved tip, is placed into the aorta.

3

A full heparinization of the patient is started by administering 5000–10 000 international units of heparin. The level of anticoagulation is maintained at 250–300 seconds of activated clotting time.

A catheter with a suitable shape, either with a so called 'shepherd's hook' shape or a 'cobra-head' shape, is used to catheterize the stenotic renal artery. Often, the catheterization is facilitated by using a soft-tip hydrophilic wire.

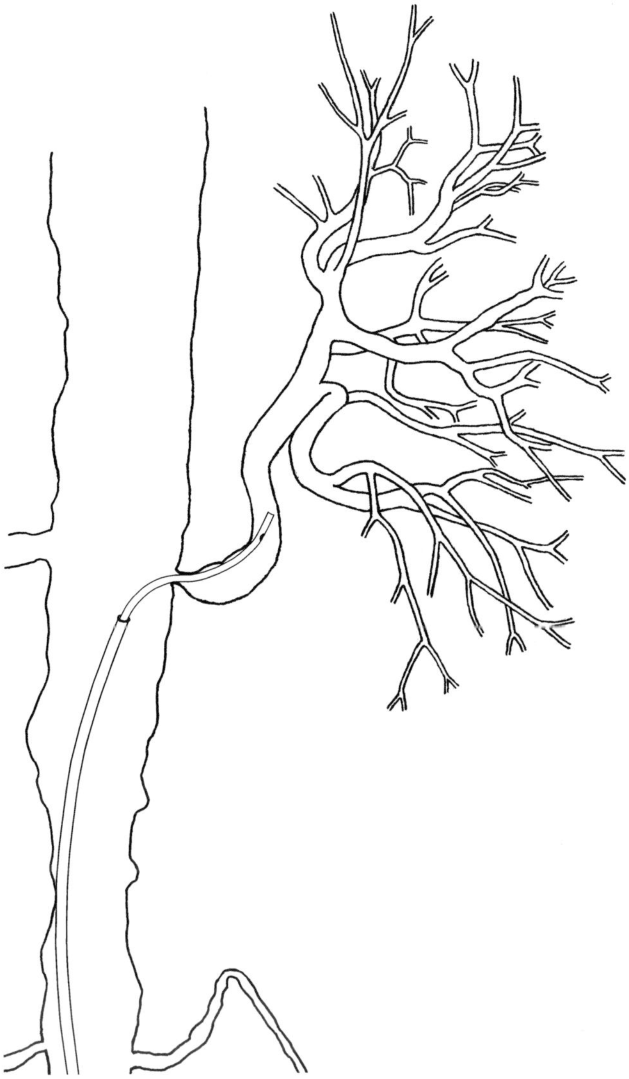

4

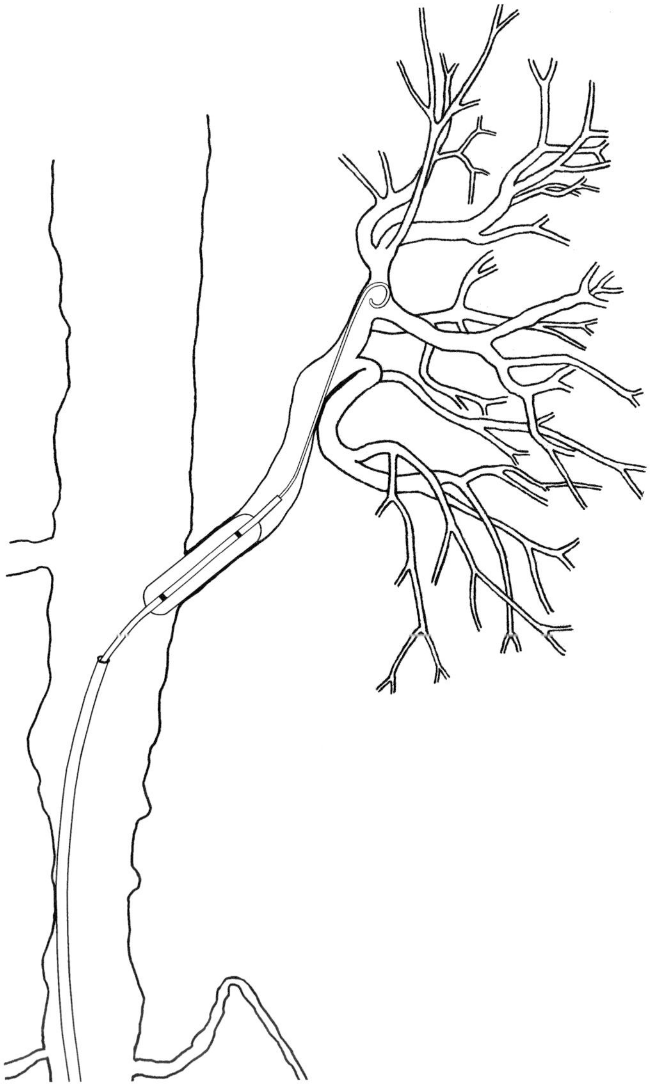

5

4

Once the stenotic lesion is catheterized, the catheter is enforced over the wire into the main renal artery. A pressure gradient can then be recorded, either using the same angiographic catheter (5F) or exchanging over the wire to a 4F catheter. If there is no pressure gradient, i.e. less than 4–5 mmHg mean pressure gradient between the main renal artery and the aorta (the aortic pressure is measured through the side port of the 6F introducer), then there is no indication for further intervention, regardless of the degree of stenosis seen on angiography. In other words, if there is no peripheral bed to accommodate enough flow to create a pressure gradient, then such a kidney is not functional enough to benefit from any further intervention. The catheter in the main renal artery is also used for delivering 0.15–0.2 mg nitroglycerin to prevent peripheral spasm.

5

Over a guidewire which is rigid enough, a balloon of appropriate size is placed across the renal ostial stenosis. The most commonly used wires are Rosenwire (Cook Europe, Bjaeverskov, Denmark) or TAD wire (Mallinckrodt, St Louis, USA). The balloon size is approximately the same or 1 mm larger than the diameter of the normal renal artery. Percutaneous transluminal renal angioplasty is performed under close supervision of the patient, giving rise to a mild discomfort in the back of the patient but no severe pain. After this, an angiography is repeated through the introducer sheath to demonstrate the effect of the percutaneous transluminal renal angioplasty and pressure measurement is again recorded. If there is a persistent gradient of at least 5–8 mmHg mean pressure, the procedure continues with placement of a stent in the stenotic renal ostium.

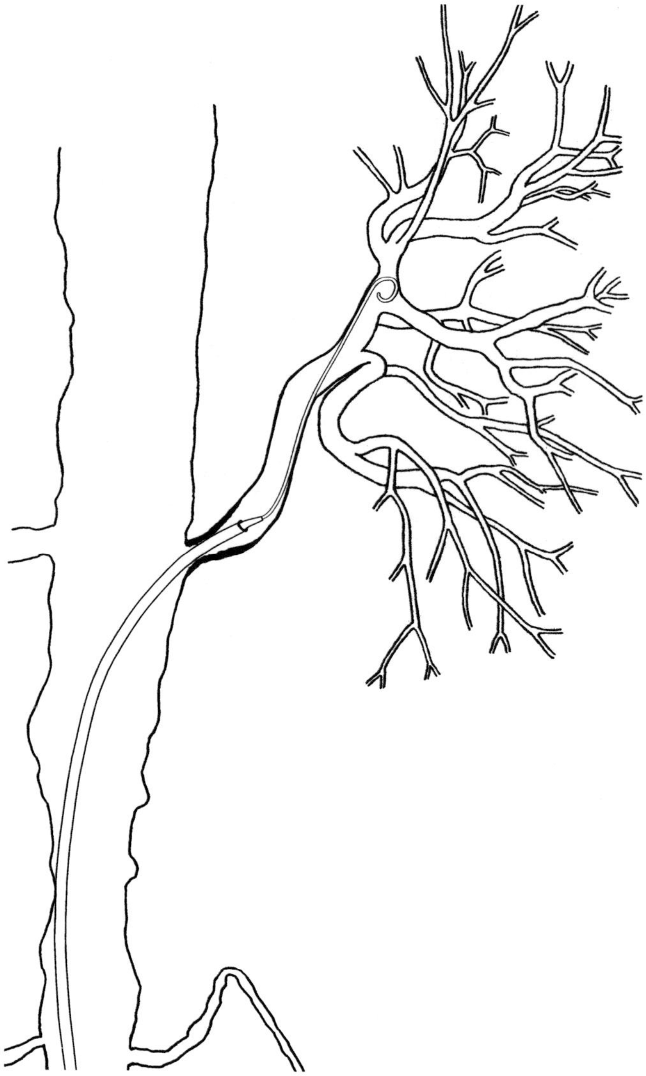

6

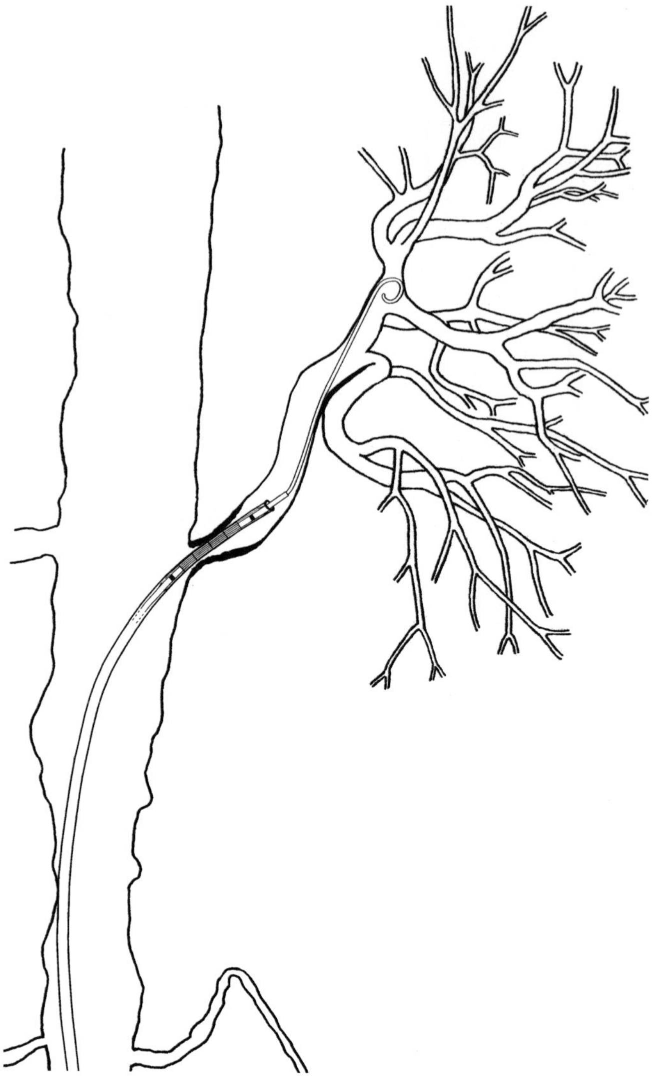

7

6

Over a relatively rigid guidewire, the balloon is exchanged for the curved 6F introducer, which is placed with the tip inside the main renal artery.

7

The dilator of the introducer is removed and over the guidewire is placed the same balloon used for percutaneous transluminal renal angioplasty, on which a stent is mounted. A pre-mounted stent on a balloon may obviate the need for introducing a 6F introducer into the artery.

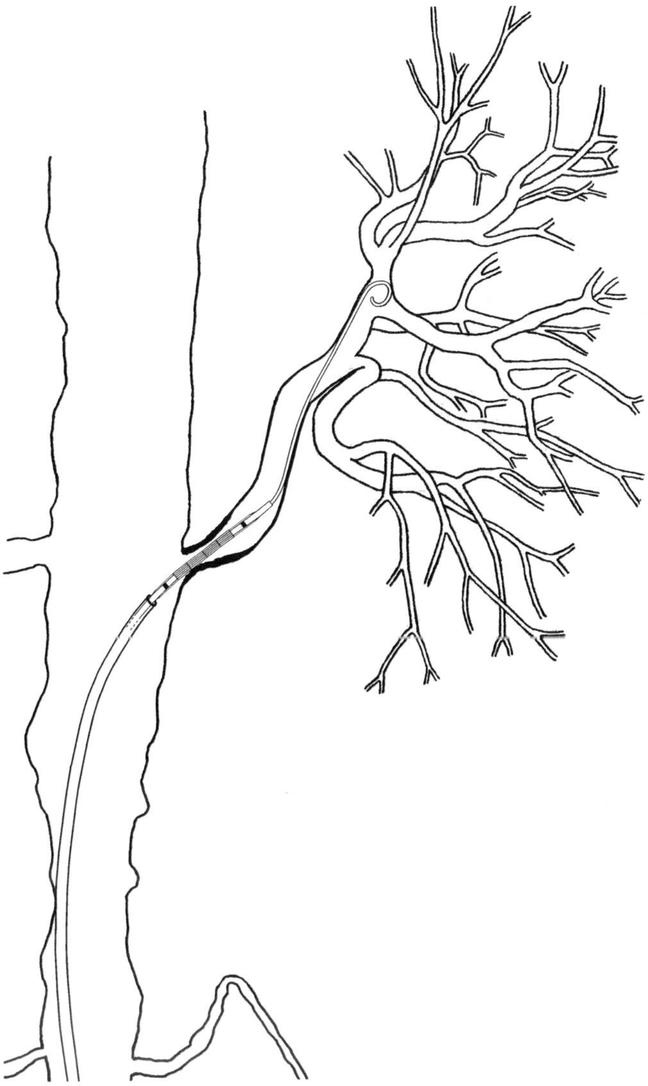

8

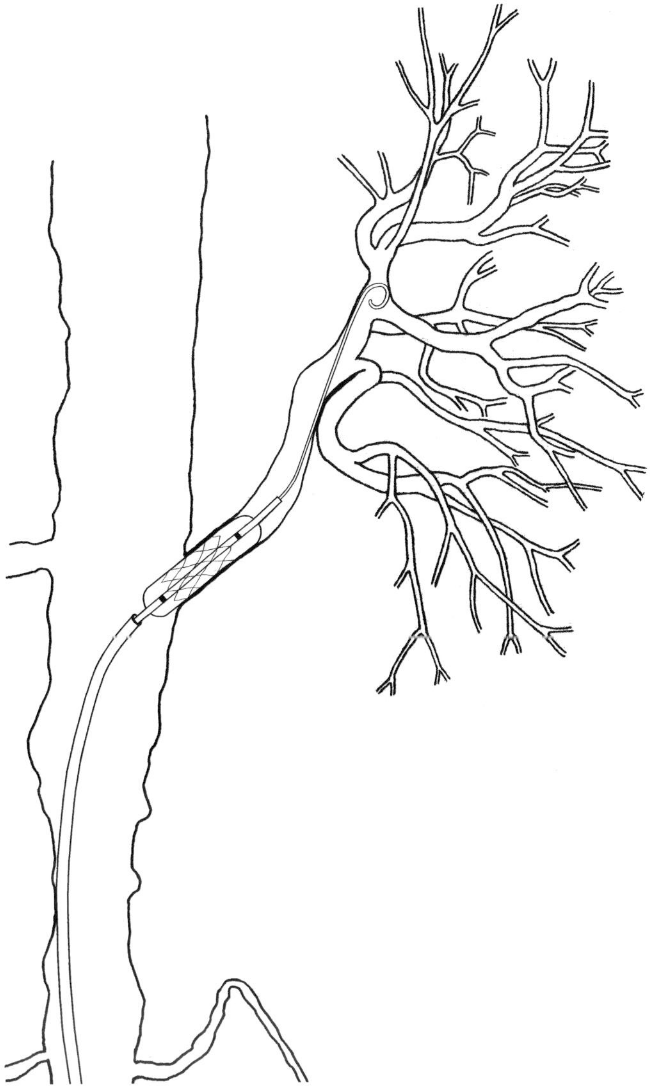

9

8

The introducer is pulled back just enough to uncover the balloon mounted with the stent. Repeated angiography is performed to define the exact positioning of the stent, i.e. protruding no more than 2 mm into the aortic lumen. The appropriate length of the stent has been chosen based on the length of the stenosis.

9

Once the correct position of the stent is achieved, the introducer sheath is pulled further down, to uncover the complete length of the balloon, and the stent is deployed. Once the stent is placed, the balloon is deflated and withdrawn and a 4F catheter is again placed over the guidewire to record pressure gradients. If necessary, further dilatation or further stent placement is performed.

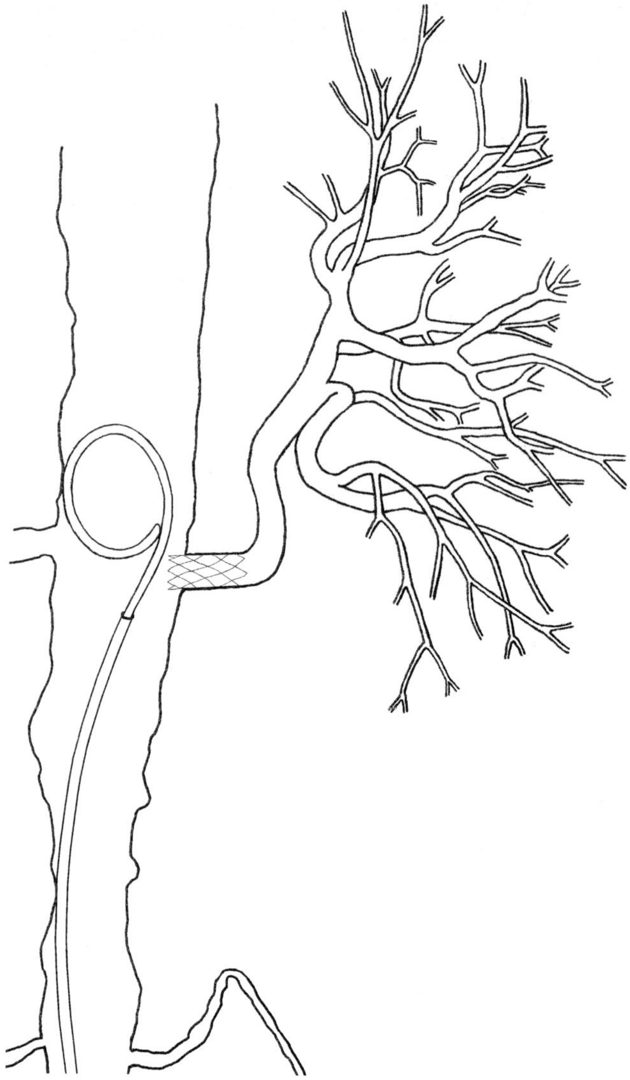

10

10

Completion angiography is performed, either using a pigtail catheter or by injection of contrast medium (iodinated or CO_2) through the introducer sheath, to demonstrate the final position of the stent and the peripheral renal circulation. A stent-graft can be used, instead of a stent, through the same 6F introducer. Finishing up the procedure is closing the access site, usually with a suturing device, such as the Perclose device (Abbott, Redwood City, USA).

References

Darling RC 3rd, Kreienberg PB, Chang BB *et al.* (1999). Outcome of renal artery reconstruction: analysis of 687 procedures. *Ann Surg* **230**: 524–532.

Rees CR (1999). Stents for atherosclerotic renovascular disease. *J Vasc Interv Radiol* **10**: 689–705.

Rocha-Singh KJ, Mishkel GJ, Katholi RE *et al.* (1999). Clinical predictors of improved long-term blood pressure control after successful stenting of hypertensive patients with obstructive renal artery atherosclerosis. *Catheter Cardiovasc Interv* **47**: 167–172.

Rodriguez-Lopez JA, Werner A, Ray LI *et al.* (1999). Renal artery stenosis treated with stent deployment: indications, technique, and outcome for 108 patients. *J Vasc Surg* **29**: 617–624.

Soulez G, Oliva VL, Turpin S *et al.* (2000). Imaging of renovascular hypertension: respective values of renal scintigraphy, renal Doppler US, and MR angiography. *Radiographics* **20**: 1355–1372.

van de Ven PJ, Kaatee R, Beutler JJ *et al.* (1999). Arterial stenting and balloon angioplasty in ostial atherosclerotic renovascular disease: a randomised trial. *Lancet* **353**: 282–286.

Weibull H, Bergqvist D, Bergentz SE *et al.* (1993). Percutaneous transluminal renal angioplasty versus surgical reconstruction of atherosclerotic renal artery stenosis: a prospective randomized study *J Vasc Surg* **18**: 841–852.

Xue F, Bettmann MA, Langdon DR, Wivell WA (1999). Outcome and cost comparison of percutaneous transluminal renal angioplasty, renal arterial stent placement, and renal arterial bypass grafting. *Radiology* **212**: 378–384.

Abdominal aortic aneurysm

John A Mannick, Anthony D Whittemore

Introduction

The indication for repair of an abdominal aortic aneurysm is the presence of an aneurysm of significant size in a patient of any age who does not have another non-correctable, life-threatening condition. It is generally conceded that aneurysms which have reached 5 cm in diameter are in danger of rupturing and surgery for such aneurysms is clearly indicated. There is some debate as to whether aneurysms of smaller diameter than 5 cm are likely to rupture. Our own practice has been to operate selectively on aneurysms between 4 and 5 cm in diameter. The decision to operate is based upon evidence of recent expansion in aneurysm size by ultrasound or computed tomography, the ratio of the aneurysm diameter to that of the uninvolved aorta and the age and fitness of the patient. We rarely operate on aneurysms smaller than 4 cm. Patients with tender aneurysms or with symptoms of back pain or abdominal pain suggesting acute expansion of the aneurysm require urgent surgery. Obviously, a patient with the diagnosis of a ruptured abdominal aortic aneurysm should be taken to the operating room immediately.

In addition to standard preoperative preparation, it has been our practice for the past decade to study every patient undergoing elective or urgent aneurysm repair by inserting a Swan-Ganz catheter preoperatively (Whittemore *et al.*, 1980). Several points on the left ventricular performance curve are then determined for each individual so that a pulmonary capillary wedge pressure can be selected which will result in a desirable cardiac index. Volume replacement during surgery can be regulated to maintain this optimal pulmonary capillary wedge pressure and thus ensure adequate tissue perfusion throughout the operation. Declamping hypotension can also be minimized with this technique.

We routinely perform preoperative aortography using the retrograde Seldinger technique in order to define the upper extent of the aneurysm better in relation to the renal arteries and to ensure that there are no anomalous renal arteries arising from the aneurysm itself. We obtain biplane views to ensure patency of the superior mesenteric artery and coeliac axis since aneurysm repair will involve ligation of the origin of the inferior mesenteric artery.

We believe that it is helpful to recover shed blood during the course of aneurysm surgery by the use of a Cell Saver. Since we began using this device 10 years ago, approximately 35% of patients undergoing elective abdominal aneurysm repair have not required banked blood transfusions.

The operation

The technique of aneurysm repair employed by our service is a modification of the graft inclusion technique previously described by Creech (1966) and Javid *et al.* (1982).

1

The abdomen is opened and explored through a midline incision extending from the pubis to the xiphoid. The small bowel is lifted superiorly and to the right, and is packed into the right upper quadrant of the abdomen. Exposure of the operative field is greatly facilitated by a multi-armed mechanical retractor fixed to the operating table. The peritoneum is incised with scissors along the inferior border of the third and fourth portions of the duodenum, and the duodenum is retracted superiorly. The peritoneum and areolar tissue overlying the aorta are opened longitudinally with the scissors or cautery, exposing the anterior surface of the aneurysm.

2

The incision is carried superiorly to the level of the left renal vein and inferiorly 2.5–5 cm beyond the aortic bifurcation. The aorta just above the aneurysm and below the left renal vein is freed up from its surrounding tissues by sharp dissection anteriorly and laterally. No

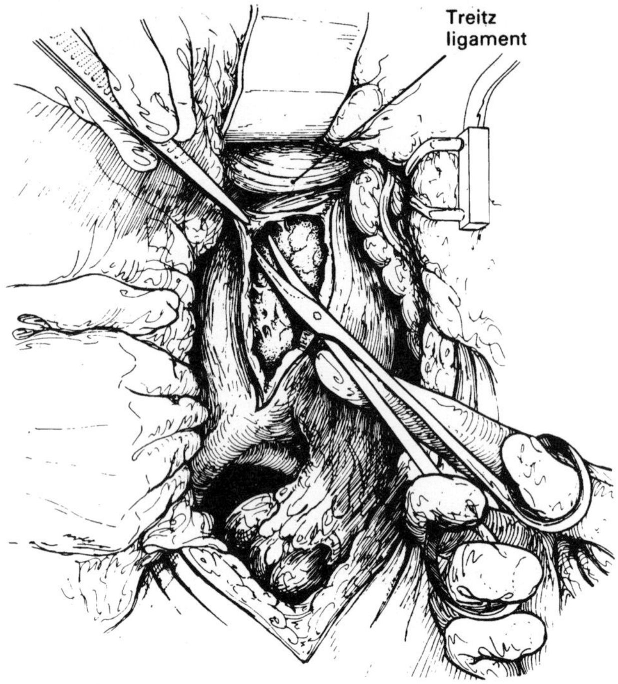

1

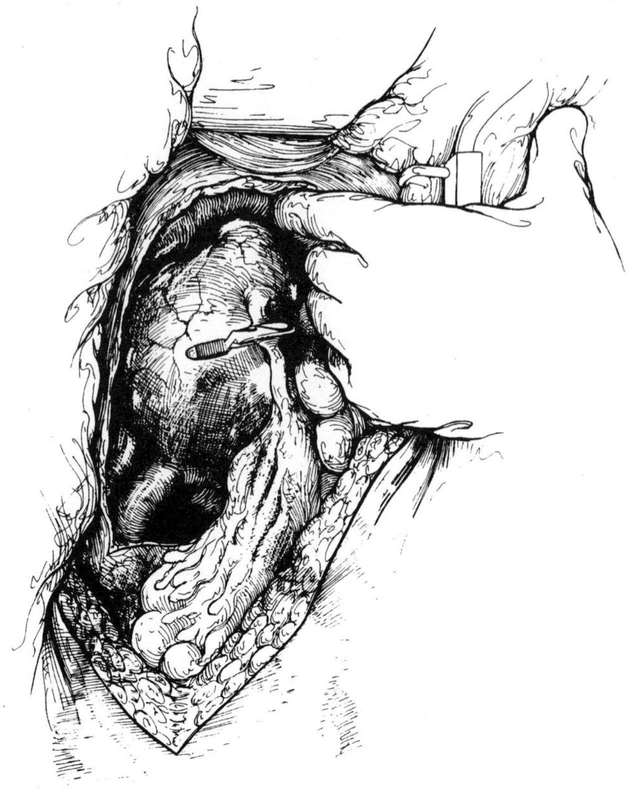

2

attempt is made to dissect behind the aorta at this level, nor is the neck of the aneurysm encircled with tape. However, the dissection along each lateral wall of the aorta is continued far enough posteriorly so that the neck of the aneurysm can be compressed easily by an occluding clamp which will be applied at this level.

Inferiorly, the anterior and lateral walls of both common iliac arteries are freed by sharp dissection in a similar fashion without separating these vessels from their attachments to the common iliac veins posteriorly. If it is convenient at this point, the inferior mesenteric artery is temporarily controlled with a bulldog clamp near its origin from the aorta as illustrated. In most instances, the origin of the inferior mesenteric artery is ligated from inside the aneurysm at a later stage. Ligation and division of the inferior mesenteric artery away from its origin is avoided for fear of damage to vital collateral branches which feed the sigmoid colon. Dissection of the lateral walls of the aneurysm is kept to a minimum to eliminate the necessity for ligating multiple small vessels that traverse the surrounding lymphatic and areolar tissue. Dissection of the aneurysm wall from the inferior vena cava is particularly avoided to reduce the risk of injury to that structure.

Heparin is administered to the patient systemically intravenously, 4000–5000 units in an average adult. While it is possible to repair many, if not most, abdominal aortic aneurysms successfully without the use of heparin, it is advisable to heparinize the patient partially when the aorta and iliac arteries are clamped; otherwise, extensive distal thrombosis can occur in patients who have severe distal arterial occlusive disease and in those instances where mural thrombus or arteriosclerotic debris from the aneurysm is inadvertently embolized distally. It has been our experience that retrograde thrombosis is kept to a minimum in such instances before the embolic debris is retrieved if the patient has been prophylactically heparinized.

3

After heparinization, large straight Fogarty vascular clamps are applied to both common iliac arteries and a deBakey reverse-angle aortic clamp is applied to the aorta above the aneurysm. The aneurysm is then opened longitudinally with a knife or cautery.

4

The incision in the aneurysm is completed with Mayo scissors.

5

All mural thrombus and loose arteriosclerotic debris is evacuated from the lumen of the aneurysm.

6

The origins of bleeding lumbar arteries are oversewn with figure-of-eight sutures of 3/0 polypropylene. The origin

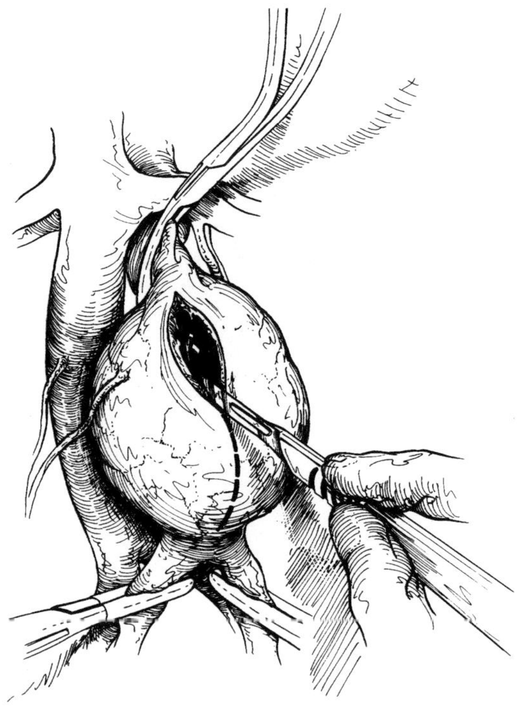

3

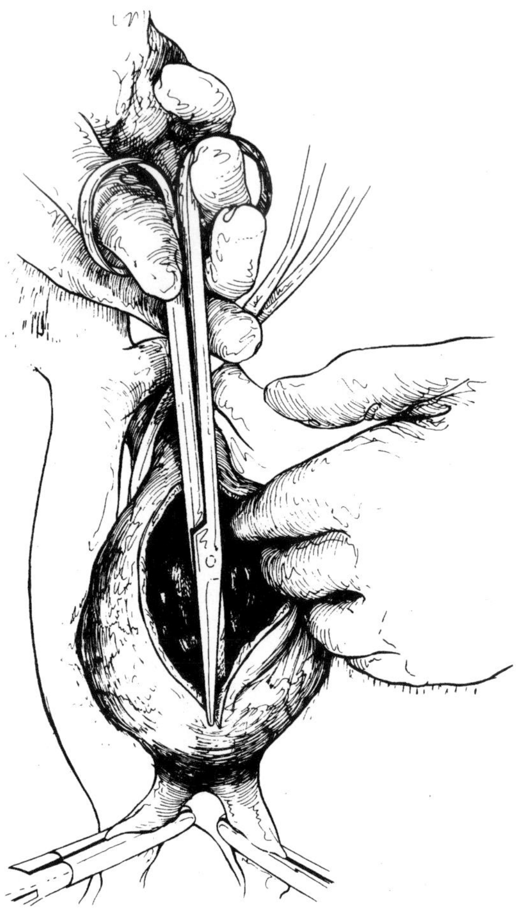

4

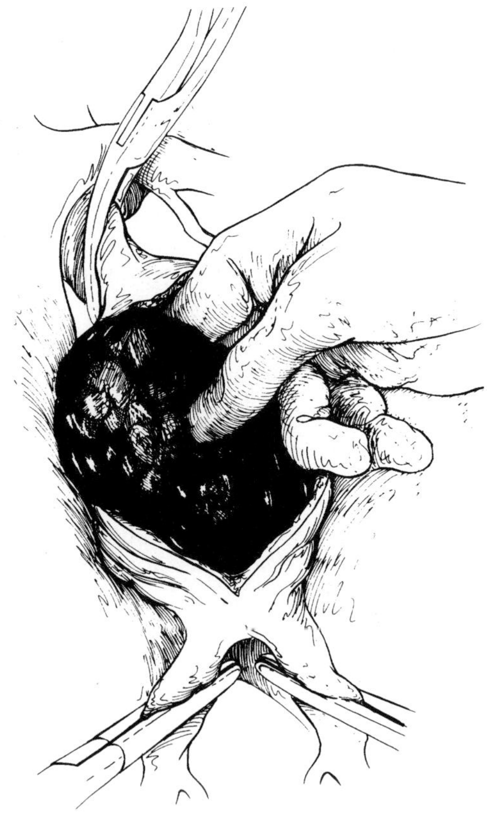

5

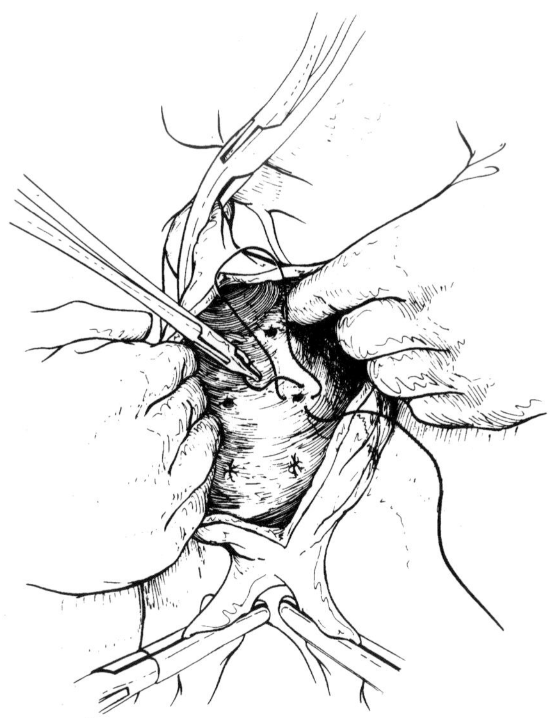

6

of the inferior mesenteric artery is similarly sutured if this vessel is still patent and the backbleeding is vigorous. If the inferior mesenteric is widely patent and backbleeding is sluggish, reimplantation of the artery into the aortic prosthesis should be considered, particularly if preoperative angiograms show disease of the superior mesenteric and/or hypogastric arteries.

7

In patients with no significant iliac aneurysms, a tube graft of woven or collagen-impregnated knitted Dacron is preferred for aneurysm replacement. This graft will be sutured distally to the aortic bifurcation which usually remains of reasonably normal size even when the aneurysm involves the entire infrarenal abdominal aorta. Cuffs may be cut proximally and distally extending partially down each side of the aorta at the neck of the aneurysm above and at the aortic bifurcation below. However, in large aneurysms, we have found it just as convenient to avoid this step and simply to suture the graft to the ring of normal vessel superiorly and inferiorly.

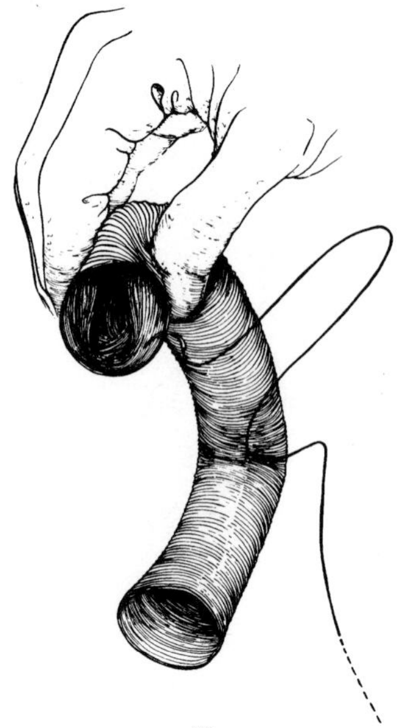

7

8

The posterior wall of the aorta is not divided either proximally or distally. The posterior aortic wall is often a rather tenuous structure and we prefer to add strength to the posterior suture line by including the surrounding fascial tissue in the posterior stitches of the anastomosis. A Dacron tube graft of appropriate size is sewn with a double-armed polypropylene suture to the posterior wall of the aorta at the neck of the aneurysm. A double-thickness of aortic wall is included in each bite posteriorly.

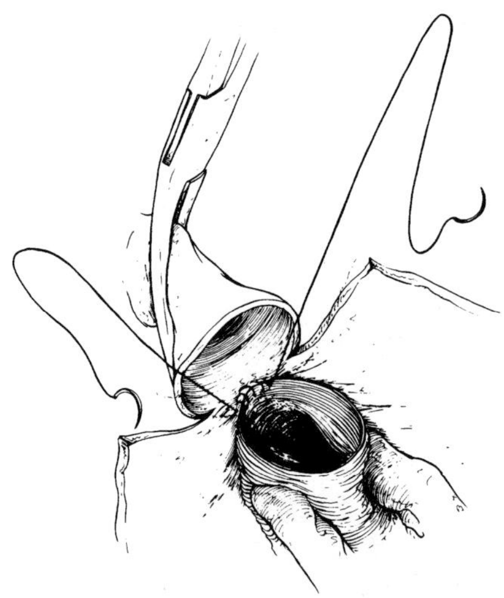

8

9

The suture is carried around each side of the neck of the aneurysm and tied anteriorly.

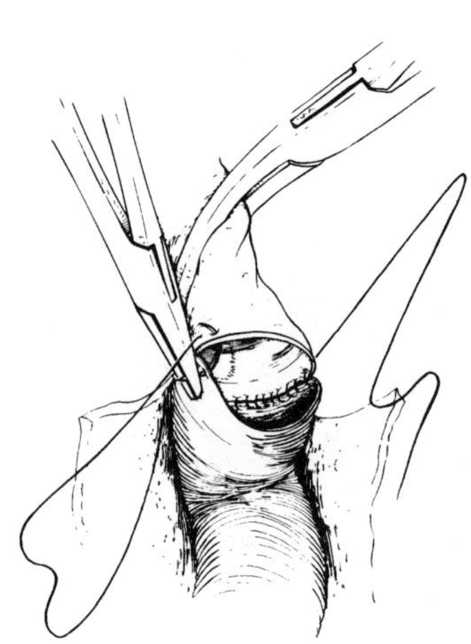

9

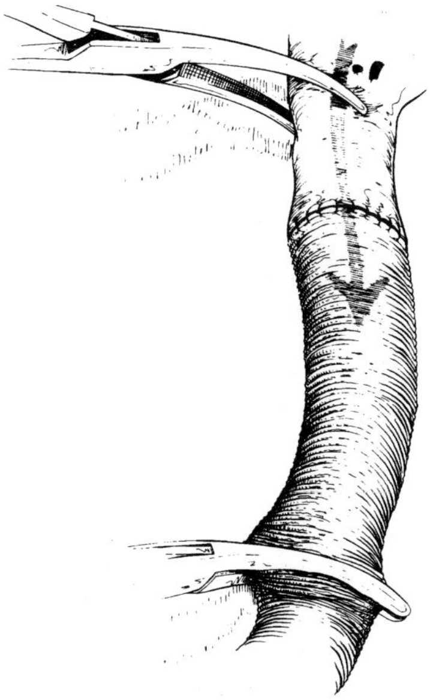

10

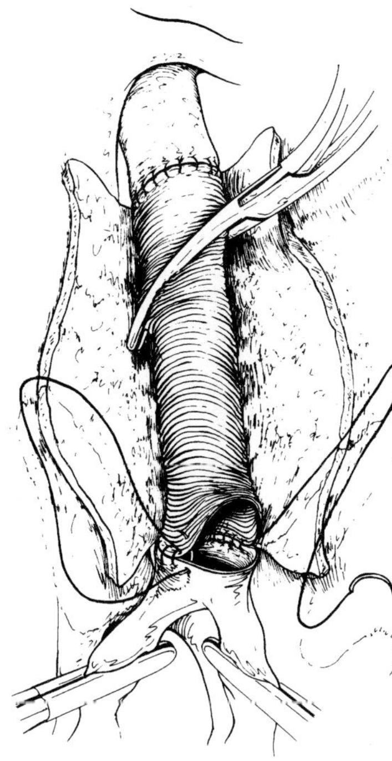

12

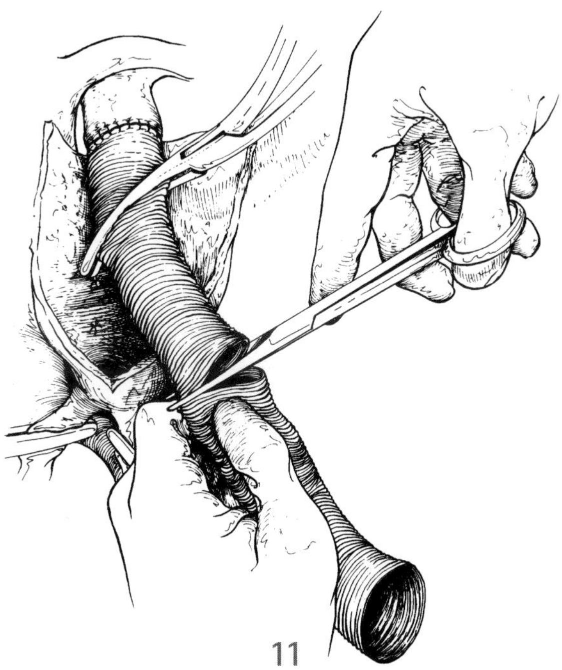

11

10

The proximal anastomosis is then tested for leaks by clamping the tube graft and releasing the aortic clamp briefly. If any leaks are noted in the anastomosis they are repaired with simple or figure-of-eight sutures of 3/0 polypropylene. The aortic clamp may then be reapplied or, if preferred, the graft may be clamped just distal to the proximal anastomosis.

11

After being evacuated of all blood with a sucker, the graft is placed under slight tension and cut to the appropriate length for anastomosis with the aortic bifurcation.

12

The lower anastomosis is performed using a double-armed suture of 3/0 polypropylene.

All vessels are flushed before completion of this suture line. If there is adequate backbleeding from both iliac systems no attempt is made to pass Fogarty catheters distally to retrieve possible emboli. The suture line is then completed and tied anteriorly as for the proximal anastomosis. The iliac clamps are released and the lower anastomosis is inspected for leaks which are repaired as for the proximal anastomosis. The proximal aortic clamp is then gradually released while the anaesthetist carefully monitors the patient's blood pressure and infuses extra volume intravenously if needed. If the patient has been maintained with an optimal pulmonary capillary wedge pressure, declamping hypotension is ordinarily not observed. After release of clamps the iliac arteries are inspected for adequate pulsations and the presence of good femoral pulses in the groin is determined by palpation. We seldom find it necessary to neutralize the heparin with protamine.

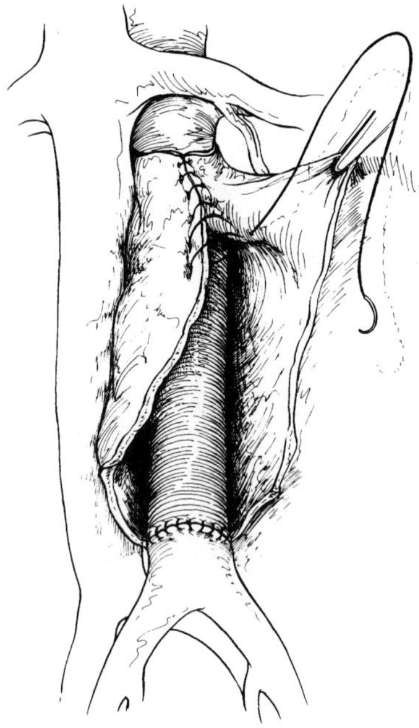

13

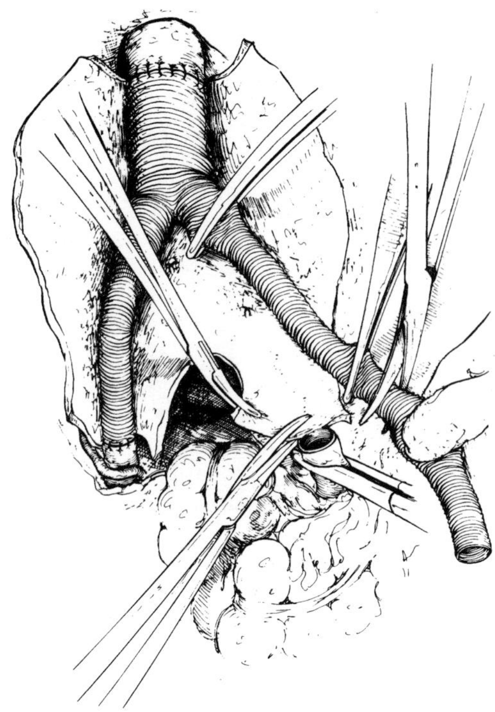

14

13

Any residual bleeding points in the aneurysm wall are sutured, ligated or electrocoagulated and the aneurysm wall is sutured back over the prosthesis with a running stitch of polypropylene. This manoeuvre ordinarily covers both the proximal and distal suture line with residual aneurysm wall.

If the wall is too large to fit snugly around the prosthesis it may be overlapped in vest-over-pants fashion as a double suture line. We have found that this is usually more convenient than trimming the wall, since trimming often produces further bleeding which must then be controlled. The periaortic tissues are then approximated over the aorta, and if possible, over the resutured aneurysm wall by a second running suture of polyglycolate in order to provide further retroperitoneal haemostasis. This also has the advantage of placing yet another layer between the prosthesis and the posterior wall of the duodenum. The posterior peritoneum is then closed over the aorta and resutured aneurysm wall with a running suture of polyglycolate. It is ordinarily possible to interpose the peritoneum as an additional layer between the posterior wall of the duodenum and the aorta. The abdomen is then closed with a continuous suture of #2 polypropylene to the rectus fascia and staples to the skin.

14

Iliac aneurysms

If common iliac aneurysms are present, a similar operative procedure is followed. However, the iliac clamps are applied to the iliac bifurcations, taking care to avoid injury to the ureters which usually cross the common iliac arteries distally. Iliac aneurysms are opened longitudinally. A bifurcation graft of Dacron is used and the upper anastomosis is performed as described. The iliac limbs are sutured on either side to the distal common iliac arteries, again from inside the iliac aneurysms. The aneurysm walls may also be sutured back over the graft limbs to provide an extra layer of host tissue between the graft and the abdominal viscera. In the case of a large left iliac aneurysm it may be more convenient to exclude the aneurysm and suture the left limb of the graft end-to-side to the external iliac artery inferior to the sigmoid mesentery.

Juxtarenal abdominal aortic aneurysms

In cases where the abdominal aortic aneurysm extends more proximally than usual and there is little or no neck of normal aorta between the aneurysm and the renal arteries, it is helpful to place the aortic clamp at the level of the diaphragm while the proximal anastomosis is performed.

15

The aorta at the level of the diaphragm can be exposed by incising the attachments of the left lobe of the liver to the diaphragm and retracting the liver to the right. The lesser sac is entered and the aorta is exposed as it passes underneath the crus of the diaphragm.

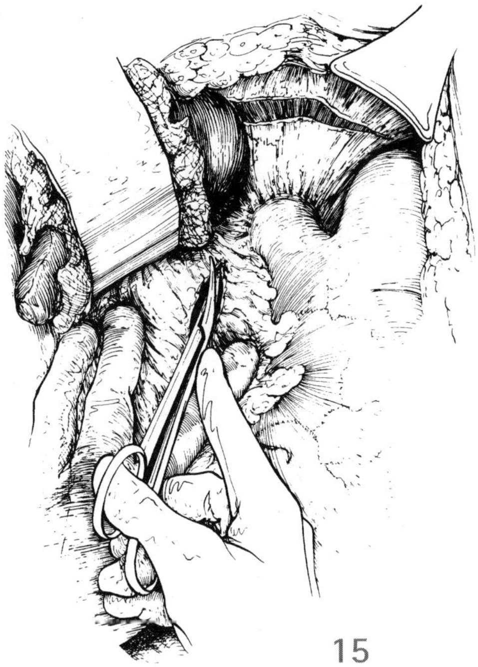

15

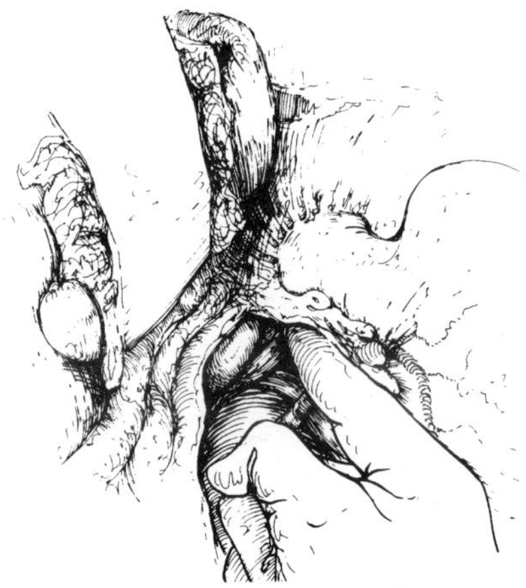

16

16, 17

With finger dissection, the crus can be stretched and split enough so that a clamp can be applied to the aorta at the hiatus, where this vessel is usually of normal calibre and free of branches.

Backbleeding from the coeliac axis and superior mesenteric artery can be controlled with an intra-aortic balloon catheter inserted from below, and the graft can be anastomosed proximally with excellent visibility from inside the aneurysm into the normal aorta just distal to the renal artery orifices. After completion of the proximal anastomosis, the aortic clamp is released and the prosthesis is clamped, restoring flow to the viscera and to the renal arteries. We believe that this manoeuvre is much less hazardous to the kidneys than attempts to clamp the aorta close to the renal artery orifices which may result in arteriosclerotic embolization to one or both kidneys.

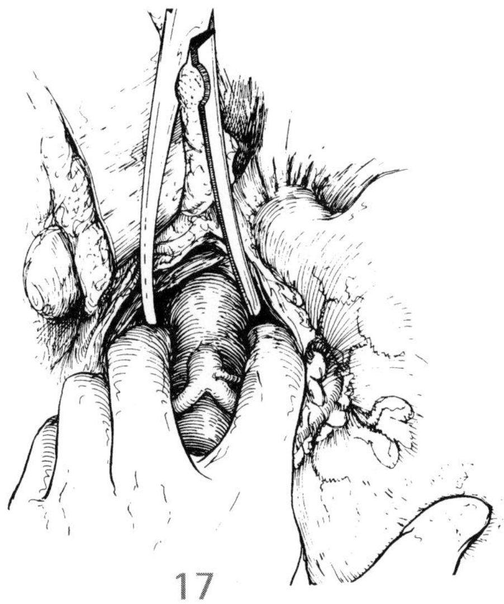

17

Some patients with juxtarenal aneurysms have a considerable, 2 cm or more, distance between the renal artery orifices and the origin of the superior mesenteric as indicated by angiography. In such individuals it may be more convenient to free up the aorta just above the renal arteries and left renal vein. The aorta can then be safely clamped below the superior mesenteric thus avoiding even a brief period of visceral ischaemia.

The retroperitoneal approach

In some patients (about 15% of those in our practice) the retroperitoneal approach (Williams *et al.*, 1980) to abdominal aortic aneurysms is preferable. We believe this approach is especially indicated in patients who have had multiple prior abdominal operations in order to avoid the lysis of adhesions which would be necessary in the transabdominal approach. We believe the retroperitoneal approach is also indicated in those rare individuals with a horseshoe kidney and an abdominal aneurysm, and in patients with inflammatory aneurysms since the attachment of the duodenum to the inflammatory aneurysm is not an issue with this approach. We have also found that the thick inflammatory aneurysm wall is usually thinner posteriorly than anteriorly. We now prefer the retroperitoneal approach in many patients with juxtarenal abdominal aneurysms since the crus of the diaphragm is readily visualized by this approach and can be divided with ease for application of a clamp to the supracoeliac or suprarenal aorta.

18

For the retroperitoneal approach, the patient is placed in the left lateral thoracotomy position with the hips rotated back toward the supine position. The positioning of the patient is greatly aided through the use of a 'bean bag'

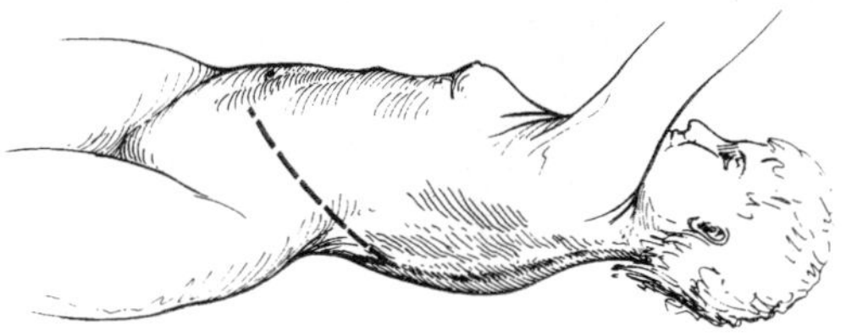

18

moulded by suction. The incision is placed in the left flank beginning at the lateral border of the rectus muscle just below the umbilicus and extending out into the 11th interspace. The abdominal muscles are cut in the line of the incision and the peritoneum and left kidney are retracted medially and to the right. This allows easy visualization of the left posterolateral wall of the aorta, the left common iliac artery, and the origin of the left renal artery.

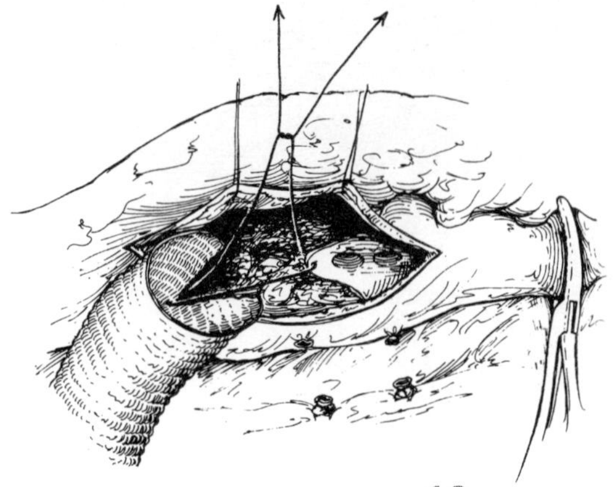

19

19, 20, 21

The neck of the aneurysm can be exposed without difficulty below the left renal artery for application of a clamp. In those instances where aneurysmal disease extends to the region of the renal vessels, this approach can be ideal. It enables easy suprarenal control and the Dacron is tailored to enable a single oblique suture line to incorporate the origins of the renal arteries as shown. Exposure of the right common iliac artery is sometimes difficult with this approach and control of the vessel with a balloon catheter after the aneurysm has been opened is sometimes preferable. The operation is otherwise conducted as in the anterior approach. The aneurysm wall is closed back over the prosthesis at the completion of the procedure. Obviously, no closure of the periaortic tissues or the parietal peritoneum is possible or necessary.

We have not found retroperitoneal exposure to reduce operative time, operative blood loss or postoperative hospital stay, as has been claimed by some authors. In fact, postoperative discomfort, in our experience, is greater with this incision than with the midline abdominal incision. However, bowel function does appear to return earlier in the postoperative period with this approach.

We believe the retroperitoneal approach is relatively contraindicated in patients with right iliac aneurysms. These aneurysms would otherwise need to be dealt with through a separate right lower quadrant transperitoneal or retroperitoneal incision. We also believe that adequate exposure with this approach is difficult to achieve in patients with a high narrow costal arch in whom the distance from the incision to the diaphragm is great, mandating that the operation take place almost entirely underneath the shelf of the rib cage.

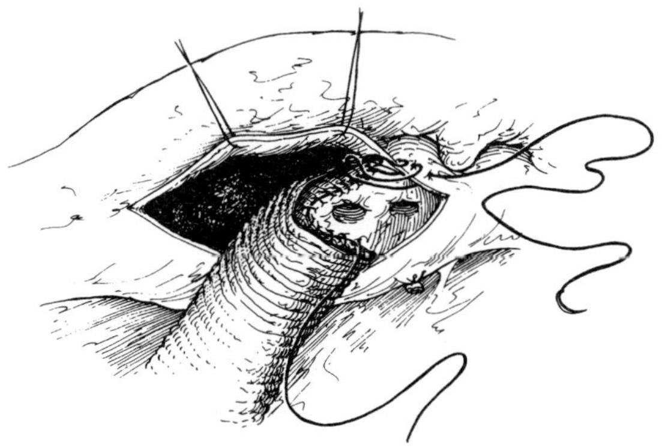

20

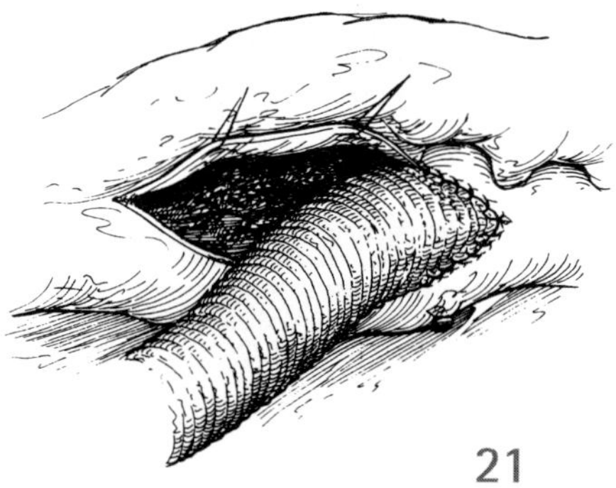

21

Acknowledgement

Illustrations by B Hyams.

References

Creech O Jr (1966). Endo-aneurysmorrhaphy and treatment of aortic aneurysm. *Annl Surg* **164**: 935.

Javid H, Julian OC, Dye WS *et al.* (1982). Complications of abdominal aortic grafts. *Arch Surg* **85**: 650.

Whittemore AD, Clowes AW, Hechtman HB, Mannick JA (1980). Aortic aneurysm repair. Reduced operative mortality associated with maintenance of optimal cardiac performance. *Annl Surg* **192**: 414.

Williams GM, Ricotta J, Zinner M, Burdick J (1980). the extended retroperitoneal approach for treatment of extensive atherosclerosis of the aorta and renal vessels. *Surgery* **88**: 846.

Juxtarenal aortic occlusion

R Courbier, J M Jausseran

Introduction

In the Leriche syndrome, progressive atherosclerotic disease involves the origin of the inferior mesenteric artery. When this artery becomes completely occluded the clot proceeds up to the level of the renal arteries; this is known as a juxtarenal aortic occlusion. Many reports have pointed to the technical problems involved in treating this (Courbier *et al.*, 1974; 1979; Liddicoat *et al.*, 1975; Starrett and Stoney, 1974; Traverso *et al.*, 1978). A classic thromoendarterectomy (Vollmar *et al.*, 1970) necessitates extensive exposure of the aorta and renal branches, which all have to be clamped.

A limited thromboendarterectomy is simpler and avoids extensive dissection, so that the aorta can be clamped at a lower level. Since 1963 we have used this technique in 102 cases (5.4% of cases of aortic reconstruction). Only in a few cases, when there is a high risk to the patient because of renal or respiratory insufficiency or when extensive disease of the visceral arteries cannot be treated, an extra-anatomical bypass is used.

Lower limb revascularization from coeliac or thoracic aorta can be indicated when subrenal aorta or abdominal wall condition prevents direct access (Barral *et al.*, 1991).

Operative technique

The patient is placed in a supine position with the left arm raised, so that a left thoracotomy can be done in case of technical problems.

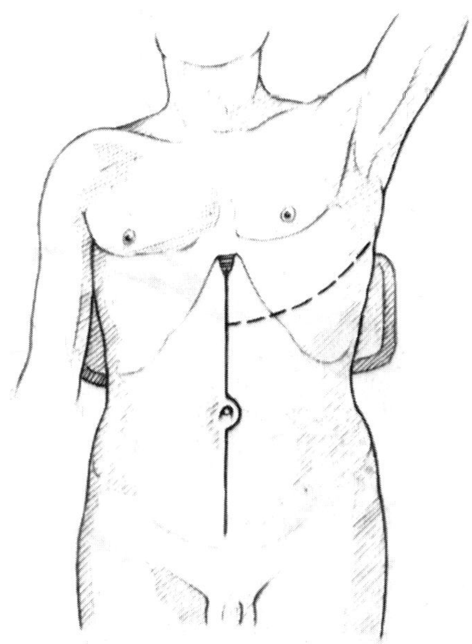

1

1

Incision

A vertical midline incision is made. Additional resection of the xyphoid increases the exposure of the upper part.

If it is not possible to expose the upper part or there is a wound in that area, a thoracoabdominal approach through the 8th intercostal space can be used.

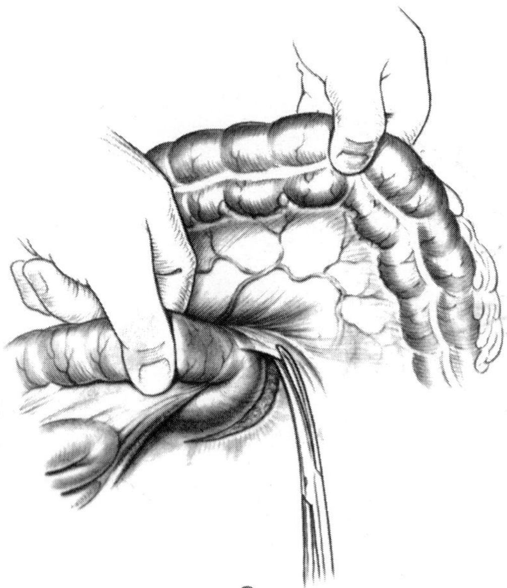

2

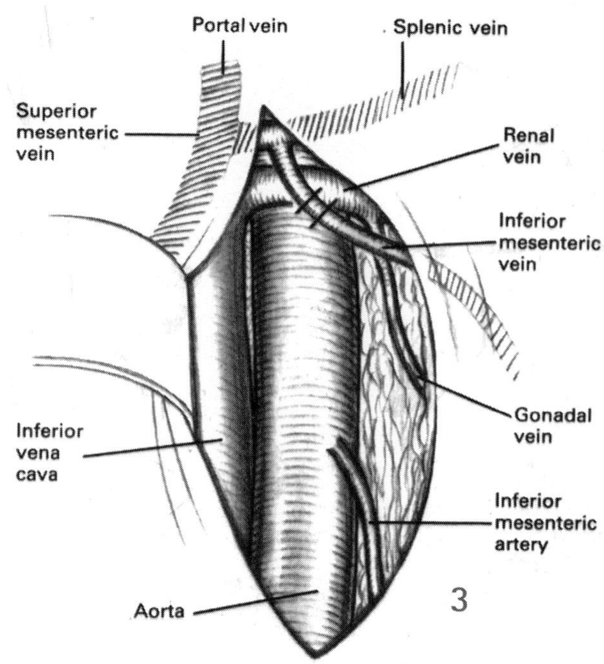

3

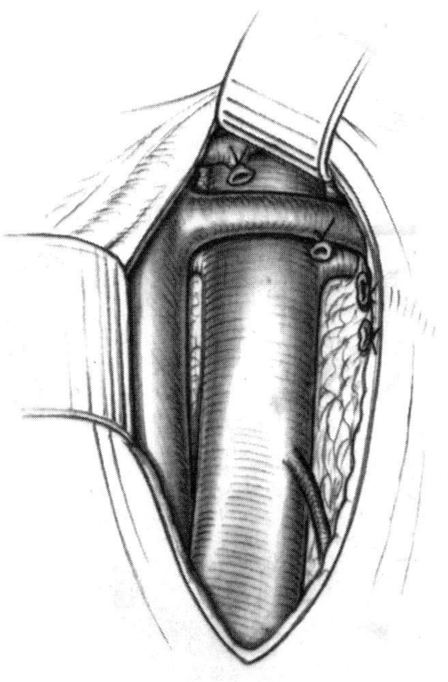

4

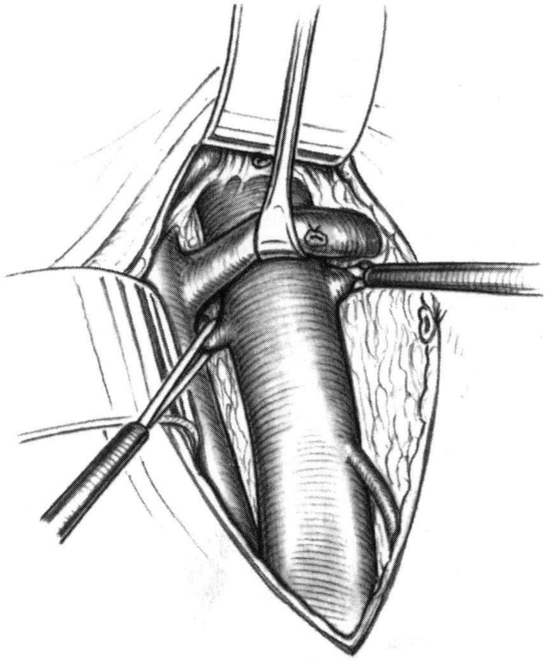

5

2

Dissection of ligament of Treitz

After incision of the posterior peritoneum, the duodenum is retracted to the right and the ligament of Treitz is incised.

3

Limited exposure of the aorta

It is necessary to divide the inferior mesenteric vein, avoiding any arterial anastomotic branch.

4

The left gonadal vein and capsular vein must also sometimes be divided.

5

Extended exposure of the aorta

This approach is used in case of arterial disease involving the origin of the renal arteries. The left renal vein is retracted and moved up or down so that a tape and a tourniquet can be placed on both renal arteries.

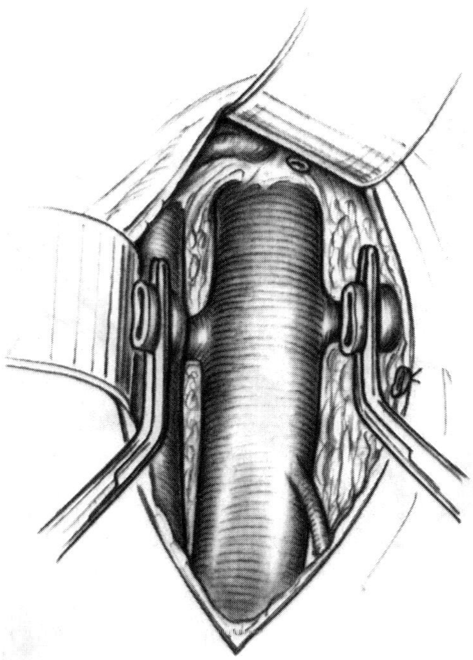

6

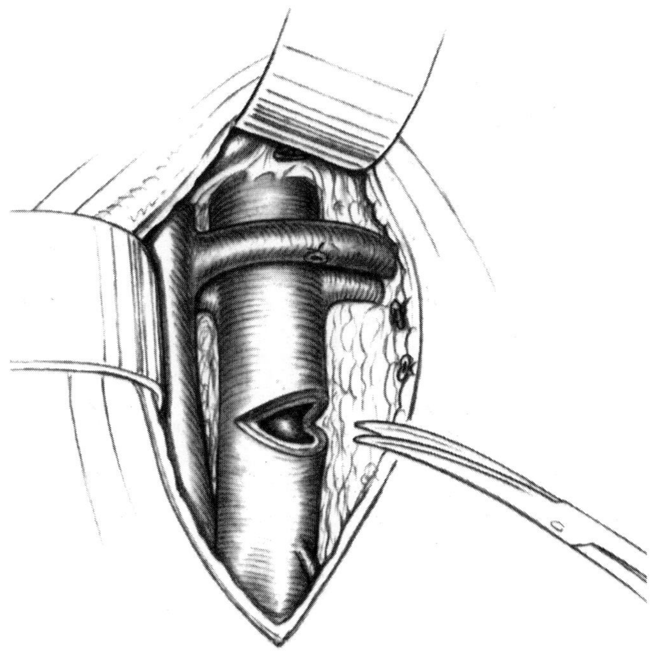

7

6

The left renal vein is divided between two arterial clamps and reconstructed later. The upper limit of the dissection is the origin of the superior mesenteric artery which does not need to be demonstrated. (With this extended dissection it is possible to perform endarterectomy of the aorta, and origins of the renal arteries. The clamp is placed across the aorta above the renal arteries. No clamp is required on the lower end.)

7

Illustration **7** shows the usual procedure where it is unnecessary to divide the left renal vein or to control the renal arteries with slings. The aorta is opened transversely, using scissors, 3 cm below the level of the renal arteries, without any posterior dissection. Clamping of the aorta is not necessary.

8

A small part of the clot is removed from the lower part of the aorta, and the artery is then occluded with a continuous suture.

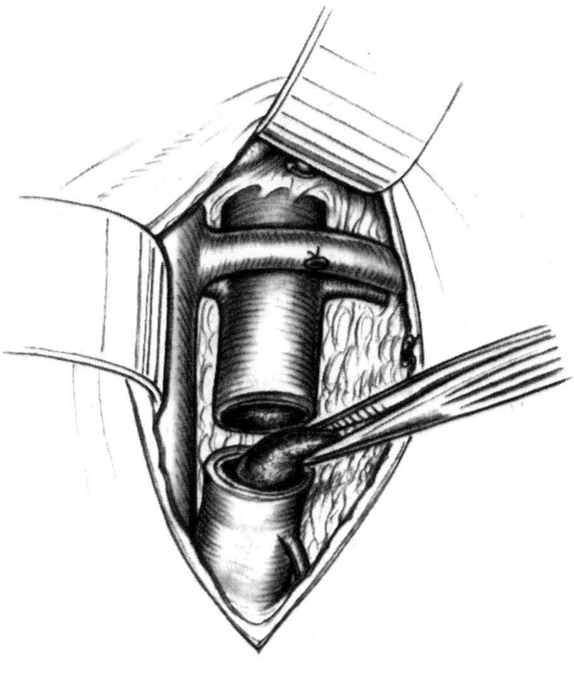

8

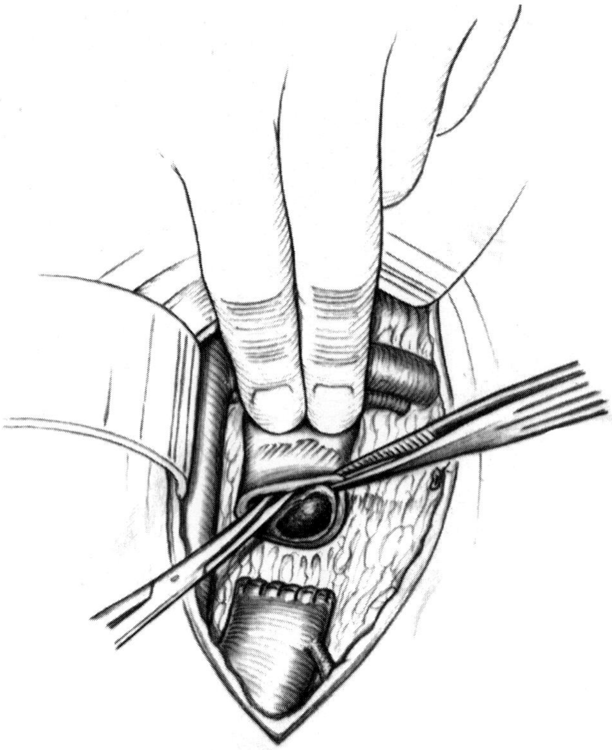

9

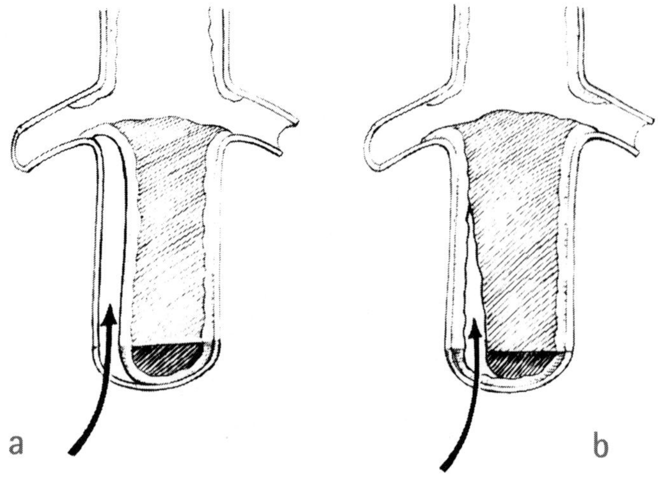

10

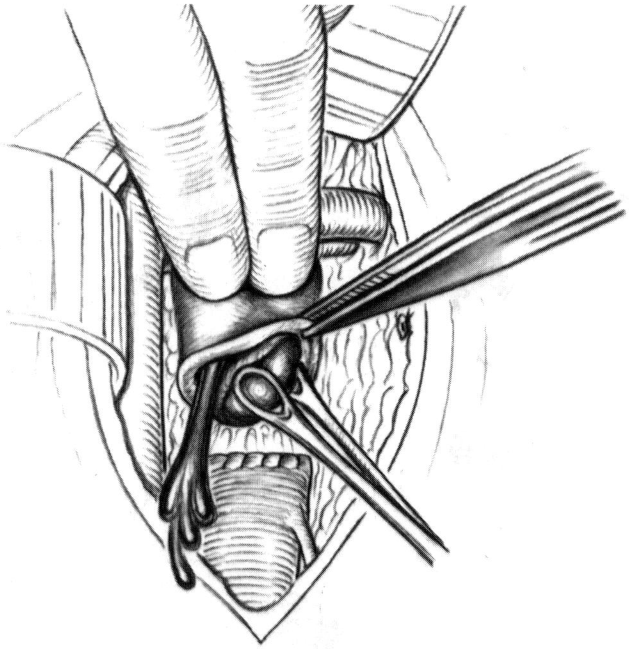

11

Thrombectomy

9

This is performed on the upper part of the aorta. The surgeon's second and third left fingers are applied to the pulsating part of the aorta just beyond the upper limit of the thrombus.

Dissection is made with a dissector or with thin scissors. It is very important to avoid the plane of thromboendarterectomy, which is too near the exterior of the artery wall, but to use the plane of thrombectomy which leaves enough artery wall behind. Dissection begins anteriorly and posteriorly and continues upward.

10a, b

The two different dissecting planes

The dissecting plane for thromboendarterectomy cannot be used in a retrograde manner because of the risk of a dissection on the origin of the renal arteries (10a).

Thrombectomy can be done without any risk. The high flow after reconstruction allows a small part of the aorta to be left without risk of rethrombosis (10b).

11

When bleeding occurs the two fingers create a temporary haemostasis and feel at the same time the tips of the dissecting scissors.

The total clot is removed *en bloc* with forceps. The finger's pressure is released to permit a flush of blood.

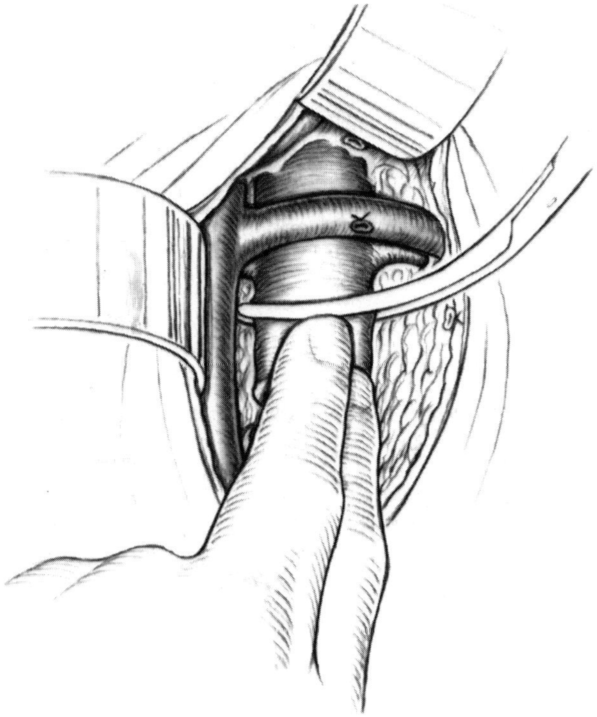

12

12

An aortic clamp is placed between the fingers and the origin of the renal arteries.

The operation can then be continued as for an ordinary aortic occlusion.

13

Supracoeliac aortic access is required for multiple aortic procedures.

A transxiphisternal laparotomy leads to an approach through the lesser sac to the right crus of the diaphragm.

A horizontal clamp of aorta at this level allows the exposure of 4–6 cm above the coeliac axis.

A prosthesis can be passed in front or behind the pancreas.

14

On occasions it is better to approach the thoracic aorta than to seek the aorta below the diaphragm, e.g. after recent infection or when much scarring is anticipated, the thoracotomy is via the 7th intercostal space. A tunnel can be made behind the diaphragm to pass a prosthesis below in the retroperitoneal space and the right limb can pass in front of the pubis.

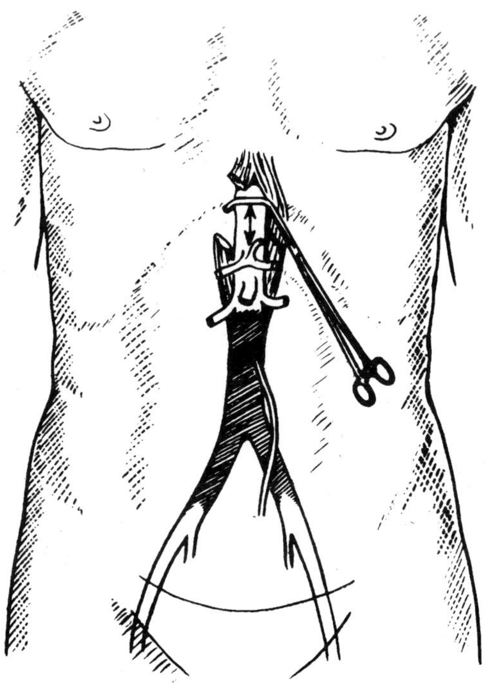

13

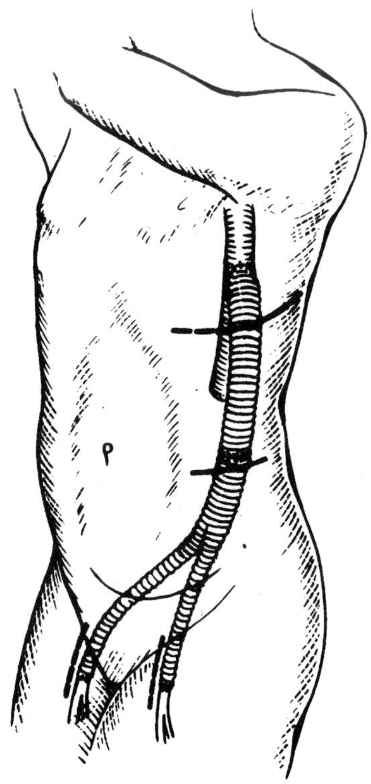

14

Acknowledgement

Illustrations by R N Lane.

References

Barral X, Gournier JP, Favre JP, Rosset E (1991). Revascularisation des membres inférieurs a partir de l'aorte thoracique. In *Les lésions occlusives aorto-iliaques chroniques*. Kieffer E ed. Paris: AERCV.

Courbier R, Jausseran JM, Reggi M (1974). Les thromboses aortiques juxtarénales. *J Chirurgie* **107**: 281.

Courbier R, Jausseran JM, Reggi M *et al.* (1979). Traitement chirurgical des thromboses aortiques juxtarénales – Résultats à long terme. *J Chirurgie* **105**: 545.

Liddicoat J, Bekassy S, Dang M, De Bakey M (1975). Complet occlusion of the infrarenal abdominal aorta: Management and results in 64 patients. *Surgery* **77**: 467.

Starrett R, Stoney R (1974). Juxtarenal aortic occlusion. *Surgery* **76**: 890.

Traverso LW, Backer JD, Dainko EA, Machleder HF (1978). Infrarenal aortic occlusion. *Ann Surg* **187**: 397.

Vollmar J, Gruss J, Lauback K (1970). Technique de la thromboendartériectomie. *J Chirurgie* **100**: 67.

Aortic bifurcation grafting for stenosing arterial disease

Michael E DeBakey

Introduction

Occlusive disease of the terminal abdominal aorta and common iliac arteries is usually well localized to this segment. The occlusive process may be complete or incomplete (stenosis) with the underlying pathologic lesion being arteriosclerotic or atherosclerotic. Whereas other diagnostic studies may be useful, arteriography is essential in order to obtain precise information regarding the site and extent of the disease, both proximally and distally, and is therefore important in planning the surgical procedure and in identifying associated occlusive disease of the renal and visceral arteries and unsuspected aneurysmal disease. In our experience, about 30% of patients have secondary segmental occlusion of the distal arterial tree. Preoperative evaluation of the patient's condition should include studies for possible concomitant occlusive vascular disease in the extracranial carotid and coronary arteries. This is emphasized by the fact that about one-third of our patients were found to have significant disease in these arterial segments.

Several methods of surgical treatment or a combination of these methods are available: 1) bypass surgery, 2) thromboendarterectomy, 3) patch-graft angioplasty, and 4) excision with graft replacement. Selection of the appropriate method or combination of methods in an individual case depends upon a number of factors, including the extent and nature of the occlusive process and involvement of the aortic wall. In some occasional patients, for example, usually young women in whom the atheroma is extremely well localized to the abdominal aorta, thromboendarterectomy with patch-graft angioplasty may be employed. In other patients in whom the wall of the abdominal aorta is extensively diseased, as in the presence of periaortic fibrosis, intense inflammatory reaction, or aneurysmal formation, resection of this segment with graft replacement is required.

On the basis of our experience extending over a period of about 40 years, the bypass operation with certain variations according to the extent and nature of the disease, has become our procedure of choice because of its simplicity, avoidance of injury to adjacent structures, and its long-term good results. The technical application of the bypass principle and its modifications or combination with other procedures, depending upon certain factors influencing its use, will be described and illustrated in this presentation.

1a–o

In patients with complete occlusion of the abdominal aorta extending up to the origin of the renal arteries, the following procedure is employed. The peritoneal cavity is opened through a midline incision (**1a**). The abdominal aorta is exposed by retraction of the small intestines to the right. A vertical incision is then made in the peritoneum overlying the aorta and separated from the aortic wall on each side, and the renal arteries are exposed. Occluding clamps are then placed on the renal arteries to prevent embolic debris into the renal arteries during the subsequent manoeuvres. The abdominal aorta immediately above the origin of the renal arteries is temporarily occluded manually, and a 4- to 5-cm vertical incision is made through the anterior aortic wall several centimetres below the origin of the arteries (**1b**).

The fairly firm thromboatherosclerotic process is recognized, and thromboendarterectomy is performed after the proper cleavage plane in the aortic wall has been identified (**1b**). The occlusive lesion is then dissected free proximally and removed. Intermittent release of pressure on the aorta permits flushing of any retained debris (**1c**). Careful visualization of the ostia of the renal arteries is important to be certain that no debris is left in the renal arteries and that dissection of the ostia of the renal arteries has not occurred. An aortic clamp is then applied to the abdominal aorta just below the origin of the renal arteries. The clamps on the renal arteries are removed, and the temporary occlusion of the aorta above the

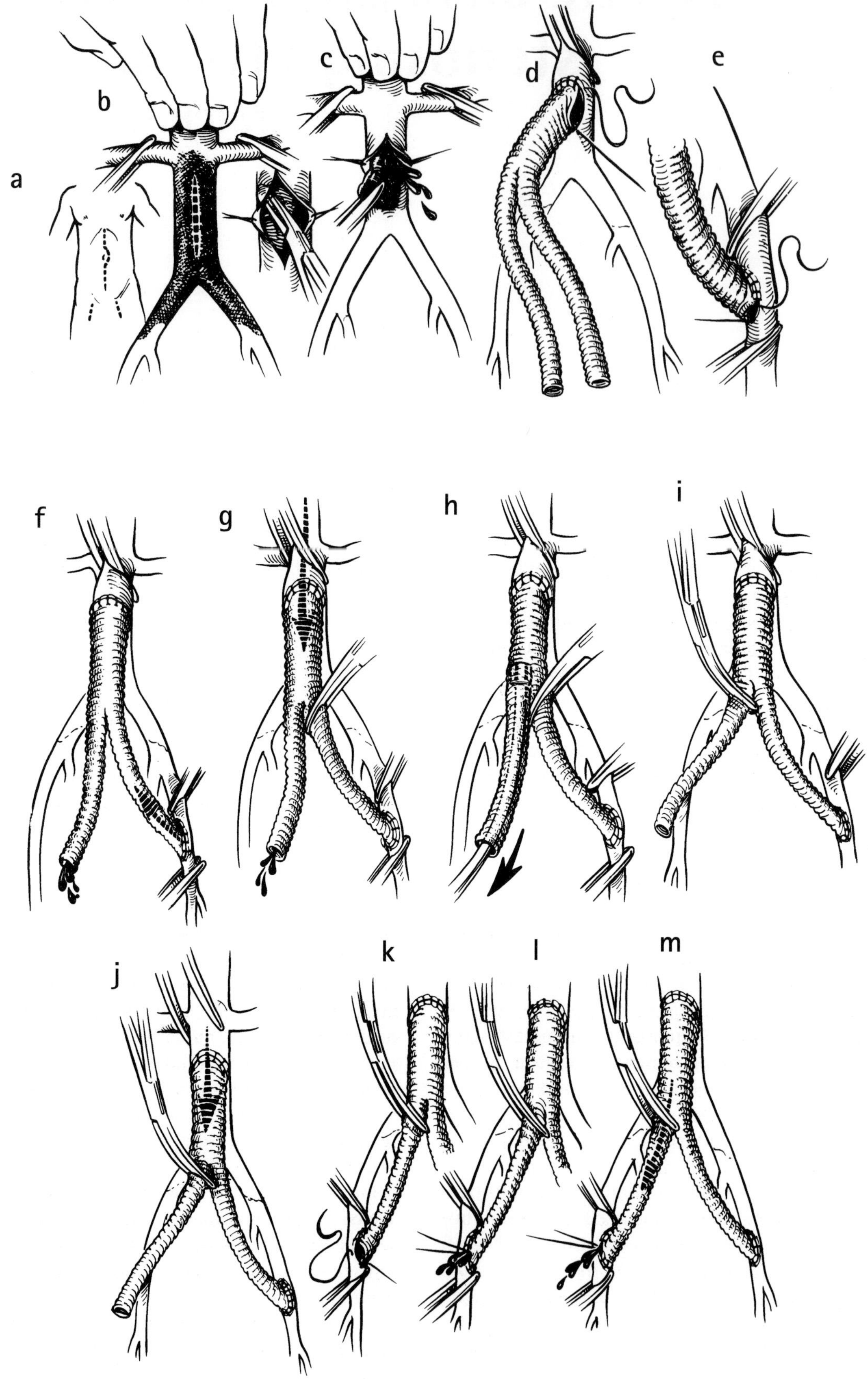

1a–m

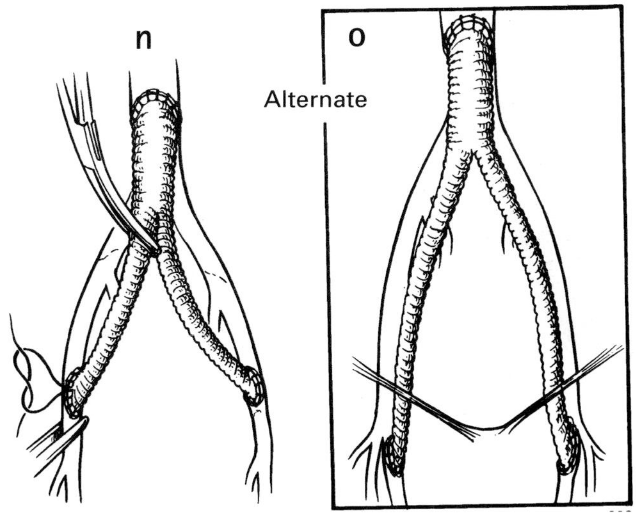

1n, o

renal arteries is released allowing restoration of renal artery perfusion (1d). This is verified by palpation of good pulses in both renal arteries.

A suitable-sized DeBakey albumin-coated Dacron bifurcation graft is selected, and the aortic end of the graft is anastomosed end-to-side to the opening in the abdominal. aorta (1d). In some cases this may be done as an end-to-end anastomosis to the opening in the abdominal aorta just below the renal arteries. The site for the distal anastomosis is then determined on the basis of the arteriogram and observation and palpation of the distal arteries. If these findings suggest that the external iliac artery is suitable, the anastomosis (end-to-side) is done at this level within the abdominal cavity (1e). If, however, there is significant disease in the external iliac artery, the distal anastomosis must be performed in the common femoral artery in the groin (1o).

The external iliac artery is exposed through an opening in the peritoneum overlying this artery in the pelvis. The appropriate limb of the previously inserted Dacron graft is passed retroperitoneally to the area of the external iliac artery. Occluding clamps are applied proximally and distally on the external iliac artery, a 1.5- to 2-cm vertical incision is made on the anterior wall of the external iliac artery, and the limb of the bifurcation is then cut at the appropriate length in a bevelled fashion and anastomosed by a continuous suture of 0000 prolene to the opening in the artery (1e). After completion of this anastomosis and just before closing to the final suture, the proximal and then the distal occluding clamps are temporarily released to flush the artery from any clot or debris (1f). The occluding clamps are then reapplied to the external iliac artery, an occluding clamp is applied to the proximal part of this limb of the graft, and the aortic occluding clamp is released for one or two pulses to wash out any clot or debris in the graft (1g). The end of a suction tube is then inserted into the open limb of the graft to remove any remaining clot or debris (1h). The occluding clamps on the external iliac artery are then removed, an occluding clamp is applied to the proximal end of the open limb of the graft (1i), and the occluding clamp in the aorta is removed, a manoeuvre that permits circulation through the anastomosed limb of the graft into that extremity (1j). The remaining limb of the bifurcation graft is then brought retroperitoneally to the exposed portion of the external iliac artery and is anastomosed to an opening in this artery as previously described (1k). Just before the suture of this anastomosis is closed, the occluding clamps on the external iliac arteries are temporarily released to flush the graft (1l), and then the occluding clamp on the graft is temporarily released to flush the graft (1m), following which the anastomotic suture is tied and all clamps are removed to permit restoration of circulation into this extremity (1n). In patients in whom the limbs of the graft must be attached to the common femoral artery, this artery is exposed by a vertical incision in the groin, and the graft is tunnelled posterior to the inguinal ligament into the groin (1o).

In patients in whom the distal limbs of the graft must be attached to the common femoral artery, it is important to determine that there is good outflow through the superficial femoral or profunda femoris or both arteries. This assumes great significance in regard to the profunda femoris when the superficial femoral artery is occluded. In such cases the profunda femoris may require profundaplasty.

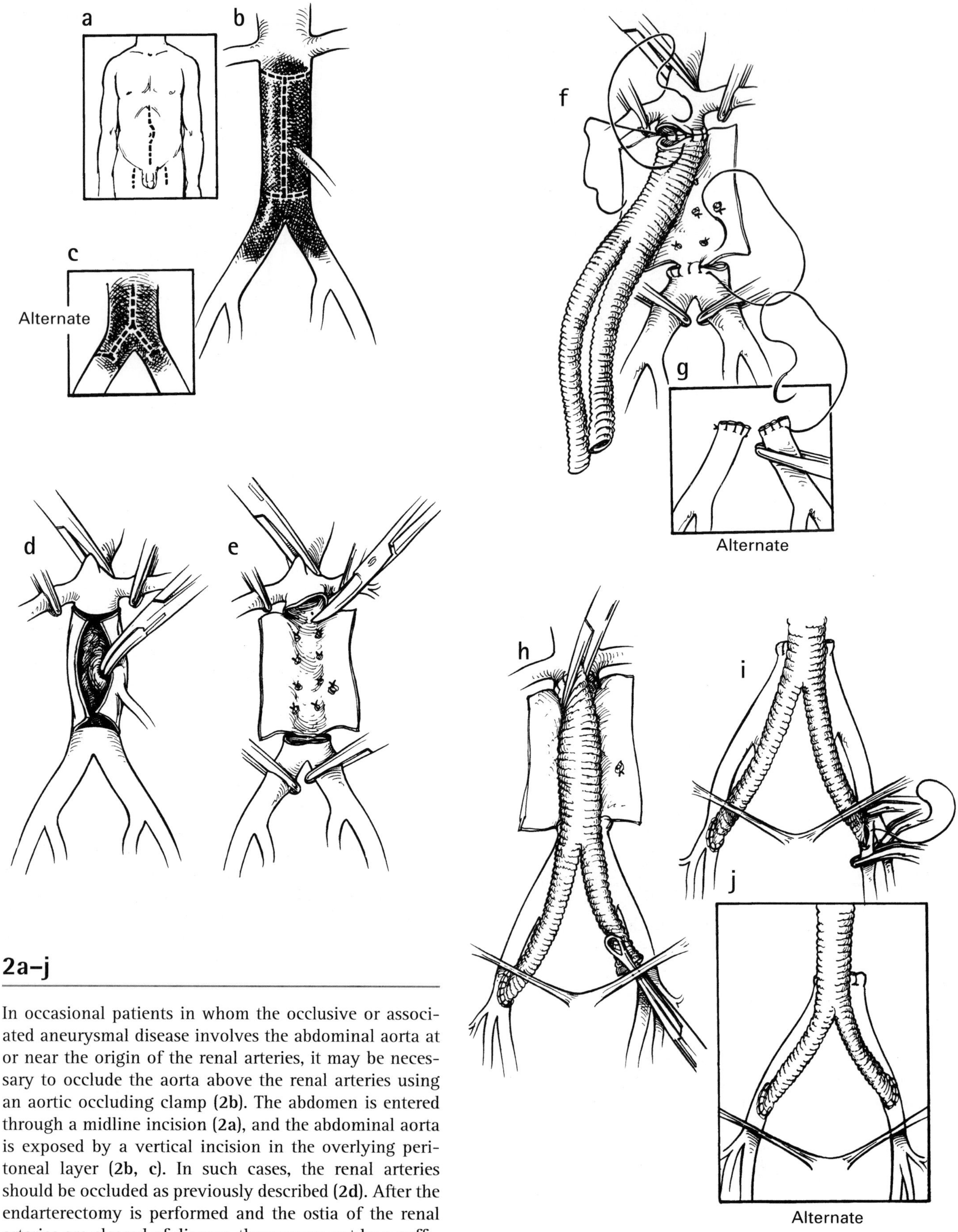

2a–j

2a–j

In occasional patients in whom the occlusive or associated aneurysmal disease involves the abdominal aorta at or near the origin of the renal arteries, it may be necessary to occlude the aorta above the renal arteries using an aortic occluding clamp (**2b**). The abdomen is entered through a midline incision (**2a**), and the abdominal aorta is exposed by a vertical incision in the overlying peritoneal layer (**2b, c**). In such cases, the renal arteries should be occluded as previously described (**2d**). After the endarterectomy is performed and the ostia of the renal arteries are cleared of disease, there many not be a sufficient amount of aorta below the renal arteries to permit the placement of an occluding clamp below the renal arteries. Under these circumstances, after completion of the endarterectomy (**2d**), the aorta is cirumferentially incised just below the ostia of the renal arteries, and the opening of the lumbar and inferior mesenteric arteries are oversewn (**2e**). In order to prevent retrograde bleeding, occluding clamps are also placed upon the common iliac arteries (**2e**).

The aortic limb of the graft is then sutured as an end-to-end anastomosis to the proximal opening in the aorta, care being taken to avoid compression of the ostia of the renal arteries (**2f**). This may be assured by placing an appropriate sized dilator into the ostia of the renal arteries during the anastomosis. After completion of this anastomosis, the aortic clamp is temporarily opened to flush the aorta and remove any clots or debris, following which the occluding clamps on the renal arteries are similarly flushed. An occluding clamp is then applied to the Dacron graft just below the anastomosis, and the occluding clamps on the aorta and both renal arteries are removed to permit restoration of circulation to the kidneys (**2h**). The attachments of the limbs of the bifurcation to the external iliac or common femoral arteries are then performed as previously described (**2i, j**). The distal opening in the abdominal aorta just above the bifurcation is closed by suture (**2f**) or the common iliac arteries are closed by suture (**2g**) depending upon local circumstances.

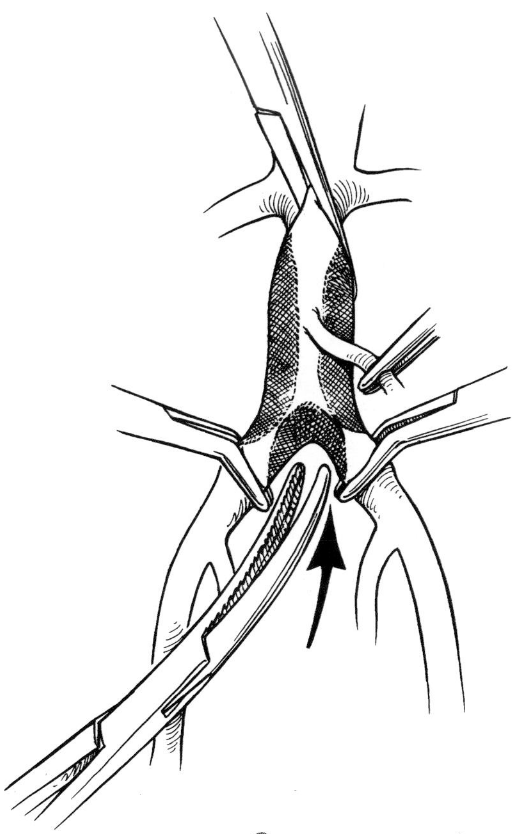

3a

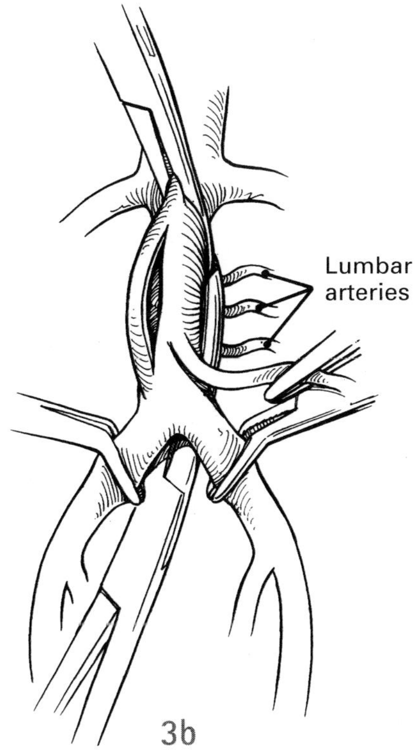

3b

3a, b

In still other patients who have incomplete occlusion but significant stenosis, the bypass procedure is usually preferred. In such cases, the abdominal aorta just distal to the renal arteries may be relatively free of disease, and endarterectomy is thus not required. After an occluding clamp is applied to the abdominal aorta just below the origin of the renal arteries and to both common iliac arteries and inferior mesenteric arteries, an aortic occluding clamp is passed under the common iliac arteries to occlude the posterior wall of the abdominal aorta to prevent retrograde bleeding from the lumbar arteries (**3a**). A longitudinal incision is then made in the abdominal aorta as close as possible to the proximal aortic occluding clamp (**3b**). The aortic limb of the Dacron graft is attached to this opening by end-to-side anastomosis, and the two limbs of the graft are attached to the external iliac or common femoral arteries as previously described.

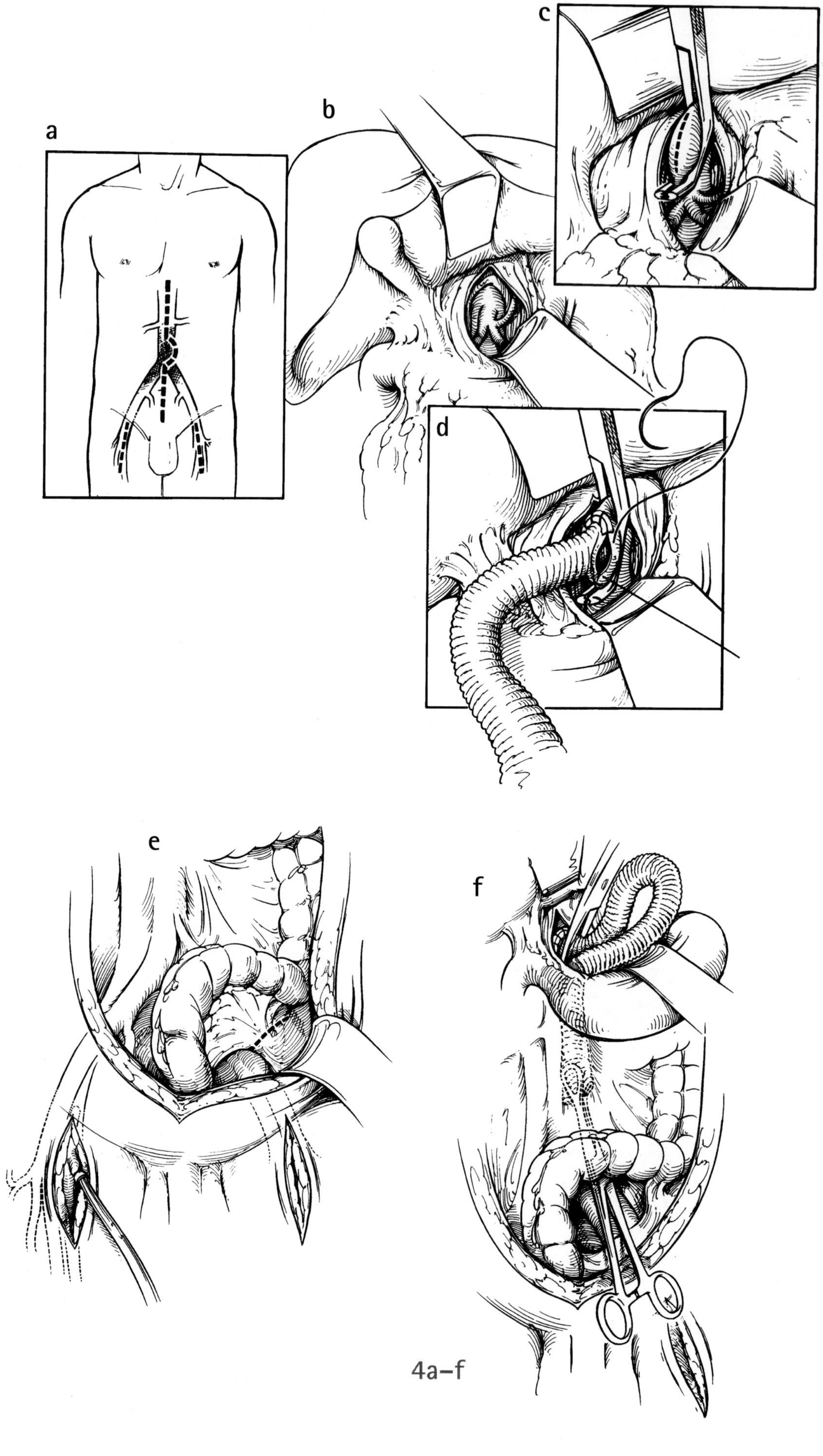

4a–f

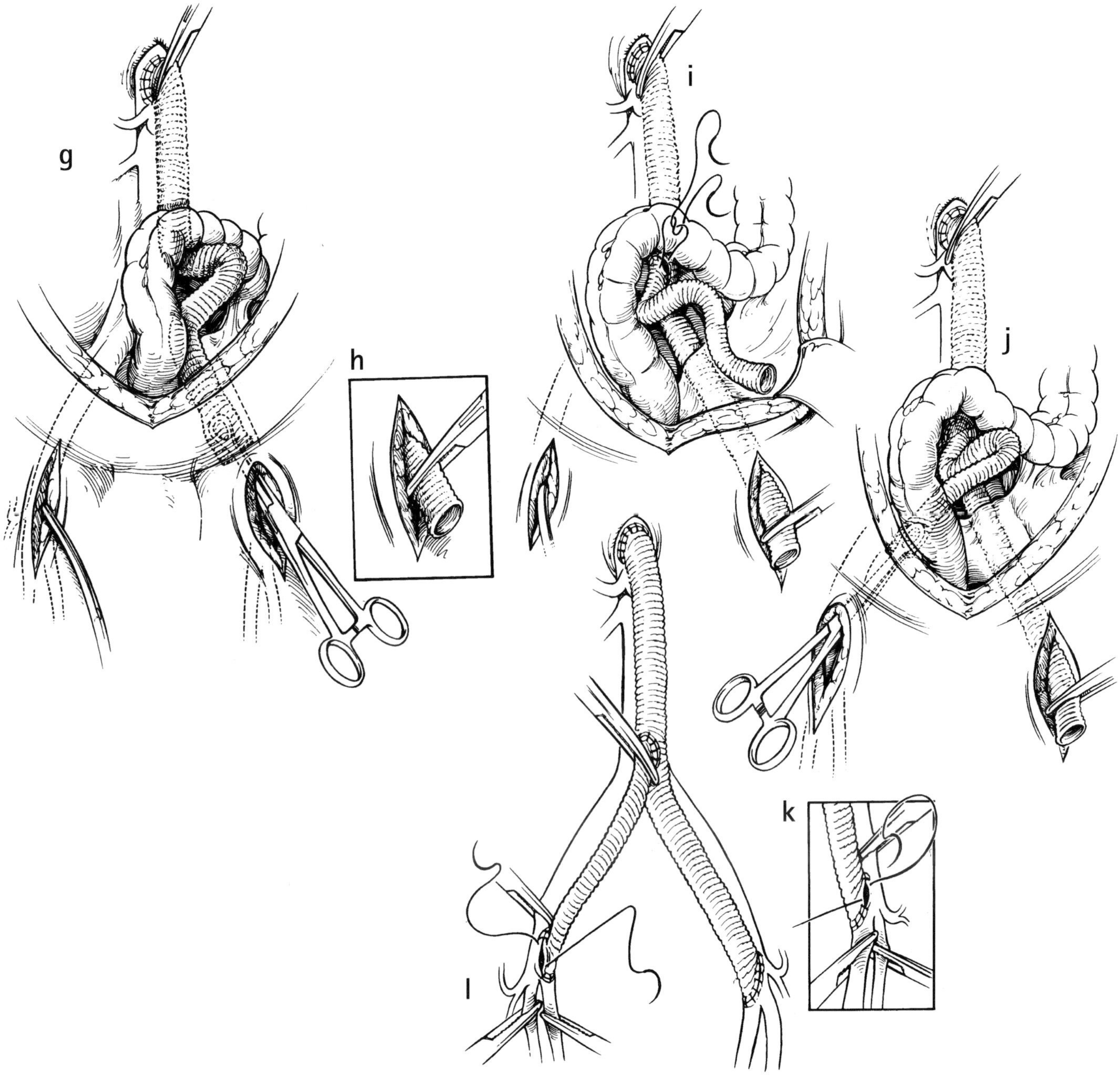

4g–l

4a–d

There are still other more complicated cases, fortunately encountered only occasionally, that require a different approach. These may be exemplified by patients in whom the infrarenal aorta is densely adherent to surrounding structures owing to previous operation or is associated with intense inflammatory reaction or periaortic fibrosis, thus creating great difficulty or even jeopardy in dissection and exposure of the infrarenal abdominal aorta. In such cases, after the peritoneal cavity is opened through a midline incision (extending up to the xyphoid) (**4a**), the abdominal aorta is exposed just below the diaphragm as it passes through the diaphragmatic hiatus by entering the lessor sac and retracting the left lobe of the liver (**4b**). A partial occluding clamp is then applied to the aorta just above the coeliac axis and a vertical incision is made in the anterior wall of the occluded portion of the aorta (**4c**). An appropriate-sized (usually ranging between 10 and 16 mm in diameter) albumin-coated tubular DeBakey Dacron graft is attached to the opening in the aorta by end-to-side anastomosis (**4d**).

4e–h

After completion of this anastomosis, an occluding clamp is applied to the Dacron graft just distal to the anastomosis and the partial occluding clamp on the abdominal aorta is removed. An incision is then made in the peritoneum overlying the iliopsoas muscle to permit entrance into the retroperitoneal space (**4e**), and by careful sharp and blunt dissection, a long sponge holder or other comparable clamp is inserted through this retroperitoneal space to the opening in the lessor sac at the site of the graft anastomosis to the aorta, and the distal end of this graft is brought out into the distal retroperitoneal opening (**4f**). The left common femoral artery is exposed through a vertical incision, and the Dacron graft is then tunnelled under the inguinal ligament (**4g**) and brought into the groin incision (**4h**).

4i–l

Here, again, as previously noted, if the distal portion of the external iliac artery is relatively normal, it is preferable to the common femoral artery for anastomosis. Another appropriate-sized (approximately 8–10 mm) albumin-coated tubular DeBakey Dacron graft is then attached by end-to-side anastomosis to a vertical opening on the right side of the previously placed aorta to right femoral graft (**4i**). This graft is then tunnelled retroperitoneally through an opening exposing the right common femoral artery (**4j**). The distal end of the graft that is brought into the left groin incision is then attached to the left common femoral artery by end-to-side anastomosis (**4k**). An occluding clamp is then applied to the Dacron graft going to the right groin just distal to its anastomosis to the main graft, and the occluding clamps on this main graft and the common femoral artery are sequentially temporarily released to flush any clots or debris, following which these clamps are removed and circulation is permitted to pass through the main graft into the legs (**4k**). The right limb of the graft is then anastomosed to the right common femoral artery as previously described (**4l**).

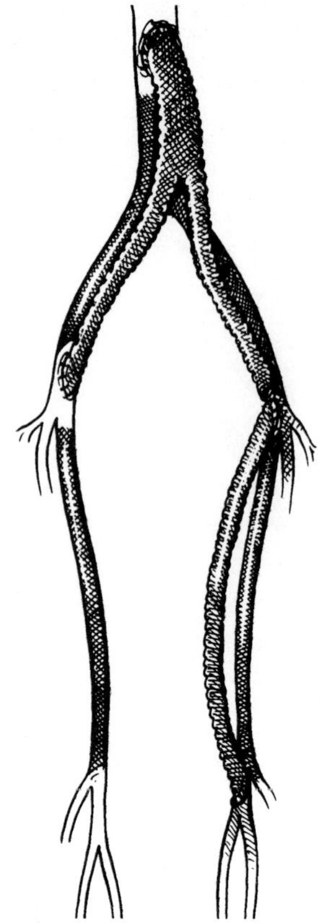

5

5

Occasionally in such cases as just described, it may be necessary to attach the proximal end of the graft to the lower part of the descending thoracic aorta rather than the abdominal aorta just below the diaphragm (**5a**). A separate lower left intercostal incision is used to expose the lower descending thoracic aorta. A partial occluding clamp is then placed on the descending thoracic aorta and a vertical incision is made along the left lateral wall of the aorta to which the graft is attached by end-to-side anastomosis. The peritoneal cavity is opened through a separate midline incision, and the graft in the left pleural cavity is tunnelled retroperitoneally through an opening in the diaphragm along the left side of the aorta as it passes through the aortic diaphragmatic hiatus.

Acknowledgement

Illustrations by Jan Redden: © Baylor College of Medicine 1989.

Management of aortic graft infection

Larry H Hollier

Introduction

Aortic graft infection is a complication that is universally dreaded by vascular surgeons since it often represents not only a breakdown in surgical technique but also a potentially lethal problem. The natural history of aortic graft infection can vary from a chronic draining fistula to acute arterial wall necrosis with false aneurysm, sepsis, or exsanguinating haemorrhage. Obviously, the management of graft infection is influenced by multiple factors, the most prominent of which are time of onset in relation to surgery, site of infection, extent of infection, location of the graft, aortoenteric fistula, and run-off vessels.

In general, aortic graft infections that occur shortly after surgery should be considered as diffuse infections that will involve the entire graft, since true tissue incorporation and obliteration of perigraft spaces have not yet occurred. These almost invariably require removal of the entire graft. Infections occurring months or years after graft implantation, however, will often be found to be localized to a specific segment of the graft which may allow extra-anatomic revascularization with salvage of most of the previous graft and excision of only the area infected. This technical discussion relates to this aspect of segmental excision of graft infection with preservation of the uninfected graft segments.

Evaluation

Although the literature is replete with multiple modalities used for identifying graft infection, we find only a few tests of significant value.

The physical examination

The presence of a draining sinus in the groin in a patient who has a previous aortofemoral graft should be sufficient evidence to suggest the diagnosis of graft infection. The only question to be answered subsequently relates to the extent of the infection. In this situation, performance of a sinugram with thin barium or Hypaque is often sufficient to delineate any proximal extension of the infection. A more subtle sign of intra-abdominal graft infection is unilateral lower extremity osteoarthropathy with joint swelling and clubbing of the toes that are indicative of bowel erosion by one limb of an aortic bifurcation graft.

Computerized tomography

Computerized tomography (CT scan) is a valuable tool in the evaluation of patients with suspected aortic graft infection and particularly in the evaluation of upper gastrointestinal bleeding in a patient with previous placement of an aortic graft. A CT scan may uncommonly show inflammatory changes and fluid around an aortic graft, though these do not necessarily indicate graft infection. However, perigraft air that is present more than 3 months after aortic graft placement should be considered diagnostic of graft infection. Although one cannot definitively make a diagnosis of aortoenteric fistula on a CT scan, the presence of a continuous and uninterrupted fat line separating the graft line from the overlying bowel is presumptive of there being no aortoenteric fistula if the CT sections are taken at 0.5-cm intervals.

Endoscopy

Upper gastrointestinal endoscopy should be performed routinely in patients with a prior aortic graft who present with gastrointestinal bleeding. Attempts should be specifically made to examine the entire duodenum since graft erosion commonly occurs in the third or fourth portion of the duodenum. While endoscopy may be helpful if a graft is visualized through the distal duodenal wall, failure to identify a bleeding point does not necessarily exclude the possiblity of aorteoenteric fistula. Additionally, identification of other bleeding sites, such as gastric erosion or duodenal ulcer, likewise does not exclude aortoenteric fistula but does mandate the need for further evaluation.

Leukocyte scan

Indium-labelled leukocyte may be injected intravenously and used for identification of indolent graft infection. Although this can occasionally provide some false-positive or false-negative findings, if the scan does show a 'hot spot' along the course of the graft or one of its limbs, it may be helpful in localizing and identifying the extent of infection.

Angiography

Angiography is generally not useful in determining the presence of graft infection or aortoenteric fistula. Nonetheless, we routinely recommend angiography in patients with graft infection, primarily for full delineation of the status of run-off vessels. We believe that this allows better planning for operative intervention for removal of the graft, assessment of collaterals, and revascularization of the lower extremities.

Management

1a, b, c

Unilateral groin infection

Under general anaesthesia, the draining site in the groin is carefully sealed with an occlusive dressing and the abdomen and lower extremity is prepped with providone-iodine solution and draped in a sterile fashion. A vertical transabdominal incision is made and the peritoneum over the aortic graft bifurcation is incised transversely. The graft limb to the involved side is dissected proximally just beyond the bifurcation of the graft. Good incorporation of surrounding tissues suggests that the graft in this area is free of infection. Even though some perigraft fluid may be present, if the perigraft space does not obviously connect to the groin and if the perigraft fluid is free of bacteria (as evidenced by Gram stain), we would proceed with proximal graft preservation and distal revascularization through the obturator canal. The involved limb is doubly clamped, transected and oversewn distally. That end of the graft is then pushed distally and the peritoneum overlying it is closed to the retroperitoneal space with running sutures of 3/0 prolene to separate the distal graft limb completely from the proximal graft. An 8-mm thin-wall ringed Gore-Tex graft is then sutured end-to-end to the proximal limb of the bifurcation graft and a separate retroperitoneal tunnel is made down to the obturator foramen. A vertical incision is then made distally on the medial thigh and the popliteal artery at this level is exposed and isolated. Using a long metal tunneller, the Gore-Tex graft is passed through the obturator foramen to lie in the space posterior to the pectineus, adductor longus and adductor brevis, and anterior to the adductor magnus. The graft is then anastomosed to the

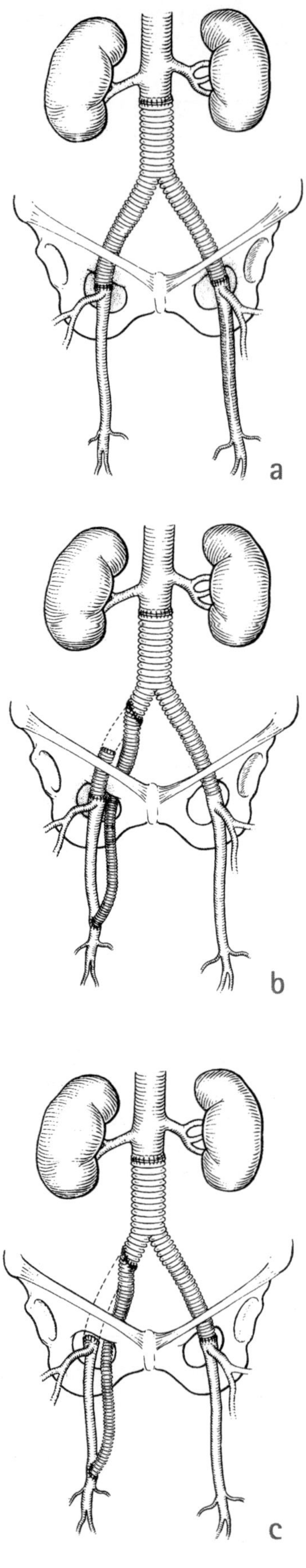

1

popliteal artery above the knee and flow is restored through the graft (**1b**).

The abdominal incision and medial thigh incisions are then closed in standard fashion and sterile dressings are applied. The patient is then redraped and the infected groin is exposed and again prepared with povidone-iodine solution. The fistulous tract is excised and the graft is exposed. The graft is then disconnected from its anastomosis to the femoral artery and arterial back bleeding is controlled with balloon catheters and three-way stopcocks. Simple running closure of the femoral artery is performed with 3/0 prolene. The graft is then gently dissected proximally and forcefully withdrawn from its retroperitoneal tunnel. The entire area is then irrigated copiously with antibiotic solution (neomycin-bacitracin-polymyxin) and a suction catheter is left in the tract from which the graft was removed. The wound is then loosely reapproximated to cover the femoral vessels and the skin is packed open with iodoform gauze (**1c**).

All patients undergoing such reconstruction for graft infection are administered intravenous antibiotics preoperatively which are continued for 4–5 days postoperatively. The suction catheter is generally removed after 24 hours and local wound care is continued until healing is complete.

2a, b, c

Isolated bilateral groin infection

The development of bilateral groin infection should strongly suggest that the entire aortic graft is infected. However, if careful evaluation by sinugram, leukocyte indium scan and computerized tomography are all indicative of infections isolated to the groins alone and not the body of the graft, selective proximal graft preservation may be indicated (**2a**).

In a fashion similar to the management of unilateral groin infection, the draining sinuses in the groin are carefully sealed, usually by placing a povidone-iodine soaked sponge over the draining sinus and suturing it circumferentially to the skin. The abdomen and lower extremities are then prepared and draped and a midline incision is made in the abdomen. The distal area of the graft bifurcation in each limb is isolated proximally. Again, a Gram stain is made of any perigraft fluid and routine cultures are submitted. The graft is doubly clamped, transected, and the distal portion oversewn. Each limb is then pushed distally into its retroperitoneal tunnel and the distal portion of the tunnel is sealed. Externally supported thin-wall 8-mm Gore-Tex grafts are then sutured end-to-end to the proximal limbs of the bifurcation graft and, as described for unilateral groin infections, the grafts are passed through the obturator tunnel and sutured distally to the popliteal arteries (**2b**). The abdominal and thigh incisions are then closed and sterile dressings are applied.

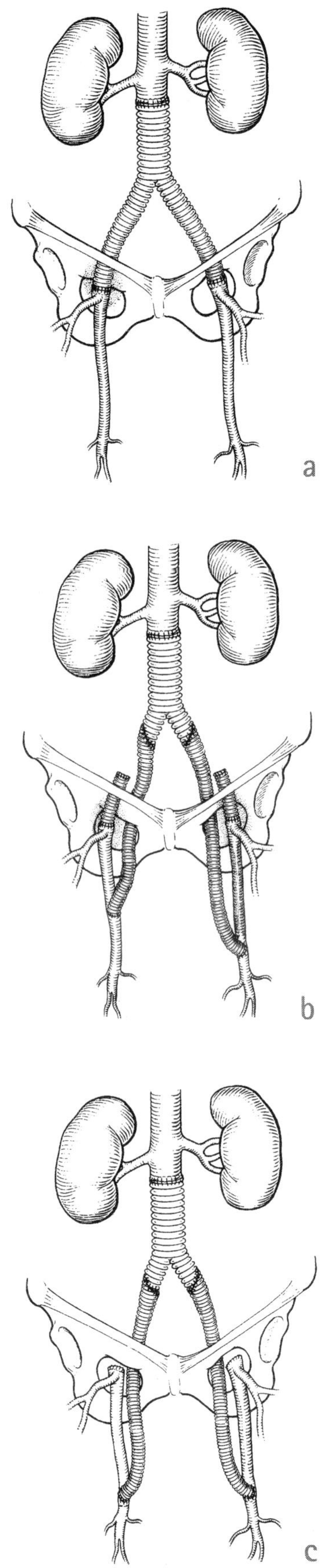

2

Adhesive drapes are then placed on the patient to completely seal away these previous operative sites. The groin areas are left exposed and the occlusive dressings on the groins are removed. The groins are then prepared with povidone-iodine solution and vertical incisions are made in each groin exposing the infected graft segments. The anastomosis is taken down on each side, with control of bleeding from the femoral vessels obtained by balloon catheters with three-way stopcocks. The femoral arteries are closed primarily with running sutures of 3/0 prolene. The proximal extension of the infected graft segments are then gently mobilized and forcefully removed from their tunnel proximal to the inguinal ligament. The areas of dissection are then copiously irrigated with antibiotic solution and suction catheters are left in each tract and brought out through separate stab incisions in each groin. Deep tissue is closed over the femoral vessels themselves and superficial layers are generally packed open with iodoform gauze. The suction catheters are removed after 24–48 h and the wounds are allowed to heal by secondary intention.

3a, b, c

Proximal graft infection

Aortic graft infection may occur but may be confined to the abdomen if a straight aortic graft has been placed, or

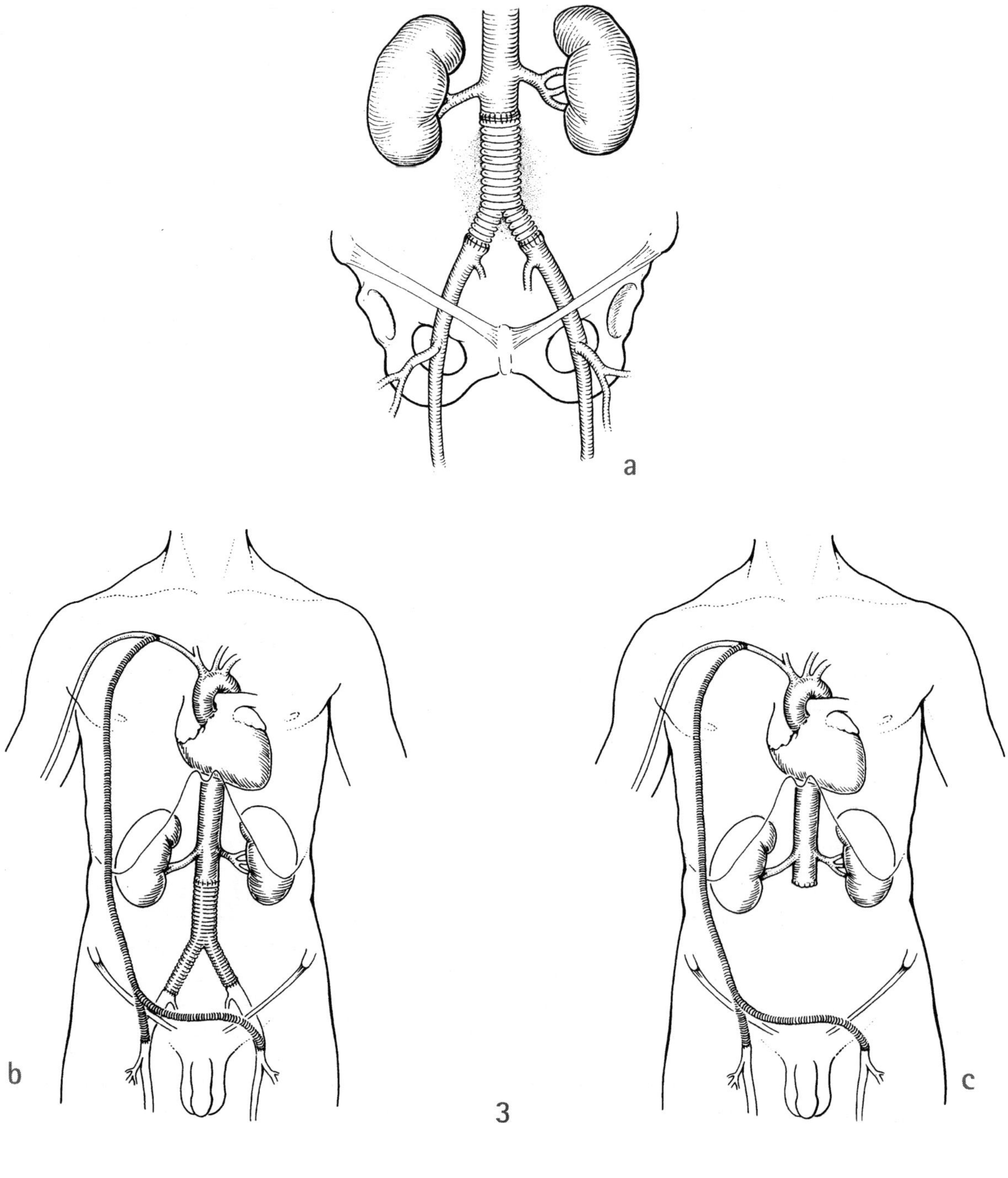

3

if a bifurcation graft has been anastomosed distally to the common iliac or external iliac arteries. In these situations, the groins and the vessels distal to the inguinal ligament are considered to be uninfected (**3a**). Occasionally, patients with aortobifemoral grafts develop isolated proximal graft infections, but with the distal limbs, i.e. the femoral anastomoses, free of infection. This is perhaps most commonly seen in patients who develop aortoenteric fistula from simple graft erosion. Although one might selectively treat some of these patients by removal of the infected graft and direct reimplantation of another Dacron graft, we would generally perform extra-anatomic bypass and complete removal of the infected intra-abdominal graft.

In patients with aortic graft infection isolated to the abdomen, we prefer to do preliminary axillofemoral–crossfemoral bypass as the initial procedure, followed by graft excision either at the same operation or with an interval of 1–2 days, depending upon the stability of the patient. For axillofemoral–crossfemoral bypass, the patient is generally placed under general endotracheal anaesthesia. However, in very high-risk patients, we have performed this procedure under local infiltration anaesthesia for the axillary dissection and epidural anaesthesia for the groin dissection.

The patient is placed on the table in a supine position and prepared from the chin to the knees with povidone-iodine solution. Determination of which axillary artery to use as the donor or inflow vessel is made preoperatively by measuring blood pressure in each arm and selecting the axillary artery with the higher blood pressure. In most cases, the right axillary artery is used. A small roll is placed vertically under the right posterior hemithorax to elevate that side of the chest slightly off of the table and to allow more thorough prepping. The arm is placed outward on an armboard. In these patients, we frequently use a multi-team approach with one surgeon exposing the axillary artery and other surgeons exposing each femoral artery.

The axillary incision is made transversely in the intraclavicular area and the underlying pectoralis major muscle is split in the direction of its fibres. The pectoralis minor muscle is identified and, after dividing the clavipectoral fascia, the insertion of the pectoralis minor on the coracoid process is divided with the electrocautery unit. The underlying axillary artery is thus exposed. The axillary artery at this level must be carefully dissected away from the adjacent nerve trunks. Small bridging veins will sometimes run across the axillary artery in this area and these should be doubly ligated and divided. It is sometimes helpful to divide the artery to the pectoralis major muscle as it arises from the axillary artery. This allows better mobilization of the axillary artery and a more proximal placement of the graft anastomosis can be accomplished. An 8-mm or 10-mm thin-walled externally supported Gore-Tex graft is then sutured end-to-side to the axillary artery. A long metal tunneller is passed cephalad from the right groin without any counter-incision being made in the skin laterally. Every attempt is made to place this tunnel in the mid-axillary line rather than directly anterior over the chest and abdomen. Several rings of the externally supported graft are removed in the most proximal portion of the femoral incision and a tangential segment of the graft is excised medially. Another segment of externally support 8-mm Gore-Tex graft is then sutured end-to-side to the axillofemoral graft at this level and this side limb is then tunnelled subcutaneously just above the level of the pubis and brought into the opposite groin. Each limb is then sutured end-to-side to the femoral artery and flow can be restored to both lower extremities in this fashion. If the patient has had a previous aortobifemoral graft placed but the femoral portions are free of infection, the previous Dacron graft on each side is simply transected and the proximal portions are oversewn. The proximal graft limbs are then pushed cephalad into their tunnel and are made to lie proximal to the inguinal ligament. The inguinal ligament is then sutured posteriorly to the underlying tissue to separate these tunnels completely from the groin. The axillofemoral–crossfemoral limbs can then be sewn directly, end-to-end, to the previous graft just proximal to their femoral anastomoses (**3b**). These wounds are then closed in layers and sterile dressings are applied.

Removal of the infected abdominal graft may be performed either at this time or deferred to a separate operation 24–48 hours later. At that time, the abdomen is prepared and draped in the usual fashion and a midline incision is performed. The infected graft is exposed and removed completely (*c*). Proximally, the aorta is debrided back from the original suture line and closed with interrupted mattress sutures of 3/0 or 0 prolene. A pedicle of omentum is then mobilized and passed through the transverse mesocolon so that it can be carefully wrapped around the aortic stump. If there has been extensive purulence in the peritoneal perigraft space, irrigating and suction catheters may be placed and brought out through separate stab incisions in the flank opposite the axillofemoral crossfemoral graft (**3c**).

4a, b, c

Aortoenteric fistula

Aortoenteric fistula may present as a sudden, severe, near-exsanguinating haemorrhage or may present as several minor episodes of gastrointestinal bleeding. If the patient has an unequivocal diagnosis and remains relatively stable, we would prefer to do an axillofemoral–crossfemoral bypass as the preliminary step followed by immediate graft removal and repair of the fistula. However, if exsanguinating haemorrhage is the overriding clinical feature, or if the diagnosis is in ques-

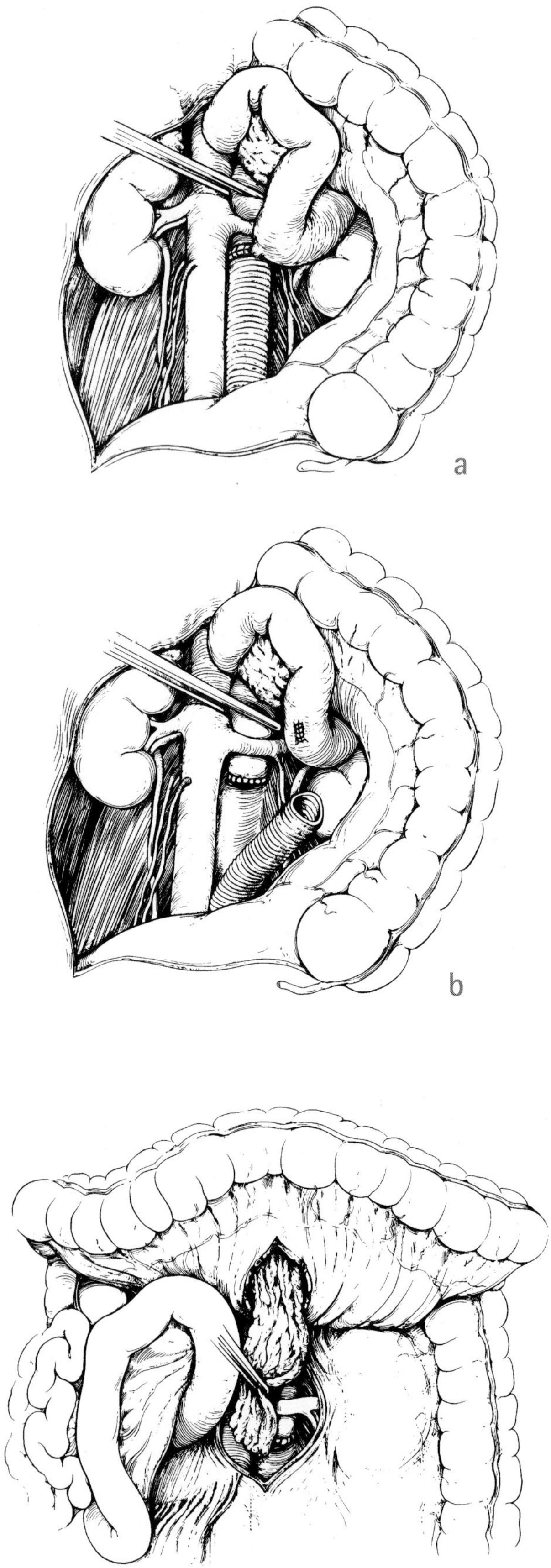

a

b

c

4

tion, primary laparotomy would be preferred, with revascularization by axillofemoral–crossfemoral graft deferred until after removal of the infected abdominal graft.

For repair of aortoenteric fistula, a transperitoneal approach is made. After entering the abdomen, the peritoneal reflection on the right lateral aspect of the ascending colon is incised and continued medially around the ciecum and extended cephalad to mobilize the hepatic flexure of the colon. A Kocher manoeuvre is then performed mobilizing the second portion of the duodenum and the head of the pancreas. This approach allows rapid dissection in previously undissected planes and minimizes the amount of time required to expose the aorta for control. By mobilizing the abdominal viscera to the left, one exposes the inferior vena cava and easily approaches the aorta above the level of the left renal vein where, in most cases, it has been spared the extensive scarring that would be evident in the infrarenal portion. This allows rapid placement of a clamp, suprarenally if necessary (**4a**). After proximal control is obtained, the duodenum can be further mobilized and the site of erosion of the duodenum by the graft can be approached in this fashion. Once the aortoenteric fistula is adequately exposed the clamps may be moved to the infrarenal position if adequate infrarenal aorta remains. If not, the aorta may be locally debrided and closed at this point so that the aortic clamp may be removed and flow restored to the renal arteries.

The opening in the duodenum is then gently debrided and the duodenum is closed in two layers. The distal graft is then removed entirely. If the distal anastomoses had been made to the common iliac or external iliac arteries, the anastomotic sites are simply oversewn with 3/0 prolene sutures (**4b**).

After closure of the aortic stump and removal of the graft, the right colon is returned to its normal anatomic position. A pedicle of omentum is mobilized and passed through the transverse mesocolon. The omental pedicle is then carefully tacked around the aortic stump to help in the prevention of stump blow-out. Irrigating and suction catheters are then left in the retroperitoneum and brought out through a flank incision opposite to the side of the previous or planned axillofemoral–crossfemoral graft (**4c**).

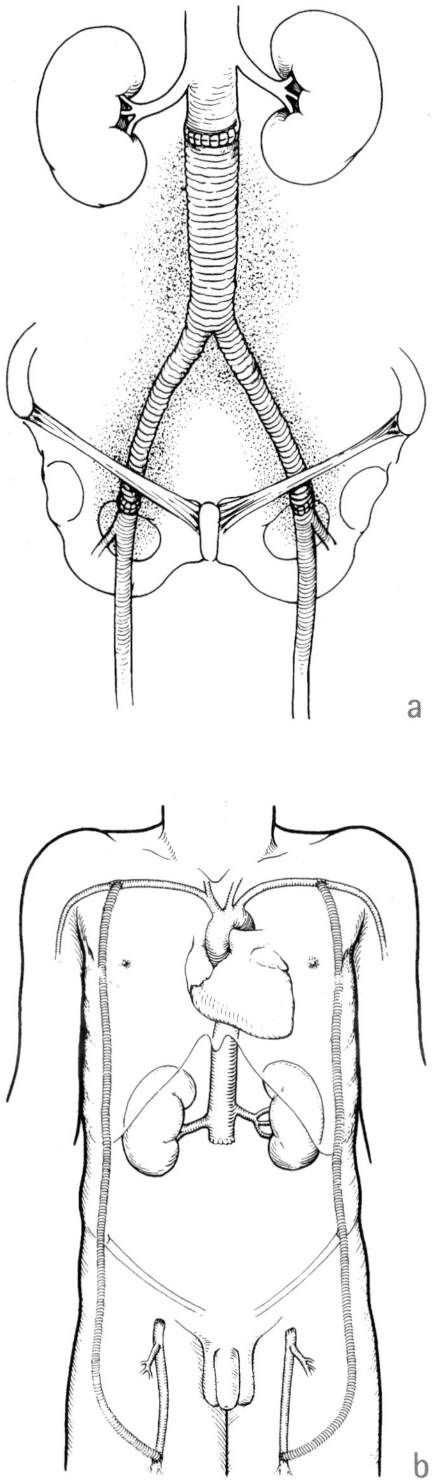

5

5a, b

Aortofemoral graft infection

When an aortobifemoral graft infection is identified with infection evident both in the groin and intra-abdominally, we generally manage this by bilateral axilloprofunds or axillopopliteal bypasses with subsequent removal of the entire aortobifemoral graft. Any draining sinuses are carefully sealed as previously described and the patient is placed in a supine position with both arms extended laterally on armboards (**5a**). The patient is prepared with povidone-iodine solution from the chin to toes so that complete exposure can be facilitated. Since both groins are infected, we avoid any incision in those areas and plan to bring the graft more laterally down to the popliteal artery.

Occasionally, however, if the superficial femoral arteries are patent and the infected graft is placed high on the common femoral artery, one might perform a distal anastomosis to the profunda vessels with expectation of a retrograde filling of the profunda and the superficial femoral artery after ligation of the common femoral artery. If the infected graft is anastomosed to the femoral bifurcation or if the superficial femoral arteries are occluded, the lower extremities are revascularized by bilateral axillopopliteal grafts.

Bilateral infraclavicular incisions are made and the axillary arteries are exposed as previously described. Bilateral incisions are then made laterally just above each knee and the popliteal arteries are exposed and isolated. Because of the distance between the axillary and popliteal incisions, a small counter-incision is usually required to facilitate passage of the graft. This counter-incision is made lateral to the posterior superior iliac spine and a tunnel is made subcutaneously cephalad and caudad from this area. Externally supported 8-mm thin-wall Gore-Tex grafts are then obtained and a graft is sutured to each axillary artery as previously described. Each graft is then passed through the subcutaneous tunnel with the graft placed along the mid-axillary line and lateral aspect of the thigh. The grafts are then sutured to the popliteal artery above the knee in each thigh and flow is restored to the lower extremities. These incisions are closed and sterile dressings are applied (**5b**).

The groins are then opened and the infected grafts are removed from their anastomosis to the femoral vessels. The femoral arteries are closed with prolene and every attempt is made to maintain a patent femoral bifurcation if possible. The abdomen is then opened and the graft is removed as previously described. As always, an attempt is made to provide coverage of the aortic stump by a pedicle of omentum.

Additional approaches

Obviously, many techniques have been devised for the management of aortic graft infection. These include direct replacement of the infected graft with a new prosthesis, rotation of muscle flaps to cover the infected graft, replacement of infected graft with autogenous tissue, and graft removal without any revascularization whatsoever.

While each of these techniques is occasionally applicable to a specific patient, they are not always feasible. Thus, this discussion has centred primarily on extra-anatomic revascularization and graft removal.

We have inadequate experience with direct replacement of an infected graft by a new prosthesis and are unable to comment about its safety. We have used rotation of muscle flaps to cover grafts in approximately 30 patients, but have been disappointed with the results. Although one can occasionally get healing of a graft that has been exposed by breakdown of overlying tissues, we have found it less helpful in eradicating established graft infection. Similarly, we have used autogenous reconstruction on several patients and found that it is satisfactory for revascularization in contaminated fields, but, unfortunately, blow-out of autogenous tissue may occur when it has been placed in areas of established infection. Because of the high incidence of lower extremity ischaemia following simple removal of an infected aortic graft without revascularization, we have abandoned that technique entirely.

Although specific situations may allow the vascular surgeon to utilize a lesser procedure for the management of graft infection, we believe that most patients with established aortic graft infection are best managed by preliminary revascularization by an extra-anatomic route, followed by removal of all infected graft material.

Editorial note

No firm evidence for the optimum technique is available (Bandyke, 1999). The potential benefits of either graft soaked in antibiotics (e.g. Rifampicin bonding) or silver impregnated grafts needs to be fully evaluated.

References

Bandyk DF (1999). Vascular graft infection. In *Vascular Surgical Highlights 1988–1999.* Davies A H ed. Oxford: Health Press. pp. 21–28.

Brown OW, Stanson AW, Pairolero PC, Hollier LH (1982). Computerized tomography following abdominal aortic surgery. *Surgery* **91**: 716.

Cherry KJ, Hollier LH (1982). Prophylactic antibiotics in vascular surgery. In *Extra-anatomic and Secondary Arterial Reconstruction.* **Greenhalgh R M** ed. London: Pitman.

Goldstone J, Moore WS (1974). Infection in vascular prostheses. *Am J Surg* **128**: 225.

Paaske WP, Buchart Hansen JH (1985). Graft enteric fistulas and erosions. *Surg Gynecol Obstet* **161**: 161.

Perdue GD, Smith RB, Ansley JD, Constantine MJ (1983). Impending aorto-enteric hemorrhage: The effect of early recognition on improved outcome. *Annl Surg* **192**: 237.

Shue WB, Worosilo SC, Donetz AP *et al.* (1988). Prevention of vascular prosthetic infection with an antibiotic-bonded Dacron graft *J Vasc Surg* **8**: 600.

Szilagyi DE, Smith RF, Elliot JP, Vrandecic MP (1972). Infection in arterial reconstruction with synthetic grafts. *Annl Surg* **176**: 321.

Reilly LM, Altman H, Lusby RJ *et al.* (1984). *J Vasc Surg* **1**: 36.

Reilly LM, Stoney RJ, Goldstone J, Ehrenfeld WK (1987). Improved management of aortic graft infection: The influence of operative sequence and staging. *J Vasc Surg* **5**: 421.

Wilson SE, Wang S, Gordon HE (1977). Perioperative antibiotic prophylaxis against vascular graft infection. *S Med J* **70**: 68.

Surgical management of secondary aortoenteric fistulae

Roger N Baird

Introduction

Anaemia from gastrointestinal blood loss, whether of clinically silent onset, or following haematemesis or melaena, in a patient with an intra-abdominal arterial prosthesis, is caused by an aortoenteric fistula until proved otherwise. This truth is self-evident to all vascular surgeons, but not, it seems, to those whose lack of awareness leads to numerous expensive and usually fruitless investigations, delaying the diagnosis and causing more than necessary blood loss and subsequent replacement (Thomas and Baird, 1986). Upper gastrointestinal endoscopy detected only two-thirds (8 of 12) of fistulae in a recent series (Tilanus *et al.*, 1988), and arteriography and comuted tomography (CT) will show extravasation of contrast into the duodenum only if bleeding is brisk when the investigation is being done. The presence of perigraft gas bubbles on CT can clinch the diagnosis of graft infection. The decision to do a laparotomy is usually taken on clinical grounds.

Pathophysiology

1

Most fistulae arise between an aortic/Dacron anastomosis and the fourth part of the duodenum. Occasionally, the abnormal communication is between an iliac/Dacron anastomosis and the small bowel or the appendix or colon, and from the suture line of an aortoiliac endarterectomy. Isolated examples have been reported in which a length of prosthesis remote from anastomoses erodes through the bowel wall, described as 'cannibalization' (Monson *et al.*, 1985), paraprosthetic-enteric sinus' (Williams *et al.*, 1987), and as graft-enteric erosions.

The overall incidence of aortoenteric fistulae following Dacron aortic bypass is low (0.7%) and gastrointestinal blood loss occurs without warning 6 months to 5 years or more after the original operation (Bergqvist *et al.*, 1987).

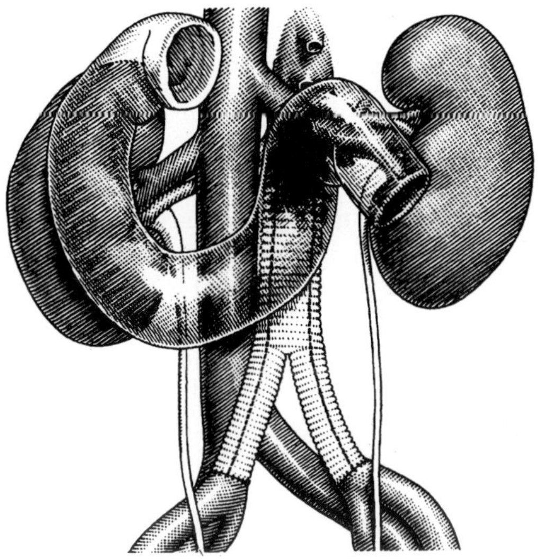

1

The pathogenesis is unknown, but the routine use of antibiotic prophylaxis and the substitution of prolene for silk as the suture material have been associated with fewer reported cases. There is disturbing association between bowel perforation at the primary aortic operation and secondary aortoenteric fistula. This suggests that Dacron grafting in elective cases should be deferred if the gut is inadvertently opened during operative exposure of the aorta.

2

At laparotomy, three separate categories can be recognized from the operative findings. First, a rupture of a false aneurysm into the bowel and, second, a simple fistula between the anastomosis and the duodenum. In both instances, there is no pus around the prosthesis, which remains well incorporated. In the third category, the infective process is advanced and the prosthesis lies slackly and unincorporated in a bed of pus throughout its length.

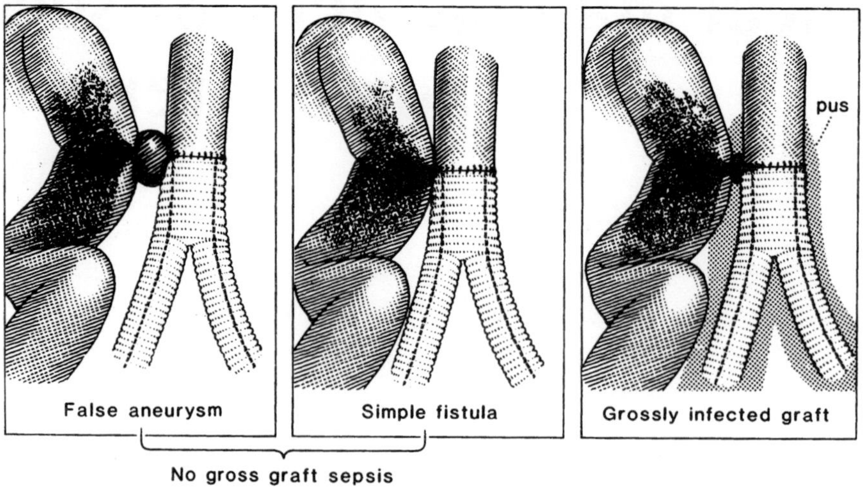

2

The operation

3

Full cardiovascular monitoring including arterial and central venous lines is mandatory. Wide bore venous access for rapid blood replacement is needed and at least 6 units of blood should be available. The abdomen is opened under antibiotic cover with a combination such as cefuroxine, metronidazole and gentamicin, and the fistula is disconnected.

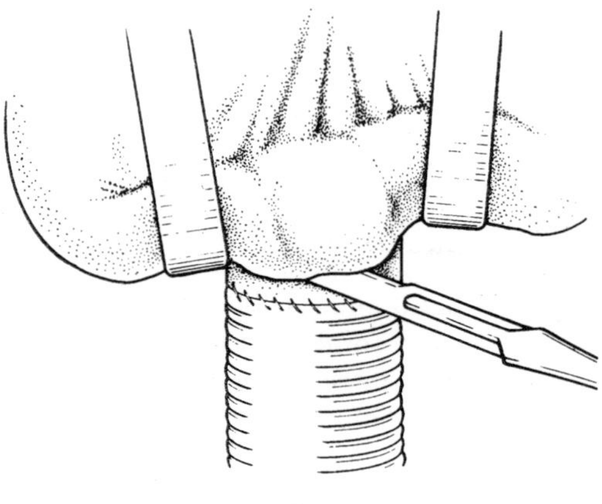

3

4

The duodenal defect is repaired using two layers of catgut or vicryl. Attention is then turned to the aortic prosthesis and suture line. Provided that the aortic wall is not discoloured the prosthesis is well incorporated, and no obvious pus is present, the fistula is likely to be caused by mechanical weakness of the aortic wall.

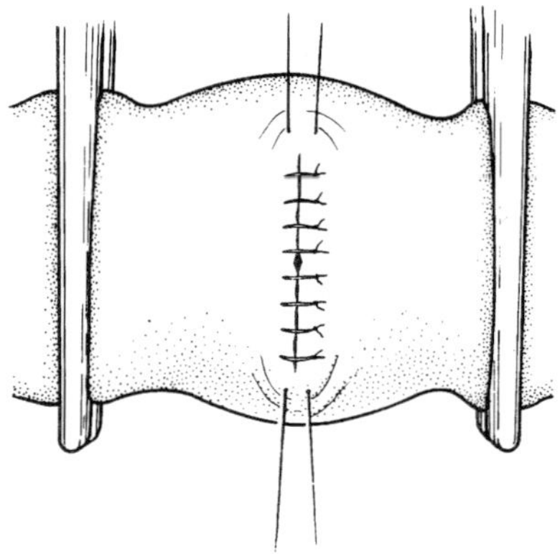

4

5

Consideration is then given to a local repair, either by inserting 2–3 prolene sutures to close the defect, or by inserting a short Dacron tube to link the prosthesis to a

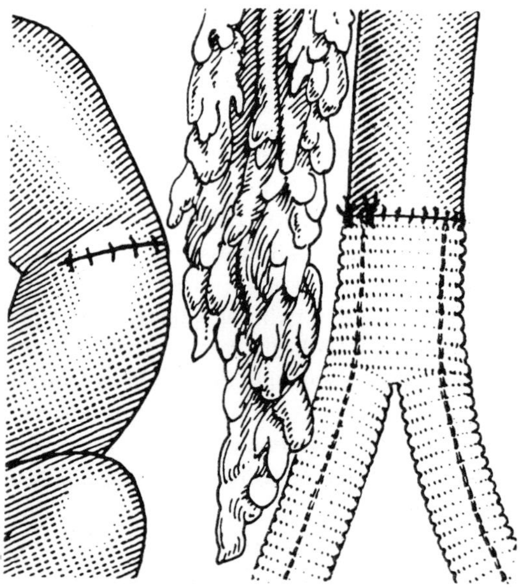

5

more proximal aortic suture line without tension (Robinson and Johansen, 1991; Thomas and Baird, 1986; Eastcott, 1982).

6

If, on the other hand, the prosthesis is unincorporated and lies in a bag of pus encased by fibrous tissue, then it should be removed. Usually, the aortic stump is oversewn and an axillobifemoral bypass performed.

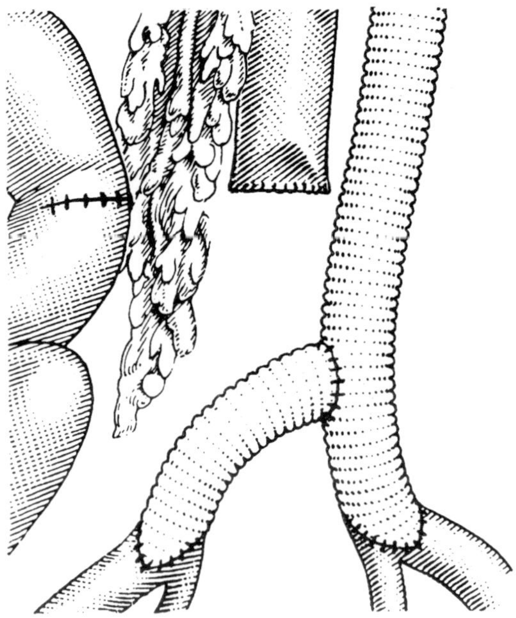

6

7

Added measures can help to reduce the risk of aortic stump blowout. These include double layers of sutures covering the closure with a flap of the anterior spinous ligament, and covering the omentum. However, Walker *et al.* (1987) have reported an alternative – placing a new prosthesis in the same location by primary exchange similar to the replacement of an infected heart valve. Robinson and Johansen (1991) have reported 11 *in situ* aortic Dacron replacements of five mycotic aneurysms, one secondarily infected aortic aneurysm and five aortoenteric fistulae (one primary; four secondary). They emphasize the need for aortic debridement to clinically uninvolved tissue, and for omental wrapping of anastomoses.

The advocates of extra-anatomical bypass typically acknowledge a high operative mortality of 49% and an amputation rate of 27% resulting from this approach (O'Hara *et al.*, 1986). In an attempt to reduce the magnitude of the undertaking, staged operations for patients

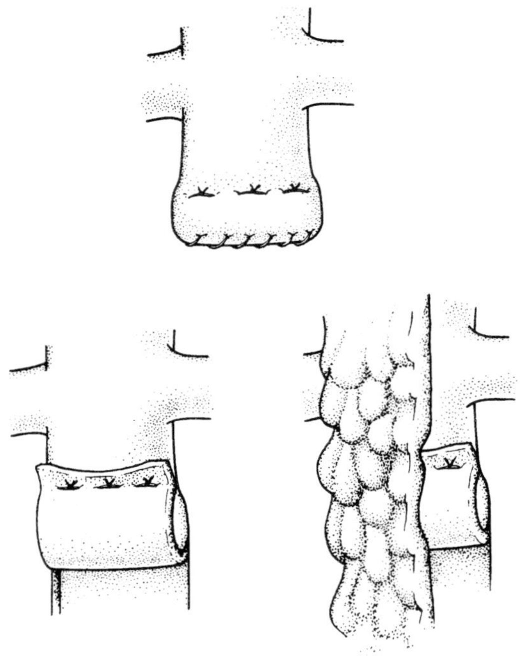

7

not actively bleeding are proposed. The axillobifemoral bypass is inserted first, and the infected prosthesis is removed later (Reilly *et al.*, 1987). The results have gradually improved in the last 20 years (Bouhoutsos *et al.*, 1974; Umpleby *et al.*, 1987). Whichever procedure is done, the duodenum and aorta should be separated as far apart as possible to minimize the risk of a further aorto-duodenal fistula. The omentum, mobilized if necessary, is used to wrap the aortic anastomosis or stump. In Bergqvist's series of 42 secondary aortoenteric fistulae, half had further gastrointestinal bleeding postoperatively from the aorto-Dacron anastomosis or from the aortic stump; and few survived for more than 5 years. Such is the anxiety about further gastrointestinal bleeding that there is even a report demonstrating that the duodenum can be transected and relocated in an antecolic position (England and Simms, 1990).

Less frequently, the fistula occurs between the distal anastomosis to the iliac arteries and the small bowel, appendix or colon or the mid-portion of the prosthesis erodes into the gut without anastomotic involvement. In these circumstances a local repair is usually done.

Conclusions

The general risks of treating secondary aortoenteric fistulae are those of major vascular surgery in arteriopaths rendered weak from blood loss. The likelihood of perioperative death and limb loss is increased if operation is precipitated by a major gastrointestinal bleed or if infection is a problem. Specifically, rupture of the aortic stump and infection of the axillofemoral bypass by cross-contamination are unsolved problems, as is recurrence of the aortoenteric fistula leading to further haematemesis and malaena. Further thrombosis without premonitory symptoms after months or years is a frequent problem with axillofemoral bypass and the patient should not stray too far from access to skilled hospital care, since urgent embolectomy may be required.

Acknowledgements

Illustrations by Gary M James and A George.

References

Bergqvist D, Alun A, Claes G, *et al.* (1987). Secondary aortoenteric fistulas – An analysis of 42 cases. *Eur J Vasc Surg* **1**: 11.

Bouhoutsos J, Chavatzas D, Martin P, Morris T (1974). Infected synthetic arterial grafts. *Br J Surg* **61**: 108.

Busuttil RW, Rees W, Baker JD, Wilson SE (1979). Pathogenesis of aortoduodenal fistula: Experimental and clinical correlates. *Surgery* **85**: 1.

Eastcott HHG (1982). Aorto-enteric fistula: Possibilities for direct repair. In *Extra-anatomic and Secondary Arterial Reconstruction.* Greenhalgh R M ed. London: Pitman.

England DW, Simms MH (1990). Recurrent aorto-duodenal fistula: a final solution? *Eur J Vasc Surg* **4**: 427.

Monson JRT, Courtney DG, Jones NAG, Kester RC (1985). Cannabilization of a Goretex aortohepatic graft by the duodenum. *Br J Surg* **72**: 101.

O'Hara PJ, Hertzer NR, Beven EG, Krajewski LP (1986). Surgical management of infected abdominal aortic grafts: Review of a 25 year experience. *J Vasc Surg* **3**: 725.

Reilly LM, Stoney RJ, Goldstone J, Ehrenfeld WK (1987). Improved management of aortic graft infection: The influence of operation sequence and staging. *J Vasc Surg* **5**: 421.

Robinson JA, Johansen K (1991). Aortic sepsis: Is there a role for *in situ* graft reconstruction? *J Vasc Surg* **13**: 677.

Thomas WEG, Baird RN (1986). Secondary aortic-enteric fistulae: Towards a more conservative approach. *Br J Surg* **73**: 875.

Tilanus HW, Terpstra OT, de Smit P *et al.* (1988). Diagnosis and management of graft-enteric fistulae. *Br J Surg* **75**: 915.

Umpleby HC, Britton DC, Turnbull AR (1987). Secondary arterio-enteric fistulae: A surgical challenge. *Br J Surg* **74**: 256.

Walker WE, Cooley DA, Duncan JM, *et al.* (1987). The management of aortoduodenal fistula by *in situ* replacement of the infected aortic graft. *Annl Surg* **205**: 727.

Williams GT, Charlesworth R, Jones DL (1987). Enterovosical fistula due to a Dacron aortic graft. *Br J Surg* **74**: 645.

In situ replacement of infected aortic graft

P Fiorani, F Speziale,
L Rizzo, G F Fadda

Introduction

Aortic graft infection can be considered the most serious complication in reconstructive aortic surgery. Although rare (0.8–6%) this continues to be responsible for a high rate of morbidity and mortality and is not influenced by any surgical treatment (Hoffert *et al.*, 1965; Szilagyi *et al.*, 1972; Goldstone and Moore, 1974; Bunt, 1983; Reilly *et al.*, 1984; Pons and Wurtz, 1991). Despite improved surgical methods and techniques the poor surgical outcome reported is mostly dependent upon major complications of advanced graft infection including sepsis, suture line disruption and gastrointestinal haemorrhage when aortoenteric fistula or aortoenteric erosion is associated.

The present standard treatment for aortic graft infection is a preliminary revascularization of the lower limbs by axillobifemoral bypass with subsequent graft excision, aortic stump ligation and suture of intestinal lesion when present (O'Hara *et al.*, 1986; Reilly *et al.*, 1987). However, a mortality rate of 25–75% can be expected according to a number of reports and the principal complication and cause of death is blow-out of the aortic stump. In addition there is a high risk of lower limb amputation of up to 50% in some reports because of occlusion of the axillobifemoral bypass which is not a durable procedure (Eugene *et al.*, 1974; Inahara, *et al.*, 1985; Yeager, *et al.*, 1990).

Recently, Walker *et al.* (1987) and others (Vollman and Kogel, 1987; Bandyk *et al.*, 1991; Robinson and Johansen, 1991; Jacobs *et al.*, 1991), reported better early and late results with an '*In situ* replacement of a new aortic graft'. These reports suggest lower operative mortality, limb salvage and documented extended survival with better quality of life, in cases without retroperitoneal abscess or septicaemia, introducing the concept of 'low-grade infection' (Walker *et al.*, 1987; Bandyk *et al.*, 1991; Fiorani *et al.*, 1993). This definition implies, from a clinical point of view, the absence of advanced graft infection symptoms (septicaemia, haemorrhagic shock) and from an anatomical point of view, the absence of gross retroperitoneal abscess or dehiscence of aortic anastomosis.

Preoperative management

Preoperative evaluation consists of routine laboratory tests, blood cultures and bacterial cultures of groin sinus secretion when present. Prophylactic therapy with specific antibiotics must be performed in those cases in which the microorganism, potentially responsible, is isolated preoperatively (groin sinus tract or groin abscess needle aspiration). In the other cases prophylaxis is performed by wide spectrum antibiotic therapy with second generation cephalosporins and aminoglycosides at least 72 hours before operation. In patients with preoperative diagnosis of aortoenteric fistula or artoenteric erosion a total parenteral nutrition is mandatory for at least 3–4 days before surgery.

Surgical techniques

Full cardiovascular monitoring including arterial and central vein lines are mandatory. The patient is placed in the supine position and general endotracheal anaesthesia is administered. The abdomen is opened and explored through a midline incision extending from the xiphoid to the pubis. The peritoneum over the aortic graft is incised longitudinally. Aortic control below the proximal anastomosis may be obtained by two principal approaches.

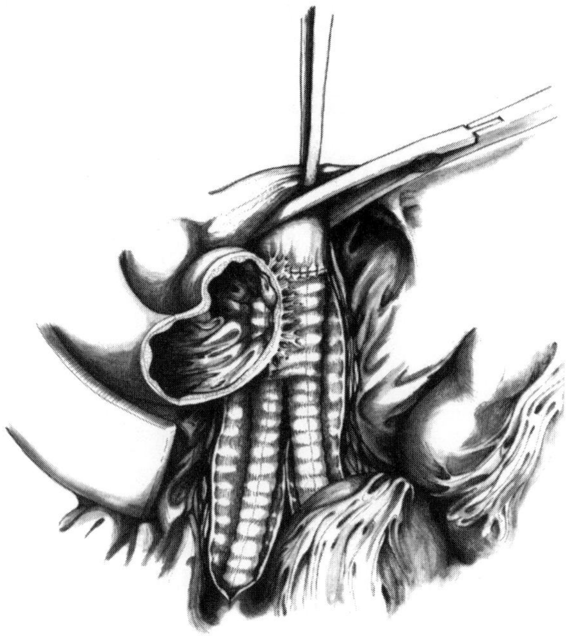

1

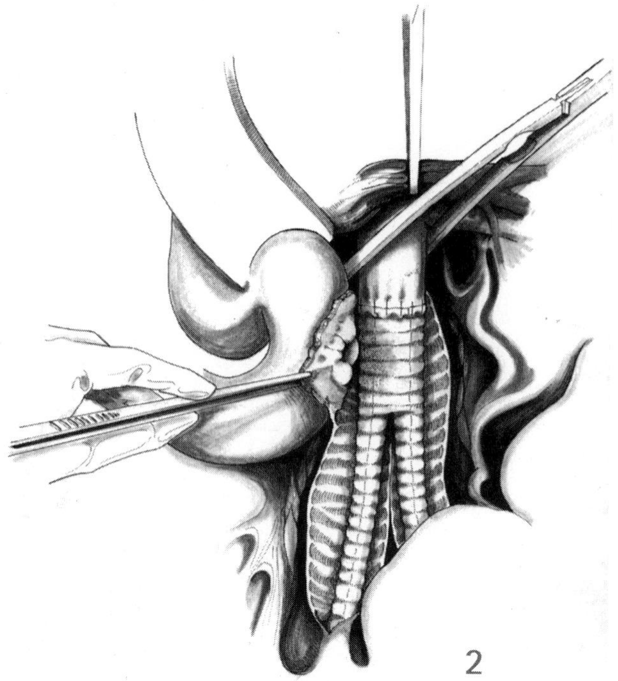

2

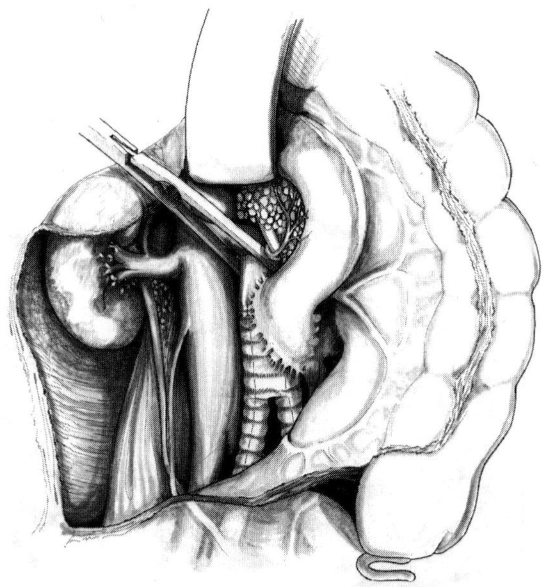

3

1, 2

Anterior transperitoneal approach

This approach can be difficult because of frequent retroperitoneal and duodenal adherences around the Ligament of Treitz and left renal vein which can make infrarenal aortic control a problem.

3

Right transperitoneal approach

This approach is possible and preferred in the majority of cases with associated aortoenteric fistula or aorto-enteric erosion. After peritoneal incision, the peritoneal reflection on the right lateral aspect of the ascending colon is incised and continued medially around the caecum and extended cephalad to mobilize the epatic flexure of the colon. A Kocher manoeuvre is then performed mobilizing the second portion of the duodenum and the head of the pancreas. This approach permits a rapid dissection in previously undissected planes. After mobilization of the abdominal viscera to the left, the inferior vena cava is exposed facilitating aortic control.

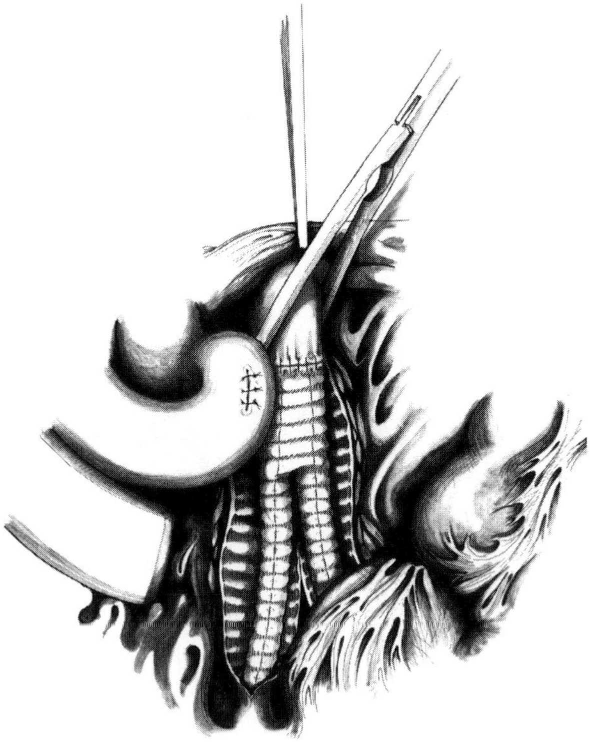

4

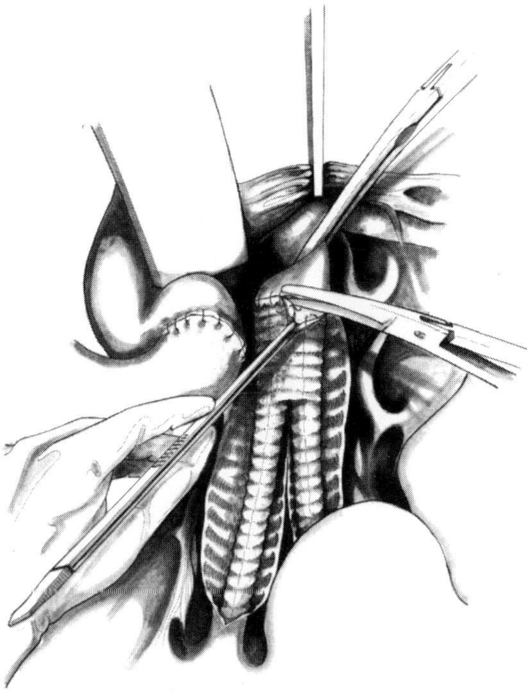

5

4, 5, 6

Graft explantation

In the presence of aortoenteric fistula or aortoenteric erosion, the first priority is to perform intestinal repair, by either simple suturing and deepening of the erosion (4) or by a segmental duodenal resection with an end to end anastomosis (5).

After aortic clamping, the infected aortic graft is removed followed by irrigation of the retroperitoneal area by antiseptic solution of 2% povidone-iodine. Explanted graft material is collected for bacteriological cultures. Illustration 6 shows completion with an *in situ* new graft replacement. The choice of the type of reimplanted graft is debated. We prefer a polytetrafluoroethylene (PTFE) graft, because of the demonstration of suggested higher resistance for those strains more frequently implicated in low-grade infection (Schmitt *et al.*, 1986; Bandyk *et al.*, 1991). Other authors report successful reimplantation with Dacron graft or homologous tissue (Kieffer *et al.*, 1993) and recently with rifampicin-soaked Dacron grafts (Torsello *et al.*, 1993).

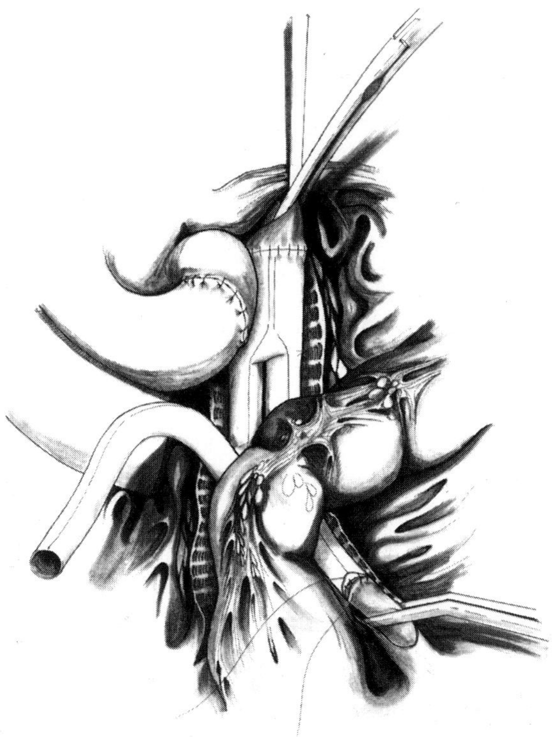

6

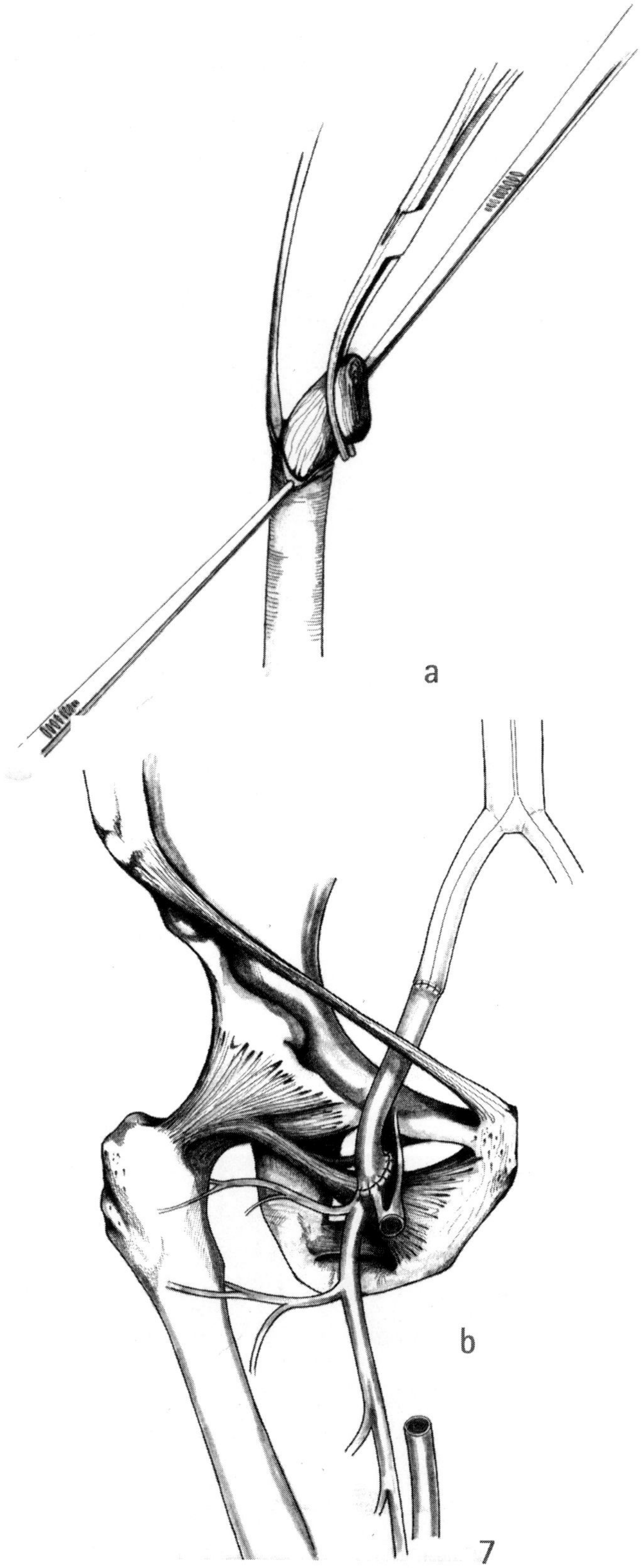

7

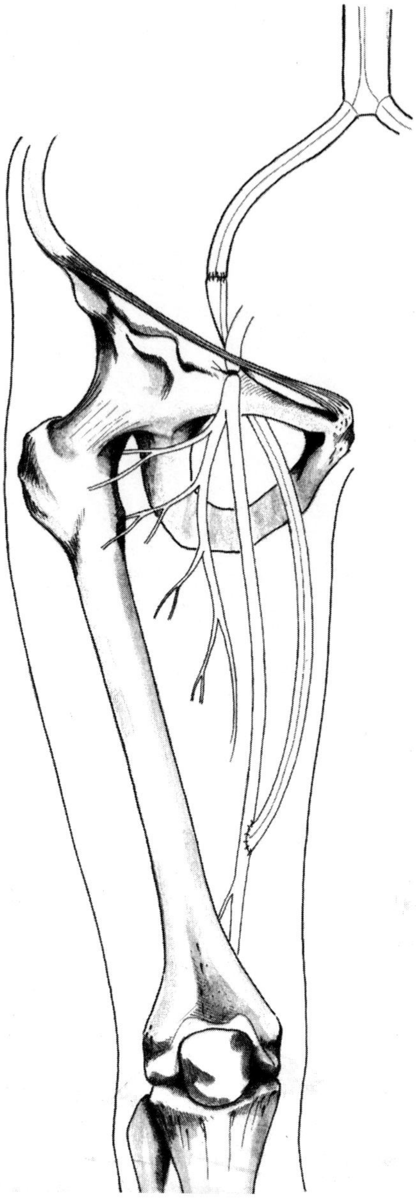

8

7a, b

Inguinal replacement

In the presence of groin sinus or abscess, the replacement of a prosthetic vascular graft is not recommended. In these cases it seems more appropriate to use autologous tissue such as inverted saphenous vein or endarterectomized superficial femoral artery shown here (**7a**) anastomized intra-abdominally with a reimplanted prosthetic graft (**7b**).

8

Another possible alternative to avoid the infected groin is to perform a transobturatory bypass to the inferior third of the superficial femoral artery with avoidance of the infected inguinal area.

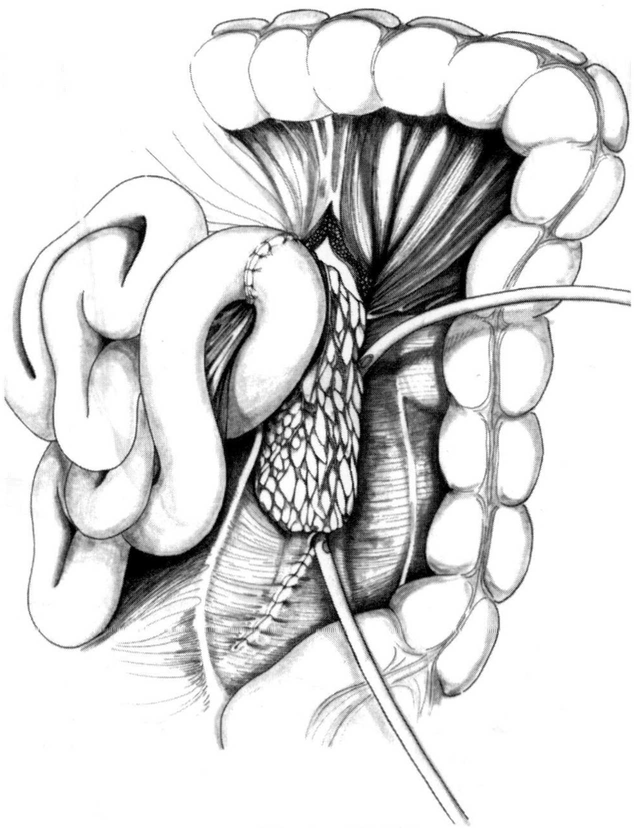

9

9

At the end of whatever procedure a pedicle of omentum is mobilized and passed through the transverse mesocolon to cover the new aortic graft, and two drainage tubes are positioned to permit postoperative antiseptic irrigation and monitoring of bacterial culture.

Conclusions

Postoperative mortality ranges from 0 to 20% with no amputations. Walker *et al.* (1987) in a paper dealing with the selection of patients as candidates for an *in situ* replacement showed a significant correlation between the presence of retroperitoneal abscess and mortality; the perioperative mortality following *in situ* replacement in patients with extensive purulent graft infection (retroperitoneal abscess) was 60% vs 22% in patients with low grade infection.

Bandyk *et al.* (1991), in a more recent experience, recommended *in situ* PTFE replacement for late graft infections in those patients in which no systemic (septicaemia) or local signs (perigraft abscess, dehiscence of the anastomosis) of infection are present. From these experiences the concept of 'grade' of infection should determine the choice of management. Reinfections among survivors are rare.

However for severe and acute onset infection *in situ* replacement seems contraindicated, but in patients with low-grade infection a better prognosis for life and limb is claimed.

References

Bandyk DF, Bergamini TM, Kinney EV *et al.* (1991). *In situ* replacement of vascular prostheses infected by bacterial biofilms. *J Vasc Surg* **13**: 575.

Bunt TJ (1983). Synthetic vascular graft infections: I. Graft infections. *Surgery* **93**, 733.

Eugene J, Goldstone J, Moore WS (1974). Fifteen-year experience with subcutaneous bypass grafts for lower extremity ischemia. *Annl Surg* **186**: 177.

Fiorani P, Speziale F, Rizzo L *et al.* (1993). Detection of aortic graft infection with leukocytes labeled with Technetium 99m hexametazine. *J Vasc Surg* **17**: 86.

Goldstone J, Moore WS (1974). Infection in vascular prostheses: Clinical manifestation and surgical management. *Am J Surg* **128**: 225.

Hoffert PW, Gensler S, Haimovici H (1965). Infection complicating arterial grafts. *Arch Surg* **90**: 427.

Inahara T, Geary GL, Mukherjee D *et al.* (1985). The contrary position to the non-respective treatment of abdominal aortic aneurysm. *J Vasc Surg* **4**: 42.

Jacobs MJHM, Reul GJ, Gregoric I, Cooley DA (1991). *In situ*-replacement and extranatomic bypass for the treatment of infected abdominal aortic grafts. *Eur J Vasc Surg* **5**: 83.

Kieffer E, Bahnini A, Koskas F *et al.* (1993). *In situ* allograft replacement of infected infra-renal aortic prosthetic graft: Results in forty-three patients. *J Vasc Surg* **17**: 349.

O'Hara PJ, Hertzer NR, Beven EG, Krajewski LP (1986). Surgical management of infected abdominal aortic grafts: Review of 25-year experience. *J Vasc Surg* **3**: 725.

Pons VG, Wurtz R (1991). Vascular grafts infections: A 25-year experience of 170 cases. *J Vasc Surg* **5**: 751.

Reilly LM, Altman H, Lusby RJ *et al.* (1984). Late results following surgical management of vascular graft infection. *J Vasc Surg* **1**: 36.

Reilly LM, Stoney RJ, Goldstone J, Ehrenfeld WK (1987). Improved management of aortic graft infection: The influence of operative sequence and staging. *J Vasc Surg* **5**: 421.

Robinson JA, Johansen KJ (1991). Aortic sepsis: Is there a role for an *in situ* graft reconstruction? *J Vasc Surg* **13**: 677.

Schmitt DD, Bandyk DF, Peuqet AJ, Towne JB (1986). Bacterial adherence to vascular prostheses. A determinant of graft infectivity. *J Vasc Surg* **5**: 732.

Szilagyi DE, Smith RF, Elliot JP, Vrandecic MP (1972). Infection in arterial reconstruction with synthetic grafts. *Annl Surg* **176**: 321.

Torsello G, Sandmann W, Gehrt A, Jungblut RM (1993). *In situ* replacement of infected vascular prostheses with rifampin-soaked vascular grafts: Early results. *J Vasc Surg* **17**: 768.

Vollmar JF, Kogel H (1987). Aortoenteric fistulas as postoperative complications. *J Cardiovasc Surg* (Torino) **28**: 479.

Walker WE, Cooley DA, Duncan JM (1987). The management of aortoduodenal fistula by *in situ* replacement of the infected abdominal aortic graft. *Annl Surg* **205**: 727.

Yeager RA, Moneta GL, Taylor LM *et al.* (1990). Improving survival and limb salvage in patients with aortic graft infection. *Am J Surg* **159**: 466.

Section fourteen EXTRA-ANATOMIC OPEN VASCULAR TECHNIQUES

Axillofemoral bypass

Sven-Erik Bergentz

Introduction

Axillofemoral bypass was first performed in 1962 by Blaisdell and Hall (1963) in the USA and by Louw (1963) in South Africa. The former operation was performed for an occluded abdominal aortic aneurysm, the latter for arteriosclerotic occlusive disease.

The technique for this operation should be known by all vascular surgeons, but it should not be used very often. The most important indication is when a standard aortic reconstruction is precluded due to aortic graft infection, an aortoenteric fistula, or intra-abdominal sepsis (Bergqvist *et al.*, 1987). The operation may also be used when there is a colostomy-ileostomy, or other types of enterocutaneous fistula. Another indication is dense abdominal adhesions, following previous surgery or irradiation. Threatening limb loss in high-risk patients due to severe cardiac or pulmonary disease is a rare indication in our institution. A rare and controversial use of axillofemoral bypass is for non-resective treatment of an abdominal aortic aneurysm after induction of acute thrombosis of the aneurysm by bilateral iliac artery ligation (Schwartz *et al.*, 1986).

Axillofemoral bypass is contraindicated in extensive subclavian or axillary artery occlusive disease. As outflow vessel, a patent deep femoral artery, and/or superficial femoral artery, is mandatory.

Preoperative evaluation

With regard to the inflow vessels, preoperative blood pressure measurements in both arms and auscultation over subclavian and axillary arteries are important. The right axillary artery is usually preferred as inflow vessel since stenotic lesions in the subclavian artery are three to four times more common on the left than on the right side. If, however, the blood pressure is more than about 20 mm Hg higher on the left side, this side should be preferred. If the blood pressure is low bilaterally, or if there are murmurs to be heard over the subclavian and axillary arteries, arteriography of the aortic arch and its branches should be performed.

If an axillofemoral graft is indicated, there is usually a need to vascularize both legs. Originally, this was done by performing one axillofemoral bypass on each side, but now we prefer to use axillofemoral bypass on one side, and add a crossover graft to the contralateral groin ('axillobifemoral bypass'). This will increase the flow in the long axillofemoral graft, which decreases the risk of occlusion.

The operation

1

Anaesthesia, positioning and draping

Axillofemoral bypass may be performed under local anaesthesia, but light general anaesthesia is preferable.

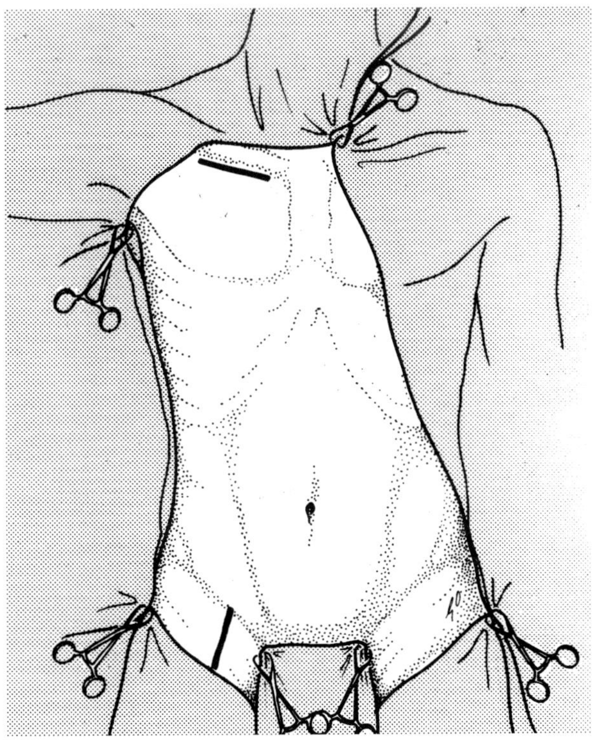

1

This gives better airway control and ventilation and is usually well tolerated even by debilitated patients.

The patient lies in a supine position with the arm on the ipsilateral side placed on an armboard, at right angles to the body. This arm is draped free and is mobile during the operation. Abduction of the arm moves the clavicle upwards, facilitating access to the first part of the axillary artery. Chest, neck, upper arm, abdomen, both groins, and upper parts of the thighs should be draped. The contralateral arm is used for blood pressure recording, sampling and infusions.

It is sometimes recommended to use two teams to speed up the operation. We prefer using one team, although the dissection of the axillary and femoral vessels may sometimes be carried out simultaneously by two surgeons.

2

Axillary artery dissection

The axillary artery lies behind and slightly above the axillary vein. It is divided into three parts, in relation to its relation to the pectoralis minor muscle. The first is located medial to, the second behind and the third lateral to this muscle. The axillary artery is crossed by the lateral and medial anterior thoracic (pectoral) nerves, innervating the pectoralis major muscle. The first part of the axillary artery gives off one branch, the highest thoracic artery. The second part, behind the pectoralis minor, usually gives off two branches. The first and, to some extent, the second part of the artery should be used for the anastomosis, since this is the fulcrum when the arm is abducted. Therefore, traction of the axillary artery by the graft is minimized.

If at least one of the common, deep or superficial femoral arteries are known to be patent, the operation starts by exploring the axillary artery. An incision is made about 2 cm below and parallel to the clavicle. Its length should be about 8 cm. The transversely running fibres of the pectoralis major muscle are split between its clavicular and sternal heads. The pectoralis minor muscle is identified behind the costoclavicular fascia. This muscle might be divided close to the clavicle, but sometimes it is possible to retract at least part of it laterally. The axillary vein is now exposed, lying anterior and inferior to the artery.

Ligation of branches to the vein, particularly those crossing in front of the axillary artery, is necessary for the mobilization. The middle part of the axillary artery now emerges below the clavicle. There are usually two branches from this part, and one from the first part of the artery which should be divided. Polyethylene tubing around the artery facilitates its mobilization. About 5–6 cm of the axillary artery should be mobilized.

3

Femoral artery dissection

The femoral artery is now dissected via a longitudinal incision over the common femoral artery. If it is not

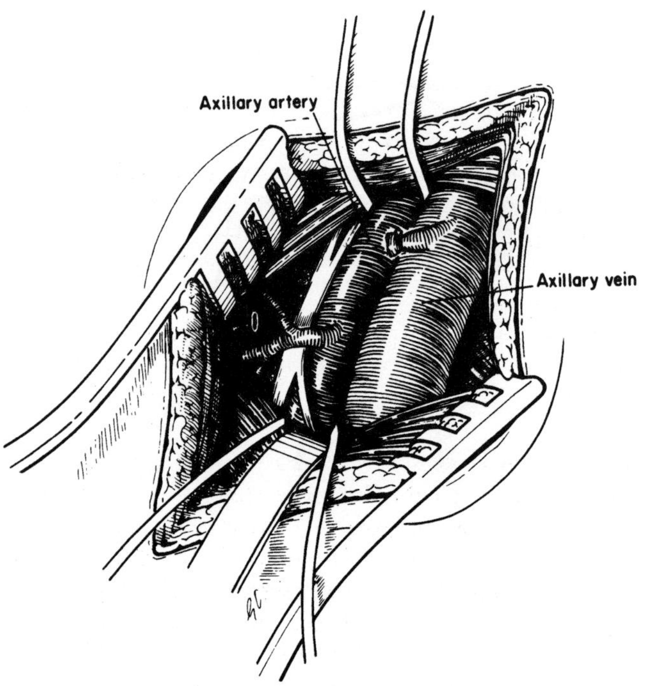

2

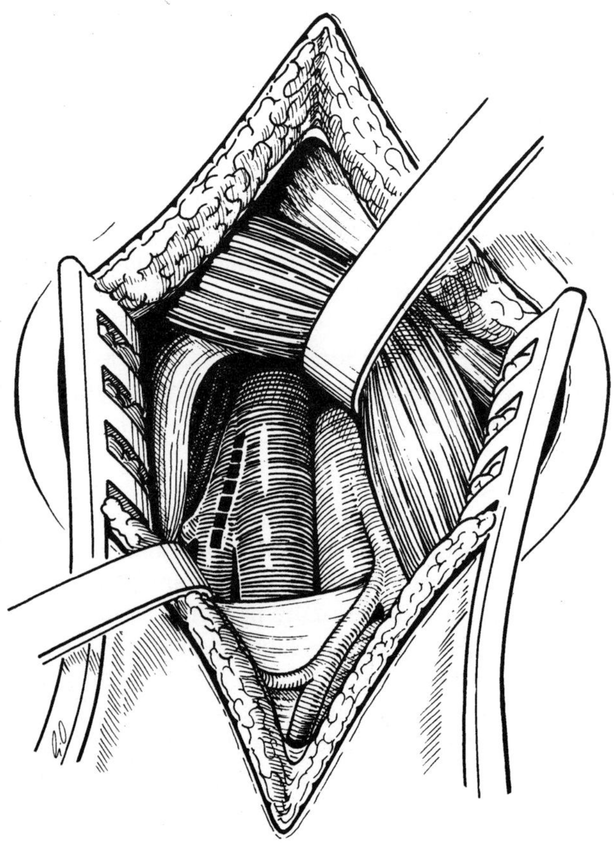

3

known that the common femoral artery or at least one of its branches is patent, the operation should start with a groin dissection. The common, superficial and deep femoral arteries are mobilized. A part of the inguinal ligament may be divided to facilitate a proximal dissection of the common femoral artery if necessary. In the relatively uncommon situation, when it is known from a good angiography that both the superficial and deep femoral arteries are patent and without stenosis in the beginning, the anastomosis may be performed to the common femoral artery. Usually, the superficial femoral artery is occluded and the deep femoral artery is often stenotic at its beginning. In these situations the deep femoral artery must be dissected to, or even beyond, its first muscular branches, thereby also dividing the lateral circumflex vein.

If the groin has been used for previous anastomosis, or is infected, the deep femoral arteries may be approached by incisions a few centimetres lateral and distal to the original groin incision. The sartorius muscle is drawn medially, exposing the deep femoral artery, which can be mobilized to a length of several centimetres.

4

Axillofemoral tunnel

The tunnel for the graft starts from the axillary incision deep to the pectoralis major muscle. In the beginning it should go in a lateral-caudal direction, the angle to the axillary artery being between 30 and 40 degrees. When the tunnel reaches the mid-axillary line (where an incision might be necessary to facilitate the formation of the tunnel), it should be directed caudal to the anterior superior iliac spine, and from there it should continue to the groin. It is important to avoid having the prosthesis anteriorly. This may result in compression of the prosthesis to the costal margin, or kinking when the patient bends.

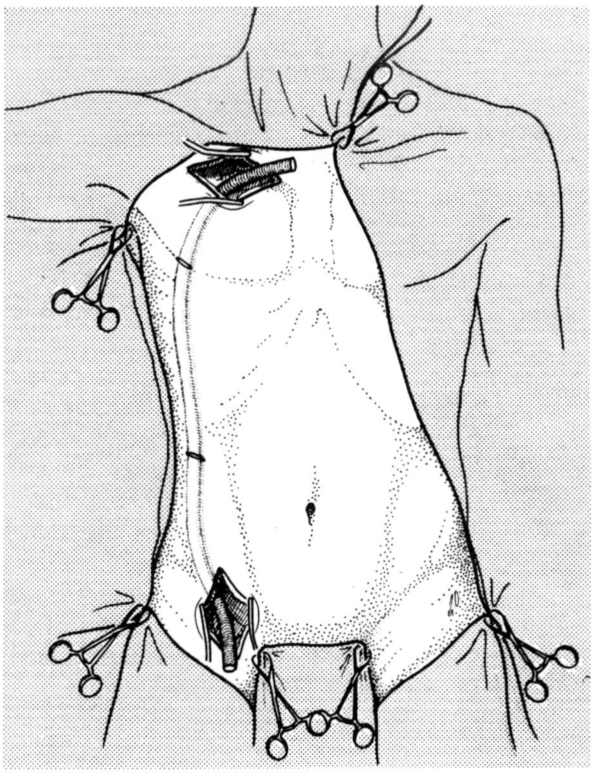

4

Selection, preparation and placement of graft

We prefer an 8–10 mm knitted Dacron graft. Careful preclotting is important to avoid haematoma formation in the long tunnel. At least 50 ml of blood is necessary for this long graft. Excellent results have been reported by the use of externally supported grafts but no randomized trial has been performed to prove the superiority of this type of graft. The polytetrafluoroethylene (PTFE) graft has the advantage of precluding preclotting, and it also makes thrombectomy easier. It is, however, non-elastic, which might possibly contribute to disruption of the axillary anastomosis when the patient raises the arm.

5a, b

Bifemoral grafts are preferable whenever feasible. These can be done with a single graft to the femoral artery with the addition of a femorofemoral graft from the groin of the donor side. This technique allows high flow throughout the length of the main stem of the axillofemoral graft. The femorofemoral graft should be 2 mm narrower than the main graft to obtain a reasonable high flow rate.

There are alternatives to the technique shown in **5b**. The femorofemoral branch can be anastomosed to the axillofemoral graft at a right angle or higher up with a more sloping angle. Experimental comparisons between these two techniques have shown that the latter gives a higher flow in the crossover branch, and also avoids turbulence in the bifurcation. A prospective randomized trial has been performed comparing these techniques. There was no difference regarding the effect on ankle pressure, nor regarding the 2-year patency of the main stem of the axillofemoral graft or the ipsilateral extension of the graft. There was, however, a two-fold increase in the occlusion rate of the crossover branch when the 90 degrees branching was used, compared with the more sloping technique with a higher anastomosis (Wittens *et al.*, 1992). Alternatively a ready made axillobifemoral graft, commercially available, can be selected. This avoids the need for the additional Dacron-Dacron anastomosis shown in **5a** and **5b**. The ready made axillobifemoral grafts have 90 degrees and also more sloping crossover angles to meet the surgeon's preference.

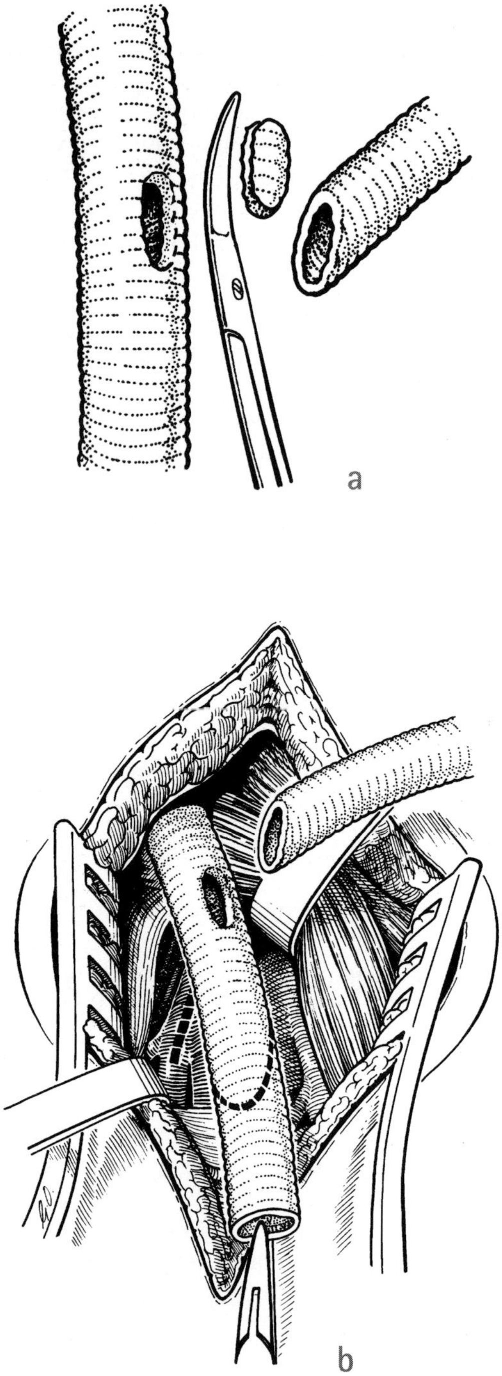

5

The proximal anastomosis

6

The axillary artery is elevated into the field by traction of the slings encircling the artery. A 2-cm long arteriotomy is made in the anterior and inferior aspect of the axillary artery as far medially as possible. The graft is bevelled at an angle of 30–40 degrees. A 5/0 synthetic double-armed vascular suture is used. The prosthesis is placed anterior to the axillary vein. The sutures are started at the lateral and at the medial ends of the arteriotomy. The back wall of the graft is sutured to the inferior part of the artery from the inside, using one end of the lateral and one end of the medial suture. These two ends are tied together at the midpoint of the back wall.

The other ends of the two sutures, the lateral and the medial, are then used to complete the anterior part of the anastomosis and meet at its midpoint. The clamps on the axillary artery are released. The graft is occluded close to the anastomosis, using a hydrogrip Fogarty clamp before the clamps on the axillary artery are released.

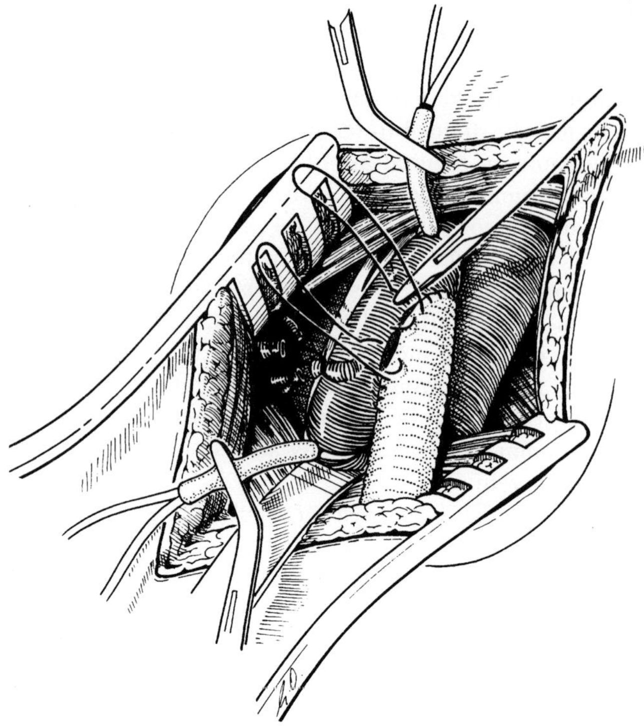

6

7

The distal anastomosis

The prosthesis is drawn from the groin incision, care being taken to avoid any twists and kinks. It is also important to avoid too much tension on the graft, which may draw the axillary artery into a Y configuration. This may result in a thrombosis of the axillary artery, or even disruption of the anastomosis, or a formation of a pseudoaneurysm.

The anastomosis between the graft and the (ipsilateral) femoral artery is made according to the principles described for aortofemoral grafting. If the common femoral artery and the superficial and/or deep femoral arteries are widely patent and without stenosis, the anastomosis is made to the common femoral artery. Very

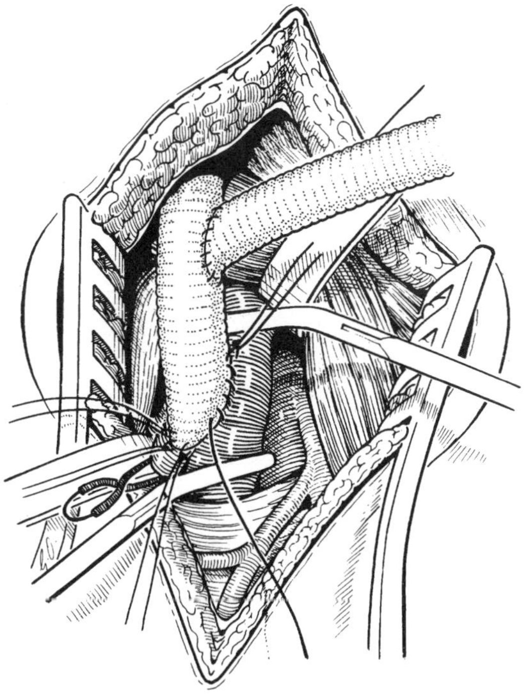

7

often, however, the superficial femoral artery in these patients is severely diseased or even occluded. The deep femoral artery is often stenotic at its origin. In these cases the arteriotomy of the common femoral artery is carried down 1–2 cm or even further into the deep femoral artery. The graft is formed as an onlay patch in the deep femoral artery. Endarterectomy should be avoided if possible. It it has to be done, it is important to prevent a distal flap development by using several intima-tacking sutures. Several interrupted sutures should be used to prevent purse string constriction when suturing the distal end of the patch on to the rather delicate deep femoral artery.

After completion of the distal anastomosis, the Fogarty clamp on the proximal part of the graft is released. The clamp on the proximal part of the common femoral artery is then removed, forcing the initial blood flow, with any remaining thrombotic material, debris and air bubbles, in the proximal direction. After a few pulses, the superficial and deep femoral artery clamps are removed. If a graft-to-graft anastomosis has been prepared to a femorofemoral graft, this can be used for flushing the axillofemoral graft. After that, a Fogarty clamp is placed on the crossover graft close to the graft-to-graft anastomosis.

The anastomosis between the crossover graft and the (contralateral) femoral artery is then performed, following the principles just described.

Wound closure

Before closing the wounds, the feet should be inspected. It is usually not possible to feel any ankle pulses, but the colour and the vein-filling in the feet can give some preliminary information about the limb perfusion.

Arteriography is considered if there is any question of distal perfusion. A total of 30 ml of contrast medium is injected through a catheter threaded into the prosthesis proximal to the graft-to-graft anastomosis.

The axillary incisions are closed in two deep layers, approximating the fascia of the pectoralis major muscle, and the subcutaneous tissue. We prefer 3/0 synthetic absorbable suture material. The groin wounds are similarly closed in two layers of subcutaneous synthetic absorbable material. The skin is closed with interrupted 3/0 synthetic suture material.

Intra- and postoperative care

Antibiotics

Prophylactic broad spectrum antibiotics, active against staphylococci, are started before surgery and continued for 48 hours.

Anticoagulation

We do not use systematic heparinization during these operations. Before occluding a vessel, we irrigate carefully with heparinized saline, and inject 20–40 ml of the solution peripherally. Furthermore, we give dextran 40 in a 10% solution continuously during the operation. The dose is 500 ml during surgery, 500 ml after surgery on the day of surgery, and 500 ml a day for the first 3 postoperative days. We strongly advise the patient to stop smoking. We see no reason to recommend aspirin since it has not been shown to decrease the risk of graft occlusion.

Graft compression

It is not quite clear whether or not compression of the graft plays a role in occlusion. Nevertheless, the patient should be encouraged to avoid constricting clothing and, if possible, lying on the graft. If the patient can cooperate, he may be encouraged to palpate the pulse daily to detect graft occlusion early, which otherwise may be difficult.

Postoperative care and complications

The lifespan of an axillofemoral graft can be prolonged by careful monitoring, and early intervention in the case of occlusion. Declotting of an occluded graft is usually a simple procedure, which can be performed under local anaesthesia. An intraoperative angiogram may facilitate complete removal of thrombotic material. Thromboembolic occlusion of the axillobrachial arteries may occur when the graft occludes.

Disruption of the proximal anastomosis, or formation of an anastomotic aneurysm, may occur if this anastomosis is placed too far laterally, and under too much tension.

Editorial note

The procedures are now often done using a purpose-built graft with external support. The grafts are designed to allow 'equi-flow' due to the configuration. Furthermore with the use of tunnelling devices (e.g. Impra Tunneller), no additional incision is required between the infraclavicular and groin incision.

References

Bergqvist D, Alm A, Claes G *et al.* (1987). Secondary aortoenteric fistulas – an analysis of 42 cases. *Eur J Vasc Surg* **1**: 11.

Blaisdell FW, Hall AD (1963). Axillary-femoral bypass for lower extremity ischemia. *Surgery* **54**: 563.

Louw JH (1963). Splenic-to-femoral and axillary-to-femoral bypass grafts in diffuse atherosclerotic occlusive disease. *Lancet* **1**: 1401.

Schwartz RA, Nichols KW, Silver D (1986). Is thrombosis of infrarenal abdominal aortic aneurysm an acceptable alternative? *J Vasc Surg* **3**: 448.

Wittens CHA, van Houtte HJKP, van Urk H (1992). European prospective randomised multi-centre axillo-bifemoral trial. *Eur J Vasc Surg* **6**: 115.

Femorofemoral bypass

P Fiorani, V Faraglia,
M Taurino, F Speziale, M Colonna

Introduction

Crossover femorofemoral bypass was first proposed in clinical practice by Vetto in 1966 for the treatment of unilateral iliac obstructive lesions. Its indications were subsequently extended to an increasing number of patients with unilateral iliac lesions, obtaining satisfactory immediate and long-term results.

Clinically, there seems to be no doubt about the indications, while special attention should be paid to the haemodynamic assessment of the donor iliofemoral axis due to its involvement with immediate patency and long-term evolution.

Indications

The clinical indications for revascularization by crossover femorofemoral bypass include unilateral stenotic-obstructive lesions of the iliac axis with claudication of limited autonomy or with rest ischaemia, showing general or local contraindications for conventional revascularization (Eugene *et al.*, 1977; Whittemore *et al.*, 1980).

General contraindications are represented by advanced age, severe cardiorespiratory failure, or of other systems, the presence of metabolic imbalance or limited life-expectancy (Vijayanager *et al.*, 1982). This procedure is extra-abdominal, feasible under local anaesthesia, requires a short operative time and involves only a minor surgical trauma. Local contraindications are represented by the presence, near the aorta, of an infected area or marked sclerosis due to previous surgery, retroperitoneal fibrosis or possible onset of septic foci because of iatrogenic lesions from abdominal surgery as well as from possible peripheral trophic lesions. The presence of extensive lesions of the host femoral axis which may affect the immediate result in terms of patency, can be considered a further local contraindication for major abdominal surgery. Moreover, crossover femorofemoral bypass is indicated for acute thrombosis of the iliac axis and for occlusion of the branch of a previous aortofemoral bypass (Rutherford *et al.*, 1987).

Special indications for this procedure include the need to preserve the erectile function by preventing iatrogenic lesions of the pelvic splanchnic nerves of the preaortic plexus, in patients affected by morbid obesity (De Laurentis *et al.*, 1978) or previously treated with radiation therapy at the level of the pelvis or retroperitoneum. Together with clinical indications, problems related to haemodynamic performance should also be considered. They concern both the host and donor limbs. The host artery frequently shows a femoropopliteal lesions, and thus it should be assessed whether the deep femoral artery is able to ensure adequate perfusion of the limb or not (Nelelsteen *et al.*, 1980; Martinez *et al.*, 1980). As for the donor limb, the problem is more complex because obstructive lesions present at this level can be the cause of flow diversion which leads to distal ischaemia (the steal phenomenon).

The steal phenomenon

In 1968, based on observations of patients treated with a crossover femorofemoral bypass for unilateral iliac obstructive lesions, and who developed ischaemia of the donor limb, explained by a diversion of blood flow between the lower limbs (i.e. the steal phenomenon), and based on other evidence (Harper *et al.*, 1967), Ehrenfeld carried out a canine experiment to try to understand the problem more fully. By modifying the inflow pressure of the donor axis and the peripheral resistance by the creation of an aortovenous fistula, Ehrenfeld was able to demonstrate that lesion-free iliac arteries are able to increase their flow tenfold, allowing them to perfuse proximally as well as contralaterally.

When an iliac artery is significantly stenosed, the flow required by both limbs cannot be satisfied. If distal to the donor axis the peripheral resistance is higher than in the contralateral axis due to femoropopliteal lesions, a femorofemoral revascularization would result in ischaemic symptoms in the donor limb. Therefore, it is important to determine whether a stenotic lesion is present or not. However, even in the presence of a 50% stenosis, this procedure can still be indicated for elderly and non-ambulatory patients. On the other hand, 30% stenosis is considered the limit for young patients with patent infrainguinal arteries who are likely to experience vasodilatation during exercise, and who therefore require an additional blood flow (Hill *et al.*, 1982).

However, in some cases postoperative ischaemia of the donor limb can be ascribed to a faulty surgical technique (stenosed anastomosis or embolization) or to a progressive distal atherosclerosis.

Preoperative assessment

The integrity of the donor iliac axis is mandatory to ensure perfusion of both limbs. Therefore, clinical, morphological and haemodynamic testing is proposed, both while the patient is at rest and while exercising the lower limbs.

Clinical testing is based on a normal femoral pulse and the absence of bruits both in the iliac artery and iliac fossa, an indication of the integrity of the donor iliac artery, especially when associated with an obstructive lesion of the ipsilateral femoral bifurcation.

The Doppler system is used to detect and assess possible pressure gradients, to examine the iliac vessels and any lesions, and to measure directly the pressure in the iliac and femoral arteries. The criteria proposed are that the Doppler thigh pressure should be equal to but not greater than the brachial pressure, and that the Doppler ankle pressure should be equal to or no more than 15 mmHg below the brachial pressure (McDonald *et al.*, 1978). The iliac axis is considered normal when the pressure in the femoral artery is not more than 10 mmHg below the brachial pressure. A further noninvasive procedure is to study waveform using a Doppler zero-crossing detector.

Nicolaides and Angelides (1981) modified the wave peak of a haemodynamically effective proximal stenosis to determine the pulsatility index. However, in the presence of a diffuse lesion, this procedure is not totally reliable. In the presence of a mildly stenosed lesion which might result in the steal phenomenon after maximal peripheral dilatation, active-passive or intra-arterial papaverine-induced hyperaemia tests have been proposed to stimulate this response (Flanigan *et al.*, 1984).

Angiography is considered the best form of assessment which, when adequately performed, is able to detect with lateral and oblique projections the presence of iliac stenoses not shown up by standard anteroposterior angiography, due to frequent posterior atherosclerotic plaque. Moreover, lesions at this level of the aortic and iliac bifurcation, i.e. where overlapping bone segments can block the view, can also be detected by these projections.

Surgical techniques

1, 2

The patient is placed in the supine position and general, local or spinal anaesthesia is administered. Most surgeons make an inguinal incision along the projection of the host femoral vessels, preparing and locating with loops the common femoral, superficial and deep femoral arteries, from the orifice to the lateral femoral circumflex vein, which is ligated to expose a portion of healthy artery suitable for the anastomosis or profundaplasty (De Laurentis *et al.*, 1978). The donor femoral artery is then prepared using a similar incision, but more limited downwards and more extended upwards to allow the best possible exposure of the common femoral artery.

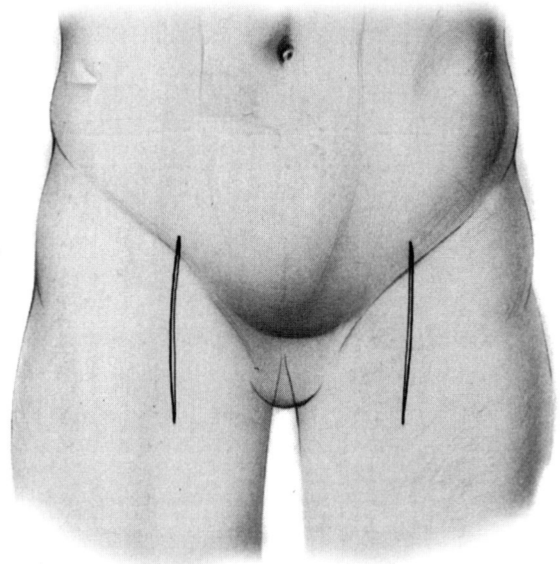

1

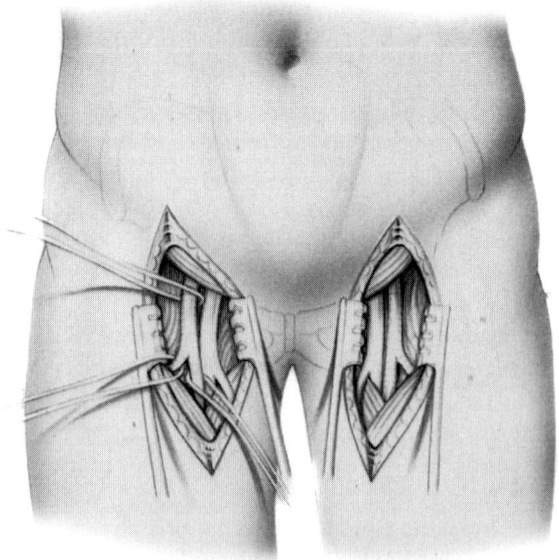

2

3, 4, 5

The patient is heparinized and preclotted knitted Dacron is used as the prosthesis. PTFE or autologous saphenous vein can also be used, provided that their calibre is not less than 6 mm. In particular instances, it should be possible to use an autologous artery such as an endarterectomized superficial femoral artery (Blaisdell *et al.*, 1970).

Arteriotomies should be performed on the anteromedial aspect of the host vessels to avoid kinking and twisting of the graft. An oblique inflow orifice is also advisable to prevent inflow stenosis (Tyson and Reichle, 1972).

After completion of the donor anastomosis, the prosthesis is canalized bluntly up to the contralateral groin following a subcutaneous course. This is then reversed to form a 'U'-shaped subcutaneous bypass.

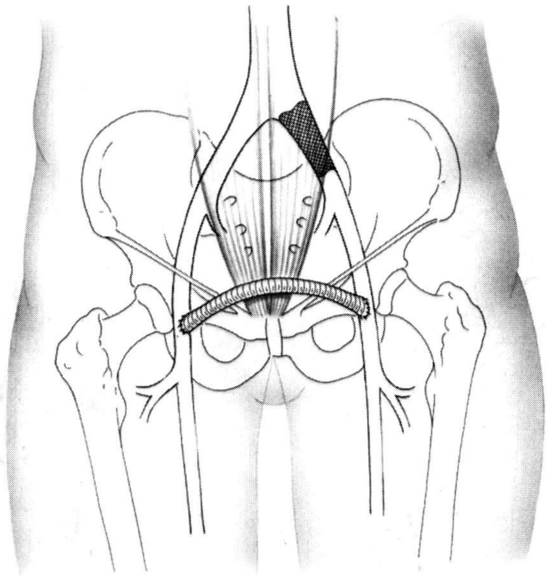

5

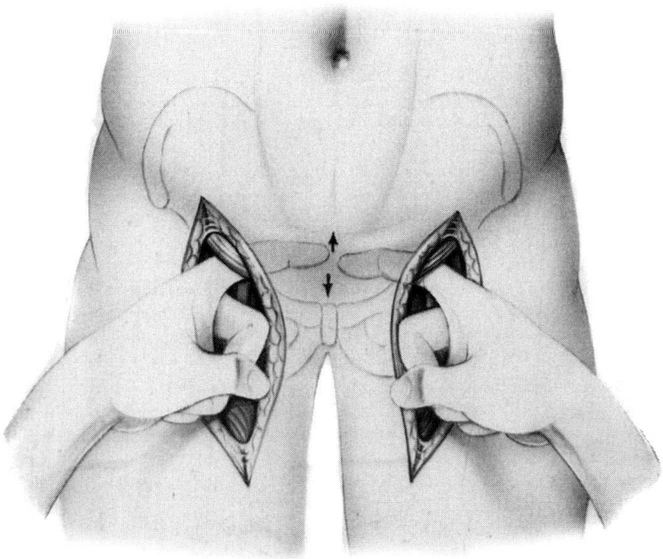

3

6

Other surgeons prefer a deeper positioning of the prosthesis and improved bypass haemodynamics (Courbier *et al.*, 1982). Donor vessels are prepared using an oblique incision parallel to the inguinal ligament, approximately 2–3 cm proximally to permit proximal anastomosis to the external iliac artery. The prosthesis is canalized more deeply behind the rectal muscle in the space of Retzius and below the inguinal ligament, resulting in a 'S'-shaped bypass.

With this procedure, the prosthesis is better protected against external compression, though there is a greater

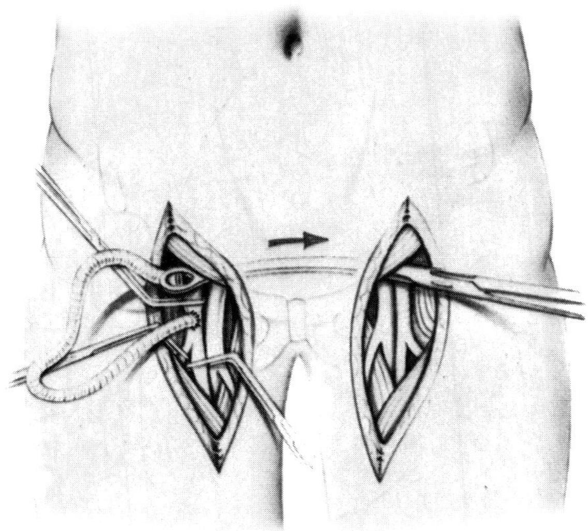

4

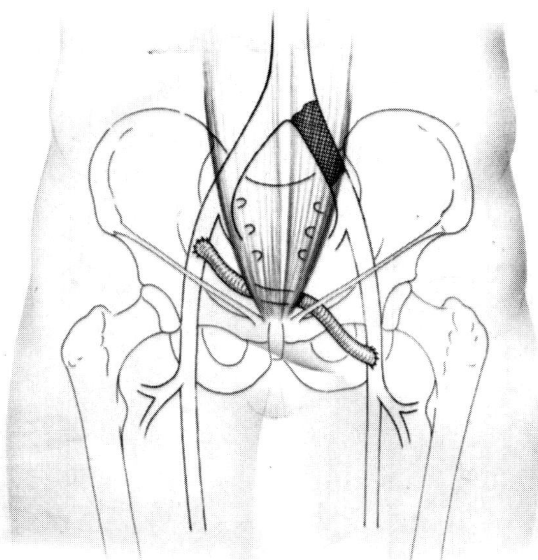

6

risk of bleeding due to the presence of a rich venous plexus. This crossover iliofemoral bypass is thus very different from the simple crossover femorofemoral bypass.

Iliofemoral bypass allows the prosthesis to be positioned outside the donor inguinal region, with its consequent lower risk of bacterial contamination from the the contralateral groin. Canalization in the space of Retzius, which lies at a deeper level than the inguinal ligament, involves the section of the fibrous layer of the ligament. This avoids compression of the prosthesis and traction on the suture line, which is frequently responsible for the formation of anastomotic aneurysms.

In the case of an infected groin, crossover transperineal bypass can be carried out. This entails a subcutaneous route at the level of the inguinoscrotal folds close to the spongy body, from the common femoral artery to the contralateral superficial or deep femoral artery, far from the site of infection. Autologous saphenous vein is the prosthesis of choice, otherwise PTFE.

Anastomoses are usually performed end-to-side, but with extended lesions of the host deep femoral artery requiring endarterectomy, at this level the anastomosis can be performed end-to-end. The suture material is usually 5/0 or 6/0 monofilament. After completion of the anastomoses with flush to prevent possible distal embolizations, the clamps are released and the pulsatility of the prosthesis and the proximal and contralateral vessels is controlled. Immediate postoperative control is performed by Doppler evaluation of the ankle pressure index (Winsor index) and by intraoperative angiography to evidence possible technical errors, e.g. torsion of the prosthesis or the intimal flap, which can be repaired immediately. After tubular drainage of the area, the groins are sutured by reconstruction of the fascia and section planes. Postoperatively, the antibiotic prophylaxis of infection plays a major role, especially in patients who show trophic lesions.

Contraindications

If adequate haemodynamic testing is carried out, there are no absolute contraindications for crossover femorofemoral bypass, though particular attention should be paid to the prophylaxis of infection, because the areas involved with the prosthesis are rich in lymphatic vessels and lymph-node stations, and are thus at risk.

In conclusion, femorofemoral bypass should be considered the procedure of choice in the treatment of unilateral iliac occlusion in high-risk patients. An accurate preoperative and haemodynamic assessment provides useful information for obtaining good long-term patency and haemodynamic function.

Editorial note

In the case where a long exposure of the profunda artery is not anticipated then an alternative incision should be considered. Chester *et al.* (1992) have shown that by performing a transverse/groin crease incision that the incidence of wound infection is markedly reduced.

References

Blaisdell RW, Hall AD, Lim RC Jr, Moore WC (1970). Aortoiliac arterial subcutaneous grafts. *Ann Surg* **172**: 775.

Chester JF, Butler CM, Taylor RS (1992). Vascular reconstruction of the groin . . . oblique or vertical incisions? *Ann R Coll Surg Eng* **74**: 112–114.

Courbier R, Larranaga J, Ferdani M *et al.* (1982). Le faux aneuvrismes sur prothèse artérielle. *Chirurgie* **108**: 459.

De Laurentis DA, Sala LE, Russell E, McCombs PR (1978). A twelve years experience with axillofemoral and femorofemoral bypass operations. *Surg Gynecol Obstet* **147**: 881.

Eugene J, Goldstone J, Moore WS (1977). Fifteen years experience with subcutaneous bypass grafts for lower extremity ischemia. *Ann Surg* **186**: 177.

Flanigan PD, Ryan TJ, Williams LR *et al.* (1984). Aortofemoral or femoropopliteal revascularization? A prospective evaluation of the papaverine test. *J Vasc Surg* **1**: 215.

Harper SA, Goldin AL, Mazzei EA, Cannon SA (1967). An experimental hemodynamic study of the subclavian steal syndrome. *Surg Gynecol Obstet* **124**: 1212.

Hill DA, Lord RSA, Tracy GD (1982). Haemodynamic consequences of cross femoral bypass. In *Extra-anatomic and Secondary Arterial Reconstruction.* **Greenhalgh** RM ed. London: Pitman.

Kalman PG, Hosang M, Johnston KW, Walker PM (1987). The current role for femorofemoral bypass. *J Vasc Surg* **6**: 71.

McDonald PT, Rich NM, Collins JG *et al.* (1978). Femorofemoral grafts: The role of concomitant extended profundaplasty. *Am J Surg* **136**: 622.

Martinez BB, Hertzer NR, Bevan EG (1980). Influence of distal arterial occlusive disease on prognosis following aortobifemoral bypass. *Surgery* **88**: 795.

Nelelsteen A, Suiw R, Daeneen W *et al.* (1980). Aortofemoral grafting: Factors influencing late result. *Surgery* **88**: 342.

Nicolaides AN, Angelides NS (1981). *Waveform Index and Resistance Factor Using Directional Doppler Ultrasound and Zero-crossing Detector.* New York: Churchill Livingstone.

Rutherford RB, Patt A, Pearce WH (1987). Extra-anatomic bypass: A closer view. *J Vasc Surg* **6**: 437.

Tyson RR, Reichle F A (1972). Retropubic femorofemoral bypass: A new route through the space of Retzius. *Surgery* **72**: 401.

Vijayanagar R, Bogudo DA, Eckstein PF (1982). Extra-anatomic bypass operation for aorto-iliac disease in poor risk cardiopulmonary patients. *Angiology* **33**: 69.

Whittemore KE, Billig PM, Pavlides C, Matsumoto T (1980). Special considerations in the revascularization for aortoiliac occlusive disease: Anatomic and extra-anatomic bypass. *Ann Surg* **46**: 279.

Subscrotal bypass for the infected groin

Roger N Baird

Introduction

Subscrotal femorofemoral bypass was described by Hardy and Bane in 1975. They reported on the management of a pelvic gunshot injury with massive blood loss by femoral-subscrotal-femoral bypass and 116 units of blood. The bypass was patent 1 year later. The following year, Kieffer *et al.*, in Paris, reported six subscrotal bypasses, aptly describing their route as 'pontages perineaux'.

Five were for infections following proximal Dacron prostheses implanted to the femoral arteries in the groin; one followed erosion of an external iliac artery by a vesical prosthesis. All were patent during follow-up of up to 8 months. Following this report, Cormier's group, also from Paris, reported 12 subscrotal bypasses for septic complications of Dacron prostheses and endarterectomy. Early graft thromboses occurred in three patients, two required further vascular operations and seven were patent with follow-up of up to 4 years.

In 1982 and 1986, Taylor and Massouh described four cases in which the indication was infection in the groin. Three arose from an infected Dacron prosthesis and one from tuberculous sinuses associated with an ischaemic leg. Two saphenous veins and two polytetrafluoroethylene (PTFE) conduits were used. In three instances the distal anastomosis was to a patent superficial femoral artery; and one to the above-knee popliteal artery. One saphenous vein bypass became stenosed at 2 years and required a patch repair. At the latest report, all four bypasses were patent at 3, 4, 6, and 7 years.

In 1985, Lawrence and Albo published a case report on the use of a subscrotal bypass of an infected groin following an aortofemoral Dacron graft, which was patent at 6 months follow-up. In 1991, Newington *et al.* included a subscrotal bypass in a report of 19 patients with deep groin wound infections.

Indications

With the exception of the first reported case, the indication for subscrotal bypass has been to bypass the infected groin. In many instances, a more conservative approach will succeed, including wound irrigation (Kwaan and Connolly, 1981) and rotational muscle flaps (Perler *et al.*, 1993). However, when the strength of the arterial wall is lost from bacterial arteritis, so that the anastomotic sutures lie slackly causing the discharging sinus to be complicated by haemorrhage, recourse has to be to local removal of the Dacron and ligation of the femoral arteries with revascularization by remote bypass. The subscrotal route is an alternative to oburator bypass, described in the following chapter. The procedure is unsuitable for women.

The distal attachment of a remote bypass is to the superficial femoral artery above the adductor hiatus, or the popliteal artery below it. The proximal attachment is to the contralateral common femoral artery. An arteriogram may be required to confirm the adequacy of the inflow and outflow arteries.

Operative technique

1

The diagram illustrates a subscrotal bypass from the left common femoral to the right superficial femoral artery. Note the infected right Dacron/femoral artery anastomosis. The patient lies supine with the legs abducted, a urethral catheter in place, the infected groin sealed with op-site, and the scrotum taped to the anterior abdominal wall. Intravenous antibiotics are administered, and the inflow common femoral artery, or uninfected limb of an aortobifemoral prosthesis, is mobilized, followed by the outflow superficial femoral or popliteal artery.

A subcutaneous tunnel is developed retroscrotally to

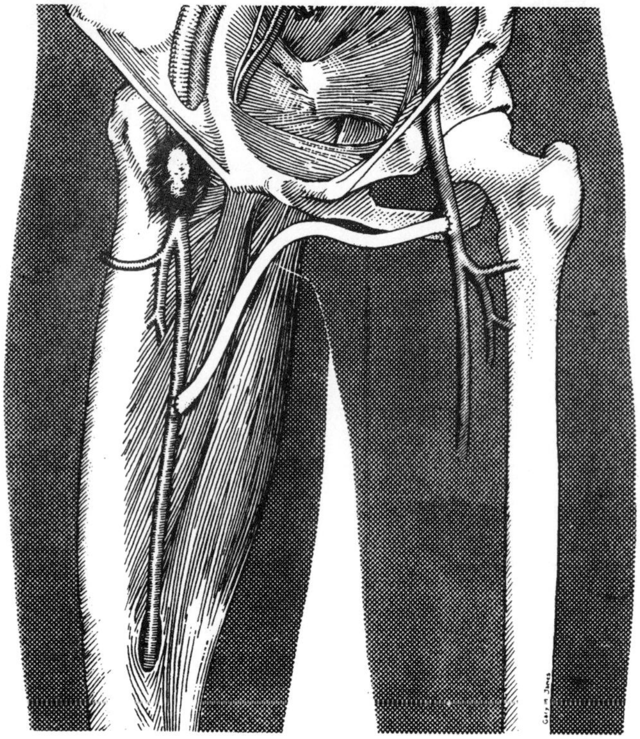

1

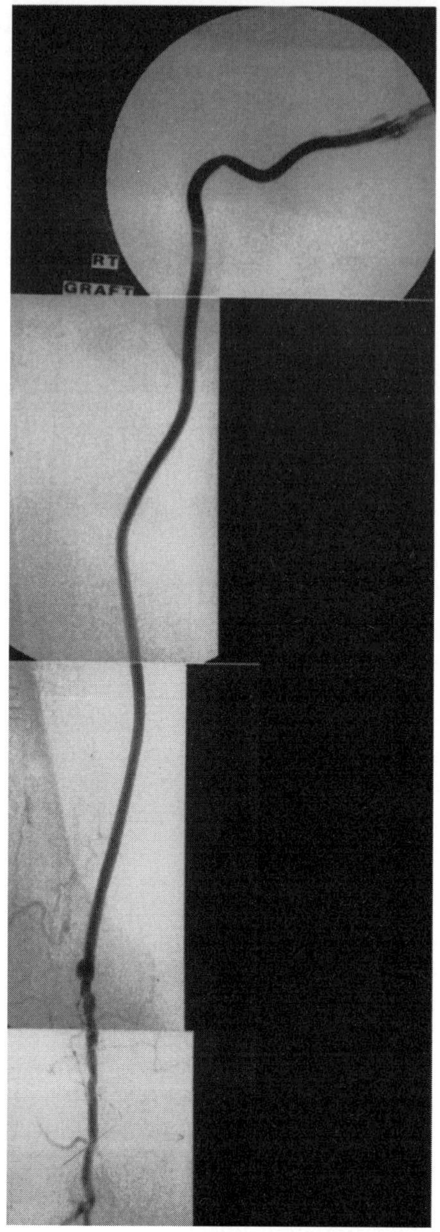

2

link the two incisions. Care is taken to avoid the urethra, which is easily identified by the urinary catheter. The bypass conduit, usually saphenous vein or PTFE is placed avoiding kinking and twisting. Excessive tension is avoided. The anastomoses are made end-to-side with 5/0 polypropylene sutures following systemic heparinization and the wounds are closed, and dressings applied.

Attention is then turned to the infected groin. As much as possible of the infected Dacron limb is ligated, excised and sent for culture. The common, superficial and deep femoral arteries are ligated and the wound edges are approximated, with wound drainage if necessary.

Postoperative care

2

Illustration 2 shows postoperative digital subtraction arteriogram of a PTFE subscrotal bypass to the above-knee popliteal artery. Note the rounded perineal arch.

Bypass patency is checked by pulse palpation, Doppler ankle pressure measurements and by digital subtraction angiography. The bypass incisions require little attention. However, it may take some time for healthy granulation tissue to appear in the infected groin wound. Routine graft follow-up for infrainguinal bypasses is undertaken. Cycling is best avoided.

Conclusions

The subscrotal route from the contralateral groin is a useful, and some would say technically easier alternative to the obturator route from the ipsilateral iliac artery, as a remote bypass of an infected groin.

References

Hardy JD, Bane JW (1975). Arterial injury and massive blood loss: a case report of management of pelvic gunshot injury with femoro-subscrotal-femoral bypass and 116 units of blood. *Ann Surg* **181**: 245.

Kieffer E, Laurian C, Surugue P, Natali J (1976). Pontage veineux fémoro-fémoral par le perinée. *Chirurgie* **102**: 420.

Kwaan JHM, Connolly JE (1981). Successful treatment of prosthetic graft infection with continuous povidone-iodine irrigation. *Arch Surg* **116**: 716.

Laurian C, Martino A, Courmier JM (1981). *Ann Chirurgie* **35**: 455.

Lawrence PF, Albo D (1985). Femoro-femoral bypass with an infrascrotal perineal approach for the patient with an infected groin wound. *J Vasc Surg* **2**: 485.

Newington DP, Houghton PWJ, Baird RN *et al* (1991). Groin wound infection after arterial surgery. *Br J Surg* 78: 617.

Perler BA, Vander Koek CA, Manson PM, Williams GM (1993). Rotational muscle flaps to treat localised prosthetic graft infection: longterm follow-up. *J Vasc Surg* **18**: 358.

Taylor RS, Massouh F (1982). The transperineal graft – an alternative route for femoro-femoral bypass. In *Extra-anatomic and Secondary Arterial Reconstruction*, Greenhalgh RM, ed. London: Pitman, pp. 237–243.

Taylor RS, Massouh F (1986). Femoro-femoral bypass with an infrascrotal approach for the patient with an infected groin wound. (letter) *J Vasc Surg* **3**: 555.

Obturator canal bypass

G Kretschmer,
B Niederle, M Wunderlich

Introduction

Since obturator canal bypass was introduced by Shaw and Baue in 1963, its indications and techniques have been precisely defined. Today the method is an established standard procedure in vascular surgery, with the results of 250 patients being published. In general, more or less anecdotal reports are available; the largest series comprise 13 and 27 patients, respectively (Van Det and Brands, 1981; Niederle *et al.*, 1988). A survey of the literature concerning long-term results and an evaluation of their own results has been published. Guidelines and conclusions are drawn from these reports and our own experience (Van Det and Brands, 1981; Prenner and Rendl, 1982; Buchardt-Hansen *et al.*, 1982; Cotton, 1982; Geroulakos *et al.*, 1988; Niederle *et al.*, 1988).

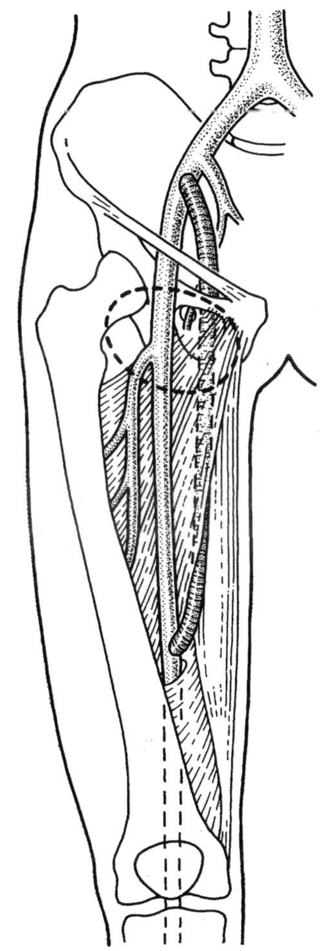

1

1

Concept

The basic principle is to create an extensive extra-anatomical bypass from the pelvic to the distal femoral or infragenicular arteries, the site of distal anastomosis depending on the respective morphological conditions.

Graft-conduction through the foramen obturatum, dorsal to hip-joint and adductor muscle group, avoids the femoral triangle so as to prevent any contamination. Accordingly, the procedure allows thorough separation of the graft from the obviously or potentially infected inguinal area through an uncompromised barrier of normal tissue.

Principally, any vascular substitute of adequate dimensions may be acceptable and most have been tested. As would be expected, autologous saphenous vein has been employed in 16% of patients. Although autologous grafts give the most satisfying long-term results, the limited diameter of these conduits often precludes their use. In the remaining patients, the greater distance to be bridged usually requires the use of fabric grafts.

We have found polytetrafluoroethylene (PTFE) prostheses (21 of 27 cases) to have been most satisfactory. Our initial experience with externally reinforced grafts has been promising, due to their greater resistance against kinking and compression.

Indications

Throughout the literature there is unanimous agreement that the most frequent indication (58%) is unilateral deep infection, strictly confined to the groin (type III according to Szilagyi *et al.*, 1972) as a sequel of vascular surgery of any kind (Brücke and Piza, 1968; Prenner and Rendl, 1982). Less frequent indications are rather evenly distributed between infections subsequent to vascular access surgery (12%; Prenner and Rendl, 1982), inguinal skin and subcutaneous tissue defects after extensive tumour surgery and/or therapeutic irradiation (17%; Niederle *et al.*, 1988) and, finally, complicated (non-arteriosclerotic) aneurysms and severe inguinal scarring (13%; Buchardt-Hansen *et al.*, 1982; Cotton, 1982).

Angiography

The value of preoperative arteriography to identify suitable areas for proximal and distal anastomoses is undisputed. However, in the case of massive bleeding as an emergency indication, valuable time can be wasted waiting for preoperative information. the site of distal anastomosis may then be chosen on grounds of radiology, obtained prior to the primary procedure, or by distal exploration, if necessary with adjunctive on-table angiography during the present bypass procedure.

2

Instrumentation

In addition to the standard instruments for vascular surgery, we use a slim, long-bladed grasping-forceps, 65cm in length and with a slight bend of 20 degrees for boring the tunnel and guiding the graft into place (i.e. sponge and dressing clamp according to Sims-Meier (Brücke and Piza, 1968). Of course, any other forceps of adequate length with long blunt jaws will be adequate.

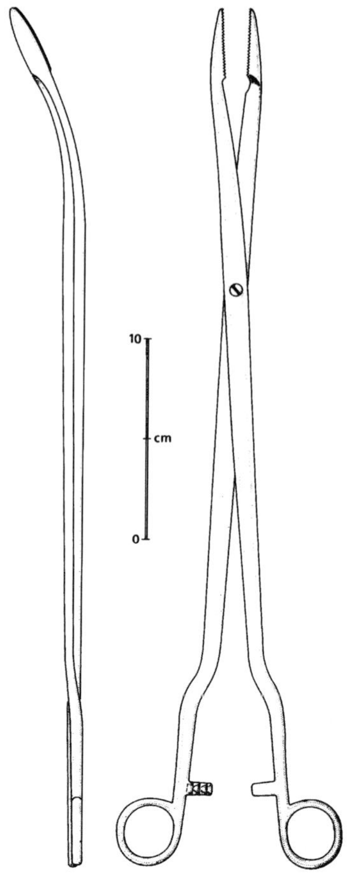

2

3

Positioning and preparation of the patient

With the patient in the prone position, the spine and hip-joints are slightly overextended to allow the grasping-forceps to be directed through the obturator canal behind the superior branch of the public bone without impediment from the abdominal wall – an obstacle most likely to be met in obese patients.

The entire abdomen and the limb concerned are disinfected and draped in such a way as to permit good access to the abdominal and distal incisions at the medial aspect of thigh and calf. Our practice is to use incisive drapes covering the skin, paying particular regard to the crucial femoral triangle so as to avoid any contamination therefrom.

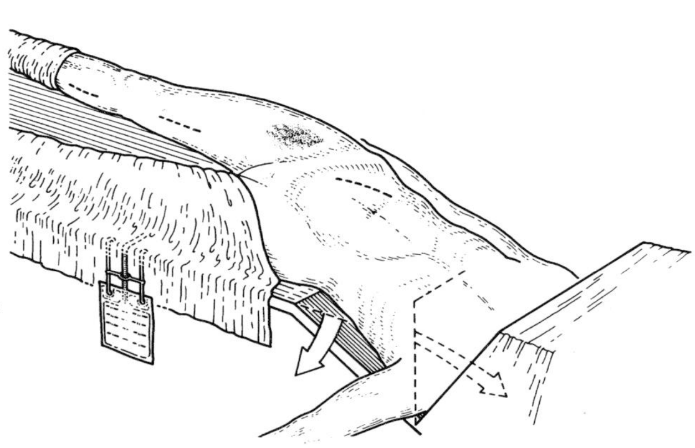

3

Anaesthetic management

Surgery is performed under general anaesthesia, with the use of at least one or two major intravenous lines, preferably a central venous catheter. A urinary catheter is essential (see Illustration 3). The operative strain on the patient can be estimated by using a mean duration of anaesthesia of 3½ hours and a mean quantity of blood loss corresponding to 3 units (Kretschmer *et al.*, 1989).

Surgical procedure

4

Standard approaches are used for extraperitoneal exposure of the pelvic arteries as well as for medial exposure of the femoral, popliteal or even crural vessles (Leitz, 1981). As a rule, we prefer the extraperitoneal (n = 17) to the transperitoneal (n = 10) approach, the latter being reserved for re-do surgery.

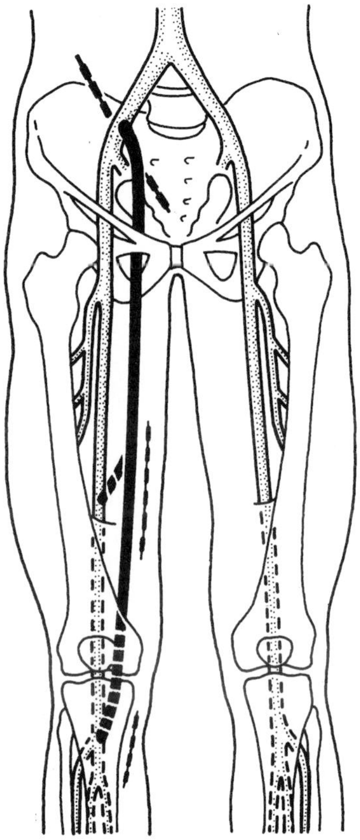

4

5,6

Gentle sweeping of the peritoneal sac, ureter and bladder to the midline gives access to the foramen obturatum. In male and obese patients in particular, the foramen is often better identified by mere digital palpation of its sharp fascial circumference than by actually viewing it during deep pelvic dissection (Brücke and Piza, 1968). It is our practice to penetrate the membrana obturatoria from the proximal distally, and then bore the tunnel and place the graft, taking care to leave the obturator vessels and the nerve unharmed. In order to avoid blind tunnelling in a heparinized patient, systemic heparin (100 international units/kg body weight) is administered after graft placement only. Alternative sites for the anastomosis are shown in Illustration **6**. The proximal anastomosis is constructed by using the side-to-end technique. Cross-clamping of externally supported grafts is not advisable. The distal end of the graft is cut to shape during full extension of the knee joint. After completion of the distal anastomosis, the vascular clamps are released.

If possible, the external iliac artery should not undergo preliminary ligation from within the pelvis in order to preserve a maximum of collateral circulation to the leg. Suction drains are left in place for 2 days.

Some authors prefer boring the tunnel from the distal proximally (Pearce *et al.*, 1983; Prenner and Rendl, 1982), suggesting that lesions of the obturator artery and vein are better avoided; however, we cannot confirm this.

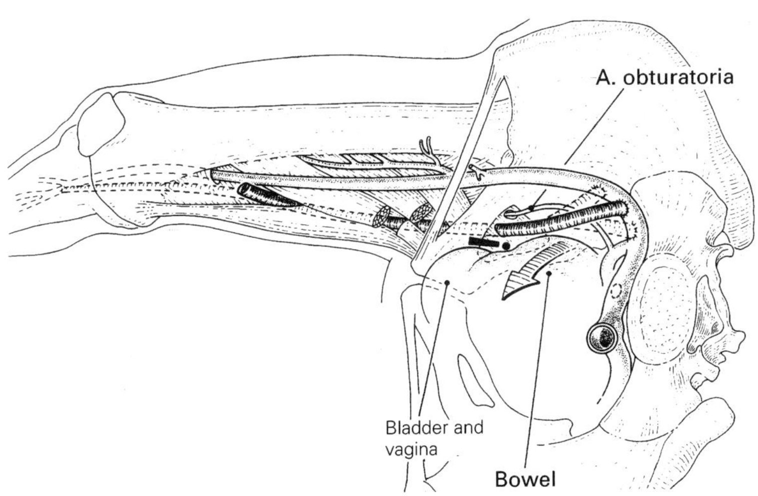

5

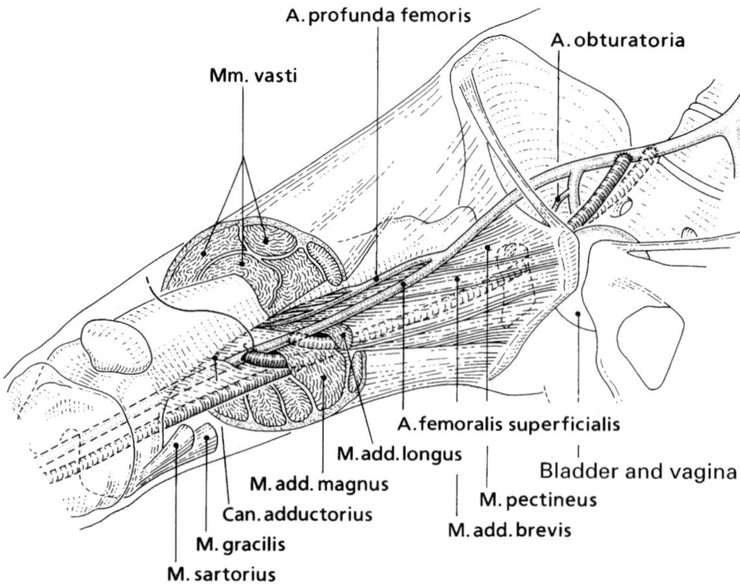

6

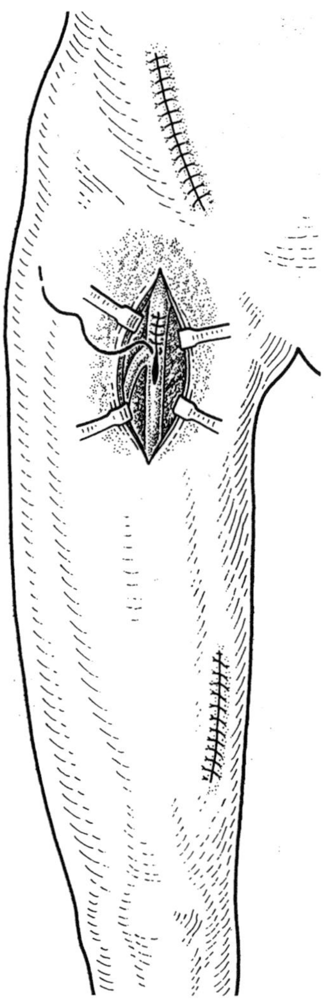

7

7

If it is felt necessary, the bypass procedure is followed by debridement of the inguinal wound by removing the remaining alloplastic material and local suturing of vascular defects, to secure haemostasis. At the same time, swabs are taken to prescribe antibiotic therapy accordingly.

The operation is rarely indicated; only limited series of patients and/or case reports are available. An evaluation of the operation with the usual techniques of estimating patency, limb salvage and finally patient survival is difficult to obtain. Data from two centres in Austria as well as results derived from the literature were pooled and comparatively assessed. The procedure was found to be reliable and durable, but demonstrated the known disadvantages like other operations, in which alloplastic vascular substitutes necessarily bridge long distances thereby crossing a major joint.

Complications

The usual complications following implantation of long-distance fabric grafts are encountered. In the absence of underlying arteriosclerotic disease, long-term graft performance is excellent. However, patency rates cannot be reliably derived from the literature, as most reports do not distinguish if lesions requiring obturator canal bypass have originally been related to chronic occlusive vascular disease or not.

As circulation along the deep femoral artery has to be sacrificed, or is at least severely compromised, graft occlusion will inevitably threaten the entire extremity. Unless prompt surgical correction is feasible, the ischaemic syndrome will necessitate major, if not above-knee, amputation. Therefore, thrombectomy should be attempted without delay, the long-term performance of the graft depending on the availability of the more favourable distal anastomotic site above the knee, the peripheral run-off conditions and the progression of the underlying disease.

The preservation of the collateral circulation in the inguinal area may become of vital importance. If the collateral blood supply is insufficient following preliminary ligation of the external iliac artery, eradication of the common femoral and the superficial and deep femoral at the origin will lead to necrosis of the thigh musculature, the graft remaining obviously patent (Rudich *et al.*, 1979).

If a combination of infection plus haemorrhage demands an extra-anatomical bypass, the procedure will reliably eradicate the danger of exsanguinating haemorrhage while preserving the limb's blood supply (Kretschmer *et al.*, 1989). However, in our series, this combination of events caused two fatalities, the patients with viable limbs having finally succumbed to irreversible sepsis (Kretschmer *et al.*, 1989). Topographical misplacement of the graft was observed, leading to perforation of the bladder or vagina (Szilagyi *et al.*, 1972) with subsequent infection and ultimate loss of limb.

Obturator canal bypass may be considered as a valuable addition to the armamentarium of vascular surgery, designed as it is for the treatment of isolated lesions concerning the femoral triangle. The procedure permits generous bypassing of the inguinal risk area and warrants surgery within operative fields as yet untouched. However, it is not devoid of the disadvantage of alloplastic grafts over long distances, with an increased risk of infection.

References

Brücke P, Piza F (1968). Zur Indikation des Obturator-Bypass. *Zbl Chir* **93**: 489.

Buchardt-Hansen HJ, Holstein P, Krogh-Christoffersen J (1982). Obturator canal bypass to avoid an infected or scarred groin. In *Extraanatomic and Secondary Arterial Reconstruction.* Greenhalgh R M ed. London: Pitman.

Cotton LT (1982). Obturator canal bypass for aneurysms in the thigh. In *Extraanatomic and Secondary Arterial Reconstruction.* Greenhalgh R M ed. London: Pitman.

Geroulakos G, Parvin SD, Bell PRF (1988). Obturator foramen bypass, the alternative route for sepsis in the femoral triangle. *Acta Chir Scand* **154**: 111.

Kretschmer G, Niederle B, Huk I *et al.* (1989). Groin infections following vascular surgery: Obturator bypass (BYP) versus biologic coverage (TRP) – a comparative evaluation. *Eur J Vasc Surg* **3**: 25.

Leitz KH (1981). *Zugangswege in der Gefäbchirurgie.* Heidelberg: Springer.

Niederle B, Polterauer P, Kretschmer G, Piza F (1988). Der Obturatorbypass – Indikation und Ergebnisse bei 27 Patienten. *Angio Arch* **16**: 90.

Pearce WH, Ricco JP, Yao JST *et al.* (1983). Modified technique of obturator bypass in failed or infected grafts. *Annl Surg* **197**: 344.

Prenner KV, Rendl KH (1982). Indications and technique of obturator bypass. In *Extraanatomic and Secondary Arterial Reconstruction.* Greenhalgh RM ed. London: Pitman.

Rudich M, Gutierrez IZ, Gage AA (1979). Obturator foramen bypass in the management of infected vascular prosthesis. *Am J Surg* **137**: 657.

Shaw RS, Baue AE (1963). Management of sepsis complicating arterial reconstructive surgery. *Surgery* **53**: 57.

Sheiner NM, Sigman H, Stilman A (1969). An unusual complication of obturator foramen arterial bypass. *J Cardiovasc Surg* **10**: 324.

Szilagyi DE, Smith RF, Elliott JP, Vrandecic MP (1972). Infection in arterial reconstruction with synthetic grafts *Annl Surg* **176**: 321.

Van Det RJ, Brands LC (1981). The obturator foramen bypass: An alternative procedure in iliofemoral artery revascularization. *Surgery* **89**: 543.

Imaging for endovascular abdominal aortic aneurysm repair (EVAR): Considerations, techniques and pitfalls

David Kessel, I Robertson, J Scott

Introduction

Not all patients with abdominal aortic aneurysm are suitable for endovascular stent-grafting. Pre-procedural assessment must reliably reject unsuitable patients, identify potential difficulties and allow selection of an appropriate stent-graft. Attention must be paid to the factors which most commonly prevent endovascular abdominal aortic aneurysm repair (EVAR). A local audit of spiral computed tomography (CT) in 100 consecutive patients with abdominal aortic aneurysms revealed that 35 (35%) could immediately be excluded from EVAR using contemporary commercially available devices. The most common reasons for rejection related to the proximal neck:

1. Proximal neck diameter more than 27 mm (52%).
2. Proximal neck length less than 15 mm (24%).
3. Proximal neck thrombus or plaque (17%).

Difficult arterial access (3%) and other factors (15%) were much less frequent; 13% of patients were precluded by more than one factor. Of the 65 patients suitable for EVAR roughly half would be considered straightforward; the remainder would be technically challenging due to complex anatomy. There are three essential requirements for successful EVAR.

1. **Access**. The introducer systems are large (16–28F in diameter) and relatively inflexible. If the iliac arteries are small, severely diseased or tortuous then it will be impossible for the delivery system to pass through them. In practical terms if the iliac arteries are less than 7 mm EVAR is unlikely to succeed.
2. **Anchorage**. All stent graft systems need to achieve a seal between the proximal and distal ends of the device and the aortic or iliac wall. This requires snug apposition over a length of at least 15 mm. The graft is oversized by 10–20% compared with the diameter of the proximal neck. The largest commercially available grafts are 31 mm, thus the upper limit of diameter of the proximal neck is 27–28 mm. Distal attachment needs to be equally secure.
3. **Adequate visceral blood supply**. EVAR is only an option if the stent graft does not occlude vital blood supply to the bowel or pelvic organs. The inferior mesenteric artery can only be covered if the superior mesenteric artery SMA is patent. Similarly at least one internal iliac artery should be preserved to minimize the risk of pelvic ischaemia.

Imaging

1, 2

Almost all imaging modalities have been used in the patient work-up. Ultrasound is used to establish the diagnosis of abdominal aortic aneurysm. Spiral CT is the mainstay of imaging in most centres and can reliably categorize most patients as suited or unsuited to EVAR. Angiography with a calibrated pigtail catheter is also widely used to assess lengths; it is indispensable when three-dimensional (3D) CT reformats are not available. Magnetic resonance imaging (MRI) has the advantage of not involving ionizing radiation or requiring iodinated contrast and is likely to become more important as availability increases (1, 9). Illustration 1 shows anteroposterior (AP) and lateral maximum intensity projections from a magnetic resonance angiogram of same patient as (9). Patent lumbar arteries are clearly seen. Like conventional angiography the true extent of the aneurysm is unclear as only the lumen is displayed.

Whichever form of imaging is chosen, the assessment of the aneurysm and choice of device remains an imprecise science and demands a pragmatic approach. Simple algorithms can be devised based on the local expertise.

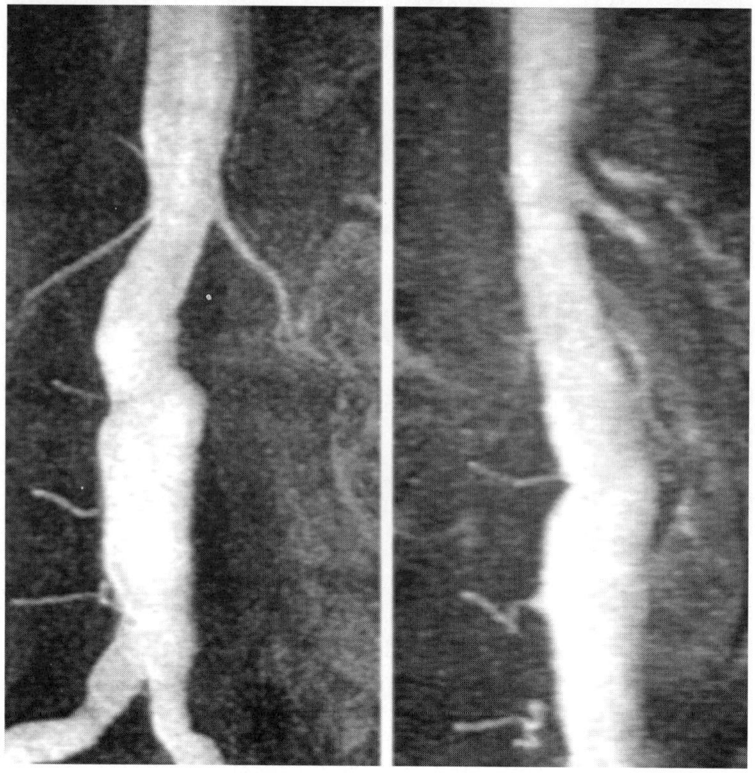

1

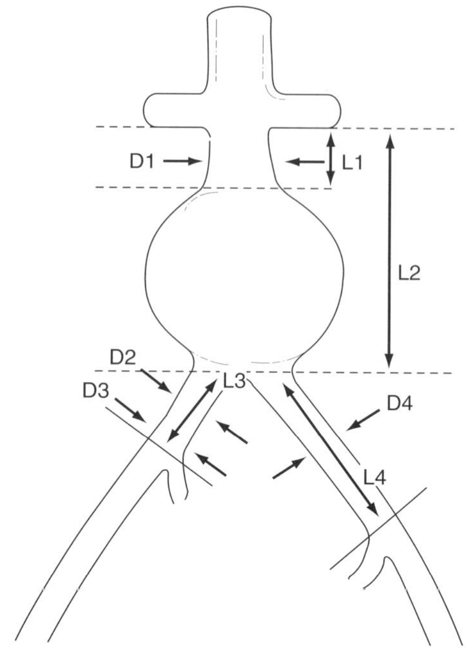

2

Regardless of which stent graft is to be used a similar series of measurements must be obtained for each patient. Lengths and diameters required for successful EVAR are shown (2). Note that when there is discrepancy in diameter e.g. right common iliac artery D2 and D3 the maximum and minimum values are recorded. These measurements are usually based on a combination of CT and calibrated angiography. A simple worksheet can be filled out to record the relevant details.

Spiral CT

3

High quality contrast-enhanced spiral CT is essential. The patient should not have oral contrast as this may interfere with 3D reconstruction. The scan must include from the coeliac axis to the common femoral arteries. The study is performed during a single breath hold. Typically 100–150 ml of iodinated contrast (350 mg/ml) is infused at 3 ml/second. A timing bolus can be performed but in practice starting scanning after 30 seconds gives excellent arterial enhancement in most cases. Collimation should be no more than 5 mm with slice reconstructions at 3-mm intervals at the proximal neck and 5 mm distal to this; 3D reconstructions are very helpful but are not available on all machines. The 3D reformat allows a much better appreciation of the arterial morphology but step artefacts can degrade images of the iliac arteries and give the impression of stenosis (3).

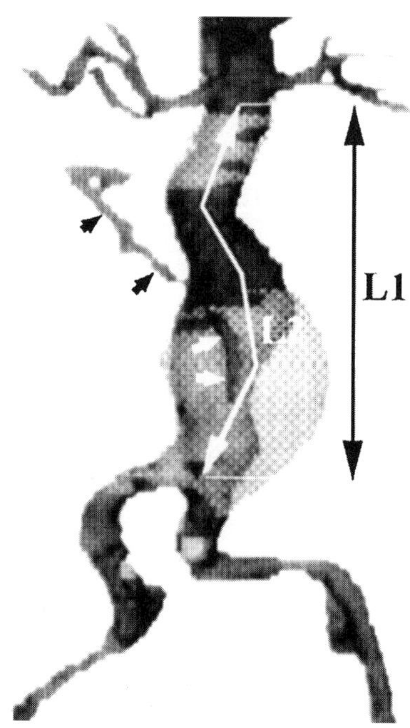

3

A 3D CT reconstruction (3) shows an aneurysm with a tortuous neck. The lumen is seen through the thrombus (hatched shading). The inferior mesenteric artery (white arrows) and an accessory right renal artery (black arrows) are seen. Step artefact is seen in the iliac arteries with a pseudostenosis in the left common iliac artery (L1 represents the renal artery to bifurcation length as calculated using table position. The true length is shown by the centre lumen line L2.)

Axial scans: what to look for

Anchorage

The first step is to evaluate the proximal aneurysm neck. The ideal neck is straight, parallel-sided and free of plaque and thrombus. Look for irregularity of the lumen, if there is more than a tiny amount then you are unlikely to achieve a seal and the patient should not have endovascular repair. Next, measure the neck diameter. There is no clear agreement as to whether the internal or the external diameter should be used. We use the internal diameter but tend to oversize by 20%. The neck diameter can be measured on the CT console using electronic callipers or from hard copy images with mechanical callipers. Either technique is acceptable as long as the operator understands the requirement for precision. Ideally, use a magnified view as this minimizes measurement error. Lengths of the aneurysm can also be estimated from the CT table position but is prone to underestimation if the anatomy is tortuous (3).

Table position at the lower end of the neck length = neck – table position at the level of the lowest renal artery.

4, 5

Potential pitfall

As the aorta expands it also lengthens causing the aneurysm neck to deviate anteriorly and laterally. Axial scanning does not take this into account and the vessel appears oval rather than round in cross-section (4).

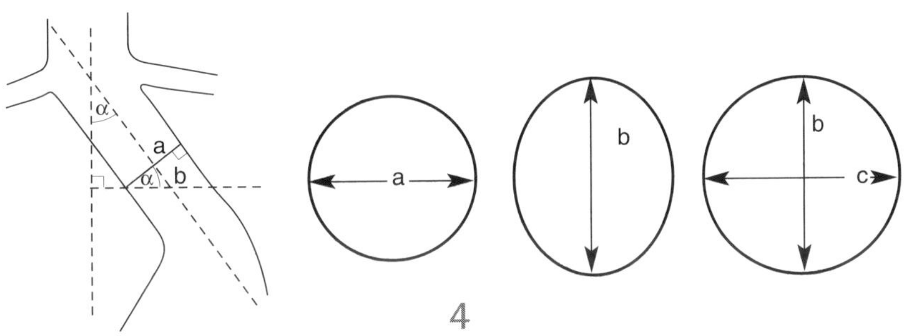

4

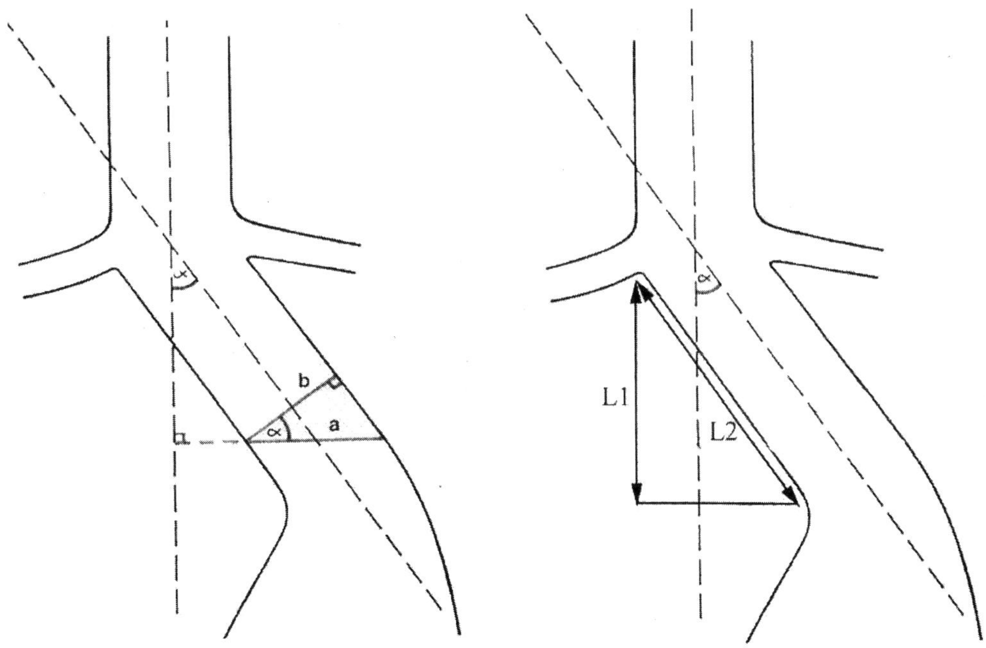

5

Illustration 4 shows the effect on the axial CT scan of neck angulation α degrees from the long axis of the aorta. The relationship between the true diameter (a) and the apparent diameter (b) is a = b cos α. When the neck deviates anteriorly and laterally the apparent diameters are increased in both the anteroposterior (b) and tranverse directions (c).

This results in a tendency to overestimate the neck diameter and to underestimate the neck length (5). Illustration 5 shows the effect of neck angulation on apparent neck diameter and length: (true diameter b = a cos α; true length L2 = L1/cos α). Neck angulation can be compensated for by angulation of the CT scanner gantry or the angiography C-arm to a plane at 90 degrees to the long axis of the neck. An angulation of 30 degrees would cause an overestimation of 4 mm in a 25 mm neck rendering the aneurysm untreatable by EVAR. The neck diameter should always be measured in the shortest axis. The only way to guarantee that there is no error is to ensure that the image is reconstructed perpendicular to the long axis of the neck.

Adequate visceral supply

Check the patency of the coeliac axis and superior mesenteric artery. Identify the renal arteries and look for evidence of renal artery stenosis. Search carefully for accessory renal arteries (3) which might be occluded by the graft. If there is any question regarding the patency of the aortic branches angiography is indicated. Identify patent lumbar arteries and the inferior mesenteric artery. These are potential collateral routes for the development of type II endoleak (1, 3).

Access

The iliac arteries are the route of access and the site of distal anchorage and should be inspected for calcification, stenosis and tortuousity. Care must be taken measuring the iliac arteries on axial scans due to the problems of slice obliquity. Focal stenosis and calcified plaques are easily overlooked.

Other

Look at the body of the aneurysm. Are there any complicating factors, mural thrombus, leak, inflammation or infection? Stent grafting should be avoided if there is any suggestion of infection. Don't forget to look for other pathology within the abdomen; cancers are common in this age group and may influence the treatment option.

If the aneurysm appears suitable for EVAR then the next issue is device-sizing. This involves measuring a series of lengths and diameters. Calibrated angiography and 3D CT reformats are essential.

Calibrated angiography

6

A 5F pigtail catheter with markers at 1-cm intervals is placed in the aneurysm and angiography performed. Both AP and lateral views are obtained (6). Anterior neck angulation causes considerable foreshortening of the neck in the AP projection. Note that the catheter does not follow the centre lumen line. Start with the proximal marker at level of the lower renal artery inject 20 ml contrast at 10 ml/second imaging at 2 frames/second. When the segment from the renal arteries has been imaged pull the pigtail back into the aneurysm sac so that the markers extend beyond the ipsilateral internal iliac artery. Now acquire AP and oblique views of the iliac arteries. This is the most reliable way of assessing stenosis and tortuousity. If the iliac arteries are tortuous and heavily calcified reject the patient. If the arteries are tortuous but non-calcified try straightening them by pasing a stiff guidewire (Amplatz super stiff or Lunderquist wire) through the pigtail catheter. If the wire will not pass or the artery does not straighten then a stent graft delivery catheter is most unlikely to succeed. Lengths and diameters can be directly measured at a workstation using the proprietary software or from the angiographic image using callipers.

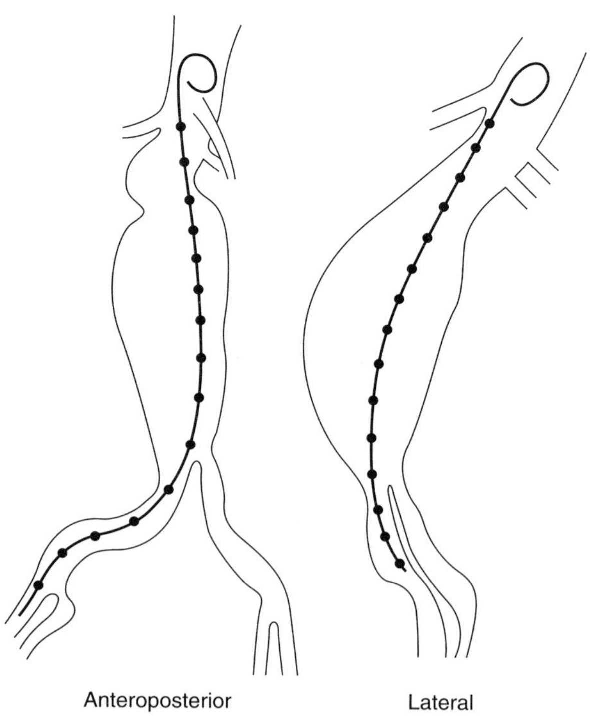

6

7, 8, 9

Pitfalls

Calibrated angiography is regarded as the gold standard but is prone to significant and predictable measurement errors caused by thrombus, magnification, parallax and catheter curvature. The angiogram only shows the vessel lumen; in the presence of extensive thrombus it is impossible to judge the size and position of the aneurysm and measurements of neck length will be unreliable (1, 7–9).

Illustration **7** shows comparison of a shaded surface 3D CT reconstruction with a calibrated angiogram in the same patient. The CT accurately reflects the anatomy. The catheter does not follow the centre lumen line and the angulation would tend to underestimate the true length. This effect can be compensated for by craniocaudal angulation of the C-arm. In contrast overall lengths are normally underestimated because the catheter takes the shortest straightest route and does not follow the central lumen line (**6–8**). Hence the length estimated by the catheter is shorter than the route taken by the stent graft. The more tortuous the anatomy the greater the error.

When calibrating from the catheter it is important to choose a projection where curvature does not cause foreshortening. Calibrate from the most widely spaced markers. The contralateral iliac artery cannot be directly measured and must be assessed on the AP projection from markers in the distal aorta (**8**).

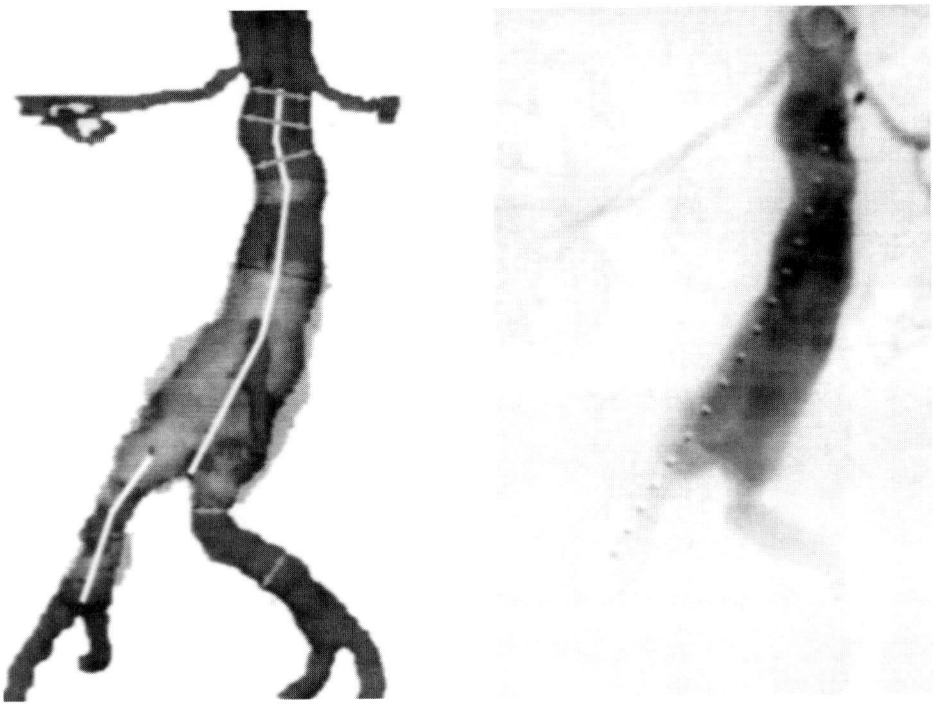

7

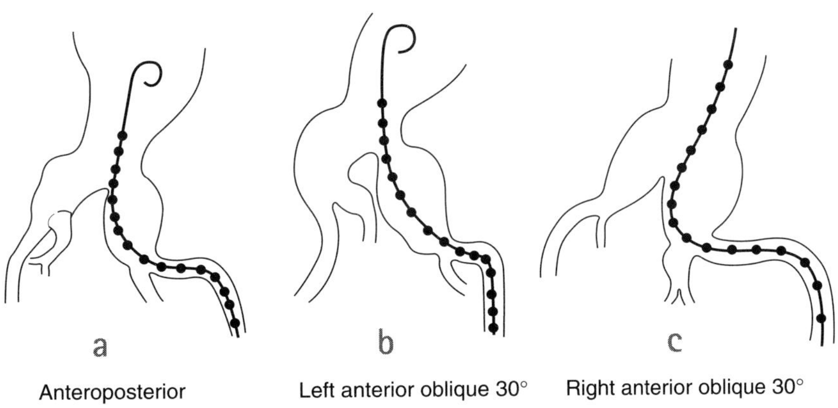

8

Illustration **8** shows tracings of calibrated angiograms showing the aortic bifurcation and iliac arteries in the AP (**8a**) and both oblique projections (Left anterior oblique 30 degrees (**8b**) right anterior oblique 30 degrees (**8c**)). Vessel curvature causes marked variation in the apparent interval between the centimetre markers. The effect is minimized in **8c**. The bifurcation to internal iliac artery distance seems to vary considerably with the projection. Measurements of the contralateral common iliac artery should be made on the AP projection and calibrated to the catheter in the distal aorta. Measure the contralateral right common iliac artery diameter on the three images above to appreciate the effects of the distortion. The effects of projection on the apparent lengths of the common iliac segments is readily appreciated.

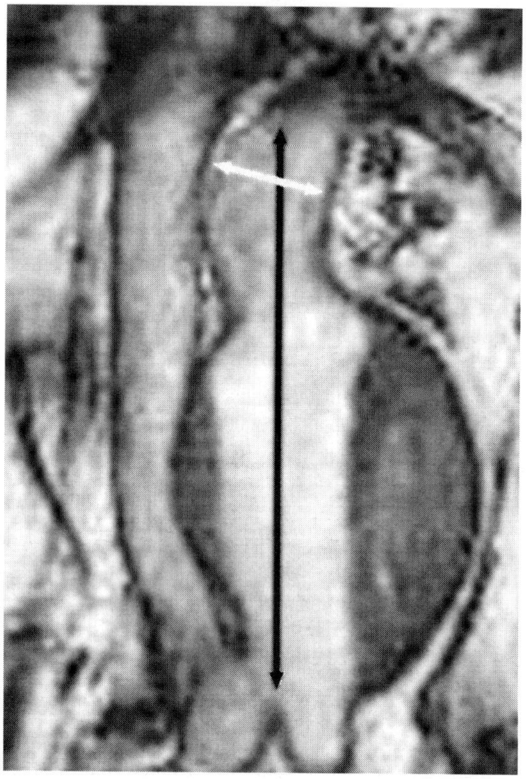

9

Many of the measurements can be made from 3D CT reformats. The capabilities of the CT scanner and workstation and local expertise will dictate which can be used. The optimal technique is a shaded surface display with a centre-line lumen measurement (**3**, **7**). Simple multiplanar reformats in the sagittal and coronal planes will allow assessment of the aneurysm neck. Illustration **9** shows coronal projection from an MRI scan of an abdominal aortic aneurysm. Lengths and diameters can be measured as long as the aneurysm does not deviate from the coronal plane. Curved planar reformats allow much of the aneurysm morphology to be appreciated. Where 3D CT has been validated it can replace calibrated angiography but it is not as accurate as catheter angiography for assessing branch vessel and iliac disease (**3**).

Deciding which device and approach

Filling in worksheets is very helpful as it allows careful planning of the entire procedure at the time of reviewing the imaging.

Computed tomography (CT) measurements of the neck usually give a greater diameter than calibrated angiogram. This is in part due to parallax errors on the angiogram. Use whichever is the larger diameter; the neck is likely to enlarge with time and there is nothing worse than using too small a graft with a resultant type I endoleak.

Lengths can be estimated from the calibrated angiogram (**7**). The catheter tends to take the shortest possible route, the graft takes a longer route and as a result often appears shorter than anticipated. The centre-line lumen length is more accurate and can be estimated from the angiogram or measured from CT or MRI reconstructions (**3**, **9**).

Iliac disease is best assessed by angiography or magnetic resonance angiography due to inherent pitfalls in CT reconstructions of small vessels especially when running in the scan plane (**3**). Take careful measurements from calibrated angiograms as there can be considerable error due to the magnification effects of obliquity (**8**).

Deciding on the size of the device requires a degree of pragmatism due to the limited range of sizes of most stent graft systems. It is always better to oversize diameters by 10–20%. Plan to leave the graft close to the internal iliac arteries at least 3 cm into the common iliac arteries. The stent graft will usually be shorter than anticipated so inadvertent occlusion of the internal iliac artery is unlikely.

Always plan the simplest approach for EVAR. Deploy the body of the graft via the straightest iliac artery. The length of modular systems can be tailored to preserve the internal iliac artery if there is concern about pelvic ischaemia.

Conclusion

Although assessment of aortic aneurysm for endovascular repair is an imprecise science careful measurement and recognition of the many pitfalls will minimize the potential for errors especially in cases with complex anatomy.

Carbon dioxide angiography 10, 11, 12

This brief section will first outline the uses of carbon dioxide (CO_2) angiography and indicate the limitations of the technique and second describe a simple system for using CO_2. Carbon dioxide angiography can only be performed on state of the art angiography equipment. Special software is required to summate minimally opacified images (**10**); this is the opposite of conventional angiography. At present this limits its use to contemporary fixed installation angiography equipment. If you are not fortunate enough to possess such a facility then read no further; CO_2 angiography is not for you. Illustration **10** is a Type II endoleak shown on CO_2 angiography. Illustration 10a shows a native non-subtracted image; **10b** shows the same image subtracted. The endoleak (black arrow) fills from the iliolumbar trunk (white arrows).

Carbon dioxide gas angiography is particularly indicated when the patient has a contraindication to conventional contrast such as a previous contrast reaction, renal or cardiac impairment. It may also be used in cases such as aortic stent-grafting where a high contrast load would be anticipated. Carbon dioxide is highly soluble in the blood and is excreted on the first passage through the lungs. There is no limit to the total volume of CO_2 that can be injected but volumes are usually restricted to 200ml per minute.

Conventional iodine-containing liquid contrast agents are of high density and opacify vessels by mixing with blood. Progressive dilution occurs as the contrast agent is carried within the bloodstream; fortunately the high contrast sensitivity of digital subtraction angiography allows visualization of peripheral vessels from a mainstream injection. Gaseous agents are low density and displace blood from a section of the vessel; as it flows along the bolus tends to float on the surface of the blood and posterior vessels may not be seen (**11**). A conventional contrast calibrated angiogram is seen in **11a** and a CO_2 angiogram during stent-grafting in **11b**. Conventional contrast fills the internal iliac arteries (white arrow), and an aortic CO_2 injection only opacifies the origin of the right internal iliac artery (short white arrow). Embolization coils are seen in the left internal iliac artery (black arrows).

Conversely, anterior vessels such as the coeliac axis, superior and inferior mesenteric arteries are readily demonstrated. The gas bolus fragments fairly rapidly and therefore best results are obtained when the gas is injected at the target level. Recent technological advances in angiographic equipment allow summation of multiple images and offset the effect of fragmentation and are essential for peripheral imaging (**12**).

Illustration **12** shows the effect of bolus fragmentation; **12a**, a single frame from the angiogram, shows multiple apparent stenoses (white arrows) due to the gas bolus breaking up. In **12b**, summation of all the frames shows that there is a single stenosis at the junction of the graft and the vein cuff (black arrow).

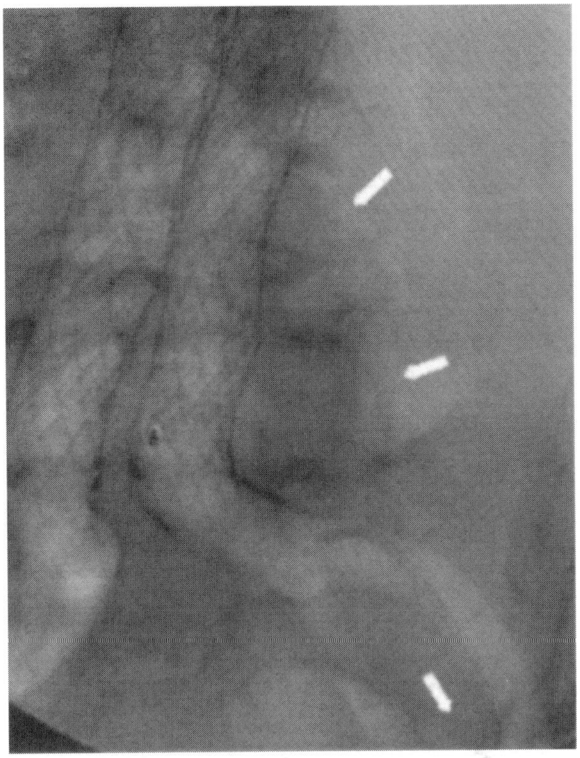

a

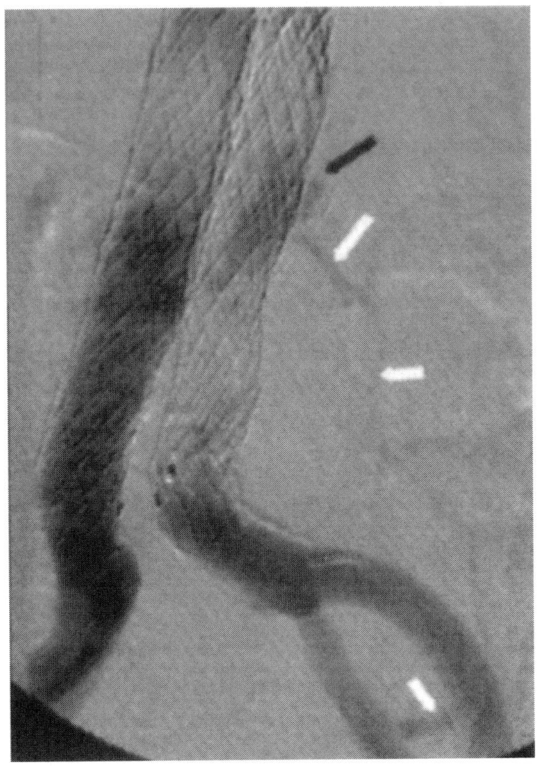

b

10

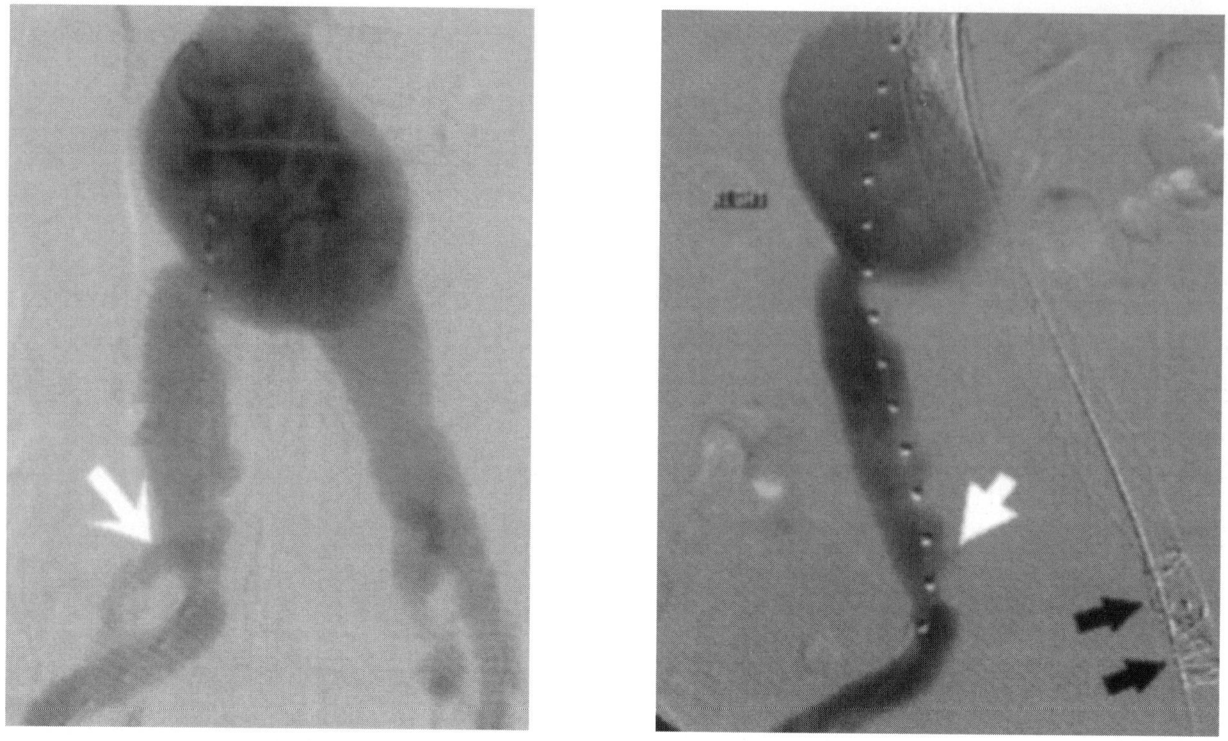

a b

11

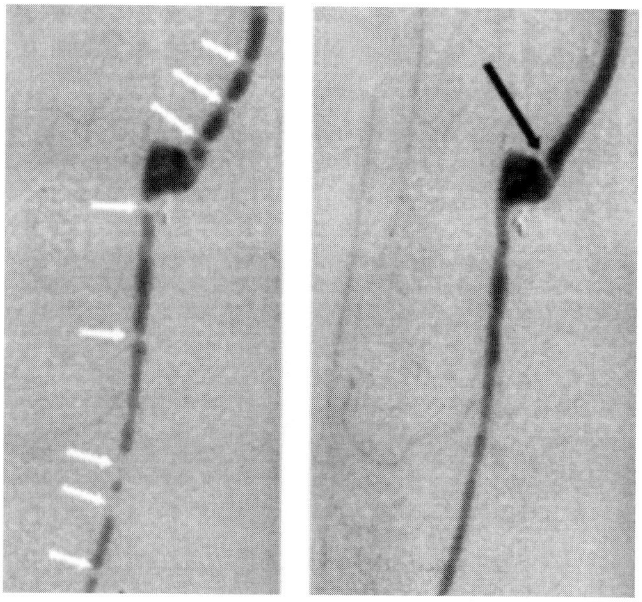

a b

12

Using carbon dioxide

13, 14

Indications

We most often use CO_2 in patients with renal impairment and have performed intra-arterial CO_2 angiography in over 200 patients including approximately 100 arterial interventions. It is now our standard practice to use carbon dioxide for renovascular intervention (**13**) and aortic stent-grafts (**14**). The mean dose of conventional iodinated contrast for endovascular aneurysm repair has fallen from about 200ml to 15ml (0-120ml). Endoleaks are particularly readily demonstrated with CO_2 (**10**).

Illustration **13** shows renal angiography and stenting in a patient with a single kidney. No conventional contrast was used during the procedure. The diagnostic angiogram (**13a**) shows hand-injection of CO_2 through a 4F cobra catheter (white arrow). The left renal artery stenosis is clearly seen (short black arrows). Note the excellent filling of the anterior visceral arteries. Completion angiogaphy is shown in **13b** with injection thorugh the balloon catheter (white arrow). The stent is seen between the black arrows.

Illustration **14** shows aortic stent-grafting following deployment of the body of the graft. Hand-injection of CO_2 through a 4F cobra catheter is seen (white arrow). The graft lies just below the renal arteries (black arrows). No conventional contrast was used during the procedure.

Limitations

Gas should only be used below the diaphragm as there is a risk of causing convulsions if it enters the cerebral circulation. A small minority of patients experience pain during CO_2 injection; this can be minimized by

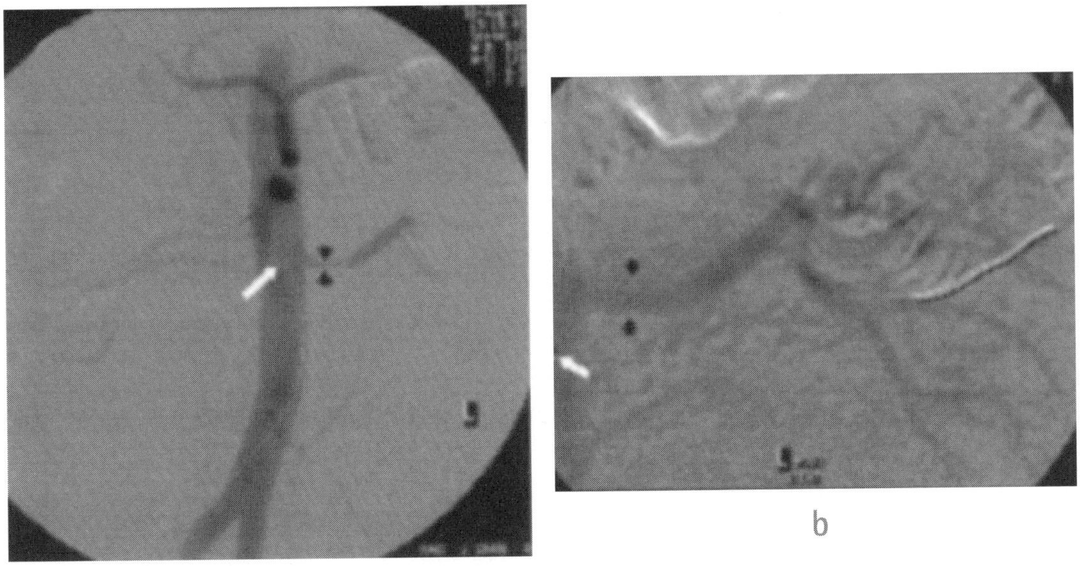

a 13 b

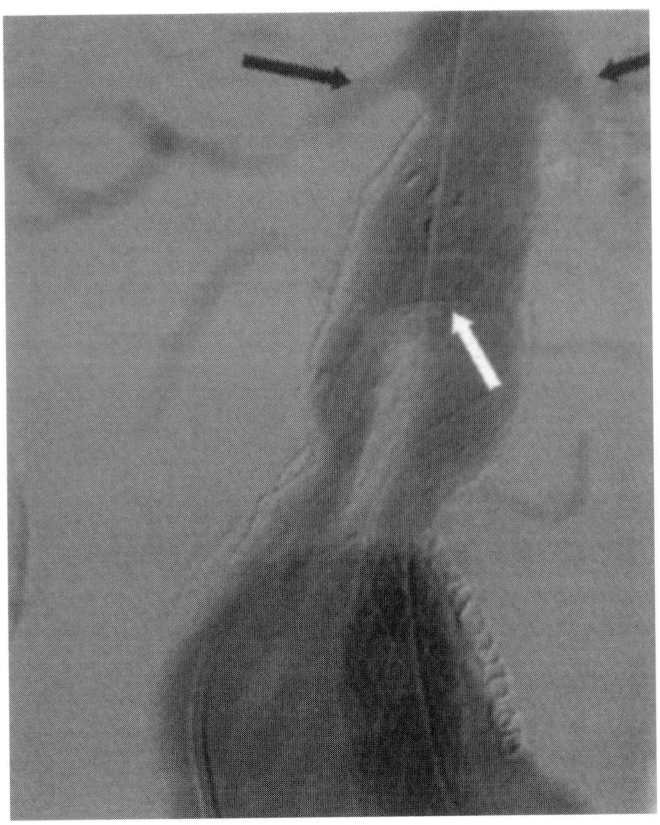

14

decreasing the volume, rate and frequency of injection. If the pain is severe it may be necessary to use conventional liquid contrast.

Carbon dioxide injection

Carbon dioxide gas can be injected either using a dedicated injector or by hand. The low viscosity of the gas makes hand-injection simple even through small catheters. The following system has proved safe and effective when used in accordance with a written protocol. It is imperative to avoid injection of air which comprises 70% nitrogen, the gas bubbles form emboli and can cause thrombosis. Because it is impossible to distinguish a syringe full of air from a syringe full of CO_2 special precautions must be taken when performing CO_2 angiography.

Equipment

15,16

We use 60-ml luer lock plastic syringes fitted with sliding two-way taps. The CO_2 circuit is represented schematically in 15 and consists of the following items:

CO_2 cylinder: make sure that you use medical grade CO_2.
Connecting tubing adapter.
Particle filter (0.2 μm syringe filter).
Two low-pressure connectors.
Three-way tap.
Underwater seal: this functions in the same way as an underwater seal with a chest drain and it is essential to prevent contamination with room air.

Filling syringes with CO_2

The aim is to fill the syringes without contamination with room air. The only way to ensure this is for the syringe to be allowed to fill actively under the pressure of gas in the cylinder (16).

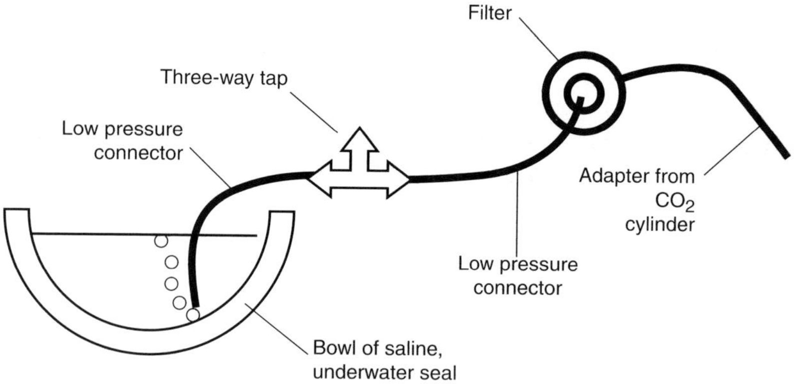

15

1) Connect the circuit as shown above and turn on the gas (flow setting between $^1/_2$ - $^3/_4$) let the gas bubble through the underwater seal.

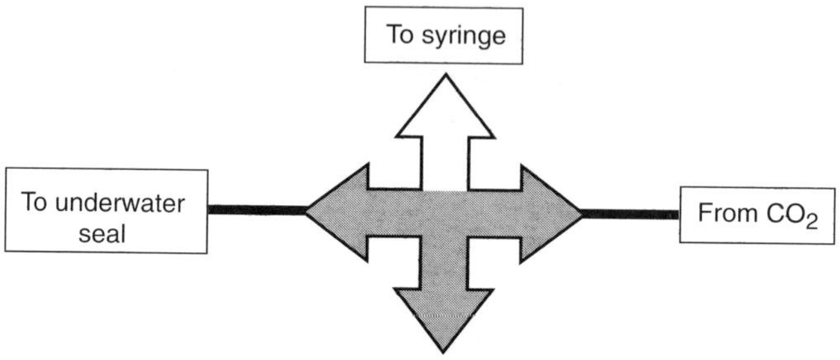

2) Connect the CO_2 syringe and open the sliding tap. Turn the three-way tap so that the syringe fills.

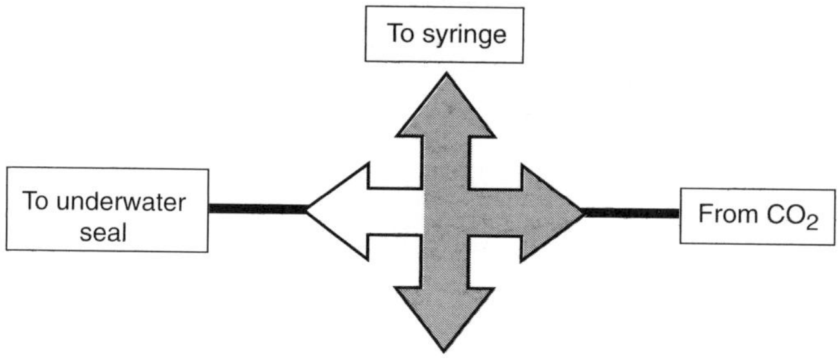

3) When the syringe has 30-40ml of gas in it turn the three-way tap to allow the syringe to be emptied through the underwater seal

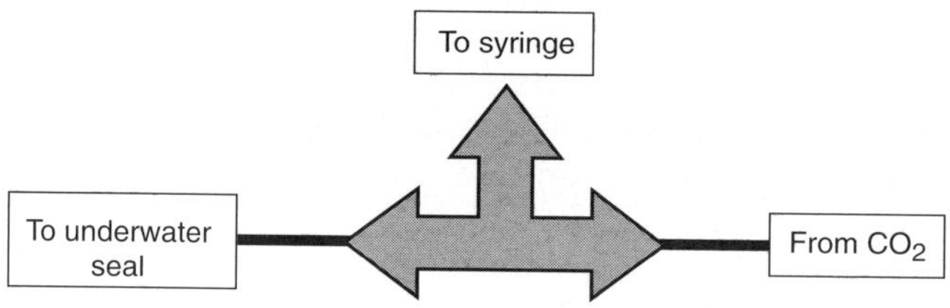

4) Fill and empty the syringe three times and then allow it to fill to 50ml before closing the sliding tap; the syringe now contains CO_2 at a greater than atmospheric pressure. Immediately turn the three-way tap to allow CO_2 to flow through the underwater drain and repeat the process to fill other syringes before turning off the gas.

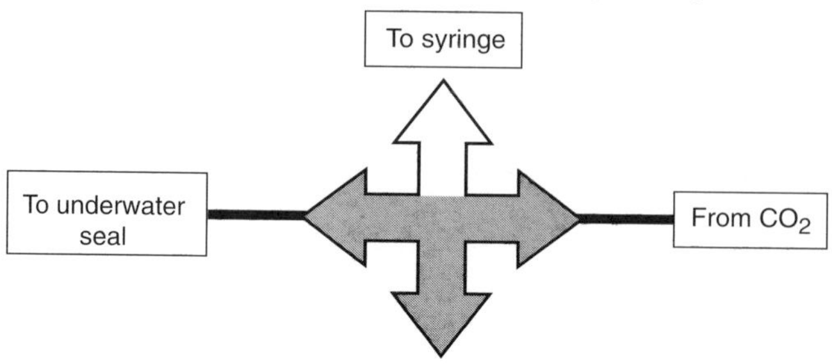

16

Injecting carbon dioxide

The syringe contains CO_2 at greater than atmospheric pressure hence the volume of gas is not known. Opening the sliding tap immediately reduces the pressure in the syringe to atmospheric pressure. Connect the CO_2 syringe to the end of the high-pressure connector and close the sliding tap.

Catheters and connecting tubes are flushed with saline as in conventional angiography. However, prior to performing angiography the catheter should be purged with CO_2. Connect the CO_2 syringe to the connecting tube and pressurize the CO_2 syringe and open the sliding tap. A fall in resistance is noted when the CO_2 has displaced the saline from the catheter. When ready to inject open the sliding tap.

Discard any syringe that is partially filled, has the tap open or if you are uncertain whether it contains CO_2 or air.

Interpreting carbon dioxide angiograms

There are well-recognized pitfalls in the interpretation of CO_2 angiograms

Bowel peristalsis

While all digital subtracted angiograms are impaired by bowel peristalsis CO_2 angiography is particularly sensitive. Use appropriate quantities of buscopan and glucagon to inhibit bowel peristalsis

Pain

Every patient experiences some sensation during CO_2 injections. This can vary from a mild peripheral tingling to intense burning. It is valuable to spend a few moments warning the patient as this is likely to improve co-operation. The exact cause of this sensation is unclear but can be reduced by trying to reduce injection volumes and rates.

Bolus fragmentation

This is inevitable after the gas has passed through several bifurcations and image summation software is invaluable to obtain completely opacified segments in peripheral angiograms (12). If fragmentation is a problem in mainstream vessels this can often be due to a slow injection. If hand-injecting it is essential to deliver the gas in one smooth rapid bolus as this causes optimal displacement of the adjacent blood

Pseudostenosis

This can be very convincing on a single image and is secondary to a combination of gas fragmentation and dependency. Always confirm stenoses by paging through the run step by step. If the morphology of the stenosis changes with each frame then regard with suspicion (12).

Failure to visualize dependent vessels

Carbon dioxide 'floats'; therefore if all the blood is not displaced within the target vessel posterior branch vessels may not be visualized (11). This can be a particular problem with the renal arteries and lumbar arteries. Ensuring that the catheter tip is at the target level, and increasing the volume of injected CO_2 are potential solutions.

Tips

Carbon dioxide angiography takes a little more effort than conventional angiography but becomes straightforward with familiarity.

High flow rates can be achieved through small catheters e.g. 3F and selective catheters (10, 13, 14).

Selective catheters are sometimes advantageous, as we have found that they generally provide better images as the bolus of gas is delivered within a smaller area. Adjust the dose of CO_2 according to the situation; 60ml is needed for aortography but much less is required when injecting into a peripheral vessel.

As CO_2 floats on blood and tends to fill anterior branches, consider rotating the patient to fill dependant vessels.

Consider higher frame rates to compensate for bolus fragmentation, in practice 2 frames per second will suffice for most applications.

Warn the patient of the potential for discomfort during and immediately after the injection, this improves cooperation.

Image processing

Image processing can be time consuming and will convince you of the worth of a good radiographer. No amount of pixel shifting or post-processing will salvage an image degraded by patient movement. Unlike conventional positive contrast the unsubtracted (10), unsummated images are rarely useful.

Summary

Carbon dioxide angiography is a useful adjunct to conventional contrast. Even complex interventions can be performed without the need for conventional contrast. It has advantages over conventional contrast for showing anterior vessels and is extremely sensitive at detecting endoleaks. However, image quality is largely dependent on angiographic hardware and software, and images will be disappointing on inferior equipment. Carbon dioxide can be injected by hand; an expensive injection pump is unnecessary. A simple and safe injection system costs very little and is readily assembled.

Intravascular ultrasound imaging during endovascular prosthesis deployment

Rodney A White,
George E Kopchok, Carlos Donayre

Introduction

Candidates for surgical and/or endovascular repair of abdominal aortic aneurysms are selected after physical examination using transcutaneous ultrasound, angiography, computed tomography (CT) and magnetic resonance imaging (MRI) to characterize the size and extent of the lesion and to plan operative strategy. Comparison of the various imaging modalities demonstrates that each provides information that is useful for pre-intervention selection of patients, for sizing of the vessel lumen and assuring accurate deployment of devices during interventions, and for follow-up assessments. Some information is complementary to that acquired by other methods and some is unique to a particular imaging modality.

The following discussion describes the techniques that enable expeditious use of intravascular ultrasound during endovascular grafting procedures, and outlines methods to enhance interpretation of intravascular ultrasound images.

Intravascular ultrasound instrumentation

1

Intravascular ultrasound catheters are available in 3–8 Fr diameters with the larger sizes typically being required to accommodate the electronics needed for lower frequencies, i.e. 8–12.5 mgHz. Three-hundred and sixty degree cross-sectional intravascular ultrasound images are achieved by either mechanically rotating the imaging elements, or by using electronically switched arrays. Illustration 1 shows schematic diagrams of prototype intravascular catheters; mechanical devices with (1) rotating and (2) fixed components (**1a**), and phase-array configuration with numerous individual transducers circumferentially placed around the tip of the catheter (**1b**).

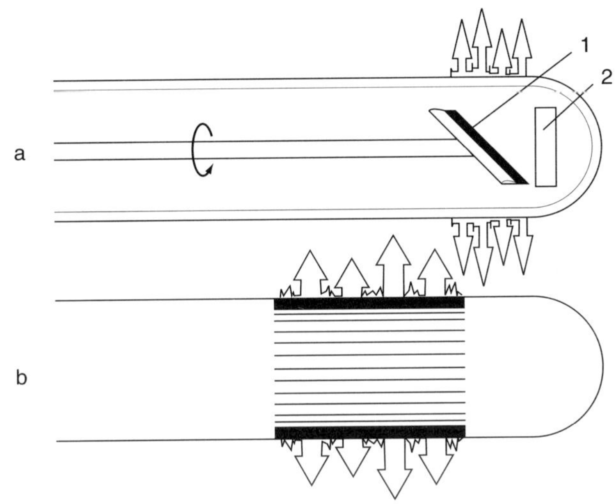

1

Current multiple element intravascular ultrasound catheters utilize frequencies in the range of 10–30 MHz. A problem of these imaging catheters, common to all high frequency ultrasound devices to some extent, is the inability to image structures in the immediate vicinity of the transducer, i.e. in the 'near field'. Because the imaging crystals in a phased array configuration are near to the structure being imaged, a bright circumferential artifact known as the 'ring down' surrounds the catheter. The ring down artifact can be electronically removed, but structures within the region that is masked will not be seen.

Mechanical transducers use one of two basic configurations; either the transducer itself or an acoustic mirror is rotated at the tip of the catheter using a flexible, high-torque cable that extends the length of the device. Some catheters use a transducer that is angled slightly forward of perpendicular and produce a cone-shaped ultrasound beam resulting in an image of the vessel slightly forward of the transducer assembly. This is done primarily to produce an image that represents the blood vessel cross-section at the tip of the catheter. Devices that utilize a rotating acoustic reflector have the mirror set at a 45-degree angle to the rotating shaft, producing an image that is perpendicular to the axis of the catheter. In both rotating transducer and rotating mirror devices, ultrasound frequencies between 10 and 30 MHz are generally used, although some experimental devices using frequencies up to 45 MHz produce excellent images of human arteries.

Intravascular ultrasound catheter introduction

2, 3, 4, 5, 6

Intravascular ultrasound imaging can be performed either by percutaneously introducing the catheters or by passage through, an arteriotomy during open conventional vessel exposures. Intravascular ultrasound catheters are introduced over a guidewire (0.009–0.038 inches diameter), which allows more controlled manoeuvreing of the device within the lumen of the vessel from a remote introduction site. Passing intravascular ultrasound catheters over wires also maintains access to the entire length of the vessel being treated, so that re-crossing of vascular segments by other devices after intravascular ultrasound removal can be easily accomplished. Introduction of the catheters through a long introducing sheath maintains haemostasis and can be very useful for passing catheters through tortuous or stenotic access vessels (2). The tortuous left external and common iliac artery (2a) are straightened to enhance passage of the intravascular ultrasound catheter (2b). Because of the configuration of mechanical rotating catheters, a central guidewire channel is not possible, and these catheters use a variety of monorail and coaxial lumens for over-the-wire applications. Multi-element array devices utilize a central guidewire channel which enhances traceability of the catheters.

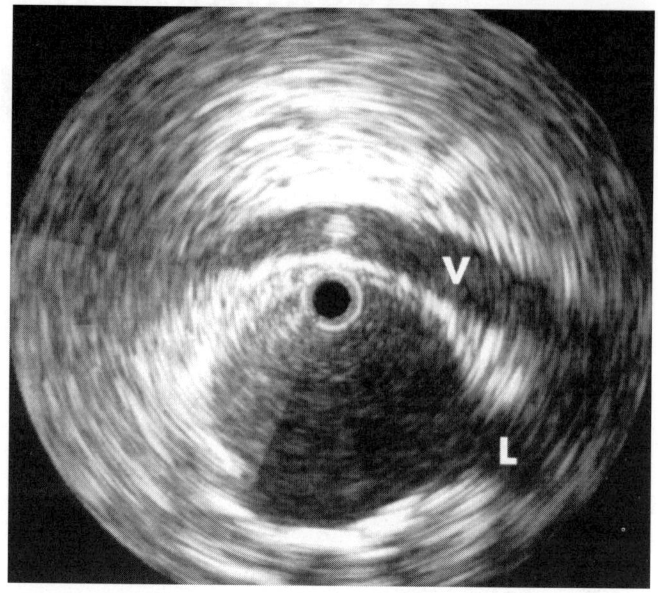

3

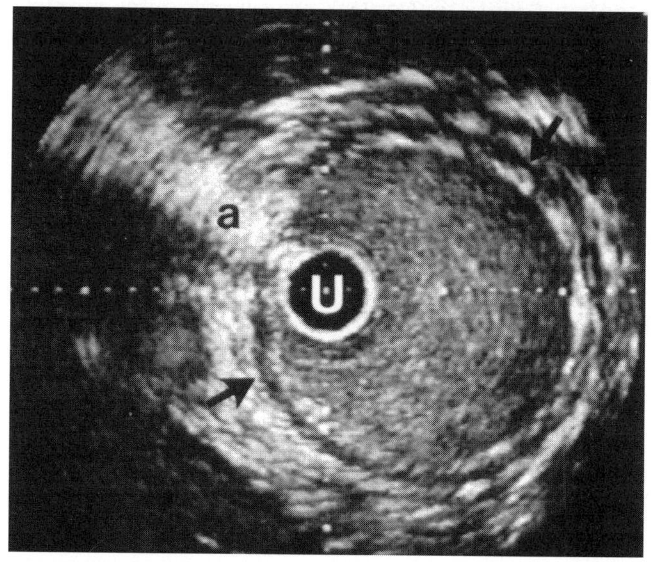

4

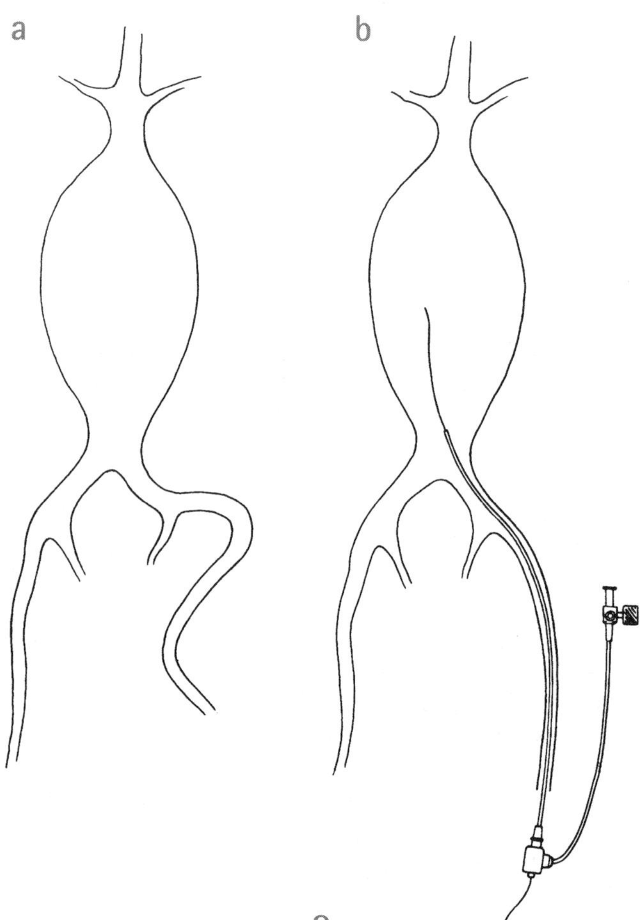

2

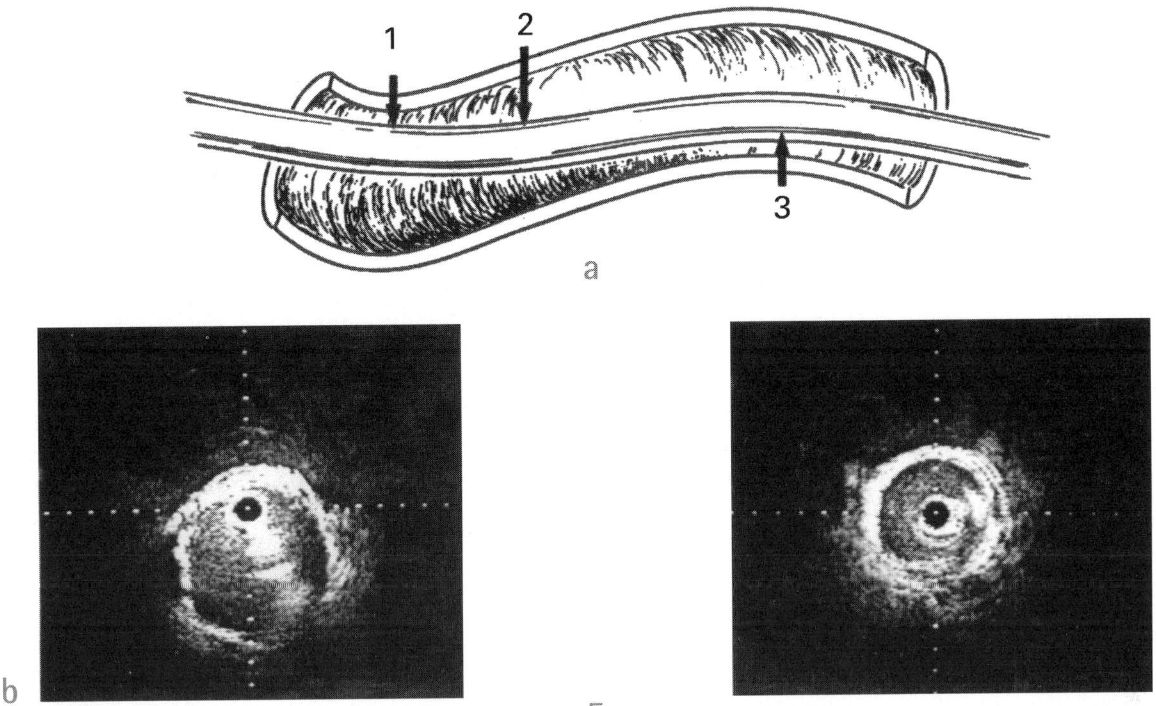

5

Successful use of intravascular ultrasound catheters in the vascular system often requires patient interrogation of the vessel segments and careful interpretation of images to yield maximum benefit. Many interventionalists are frustrated by intravascular ultrasound technology as it requires experience and interpretation skills that vary from those needed for conventional imaging methods. These problems are compounded by the relative fragility of the devices, and other technical considerations such as determining the intraluminal orientation of the cross-sectional imaging element in the vessel lumen.

One may want to align the intravascular ultrasound catheter within the vessel so that anteroposterior orientation can be achieved. When imaging the aortoiliac segments via a femoral puncture site, rotational accuracy can be confirmed by the relative position of constant anatomical landmarks (3). For example, as the catheter crosses the aortic bifurcation, the common iliac arteries should be positioned side-by-side on the screen. Occasionally this anatomical arrangement is not true, especially in tortuous, dilated vessels, and the alignment must be checked against other imaging parameters.

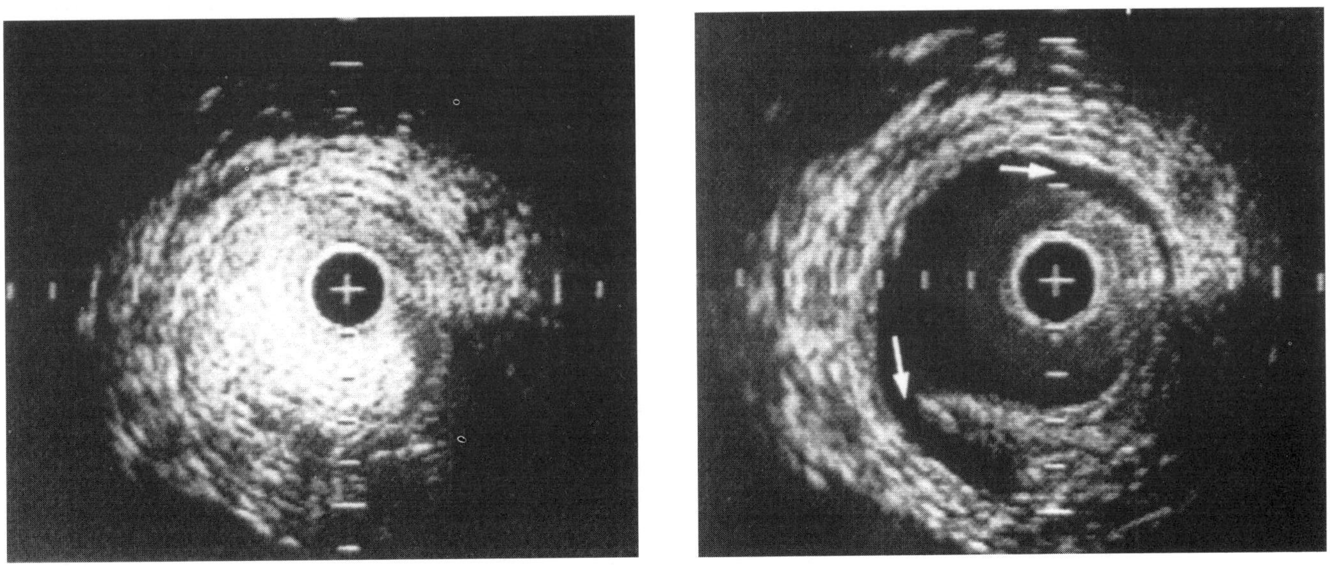

a 6 b

Illustration 3 shows the intravascular ultrasound image in the abdominal aorta at the level of the renal vein (V). Note the origin of the (L) renal artery.

The small wire connection that crosses the imaging chamber in most mechanical transducers produces a visual artifact, which can be rotationally aligned with both an external longitudinal mark on the catheter or by establishing correct alignment when the catheter is inserted (**4**). Because the catheters are rotationally rigid, there is very little loss of orientation with torquing and manipulation during imaging. Although catheters can be rotated to maintain alignment, most intravascular ultrasound imaging systems enable independent image rotation. This feature enhances image interpretation. Illustration **4** shows a cross-sectional intravascular ultrasound image of a human iliac artery. The artifact produced by the electronic transducer (a) denotes the site of the transducer connecting wire on the outside surface of the catheter. Arrows indicate the vessel wall; U indicates the ultrasound catheter.

Careful positioning of the catheter tip within the vessel and appropriate size-matching of device to the artery diameter is essential to optimize visualization. Image quality is best when the catheter is parallel to the vessel wall, i.e. the ultrasound beam is directed at 90 degrees to the luminal surface, while minor angulations may affect the luminal shape and dimensional accuracy. Catheter centreing is especially difficult in tortuous vessels, and rotational alignment may also be partly lost as the catheter meanders through the vessel. The best quality images are obtained as the catheter is withdrawn through the lumen, rather than during advancement. The slight catheter tension produced during withdrawal straightens the catheter and the distal tip tends to find the centre of the vessel if there is no gross tortuosity. As vessel tortuosity or angulation increases, the catheter tends to assume a direct course through the lumen resulting in more eccentric images (**5**). In **5a** at positions 1 and 3, the catheter lies against the vessel wall; at position 2, the catheter is centered within the lumen. Eccentric image (**5B**) produced at positions 1 and 3 causes the vessel wall nearer the imaging chamber to appear more hyperechoic than the distant wall, resulting in an artifactural difference in wall thickness. Concentric image (5c) produced at position 2 shows relatively equal echogenicity of the wall at all locations. While the off-centre position may not be an immediate problem during most intravascular ultrasound interrogations, the differences in mural echogenicity produced by eccentric catheter positioning may greatly affect the results of three-dimensional image reconstructions.

One difficulty resulting from the use of high frequency ultrasound and short imaging ranges is the echogenicity of blood which surrounds the intravascular catheter. Although this problem can be partly overcome by adjustments of the gain and use of image processing techniques such as time-gain compensation and suppression, the echogenic blood may still obscure the interface between the lumen and intima or lumen and pathologic lesion. Flushing of the vessel lumen with saline to remove echogenic blood results in 'interface enhancement' and improves the quality of the ultrasound image (**6**). **5a** shows how echogenicity of blood obscures the luminal detail; **5b** shows how during saline interrogation of vessel lumen, the intimal surface is enhanced showing plaque dissection.

The same principle of interface enhancement that is seen with saline luminal flushing can be utilized using radiographic and ultrasound contrast agents. By instilling radiographic contrast into the vessel being imaged by intraluminal ultrasound, the lumen can be rendered hyperechoic and an improved lumen/mural acoustic interface is produced. An innovation for visualizing vascular structures using current extraluminal ultrasound imaging is the use of ultrasound contrast agents. These agents include free or encapsulated gas bubbles, colloidal suspensions, emulsions and aqueous solutions.

Three-dimensional intravascular ultrasound imaging

7

The development of three-dimensional (3D) computerized intravascular ultrasound image reconstruction has offered a unique method for the viewing of normal and diseased vascular segments. This technology has developed as a result of advances in digital computer graphics technology and mass data storage capabilities of personal computers. In order to produce the 3D images, a series of consecutive 2D images obtained during imaging of a vessel segment is assembled in sequence to produce the 3D image (**7**). The 2D dimensional images (centre) acquired along the length of the vessel are 'stacked' by the computer to produce the longitudinal grey-scale image (left) and the 3D image (right).

Because the final reconstruction is dependent on the quality of the original images, the technique of acquisition of the data is very important. The images should be acquired by slowly withdrawing the intravascular ultrasound catheter through the vessel and sampling the cross-sectional images at a defined rate. The actual withdrawal of the imaging catheter is known as a 'pullback' and can be performed either manually or using a mechanical device.

A few seconds is required for the initial reconstruction of a high-resolution grey scale longitudinal 2D view of the vessel segment. This image represents a hemisection of the vessel. The plane of section can be varied at every degree of axial rotation (anteroposterior, lateral, oblique) or coronal alignment. The luminal profile can be examined, providing similar data to angiography but with almost limitless available projections. A more important feature of 2D longitudinal reconstruction is its display of

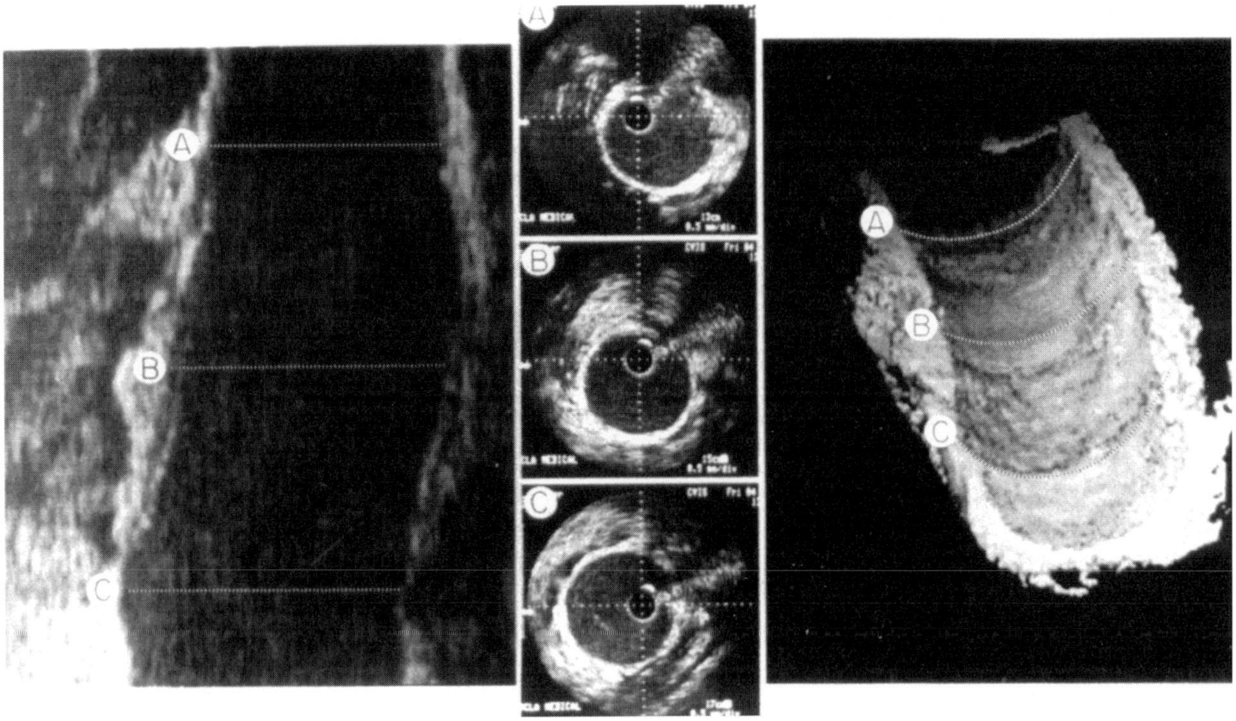

7

the transmural blood vessel morphology. The 2D grey-scale image is especially useful because it displays the luminal and transmural morphology in true multiple grey-scale. The differentiation of plaque, normal tissue, thrombus, dissections and flaps is often better appreciated in the 2D longitudinal image than in the final 3D projection.

The 3D reconstruction can be displayed as a complete vessel cylinder or as a luminal cast by removing vessel wall signals and using the lumen/intima interface as the only connected surface. The image can then be manipulated on-screen and examined in multiple orientations to allow inspection of the vessel segment in all possible projections, both from within the lumen and from the adventitial surface. Other parameters such as image sharpness, contrast and ambient light can be altered to improve the resolution of particular features being examined.

Clinical significance

In our experience, the selection and deployment of endografts is enhanced by intravascular ultrasound with it being particularly useful in assessing the candidacy of patients with complex aneurysm morphology. Although we routinely use intravascular ultrasound during procedures to confirm the anatomy of patients selected by CT or contrast angiography, there are several scenarios where intravascular ultrasound has unquestionable benefit. Patients with contrast allergy or renal compromise can be treated using intravascular ultrasound as the sole imaging modality during the procedure. This obviously applies to only a limited number of patients, but is an important addition to the interventional armamentarium.

An important aspect provided by intravascular ultrasound is identification of vascular lesions i.e. blebs, dissections, stenoses not visualized by CT or cinefluoroscopy. The information provided by an intravascular ultrasound interrogation at the beginning of each procedure alters the site of device deployment or the deployment strategy in a significant number of patients. We also find that intravascular ultrasound enhances accurate device placement near branch vessels, helps select and guide placement of modular components, and helps secure devices and preserve flow in visceral or lumbar arteries during treatment of supracoeliac and thoracic aneurysms and dissections. An additional important factor supporting the use of intravascular ultrasound in endograft deployment is that cinefluoroscopy time and contrast utilization can be significantly reduced minimizing risks to both the patient and personnel.

Acknowledgements

Illustration 5 is reproduced from Reference 1 with permission. Illustration 6 is reproduced from Reference 4 with permission. Illustration 7 is reproduced from Reference 2 with permission.

References

Cavaye DM, White RA (1993). *Intraluminal Ultrasound Imaging.* New York: Raven Press Inc., pp. 56–57.

Cavaye DM, Tabbara MR, Kopchok GE *et al.* (1991). Three-dimensional vascular ultrasound imaging. *Am Surg* **57**:751–755.

Tabbara MR, White RA, Cavaye DM, Kopchok G (1991). *In-vivo* human comparison of intravascular ultrasound and angiography. *J Vasc Surg* **14**:496–504.

Van Urk H *et al.* (1991). Assessment of arterial disease and arterial reconstructions by intravascular ultrasound. *Int J Card Imaging* **6**:157–164.

White RA, Verbin C, Scoccianti M *et al.* (1985). Role of cinefluoroscopy and intravascular ultrasound in evaluating the deployment of experimental endovascular prostheses. *J Vasc Surg* **21**:365–374.

White RA, Donayre C, Kopchok G *et al.* (1996). Vascular imaging prior to, during and following endovascular repair. *World J Surg* **20**:622–629.

White RA, Donayre CE, Walot I, *et al.* (1996). Preliminary clinical outcome and imaging criterion for endovascular prosthesis deployment in high risk patients with aortoiliac and traumatic arterial lesions. *J Vasc Surg* **24**:558–571.

White RA, Donayre CE, Walot I *et al.* (1997). Modular bifurcation endoprosthesis for treatment of abdominal aortic aneurysms. *Ann Surg* **228**:381–391.

Planning endovascular aneurysm repair (EVAR) with three-dimensional modelling

Simon C Whitaker

Introduction

Endovascular repair of the aorta (EVAR) brings many new challenges, not least in its requirements for detailed preoperative imaging. Unlike a conventional surgical graft, the dimensions of an endovascular prosthesis must be known, to a high degree of accuracy, before the procedure. For this task, the tools of calibrated angiography, spiral computed tomography (CT) and magnetic resonance (MR) angiography have been used to provide measurements of the patient's aorta. However, the three-dimensional (3D) anatomy of the aorta is complex and, in this context, measurements made from two-dimensional (2D) images have fundamental limitations.

Calculation of the required length of an endograft can be a difficult task. Longitudinal measurements of the aorta may be made from calibrated angiography, CT or MR images but will not take into account distortion of the aorta produced by the stiff guidewire and delivery system or by the endograft itself. Discrepancy between the calculated requirement and the apparent size of the endograft when it is deployed becomes greater when the vessels are tortuous. The problem is not so much that the measured lengths are wrong, but that the distances from renal arteries to bifurcation and from the aortic to iliac bifurcation have shortened because of the straight path adopted by the delivery device.

There is also uncertainty as to the exact line along which such length measurements should be made in order that they correspond to the maximum length of a cylindrical endograft. When a graft is required to follow a curved lumen, it will maintain its full length along the outer aspect of the curve but shorten along the inner aspect. In tortuous vessels, the true measurement line may spiral around the lumen edge and thus be impossible to measure from 2D images. The process of virtual reality, 3D preoperative planning, described in this chapter, has been developed to address these difficulties.

Software

Our experience is based upon the use of the StentView™ planning system (William Cook Europe A/S, Bjaeverskov, Denmark) which is designed for use with the Zenith™ and TriFab™ endografts. The AAA Preview™ package (Medical Media Systems, West Lebanon, NH, USA) provides very similar features for the Baxter Endograft (Fillinger, 1999).

Three-dimensional modelling

1, 2, 3, 4, 5, 6, 7

The aims of any preoperative planning process for EVAR should be:

1. to determine the best treatment strategy;
2. to determine accurately the correct size of prosthesis;
3. to detect important co-morbidity;
4. to predict deployment pitfalls.

Most of these aims can be met with 3D imaging, to a greater degree than is possible with 2D imaging alone. First, it is necessary to create a 3D wire-frame model of the patient's aorta from cross-sectional images. A wire-frame model consists of a mesh of interconnecting 3D coordinates, which describe the surface of the object. It can be viewed as a mesh or, more usually, in fully rendered format with appropriate lighting effects (2). Because of their nature, wire-frame models occupy little computer memory and can be drawn quickly for realistic animation effects. They are self-contained structures that have all the required information for accurate scaling.

Source data

Source images can be obtained from either contrast-enhanced CT angiography (Fillinger and Weaver, 1999) or contrast enhanced MR, angiography (Ludman *et al.*, 2000; Nasim *et al.*, 1998). For the majority of cases, CT angiography will be used because the modality clearly demonstrates important detail such as calcification, thrombus and atheroma. CT angiography protocols vary considerably but most require a large volume of iodinated contrast agent (100–150 ml), narrow collimation (3–5 mm) and reformatting of overlapping axial slices at close (2–4 mm) intervals.

Segmentation

Segmentation is the process whereby the user demarcates, in each source image, the region that will be included in the final model. This is achieved by highlighting the appropriate object (e.g. the aortic lumen) in colour (1). User input is necessary because the complexity of the aorta together with the variability of contrast enhancement between individuals render automatic segmentation processes unreliable. The model construction from segmented images is automatic.

Once a suitable model of the recipient aorta exists, established computer graphic techniques are used to construct and draw a 3D model of the proposed endograft to the same scale (3) and to superimpose the two (4, 5).

Whereas the aorta model is constructed from data acquired in the real world, the 3D model endograft is generated entirely by the computer from dimensions provided by the user. The geometric shapes of the Zenith and TriFab (Cook Inc) prostheses, both of which are constructed using a skeleton of Gianturco stents, are well suited to computer simulation. The model endograft is built, as is its real world counterpart, from a column of Gianturco subunits, which can move relative to each other to allow the endograft to adopt the curve of the vessel lumen in which it will be placed. The dimensions of each component can be changed according to the same rules and constraints that apply to the real graft. Different templates are available, allowing the operator the opportunity to experiment with different endograft types as well as with different endograft sizes.

Verification

It is important to be certain that a program for the construction of 3D models produces output that is true to life. We have validated 3D aorta models by printing life-size images of the models and comparing these directly with similar, life-sized reproductions of 3D surface rendered or maximum intensity projection images of the same aorta produced by the original CT or MR imaging equipment (2). A 3D model endograft shown in the same scene can simply be measured by hand on the printed output. Verification of accuracy of the endograft model can be confirmed after deployment by creating a 3D model of the actual graft used and comparing this with the original plan (7).

Determination of endograft length

Planning an endograft with a 3D model of the aorta relies upon the experience of the user to select the correct graft size by eye. This approach removes the need for absolute longitudinal measurements because the size of the endograft is simply altered until it is seen to fit correctly.

For the Zenith and TriFàb endograft, the user must select an appropriate body length to ensure that the bifurcation of the endograft is close to, but still above, the aortic bifurcation. The illac sections should be long enough to extend well into the common iliac arteries without occlusion of the internal iliac arteries. To try and predict the full range of positions that the endograft could adopt, the endograft is viewed in both catheter and deployment simulations.

Catheter simulation

In this view, the diameter of the endograft model is restricted so that it is shown as if constrained within a delivery sheath (6). The user can adjust the course taken by the model to simulate that taken by the device which, typically, will straighten the iliac arteries somewhat and follow the shortest path across the aneurysm sac. The length of the body section of the endograft is chosen to ensure that the graft bifurcation falls close to that of the aorta. Similarly, the iliac sections should fall just above or at the iliac bifurcations.

Deployment simulation

The same longitudinal dimensions are applied to a simulation of the deployed endograft. To ensure that the appearance of the model endograft is an accurate reflection of the final appearance of the deployed graft, its diameter is set to the *same* diameter as the aortic neck. The final graft will need to be wider than this to ensure an adequate seal at the aortic neck (we usually oversize the endograft by approximately 4 mm relative to the aneurysm neck diameter). The curve of the model endograft is adjusted so that it follows the expected course of a satisfactorily deployed device, first in a frontal (4) and then in a lateral view (5). This path can differ from that of the lumen if the aorta is tortuous, because the graft may distort and straighten the vessel. The model of an endograft in its deployed form will usually appear shorter than a model of the same dimensions viewed as a catheter simulation. In cases where the vascular channel is fairly straight, this discrepancy will be small, but increasing tortuousity produces greater and greater differences.

Diameters

In complete contrast to length assessment, 3D modelling has little, if any, role in the determination of the endograft diameters. This task requires measurement of the wall-to-wall diameter of the vessel lumen at the proximal and distal attachment sites of the endograft. Because accuracy of these measurements is critical, they should always be made from 2D cross-sectional images (i.e. CT or MR) and never from 3D reconstructions or images

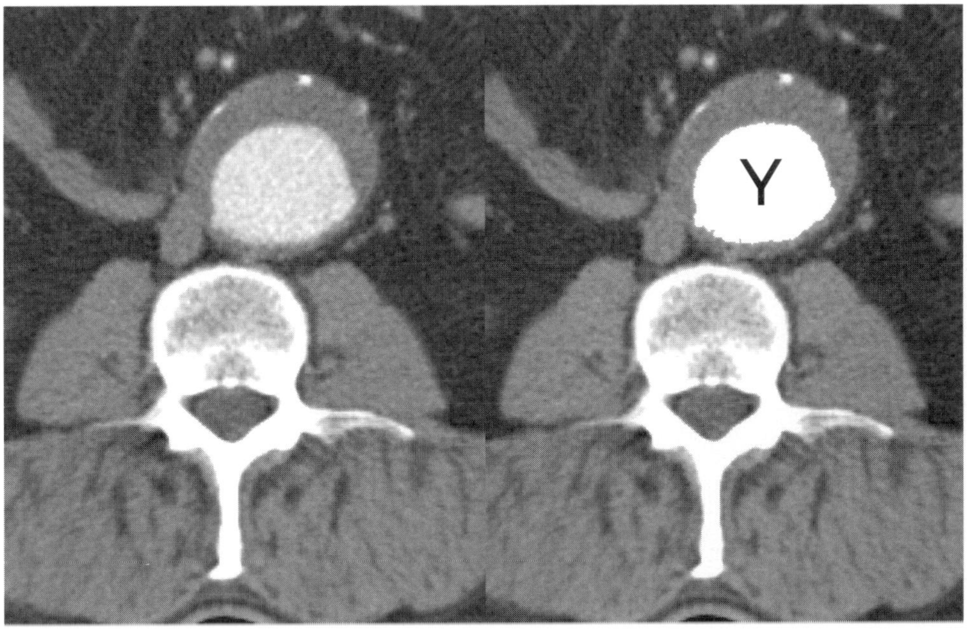

1

Illustration **1** shows a single slice from a spiral CT angiogram of the abdominal aorta in its original form (left) and after segmentation (right). The lumen has been highlighted in yellow (Y) to indicate that it should be included in the 3D model. The same process is repeated for all images in the series. The software then constructs the complete model by summating the selected regions in each slice.

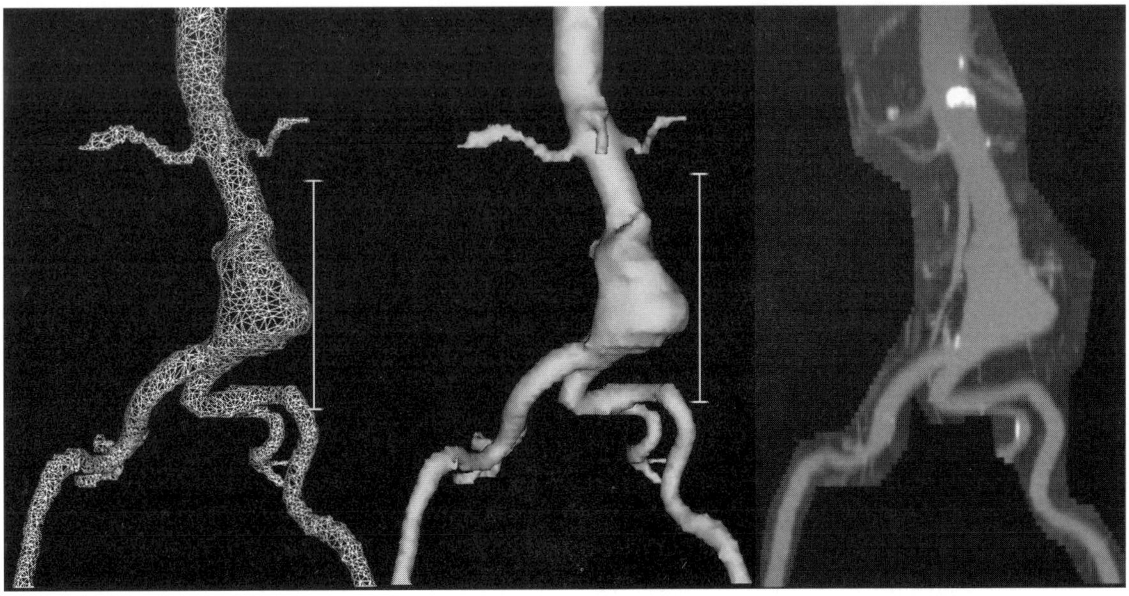

a b c

2

Illustration **2a** shows a complete 3D wire frame model of an abdominal aorta in a wire-frame format; **2b** shows the same model, fully rendered; **2c** is a maximum intensity projection image of the same aorta constructed on the CT console. It has been reproduced to the same scale as the model images to confirm that the 3D model is accurate.

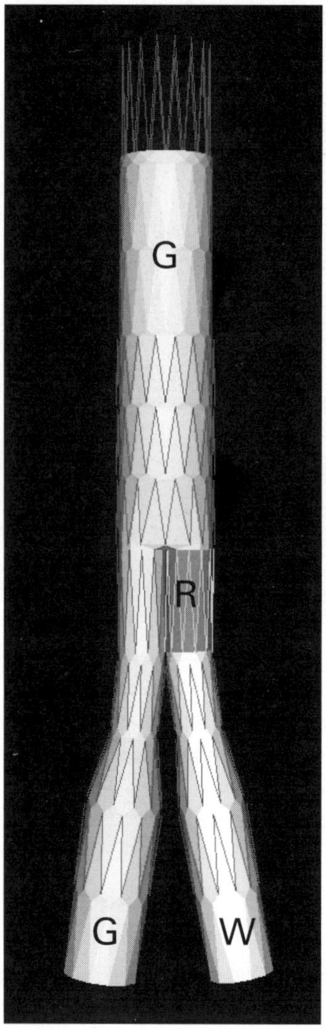

3

Illustration 3 shows a 3D computer-generated endograft model of a bifurcated Zenith™ endograft. G indicates the main component, comprising the body section and the ipsilateral iliac section. W indicates the contralateral iliac segment and R the short limb stump of the main component. This endograft is characterized by an uncovered suprarenal stent. In this particular model, the top two and the most distal stents are internal to the graft fabric.

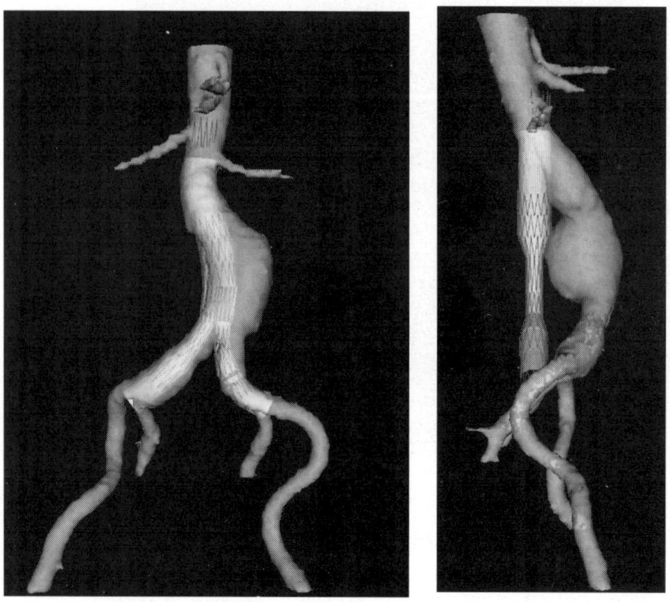

a 4 b

Illustration 4 shows the first stage of planning the endograft. The first step is to adjust the length and alignment of the endograft model so that it matches the aorta in the frontal view (4a). A lateral view of the same scene at this point (4b) shows the expected mismatch that still exists in this plane.

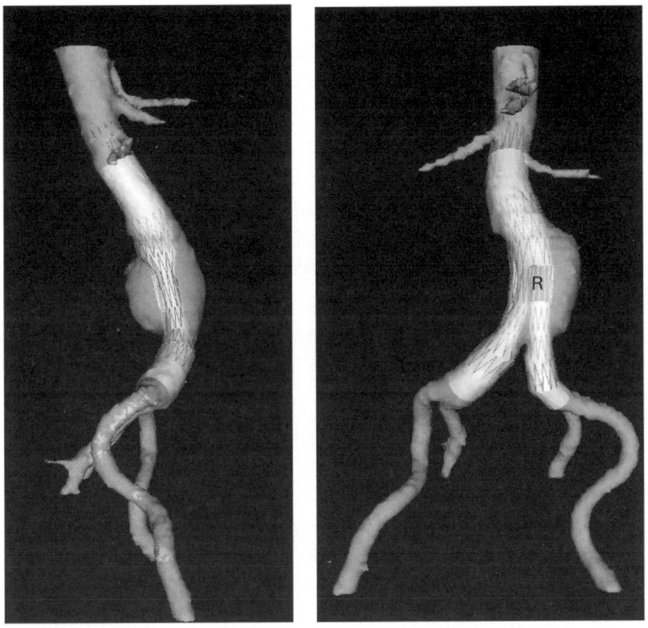

a b

5

Illustration 5 shows the second stage of planning the endograft. The alignment of the endograft model is now completed in the lateral perspective (a). Now, a frontal view of the same scene (b) or simple rotation of the scene on the console shows exact alignment of the model endograft. The position of the short limb stump (R) appears well clear of the aortic bifurcation.

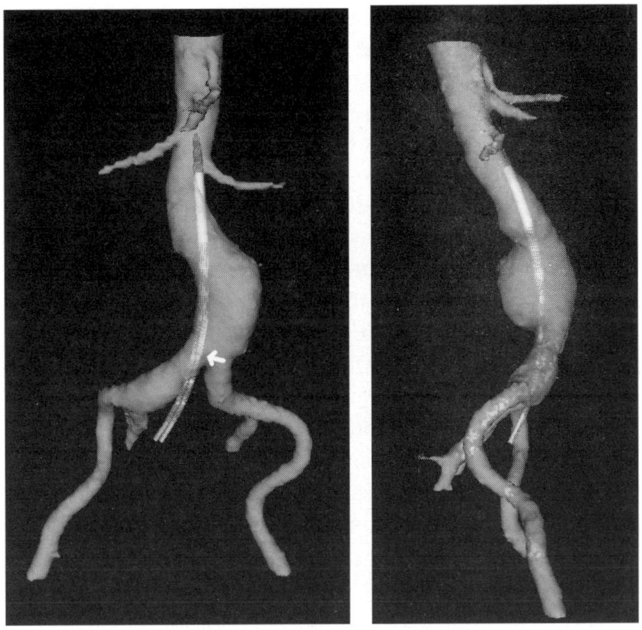

a b

6

Illustration 6 shows a catheter view. To check that the endograft will not seem unexpectedly long when introduced, an endograft model of the same longitudinal dimensions as in 4 and 5 but with a narrow diameter is constructed to simulate the appearance of the endograft within the delivery sheath. This new model is aligned along the path that the sheath might be expected to take, cutting across the corners, in both frontal (left) and lateral (right) views. This simulation shows that the orifice of the short limb stump (white arrow) will lie much closer to the bifurcation than might be expected from the appearance of the deployed endograft.

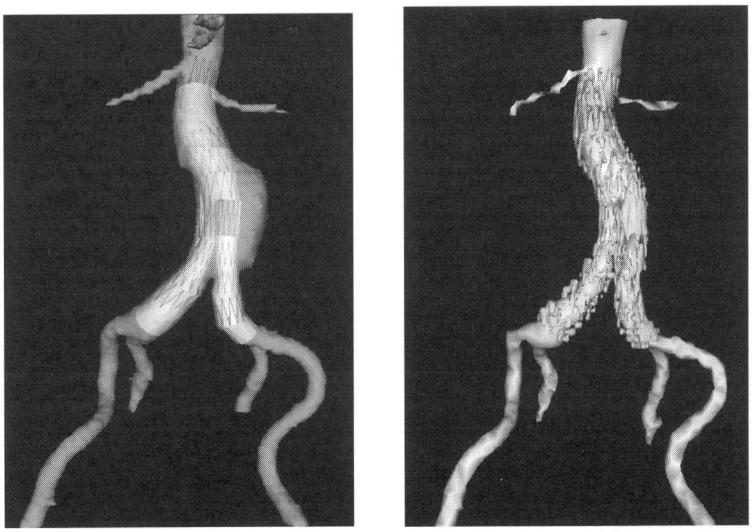

a b

7

Illustration 7 shows a follow-up comparison of the planning (a) and the follow-up CT scan (b). There is excellent agreement between the two studies. For the follow-up image, a 3D model of the deployed endograft has been constructed from the follow-up CT scan data by selecting the metal wires of the stents during segmentation. This is superimposed on a model of the lumen itself.

from calibrated angiography. Ideally, images for measurement should be true cross-sections of the vessel, at right angles to the axis of the vessel lumen, to avoid errors when the cross-section of the aortic neck is not a true circle (Armon *et al.*, 1998).

Planning and flexible deployment

Planning and dimensions of an endograft in this way is only one part of the solution to endograft sizing. Equally important is the ability to adjust the distal placement of the endograft, independently of the top, during deployment. We position 4F straight angiographic catheters in the lumen of both common iliac arteries at the start of the procedure to allow later contrast injection for demonstration of the precise position of the internal iliac arteries with the delivery sheaths in place. If the iliac section of the graft appears low, perhaps extending into the external iliac artery, its position can be adjusted before final release to prevent occlusion of the internal iliac artery.

The role of preoperative angiography

What is the current importance of preoperative calibrated angiography in the preoperative assessment protocol for EVAR now that 3D modelling techniques exist? The functions of angiography in this clinical setting are to provide measurements, to provide a road map of the anatomy and to detect relevant vascular abnormality such as iliac or renal artery stenoses.

Measurements made from calibrated angiography are fraught with problems. Direct measurements using the catheter as a tape measure within the aorta assume that the catheter follows the optimum path. Calibrated measurements can also be inaccurate – the aorta and iliac arteries show pronounced curvature so a single calibration factor is not valid for all points. By comparison, the process of 3D model generation from axial image ensures that scaling information is known for the entire scene. The intermediate stage of longitudinal measurement is removed because, rather than rely upon the indeterminate path of a calibration catheter, the endograft itself is compared directly with the aorta and adjusted until it is the correct size.

Measurements of the aortic lumen diameter made with calibrated angiography are likely to be an underestimate of the true value, not only because of errors of calibration but also because they will ignore any thrombus or atheroma lining the vessel. The same criticism can also be applied to 3D models, which are made to the lumen dimensions and may also underestimate the wall-to-wall diameter. Correct measurement of the aortic neck is critical and small errors can be very significant. Determination of the aortic neck diameter (and hence the endograft diameter) from calibrated angiography or from 3D models is likely to be inaccurate and is therefore not recommended.

The 3D environment is excellent for the purpose of anatomy demonstration. If needed, modern CT or MR scanners can image the patient from the aortic arch to the common femoral arteries in a single pass, far greater coverage than can be provided in a single angiographic view. The user can view the 3D scene from any position and suitable viewpoints can be reproduced in the operating suite using orientation information provided by the 3D system. A drawback of 3D model techniques is that fine anatomical detail such as renal or iliac artery stenosis may be lost in the final model. Conversely, spurious stenoses may be generated as a result of incomplete segmentation of the input data or excessive smoothing of the model mesh. For this reason, the 3D model of the aorta used for endograft planning should be seen as an adjunct to, not a replacement for the original CT or MR images from which it is generated. Stenoses of the iliac or renal arteries are depicted with greater reliability using CT when thin collimation and a narrow slice interval are used. The presence of vascular calcification may impair visualization of the lumen channel on CT images. Conversely, MR angiography is unaffected by calcification in this way (Ludman *et al.*, 2000).

Conclusion

3D model visualization of the aorta and 3D virtual reality simulation of endovascular aneurysm repair are valuable tools which simplify the planning process. The production of a 3D scene of the aorta and proposed endograft does not generate any extra information that does not already exist in the input images; rather it presents the data to the operator in a logical and familiar fashion. Determination of the correct size for an endograft requires both experience and intuition. Although 3D modelling does not replace these qualities, it makes it easier for the operator to transfer their real-life experience and knowledge into the planning process.

References

Armon MP, Whitaker SC, Gregson RH *et al.* (1988). Spiral CT angiography versus aortography in the assessment of aortoiliac length in patients undergoing endovascular abdominal aortic aneurysm repair. *J Endovasc Surg* **5**: 222–227.

Beebe HG, Kritpracha B, Serres S *et al.* (2000). Endograft planning without preoperative arteriography: a clinical feasibility study. *J Endovasc Ther Official J Int Soc Endovasc Spec* **7**: 8–15.

Fillinger MF (1999). New imaging techniques in endovascular surgery. *Surg Clin N Amer* **79**: 451–475.

Fillinger MF, Weaver JB (1999). Imaging equipment and techniques for optimal intraoperative imaging during endovascular interventions. *Semin Vasc Surg* **12**: 315–326.

Ludman CN, Yusuf SW, Whitaker SC *et al.* (2000). Feasibility of using dynamic contrast-enhanced magnetic resonance angiography as the sole imaging modality prior to endovascular repair of abdominal aortic aneurysms. *Eur J Vasc Endovasc Surg* **19**: 524–530.

Nasim A, Thompson MM, Sayers RD, *et al.* (1998) Role of magnetic resonance angiography for assessment of abdominal aortic aneurysm before endoluminal repair. *Br J Surg* **85**: 641–644.

The AneuRx device

Simon D Parvin

Introduction

The Medtronic AneuRx device has been available in the UK since October 1997. It is a modular system with one long and one short limb.

The main part of the device is deployed from one groin, and the contralateral iliac limb from the other, by cannulation of the open short leg from groin level. The delivery system is simple to use needing only two moves to complete deployment. This minimizes the chances of making mistakes.

Graft sizes are from 20 to 31 mm at the top with corresponding iliac limbs of 12–16 mm matching the respective body size. Grafts are 165 or 135 mm long. The contralateral iliac limb can be 1 mm larger than the main iliac limb and 20 mm cuffs can be placed inside 16 mm iliac limbs if needed. Extender cuffs are available for the top end where oversizing by 2 mm is acceptable.

There are a number of features that set it apart from others.

The whole of the graft is supported on the outside by nitinol rings 1 cm wide. The rings are cut to diamond shape from solid rings of nitinol rather than being made up from wire. This is thought to reduce the risk of stent strut fracture. Having the stent rings outside the graft is thought to reduce the risk of graft puncture (by the rings) and of graft migration (by approximation of stent rather than fabric to the arterial wall).

Every stent ring is sewn to the fabric at each diamond midpoint intersection within each stent ring. In addition the apex of each diamond on the upper and lower edge of the stent ring is sewn to the next stent ring and to the fabric. This construction technique provides both strong radial support and column strength, leading to reduced risk of kinking or buckling of the graft, and permitting enhanced conformability to different aneurysm morphologies. Adjacent stent rings can overlap a little to increase conformability.

Oversizing of the stent graft by 20% provides adequate fixation of the graft without the need for hooks or barbs (at graft tip or suprarenal). The strong exoskeleton, with enhanced radial force and column strength, is the key to maintenance of graft position within the artery.

Because the stents are self-expanding, there is generally no need to use angioplasty to seat the graft in place. This leads to a saving of time and expense.

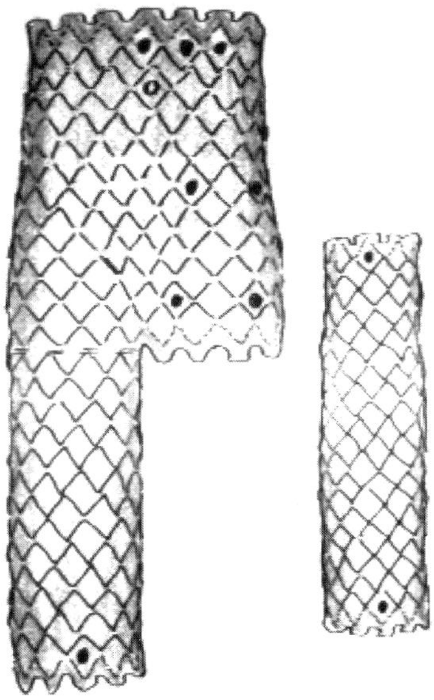

a

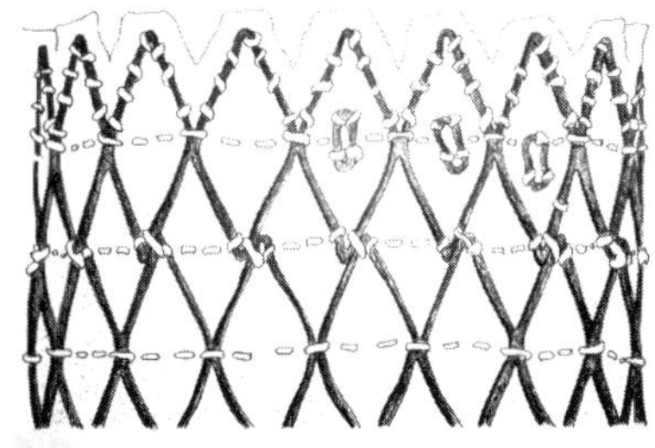

b

1

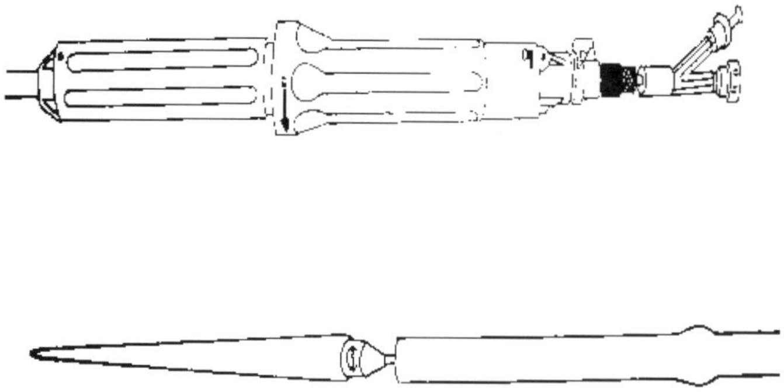

2

1

The body of the graft is 2 cm long with full diameter and another 2 cm long approaching the crutch. The gate area is 3 cm long and employs dumbell-shaped stent rings for support. At each end of the graft the fabric is crenellated and sewn continuously to the top half diamond.

2

The graft is supplied packed within a delivery system, which is introduced into the aorta from the femoral artery. Graft deployment is controlled very accurately by use of a turning handle that withdraws the outer sheath of the delivery system exposing the graft within, which springs open into place. Lying between the graft and the inside of the sheath are metal runners 1–2 mm wide, which allow the smooth passage of the sheath over the graft during deployment.

The new delivery sheath differs from the original by having an integral handle. This is activated by clockwise rotation. The tip of the delivery system is now tapered removing the need for regular use of introducer sheaths on either side.

3

To achieve a controlled deployment, the graft has metal markers sewn to it to allow both accurate vertical position within the artery and correct rotational alignment.

At the top of the graft on the front are three metal markers 5 mm from the top edge, and approximately 5 mm apart, extending from the centre of the graft towards the contralateral side. One cm below this is a single metal marker in the centre on the back of the graft. This second marker must be lined up with the centre front marker for perfect alignment.

The top three stent rings have been deployed initially above the renal arteries. The orientation of the graft is correct with the most medial of the three upper metal markers lying vertically over the lower marker. The two more lateral of the top markers and the four gate markers lie on the contralateral side.

With the top of the graft deployed above the renals, it can be pulled down accurately into position immediately below the renal arteries. The top markers are 5 mm from the top of the graft, and the top of the diamond-shaped stent can usually be clearly seen on X-ray. Control angiography can be performed during this crucial part of the process via a catheter normally placed from the contralateral groin or sometimes from the brachial artery.

Once the top of the graft is accurately placed, the remainder of the primary device can be deployed

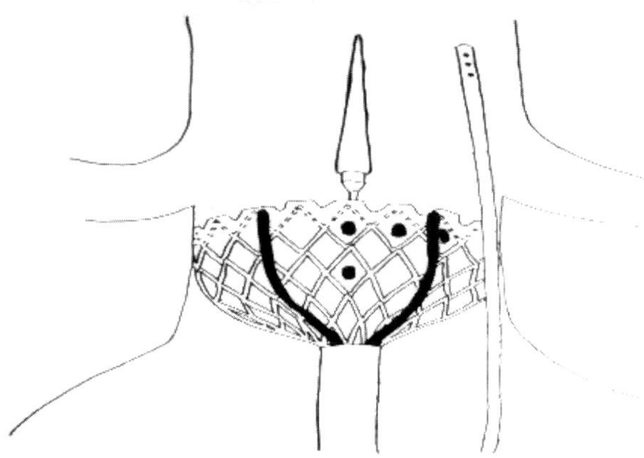

3

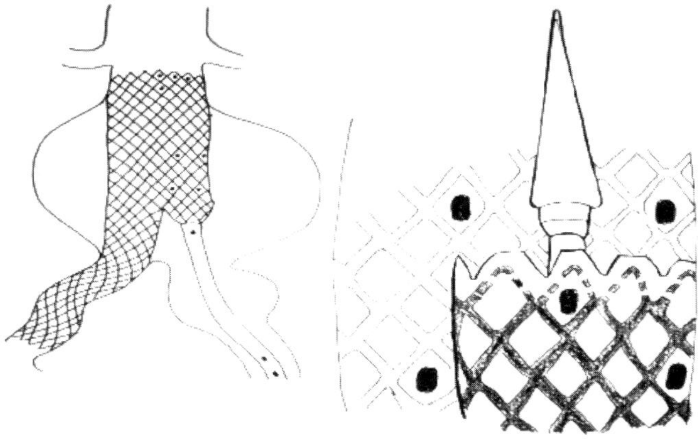

4

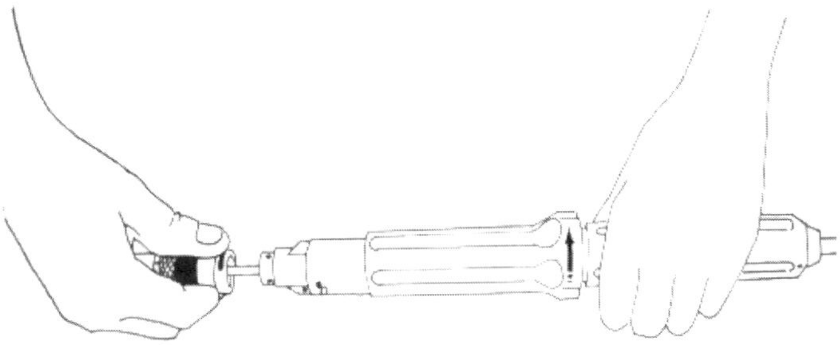

5

4

Having delivered the primary device into position and checked it by angiography, the angiogram catheter from the contralateral groin is withdrawn in to the aneurysm sac. Using a mixture of angled catheter and angle tipped wire the contralateral short limb is catheterized. Rotation of the image intensifier tube usually confirms correct placement of the wire through the short limb.

The gate area on the short limb has two metal markers at the top and two more, 2.5 cm below, which are 1 cm from the tip of the gate. The marker at the tip of the contralateral iliac limb must be placed between these markers to ensure adequate overlap.

The distal end of each iliac limb has a single marker 5 mm from the tip.

The iliac limb is introduced from the groin and deployed in the gate area.

5

Once deployment of either primary device or iliac limb or cuff has been completed, the tapered nose cone and metal runners are withdrawn through the graft. The back end of the delivery system is attached to the nose cone and runners and must be unclipped from the body of the delivery system. Gentle sustained traction then leads to withdrawal of the nose cone and runners into the iliac artery below the lower end of the graft. When beginning the withdrawal process, when the graft is tight, and sometimes when there is tortuosity in the anatomy, the whole graft and aorta may appear to be pulled down. When this happens, alternate gentle sustained traction with rests between, will gradually lead to withdrawal of the nose cone.

Acknowledgement

Illustrations by C Meriel Parvin.

The Zenith endoluminal stent-graft system: suprarenal fixation, safety features, modular components, fenestration and custom crafting

Michael MD Lawrence-Brown,
James B Semmens, David E Hartley

Introduction

The Zenith stent-graft system was developed from the H & LB Endograft which was first reported at the International Endovascular Society meeting in Sydney, 1994, as the Perth bifurcated system. The majority of infrarenal abdominal aortic aneurysms are unsuitable for straight tube grafts because of an inadequate distal neck in which to lodge the distal end of a straight tube graft securely. Femorofemoral crossover and occlusion of the contralateral iliac artery involves a significant open component to the procedure and destruction of a normal patent major vessel with subsequent dependency of both lower limbs upon one iliac artery. This compromise is contrary to best surgical principles of preservation of normal anatomy and useful tissue. Using a combination of animal experiments and life-size plastic moulds, a bifurcated self-expanding modular system was developed in June 1994, using Z stents made of stainless steel and Dacron fibre.

1, 2

Two-piece aortoiliac modular bifurcated grafts formed the basic unit for endoluminal repair. The Zenith two-piece bifurcated endoluminal graft is shown (1) on its delivery system featuring the top cap, anchor stent and long body. Extension pieces were added to the iliac limbs to treat shortfalls in the design or accompanying iliac aneurysm disease. Extension pieces have also been added to the proximal ends of endoluminal grafts, usually for the purpose of correcting deployment error, or bolstering the support to counter an endoleak. Standard three-piece units are replacing the two-piece modules because they lend themselves to addressing length assessment problems. The Zenith three-piece (Trifab) endoluminal graft for infrarenal aortic aneurysm (2) maintains the long body, and low joint close to the iliac origin for stability and ease of cannulation. It includes flared iliac ends for

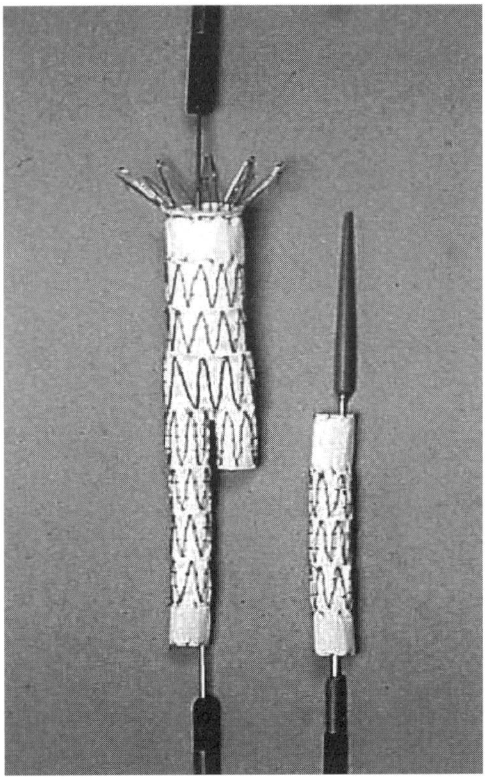

1

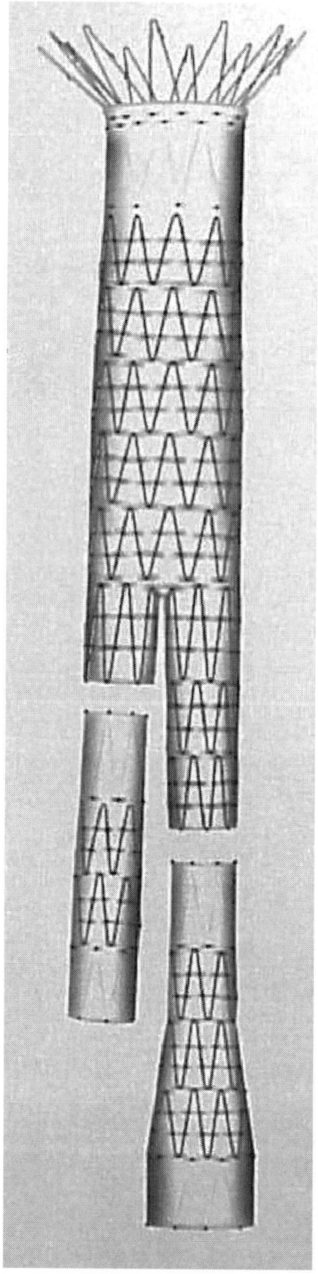

2

seal in the common iliac. It adds flexibility for length adjustment on both sides and this flexibility enables it to be an 'off-the-shelf' device. While the design of the Zenith graft has evolved, the essential features of the original graft have been preserved and include:

1. *bifurcated graft* – to restore normal anatomy perfusing both iliac conduits;
2. *self-expanding graft* – accommodates for errors in diameter assessment and variation;
3. *modular system* – allows for endoluminal building of the bifurcated system via two ports to address length assessment problems and optimize the landing zone in the iliac vessel;
4. *full length metallic skeleton* – provides for maintenance of length and some pillar (column) strength, visibility for alignment and insertion and protection against kinking and twisting.

3, 4, 5, 6

Suprarenal (transrenal) fixation with an anchor stent is an original feature of this graft with the purpose of providing secure proximal attachment to an area of aorta which is less likely to dilate or contain significant atheroma (3). The region of mesenteric and renal vessels in the aorta is the least likely to be involved in aneurysmal disease and provides the best attachment zone to resist the drag placed on a bifurcated graft by the blood flow. Illustration 3 shows the impending use of this attachment zone with a hooked, uncovered anchor stent.

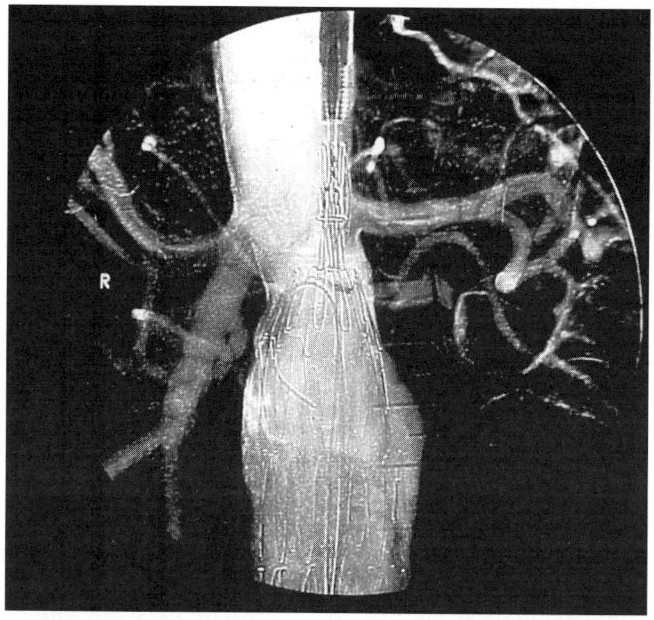

3

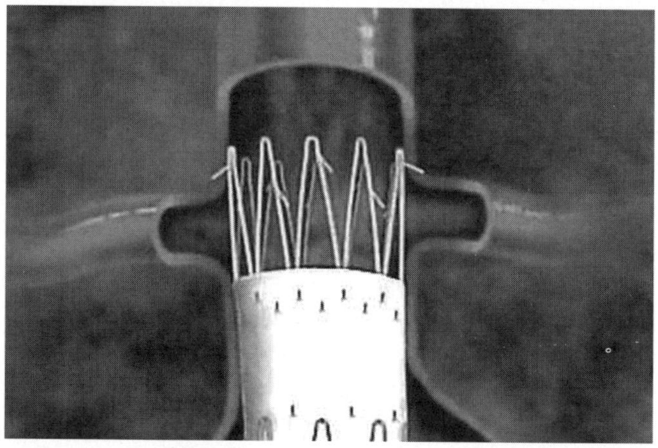

4

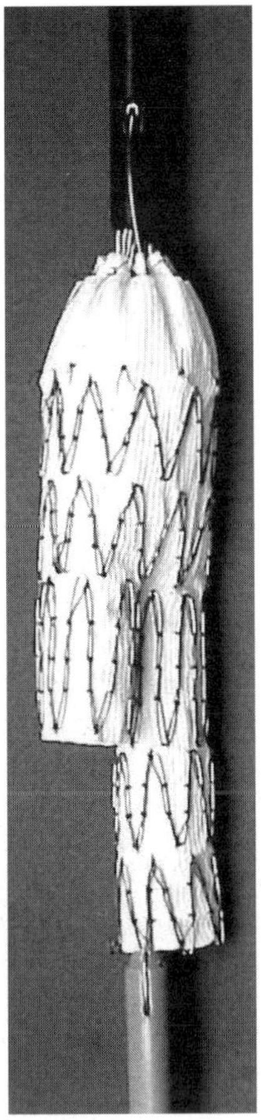

5

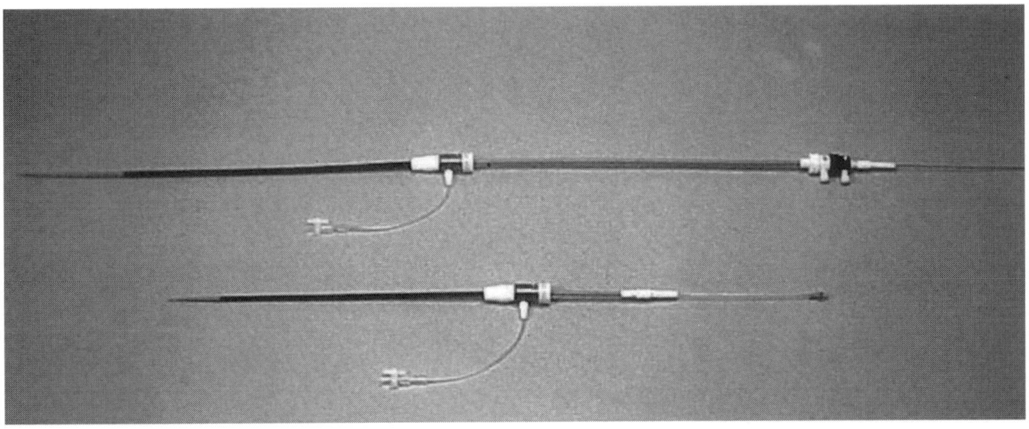

6a

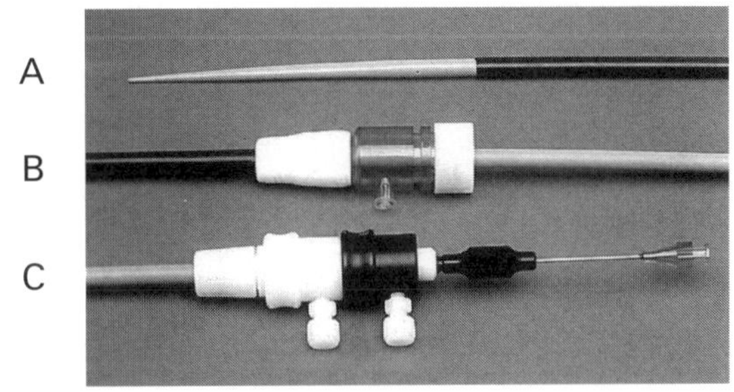

6b

The current anchor stent features hooks which embed into the aortic wall and increase the attachment strength ten-fold compared with radial attachment alone (**4**).

Safety features to contain the anchor stent and enable controlled deployment include a proximal cap for the anchor stent, safety wires and a pin-holding device to prevent premature deployment (**5**, **6**). Illustration 5 shows the graft loaded on the delivery system prior to being placed inside the sheath. The anchor stent is contained within the cap. It is prevented from premature release by the safety trigger wire positioned through a crown in the stent. The bottom stent is similarly held by a separate wire. The top cap is mounted on a central metal shaft which passes through a plastic dilator. It may move independently of the plastic dilator which holds the bottom of the graft. The graft may therefore be stretched or compressed – a position secured by the use of a pin device (see **6**: an ensheathed device with accessory extension piece).

The body of the graft was made as long as possible so that haemodynamic displacement forces and resistance to flow would be reduced to a minimum within the aneurysm chamber (Lawrence-Brown *et al.*, 1996, 1999; van Schie *et al.*, 1998). It also allowed the joint between the main body of the graft and the short limb to lie close to the iliac orifice for two reasons. The first reason was to reduce the leverage upon the joint by having the fulcrum as close to the iliac orifice as possible and the second was to make cannulation of the short limb easier by placing it close to the iliac orifice. The system was also designed so that travel through the axis conduit (iliac arteries) involved a pulling mechanism, rather than one based on pushing forces. This provides a better mechanism for delivery, particularly through tortuous vessels.

Unfavourable necks and fenestration

7

Proximal seal is dependent on a suitable infrarenal neck with straight parallel walls which is long enough (recommended 20 mm) to allow an adequate area for a complete and durable seal. Graft design, radial strength and fatigability are also important in maintaining a durable attachment and seal to overcome long-term friction and strain on the graft. The most unfavourable feature for a proximal neck is an irregular and non-parallel neck contour (**7**). Type 1 is the ideal and the others depict examples of contour change, which may lead to endoleak. Any

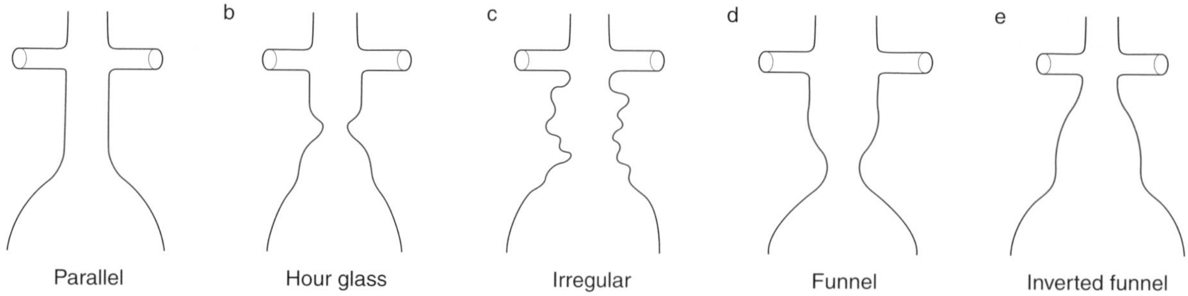

7

change in diameter greater or equal to 3 mm increases the risk of endoleak three-fold (p=0.003). As a continuous variable a neck shorter than 20 mm increases the risk of endoleak (p=0.01). Angulation of the neck increases the risk of endoleak if the neck is short. Large diameters are associated with migration because the drag force is exponentially increased with increased diameter.

8, 9

Sometimes custom crafting of the proximal end of the graft at the sealing zone can improve the ability to exclude the aneurysm. Asymmetry of the renal arteries or a significant lower pole vessel are ready examples of limited available neck which may otherwise be suitable. To overcome these problems and increase the area of the attachment zone and seal, fenestrated grafts serve a purpose (**8**). The illustration shows examples of fenestration an infrarenal aortic graft thoracic graft. The use of fenestration requires control and accuracy of deployment especially rotational manoeuvrability to allow exact positioning of the fenestration over the intended orifice. Accurate planning and construction requires high quality three-dimensional (3D) computerized tomography imaging and good angiography.

Controlled and accurate positioning of the fenestrated system is based on partial deployment of the graft to allow rotational as well as caudal and cephalic movement to position the fenestration over the orifice of the

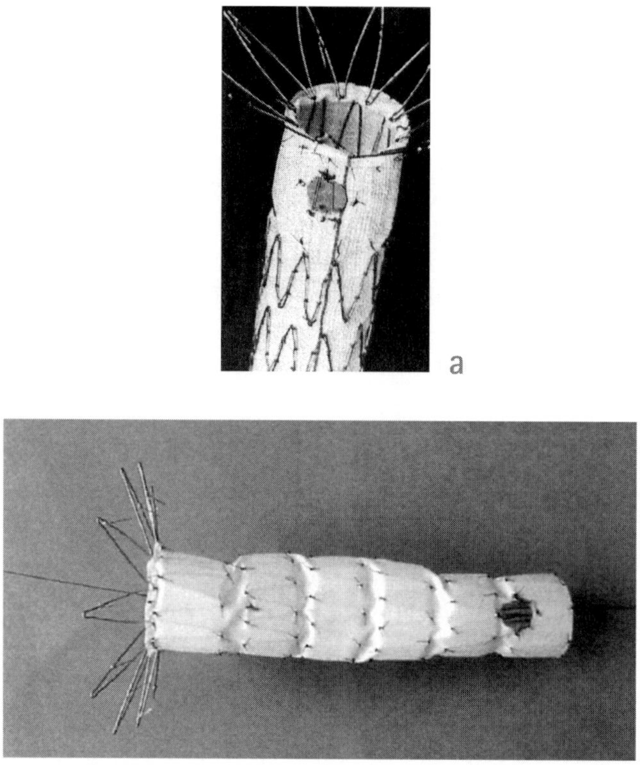

a

b

8

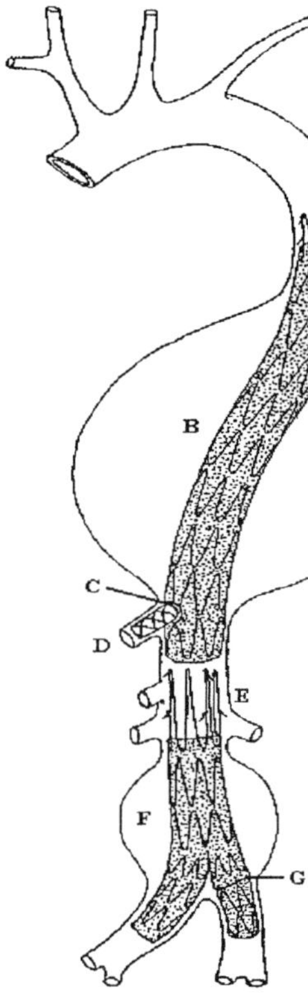

9

target vessel. Once positioned and still partially deployed the vessel is cannulated from inside the graft through the fenestration into the vessel with a guidewire. The guidewire is then given added support with either a guide catheter or inflated rigid balloon. This then acts to track the fenestration down to its orifice on completing deployment of the graft. Further fixation of the orifice through the fenestration with a stent (covered or uncovered) prevents a change in the position of the main graft from the orifice or causes the orifice to move with the graft and parent artery as a unit. This has opened the door to link the thoracic and infrarenal domains.

The feasibility of treating a thoracic aneurysm and an infrarenal aortic aneurysm with preservation of the coeliac vessel has now been demonstrated (**9**). Illustration **9** includes: A-uncovered anchor stent of thoracic graft, B-covered stent. C-fenestration, D-palmaz stent, E-open anchor stent of abdominal graft, F-covered stent, G-join.

Custom crafting of the endograft with alteration of the gaps and distances between the metal skeleton stents and the Dacron soft coating addresses some changes in direction and contour. Adherence to favourable features of the proximal neck is advised to exclude the aneurysm from direct aortic flow. These features are a neck of parallel walls (less than 3 mm diameter change), a length of 20 mm or more, an angle of less than 60 degrees from the aortic axis and a diameter of less than 28 mm.

References

Brown TF, Hartley D, Purchas S *et al.* (1999). A fenestrated covered suprarenal aortic stent. *Eur J Vasc Surg* **18**: 445–449.

Lawrence-Brown MMD, Hartley D, MacSweeny S *et al.* (1996). The Perth endoluminal bifurcated graft system – development and early experience. *J Cardiovasc Surg* **4**:706–712.

Lawrence-Brown MMD, Sleunarine K, Hartley D *et al.* (1998). Should an anchor stent cross the renal artery orifices when placing an endoluminal graft for abdominal aortic aneurysm? In *Indications in Vascular and Endovascular Surgery.* RM Greenhalgh, ed. London: WB Saunders Co. p. 261.

Lawrence-Brown MMD, Semmens JB, Hartley DE *et al.* (1999). How is durability related to patient selection and graft design with endoluminal grafting for abdominal aortic aneurysm? In *Durability of Vascular and Endovascular Surgery.* RM Greenhalgh, ed. London: WB Saunders Co. pp. 375–385.

Lawrence-Brown MMD, Semmens JB, Stanley BM *et al.* (2000). Endoluminal building of the aortic grafts for aneurysmal disease, and other members of the Zenith endoluminal stent-graft program. In *Vascular and Endovascular Opportunities.* RM Greenhalgh, AWM Mitchell, eds. London: WB Saunders Co. pp. 249–261.

Stanley B, Semmens JB, Lawrence-Brown MMD *et al.* (2001). Fenestration for endoluminal repair of aortic aneurysm: new horizons for preserving blood flow in branch vessels. *J Endovasc Ther* **8**:16–24.

van Schie G, Sieunarine K, Lawrence-Brown MMD, Hartley D (1998). The Perth bifurcated endovascular graft for infrarenal aortic aneurysms. *Semin Intervent Radiol* **15**:63–69.

The Ancure/Guidant stent-graft system for abdominal aortic aneurysm

Dieter Raithel

Introduction

Proximal and distal fixation is an important issue for any graft used in endovascular abdominal aortic aneurysm repair. This fixation renders the graft resistant to migration and prevents movement, or adjustment of its location after deployment.

Optimal fixation of the iliac limbs is also an important prerequisite to prevent long-term migration, considering the increasing elongation of the iliac axis.

Through optimal proximal and distal fixation, a large percentage of type I endoleaks (endoleaks at the attachment site) can be prevented.

An endoprosthesis should imitate, as closely as possible, the result of open surgical replacement of the aorta. This will probably only be possible using a graft that is not fully stented, as the greater flexibility of such grafts (e.g. a crimped graft), provide better long-term adaptation to the morphologic changes of the aorta and the iliac axis.

In the literature when comparing the long-term results of modular systems with unibody grafts the endoleakage rate seems to be lower for the so-called unibody grafts. This applies particularly to type III endoleaks (modular disconnection), as frequently observed using modular systems.

This demonstrates, that unibody grafts mimic surgical repair and do not carry the risk of component separation.

The Ancure™ graft was invented by H Lazarus (a vascular surgeon in Utah). It was a further development of the EVT™ (Endovascular Technologies) graft. The original EVT endovascular graft, known as EGS (Endovascular Grafting System) was a tube graft, and Dr Wesley Moore performed the first human graft at the University of California, in February 1993. That case was successful, and all subsequent clinical research was done under FDA-approval protocols.

These phase I trials for the tube and bifurcated configurations of the Ancure graft were carried out between 1993 and 1995. The phase II trials were designed to compare the safety and efficacy of endovascular repair with conventional repair. Phase II trials for the tube, bifurcated and aortoiliac Ancure systems were completed between 1995 and 1998.

Ancure graft design

1, 2, 3

The defined philosophy was to develop a graft identical to a conventional graft, which replicates long-term performance of conventional surgery.

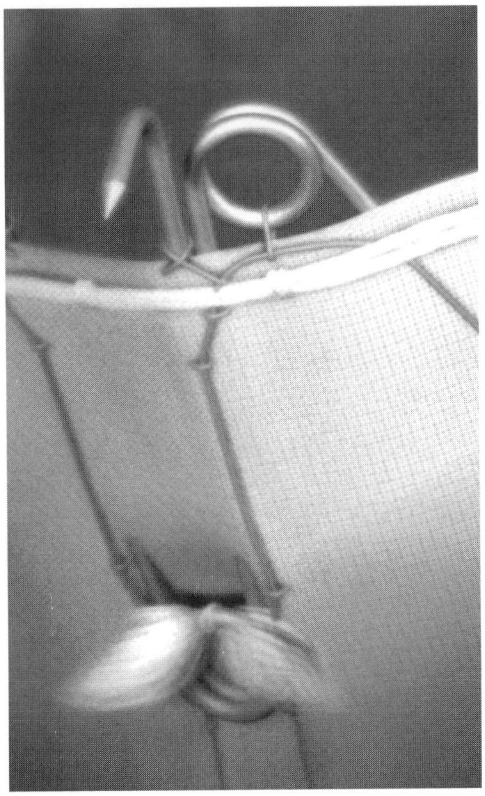

1

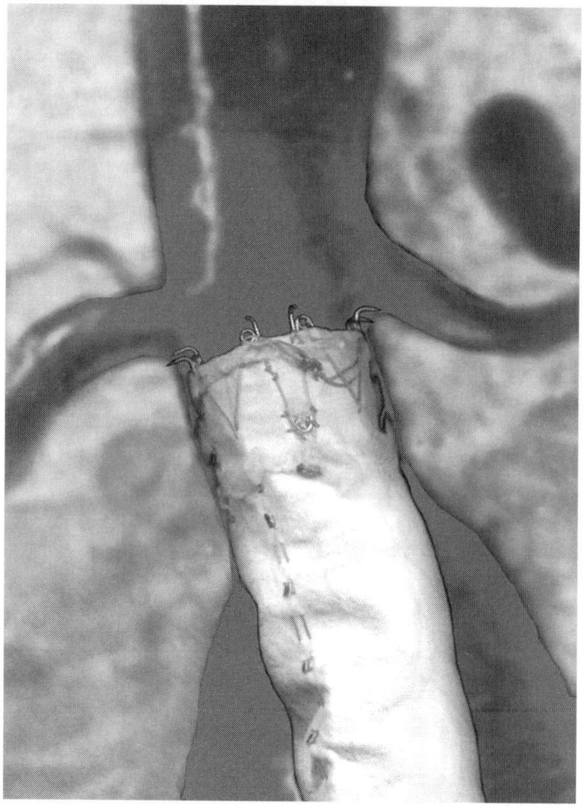

2

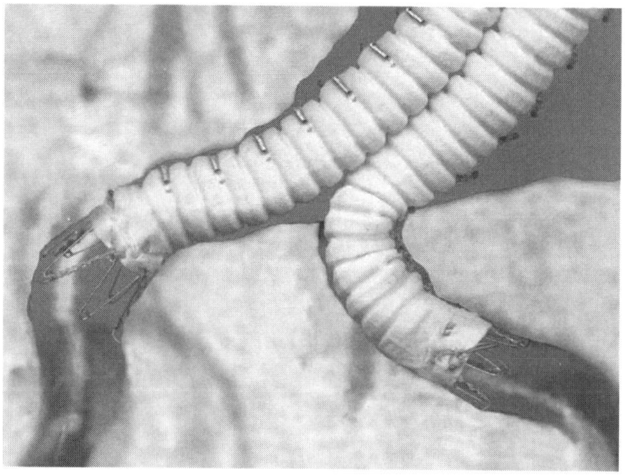

3

The graft is available in tubes, bifurcated **unibody** grafts and aortomonoiliac grafts.

The graft is made of woven polyester fabric, has an Endo-Hooks™ attachment system and 'fuzzy' tufts to promote ingrowth of the graft (1). Platinum radiopaque markers are incorporated for identification of the graft position (2: infrarenal attachment system; 3: distal). The graft is designed as flexible and has a crimping of the iliac limbs (3), for better adjusting to longitudinal shrinkage.

Furthermore, the non-stented graft adapts to changing morphology. The combination of a non-stented design with a flexible graft particularly allows an optimal placement of the graft in tortuous anatomy and angled necks. (2, 3)

The flexibility enables the adjustment of differences in length between the preoperative measurement and the intraoperative application. For example, there is the possibility of adjusting a possible overlength of long tube grafts by compression of the prosthesis.

Aortoiliac prostheses can, in the case of possible overlength – which would result in the overlapping of the hypogastric artery – also be shortened by compression of the crimped iliac limbs.

Operative technique

4a, b, 5, 6

Vascular access is achieved with a 25.5 F special expandable vascular access sheath (**4a**) with two iris-type valves, that permit a haemostatic seal. The intuitive delivery

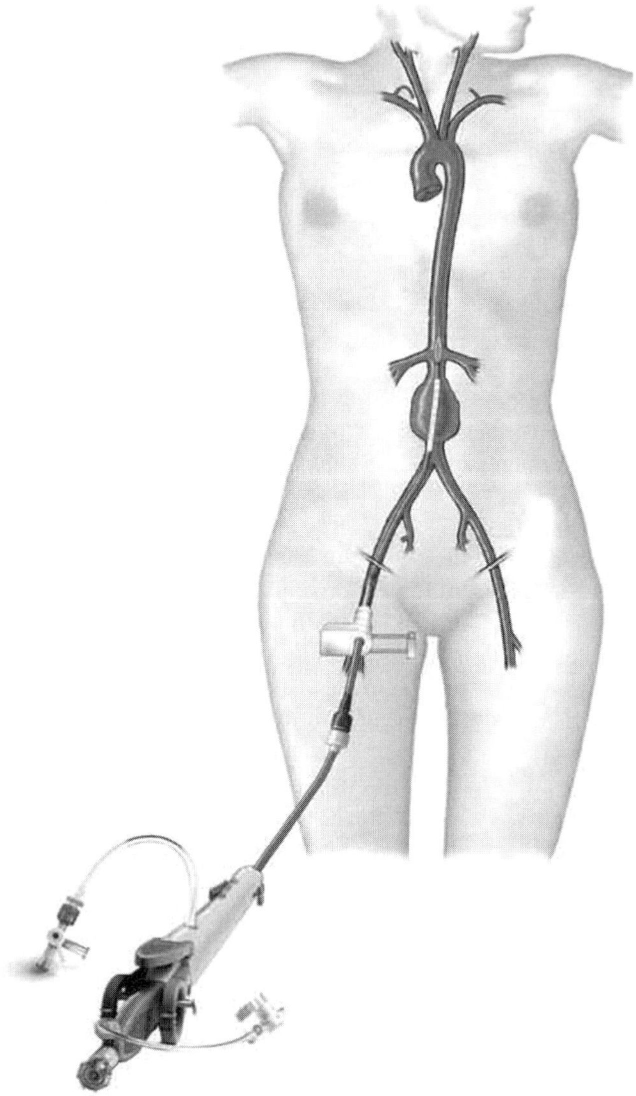

4a

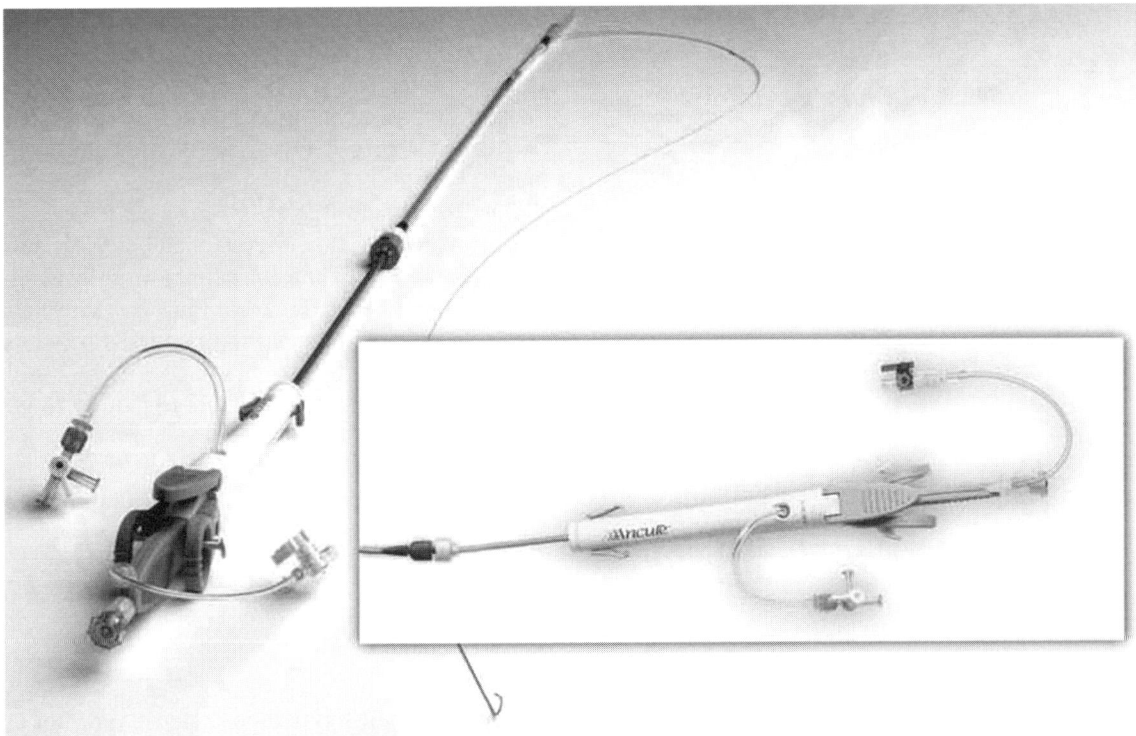

4b

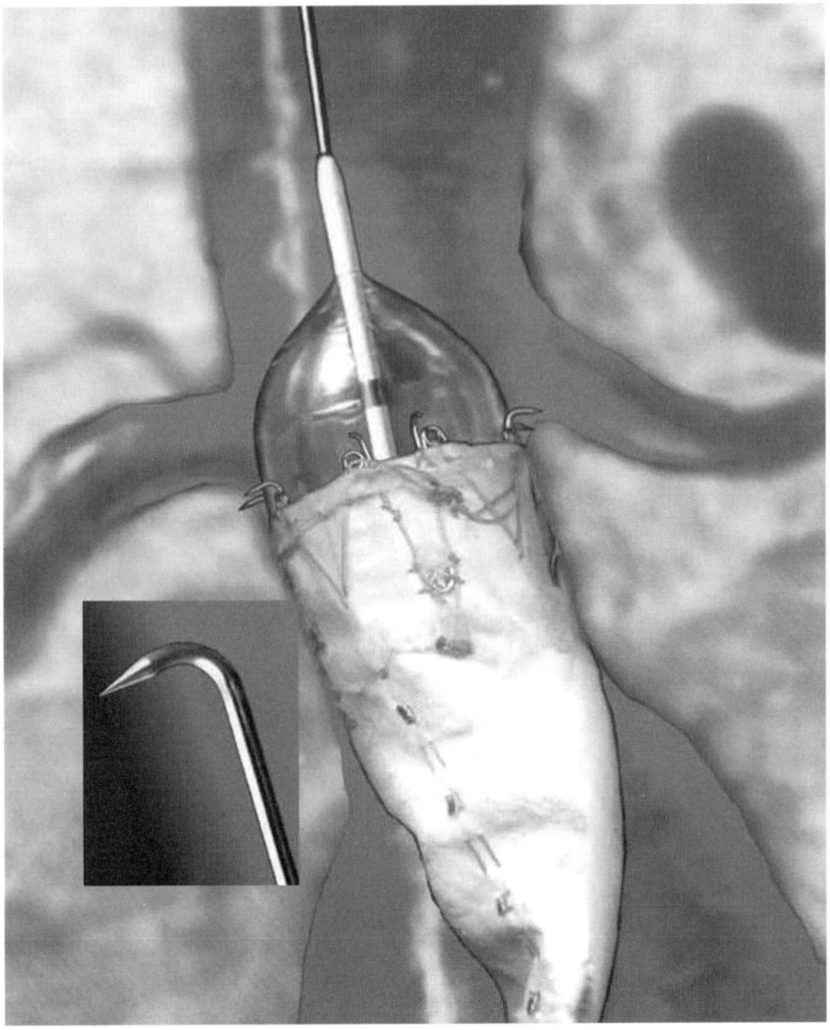

5

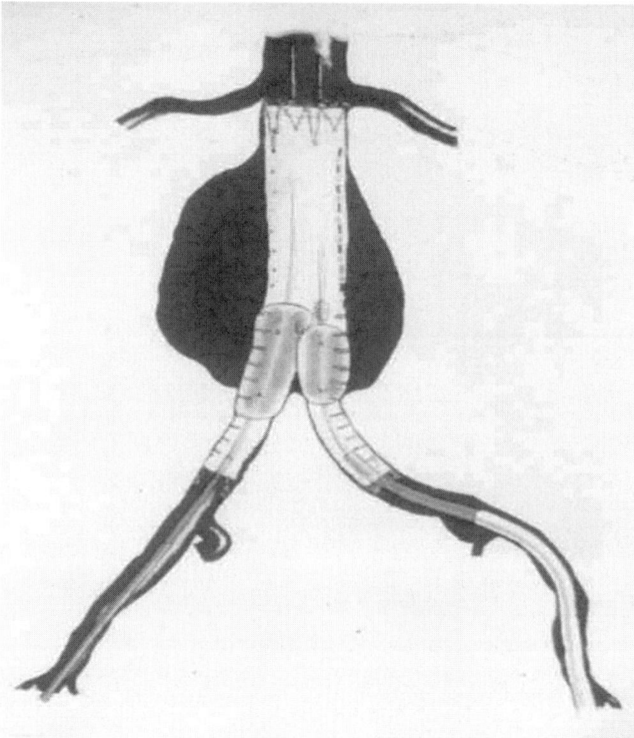

6

catheter has numbered controls for step-by-step deployment and logical interlocks to help maintain proper step sequence.

The graft delivery catheter is an over-the-wire system. The delivery system allows independent control of the aortic and iliac attachments with respect to both longitudinal and radial position. Each attachment system is locked in a metal capsule and cannot be deployed until made active by the surgeon, to prevent premature or wrong deployment.

The proximal and distal attachment system (EndoHooks) allows self-expanding initial deployment at the desired location, and is followed by balloon inflation (5).

The single-piece graft has a series of radiopaque markers along the length of the graft, which allows determination of the graft configuration and position during implantation and follow-up.

The markers on the body of the graft are orientated longitudinally, while limb markers are oriented radially (2, 3). The graft bifurcation is indicated by a single marker.

Due to the fact, that the Ancure graft is a non-stented graft (unsupported), we recommend subsequent simultaneous dilatation of the iliac limbs in a 'kissing-balloon' technique (6). Using this technique, it is very seldom necessary to support one of the iliac limbs by, for example, a Wallstent.

The largest diameter available to date is 26 mm for the Ancure tube graft, with hook-to-hook lengths of 9.0 to 16.0 cm; for the bifurcated graft the available prostheses diameters range from 20 to 26 mm. Iliac limb diameters are 10 to 13 mm, and prosthesis hook-to-hook lengths 12 to 19 cm.

Summary

The Ancure graft has demonstrated a very high degree of implantation reliability, reproducibility and accuracy. The unibody compliant design allows the graft to adapt to native anatomy and furthermore avoids the pitfalls of modular junctions. However, until now, with respect to the pathological anatomy (e.g. large common iliacs, variant iliac lengths and larger aortic necks) the graft has a limited applicability.

Acknowledgements

Illustrations by M Hellmuth.

References

Deaton DH, Bogey WM, Chiang K *et al.* (1999). Bifurcated endovascular grafting for abdominal aortic aneurysm. *Ann Vasc Surg* **13**: 23–31.

Makaroun M, Zajko A, Sugimoto H *et al.* (1999). Fate of endoleaks after endoluminal repair of abdominal aortic Aneurysms with the EVT® device. *Eur J Vasc Endovasc Surg* **18**: 185–190.

Raithel D (1999). Which industry-made endovascular grafts are best for abdominal aortic aneurysm repair and why. In *Perspectives in Vascular Surgery*. Gloviczki P. ed. Vol. 12, No 1. New York, Stuttgart: Thieme. pp. 1–10.

The Vanguard III aortic stent-graft

Hugh G Beebe,
Svante Horsch, Steven S Gale

Introduction

The origin of Vanguard I

Evolution of the Vanguard aortic stent-graft illustrates many aspects of endovascular device development that seem to apply generally to all such devices as well as specifically to this endograft type. By considering briefly the evolution of the design into its current version, we can see the influence of the properties of both the endograft itself, and delivery system for inserting it, upon the technique used for treatment of aneurysm patients by this still evolving method.

The basic endograft design evolved from the MinTec Stentor endovascular prosthesis conceived in the early 1990s. The Stentor endograft had begun clinical application in Europe under investigational circumstances but without the strict controls necessary to allow accumulation of best quality outcome data. By analysis of individual institutional experience where careful follow-up information was known, it was possible to identify aspects of the original design that suggested opportunity for improvement. Following acquisition of that technology by Boston Scientific Corporation in 1996, the design was altered to eliminate known failure risks.

The general concept of the Vanguard stent-graft was a modular endoprosthesis that was assembled *in situ* through bilateral remote arterial access and insertion of modular components. These components were held in position within each other and the entire assembled endograft held in position within the aortoiliac anatomy through friction applied by self-expanding metal stents. The nitinol alloy metal used for manufacturing the stents was thermally activated such that it exerted maximum force when exposed to body temperature. The metal stents were located on the inside of the fabric tube to expand it, except at the proximal end where there was a small, 10 mm, but significant length of exposed stent material above the upper end of the fabric.

The stent-graft was compressed and contained within a series of concentric round tubes comprising the delivery system for insertion above and below the arterial segment. The basic operation of the delivery system allowed deployment of the endoprosthesis, after fluoroscopically guided positioning, by withdrawing an outer sheath to expose the self-expanding stent while holding the stent-graft in position by resistive pressure of a central catheter.

Among the early changes that were incorporated into the design of the Vanguard I prosthesis were changes in the polyethylene fibre and weaving process to increase strength. Also the full-length sutured seam that had been a part of the original design was eliminated because this had, in a few cases, been observed to cause late failure from fabric tearing along this long suture line.

The delivery system turned out to be more important than had been fully realized in the early clinical application. One aspect of this was that the leading edge of the delivery system being advanced into the iliac artery consisted of a latex balloon held in position by friction within the outer sheath. If this moved backward from increased frictional load when inserted into a small iliac artery, it exposed a sharp leading edge on the sheath that could induce arterial trauma. Also the backward motion of the balloon could transmit pressure to the endoprosthesis by inducing compression loads within the sheath. Passage of the delivery system catheter through tortuous iliac vessels induced torque. But this rotational force was not easily resisted because the original endograft delivery system was constructed of a circular section tubing within a circular section tubing. Thus the torque applied during delivery system passage upwards into the aorta, especially in narrow and highly convoluted iliac arteries, could induce rotation and distortion of the endograft contained within.

Evolution into Vanguard II

A controlled clinical trial, known as the US Investigation Device Exemption study of the Vanguard I aortic stent-graft, was launched in the USA in 1997 and widespread use in European sites was also begun. This clinical experience produced observations on differences between features of Vanguard I and Vanguard II and illustrates the impact of design changes upon endovascular surgery technique. For example, the operation of the original delivery system often required the manual application of significant physical force by the operator to get the contralateral limb to pass upward. This is inimical to the requirement for gentle movements of any object within the arterial wall that can induce trauma and to maintaining precise location while positioning a device to exclude parts of the arterial circulation.

The Vanguard II endograft system employed the same implanted endoprosthesis but a redesigned and substantially improved delivery system. Features of the new delivery system had a significant impact on technique for using this endograft. Chief among them were: a redesign of the leading end of the outer sheath ('nose cone'), effective antitorque control of rotational forces, simplicity of deployment steps with intuitive controls and end-loading of the contralateral limb component. Since this delivery system is the one used for the Vanguard III endograft, these features are described and illustrated in detail subsequently.

Other design changes were based on results of the Vanguard I/II device as previously reported and extensive bench testing with simulation of the physical forces that stent-grafts must withstand. The original Vanguard I and II trial was begun in the USA in 1997 and accrual of follow-up data is ongoing (Beebe *et al.*, 2001). Some adverse events in that trial deserve a brief summary because they became a focal stimulus for consideration of design changes. Limb occlusions occurred in 4.6% of bifurcation endografts within 12 months increasing to 9% with longer follow-up. The incidence was skewed toward the side of the contralateral limb module. A variety of reasons for this were postulated, including the effect of asymmetrical distribution of patient arteriosclerotic disease. Component dislocation resulting in endoleak was observed in approximately 2% over a span of 2 years. This was usually associated with major change in endograft alignment due to changing aortoiliac morphology in response to aneurysm exclusion. Fabric erosion occurred in 2.2% within a 30-month follow-up interval thought to be due to relative motion between fabric and the underlying stent framework. This was especially associated with the apex of an angled stent presenting a focal point for repetitive impact between it and the fabric.

Impact of Vanguard III on technique and patient selection

1

Although the Vanguard III aortic stent-graft is properly considered a new device and will need clinical trial validation as such, there are lessons to be learned from understanding the changes from Vanguard II resulting from carefully analysed clinical observations and data from bench testing using deliberately stressed models (**1**). Illustration **1a** shows Vanguard II and **1b** shows Vanguard III. The larger diameter nitinol wire results in greater radial force in the Vanguard III endoprosthesis. The result is a tighter fabric fit on the stent structure with decreased motion potential and greater resistance to kinking as shown in these views of a model being stress-tested in compression.

2

The configuration of the Vanguard III aortic stent-graft eliminates large zigzag stents in the middle of the aortic trunk portion and thereby also tends to eliminate unopposed stent angles that could present an isolated apex to impact on prosthesis fabric. The radius of the supporting nitinol wire stent was increased from 0.011 inches to 0.015 inches thus resulting in greater radial force applied by the stent. The result of this change was to inhibit fabric motion by stretching the surrounding fabric more

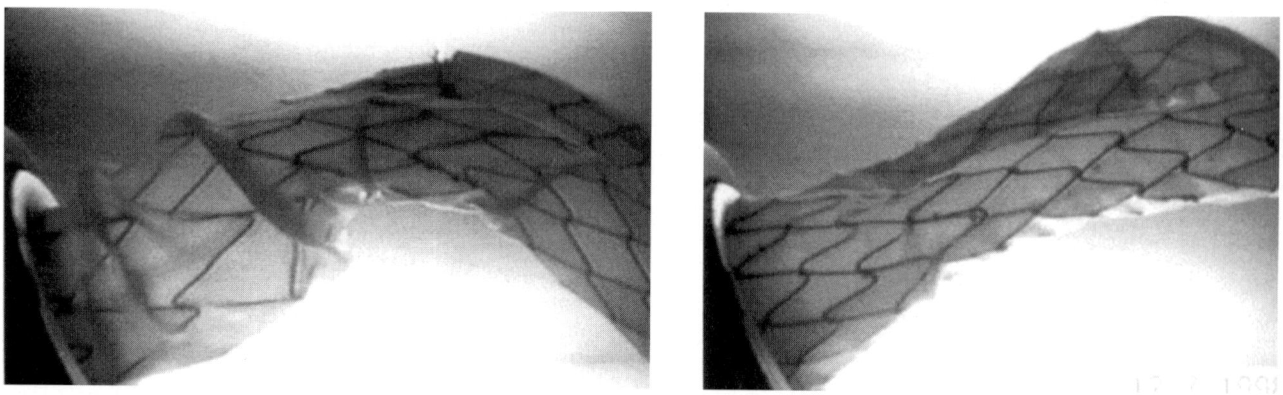

a b

1

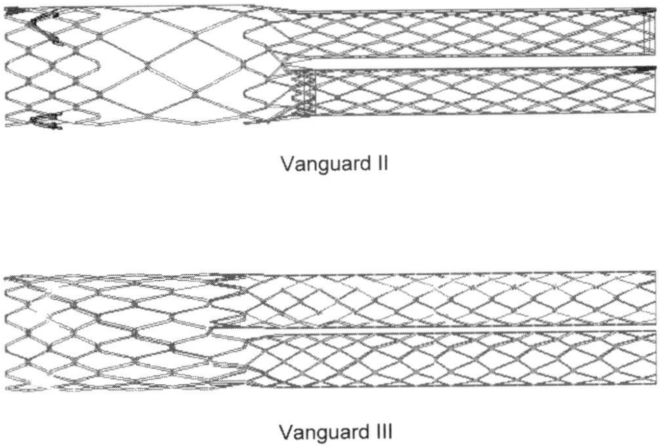

2

tightly over the underlying frame when the endograft is not constrained by apposition to the arterial wall. Together these elements of the new design may increase resistance to fabric erosion that was observed in a small percentage of earlier cases (2).

3

Another aspect of the Vanguard III design addresses some probable causes of the observed incidence of late endograft limb occlusions. This problem has been greater on the contralateral limb side than that of the ipsilateral limb which suggests that iliac stenosis, femoral arterial occlusive disease or other anatomical factors play a role. But structural features of the Vanguard II endograft have been changed to reduce whatever contribution to limb occlusion was being made by the endoprosthesis. The changes here include increase in the size of the iliac limbs to 50% of the aortic trunk diameter in all cases rather than only in the 22 mm stent-graft and a generally smoother contour that results from the reconfigured stents as can be seen in Illustration 3, which shows Vanguard II (**3a**) and Vanguard III (**3b**). Changes in the shape of the stent-graft bifurcation can been seen in this luminal view looking distally from within the aortic trunk. The contralateral limb is inserted on the right in both.

Regarding the technique for insertion of the endograft, there are at least eight elements of the redesigned Vanguard III system that are a significant influence on early technical results as described below.

1. The lumen-seeking graduated stiffness nose cone.
2. Torque-resistant catheter containing the endoprosthesis.
3. Intuitive, simple operating controls for stent-graft deployment.
4. Controlled partial deployment of the upper stent-graft.
5. Uncovered proximal stents of the endograft.
6. Contralateral iliac limb stump features.
7. End-loaded contralateral limb sheath.
8. Range of endograft component sizes.

Early results of Vanguard III usage are available from the European trial started in June 2000. This trial was

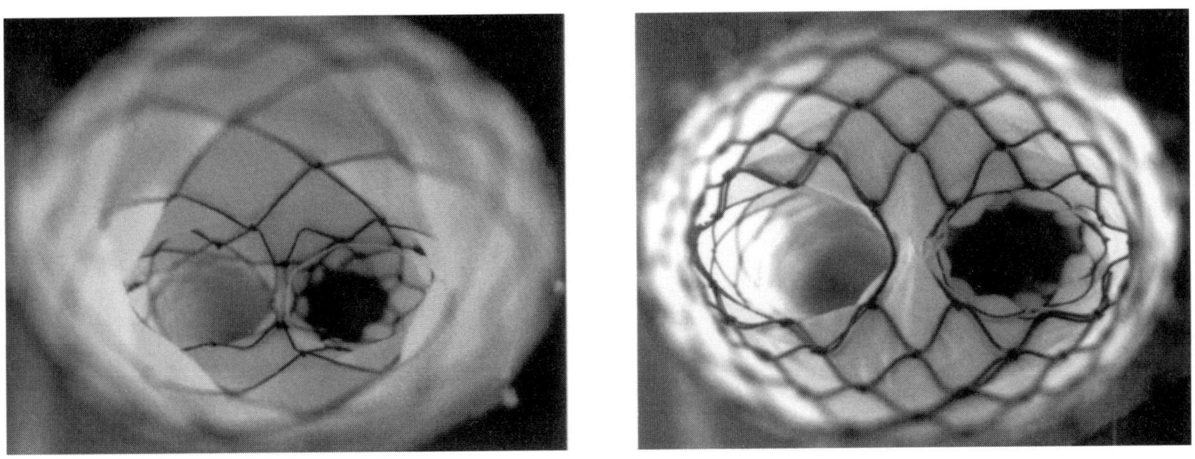

a 3 b

designed as a multicentre, consecutive enrollment study of infrarenal aortoiliac aneurysm among 14 European investigational centres. At the time of this writing, 42 patients had been enrolled from six clinical sites and follow-up data at 30 days were already available in 33 cases. Device sizes implanted included 24 mm in 13 patients, 26 mm in 24 patients, 28 mm in three patients and 30 mm in two patients. Among the 33 patients with 30-day follow up, mean age was 68.9 years and 84.8% (28) were male.

Technical success in device placement was accomplished in 100% without significant device-related deployment events. One early endoleak of unknown type, but probably type II, was observed. In two cases, arterial wall dissection of a transit iliac vessel was seen but resolved without treatment.

The lumen seeking graduated stiffness nose cone

4, 5

In the earliest days of endograft use, early delivery systems were crude by comparison with current devices. An important source of procedural morbidity that resulted was iliac artery injury from the upper (proximal) end of the delivery system being traumatic.

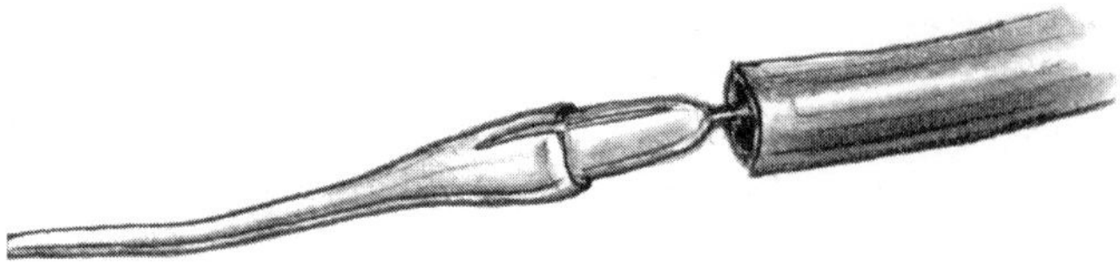

5

Sometimes passage of the delivery system was impossible because of its size and resultant friction and in tortuous vessels short blunt-ended catheters added to the difficulty. The Vanguard III delivery system has a long tapered nose cone that provides a gradual transition from flexible to stiffer deformation resistance that results in ease of insertion due to the lumen-seeking quality when advanced over a guidewire, even through relatively angled access vessels (4). The importance of applying consistent pressure to the delivery system during passage through iliac vessels is real. Extremely

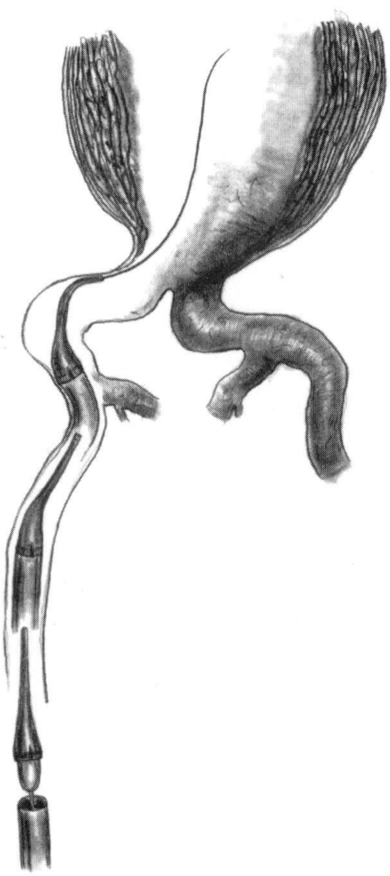

4

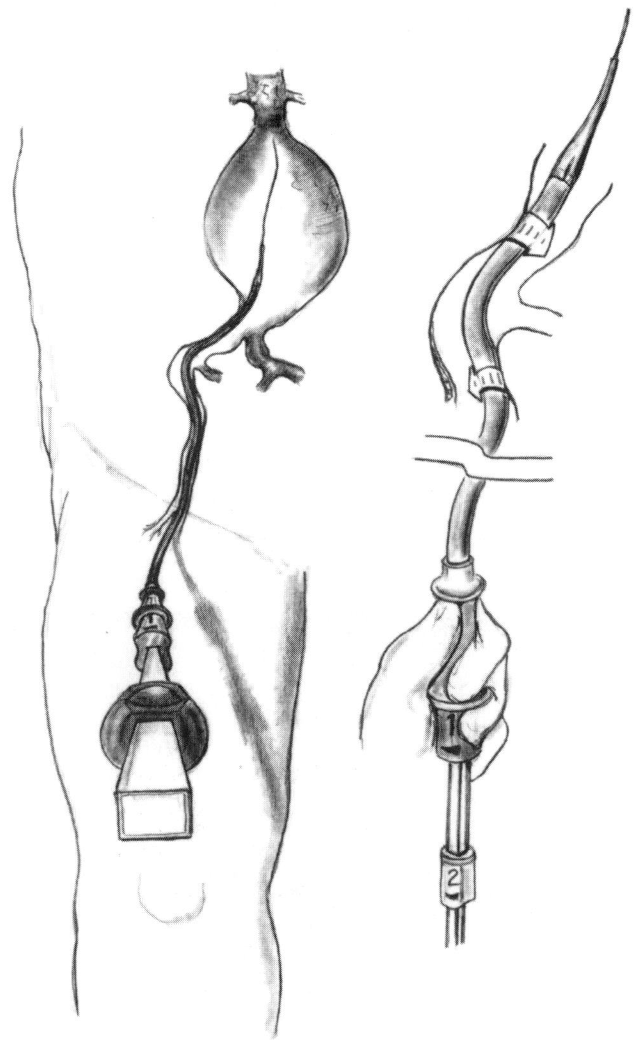

6

high pressure, or sudden variance in resistance to passage, puts stress on the arterial wall and on iliac artery fixation points which are centered around the internal iliac artery and has resulted in haemorrhage from avulsion of the origin of this vessel when misapplied. The new delivery system also eliminated the leading edge balloon and replaced it with a long, tapered, lumen-seeking nose cone that resisted frictional back pressure during insertion by an indented step. This indented step sits on the upper end of the outer sheath and creates an immobile transition between leading edge parts that presents a smooth surface to the arterial wall. In addition this design prevents transmission of backpressure to the contents of the sheath (5).

Torque-resistant catheter containing the endoprosthesis

6

The torque problem was also dealt with by an ingeniously simple method. While tubes are usually circular and thus can easily rotate within each other, a tube within a tube that has a square section cannot rotate because the angles lock them in position (6). A common experience analogy would be to consider the forces involved when pliers are used to rotate a round object as contrasted with a flat-sided wrench used to rotate a flat-sided nut. Thus when the delivery system receives asymmetrical frictional forces that are torque inducing, this is resisted and provides protection from misalignment of the endoprosthesis during insertion.

Intuitive, simple operating controls for stent-graft deployment

7

The value of precise control of endograft placement is very high at the proximal end because this determines the position of the remainder of the endograft and, as is usually true, allows utilization of all of a limited attachment zone within the infrarenal neck to achieve an effective seal. One of the elements of easy, facile control is having a simple, intuitively obvious method of accomplishing the steps to deploy the stent-graft through use of natural, ergonomically correct manual operation. A single grasping point for one hand of the operator through all steps and obvious, sequential unlocking controls aid this process (7).

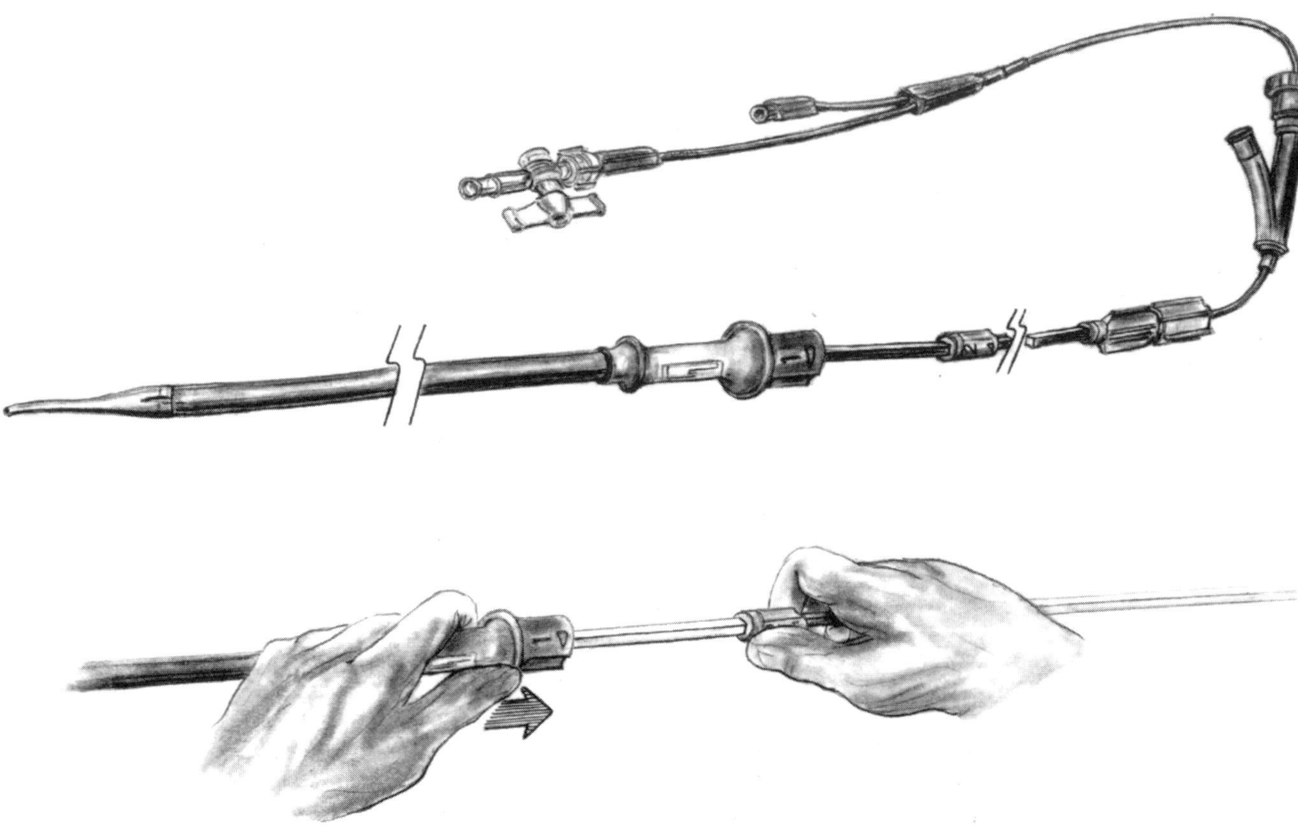

7

Controlled partial deployment of the upper stent-graft

8

Another aspect of operator control that results in accurate deployment of endovascular devices is the ability to make last minute, fine-tuning adjustments before irrevocable steps are taken. Thus there is outcome value in having a device that permits partial deployment under visualization while still permitting movement proximally or distally within the infrarenal aortic neck. While the Vanguard III prosthesis cannot be recovered once it is partially released from the outer sheath, it can be stopped at a point during the initiation of deployment that permits the operator to move the most proximal limit of the stent-graft very precisely (8).

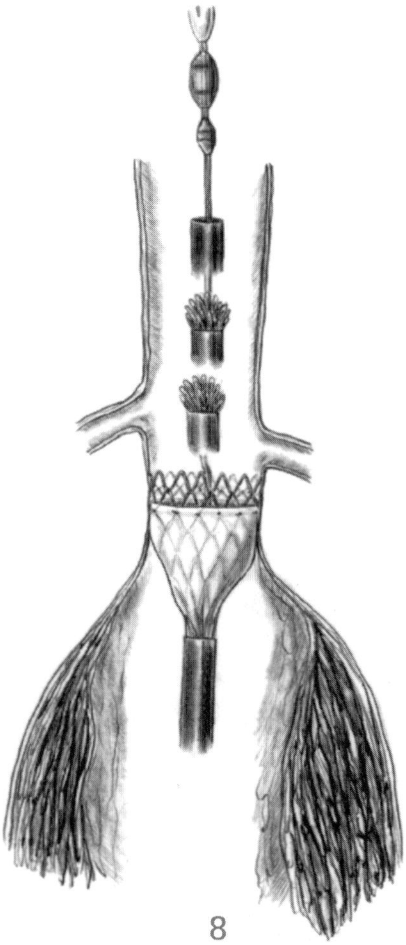

8

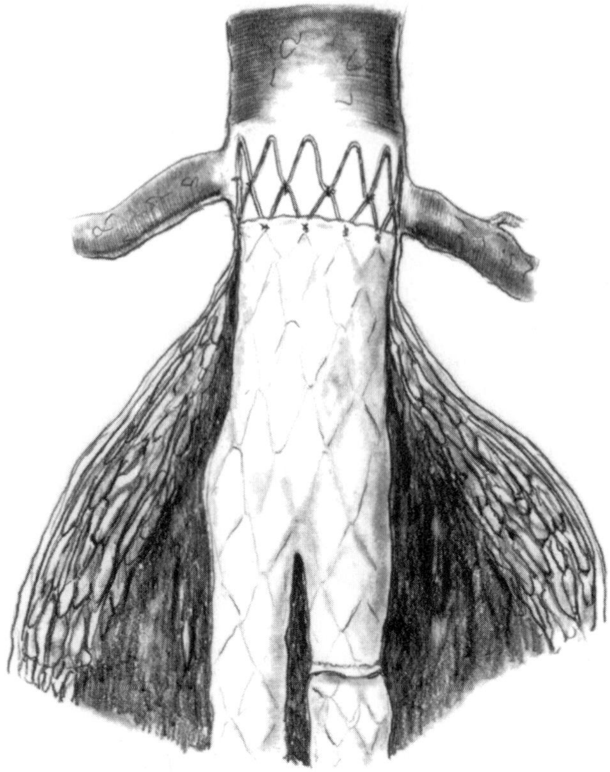

9

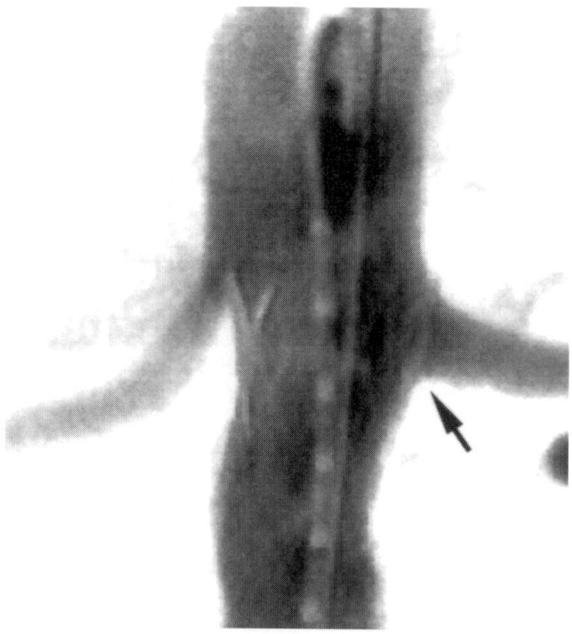

10

Uncovered proximal stents of the endograft

9, 10

When the infrarenal aorta presents a sufficient length of undilated diameter to make proximal attachment of a stent-graft an easy technical step, there is little need for deployment of an endograft in a suprarenal position. When the proximal neck is short, in the range of 10 mm or less, the value of suprarenal fixation has been suggested by an increasing number of reports (Greenberg *et al.*, 2000; Malina *et al.*, 1999). Thus the provision of two rows of zigzag stents in the Vanguard III stent-graft allows the operator a limited choice in this regard: **9** and **10** illustrate this point.

Contralateral iliac limb stump features

11

The Vanguard III stent-graft has a larger stump that is flared at its distal extent to provide a larger diameter for retrograde access and guidewire cannulation. Since this step in modular endograft insertion is accomplished by fluoroscopic guidance, the quality and positioning of radio-opaque markers has a leveraged and significant influence of results. Fluoroscopy is a two-dimensional medium used in performing the three-dimensional task of inserting a contralateral limb.

Anything that makes this easier will save fluoroscopy time, a safety and cost-saving enhancer, and reduce the need for manipulation of equipment within a vascular space that usually contains potential emboli. One of the complications of aortic endografting by modular prostheses that are assembled within the treated anatomy is late dislocation of the elements resulting in repressurization of the aneurysm sac. Two changes have been made aimed at reducing the risk of this late problem. One was extending the length of the contralateral limb stump from 11 mm to 22 mm which provides not only a more forgiving location in which to insert the additional component, but when placed in the nominal position a greater surface area of contact for friction-induced stability. Also, matching a tapered shape of the contralateral limb proximal extent and the aortic stump provides additional security of attachment (**11**).

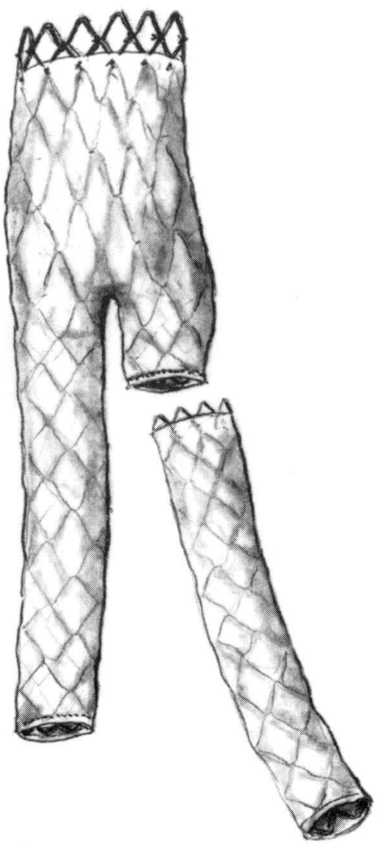

11

End-loaded contralateral limb sheath

Another major change in delivery system design between Vanguard II and Vanguard III had important implications for technique of endografting. The original Vanguard I delivery system required the contralateral limb module to be pushed up within the full length of an empty sheath inserted through the 'stump' into the aortic trunk. This was always an awkward step, made more so if the prosthesis was not kept chilled to reduce friction caused by warming nitinol stents, and was sometimes made impossible by kinking of the sheath within adverse iliac arteries. The Vanguard II delivery system provided a preloaded contralateral limb delivery system with the prosthesis already placed in the proximal part of the delivery sheath ready to deploy without a separate manoeuvre to position it.

Range of endograft component sizes

The range of standard sizes, variable in length, diameter and shape, is an important influence on patient selection and, in some cases, on cost of the procedure. This latter point is specific to the manufacturer's pricing structure to hospitals, a factor subject to market-driven forces without doubt. But, considering the emphasis evidenced in recent publications in the medical literature (Seiwert *et al.*, 1999; Sternbergh and Money, 2000; Abbott, 2000; Quinones-Baldrich *et al.*, 1999), device cost is directly acknowledged as an element influencing acceptance of this developing method of treating aortic aneurysm. If unit pricing for endografts were to prevail, as distinct from charges for each endograft component, then the importance of size range becomes more influential as a factor in overall procedural cost. The availability of Vanguard III sizes planned as of October 2000 includes proximal aortic diameter ranging from 22 up to 30 mm and iliac artery diameters from 12 mm to 16 mm – significant increase in ranges from Vanguard II.

It should be mentioned that making larger diameter sizes available might provide a subtle basis for influencing late results by allowing inclusion of patients with necks that are destined to show instability of size after short-term successful exclusion. The late diameter change of the proximal neck attachment zone has been a source of concern from the beginning of endograft treatment of abdominal aortic aneurysm and remains so today. On the other hand, especially when treating patients with unacceptable risk for conventional open surgery, the ability to include patients with larger diameter necks and larger iliac artery diameters makes endovascular methods more widely applicable and thus enhances protection from rupture risk for more patients.

The attempt to exclude aortic aneurysms from the circulation by minimally invasive, remote access methods that provide protection from life-threatening rupture risk is a valuable contribution to vascular surgery. But this is still emerging technology after the first decade of only limited investigation of the procedures. The techniques are not yet refined, and all observers and active participants in the field agree that much remains to be learned that will result in changes in both the devices and techniques for using them. A major influence in this evolution is the lack of suitable animal models or truly sophisticated *ex vivo* simulation because we are left to conduct the investigation of what works and what does not in the clinical setting. Thus an active dialogue between physicians attempting to bring increased benefit to patients and device manufacturers with a shared goal will continue to result in changes of devices and techniques for using them. This chapter has attempted to show how the interaction between clinicians and device developers influences both participants with practical clinical results.

References

Abbott WM (2000). Robert R Linton Distinguished Address. 'The Science of Arterial Prosthesis: Past Frustrations and Future Promise.' 27th Annual Meeting, New England Society for Vascular Surgery, Boston, Massachusetts, Oct. 4–6, 2000.

Beebe HG, Cronenwett JL, Katzen BT *et al.* (2001), for the Vanguard Endograft Trial Investigators. Results of an aortic endograft trial: impact of device failure beyond 12 months. *J Vasc Surg* (in press).

Greenberg R, Fairman R, Srivastava S *et al.* (2000). Endovascular grafting in patients with short proximal necks: an analysis of short-term results. *Cardiovasc Surg* **8**: 350–354.

Malina M, Brunkwall J, Lindblad B *et al.* (1999). Endovascular management of the juxtarenal aortic aneurysm: can uncovered stents safely cross the renal arteries? *Semin Vasc Surg* **12**: 182–191.

Quinones-Baldrich WJ, Garner C, Caswell D *et al.* (1999). Endovascular, transperitoneal, and retroperitoneal abdominal aortic aneurysm repair: results and costs. *J Vasc Surg* **30**: 59–67.

Seiwert AJ, Wolfe J, Whalen RC *et al.* (1999). Cost comparison of aortic aneurysm endograft exclusion versus open surgical repair. *Am J Surg* **178**: 117–120.

Sternbergh WC 3rd, Money SR (2000). Hospital cost of endovascular versus open repair of abdominal aortic aneurysms: a multicenter study. *J Vasc Surg* **31**: 237–244.

Stent-graft for abdominal aortic aneurysm: the Endologix device

Edward B Diethrich

Introduction

Worldwide experience with endoluminal devices that exclude abdominal aortic aneurysms continues to grow at a somewhat frenzied pace – although we have yet to make a definitive statement about anything more than the future importance of the technology. There is a paucity of mid- to long-term data and many unanswered questions, making it impossible to draw educated conclusions about this exciting technology. For scientists, investigators, and investors, lack of information about the performance of a new device may be extremely frustrating. Nevertheless, there is a great opportunity for exploration. While we acknowledge the imperfections of the present Endologix™ endoluminal graft for exclusion of abdominal aortic aneurysms, we believe that those involved in the future will continue with the zeal and commitment of the team that brought the device from an idea to its present state-of-the-art design.

Brief history

The Vascular Surgery Department at the Arizona Heart Institute and Arizona Heart Hospital in Phoenix, USA has been involved in endoluminal grafting for over a decade. Working within the framework of a single-centre, Investigational Device Exemption (IDE), protocols were approved by our Investigational Review Board (IRB) and the Food and Drug Administration (FDA), lending support and opportunity for clinical investigations of a variety of concepts. Disappointed by early results with Dacron grafts supported at each end by Palmaz stents, research efforts turned to polytetrafluoroethylene (PTFE)-covered devices that were either partially or fully supported by a stent. The latter appeared to provide superior clinical results, and the current prosthetic, which is fully supported, incorporates a PTFE-covered stainless steel stent. Grafts were initially constructed at our campus, but as the complexity of the delivery system increased, outside engineering expertise was required. Thus, a team of Endologix™ engineers, designers, and regulatory experts was assembled to move the project forward.

Design considerations

1

The advantages and disadvantages of current endoluminal graft configurations are being debated worldwide – a discussion that is likely to continue for a number of years. A few points about the design rationale for the Endologix graft are worthy of comment. We wanted the delivery system for the prosthesis to be as user-friendly as possible. Complex delivery systems seem only to enhance the opportunity for failure. A unibody graft configuration is appealing because it is simple and minimizes modular attachment site problems. It also allows the device to 'rest' on the bifurcation, rather than having the body of the graft floating within the aneurysm sac. Whether or not these design features will prove successful in the long-term requires further study. We have yet to answer questions about suprarenal fixation; however, evidence is accumulating in its support, and one configuration of the Endologix graft (1) incorporates it. The graft does not have hooks, barbs, or other anchoring techniques at present, but future configurations may incorporate them.

The Endologix graft is self-expanding and lends itself well to both cephalad and caudad post-deployment ballooning should the need arise. Re-crossing a limb or the body of the graft with a 'J' wire or other flexible wire is not a problem. Suprarenal cuffs and limb extenders provide additional assurance of successful aneurysm exclusion. Straight aortic tube grafts and an aortomonoiliac configuration with a contralateral iliac excluder complete the array of devices presently available. Delivery of

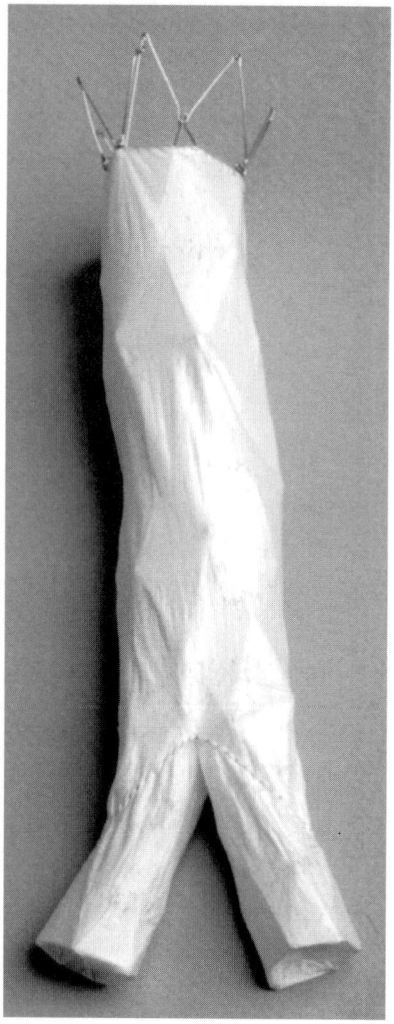

1

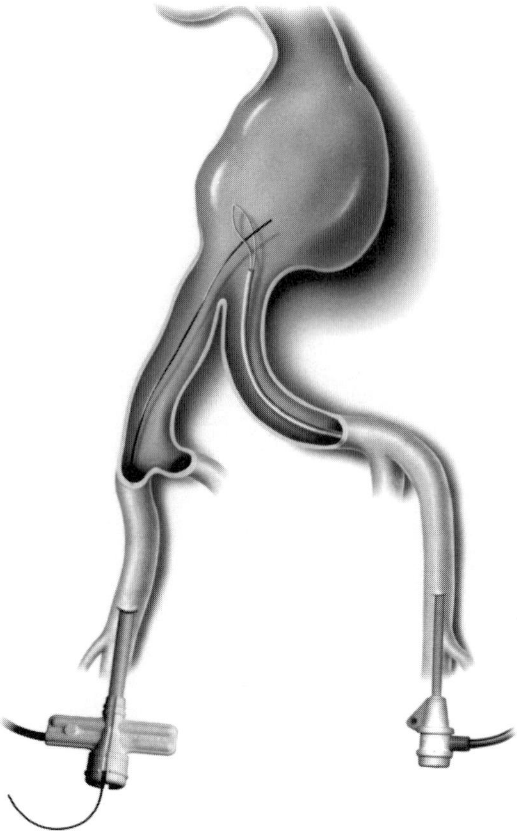

2

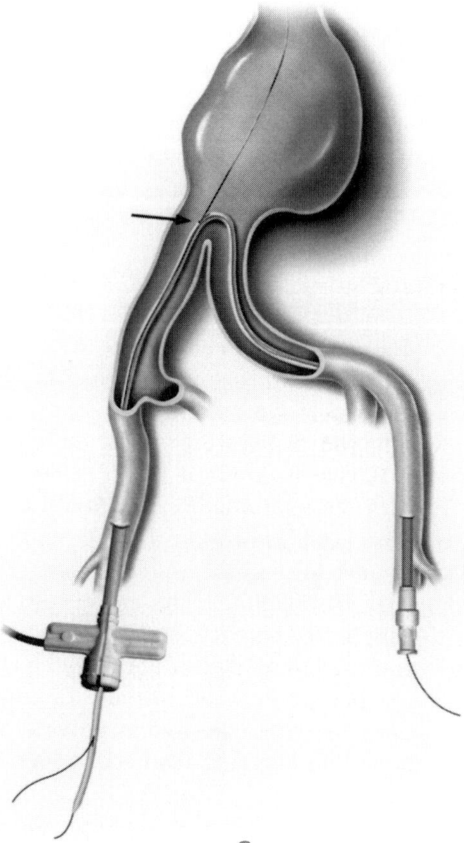

3

the unibody bifurcated system has generally been accomplished by open exposure of one common femoral artery and percutaneous deployment of the contralateral limb. A few bifurcated systems have also been deployed percutaneously, as have the aortic tube grafts. The aortomonoiliac design requires bilateral common femoral artery exposure to complete the procedure with a femorofemoral bypass graft.

The procedure

2, 3, 4, 5, 6, 7, 8

The right common femoral artery is exposed using an oblique incision just below the inguinal ligament. If the common femoral artery is small, the external iliac artery is exposed beneath the inguinal ligament and used for entry of the delivery device. A 12.5F peel-away sheath (Safe Sheath, Pressure Products Inc., Rancho Palos Verdes, CA) is inserted.

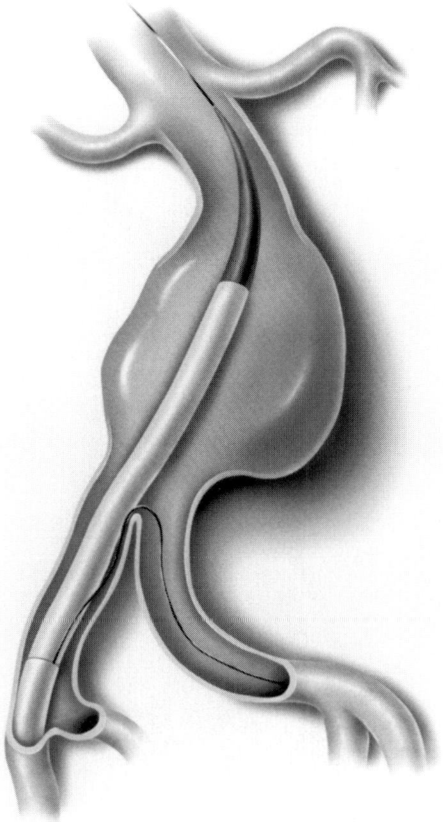

4

The left common femoral artery is cannulated with a 9F sheath. Heparin (5000 units) is injected.

Contrast is injected bilaterally to access the iliac arteries, the origin and nature of the internal iliac arteries, and the degree of iliac tortuosity are assessed.

Bilateral 0.035-inch angled Glidewires (MediTech/ Boston Scientific, Natick, MA) are passed into the lower abdominal aorta.

A Microvena snare (Microvena Corp., White Bear Lake, MN) is used to pull one of the Glidewires (does not matter which one) to the appropriate sheath where it exits (**2**).

An aortogram is performed using a pigtail catheter. The image intensifier is positioned so that the renal arteries are seen at the top of the fluoroscopic screen, and the crossover wire is seen below them. A needle is placed transversely on the skin to identify the level of the renal arteries (optional). Once the image is obtained, the image intensifier is not moved, thereby eliminating the problem of parallax.

A crossover catheter is passed from the left (contralateral) to the right (ipsilateral) side (**3**). The catheter is positioned on the fluoroscopic screen so that the radiopaque beads (arrow) are located at about the 11 o'clock position. This ensures that the stiff wire (Nitinol Guidewire, Microvena Corp.), over which the prosthesis will be delivered, can pass into the suprarenal position through the hole in the crossover catheter marked by the beads.

The Endologix device is placed on the table and prepared for delivery.

The stiff delivery wire is passed through the device, and the contralateral pullwire is loaded into the crossover catheter and pulled through until it appears on the opposite side.

The crossover catheter is removed while the crossover wire is firmly held at its junction on the delivery sheet; this prevents premature disconnection of the wire and contralateral limb.

The prosthesis is advanced to the common femoral artery sheath (**4**). The sheath is withdrawn, and the common femoral artery is squeezed between the thumb and index finger to prevent bleeding while the peel-away sheath is removed.

The prosthesis is advanced into the common femoral artery as the contralateral pullwire is pulled gently.

In order to ensure proper alignment from the contralateral sheath and avoid wire twist, the orientation is always pullwire-medial and guidewire-lateral at the groin level. Additionally, the irrigation port on the delivery sheath should always point towards the contralateral side.

The prosthesis is delivered under fluoroscopic control *above* the aortic bifurcation.

The contralateral pullwire is withdrawn into the left groin in order to remove excess 'slack.'

The contralateral limb (**5a, b**) is freed by retracting its retaining sheath while the contralateral pullwire is gently pulled from the groin.

The main body of the prosthesis is re-sheathed (**5c**). The cephalad end of graft is lowered and positioned at the renal artery level (**5d**).

The body of the graft is deployed up to the last cephalad stent (**6**). This deployment is caudad to cephalad. Until the body is completely deployed by releasing the most cephalad stent, the graft can be moved in relation to the renal arteries.

The prosthesis is held in position (**7a**) as the contralateral pullwire is pulled to release the contralateral limb, and (**7b**) the last stent is released to complete the deployment of the main body.

The pusher rod is further advanced until it encapsulates the nose cone.

The nose cone is withdrawn through the body of the graft down to the ipsilateral limb still covered by the sheath (**8a**).

The ipsilateral limb is deployed (**8b**), and the nose cone is withdrawn into the sheath; the entire assembly is removed (**8c**).

A 9F sheath is inserted into the right common femoral artery, and a control angiogram is obtained.

Bilateral femoral sheath angiograms are performed to confirm the absence of a distal endoleak.

The right common femoral artery is repaired. The incision is closed, and the patient is returned to the recovery unit; the left common femoral artery sheath is removed when the activated coagulation time returns to normal range.

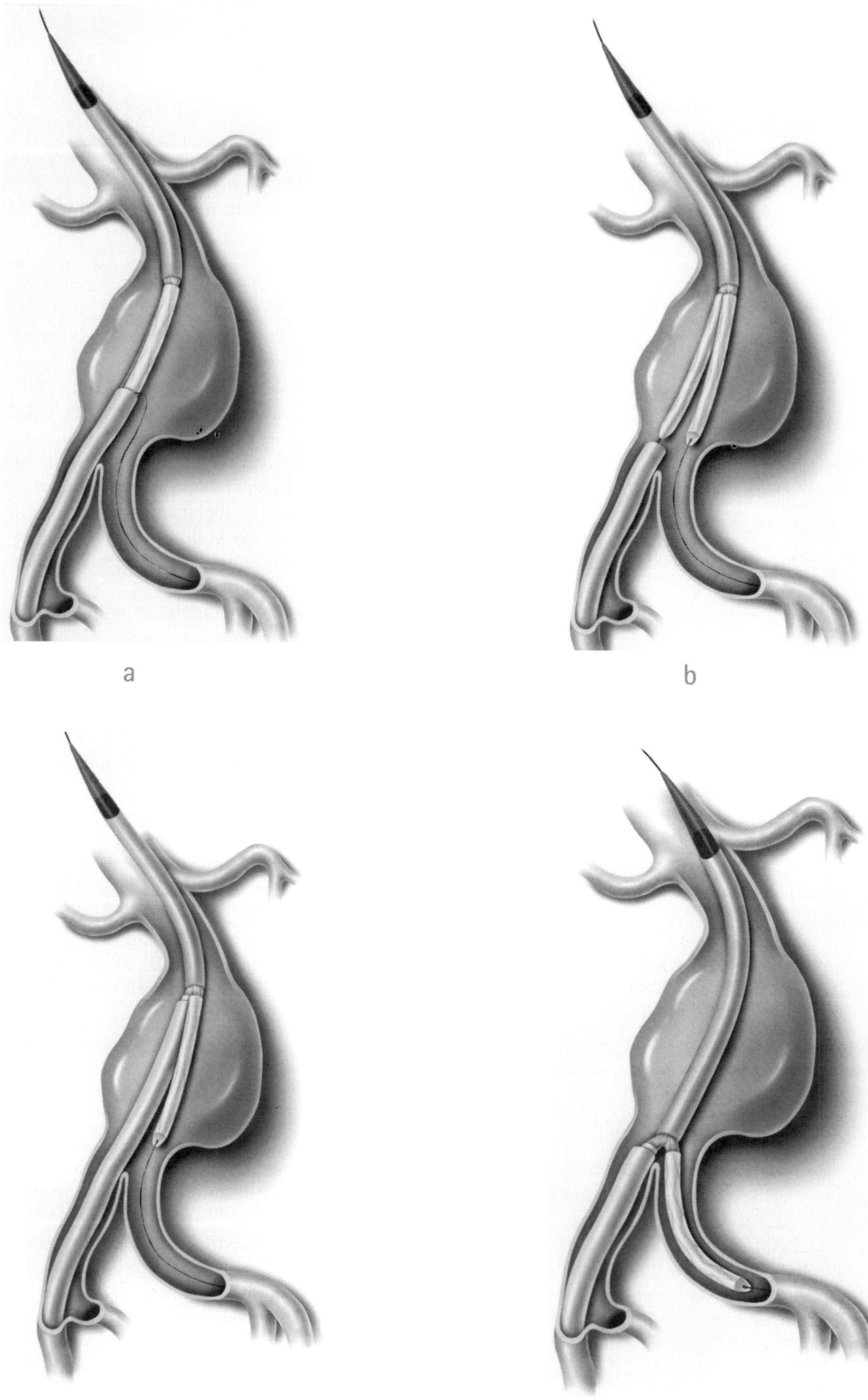

a b c d

5

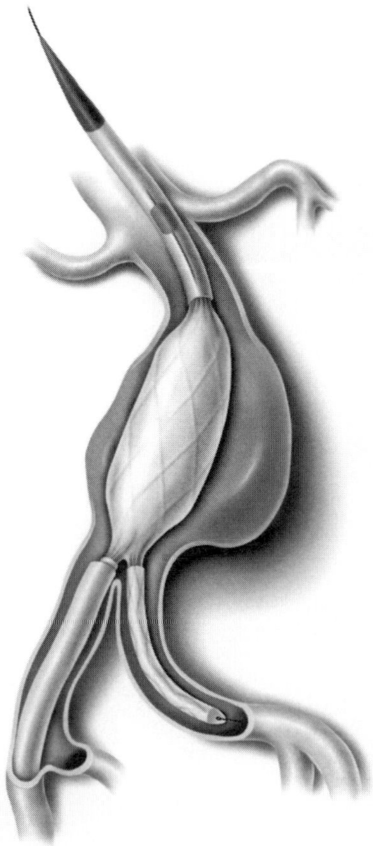

6

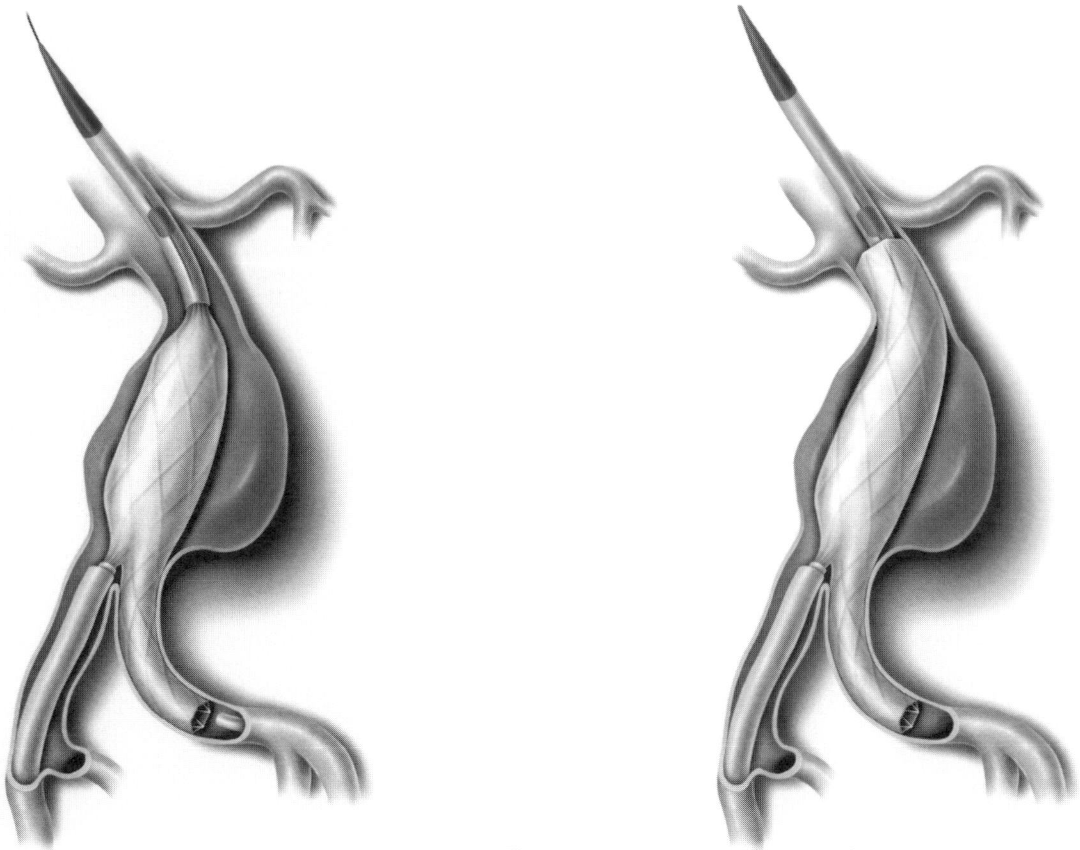

a 7 b

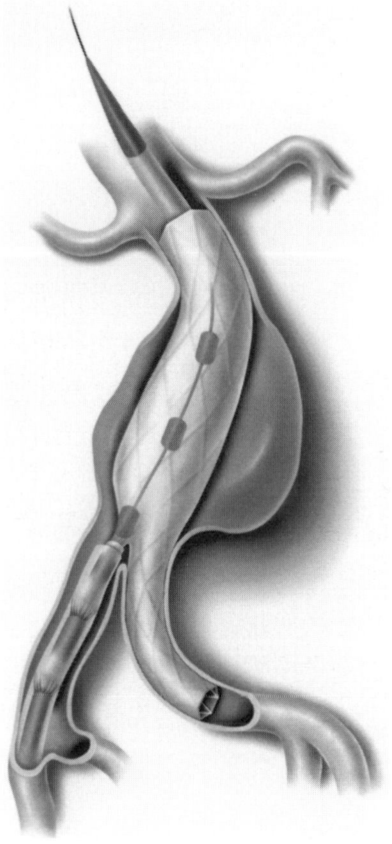

a

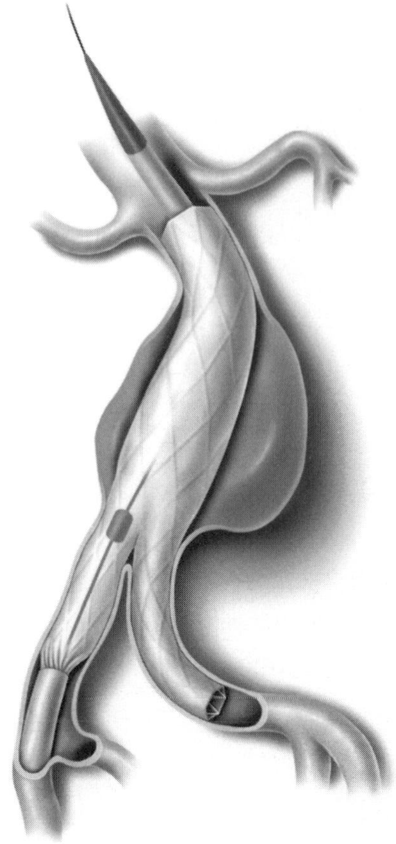

b

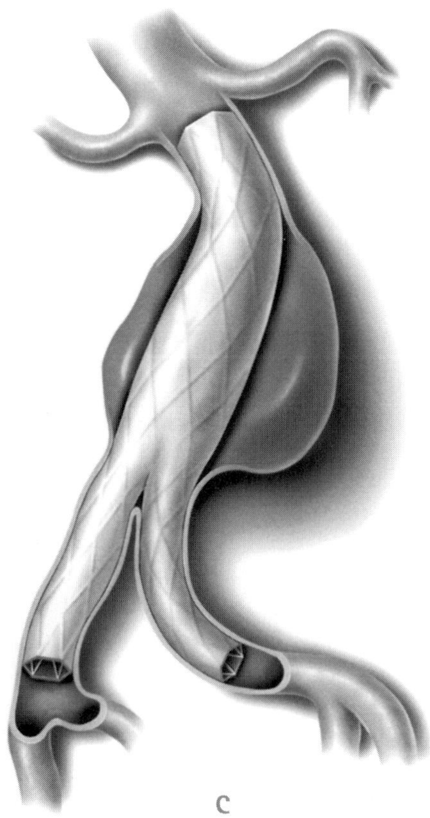

c

8

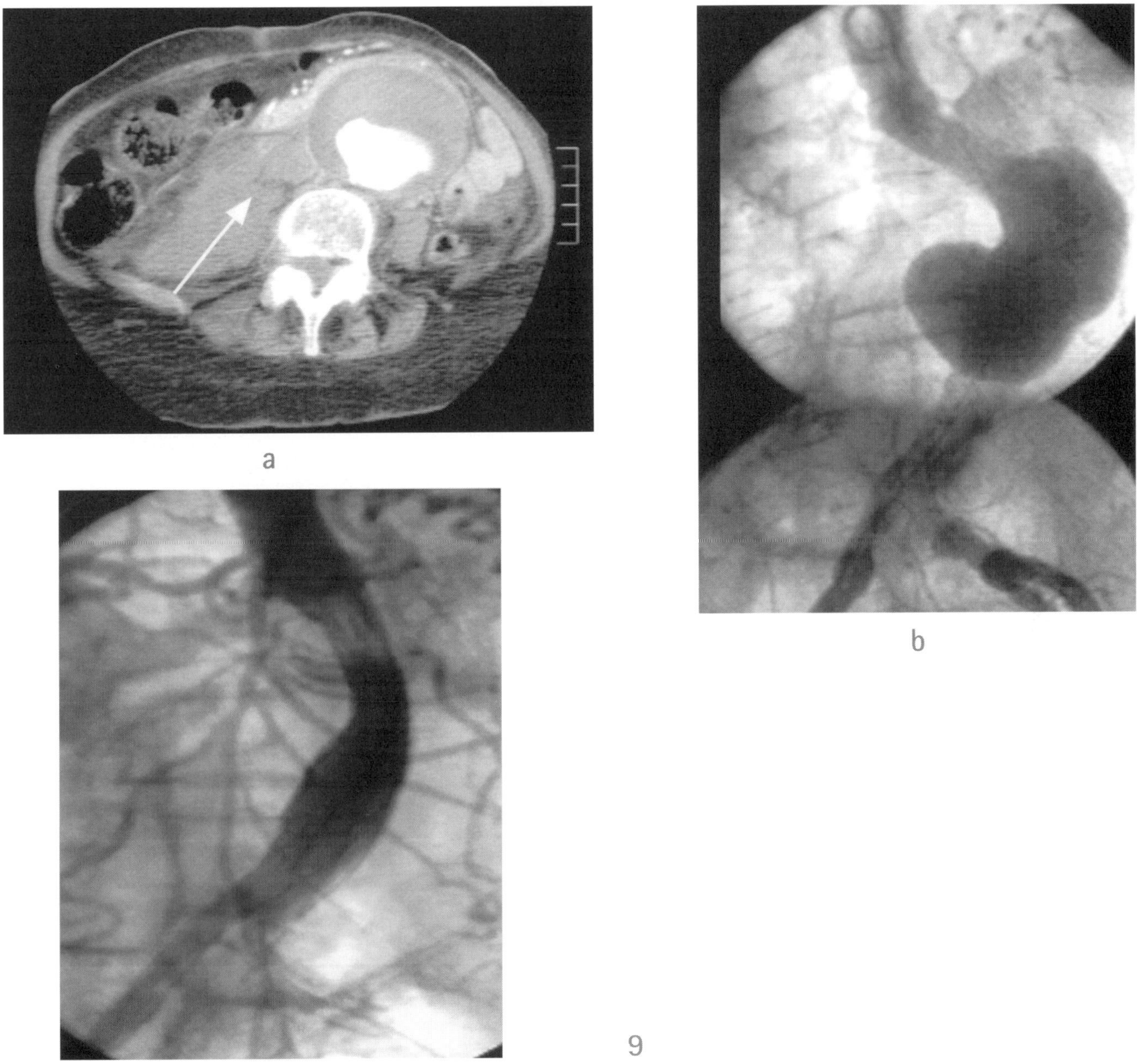

a

b

c

9

Discussion of early results

The Endologix graft has been used in approximately 500 patients worldwide. The United States Phase II FDA trials are under way after a 100% success rate in the Phase I study. Technical success has been achieved in 98% of the cases in the Phase II trials. The endoleak rate at the 30-day mark is approximately 2%. There have been no deaths related to the device itself.

Clearly, the investigative trials of the device are in the early stages, however, the results to date have been satisfactory. A recent case in our institution, where we have a separate investigator IDE that extends our indications for treatment with the device, is interesting to note. A patient arrived at our hospital by air ambulance 6 hours after an abdominal aortic aneurysm rupture with a massive retroperitoneal haemorrhage (**9a**) (arrow). The angiogram demonstrated an 8-cm infrarenal aneurysm (**9b**). The patient was successfully treated by a percutaneous deployment of the bifurcated graft (**9c**) just 35 minutes after arriving in the endovascular suite and made a complete recovery.

This case illustrates the simplicity and flexibility of Endologix graft and deployment system. Further experience should lead to added refinements and improvements. As with all of the current endoluminal grafts, long-term data will assist us in determining the proper indications for these devices.

Exclusion of abdominal aortic aneurysm utilizing the Gore Excluder bifurcated endoprosthesis

Barry T Katzen

Introduction

Endovascular repair of abdominal aortic aneurysms has become a viable alternative in many patients, provided the infrarenal anatomy is suitable. Some patients have anatomy that may not be suitable for treatment with endografts due to severe tortuousity, calcification or stenoses of the iliac arteries. Some devices lack longitudinal support limiting tractability of the device through difficult pelvic access. The ideal endograft would be uncomplicated to use, accommodate difficult iliac anatomy, be impermeable to blood, and require a minimal of adjunctive or subsequent procedures. All of this should be associated with an initial technical and long-term success rate.

The Gore Excluder™ bifurcated endoprosthesis is a device that allows for exclusion of infrarenal abdominal aortic aneurysm using an endovascular modular system. It consists of a trunk-ipsilateral leg endoprosthesis, and a contralateral leg endoprosthesis, and may be complimented to additional components, including distal and proximal extensions. It currently can be used in patients who have proximal neck lengths of greater than or equal to 15 mm and proximal neck diameters of 18–26 mm. Common iliac artery diameter sizes range from 8 mm to 14 mm, with extensions available to cross the hypogastric artery into the external iliac artery. As with all endovascular therapy, careful preoperative assessment, using spiral computed tomography examination with two-dimensional and three-dimensional reconstruction, as well as preoperative marker catheter angiographic (anteroposterior and lateral) assessment is critical to ensuring high initial technical success rates.

Device description

1

The Gore Excluder device is unique among endografts in that it is made of expanded polytetrafluoroethylene (ePTFE) tubing with an external nitinol supporting stent structure (exoskeleton) (1). The exoskeleton is made of thermosensitive nitinol, which provides radial strength to prevent kinking, and also assists in fixation to the arterial wall. At the craniad end of the trunk-ipsilateral leg component, there are seven pairs of anchors to improve fixation to the infrarenal aortic neck. The excess skeleton sinusoidal pattern is designed to accommodate longitudinal shortening in a large degree of tortuousity. The ePTFE graft materials are bonded to the nitinol with PTFE–FEP film-tape so that no sutures or suture holds are present in the graft material that lines the endoluminal surface. Unique ePTFE technology permits the manufacturer of the endoprosthesis the tapered configurations that allow the design of a modular system in which components are universally compatible, thus expanding the available configurational options. This is in contrast to standard aortografts which come with equal iliac diameters, roughly one half of the aortografts. Tapered grafts also allow long and wide diameter junctions between components that may reduce late dislocation and improve limb patency.

2a, b

A gold wire ring is embedded into the ePTFE layers of the trunk component, marking the contralateral leg opening. This is quite visual under fluoroscopy, and simplifies catheterization of the contralateral short limb. The flow splitter is located approximately 4 cm from the proximal end of the endoprosthesis (**2a**). It is designed to direct flow towards the continuous ipsilateral leg and the contralateral leg opening. Three short radiopaque marker bands are attached to the stent graft at the aortic end, and one radiopaque marker band is attached at the iliac end. To facilitate proper orientation of the trunk component in the aorta, one long marker band is placed in the contralateral side, and one short marker band is placed on the ipsilateral side at the level of the flow splitter (**2b**).

The entire device is constrained in a unique sleeve,

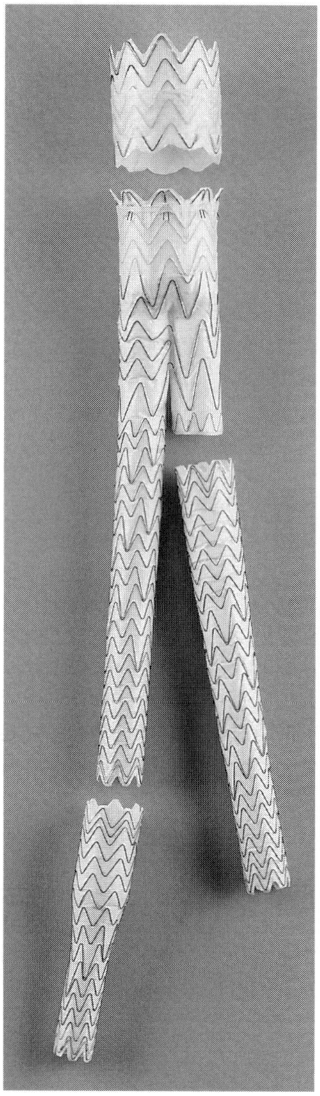

1

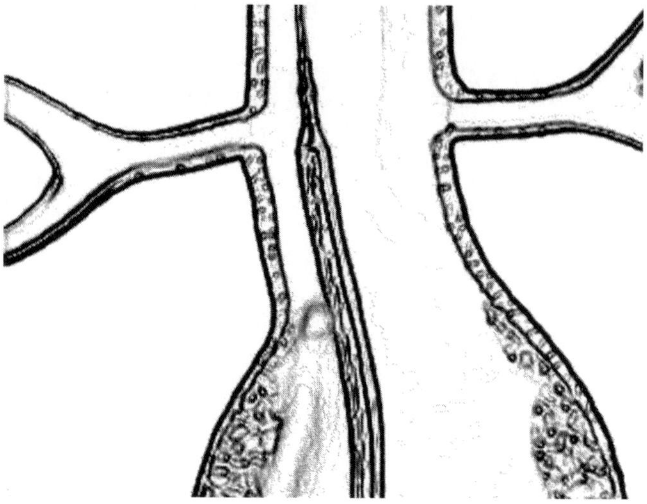

2a

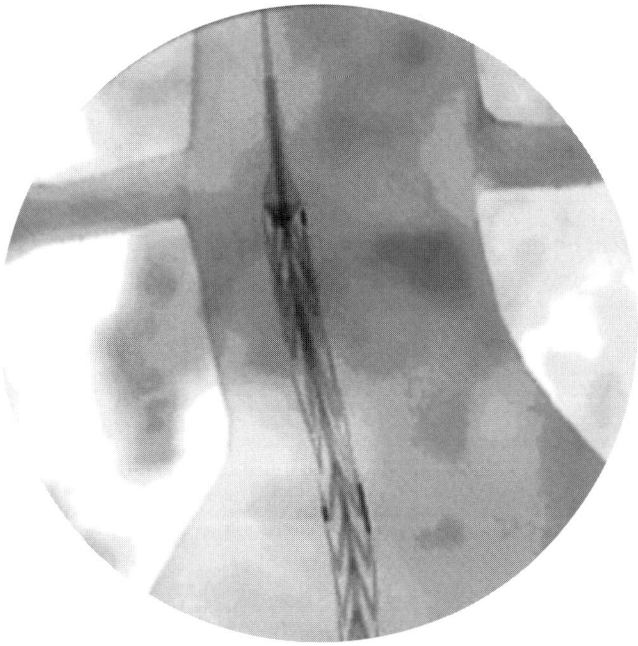

2b

which is made of ePTFE and FEP films. The sleeve is attached to the endoprosthesis with ePTFE fibre material. The sleeve is closed around the endoprosthesis and sewn closed using ePTFE fibre material. Following deployment, the sleeve remains in place between the endoprosthesis and the vessel wall.

3

To facilitate introduction of the trunk-ipsilateral delivery system, a 30-cm 18f Teflon sheath is used, and to deploy the contralateral limb a 12f, 30-cm sheath is used (3).

4a–f

Deployment of the Excluder endograft may be accomplished through a unilateral arteriotomy, and either percutaneous or surgical exposure of the contralateral common femoral artery. Once access to the arterial system has been obtained a super-stiff guidewire is ultimately passed into the lower thoracic aorta (**4a**) and used to guide an 18F 30 cm Teflon sheath (Cook, Inc., Bloomington, Indiana). This sheath protects the endoprosthesis during delivery, and facilitates delivery utilizing standard angiographic techniques. Once the sheath has been positioned, the delivery device is inserted

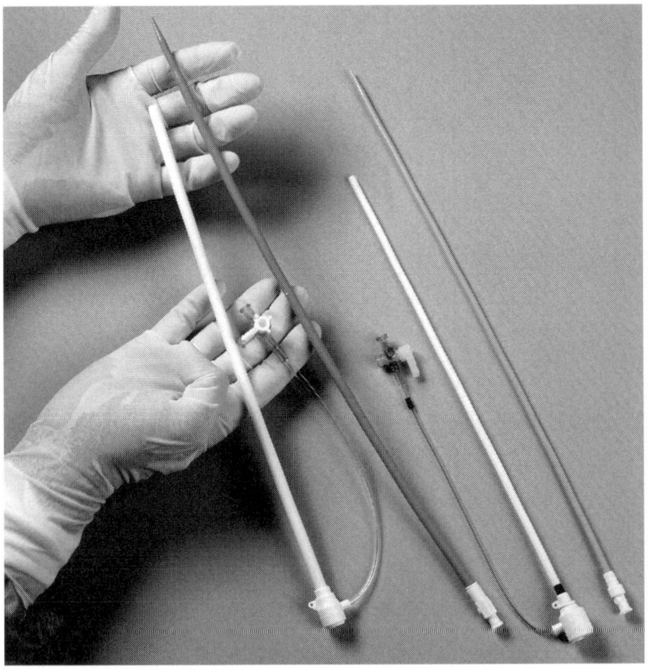

3

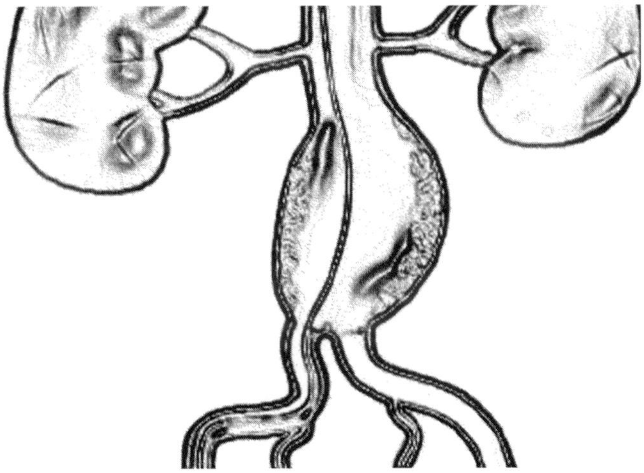

4a

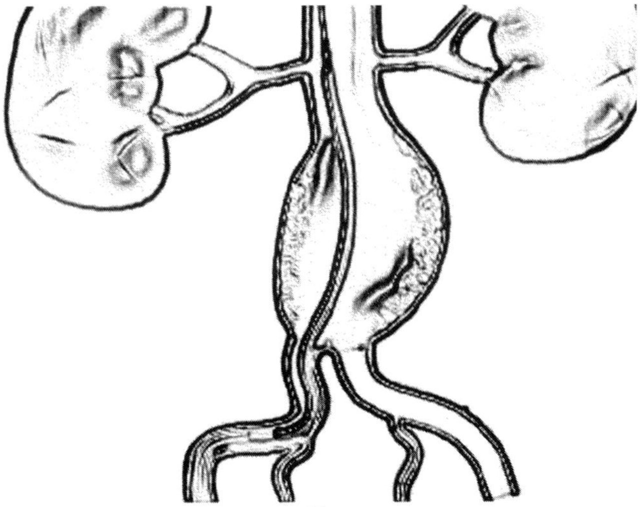

4b

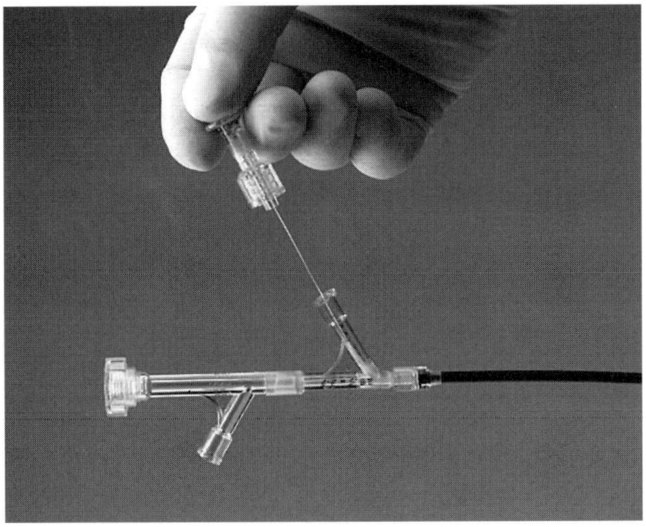

4c

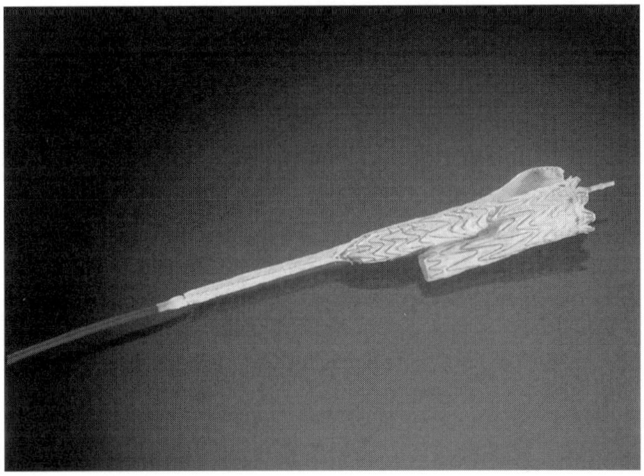

4d

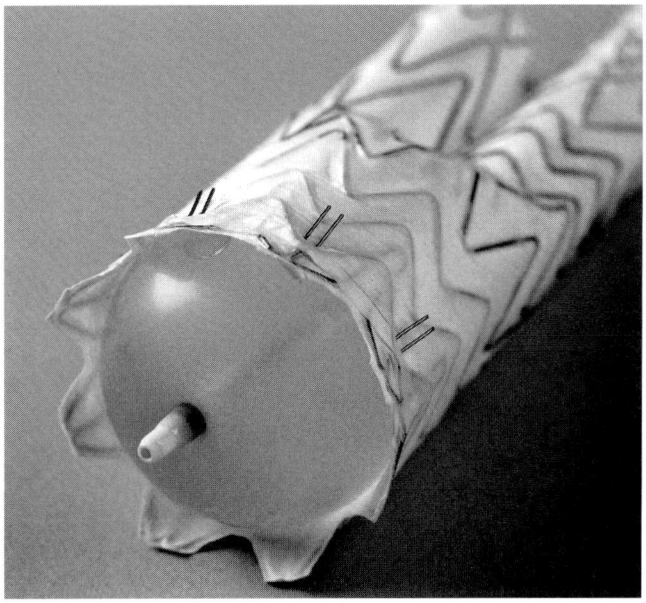

4e

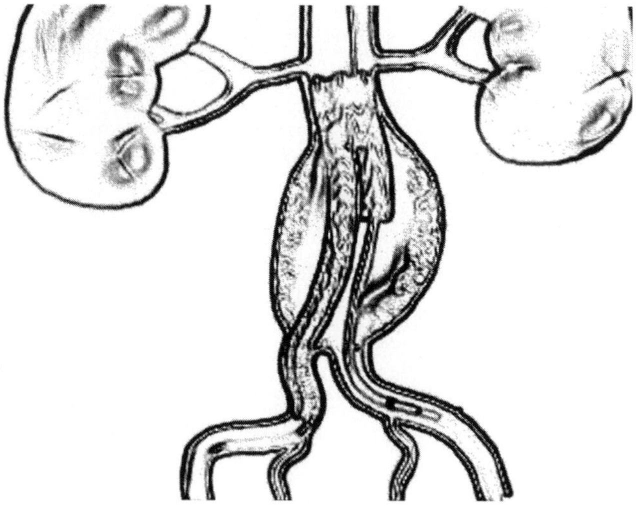

4f

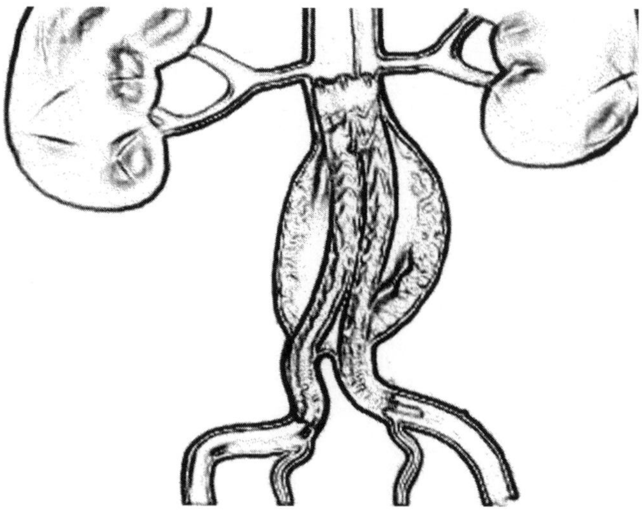

4g

through the sheath, and positioned in the proximal aortic neck. Injection of contrast may be performed using a diagnostic catheter placed on the contralateral approach.

When appropriately positioned, the introducer sheath is then withdrawn to a level indicated by a predetermined white marker on the catheter shaft (**4b**). Under magnification fluoroscopy, the trunk delivery catheter can be rotated to maximize separation between the long (contralateral) and short (ipsilateral) radio-opaque markers. The long markers are oriented towards the contralateral side. The trunk delivery catheter is then stabilized at the introducer sheath. The deployment knob on the proximal end of the catheter (**4c**) is then released by counterclockwise rotation, and the deployment is accomplished by pulling the knob straight out from the catheter side arm. Deployment is relatively sudden and complete, and reposition of the endoprosthesis should not be attempted (**4d**). No significant migration or movement of the device has been noted during deployment. Once deployment is complete, the delivery catheter is then withdrawn under fluoroscopic control.

An aortic balloon is then advanced until it is approximately 1 cm inferior to the proximal end of the prosthesis (**4e**). The balloon is inflated to fully contour the aortic end of the prosthesis. Appropriate balloons may also be used to inflate and seat the iliac limbs of the endoprosthesis. Once the body and ipsilateral limb have been deployed, the contralateral limb is easily catheterized using standard angiographic techniques. The radio-opaque ring is easily identified under fluoroscopy, and used as a target for catheterization. Shaped catheters, such as 'Cobra' and 'Sidewinder', are valuable depending on specific aneurysm shape and tortuousity in the iliac arteries.

Once the contralateral limb is catheterized (**4f**) appropriate exchanges are made for super-stiff guidewire, and a 12F × 30 cm introducer sheath is then passed through the contralateral limb. This allows for stabilization and protects the contralateral sheath during subsequent limb placement. Once the sheath has been placed, the contralateral leg is positioned, and the introducer sheath moves to the white marker on the delivery catheter. No rotation of the limb should be attempted.

The radio-opaque marker, which is at the proximal end of the contralateral leg prosthesis, should be aligned with the radio-opaque marker on the trunk of the implant, allowing maximum overlap at the contralateral short limb.

Once positioning is idealized, the deployment knob is loosened, and the contralateral limb is deployed by using steady continuous pull of the deployment knob to release the prosthesis (**4g**). Fluoroscopic guidance is used to withdraw the delivery catheter. A 14-mm percutaneous transluminal angioplasty balloon catheter, or other size balloon catheter is used to seat the proximal end of the contralateral limb within the trunk, and also to iron out the distal attachments.

Once the procedure has been completed, angiography is performed utilizing a power injector and delayed imaging is obtained to confirm exclusion of the aneurysm, as well as detection of any type of endoleaks. Arterial access sites are closed according to standard practice.

Summary

The bifurcated Excluder endoprosthesis has been demonstrated to successfully exclude infrarenal aortic aneurysms. Although late US multicentre trials are still under way, initial experience has confirmed the advantages of reduced profile, high flexibility and ease of deployment to be of significant benefit in treating patients with abdominal aortic aneurysms.

References

Abn SS, Rutherford RB, Johnston KW *et al.* (1997). Reporting standards for infrarenal endovascular abdominal aortic aneurysm repair. *J Vasc Surg* **25**: 405–410.

Blum U, Voshage G, Lammer J *et al.* (1997). Endoluminal stent grafts for infrarenal abdominal aortic aneurysms. *New Engl J Med* **336**: 13–20.

Brewster DC, Geller SC, Kaufman JA *et al.* (1998). Initial experience with endovascular aneurysm repair: comparison of early results with outcome of conventional open repair. *J Vasc Surg* **27**: 992–1005.

Davidian MM, Benenati JF, Powell A (2000). Endovascular grafts for the treatment of abdominal aortic aneurysms development of stent grafts, design of devices and technical results. In *Stent-Grafts Current Clinical Practice.* Dolmatch BI, Blum U eds. New York: Thieme. pp. 55–68.

Food and Drug Administration (1999). National Institutes of Health. Circulatory system devices panel meeting: 23 June 1999; Gaithersburg, Maryland.

Matsumura JS, Katzen BT, Hollier LH, Dake MD (2001). Update on the bifurcated EXCLUDER endoprosthesis: phase I results. *J Vasc Surg* (in press).

May J, White GH, Yu W *et al.* (1998). Concurrent comparison of endoluminal versus open repair in the treatment of abdominal aortic aneurysms: analysis of 303 patient by life table method. *J Vasc Surg* **27**: 213–221.

Zarins CK, White RA, Schwarten D *et al.* (1999). AneuRx stent graft versus open surgical repair of abdominal aortic aneurysms: multi-center prospective clinical trial. *J Vasc Surg* **29**: 292–308.

LifePath Abdominal Aortic Aneurysm Graft System: the only balloon-expandable type

Geoffrey H White
Weiyun Yu, James May

Introduction

The Edwards LifePath Abdominal Aortic Aneurysm Graft System is currently the only commerially manufactured endovascular graft device which uses balloon expansion of its components as the primary mode of device deployment. The basic graft is a modular three-piece design which is constructed within the aorta by overlap technique of the two iliac limb grafts within the legs of the bifurcated trunk component. The graft components are compressed over balloon catheters which are integral with the delivery catheter. The graft is preloaded into a loader which interlocks with the delivery sheath during the deployment procedure.

Balloon-expansion conveys the advantages of precise, controlled positioning of the graft during deployment, firm attachment to the aortic wall and full expansion of the attachment components.

Device development

The graft system is based on an endoluminal technique reported by White and colleagues in 1994. They described a balloon-expandable prosthesis custom-made from a commercially available woven Dacron graft material with metallic wireform graft attachment devices incorporated into the fabric of the graft and extending throughout its length. The prosthesis had been tested in the laboratory and extensively trialled in the clinical situation by the group. In 1996 the vascular division of Baxter Healthcare Corporation (now Edwards Lifesciences) commenced the task of turning the 'home-made' product, which had been limited in its use to the originators, into a commercially available device which could be used by others. A series of benchtop studies, animal implants and clinical feasibility studies were undertaken before commencement of phase I and phase II comparative clinical trials.

Device design

The LifePath Abdominal Aortic Aneurysm device design features polyester prosthetic fabric, supported by a series of intermittent, balloon-expandable, curvilinear wireforms which are interwoven with the graft material. The bifurcated graft consists of three individual units: a bifurcated graft trunk and two iliac limb grafts. There are also two introducer sheaths: a 19F sheath which is used for passage of the bifurcated graft trunk, and a 16F sheath for introduction of the iliac limb.

The graft delivery systems contain the prosthetic device mounted on a deployment balloon and housed within a loader. When the sheath has been positioned within the aorta, the loader interlocks with the introduced sheath unit, facilitating transfer of the device into the sheath for deployment into the aorta by passage through the length of the sheath. The delivery system is supported by an integrated pusher catheter component which serves to hold the graft in its position on the balloon, and support the positioning of the system during deployment. Additional self-expanding wireforms on the legs of the trunk graft open spontaneously when the graft is exposed by retraction of the delivery sheath.

Graft material

The fabric of the graft is woven polyethylene terepthalate (PET), with standard wall-thickness (0.3 mm). The material is identical to off-the-shelf woven PET grafts used in conventional open repair. Porosity of the fabric is sufficient to allow healing, but does not lead to porosity blush on completion angiography.

Wireform (stent) material

The wireform support is composed of annealed Elgiloy® wire, which is a corrosion-resistant alloy that has excellent fatigue-resistant characteristics. The material has an extensive clinical history as a long-term implantable material, including many years use in heart valves. Annealing, or tempering, of the Elgiloy wireform results in increased ductility, which is necessary to allow balloon-expansion of the device. The wireforms are separate from each other to add flexibility, and are woven into the graft material in a curvilinear configuration, running in series around the graft without attachment sutures. These segments are woven into the graft wall such that alternate crests of each wire are outside the graft, and the remainder of the wire material is inside the graft. The free ends of each segment are mechanically connected with a crimped Elgiloy splice to create the wireform.

Device deployment

1

With the patient appropriately anaesthetized and lying supine, the operative fields are prepared and bilateral groin incisions are performed to expose the common femoral arteries. The patient is then anticoagulated with 5000 units of intravenous heparin. The common femoral artery on the side of the widest diameter and least tortuous iliac arteries is usually chosen for ipsilateral access with the larger deployment sheath. The shape of the abdominal aortic aneurysm and the perceived risk of dislodging mural thrombus are other factors which influence the side chosen for access. An 8Fr sheath is inserted into the ipsilateral common femoral artery using the Seldinger needle technique. A guidewire and angiographic catheter are advanced to the level of the renal arteries in the abdominal aorta. An aortogram is then performed. An Amplatz 0.035 inch super-stiff guidewire is exchanged and the angiographic catheter and the 8Fr introducer sheath are removed.

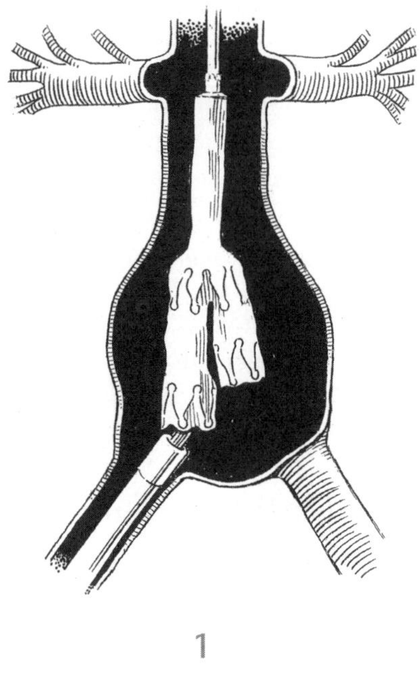

1

2

A 19Fr main introducer sheath assembly is inserted over the guidewire from the ipsilateral side and the tip of the introducer sheath is advanced until it is above the proximal neck of the aneurysm and passes renal artery level on fluoroscopy. The introducer is removed from the assembly while leaving the introducer sheath and guidewire *in situ*. A slow-rate pressurized heparinized saline infusion is commenced via the introducer sheath side port. The bifurcated main graft delivery assembly is then connected to the sheath head over the guidewire using the loader locknut. The graft is delivered to the desired deployment position by advancing the pusher. The pusher may be rotated to allow for the correct orientation of the bifurcated graft (2). Once the graft has reached the planned level of deployment, the main introducer sheath is retracted until the bifurcated graft main trunk is fully exposed to the circulation. Self-expanding wireforms on the trunk limbs result in these opening at this stage, allowing adjustments to the orientation of the device to be made prior to deployment of the proximal attachment wireforms.

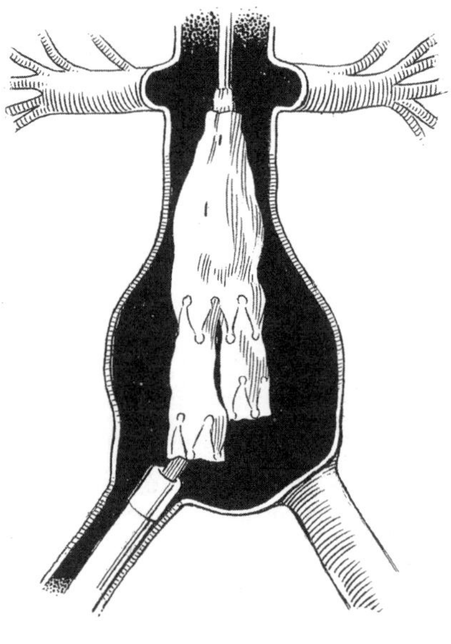

2

3

Final adjustments are made to the bifurcated graft position before deployment of the graft. The graft is deployed by inflating the main balloon to maximum inflation (2 atm) for 30 seconds (may be repeated). The balloon is then deflated and the balloon catheter is removed through the introducer sheath while leaving the sheath and guidewire *in situ*. The 19Fr introducer is reinserted into the main introducer sheath that was left in the ipsilateral limb. The entire assembly is advanced into the ipsilateral limb until the tip of the Introducer Sheath reaches above the main graft septum. The Introducer is again removed.

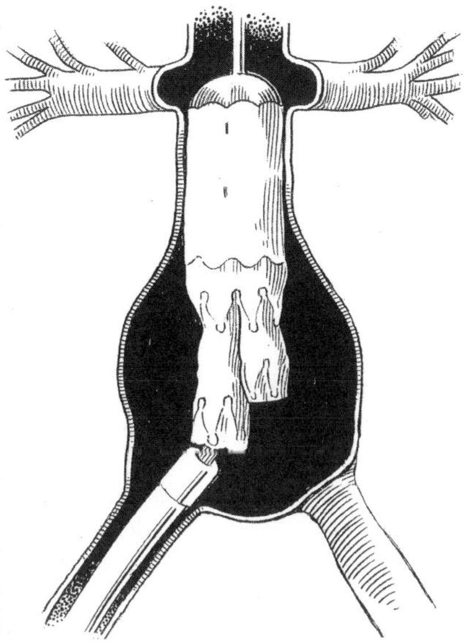

3

4

The next steps involve controlled overlap of the iliac graft limbs into the legs of the trunk segment. The sequence for deployment of the limbs is variable, and may involve deployment of either the ipsilateral or contralateral limb first. After initial access, exchange is made for a 0.035 inch Amplatz super-stiff guidewire through the contralateral access vessels and contralateral limb of the bifurcated main trunk graft to allow introduction of the contralateral iliac extension catheter. One method to obtain contralateral access is to use the Edwards directional catheter (optional procedure explained below). Other methods may include advancing a guidewire through the contralateral access vessels and through the contralateral limb of the bifurcated graft, or directing a glidewire (260 cm) from the left brachial approach.

Each iliac limb graft is positioned so that there is a minimum of 2 cm overlap within the corresponding limb of the main graft. The proximal aspect of the iliac graft is usually positioned at the septum marker of the trunk segment (provides for at least 2 cm overlap) The distal iliac graft will ideally overlap the non-aneurysmal iliac artery attachment zone by at least 1.5 cm. Once the graft has reached the planned level of deployment, its introducer sheath is retracted until the Lifepath abdominal aortic aneurysm iliac graft is fully exposed to the circulation. The graft is then deployed by inflating the iliac extension balloon.

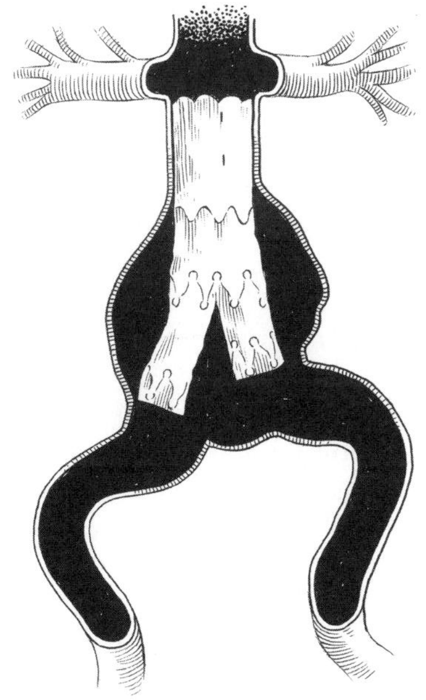

4

5

The ipsilateral and contralateral iliac grafts may be deployed simultaneously ('kissing' balloon technique). After graft implantation, the iliac balloons are removed and a completion angiogram is then performed from either sheath using an angiographic catheter. Then both sheaths are removed.

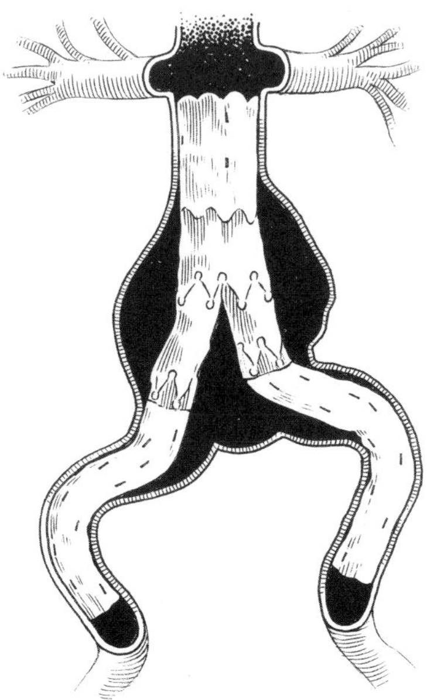

5

Deflecting catheter technique for contralateral limb cannulation

If the method using the Edwards directional catheter is selected, the Edwards directional catheter is inserted over the ipsilateral guidewire through the haemostatic valve of the main introducer sheath. The deflecting tip marker of the directional catheter is advanced 2–3 cm above the bifurcated graft septum, uncovered and the tip is manually deflected over the septum. A second guidewire (0.025–0.035 inch Terumo glidewire) is inserted into the guidewire port within the directional catheter. This wire is advanced over the graft septum to cannulate the contralateral limb of the bifurcated graft and continue into the contralateral common iliac artery until it reaches the femoral artery. The guidewire is then retrieved by snare loop or by a small transverse arteriotomy of the contralateral common femoral artery. A 0.035 inch super-stiff or Amplatz extra-stiff guidewire is then exchanged for the glidewire using an exchange catheter (e.g. contralateral exchange catheter, angiographic catheter).

After successful contralateral stump access procedure, the deflecting tip is retracted and and covered by advancing the directional catheter sheath fitting forward. Then the directional catheter is withdrawn from the 19Fr main introducer sheath.

Special features of the lifepath abdominal aortic aneurysm graft

Features specific to this device are:

1. Balloon deployed graft.
   Advantages: Allows precise controlled delivery and positioning, with adjustments during balloon expansion. Relative rigidity of the wireforms allows complete expansion of the attachment region. No separate balloon manoeuvres required to expand or dilate the deployed graft.
   Disadvantages: Potential for balloon damage to the aortic neck zone; therefore more precise sizing is required with less oversizing than self-expanding grafts.
2. Modularity.
   Advantages: A variety of graft lengths, diameters and graft limb geometries (tapered or reverse-tapered) are available for customized selection to individual patient anatomy. Avoids graft twist or kink.
   Disadvantages: Potential for late component separation (endoleak).
3. Standard thickness woven polyester graft matrix material.
   Advantages: Proven material durability and longevity, without fabric tear or holes as seen with thin-walled materials.
   Disadvantages: Thicker material increases delivery system profile.
4. Segmental, hooped, curvilinear Elgiloy wireforms.
   Advantages: Full-length graft support; device flexibility; non-kink due to wireform spacing interval.
   Disadvantages: Device bulk due to use of strong wires.
5. Wireforms woven into the graft matrix.
   Advantages: Eliminates problems with suture breakage and wireform detachment
   Disadvantages: Complexity and cost of device manufacture.
6. Separate sheath system.
   Advantages: Top of the line, flexible, atraumatic, hydrophilic sheath system. Sheath access may be assured before device chosenor opened.
   Disadvantages: Non preloaded device slightly adds to complexity of deployment procedure.
7. Over the wire, deflecting-tip catheter guidewire access system.
   Advantages: Allows simplified antegrade access to the contralateral stump without requiring removal of the ipsilateral primary guidewire.
   Disadvantages: Snare catheter required in soem cases, to retrieve guidewire down into the iliac artery.

References

Chafour X, White G H, Yu W *et al.* (2001). Evaluation of the risks of using an oversized balloon catheter in the human infrarenal abdominal aorta. *Eur J Vasc Endovasc Surg* (in press).

White G H, Yu W, May J (1994). A new non-stented balloon expandable graft for straight or bifurcated endoluminal bypass. *J Endovasc Surg* **1**: 16–24.

White G H, Yu W, May J (1997). Three-year experience with the White–Yu endovascular GAD graft for transluminal repair of aortic and iliac aneurysms. *J Endovasc Surg* **4**: 124–136.

Yu W, White G H, May J, Stephen M S (1996). Endoluminal repair of abdominal aortic aneurysms using the trombone technique. *Asian J Surg* **19**: 37–40.

Endovascular techniques with the Talent stent-graft for exclusion of abdominal aortic aneurysms

Frank J Criado,
Snehal C Patel, Vipin Bansal

Introduction

The Talent device is a self-expanding, modular stent-graft system composed of serpentine-shaped nitinol stents inlaid in woven polyester fabric (Criado *et al.*, 1999). The stents are spaced along a full-length nitinol spine that provides longitudinal support to aid transluminal delivery and deployment. The delivery system is composed of a coaxial sheath with an internal pusher rod and a compliant balloon that is sequentially inflated to maximize apposition of the graft to the vessel wall attachment zones and to insure full expansion of the device along its length. Basic components of the Talent system are a bifurcated main section and a contralateral iliac limb. The Free-Flo configuration contains a 15-mm long uncovered stent at the proximal end to allow transrenal fixation. Additional modular components include aortic cuffs and iliac extensions. The manufacturer (Medtronic World Medical) offers customization (Criado *et al.*, 2000) in a variety of configurations, lengths and diameters. Range of diameter is 16–36 mm for the aortic section and 8–22 mm for the iliac limbs. A 22F delivery sheath is used in the majority of procedures performed for endovascular exclusion of abdominal aortic aneurysms.

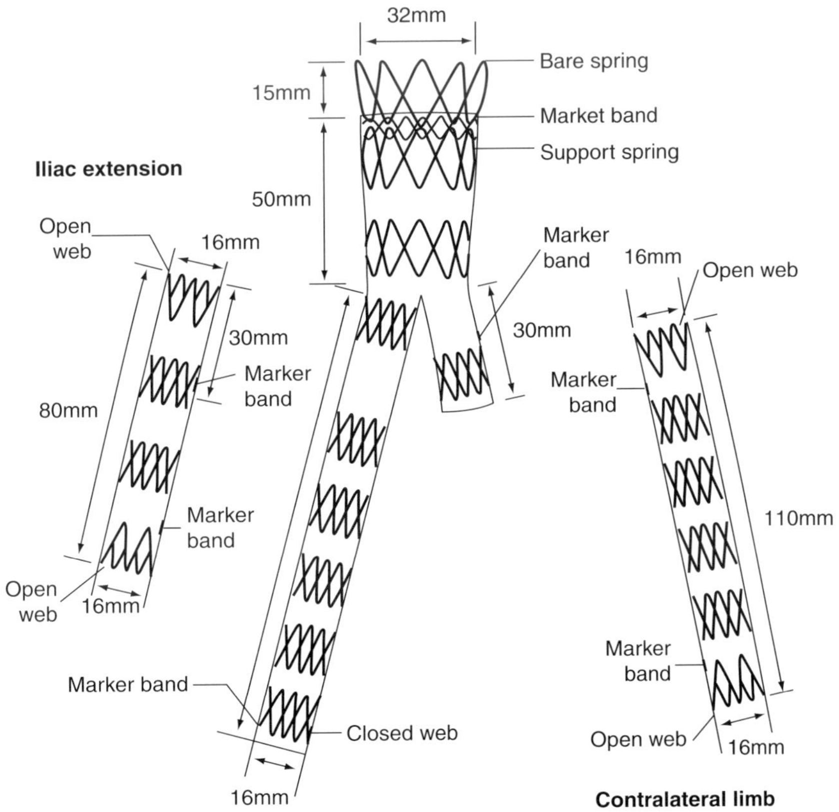

1

1

Illustration 1 shows a diagram used for design and customization of the Talent abdominal aortic aneurysm stent-graft in accordance with measurements taken by computed tomography imaging and angiography.

2

The Talent 'double short leg system' (2) offers greater design flexibility for limb length adjustments, useful for patients with very short common iliac arteries.

3

The right common femoral artery has been exposed through a short vertical (or oblique) incision (3). A 0.035-inch 260-cm long Lunderquist guidewire has been placed to the level of the aortic arch using exchange technique. The main section of the Talent stent-graft is delivered intraluminally using the 'puncture technique', without a formal arteriotomy in the common femoral artery. The puncture technique has the advantage of better haemostasis and continued blood flow.

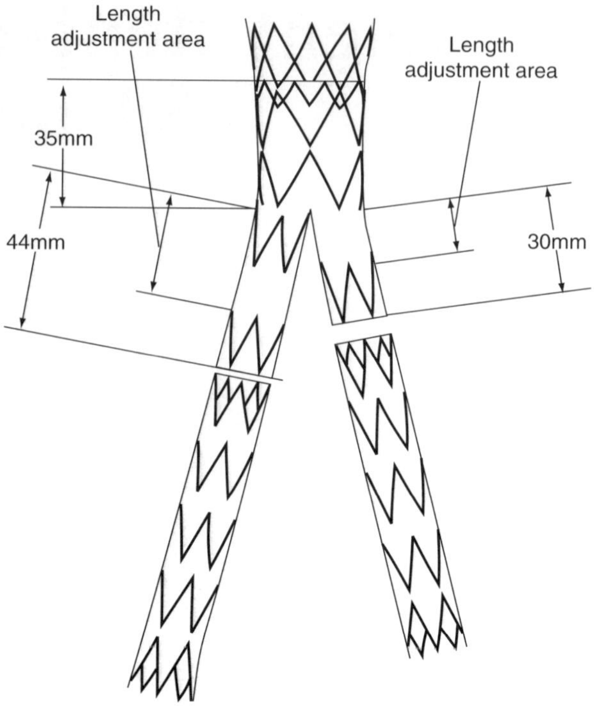

2

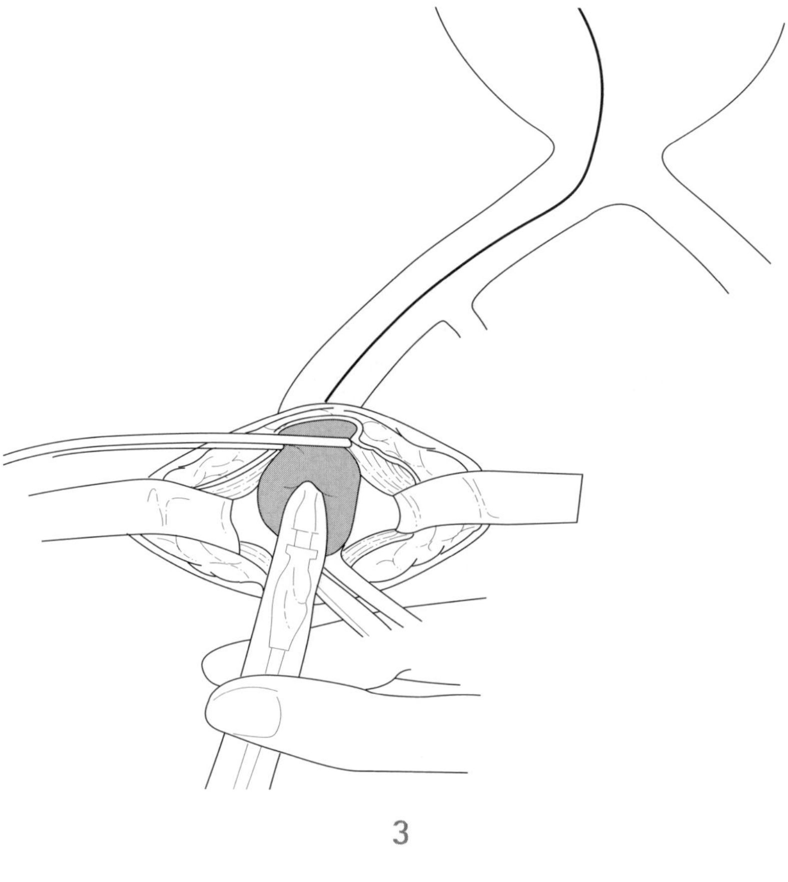

3

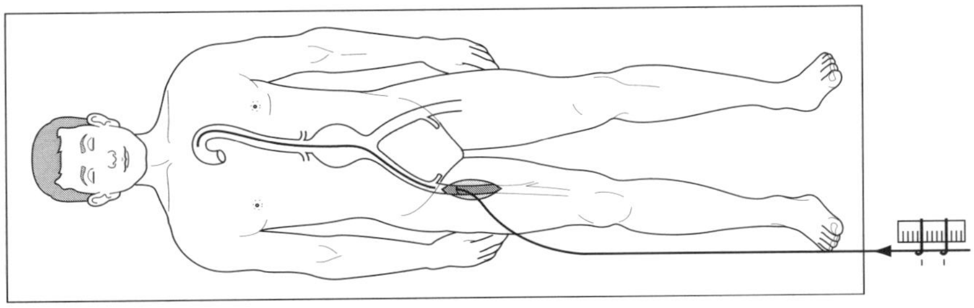

4

4

'External control' of the depth of penetration of the trans-femoral guidewire is useful to prevent inadvertent entry of the aortic arch branches or heart chambers. A 'foot extension' of the procedure table is necessary for this purpose.

5

A diagnostic 5F pigtail catheter has been placed from the left common femoral artery, and is used for repetitive 'puff' angiography during device deployment in the juxtarenal aorta (5). Deployment is initiated at (or slightly above) the level of the renal arteries, and then the graft is repositioned caudad to a level immediately below (1–2 mm) the origin of the renal arteries. Repetitive angiographic puffs through the pigtail catheter are of great help to aid precise placement. Over-the-wire removal of the pigtail catheter, after deployment of the stent-graft, has not been a problem in our experience.

6

The authors' preferred access technique for contralateral limb deployment uses a diagnostic 5F pre-shaped catheter (Universal Flush, Omni Sos, Simmons or similar) for crossover advancement of a 0.035 inch (or 0.025 inch) Glidewire (6). A 6F 15-mm nitinol wire-loop snare is used to capture the Glidewire intraluminally and extract it through the contralateral femoral artery sheath. Once this has been achieved, the approach can be simply converted to a more standard retrograde ipsilateral access through the use of an exchange catheter for placement of the Lunderquist (or superstiff Amplatz) guidewire.

7

Illustration **7** shows a completed Talent stent-graft implant, with trans/suprarenal fixation of the bare spring (uncovered stent).

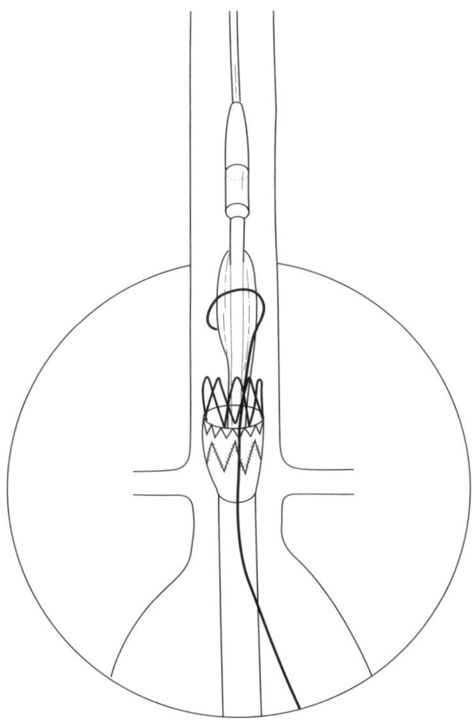

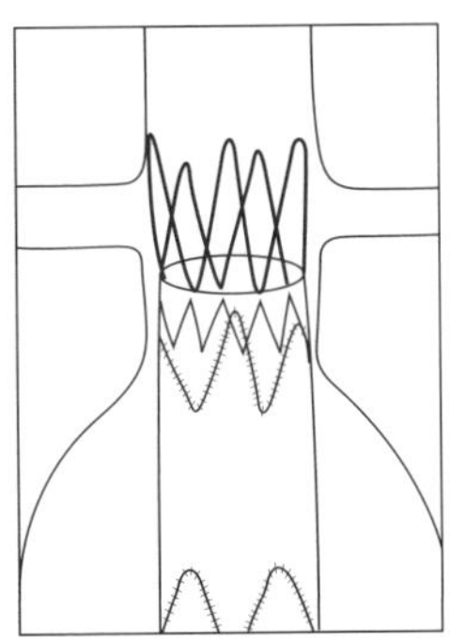

5

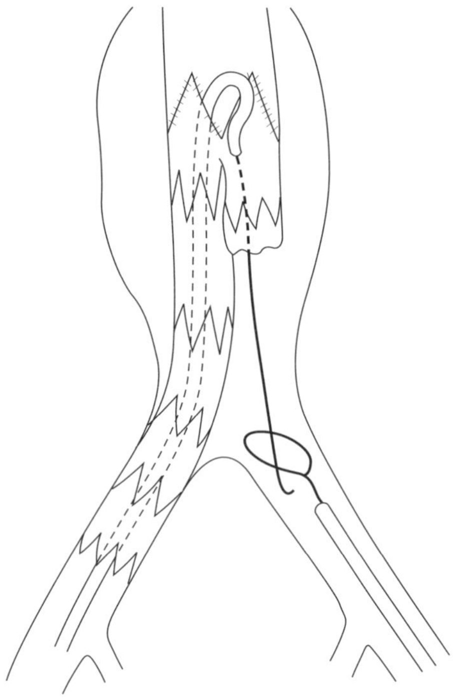

6

8

On occasion, even the Lunderquist guidewire may not be good enough to straighten a severely tortuous access iliac artery (8). The brachial-femoral 'body floss' technique is the ultimate transluminal access manoeuvre, capable of enabling placement of a stent-graft in otherwise 'impossible' situations. As illustrated, it is extremely important to protect the aortosubclavian junction with a 5F or 6F catheter that must be placed over the wire before any tension is applied. The authors' guidewire choice for this manoeuvre is the 450-cm long Microvasive Glidewire (marketed for gastrointestinal endoscopic procedures).

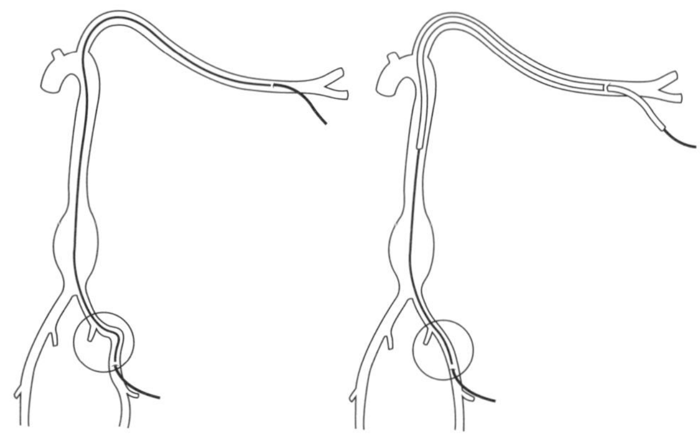

8

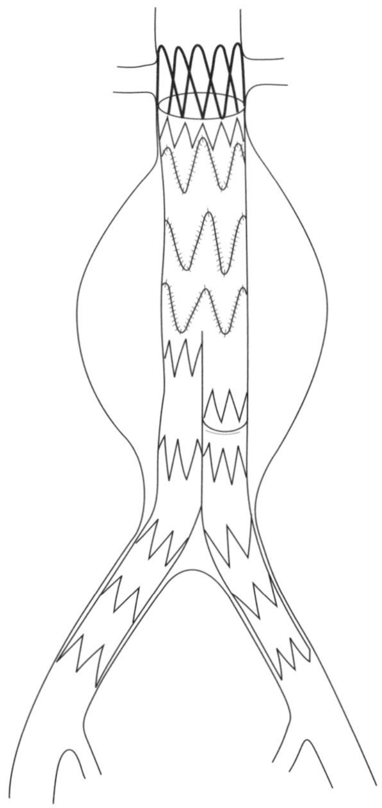

7

9

Aortouni-iliac stent-graft configurations are often required in the setting of disadvantaged iliac artery anatomy and/or concomitant severe iliac artery disease. A 10-mm synthetic iliac conduit is anastomosed to the common iliac artery exposed through a limited retroperitoneal approach. The conduit is used as a pathway for transluminal access and delivery of the stent-graft system (9). It can also serve conveniently as the distal attachment site for the iliac limb, with subsequent anastomosis of the conduit graft to the ipsilateral common femoral artery. The procedure is completed by exclusion of the ipsilateral internal and external iliac arteries and of the contralateral common iliac artery, as well as a crossover femorofemoral bypass.

Overview

Approximately 10 000 Talent stent-graft implants have been performed worldwide following initial clinical experience in December 1995. Several studies have been

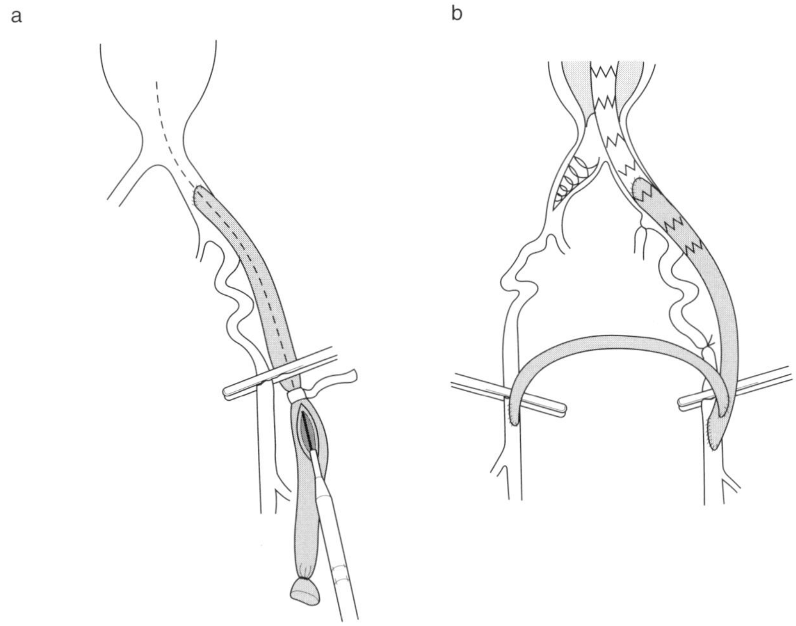

9

conducted in the USA, beginning with the Phase I feasibility study in early 1997 (Criado *et al.*, 2001) Phase II studies have been completed, and follow-up information is being gathered and audited at this time (December 2000) for Pre-Market Approval (PMA) submission to the Food and Drug Administration in 2001.

References

Criado FJ, Abul-Khoudoud O, Wellons E *et al.* (1999). The Talent abdominal aortic aneurysm stent-graft: technical approaches and results of aneurysm exclusion. In: Greenhalgh RM ed. *The Durability of Vascular and Endovascular Surgery.* London: WB Saunders Co. pp. 433–448.

Criado FJ, Wilson EP, Martin JA *et al.* (2000). Custom manufacturing of aortic stent-grafts to expand applicability of endovascular repair: In: Greenhalgh RM, Powell JT, Mitchell AW eds. *Vascular and Endovascular Opportunities.* London: WB Saunders Co. pp. 287–296.

Criado FJ, Wilson EP, Fairman RM *et al.* (2001). Update on the Talent aortic stent-graft: a preliminary report from US phase I and II trials. *J Vasc Surg* (in press).

The Anaconda stent-graft system for abdominal aortic aneurysm

F Benedetti-Valentini, PG Cao, G Coppi, M D'Addato, G Picchi, P Rossi, V Stancanelli, DG Tealdi

Introduction

1a, b

Illustration **1a** shows the polyester nitinol body of the graft with Tantalum ring markers to identify, first, the contralateral side of the body and, second, the docking zone, to allow accurate placement of the legs. The longitudinal nitinol support along the body has been designed to provide a balance between rigidity and flexibility and the body has thus been designed to have the flexibility to conform to changing anatomy over time.

Illustration **1b** shows the nitinol support legs which behave in an identical fashion to crimped graft legs used in conventional surgery. These legs have been designed to provide the optimum balance between flexibility and kink resistance. The legs also have Tantalum markers to enable accurate docking into the docking zone of the body and to visualize the position of the distal end of the leg in relation to the hypogastric artery.

2

The endograft is attached to the delivery system and can be controlled from the handle. By changing the position of the collar on the control handle the ring stent can be collapsed, thus reducing the diameter of the endograft and therefore allowing repositioning at any time during the procedure.

3a, b, c

The sequence of using the magnet system to cannulate the contralateral stump of the body is illustrated.

4a

The control handle enables fine movements of the collar which control both the reduction in diameter of the ring stent to allow repositioning and give the ability to tilt the device by rotating the collar.

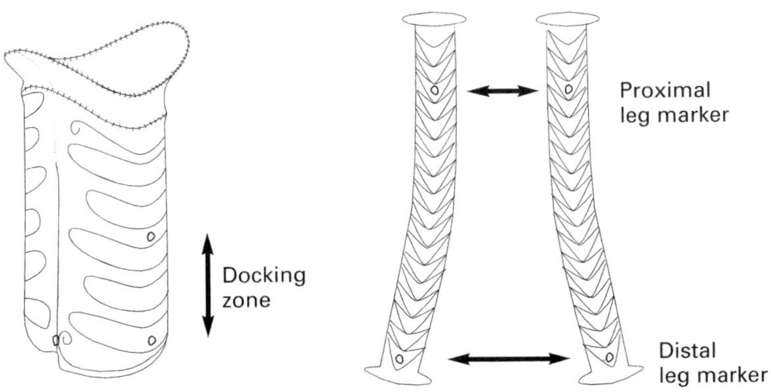

a 1 b

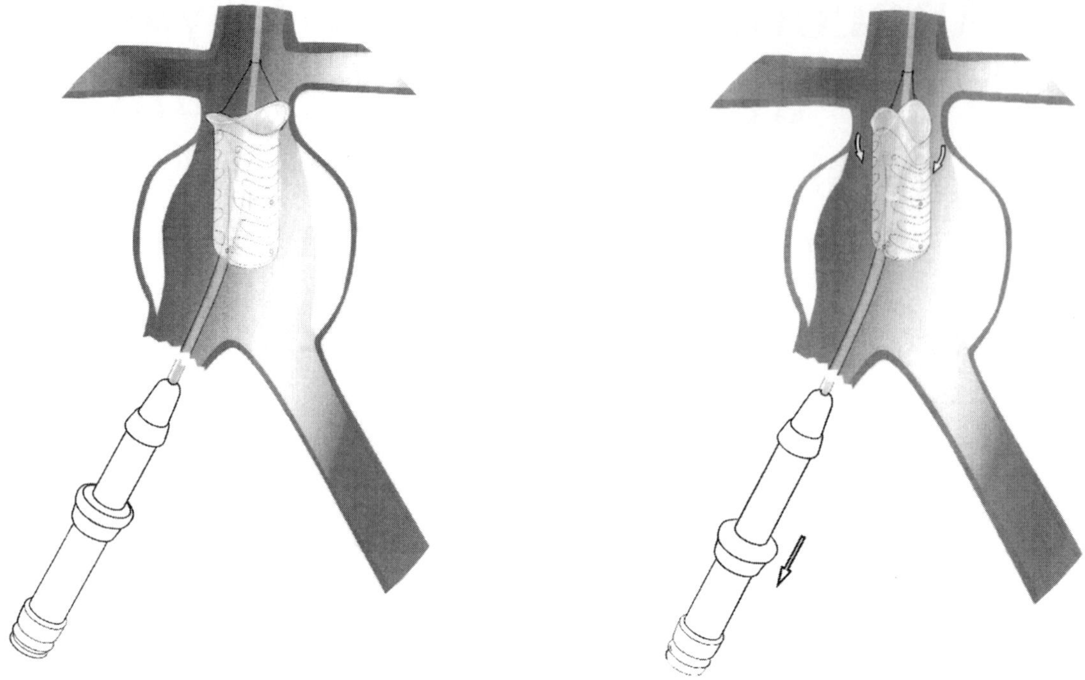

2

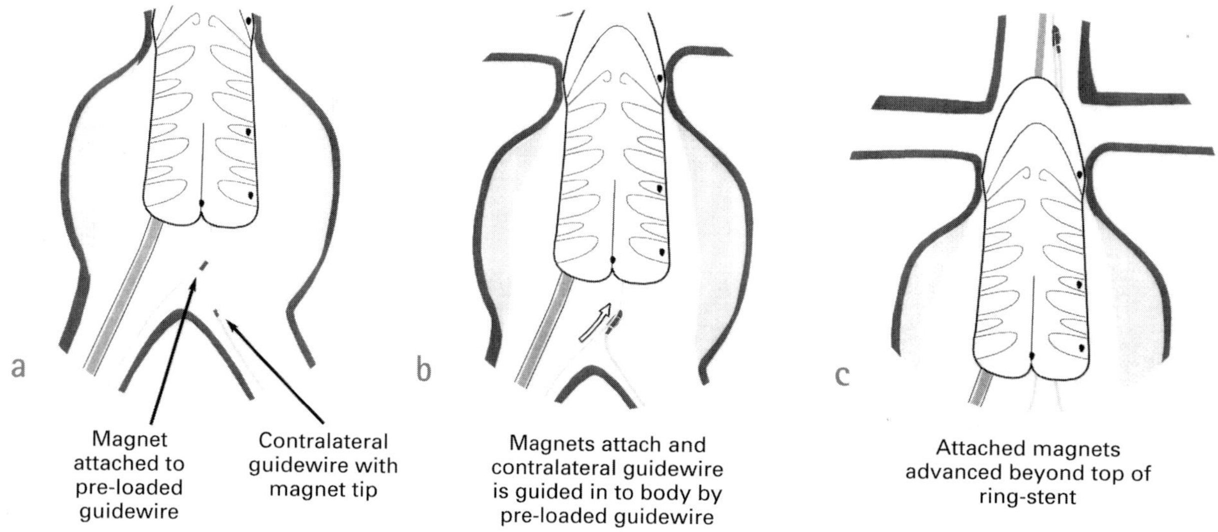
a
Magnet attached to pre-loaded guidewire
Contralateral guidewire with magnet tip
b
Magnets attach and contralateral guidewire is guided in to body by pre-loaded guidewire
c
Attached magnets advanced beyond top of ring-stent

3

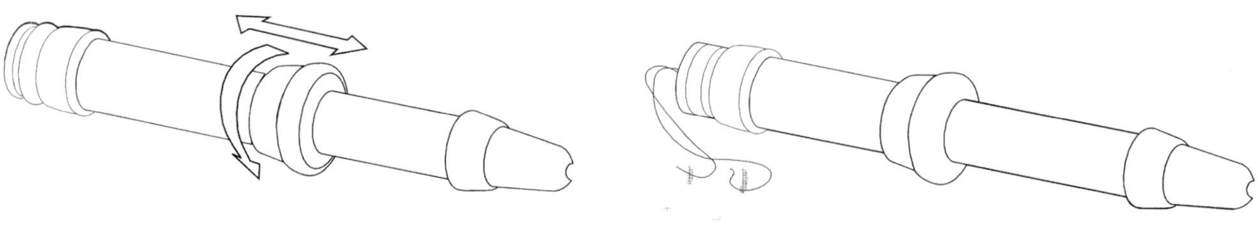
a
b

4

4b

The device can only be finally deployed, i.e. no further repositioning possible, after subsequent removal of these two release wires. This feature has been designed to prevent accidental 'snap lock' of the device before optimization of the final position.

The Italian Clinical Trial Group of authors find this a new and fine concept of endograft. Repositioning and flexibility is an advantage and the delivery system is elastic. Experience is rapidly being acquired but only short-term outcomes are available.

Acknowledgement

The editor wishes to thank Stuart Rodger of Sulzer Vascutek for help with this chapter.

Section fifteen ENDOVASCULAR STENT-GRAFT TECHNIQUES FOR ABDOMINAL AORTIC ANEURYSM
C: Special difficulties

Management of endoleak and endotension

Peter L Harris

Classification of endoleak

1

Endoleak is a condition associated with endoluminal vascular grafts defined by the presence of blood flow outside the lumen of the endoluminal graft but within the aneurysm sac or adjacent vascular segment treated by the graft (White *et al.*, 1997).

Basically there are two categories of endoleak, those related to the endograft itself including the anastomoses or fixation sites (Types 1 and 3) and those due to retrograde flow into the aneurysm sac from patent aortic side-branches (Type 2). Endoleak due to porosity of the graft material (Type 4) is a transient phenomenon only.

Proximal fixation site endoleaks (Type 1a) and those associated with defects in the endograft (Types 3a and 3b) are considered to be the most dangerous and this impression is confirmed by data from the EUROSTAR registry which indicates that they are important risk factors for later rupture of the aneurysm (Harris *et al.*, 2000). Therefore, endoleak Types 1a and 3 should be treated urgently by secondary intervention as soon as their presence is detected.

Type 2 endoleaks in isolation are rarely associated with adverse events (Harris *et al.*, 2000) and many resolve spontaneously. Therefore, it is generally accepted that they may be managed by continued surveillance in the first place. An important indication for interventional treatment of Type 2 endoleak is co-existing 'endotension' or pressurization of the aneurysm evidenced by continued or recurrent expansion of the sac (Gilling-Smith *et al.*, 1999).

In some patients it is difficult to differentiate between Type 1 and Type 2 endoleak and there is potential, particularly, to misdiagnose Type 1 endoleak as Type 2. Furthermore Type 1 and 2 endoleaks may co-exist in which case the patent aortic side-branch is likely to function as an outflow tract for the Type 1 endoleak rather than as inflow tract. If a Type 2 endoleak persists suspect either misdiagnosis or a co-existing occult Type 1 endoleak.

Classification of endoleak
Type 1a: proximal fixation site
Type 1b: distal fixation site
Type 1c: iliac occluder
Type 2a: inferior mesentric artery
Type 2b: lumbar artery
Type 3a: disjunction of modular parts
Type 3b: fabric tear
Type4: fabric porosity (up to 30 days post-op only)

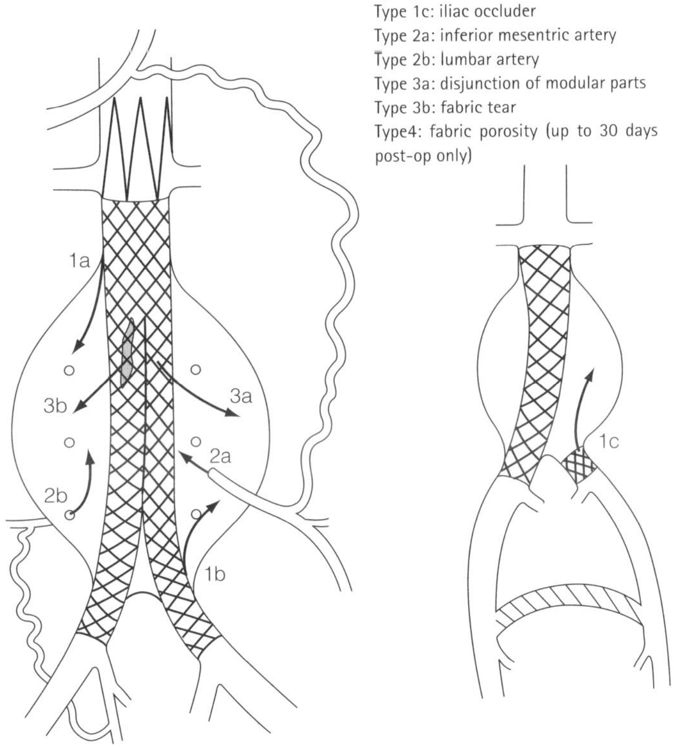

1

Classification of endotension

2

Endotension is defined as persistent or recurrent pressurization of the aneurysm sac following endovascular repair (Gilling-Smith *et al.*, 1999).

Non-invasive measurement of intra-sac pressure is not yet possible but is the subject of considerable technological investigation. In the short-term, pressure within the sac can be measured using a catheter placed alongside the endograft and brought out in the groin (Chuter *et al.*, 1997) or by translumbar puncture of the sac (Baum *et al.*, 2000). However, usually the presence or absence of endotension is inferred from postoperative changes in sac morphology. Expansion of the sac is evidence of endotension while contraction of the sack signifies absence of endotension. The significance of the sac that remains unchanged in size is uncertain.

Endotension has been classified into three grades according to the presence or absence of detectable endoleak and the type of endoleak (Gilling-Smith *et al.*, 1999). Endotension may exist in the absence of a detectable endoleak (Grade 3) either because there is no blood flow into the sack or because the rate of blood flow is too low to be detectable by current imaging techniques. It is well established that thrombus is capable of transmitting pressure without flow (Marty *et al.*, 1998). A worrying possibility is that pressure may be transmitted without flow through the fabric of some endografts.

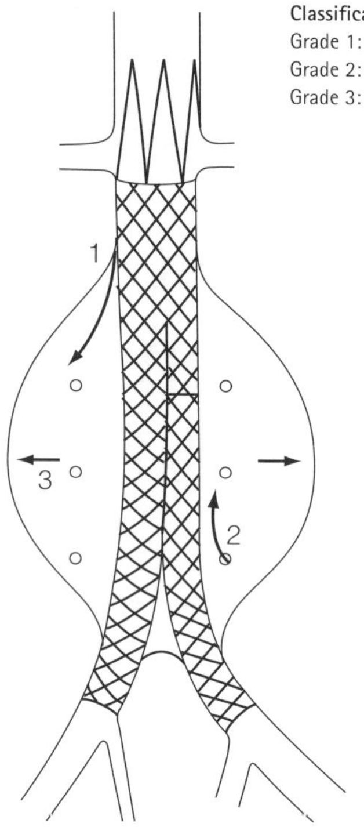

2

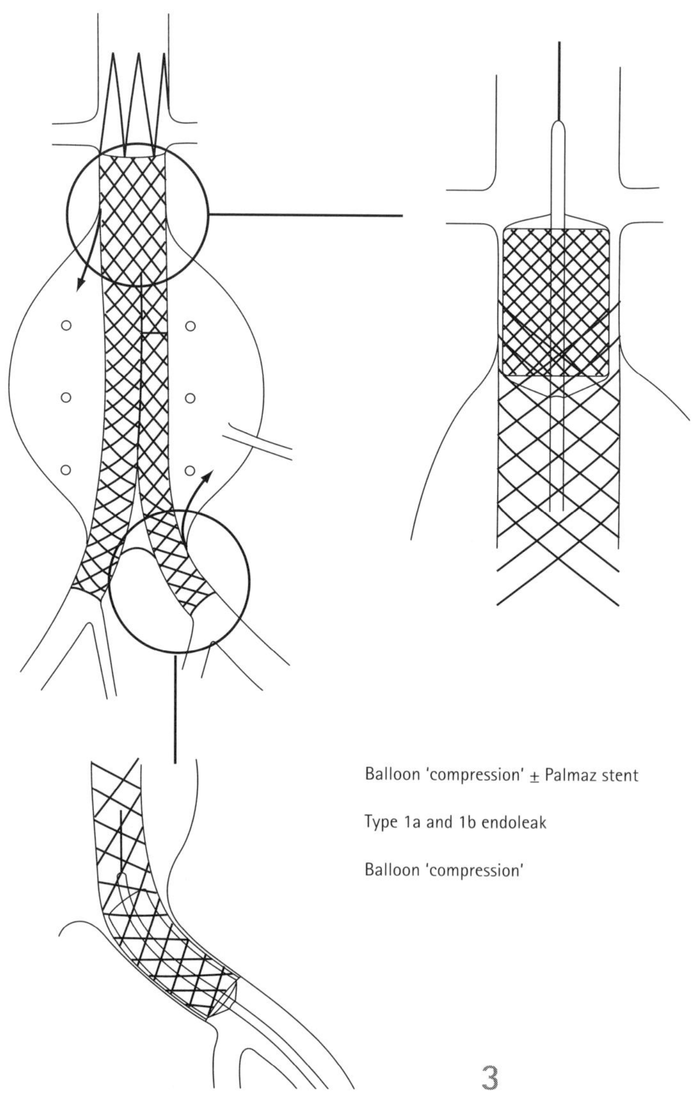

3

Type 1a and 1b endoleak: no migration of the device

3

The first and most important consideration in the management of endoleak is prevention and the key to this is patient selection. Data from EUROSTAR indicates that the risk of Type 1 endoleak exceeds 5% for each of the following anatomical factors: a) length of aneurysm neck less than 10 mm; b) diameter of aneurysm neck more than 30 mm; c) angulation of the neck greater than 50 degrees. It has been shown also, from the same source, that oversizing of the graft relative to the neck diameter by 20% is associated with a lower risk of Type 1 endoleak than oversizing by 10%, which is the accepted standard. Patient and graft selection that takes account of these factors will minimize the risk of Type 1 endoleak.

It is a generally accepted axiom that no patient should be allowed to leave the operating table with an unresolved proximal Type 1 endoleak. Although distal Type 1 endoleaks are apparently less dangerous it is good practice to eliminate these at the time of the primary procedure also.

In both cases balloon dilatation to compress the device against the aortic wall and to eliminate or reduce irregularity of the wall due to atheroma that may compromise 'seal' is the most appropriate first step. If this fails, application of a 'jumbo' Palmaz stent is likely to be successful in resolving a proximal endoleak when the device has been positioned correctly.

Endoleak associated with migration

4

Migration of the proximal or distal fixation stent or malpositioning of these stents at operation can result in endoleak as can migration with disjunction of the components of a modular stent. Secondary intervention to extend the endograft is indicated to treat endoleak from these causes as shown.

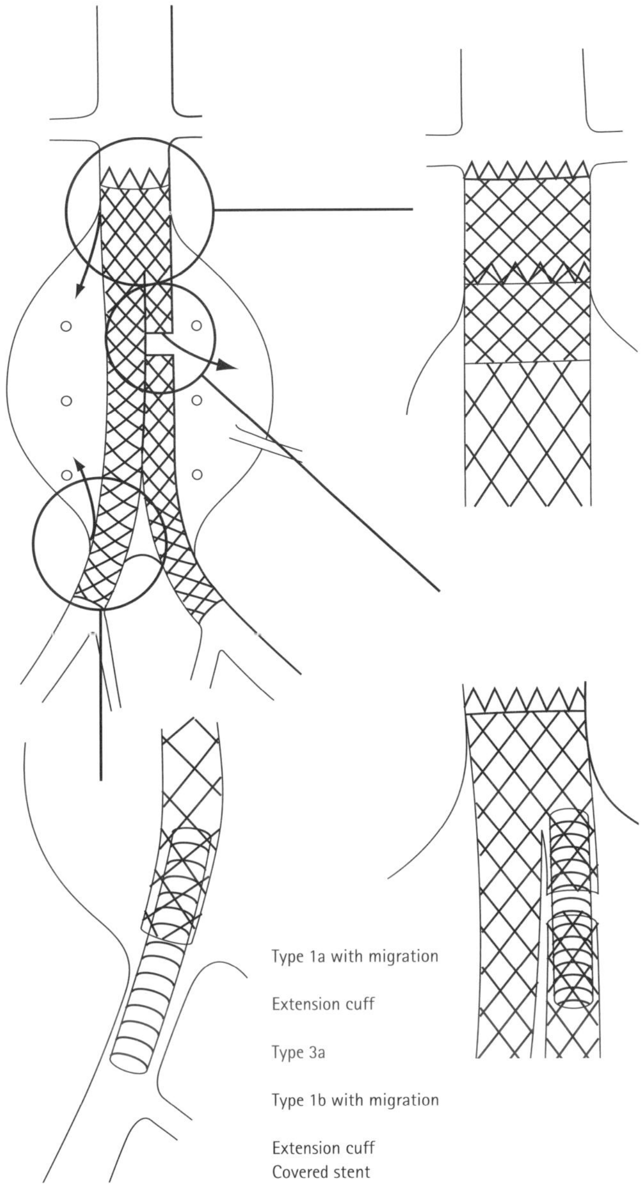

4

Type 2 endoleak

5, 6

Attempts to prevent Type 2 endoleak by preoperative coiling of aortic side-branches have proved unsuccessful (Gould *et al.*, 2001). An alternative strategy involving the placement of thrombotic sponge material within the sac at the original operation has been reported to be more effective and safe (Walker *et al.*, 1999). Given the apparently benign natural history of Type 2 endoleaks prophylactic measures to prevent them are probably not justified as a routine practice. However, it is accepted by most endovascular interventionalists that patent hypogastric arteries that are to be excluded by the endograft should be coil-embolized either preoperatively or at the time of the procedure because they are a potential source of a major Type 2 endoleak. A case may be made for similar management of large patent inferior mesenteric arteries.

If it is deemed necessary to treat Type 2 endoleak the first option attempted is usually coil embolization. The inferior mesenteric artery may be accessed from the superior mesenteric artery via the marginal artery and the lumbar arteries from the hypogastric via the iliolumbar artery using fine 'tracker' catheters. These are technically difficult procedures that carry a significant risk of complications (Gould *et al.*, 2001).

An alternative to coil embolization is laparoscopic clipping of the inferior mesenteric or lumbar arteries.

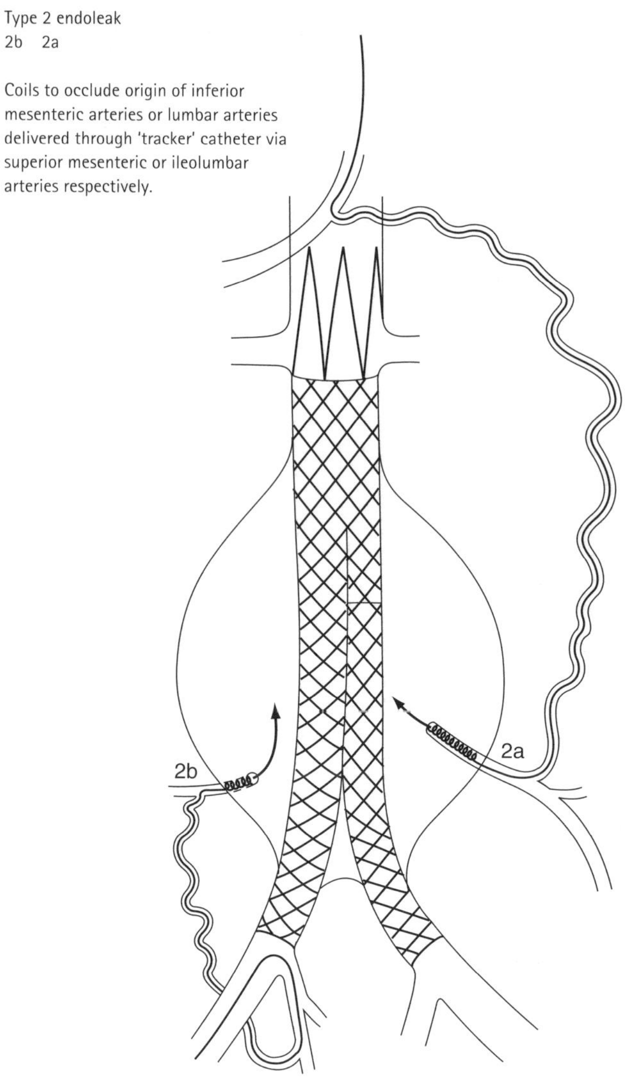

5

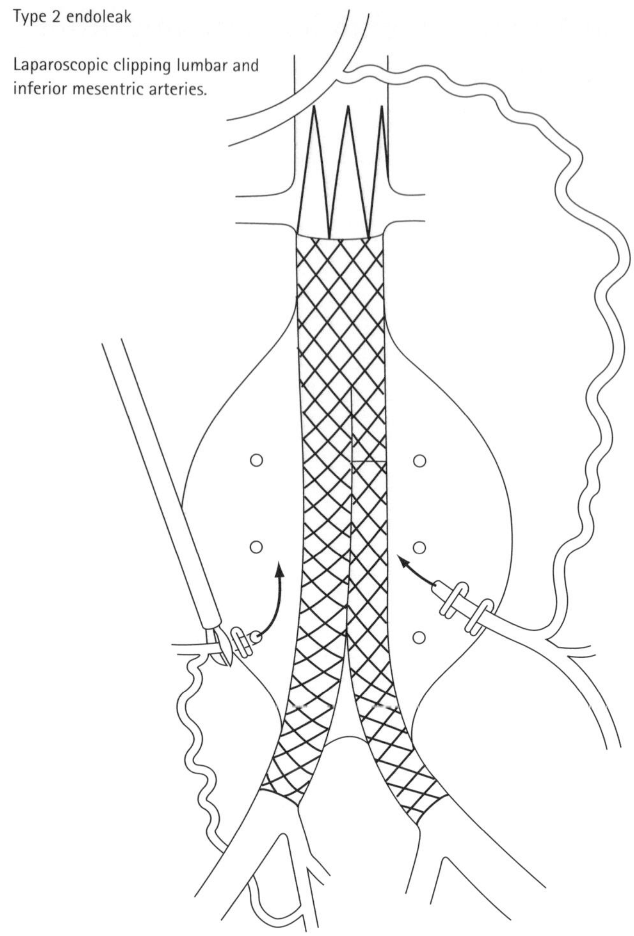

6

Because Type 2 endoleaks are associated with a low risk of adverse consequences (Harris *et al.*, 2000) it follows that secondary intervention should be undertaken selectively. Treatment is indicated when there is evidence of endotension, for example when the aneurysm sac continues to expand or when intra-sac pressure measurements approximate to systemic pressure.

Combined Type 1 to 2 and Type 2 to 2 endoleak

7

Whenever there is an exit as well as an entry point for an endoleak there is a tendency for the endoleak to persist.

Secondary intervention is usually indicated when Types 1 and 2 endoleak co-exist and treatment should be directed primarily to the anastomotic or Type 1 element by one of the methods described previously. The indications for treatment of combined Type 2 to 2 endoleak are less clear-cut.

A recently described technique for defining the sites of entry and exit of a combined endoleak and its course through the sac involves translumbar, transsac cannulation of the endoleak itself (Baum *et al.*, 2000). Direct measurement of pressure is possible by this means in addition to contrast imaging of the endoleak. Pressure within the endoleak invariably approximates to systemic pressure. Treatment can be administered by injection of thrombin or deployment of coils through the translumbar cannula. To ensure success one or both of the feeding arteries must be occluded directly. It has been shown that intrasac thrombus may transmit pressure (Marty *et al.*, 1998), for this reason placement of thrombin or coils into the intrasac track of the endoleak alone is unlikely to be effective.

Conversion to open repair

Open surgery to remove the endograft and conversion to conventional repair is the definitive therapeutic response to endoleak and endotension. It signifies failure of the endovascular technique and is associated with a mortality risk of 20%. Therefore, it is a treatment of last resort.

Conversion to open repair is indicated under the following circumstances:

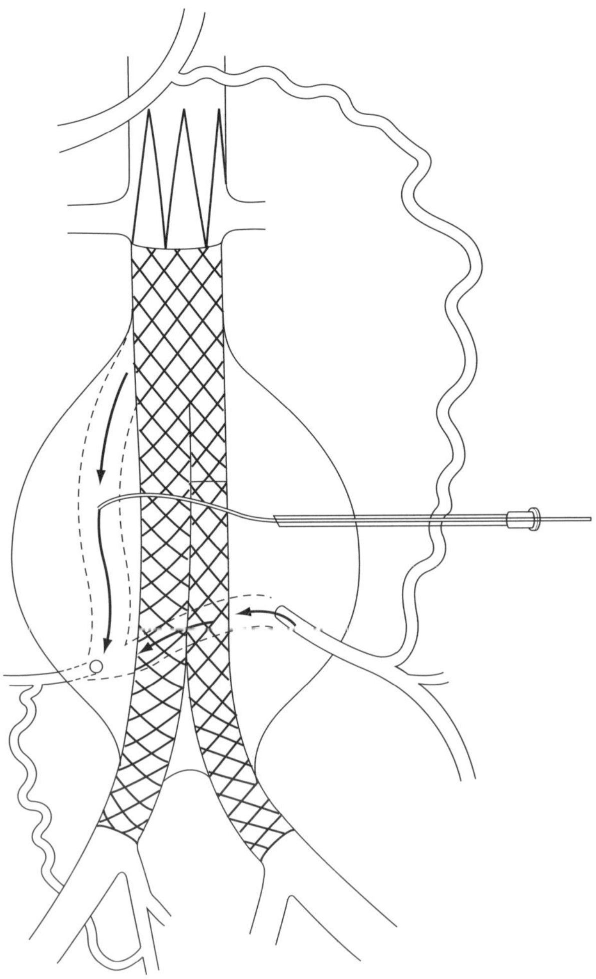

7

Type 1a to Type 2b (proximal fixation side to lumbar)
Type 2a to Type 2b (inferior mesenteric lumbar)

Direct needle puncture of the sac, injection of contrast into the track of the endoleak or placement of coils into patent aortic side-branches, with or without intraendoleak measurement of pressure.

1. Type 1a endoleak that persists despite application of other methods.
2. Type 1b or Type 2 endoleak that persists despite application of all other methods and sac expanding (endotension).
3. Expanding sac (endotension) in absence of detectable endoleak or other identifiable source of intrinsic pressure.
4. Ruptures (some ruptures associated with Type 1 or 3 endoleak are re-amenable to endovascular treatment.

References

Baum RA, Carpenter JP, Cope C, Fairman RM (2000). Direct pressure measurement of intra-sac pressure after AAA repair: Technique, results and implications. *Proceedings of 27th Global Symposium on Vascular, Endovascular, Issues, Techniques and Horizons.* New York City 2000.

Chuter TAM, Ivancef K, Malina M *et al.* (1997). Aneurysm pressure following endovascular exclusion. *Eur J Vasc Endovasc Surg* **13**: 85–87.

Gilling-Smith GL, Brennan J, Harris PL *et al.* (1999). Endotension after endovascular aneurysm repair: Definition, classification and strategies for surveillance and intervention *J Endovasc Surg* **6**: 305–307.

Gould DA, McWilliams R, Edwards R *et al.* (2001). Aortic side branch embolisation before endovascular aneurysm repair: Incidence of type 2 endoleak. *JVIR* (in press).

Harris PL, Vallabhaneni R, Desgranges P *et al.* (2000). Incidence and risk factors of late rupture, conversion and death after endovascular repair of infrarenal aortic aneurysms: The EUROSTAR experience. *J Vasc Surg* **32**: 739–749.

Marty B, Sanchez LA, Ohki T *et al.* (1998). Endoleak after endovascular graft repair of experimental aortic aneurysms: Does coil embolisation with angiographic 'seal' lower intra-aneurysmal pressure? *J Vasc Surg* **27**: 454–462.

Walker SR, Macierewicz J, Hopkinson BR (1999). Endovascular AAA repair: Prevention of side branch endoleaks with thrombogenic sponge. *J Endovasc Surg* **12**: 199–206.

White GH, Yu W, May J *et al.* (1997). Endoleak as a complication of endoluminal grafting of abdominal aortic aneurysms: Classification, incidence, diagnosis and management. *J Endovasc Surg* **4**: 152–168.

Access difficulties in endovascular aneurysm repair

P R F Bell

Introduction

Endovascular repair can only be achieved if the aortic neck above the lesion can be accessed and if the device can be deployed distally adequately. As time progresses the limitations of endovascular repair become more obvious and the results can be improved only if high risk marginal cases are not done. These are however often the patients who need treatment because they are unfit or because of hostile conditions in the abdomen for open repair. Difficulties in access can be divided into three areas, excessive tortuosity, stenosis of the iliac access sites or difficulty in inserting the contralateral leg into the modular prosthesis.

Tortuosity

Proximal aortic neck

1, 2

Tortuosity of the proximal aortic neck is not uncommon and is more often seen in patients with a large aneurysm greater than 6 cm. Whether these cases should be dealt with or not remains uncertain because device slippage and leakage appear to be more common here. If a decision is taken to insert a device in such a patient, one difficulty is getting the device or at least the sheath to enter the neck of the aneurysm because it impinges in the sac itself as shown in (1). This situation can usually be remedied by manual pressure on the aneurysm itself which will straighten out the neck and allow the device through (2).

Distal iliac arteries

3, 4, 5, 6

This can occur again usually in larger aneurysms and can make the insertion of the device difficult or impossible. There are several ways of dealing with this. First, it can be done by inserting the finger under the inguinal ligament after ligating the anterior branch of the common femoral artery. Much of the vessel can

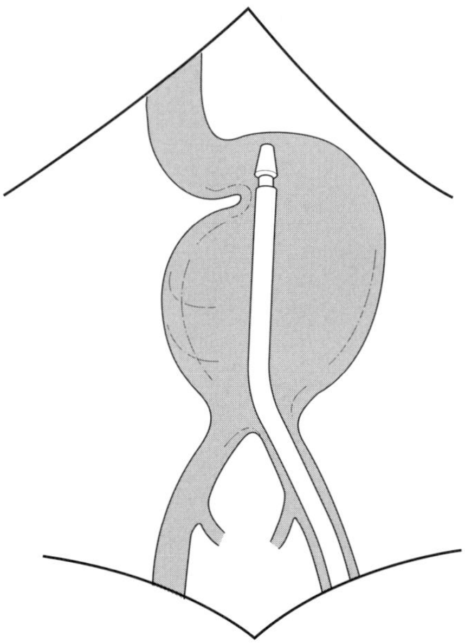

1

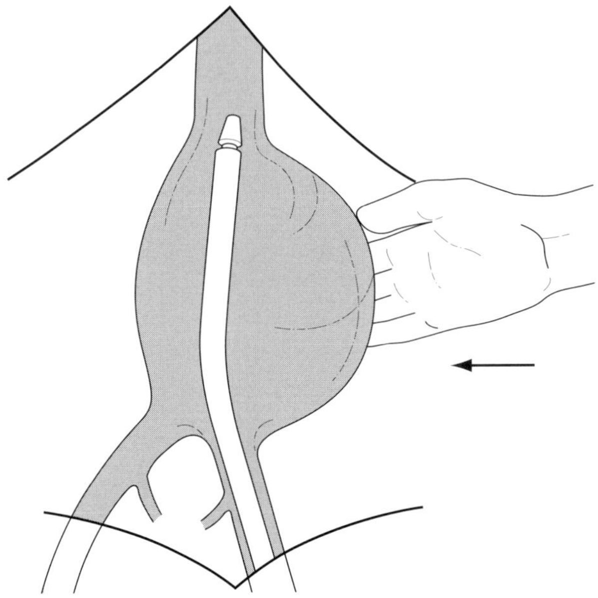

2

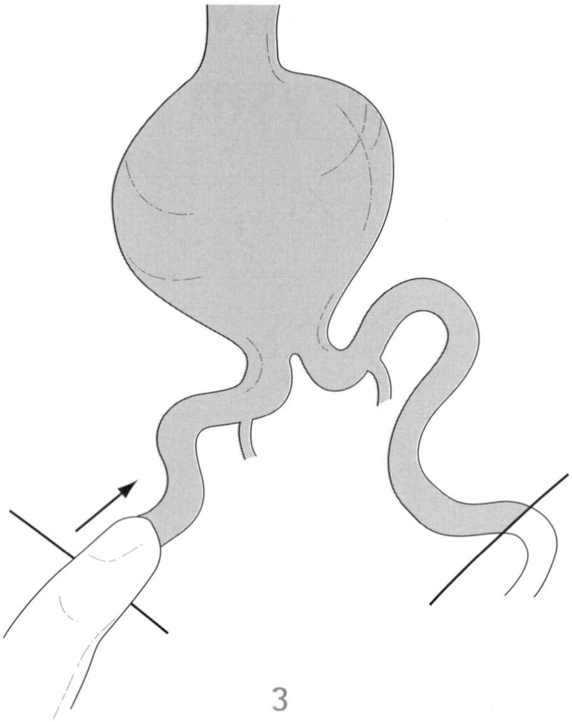

3

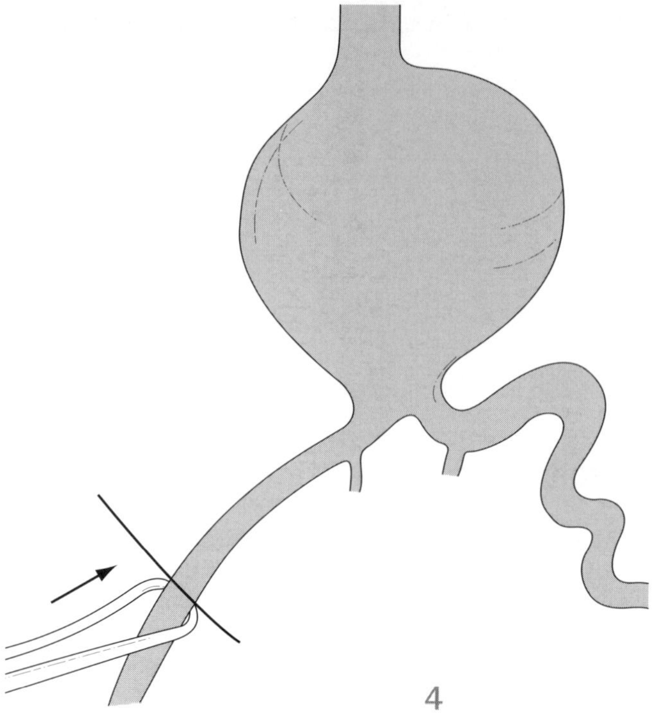

4

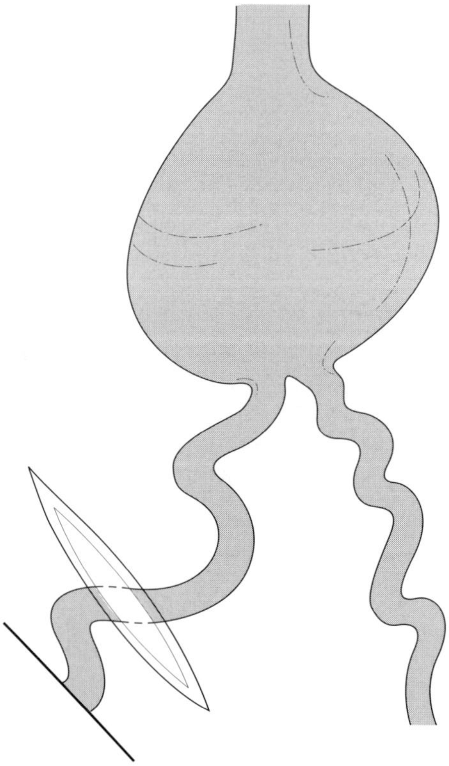

5

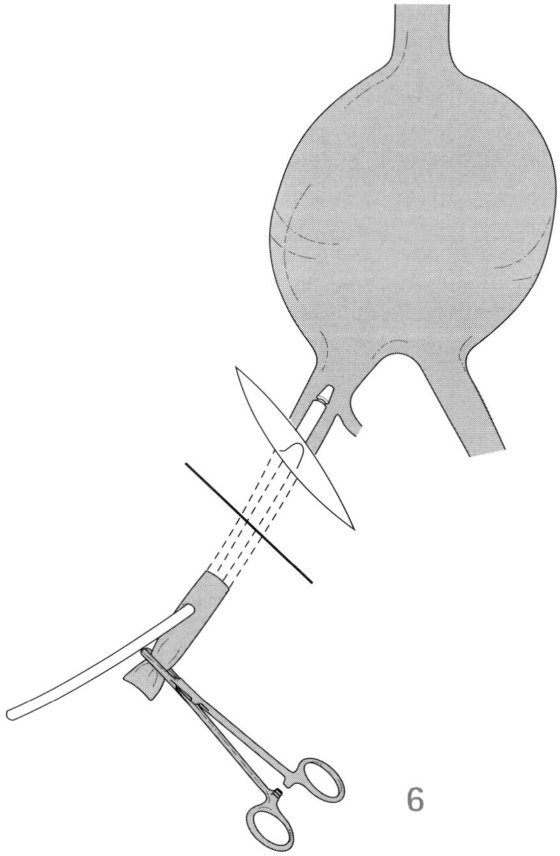

6

be mobilized as in (3). When this has been done, by placing a sling around the artery below the inguinal ligament, the vessel can be straightened out as in (4). The tortuosity of such vessels can of course be assessed preoperatively by doing an angiogram and inserting a stiff amplatz or lundeqvist wire. If, in spite of this, it is not possible to straighten the vessel this can be achieved by making a small incision above the inguinal ligament, mobilizing the external iliac artery and stitching a 10-mm Dacron graft on to the external or common iliac artery (5, 6). The graft is then brought into the groin under the inguinal ligament and the vessels straightened by gentle traction. The graft itself can then be used as an access conduit to insert the sheath. Further assistance can be obtained by placing the index finger through the incision in the abdomen and pulling the device and the sheath forward so that they enter the sac easily. Using this technique almost any device can be inserted successfully.

Stenoses of the iliac vessels

These should not be contraindication to stenting provided the other requirements such as neck length, tortuosity etc have been met. Providing the vessel is patent a wire is passed in the usual way and the iliac arteries dilated with an 8 or 9 french balloon prior to insertion of the wire followed by the sheath. If this cannot be achieved then the case should probably not be done in this way.

Difficulties in inserting the contralateral limb in a modular prosthesis

7, 8, 9

In the majority of cases it is possible to insert a wire using an appropriate catheter into the contralateral limb without difficulty. If, however, this is not possible then a wire is passed up the ipsilateral limb. Using a J or Cobra catheter the wire is then passed down the contralateral limb (7). It can be retrieved quite easily in the contralateral femoral artery through a small arteriotomy. A van Andel catheter is then passed up the wire on the contralateral side (8) and as this is done the wire on the ipsilateral side is released so that it flicks up into the aorta. The van Andel catheter can then be pushed proximally (9). This wire can then be used to insert the contralateral limb in the usual way. If there are problems in doing this, due to kinking etc, gentle traction on both arms of the wire in the groins as it passes over the graft bifurcation can lead to straightening of the iliac vessels so that the device can be inserted. This sometimes occurs when the contralateral limb is to be inserted into kinked vessels. This technique is preferable to using an arm entry point

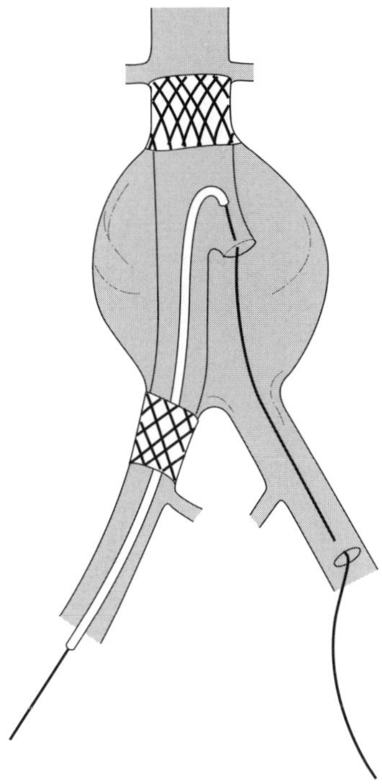

7

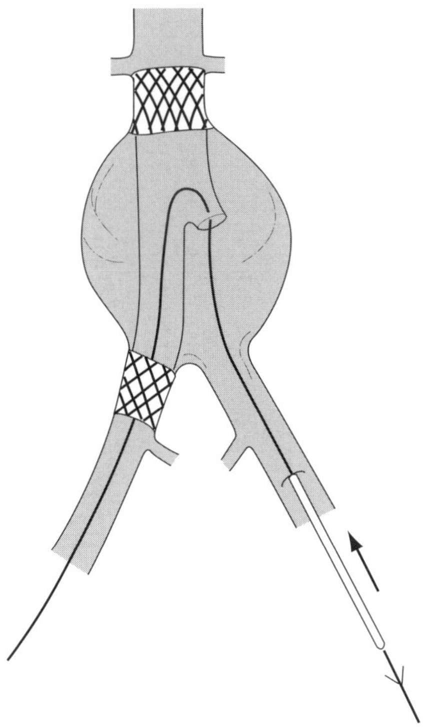

8

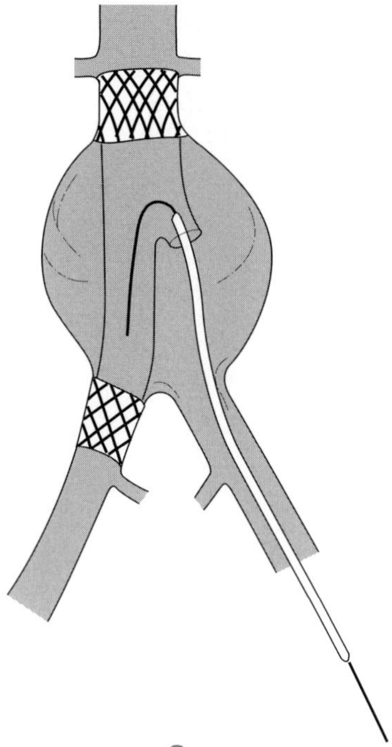

9

which is straightforward but means another puncture and exposure of the arm during the procedure. This is not usually necessary.

Access is rarely a difficulty in these cases. If they are suitable for endovascular repair by other criteria then they can usually be dealt with by using some of the methods outlined above.

Conversions

Dieter Raithel

Introduction

The endoluminal method continues to be used with increasing frequency in the management of patients with abdominal aortic aneurysms. Despite worldwide experience and improving interventional skills, mid-term results still show e.g. an overall endoleak rate of approximately 20–30%. If endoluminal abdominal aortic aneurysm repair is unsuccessful, conversion may become necessary. The technique of open repair after endografting may be more complicated than standard elective operation. Operative strategies and technical manoeuvres regarding clamp techniques and stent extraction make conversion a demanding procedure. This chapter examines our continuing experience with surgical conversion and discusses indications, strategies and techniques that may be used for performing this operation.

Definition, incidence and indications for conversion

We have to differentiate between *primary conversions* (at the original operation) and *secondary conversions* (at a later operation). The conversion rate in most vascular centres is about 2–15%; in our own institution it was 6.7%.

The current indications for *primary conversions* include access problems, i.e. iliac aortic rupture, endograft migration with obstruction of renal or iliac arteries and device-related technical problems (entrapment of the delivery catheter above the renal arteries, blocked iliac outflow by the endoprosthesis, bifurcated deployment failure etc.).

Secondary conversion is indicated in persisting and growing endoleaks, continued aneurysm expansion in the absence of endoleak (endotension), graft thrombosis and graft infection, renal artery obstruction, migration of prostheses, renal artery obstruction. In this secondary conversion detailed imaging by computed tomography and aortography using calibrated catheters were performed preoperatively in all patients.

Techniques for surgical conversion and intraoperative strategies

A clear distinction must be drawn between primary and secondary conversion. The different methods of open repair being selected are determined by the cause of failure leading to conversion, by the type of prosthesis and by the site of deployment of the device (e.g. above the renal arteries).

Conventional open abdominal aortic aneurysm repair (standard)

This is performed in patients in whom transfemoral intraluminal graft implantation for abdominal aortic aneurysm is abandoned due to access problems, device malfunction or no endograft present in the aorta. In this group infrarenal and common iliac artery clamping is therefore possible without injuring the vessels due to underlying metal stents. The operation is performed as a standard open repair mostly by tube interposition after opening the aneurysm sac.

Conventional repair has to be modified

1, 2

In cases where the endograft is deployed in the correct position below the renals or is occluding the iliac arteries the conventional repair has to be modified. In patients in whom the endoluminal approach had been abandoned due to graft thrombosis, due to difficulties in connecting the contralateral limb into the main body, due to distal stent migration or persisting endoleaks sometimes routinely infrarenal applied clamps are opened and closed in sequence, but frequently a suprarenal aortic clamp must be applied (1, 2).

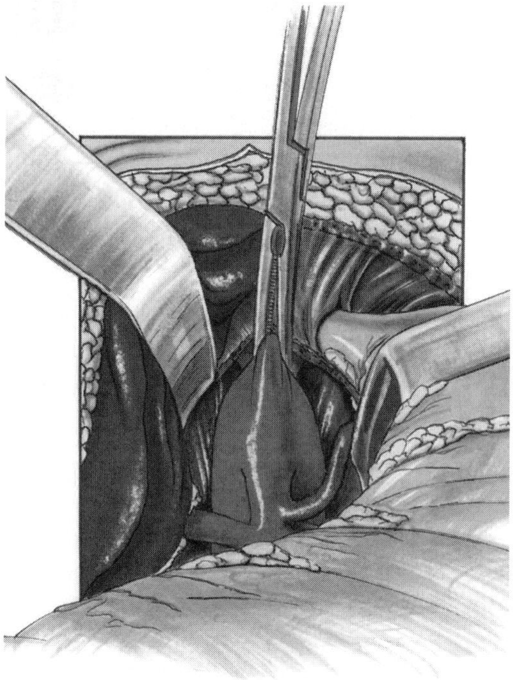

1

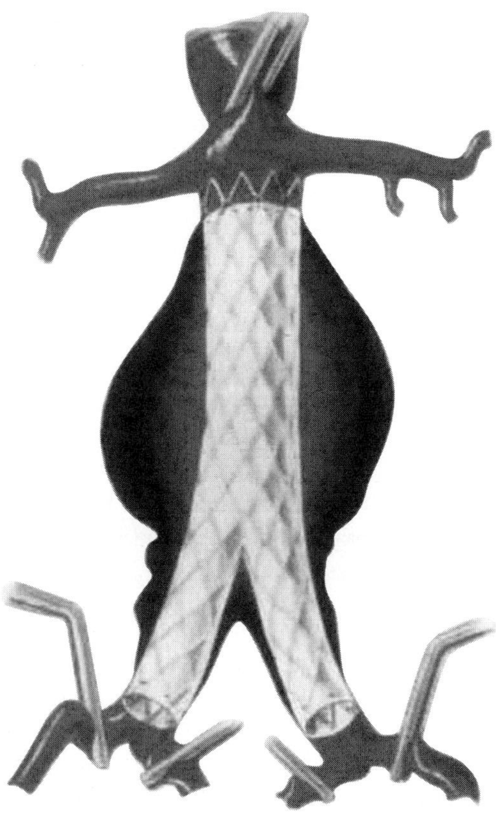

2

Illustration 2 shows suprarenal clamping of the aorta and selective clamping of the external and internal iliac arteries. The technique of gaining supracoeliac control is performed in the following steps: 1) division of the gastrohepatic omentum; 2) Display of the right diaphragmal crus; 3) Separation of this crus and definition of the distal thoracic aorta in order to guide the aortic clamp around it (1).

3, 4

The aorta can sometimes be cross-clamped within the opened sac just above the left renal vein to reduce blood loss (3), then the aortic clamp is temporarily released and the endograft is removed by traction (4). Illustration 4 shows mobilizing of the aortic stent graft in patients with incorporated aortic stent. Normally the aorta is cross-clamped at the diaphragm level and this clamp can reduce some bleeding. After removal of the graft, the clamp can be applied infrarenally and reconstruction is continued.

Due to the fact that sometimes the juxtarenal infrarenal portion of the aorta is damaged by the stent (hooks and barbs), however, we recommend keeping up suprarenal clamping until the proximal anstomosis has been finished.

Supracoeliac or subdiaphragmal control of the aorta

This will usually be required where endografts have been deployed over the renal arteries or in patients who sustained rupture of the proximal neck of the aneurysm

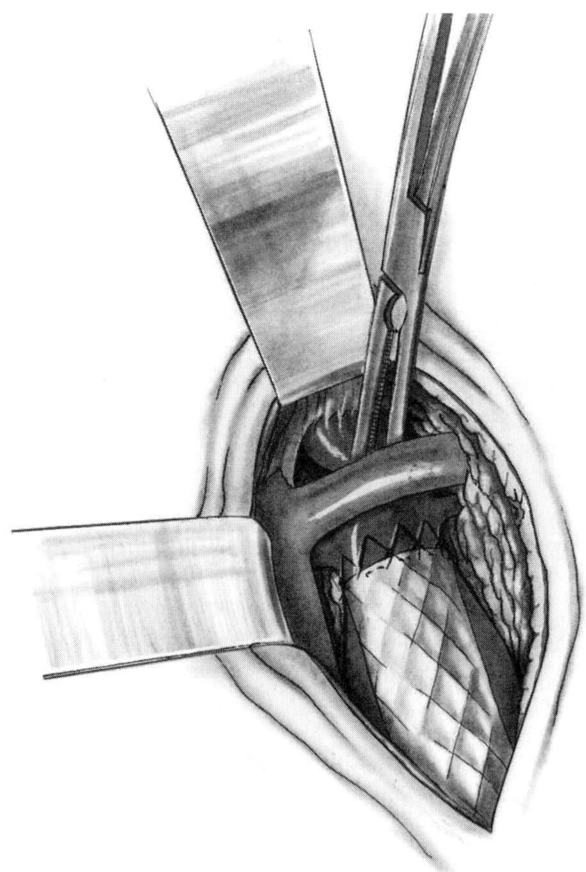

3

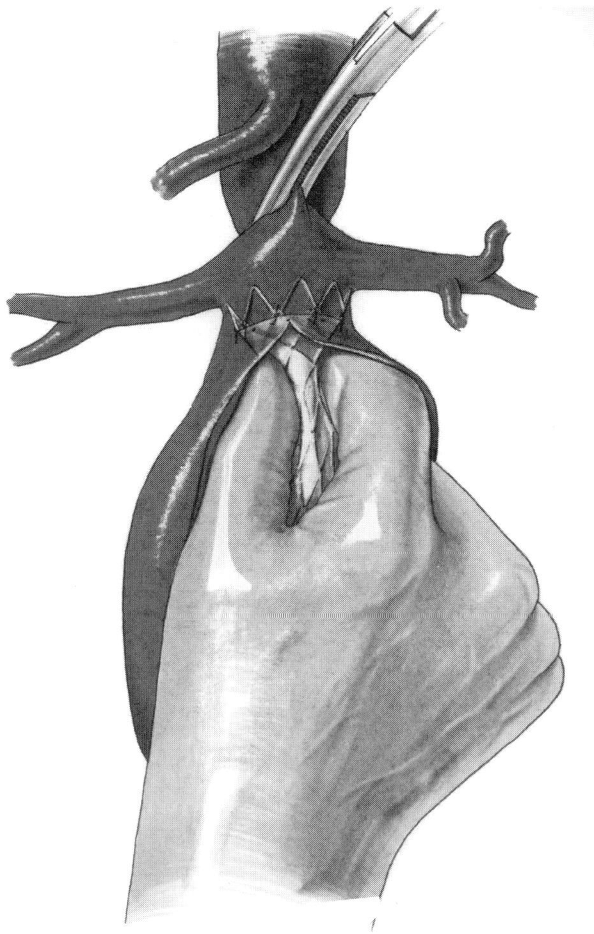

4

during deployment of the endograft by balloon inflation. Certainly subdiaphragmal clamping is recommended in patients with an overstenting of the renal area with the uncovered part of the endograft (e.g. Cook, Endologix, Vanguard).

Furthermore we recommend supracoeliac or better subdiaphragmal clamping in patients with ruptured aneurysms after endografting or in patients in whom an infected endoprosthesis has to be removed.

Subdiaphragmal control of the aorta and amputation of the infrarenal portion of the endoprosthesis

5

In cases of graft incorporation in the aortic wall during secondary conversion, amputation of the infrarenal portion of the endoprosthesis by cutting the metal frame of the para- and suprarenal attachment system has to be performed (5). The proximal amputated prosthesis remains *in situ* and is incorporated in the new anastomosis of the new graft. This technique is recommended by Lawrence-Brown and is considered to be less traumatic than removal of the entire (e.g. Cook) device. The reconstruction following removal of the endoprosthesis follows open surgery rules.

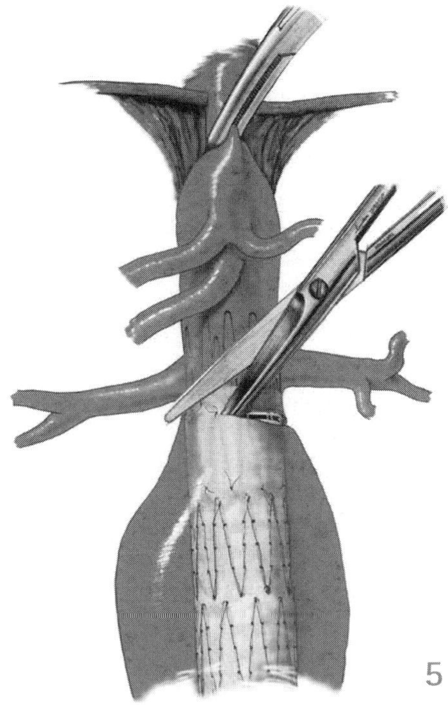

5

Special problems in conversions

Conversion needs a flexible intraoperative treatment regarding the clamping technique and stent extraction. Immediate conversion is generally carried out without problems in cases of graft misplacement, persistent endoleaks or graft thrombosis. To enable optimal reconstruction after stent-graft explantation, subdiaphragmal or suprarenal clamping far from the stent may be necessary. In particular, patients who underwent explantation after a longer postoperative period show well incorporated stents in the proximal anchoring zone.

In cases of proximal misplacement, subdiaphragmal clamping becomes necessary. In distal misplacement, endoleak and iliac artery rupture, infrarenal clamping and standard operation are sufficient and easily performed. The iliac arteries have to be dissected distally and clamped selectively (internal/external) (2). Sometimes endarterectomy of the iliac arteries becomes necessary. After incision of the aneurysm the graft has to be digitally loosened in order to avoid tears or ruptures by the anchoring hooks of some devices. Then the graft can be removed. The aorta and the iliac arteries have to be inspected for any damage, irrespective of whether the anchoring mechanism was dependent on hooks, barbs or controlled ballon expansion.

Again, the risk of dissecting or rupturing the iliac artery requires endovascular surgery to be performed in the operating room.

Some endoprostheses have a balloon as a part of the delivery system. In cases of perforation this balloon may be inflated and used for controlling the haemorrhage.

In our experience, bifurcated endografts have also been implanted; most of these patients could undergo reconstruction by open repair and by using a *tube* graft.

Summary

Conversions, being performed electively, show low complication rates and mortality, similar to conventional open aneurysm repair and can be performed with little disadvantage to the patient. Emergency stent explantations, in contrast, especially when preceded by significant retroperitoneal bleeding, carry a poor prognosis and have a high mortality rate.

For removal of the endograft, suprarenal or sometimes better subdiaphragmal clamping is recommendable.

Acknowledgements
Illustrations by M Hellmuth.

References

Lawrence-Brown MM, Hartley D, MacSweeney ST (1996). The Perth endoluminal bifurcated graft system – development and early experience. *Cardiovasc Surg* **4**:706–712.

May J, White GH, Harris JP (1999). Techniques for surgical conversion of aortic endoprosthesis, *Eur J Vasc Endovasc Surg* **18**:284–289.

Raithel D, Boeckler D (1999). Open operative conversion after failed endovascular grafting for AAAs: Strategies and technical maneuvers to make it safer. Material presented: *26th Annual Symposium on Critical Problems, New Horizons and Techniques in Vascular and Endovascular Surgery*. New York, 18–21 November, 1999.

Section sixteen **UPPER LIMB OPEN VASCULAR TECHNIQUES**

Transaxillary first rib resection

J F Thompson

1

Transaxillary first rib resection is recommended for arterial, venous and lower plexus thoracic outlet syndrome, with or without a cervical rib. If upper plexus symptoms are present, supraclavicular exploration is best. The patient is seen on the ward and the case reviewed carefully. The indications for surgery are discussed once again, along with the possible complications. Subcutaneous low molecular weight heparin is administered preoperatively (preferably the night before). Antibiotic prophylaxis is not employed. The patient is placed on a foam filled vacuum bag and positioned in the three-quarter lateral position with a pillow between the legs. A padded angled bar is positioned to elevate the limb which is gently but firmly bound to the bar using Velband and crepe bandages (1). A sterile, tubular stockinette is rolled over the arm after skin preparation and the drapes secured with Op Site strips. The surgeon and assistant stand on the ipsilateral side with the scrub nurse opposite.

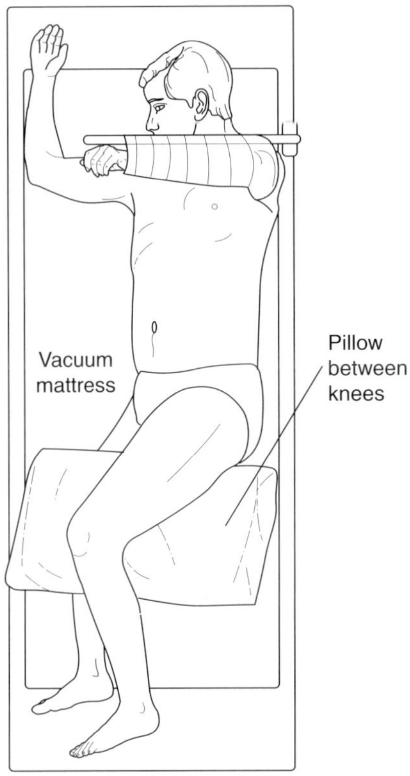

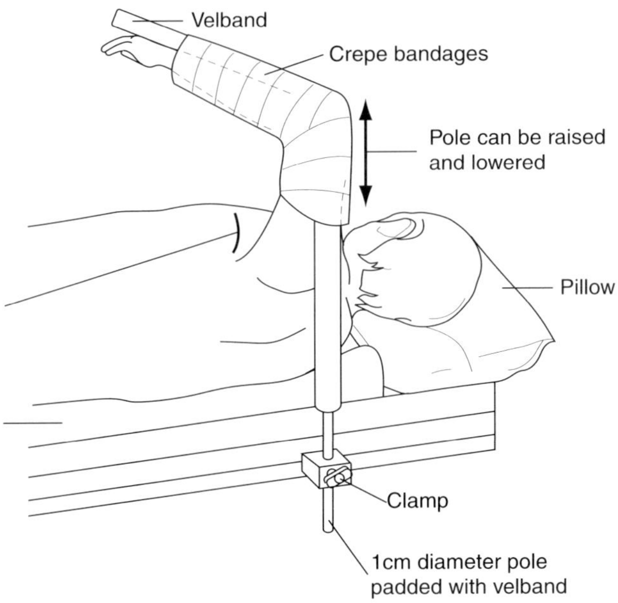

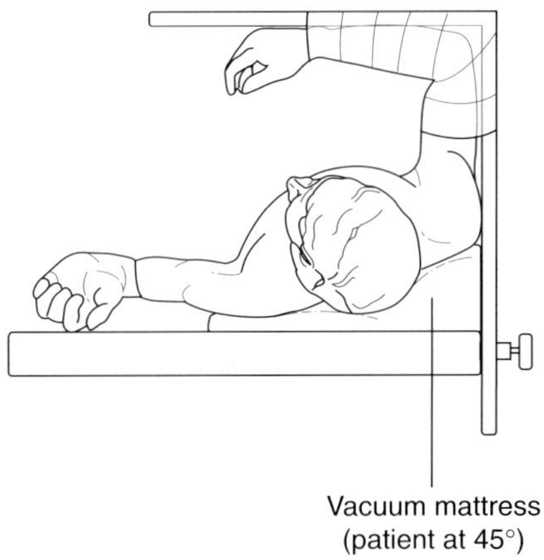

1

2

The incision is placed low in the axilla between the pectoralis major and latissimus dorsi muscles, in Langer's lines, following the axillomammary skin crease at the lower junction of the hair bearing area of the axilla. This crease is less obvious in males. The dissection is taken straight down to the chest wall, ligating and dividing the thoracoepigastric veins and the lateral thoracic artery. The dissection is posterior to the axillary tail of the breast and carries on down to the investing layer of thoracic fascia (2). The intercostobrachial nerve is variable – usually exiting via the second interspace. It is often possible to retract the nerve but if stretched or traumatized it is divided cleanly to avoid unpleasant postoperative neuralgia. Patients are counselled about this preoperatively.

3

The apex of the axilla is opened up by blunt dissection and the supreme intercostal artery and vein ligated in continuity and divided. This enables the neurovascular bundle to be elevated – the clamp is loosened and the angled bar elevated 10 cm or so, opening up the axilla but avoiding undue traction. We have not experienced nerve injury with this technique in over 200 cases. A loose swab is firmly pushed upwards to sweep the neurovascular bundle off the scalene muscles and left in place to achieve haemostasis whilst an angled retractor is inserted. An illuminated Deaver retractor is placed anteriorly. We use a 30 degree video laparoscope for illumination, teaching and dissection using conventional instruments (3). The Vital Vue suction, irrigation and light source is also useful.

4, 5

After identifying the subclavian vein and artery and the C8/T1 nerve root, the scalenus anterior muscle is cleared of its investing layer of fascia by sweeping upwards, taking the phrenic nerve with it. Lahey forceps are passed deep to the muscle and opened 2–3 cm. This elevates the subclavian artery and enables the muscle to be divided with scissors well above the rib, discouraging reattachment to the brachial plexus (4). The yellowish tendon of

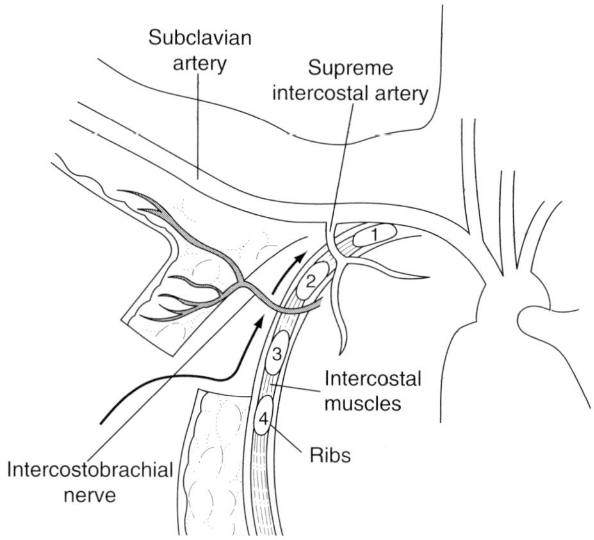

2

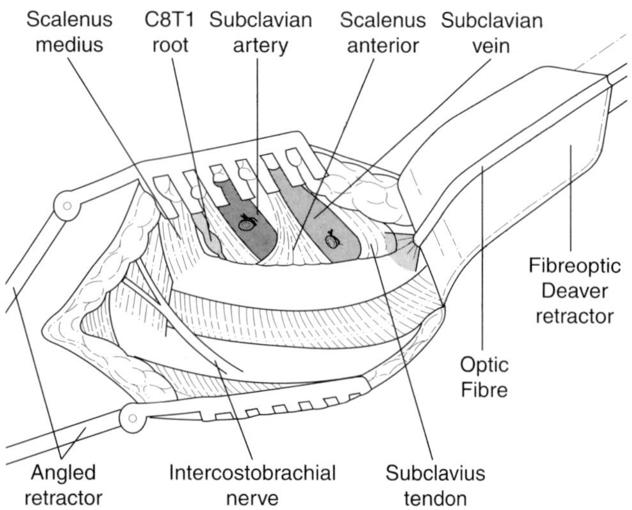

3

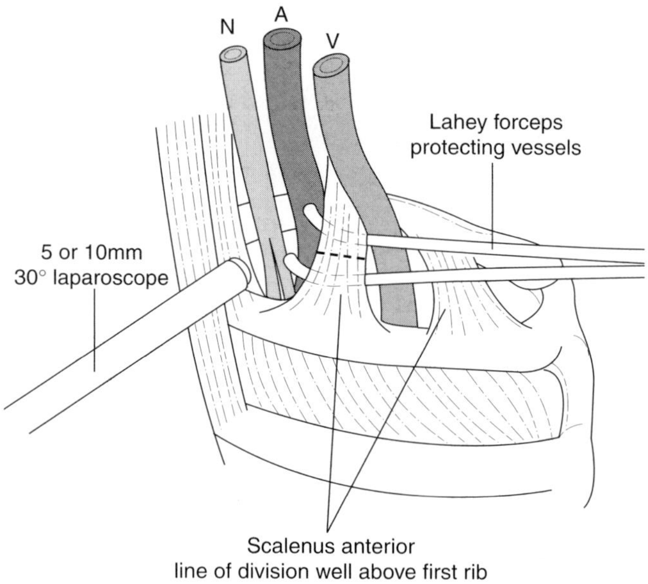

4

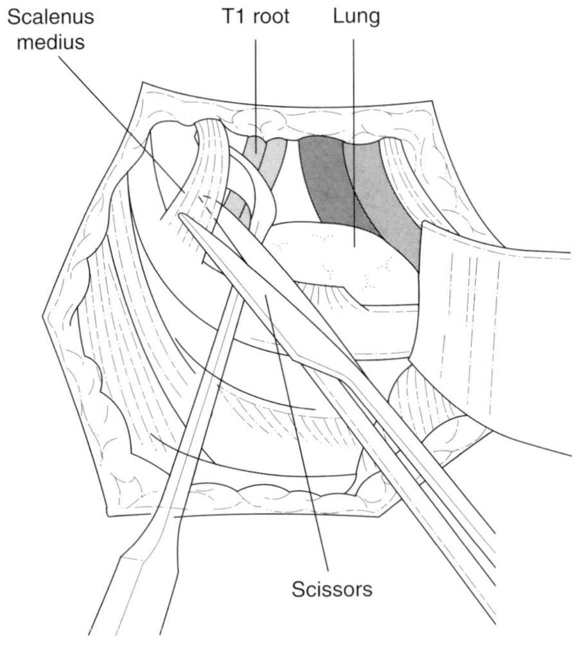

5

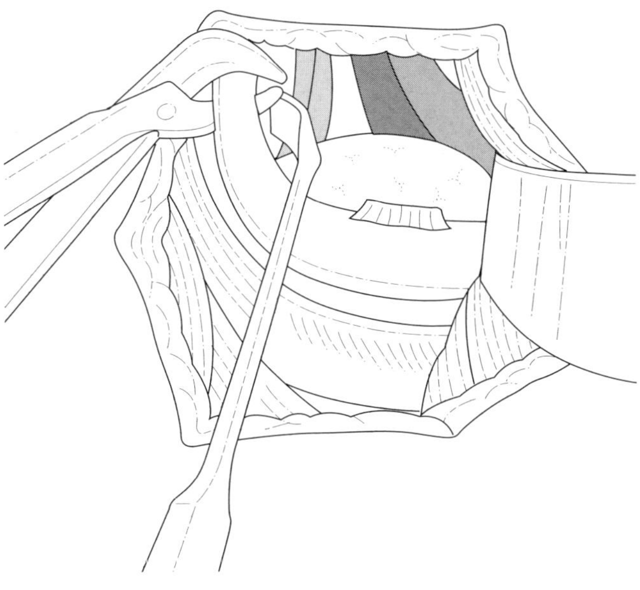

6

the subclavius muscle is seen anteriorly and the tip of a Roberts forceps used to gently separate it from the subclavian vein. It is then divided under direct vision. The C8/T1 root is gently swabbed upwards away from the scalenus medius muscle which is detached from its insertion into the upper border of the first rib using scissors and a periosteal elevator (5).

The hook of a double-edged ended raspatory is passed over the upper medial border of the rib and used to reflect the suprapleural membrane, which can be a tough structure. A large swab is then introduced and pushed into the apex of the thoracic cavity, reflecting and stripping the pleura away from the upper two ribs, assisting haemostasis and aiding visibility. The intercostal muscles are then divided with scissors just below the rib and the spatulated end of the double-ended raspatory used to clear the inferior border of the rib. Troublesome bleeding can occur at this stage, which should be left until all the anatomy has been confirmed.

6

Resection of the rib should be extraperiosteal to prevent regrowth. The rib is divided under direct vision behind the T1 root which is protected with an angled Roos spatula (6). If visibility is poor, the rib is divided more anteriorly and nibbled back after the central part has been removed. Angled rib shears are then used to divide the costal cartilage, carefully avoiding the subclavian vein. Once divided, the rib is removed very carefully using Kocher's forceps to avoid damage from bone spicules. The anterior and posterior stumps are then shortened and smoothed using nibblers. The posterior stump should be well clear of the T1 root to avoid reattachment to scar tissue. We are seldom able to cover the stump with the divided scalenus medius muscle. If a cervical rib is present it should be cleared of muscular attachments and divided as high as possible under vision using nibblers.

The neurovascular bundle is then re-examined and cleared of all possible constricting bands. Care must be exercised to avoid mistaking the transverse cervical or internal mammary arteries for bands. If bleeding does occur, the Vital Vue is invaluable as blind application of clips can result in neurological damage. Although the T2 ganglion is accessible, we prefer to perform a more precise sympathectomy using the video technique, before the rib is resected.

In cases of effort thrombosis or venous thoracic outlet syndrome, the subclavian vein is often encased in a cylindrical rind of fibrous tissue. This is gently and meticulously dissected free from the vein. A constant valve is seen within the vein at the confluence of subclavian and axillary veins, just above the first rib.

There should be no concerns over a breach in the pleura, which is probably beneficial, as blood clot will run into the chest where it is liquefied, rather than causing a haematoma around the plexus. A size 16FG suction drain is then inserted into the apex of the wound with constant suction during wound closure. Bupivicaine is instilled into the wound and cavity and the arm lowered. The wound is closed in two layers with absorbable sutures. Immediately following the operation the arm is massaged thoroughly to discourage superficial thrombosis and a postoperative chest X-ray is obtained in the recovery room.

Postoperatively the drain is removed at 24 hours. Combination analgesia with non-steroidal anti-inflammatories, codeine and paracetamol is normally sufficient. Light activities are encouraged immediately and mobilization under the direction of the physiotherapist is started to avoid shoulder joint contracture. We do not encourage aggressive or repetitive physiotherapy to discourage scar formation.

Redo surgery is a serious undertaking and should only be performed by expert operators. The principles are the same but the entire suprapleural membrane is excised to clear the T1 root which involves a painstaking dissection. The axillary fat pad is mobilized and reflected inwards to cover the brachial plexus on closing the wound to avoid adhesion formation.

Acknowledgements

This technique is a modification of that of Dr David Roos who has been a great inspiration.

Cervical sympathectomy

Giorgio M Biasi,
Paolo Mingazzini, Ugo Ruberti

Introduction

Although it is a commonly used term, 'cervical' sympathectomy is something of a misnomer, since it has never implied division of the cervical chain. The approach, which is via the neck to the upper thoracic sympathetic chain, has given rise to the term.

Indications

Since the first cervical sympathectomy performed in 1899 by Alexander for epilepsy (White *et al.*, 1952), this procedure has been applied for various indications. Nowadays the surgical ablation of thoracic (dorsal) sympathetic ganglia continues to play an important role in the treatment of a few selected pathologies.

Primary hyperhidrosis refractory to conservative treatment remains one of the main indications for the procedure with good postoperative results (Greenhalgh *et al.*, 1971). Excessive sweating of the hands frequently causes severe psychological and social problems, which can justify the surgical option if all medical measures fail. If abnormal axillary sweating is also present, a resection of the fourth thoracic ganglion, in addition to the second and the third, must be performed in order to obtain a complete sympathetic denervation of the axilla.

True causalgia and other pain syndromes like the post-traumatic sympathetic dystrophies can be relieved by upper thoracic sympathectomy, if diagnosed early and not treated sufficiently by physical therapy and nerve blocks (Witmoser, 1984; Kleinert *et al.*, 1973).

Ischaemic disorders of the upper extremity were the most common indications in the past; these can be caused by atherosclerotic disease as well as by other less common pathologies, such as Raynaud's syndrome, scleroderma, frostbite, embolism, thromboangiitis obliterans (Buerger's disease). The surgeon should always inform the patient that Raynaud's symptoms may recur in 1 or 2 years (Welch and Geary, 1984), a reason to reserve the surgical procedure for digital ulceration.

Raynaud's phenomenon is frequently associated with a collagen disease such as the CREST syndrome (calcinosis cutis, Raynaud's phenomenon, esophageal dysfunction, sclerodactyly and telangiectasia) and sympathectomy is then of limited value, but sometimes may delay the need for amputation (Harris and May, 1989). An unusual indication for cervical sympathectomy is the Long Q-T syndrome, a congenital disorder accompanied by a high incidence of sudden cardiac death. In this extremely rare disease, when resistant to the use of β-blockers, left cardiac sympathetic denervation obtained by stellectomy resulted in a marked reduction in the incidence of tachyarrhythmic syncope (Schwartz *et al.*, 1991)

Surgical approaches

Access to resect the thoracic sympathetic chain can be gained by several approaches.

The posterior approach described by Smithwick (1940), with excision of part of the third rib and transverse vertebral process, has been almost completely abandoned.

The extrapleural axillary approach through excision of the first rib (Ross, 1980) has low postoperative effects such as postoperative pain, but is technically demanding.

The transaxillary approach through the second or third intercostal space (Atkins, 1954) gives a good view of the sympathetic chain and allows extended resection to the fourth ganglion. (See following chapter – 'Transaxillary sympathectomy'.)

The supraclavicular approach is perhaps the classical route. It was proposed by Jonnesco (1923), Bruning (1923), Royle (1924) and later well described by Telford (1935) and Gask and Ross (1937). His approach has less complications for pulmonary function and less postoperative pain and is consequently preferred by many surgeons. The disadvantages are the deep and narrow surgical field which can cause difficulties (e.g. control of deep bleeding), therefore the surgeon must be very familiar with this procedure. Moreover, access to the lower part of the sympathetic chain is difficult, so if the fourth thoracic ganglion must also be resected, the transthoracic route is preferred.

The thorascopic approach is a new surgical technique since the first description dates back to 1943 by Hughes (Adams *et al.*, 1992), but recent improvements in instrumentation and technology have enhanced the possibilities of this minimally invasive approach.

In this chapter we will describe in detail the supraclavicular approach which is the one that we most frequently adopt.

Anatomy

1

The thoracic sympathetic chain passes vertically down the side of the vertebral column deep to the pleura on the rib necks.

The first thoracic ganglion fuses with the inferior cervical ganglion forming the stellate ganglion. Thoracic ganglia receive preganglionic fibres from the thoracic spinal cord via the white rami communicantes from the adjacent spinal nerve. These fibres synapse in the ganglion where postganglionic fibres commence and pass back to the nerve root via grey rami communicantes. The sympathetic outflow to the upper limb is from within the spinal cord at level thoracic 5–9. The fibres either pass up the spinal cord and then cross via rami communicantes at a higher thoracic level or near the original outflow (5–9). To interrupt the sympathetic supply to the upper limb the chain must be transected below the third ganglion and all rami cut including to the second ganglion.

Some consider it necessary to resect the thoracic component of the stellate ganglion (lower one-third), for complete sympathetic denervation of the upper limb, but it is not necessary and adds to the risk of Horner's syndrome.

The operation

2

The operation is performed under general anaesthesia with tracheal intubation, because accidental opening of the pleural dome can cause a pneumothorax. With the patient's head turned away from the side of the incision and with the neck slightly hyperextended, a horizontal incision is made 1 cm above the superior border of the clavicle, 1–2 cm lateral to the jugular fossa on the anterior face of the clavicular head of the sternocleidomastoid muscle. An incision of 5–6 cm is sufficient to facilitate division of the clavicular head of the sternomastoid. The incision passes through the platysma muscle and the external jugular vein may have to be divided.

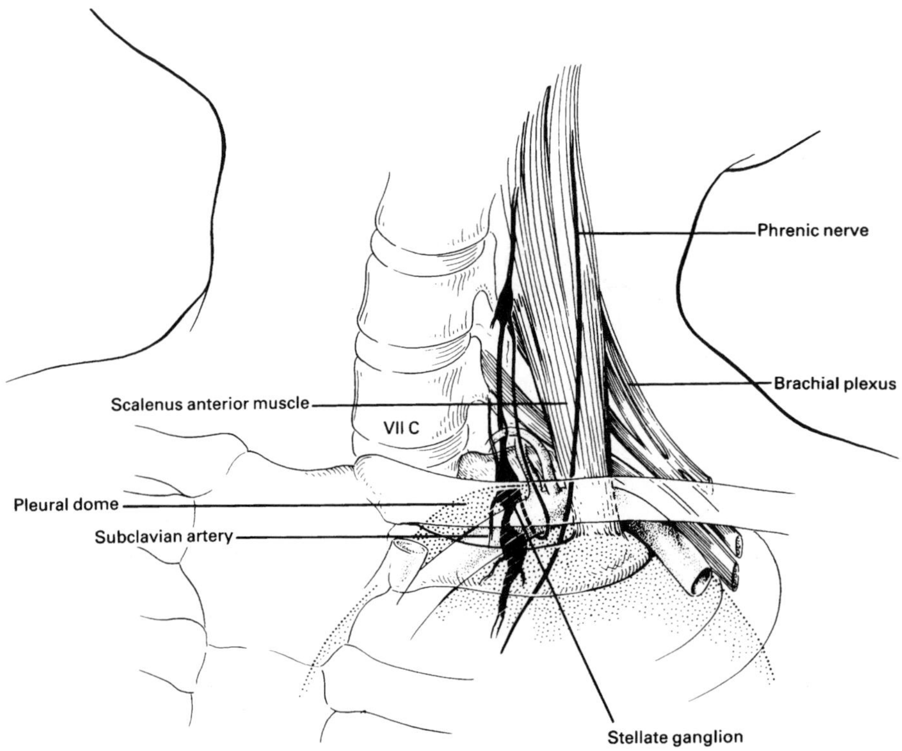

1

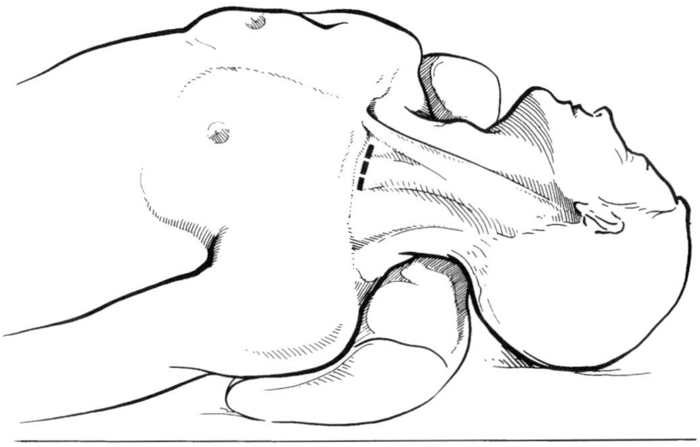

2

3

The clavicular head of the sternocleidomastoid muscle is then divided, leaving sufficient muscle below for the reconstruction. The omohyoid muscle crosses the operative field obliquely and occasionally it may have to be divided.

4

The internal jugular vein is identified and preserved. The scalene pad of fat with lymph nodes is situated in the centre of the field; this is displaced upwards and must sometimes be divided between clips. The scalenus anterior muscle is now visible. The phrenic nerve, attached to the muscle by fascia, can be seen running from lateral to medial on the muscle from above downwards. The nerve must be dissected free and isolated. Using extreme delicacy it is retracted medially with a small retractor or, preferably, with a Silastic loop. The scalenus anterior muscle is then divided very near its insertion into the first rib. Immediately behind the scalene muscle lies the subclavian artery and from it the vertebral artery branches and runs upward. It is vital, therefore, when dissecting the scalene muscle, to avoid damage to these deep vascular structures. For this reason some surgeons first pass an instrument behind the muscle before dissecting it. However, we prefer not to perform this potentially dangerous manoeuvre, and instead cautiously dissect the muscle with an electroknife, eventually inserting the index finger of the left hand behind the remaining bundles of the muscle. The muscle fibres retract as

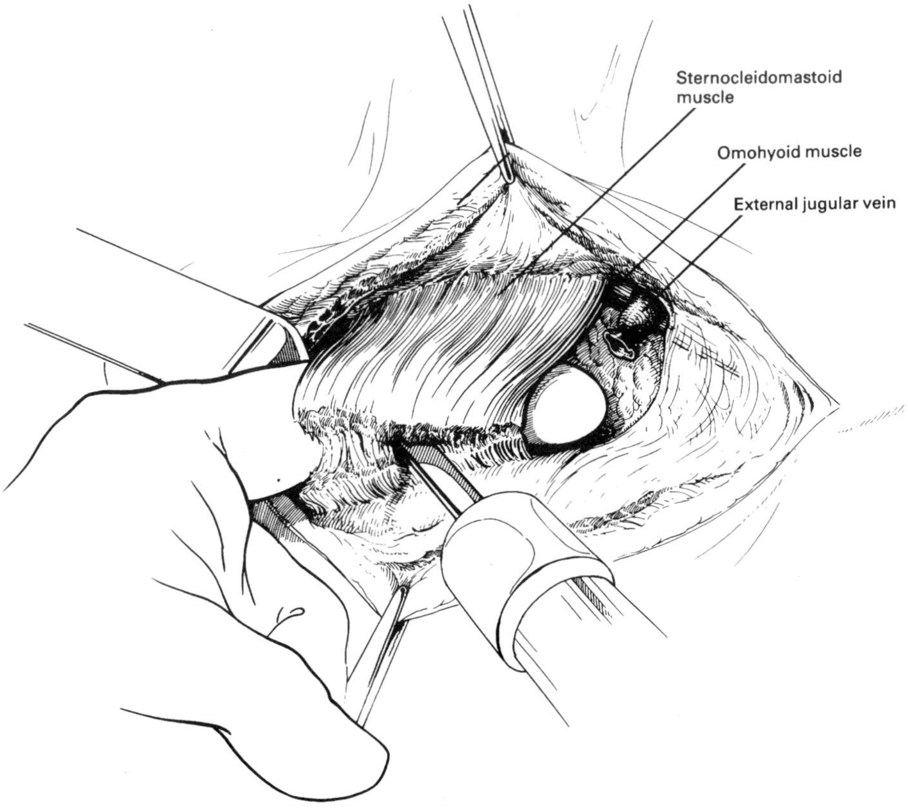

3

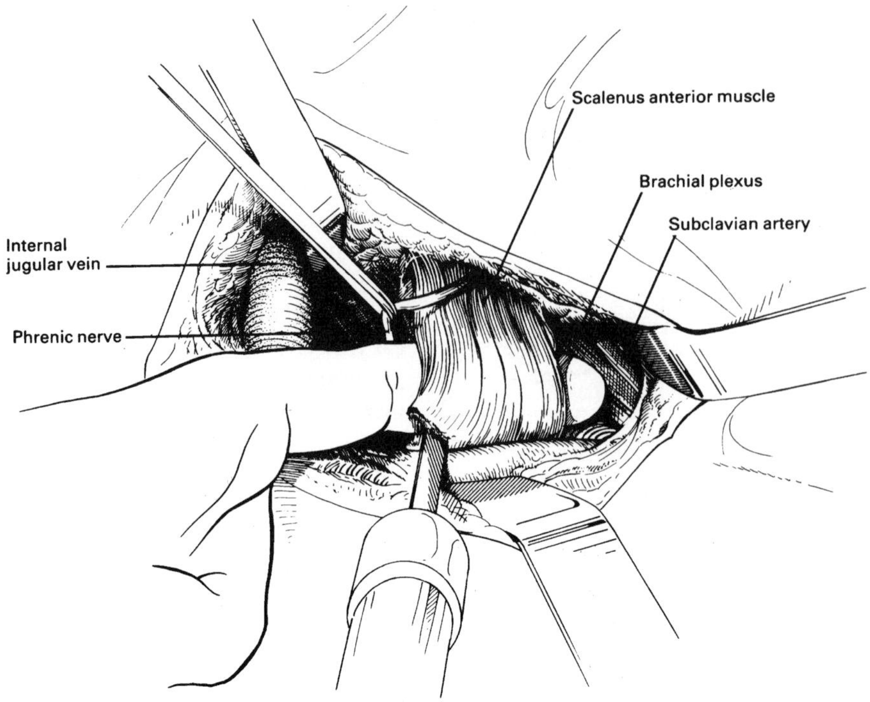

4

the dissection proceeds and, when only a few layers remain, the transparent sheath of the subclavian artery can be seen. The last muscle fibres are then cut with dissecting scissors.

5

The subclavian arch is thus isolated from the internal jugular vein and under it lies the vertebral artery. Distally the thyrocervical trunk, which may be tied, originates from the subclavian artery. Whenever a *left* sympathectomy is performed one should be aware of the presence of the thoracic duct that emerges from the mediastinum and enters the subclavian vein lateral to its confluence with the internal jugular vein. At this point, the subclavian arch is retracted upward to display the apex of the lung, the pleural dome and the suprapleural membrane (Sibson's fascia). Sibson's fascia is bluntly dissected from

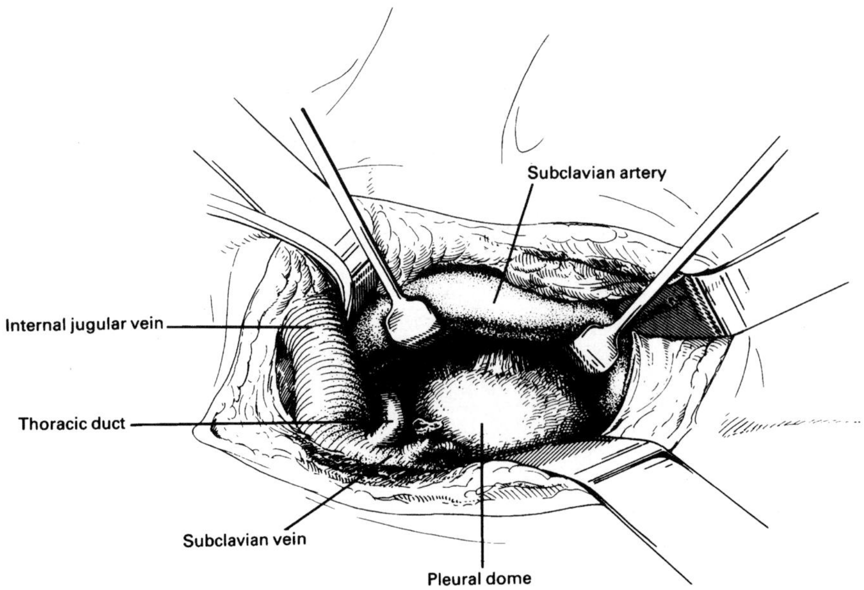

5

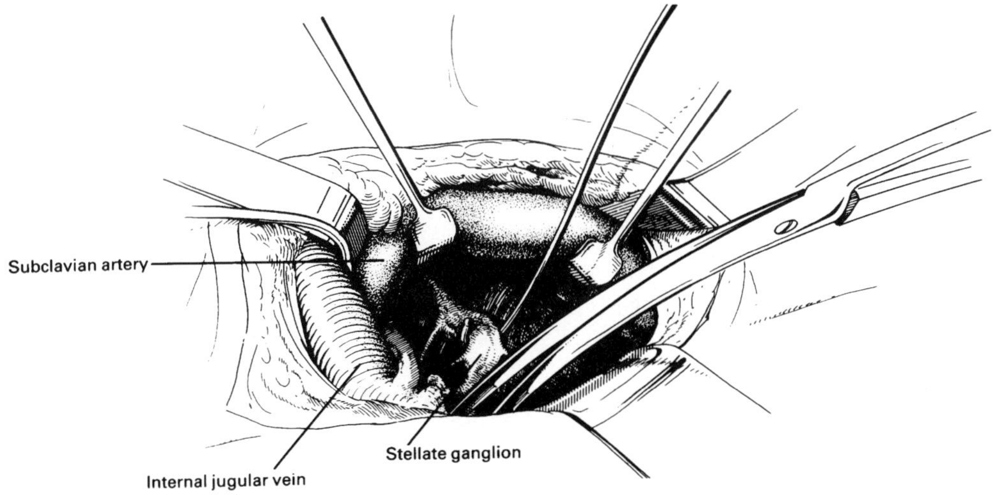

6

the rib, thus allowing entry to the retropleural space. It begins to strip more easily below on the medial side. Once the stripping begins a swab is gently pushed into the enlarging space with the index finger until the lung is fully depressed without injury to the pleura.

6

The sympathetic chain can now be seen but it is more important that the surgeon's hand be guided by a sense of touch in this deep space. The chain is like a thick corded structure that passes across the neck of the first rib. The intercostal artery and vein must be carefully avoided (the first intercostal artery is a branch of the subclavian costocervical trunk). The chain is palpated with the finger and an illuminated lighted retractor is used to view it. A hook is then used to lift the sympathetic chain which is traced as far as possible. Usually, it is easy to reach the third thoracic ganglion and below this the chain is divided and delivered upwards. All of the rami communicantes are divided between neurosurgical metal clips, but the stellate ganglion is not mobilized for fear of producing Horner's syndrome. Some surgeons divide the chain and take the lower part of the stellate ganglion, but it has been shown that embedding the cut chain into the scalenus anterior muscle with a transfixion stitch is sufficient.

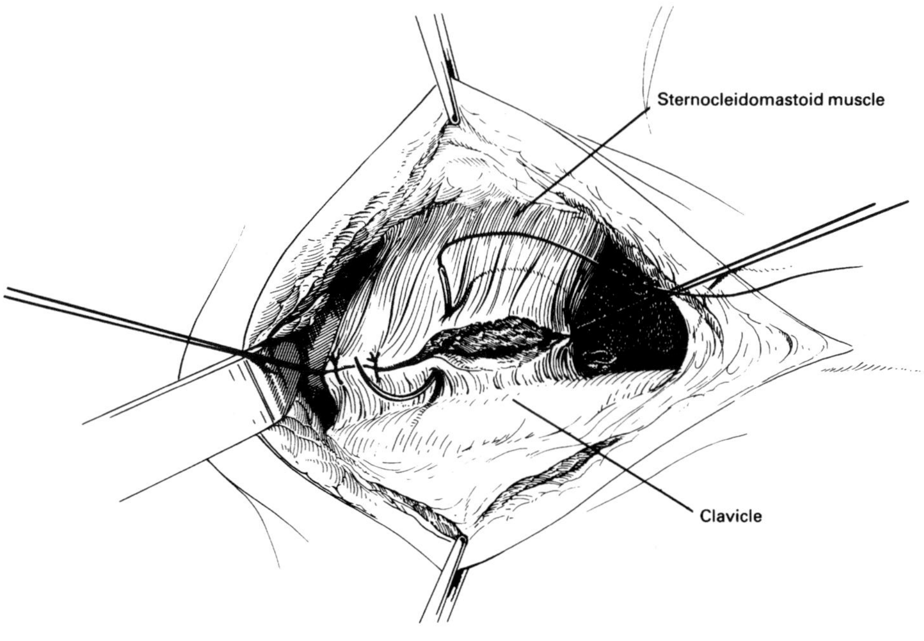

7

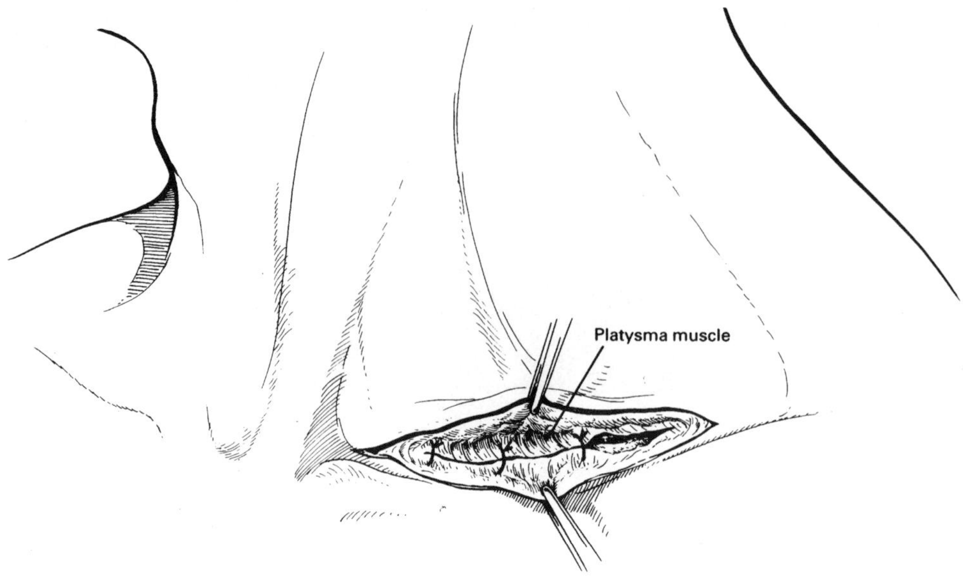

8

7, 8

Once haemostasis has been secured the incision is closed without drainage. (However, if damage to the pleural dome is suspected, it is advisable to place a slender catheter in the extrapleural space.) The edges of the clavicular head of the sternocleidomastoid muscle are brought together, followed by the platysma muscle, with fine catgut sutures. Finally, the skin is closed, either with Michelle clips or very fine nylon sutures. If a drain is used a Redivac suction drain is usually ideal.

Complications

There are complications of sympathectomy: temporary sweating of the palms in the postoperative period, usually lasts for 1–3 days only; compensatory hyperhidrosis may present on the contralateral side or in other parts of the body after sympathectomy but which reduces in time. Postoperative pain may occur, such as neuralgia of the face, shoulder or chest region; it is more frequent after axillary procedures but seldom lasts more than a few weeks. A postsympathetic neuralgia is fortunately rare, but the severe pain in the upper arm may be really debilitating and may last several months. Horner's syndrome, with ptosis of the lid, endophthalmitis and miosis is more frequent after the supraclavicular procedure, but may affect all approaches. It is mandatory to discuss this possibility with the patient before surgery, as well as other possible complications. Horner's syndrome is associated with nasal congestion and visual disturbance, or with dryness of the nasal mucosa and loss of facial sweating, but is rarely permanent.

Lymph fistula and lymphocoele may occur after the supraclavicular procedure. Chylothorax may also occasionally occur, requiring dissection and ligation of the thoracic duct and chest drainage. Incomplete re-expansion of the lung, or frank pneumothorax are possible but pulmonary complications are more frequent after the transthoracic route.

Acknowledgements
Illustrations by Greco.

References

Adams D C R, Wood S J, Tulloh B R *et al.* (1992). Endoscopic transthoracic sympathectomy. *Eur Vasc Surg* 6: 558.

Atkins H J B (1954). Sympathectomy by the axillary approach. *Lancet* 1: 538.

Bruning, F (1923). Weitere Erfahrungen uber den Sympathiens. *Klin Walkenschr* 2.

Gask G E, Ross J P (1937). *The Surgery of the Sympathetic Nervous System.* Baltimore: W Wood and Co.

Greenhalgh R M, Rosengarten D S, Martin P (1971). Role of sympathectomy for hyperhidrosis. *Br Med J* 1: 322.

Harris J P, May J (1989). Upper extremity sympathectomy. In *Vascular Surgery.* Rutherford R B ed. London: W B Saunders Co.

Jonnesco, T (1923). *Le Sympatique Cervico-thoracique.* Paris: Masson.

Kleinert H E, Cole N M, Wayne L (1973). Post-traumatic sympathetic dystrophy. *Orth Clin N Amer* 4: 917.

May J, Harris J P (1984). Upper extremity sympathectomy: A comparison of the supraclavicular and axillary approaches in evaluation and treatment of upper and lower extremity circulatory disorders. In *Operative Techniques in Vascular Surgery.* Bergan J J, Yao J S T eds. New York: Grune and Stratton.

Ross D B (1980). Transaxillary extrapleural thoracic sympathectomy. In *Operative Techniques in Vascular Surgery.* Bergan J J, Yao J S T eds. New York: Grune and Stratton.

Royle N D (1924). The treatment of spastic paralysis by sympathetic ramisection. *Surg Gynecol Obstet* 39: 701.

Schwartz P J, Locati E H, Moss E J *et al.* (1991). Left cardiac sympathetic denervation in the therapy of congenital long QT syndrome (world-wide report). *Circulation* 84: 503.

Smithwick R H (1940). The rationale of sympathectomy for the relief of vascular spasm of the extremities. *New Engl J Med* 222: 699.

Telford E D (1935). The technique of sympathectomy. *Br J Surg* 23: 448.

Welch E, Geary J (1984). Current status of thoracic dorsal sympathectomy. *J Vasc Surg* 1: 202.

White J C, Smithwick R H, Simeone F A (1952). *The Autonomic Nervous System: Anatomy, Physiology and Surgical Application.* New York: Macmillan.

Witmoser R (1984). Possibilities of using sympathectomy for treatment of pain syndromes. *Appl Neurophysiol* 47: 203.

Transaxillary sympathectomy

Harold Ellis

Preoperative

Indications

Excision of the upper portion of the thoracic part of the sympathetic chain has, as its main indication, the treatment of severe idiopathic hyperhidrosis of the hands. This has an equal sex distribution, although women with this condition are more likely to complain of the excessive associated axillary sweating. Symptoms usually commence at the time of puberty but may be seen in childhood (Law and Ellis, 1989). All four limbs may be affected but individual patients may complain that the sweating of the axillae, the hands or the feet is the principal nuisance. There is often little difference during summer or winter and the sweating is not usually aggravated by exercise. It is precipitated by emotional or mental stress and ceases during sleep. There is often an associated Raynaud's phenomenon, with the hands and feet being cold and blue as well as sweating.

The cause of this condition is unknown. The sweat glands in the involved areas are normal, both histologically and numerically. Histochemical and electron microscopic changes cannot be detected. The clinical effects of severe hyperhidrosis are most distressing; slippery objects drop out of wet hands, it may be impossible to use a pen and the patient avoids social contact.

Upper thoracic sympathectomy is also indicated in severe examples of Raynaud's phenomenon which do not respond to conservative measures. However, unlike the permanent results of sympathectomy for hyperhidrosis, there is a tendency to progressive relapse following the operation so that only some 50% of patients show persistent improvement when assessed several years postoperatively.

Advantages and disadvantages of the transthoracic approach

The advantages of the transthoracic approach are the almost invisible scar, which lies hidden in the axilla, the avoidance of Horner's syndrome in the great majority of cases, provided that the stellate ganglion is carefully preserved, and the simplicity of the anatomical approach to the chain compared with the transcervical technique.

The disadvantages of the operation are that most surgeons, including the author, consider that it is only safe to perform one side at a time. I usually leave at least a month between the two operations in bilateral cases. Some surgeons, however, have practised synchronous bilateral thoracotomy successfully. The operation is also contraindicated if there has been previous intrathoracic infection, e.g. quiescent pulmonary tuberculosis, with resultant pleural adhesions. In such cases (and I have only encountered one example of this) the transcervical approach becomes mandatory.

Where the expertise and facilities are available, transthoracoscopic diathermy coagulation of the chain is now the operation of choice. The scar is minimal, both sides can be dealt with at the same sitting and, in trained hands, the morbidity is negligible.

This is described in the following chapter – 'Sympathectomy by thoracoscopy'. It should be remembered, however, that occasionally adhesions at the lung apex make the endoscopic method virtually impossible – it is important to be familiar with the classical approach.

Surgical anatomy

1

In planning excision of the upper thoracic sympathetic chain for sympathetic denervation of the upper limb and axilla, the surgeon needs to know how much of the chain to remove in order to effect satisfactory denervation and how to prevent Horner's syndrome. The thoracic portion of the chain continues downwards from the cervical sympathetic chain and lies anterior to the heads of the ribs. It lies immediately external to the parietal pleura, almost invariably immediately anterior to the intercostal vessels. However, the chain lies uncomfortably close to the intercostal veins, which may occasionally cross in

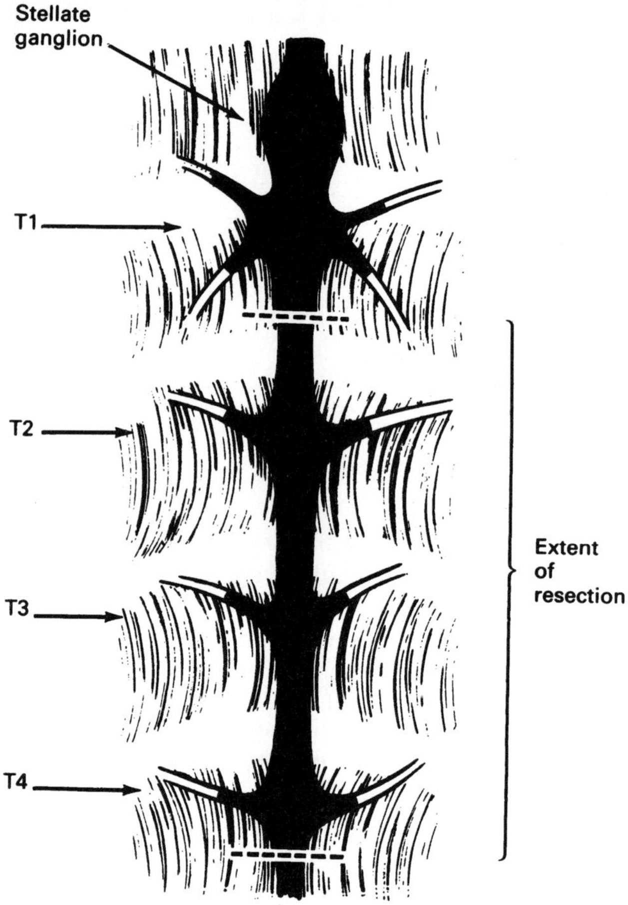

1

front of it. Each ganglion is situated fairly consistently in front of the corresponding rib head.

The first thoracic ganglion may be independent or, more usually, is fused to the inferior cervical ganglion to constitute the stellate ganglion. Occasionally, the second thoracic ganglion may be fused into this ganglionic conglomeration. Each ganglion lies below the level of the corresponding intercostal nerve to which it is connected by the white ramus communicans of preganglionic fibres and the grey (postganglionic) ramus. The grey ramus usually lies medially to the white ramus but occasionally these are combined into a single trunk and at times there may be more than two rami.

The fibres in the white ramus communicans of the first thoracic nerve ascend in the chain to the superior cervical ganglion in order to supply sympathetic fibres to the face. Interruption of the sympathetic chain at or above this first thoracic ganglion level will thus result in Horner's syndrome, comprising ptosis, pupillary constriction, flushing of the face and facial anhidrosis on the affected side.

The second thoracic nerve is the highest one to contain preganglionic fibres to the upper limb. There is much more variability to the lower limit and fibres as low as the seventh thoracic nerve may contribute fibres to the upper limb. Although there is this widespread origin of preganglionic fibres to the upper limb, division of the thoracic sympathetic chain immediately below the first ganglion will usually interrupt all fibres that traverse the sympathetic chain to reach the upper limb by distribution through the brachial plexus. In practice, removal of the thoracic sympathetic chain to include the second, third and fourth ganglia, which means removing the chain from the head of the second to the head of the fourth rib, is found to produce effective sympathetic denervation of the upper limb and axilla.

Surgical technique

2

The transaxillary approach was first described by Sir Hedley Atkins in 1949. Endotracheal general anaesthesia is used. The patient is placed in the lateral position with the arm abducted to 90 degrees. A suitable right-angled arm support is used. It is convenient to tilt the patient in the head-up position at about 20 degrees to allow adequate illumination of the depths of the wound. It is useful to have a malleable light on a probe to improve illumination if necessary, particularly in an obese patient.

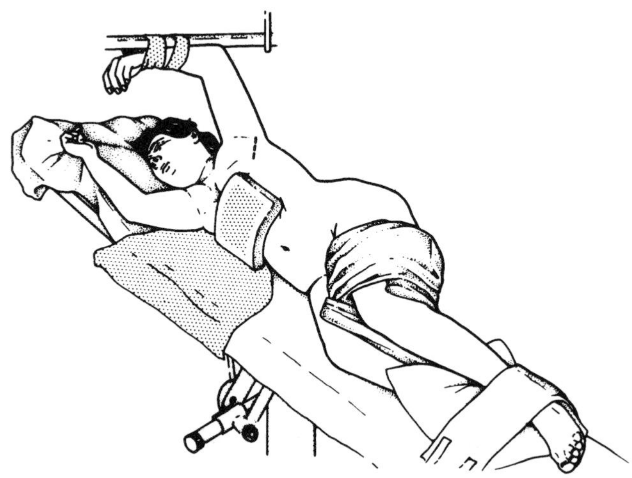

2

3

The incision is made along the line of the second intercostal space from pectoralis major in front to latissimus dorsi posteriorly. The obliquity of this incision varies quite considerably from one subject to another. Because the area is quite vascular, bleeding is controlled by preliminary infiltration of the subcutaneous tissues with a 1 : 200 000 solution of adrenaline in normal saline and by the use of the diathermy cutting needle. The incision

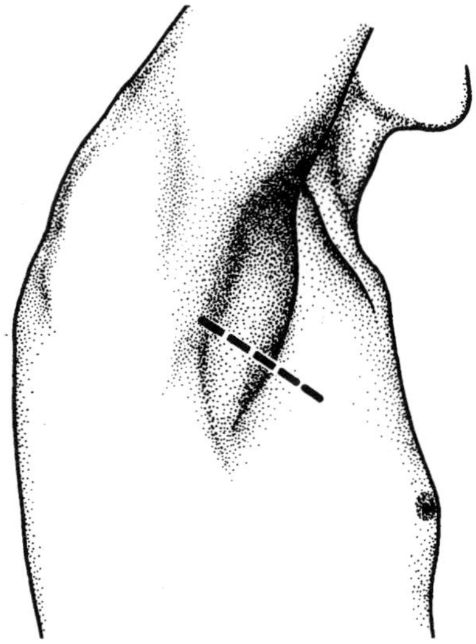

3

is made through the axillary fat down to the serratus anterior. The nerve to this muscle (the long thoracic nerve of Bell) is identified at the posterior limit of the incision and is carefully preserved. Injury to this nerve will produce winging of the scapula.

The second intercostal space is now palpated and the serratus divided with diathermy over the space. The dissection is then continued through the intercostal muscles down to the pleura. By staying immediately superior to the second rib, damage to the intercostal bundle can be avoided. The pleura is opened, the lung collapses and the intercostal space is opened for the full length of the wound. The ribs are then retracted by means of a Price-Thomas self-retaining retractor which is slowly opened to its full extent. A wet pack is placed over the collapsed lung, which is retracted downwards by means of a suitably bent malleable copper retractor.

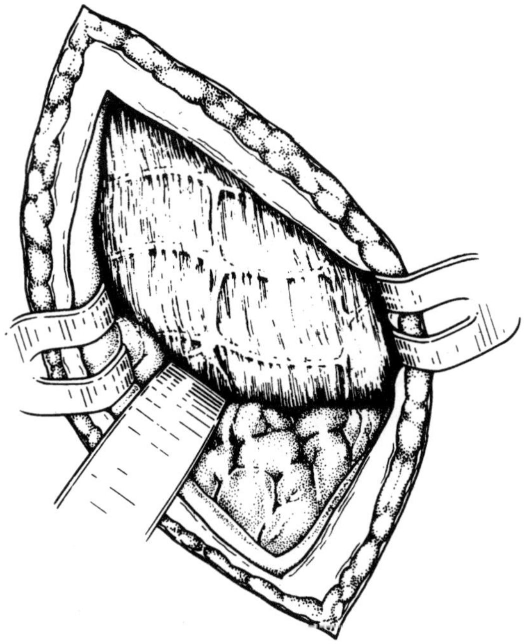

4

4

The sympathetic chain can now be easily identified as it lies beneath the parietal pleura on the heads of the upper ribs. On the right side, the azygos vein is seen lying medially to the chain, whereas on the left side, the aorta and left subclavian artery can be seen.

It is important to identify the sympathetic chain quite precisely before the parietal pleura is opened, otherwise oozing of blood may obscure the anatomy. The line of the chain is indicated on the pleura by two or three scalpel nicks and 2 or 3 ml of the dilute adrenaline solution is then injected via a fine needle beneath the pleura to free it from the underlying ribs.

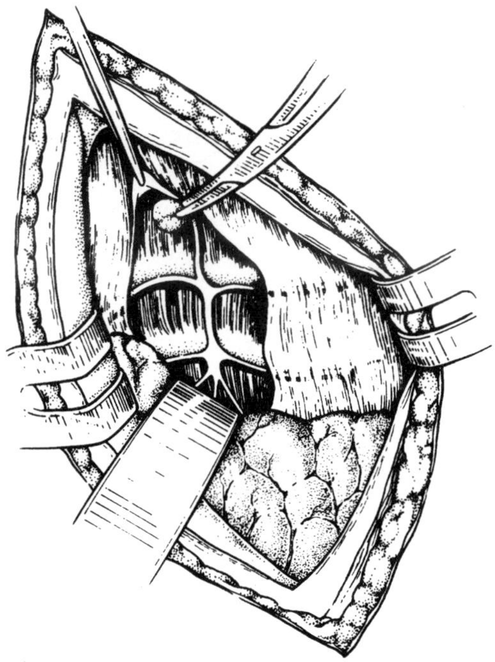

5

5

The parietal pleura is now divided longitudinally along the line of the sympathetic chain using a fine scalpel blade on a long handle. The pleura is pushed aside from the chain by means of small gauze pledgets held in long artery forceps.

The chain is caught up on a nerve hook and carefully removed from below upwards from the level of the fourth rib to just below the stellate ganglion, thus removing the fourth, third and second ganglia.

6

Bleeding may be encountered from branches of the intercostal vessels, particularly the veins, and haemostasis is effected by means of diathermy coagulation, Cushing's silver clips or a combination of the two.

It is my practice to mark the upper and lower extremities of the chain resection by means of Cushing's clips so that subsequent radiology can confirm the extent of the resection.

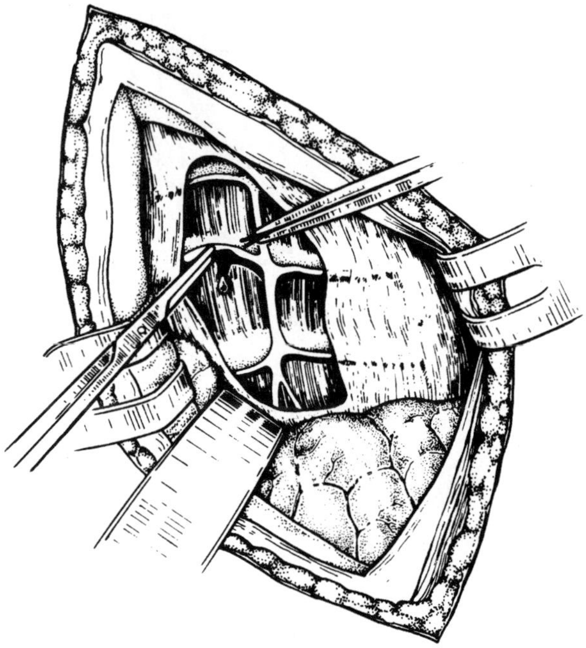

6

A check is made to ensure complete haemostasis before the anaesthetist is asked to inflate the lung.

A plastic intercostal tube is inserted through the second space and brought out through a small stab wound. The wound is closed in layers using catgut, the skin sutured and the intercostal drain connected with an underwater seal. Meanwhile, the anaesthetist continues to ensure that the lung is completely inflated in order to obliterate the pneumothorax.

The patient is transferred to the recovery room and, when conscious, a check X-ray of the chest is carried out. If this confirms that complete expansion of the lung has occurred, the chest tube can be removed in the recovery room before the patient is returned to the ward.

Postoperative care

The patient requires vigorous postoperative chest physiotherapy and a repeat chest X-ray the day following operation ensures the absence of a pneumothorax or pleural effusion. The majority of patients can leave hospital 3 or 4 days postoperatively.

References

Atkins H J B (1949). Per axillary approach to the stellate and upper thoracic sympathetic ganglia. *Lancet* **2**: 1152.

Ellis H (1979). Transaxillary sympathectomy in the treatment of hyperhidrosis of the upper limb. *Am Surg* **45**: 546.

Law N, Ellis H (1989). Transthoracic sympathectomy for hyperhidrosis in children under the age of 16. *Ann R Coll Surg Engl* **71**: 70.

Sympathectomy by thoracoscopy

Alun Davies, Gill Clayton

Introduction

Palmer hyperhidrosis is a disabling condition often affecting the young with deleterious effects on their social lifestyle and employment. Traditional open surgical techniques have been associated with significant morbidity. Thoracoscopic sympathectomy is now the most widely accepted approach to cervicothoracic sympathectomy. The upper dorsal sympathetic chain can be well visualized through a thoracoscope and successfully divided. Electrocautery (Byrne *et al.*, 1990) has also been used but there can be a danger to the stellate ganglion and for this we are in favour of staying at the neck of the second rib and below.

Preoperative

This operation should be considered in those patients whose sweating is severe enough to interfere significantly with their occupation or enjoyment of life (Blumberg, 1986). Patients selected for this procedure require preoperative chest X-ray, thyroid function tests and examination to exclude a systemic disease causing excessive sweating.

The operation

Position

1

The procedure is performed under anaesthesia with a double lumen tube. The patient is placed supine with both arms abducted to 60 degrees and supported on arm boards.

Procedure

2, 3

Both sides of the chest can be operated on under the same anaesthetic.

Using blunt dissection a size 10-mm thoracoscope is inserted through the fourth intercostal space, mid-axillary line. A second small cannula is then placed under direct vision through the second intercostal space mid-clavicular line. The insulated monopolar diathermy electrode is introduced through this port (1).

The second rib is the highest rib visible. The ribs are followed medially until the sympathetic ganglia and chain is seen overlying the neck of the ribs beneath the pleura. The sympathetic chain can be identified by using the diathermy probe to confirm its soft consistency.

On the right side the superior vena cava, azygos vein and vagus nerve should be identified.

In the left chest the subclavian artery and vagus nerve can be seen medially (2).

The diathermy probe is used to incise the pleura immediately over the sympathetic chain. The second ganglion is identified beneath the yellow fat pad overlying the stellate ganglion. The ganglion and chain immediately above and below are ablated to expose bare rib. The diathermy current is applied laterally for 2 cm along the neck of the second and third ribs to ablate the nerve of Kuntz (Kuntz, 1927).

The diathermy probe and cannula are removed under direct vision and the lung reinflated. The presence of any residual pneumothorax will be seen on withdrawal of the thoracoscope. If the lung is fully inflated the thoracoscope and cannula can be removed and the wounds sutured. A chest drain is not necessary.

A single thoracoscope inserted in the fourth intercostal space mid-axillary line, with a resectascope with a single side channel for a diathermy hook can be used as an alternative method.

Postoperative care

A postoperative chest X-ray should be performed to confirm lung inflation.

Complications

A small pneumothorax may persist for 24 hours postoperatively. Bleeding from an intercostal artery can be avoided by careful coagulation.

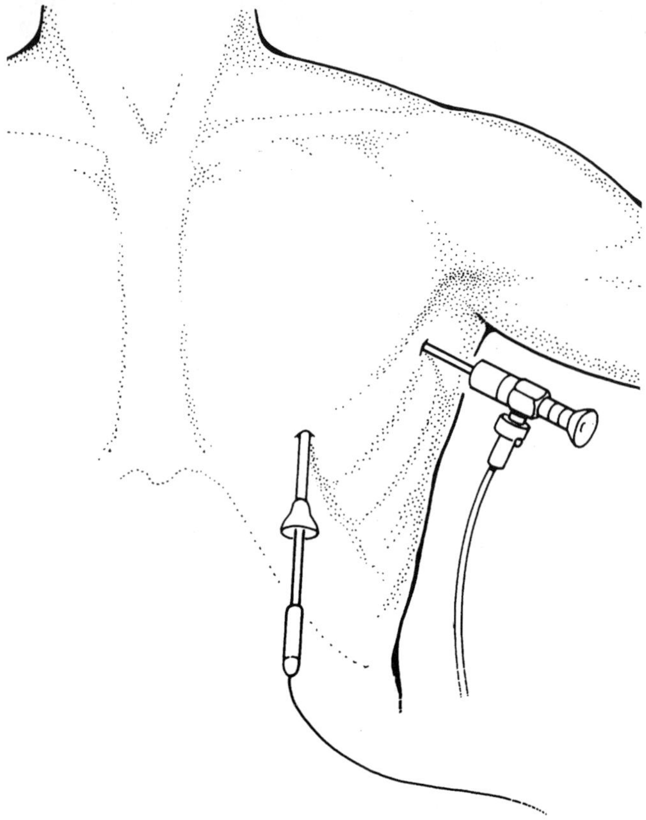

1

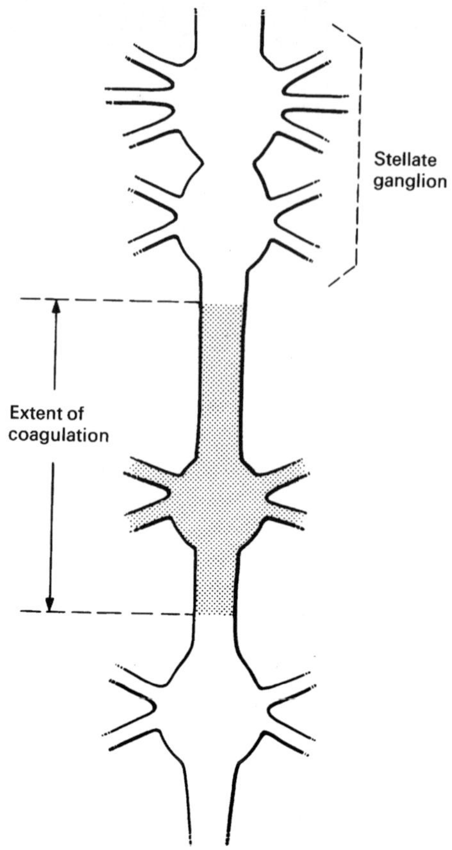

3

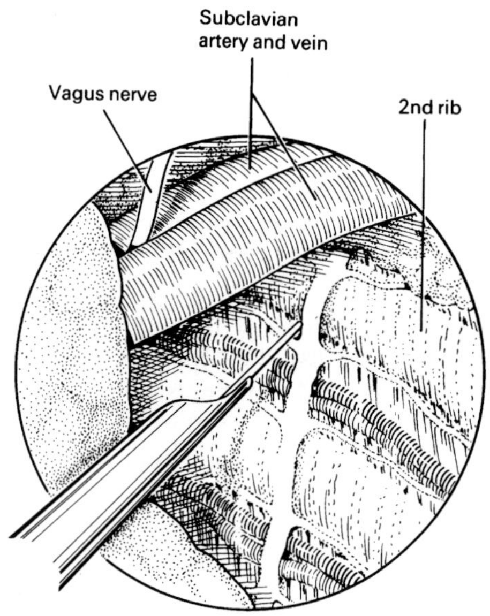

2

Horner's syndrome can likewise be avoided by using a low diathermy current and dissection only below the second rib (3).

Compensatory hyperhidrosis may occur in up to 50% of patients (Rennie, 1996). Pleuritic chest pain is common.

Acknowledgements

Illustrations 1–3 are reproduced from WP Hederman (1994). Sympathectomy by thorascopy. In *Vascular and Endovascular Surgical Techniques* 3rd edn. RG Greenhalgh ed. London: WB Saunders Co, pp. 281–284.

References

Blumberg L (1986). Endoscopic thoracic sympathectomy in the treatment of upper limb hyperhidrosis. *Ann Roy Coll Surg Engl* **68**:293.

Byrne J, Walsh TN, Hederman WP (1990). Endoscopic transthoracic electrocautery of the sympathetic chain for palmar and axillary hyperhidrosis. *Br J Surg* **17**:1046.

Kuntz A (1927). Distribution of the sympathetic rami to the brachial plexus: its relation to sympathectomy affecting the upper extremity. *Arch of Surg* **113**:264.

Rennie J. (1996). Compensatory sweating: an avoidable complication of thoracoscopic sympathectomy? *Min Invas Ther All Technol* **5**:101.

Subclavian and axillary artery angioplasty and stenting

Trevor J Cleveland

Introduction

Peripheral vascular disease affecting the legs is a common clinical problem, frequently seen in conjunction with coronary and renal artery disease. Atheromatous disease affecting the supra-aortic vessels is usually seen at the carotid bifurcation where it makes a major contribution to the aetiology of stroke. Less commonly the same disease process affects the arterial supply to the upper limbs by causing stenoses or occlusions in the brachial cephalic artery, subclavian artery or the axillary arteries. Vascular compromise to the arms is usually, but not always, due to atheroma. It may also arise from traumatic injury or inflammatory causes such as Takayasu's aortitis. The 'central' location of these lesions makes them problematic from the point of view of surgical access, in that these arteries are in intimate relationship with other structures, such as the brachial plexus, or require complicated surgical access such as sternal splitting. These factors, along with advances in endovascular technology and techniques, makes angioplasty and stenting an attractive alternative to open surgical techniques.

1

Access to upper limb lesions needs to be tailored to the individual lesion. In general, stenoses are less complex,

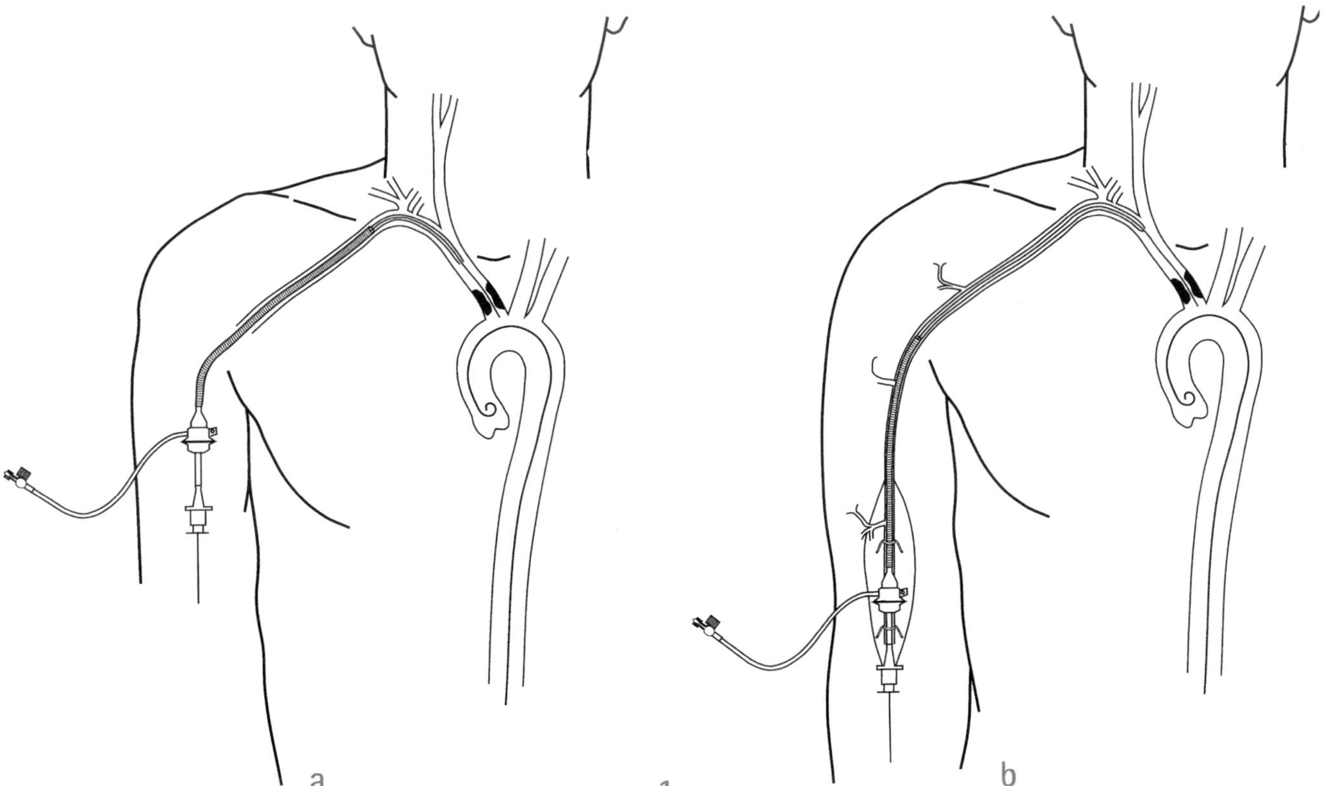

1

particularly in the left subclavian artery. The majority of endovascular procedures are performed from the transfemoral route, as the femoral artery is of sufficient size and is superficial. The route from the femoral artery to the left subclavian artery is a relatively straight one, and there is little need for catheter manipulation across the carotid artery origins. Selective catheterization of the left subclavian artery, using standard-shaped catheters (e.g. Headhunter) is therefore usually easy; however, the majority of lesions are close to the left subclavian origin and so the catheter tip may traverse the lesion in a relatively uncontrolled fashion. With modern, small diameter, soft tipped catheters, this is usually of little consequence, certainly in the left subclavian artery, where the cerebral consequences of microembolus is remote. There is also often reversed flow in the vertebral artery thereby protecting the cerebral circulation. The situation is different in the brachiocephalic artery where the right carotid territory is at risk from microemboli. In these lesions a more controlled wire and catheter traversal is recommended (**1a**). A pigtail catheter is placed in the aortic arch from the femoral artery, and the patient's vascular anatomy is roadmapped from this. A guidewire/catheter combination is then placed from the ipsilateral brachial artery and used to traverse the lesion. Percutaneous access to the femoral artery will allow introduction of all the necessary equipment, but until recently 7 French delivery devices were needed for stent placement. These were too large for percutaneous brachial access in many cases and a formal cut-down and arteriotomy were needed (**1b**). More recently, appropriately sized stents have become available which can be introduced through a 6 French sheath making arteriotomy unnecessary in many cases. A formal cut-down is more likely to be needed for the brachiocephalic artery, particularly if cerebral protection is to be used (see **5**).

2

The previous discussion relating to traversing upper limb lesions relates to patients with stenoses. Full occlusions pose a more difficult problem. Some interventionists recommend thrombolysis prior to angioplasty and stenting of iliac occlusions. Such a concept is not appropriate to the upper limb because lytic agent may cause devastating complications if delivered into the carotid or vertebral arteries. Also upper limb lesions generally present later in their evolution than lower limb occlusions, and so there is less likelihood of thrombolysis being successful. Thrombolysis should therefore not be considered. Subclavian and brachiocephalic artery occlusions usually present within 2–3 mm of the origin of the artery and extend a variable distance along it. As a result a guidewire introduced from the groin, and supported by a catheter from the same site, is often unable to gain sufficient purchase on the lesion to allow the guidewire traversal (**2a**). The morphology is usually much more favourable if approached from the brachial artery. Not only is the lesion closer to the access site, but also the artery in which the catheter is positioned is much smaller (axillary vs aorta). This makes directional control of the guidewire more accurate. Also the proximal end of these occlusions is usually a smooth dome shape, as apposed to distally where there is frequently a tapered lumen which leads the guidewire in to the lesion appropriately (**2b**). A combined approach to these difficult lesions from both the femoral and brachial arteries therefore considerably increases the likelihood of successful traversal of the lesion.

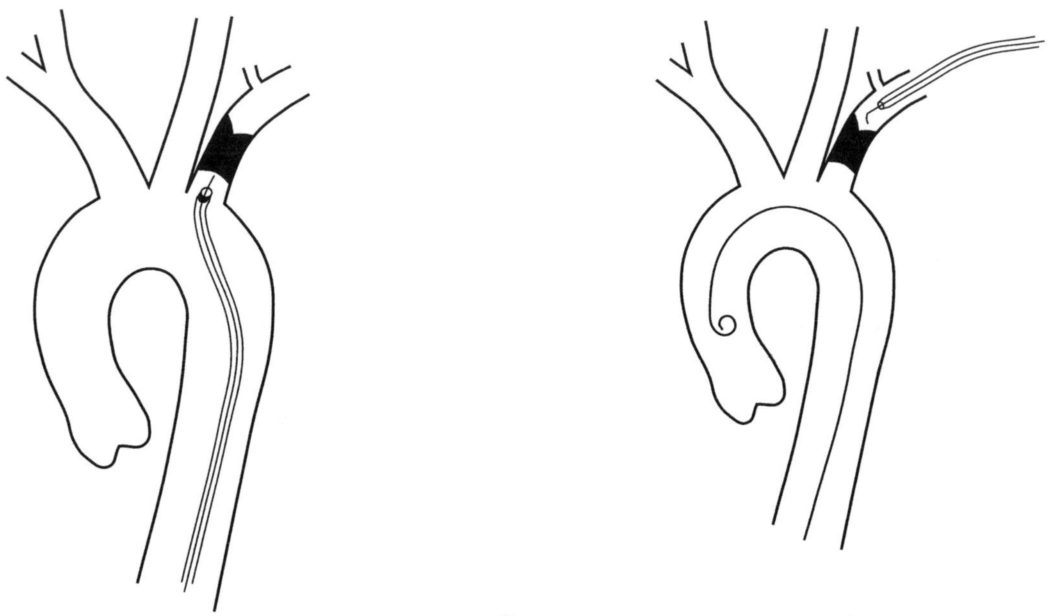

a 2 b

3

Brachiocephalic, subclavian and axillary lesions may therefore be traversed from either 'above' or 'below'. Stent placement is, however, usually more accurate if performed from the brachial approach. This is because, even if a guiding catheter or long sheath is used from the groin, the stent delivery system is in the large diameter aorta and stent placement is a relatively long way away from the access site. As a result the delivery system is less stable, making fine stent manipulation difficult. This is important, particularly in the brachiocephalic and subclavian arteries where the position of both ends of the stent are important to avoid either the stent protruding into the aorta or the stent overlying the origin of the vertebral or carotid arteries. For these reasons stent placement from the brachial artery is preferable. If the lesion has been crossed from the brachial artery then the floppy tip of the guidewire is manipulated into the descending thoracic aorta and stenting performed. However, if the lesion was crossed from the groin it is necessary to pass the guidewire to the brachial artery and out through the arterial sheath. This may be achieved in two ways:

a) The wire is manipulated into the sheath (**3a**); the sheath introducer is cut at a 45 degree angle and then passed into the sheath, with a tap on the end (**3b**). The wire is passed into the introducer and up to the tap (**3c**). The introducer is removed with the wire protruding through the arterial sheath valve.

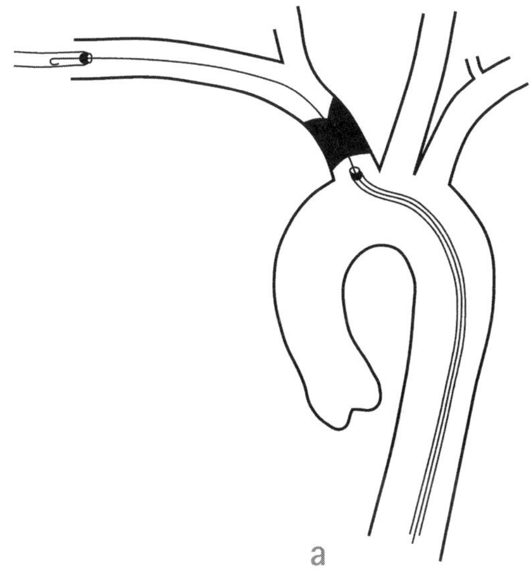

a

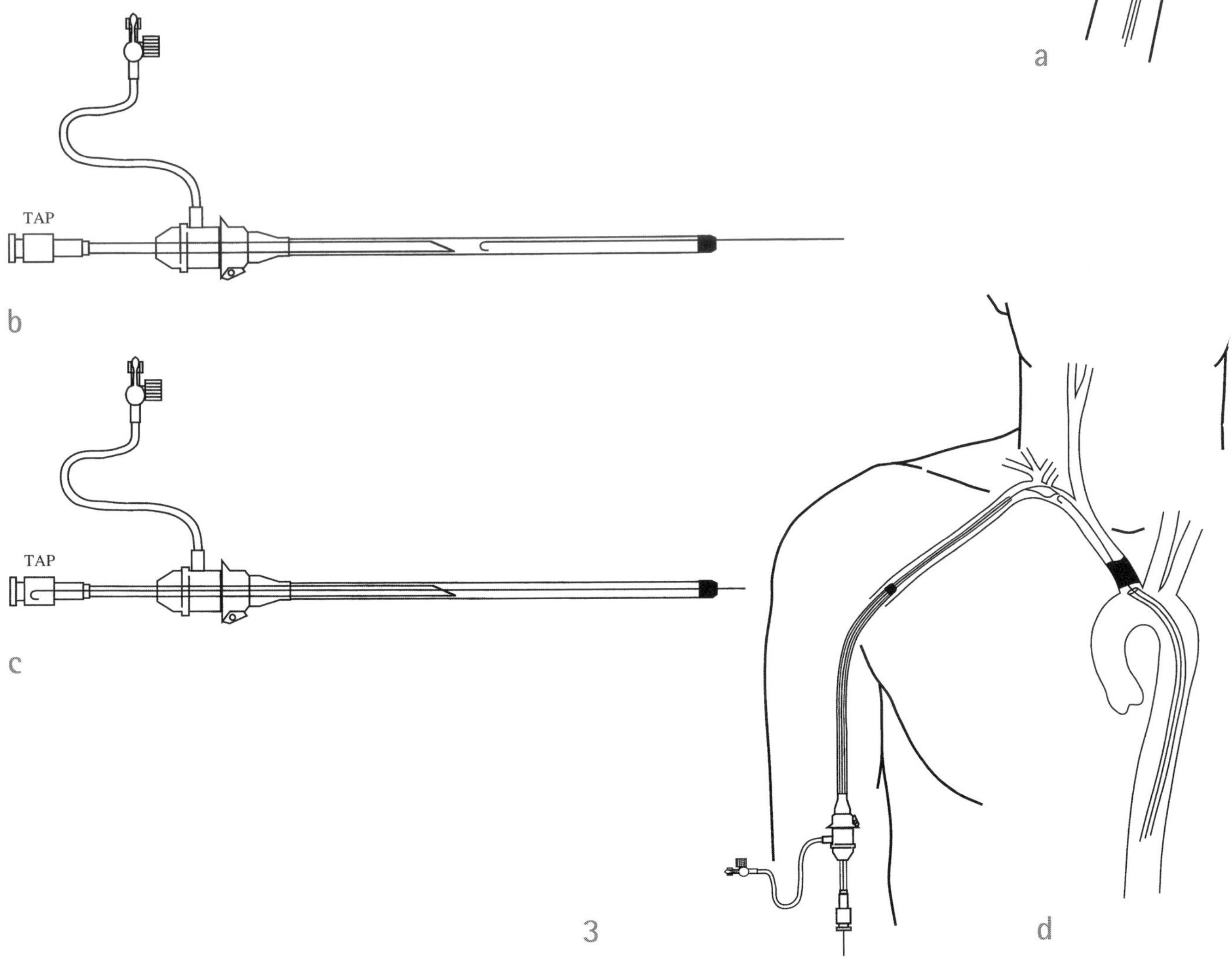

b

c

d

3

b) The above may be time-consuming and increases the radiation dose to both patient and operator. An alternative is to pass a Gooseneck snare (Microvena) into the axillary artery via the sheath (**3d**). The guidewire across the lesion is then 'caught' in the snare and withdrawn through the sheath valve.

Both of these techniques allow a guidewire passed from the groin to exit through the brachial artery sheath. The wire can then be pulled out of the brachial sheath a sufficient distance to allow the passage of a 50–60 cm catheter over the wire from the patient's arm, to cross the lesion and pass into the descending thoracic aorta. The wire may then be completely withdrawn and reversed. As a result the wire can be placed from the arm with a floppy tip in the descending thoracic aorta, and the catheter withdrawn. The lesion is then prepared for treatment.

4

Balloon placement for angioplasty is routine for stenoses, particularly if the indication for treatment is blue digit syndrome. Stent placement is recommended for complete occlusions, failed angioplasty and sometimes as a primary treatment for stenoses. Primary stenting for stenosis may be indicated in patients for whom the lesion lies proximal to an internal mammary artery, which is to be used as a coronary artery bypass conduit. The length of the stent employed is vital, as is the ability to accurately place it. The length of the stent needed can easily be

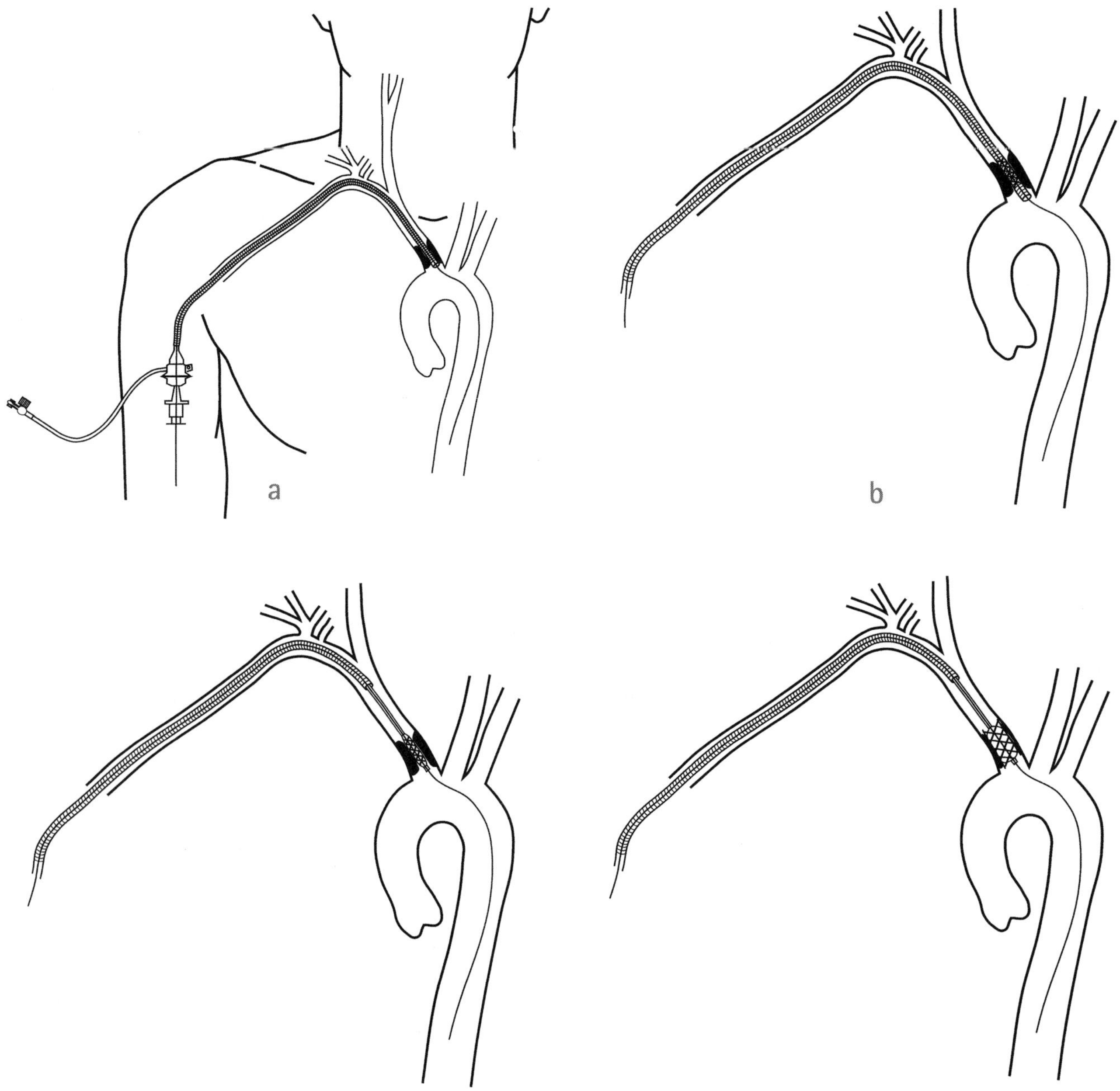

a b c 4 d

determined by the passage of a catheter with an opaque tip across the lesion. The tip is placed at one end and drawn to the other. The distance by which the catheter has been withdrawn is measured directly giving the length of the segment to be treated. The stent lengths utilized in the brachiocephalic artery and left subclavian artery are usually be between 2 and 3 cm, with diameters of 7 mm or greater. Accuracy of placement in these segments is important to ensure no encroachment over the carotid or vertebral origins, without stent protrusion into the aorta. These segments are also not subjected to compression from external sources. Balloon-expanded stents are generally more accurate to place than their self-expanding counterparts, particularly in the short lengths with large diameters. For these reasons balloon-mounted stents are usually used in the brachiocephalic and left subclavian arteries. However, delivery of these systems around the curve of the proximal subclavian artery may cause dislodgement of the stent from the balloon (even if it is factory mounted) and so a long sheath (**4a**) may be placed across the lesion, with the stent positioned within the sheath protection (**4b**), then the sheath withdrawn (**4c**) and the stent deployed (**4d**).

The situation in the axillary artery is different. Here the flexibility, crush recoverability and sufficient length of the stent are more relevant, making self-expanding stents better suited. In addition, precise placement is less critical and the stent can be easily introduced from the brachial artery, obviating the need for any catheter/wires to be across the vertebral origins.

5

A specific concern when treating brachiocephalic stenoses or occlusions is the risk of embolization into the right common carotid artery and subsequently the cerebral circulation. Until recently the only method of countering this risk was to manually compress the right common carotid artery and occlude flow. This manoeuvre is uncomfortable for the patient and also exposes the operator's assistant's hand to radiation close to the primary X-ray beam. More recently protection systems have been introduced for carotid stenting. These are discussed in more detail elsewhere, but the Percusurge™ protection balloon will inflate to sufficient size to occlude flow in most common carotid arteries, and so protect the cerebral circulation during stent placement and angioplasty (**5**). The device is delivered from brachial access route and the right common carotid artery selectively catheterized. The Percusurge™ wire is delivered, the sheath withdrawn and the balloon inflated. The brachiocephalic artery lesion is traversed. The brachiocephalic artery is then treated with the carotid artery protected, particulate matter is aspirated by the Export™ catheter, the balloon deflated and removed.

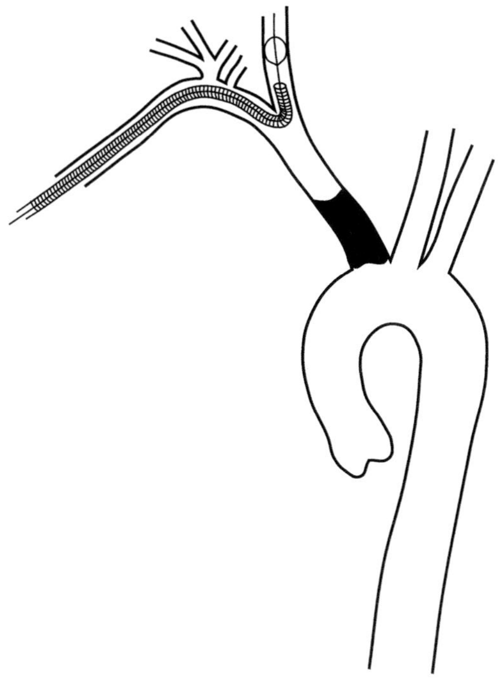

5

6

The left vertebral artery origin is potentially at risk of acute occlusion at the time of angioplasty if the lesion is close to the vertebral origin (**6a**). At the time of balloon inflation, atheromatous plaque material may be displaced across the origin (**6b**). Whilst this complication may be identified as a possibility, it is not possible to predict its occurrence with certainty and so placement of a separate balloon in to the origin of the vertebral artery is not justified in all cases. A protection balloon may itself have the potential for causing damage to the vertebral artery, and it is also costly. When treating left subclavian artery stenoses a long sheath may be placed from the femoral artery and a 0.35″ guidewire placed across the lesion and into the axillary artery. An 0.018″ guidewire can separately be placed in the vertebral artery and the lesion treated by angioplasty (**6c**). If atheromatous material does protrude across the vertebral artery origin, a low profile balloon, tailored to the vertebral artery size, can be passed over the 0.018″ wire and the vertebral artery retrieved (**6d**).

7

When occlusions are being treated and primary stenting of the subclavian artery performed, the procedure in **6** cannot be followed because once the stent has been placed, the 0.018″ guidewire would be plastered against the subclavian artery wall and no balloon passed to relieve the vertebral artery. Thus, when stents are being placed for lesions close to the vertebral origin, the safety

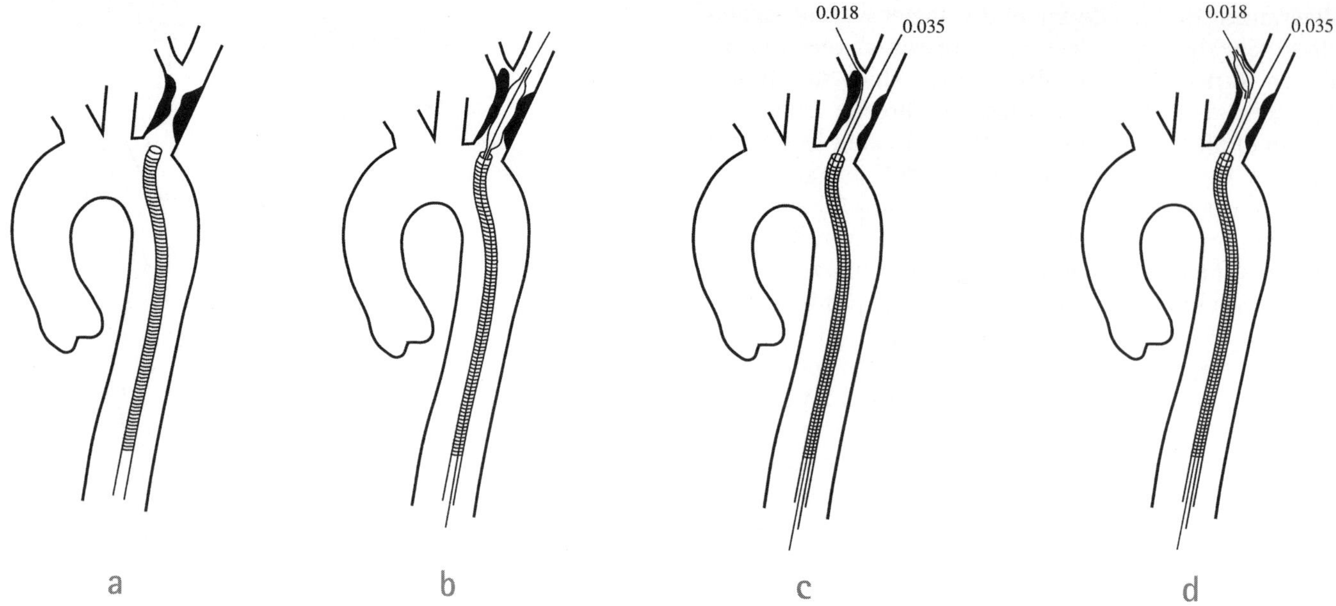

6

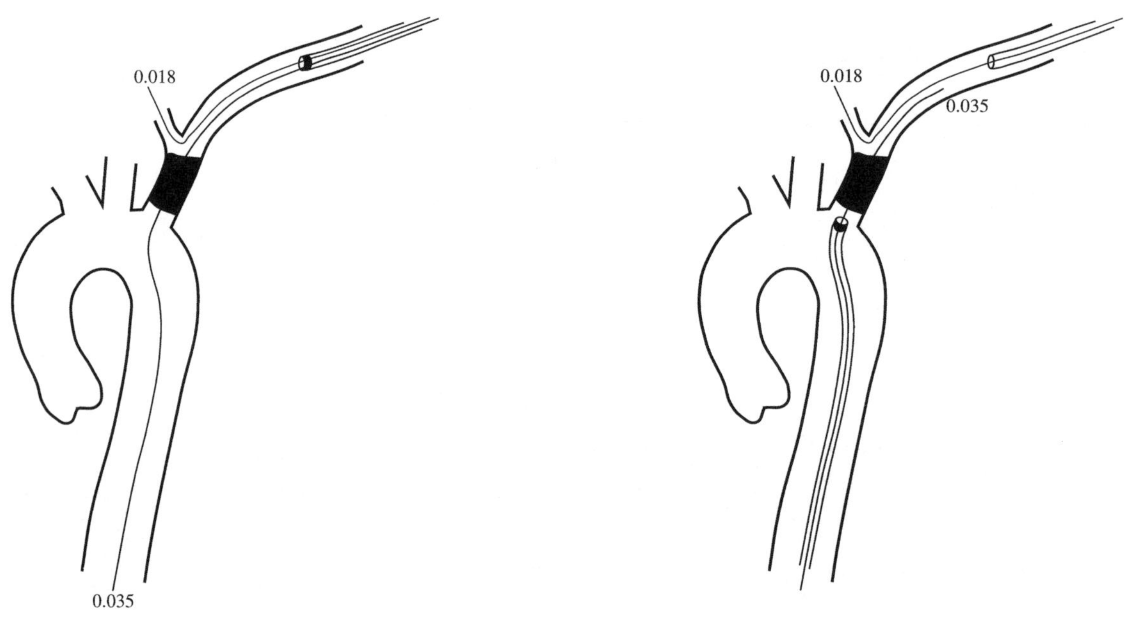

7

0.018″ guidewire should be placed from the brachial approach and the stent placed either from the brachial artery (**7a**) or from the groin with the support of a long sheath (**7b**). The protection wire has dual purpose in these circumstances. It acts as a marker for precise stent placement to ensure no stent protrudes over the vertebral artery. It also acts for subsequent placement of a vertebral balloon if necessary.

8

A 60-year-old female patient presented to another centre with symptoms considered by a neurologist to be due to cerebral hypoperfusion and a heavy feeling in her right arm after use. An arch aortogram (**8a**) shows stenoses of the brachiocephalic artery, the left subclavian artery and the origin of the left vertebral artery (which is a direct branch of the aortic arch). The acute angle of approach from the right arm to the right common carotid artery precluded placement of a protection device from the arm.

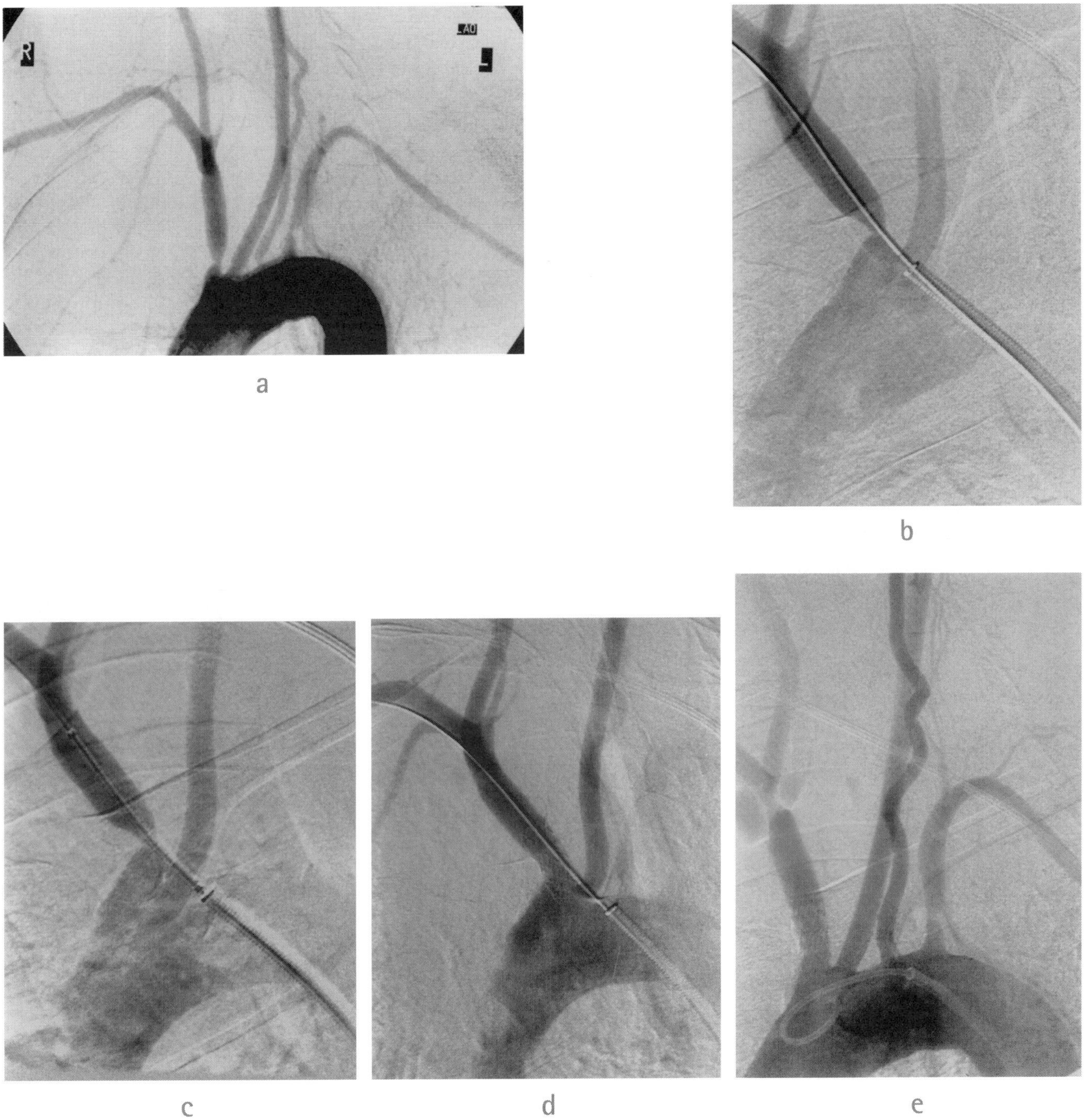

8

The brachiocephalic artery stenosis was traversed from the arm and the wire passed out through the groin. A 7F Arrow sheath (Arrow international) was placed over this wire and positioned with the tip just proximal to the stenosis (**8b**). An attempt was made to pass the PurcuSurge GuardWire (Medtronic) via this sheath, but the lesion could not be crossed, without removal of the guidewire already in place. Carotid protection was therefore obtained by pressure. A balloon mounted Saxx medium stent (Bard Peripheral Technologies) was positioned across the stenosis (**8c**). Note the distortion of the brachiocephalic artery morphology by the 'through wire'. The stent was positioned to avoid overlay of the common carotid artery origin and protrusion into the aorta. The stent was expanded to 8mm (**8d**). The left vertebral artery origin was then stented with a Saxx small stent, with an excellent result at both sites (**8e**). The apparent stenosis of the right common carotid and subclavian arteries is due to 'flare' artefact. The left subclavian artery stenosis was asymptomatic and therefore not treated.

9

A 66-year-old woman presented with dusky blue fingers on her left hand, and was noted clinically to have reduced pulse pressures in her left arm. A clinical diagnosis of a left subclavian stenosis was made, which was confirmed at arch aortography (**9a**). The major stenosis was seen to lie immediately adjacent to the left vertebral artery origin making stent placement impossible without direct compromise of the vertebral artery. The decision was made to angioplasty the lesion, with stenting as a 'bale out' option. The left subclavian origin was selectively catheterized using a Headhunter catheter (Cordis) and the lesion crossed with an 0.035 inch guidewire. A 7F Arrow sheath (Arrow International) was positioned with the tip in the proximal left subclavian artery. Using this sheath a V18 Control wire (Boston Scientific) was manipulated into the left vertebral artery (**9b**). The subclavian artery stenosis was angioplastied using a 7mm balloon (Opti-plast, Bard Peripheral Technologies) over the 0.035 inch wire (**9c**). Following balloon angioplasty there was little flow in the vertebral artery (**9d**) compared with the antegrade flow at the time of the arch aortogram (**9a**). A 3-mm balloon angioplasty (Savvy, Cordis) of the vertebral artery origin restored the vertebral flow (**9e**).

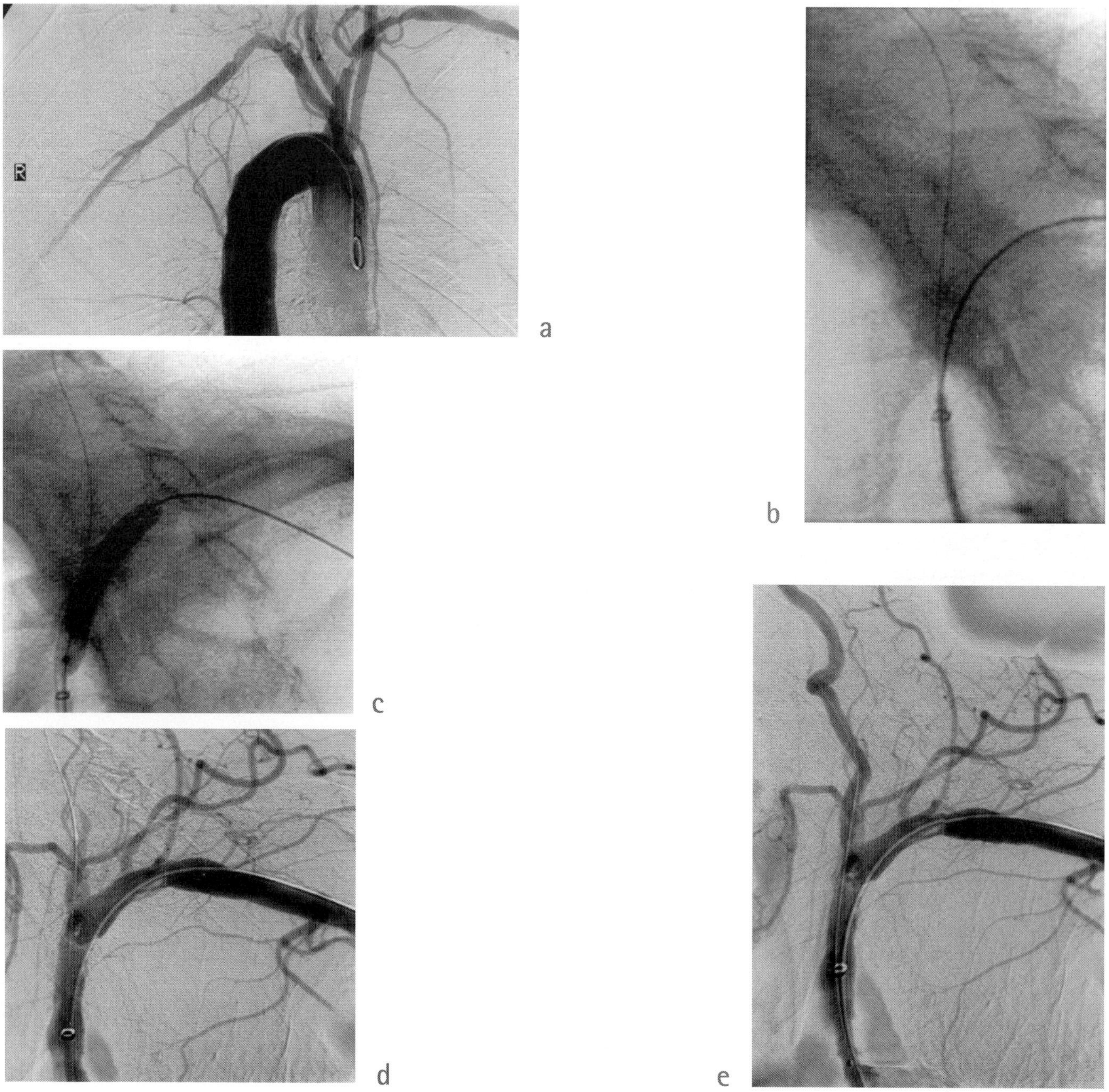

9

10

A 65-year-old man presented with left arm claudication and was found to have an occluded left subclavian artery distal to costo-cervical trunk, with a mild stenosis proximal to the left vertebral artery origin (**10a**). The occluded segment was traversed using a guidewire introduced from the left brachial approach and stented with a Wallstent (Boston Scientific) and post-dilated to 7mm (**10b**). There was no pressure gradient across the more proximal stenosis and this was not treated. The patient experienced recurrence of his symptoms 6 months later and neointimal hyperplasia was found (**10c**), which was successfully treated with re-angioplasty of the stented segment (**10d**).

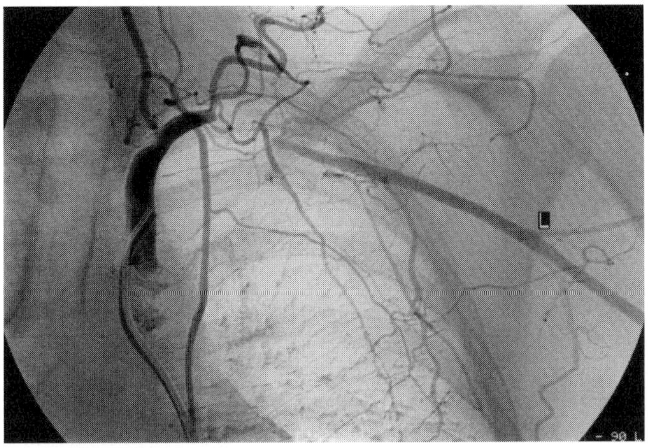

a

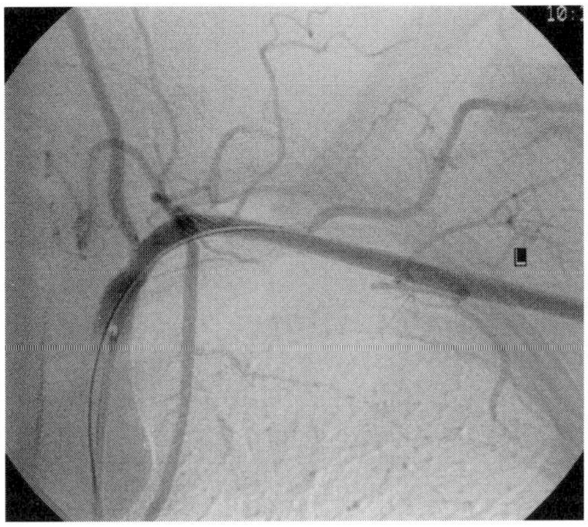

b

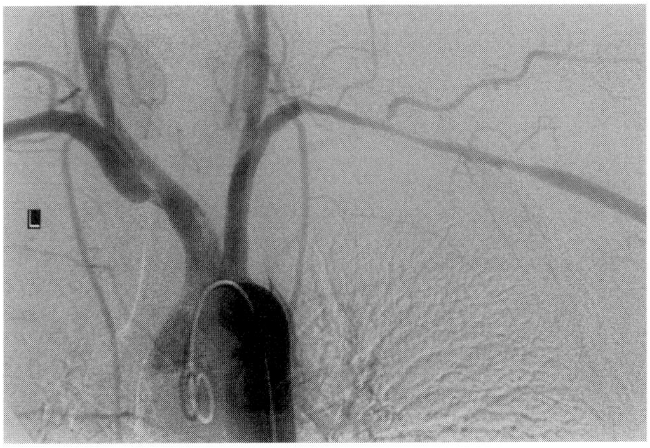

c

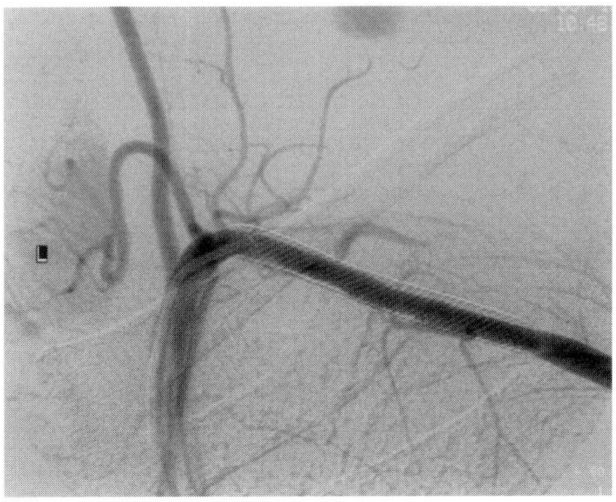

d

10

Embolization of arteriovenous malformations involving the subclavian and axillary arteries

James E Jackson

Introduction

1a, b, c

Vascular malformations of high-flow type – so-called arteriovenous malformations – involving the supraclavicular fossa and shoulder are extremely difficult to treat successfully. Surgical excision is rarely, if ever, an option because of the invariable diffuse nature of these lesions, with superficial soft tissue, muscular, neural and occasionally osseous involvement. Pain is a common symptom that may severely restrict activities.

Embolization provides the mainstay of treatment and, although a cure is exceptional, an improvement in symptoms is likely when performed correctly. The main determinant of the response to this form of therapy is the vascular anatomy within the malformation itself. Three main types of arteriovenous communication are seen within malformations and these may co-exist within the same lesion (1a–c). When arteriovenous and/or arteriolovenous shunts are present, these may be successfully occluded by catheterizing or directly puncturing percutaneously the first venous component; this form of treatment produces excellent long-term results.

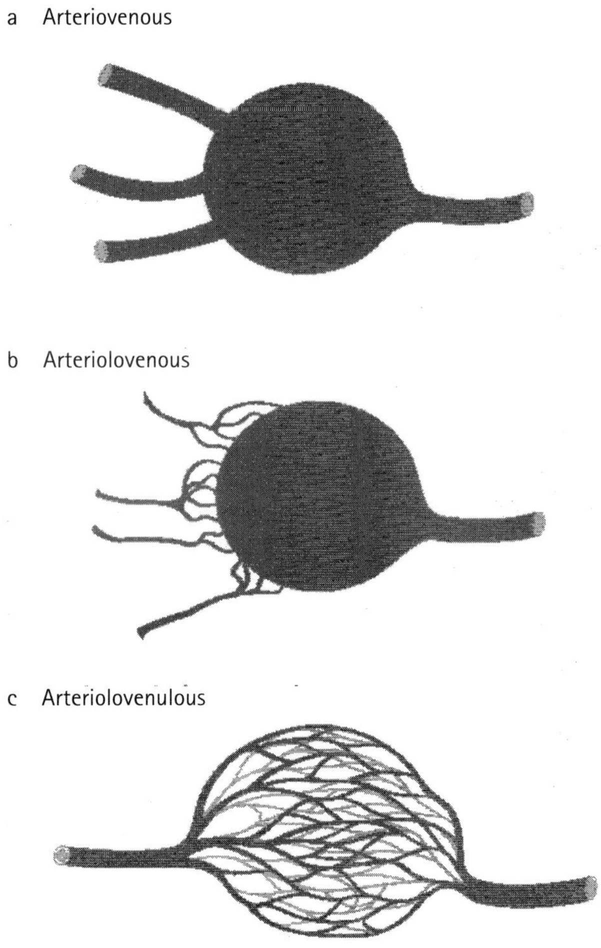

1

Technique

2

Subclavian arteriography is performed via a transfemoral arterial approach in order to demonstrate the vascular anatomy of the malformation. The types of arteriovenous communication present within a particular lesion are often very difficult to visualize on this initial arteriogram because of the presence of rapid arteriovenous shunting and the superimposition of the numerous supplying arteries and draining veins; superselective catheterization of the branch vessels supplying the malformation is almost always necessary.

In this particular malformation a central dilated venous component is present within the supraclavicular fossa (small arrows), which is supplied by multiple hypertrophied branches of the subclavian and axillary arteries. This represents an arteriolovenous anatomy.

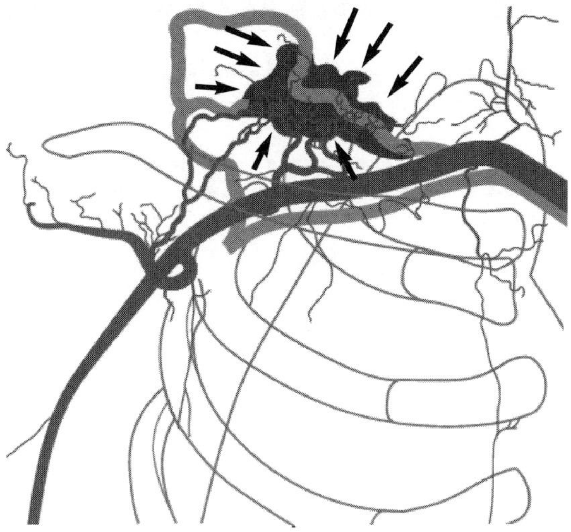

2

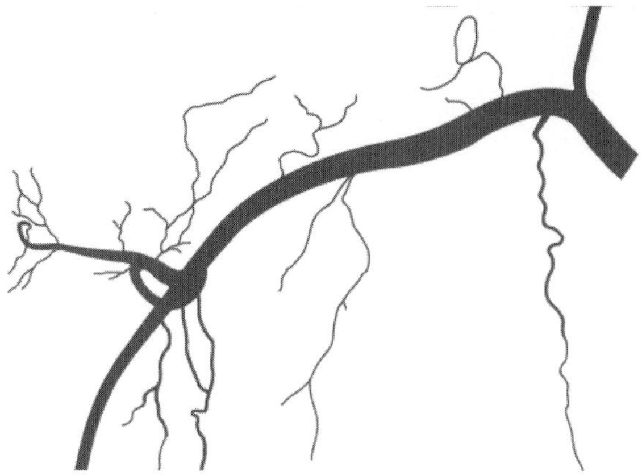

4

3

The central venous component of the malformation has now been retrogradely catheterized using a co-axial catheter (short arrow) via the dominant draining vein from a femoral venous approach. A direct percutaneous puncture of this portion of the malformation with a 22G spinal needle would have been an alternative technique in this case. With the venous catheter in position an occlusion balloon (long arrow) has been inflated within the subclavian artery proximal to any feeding vessels to the malformation to temporarily obliterate, or at least substantially slow, arterial inflow. Embolization of the venous sac was then performed using a combination of isobutyl-2-cyanoacrylate and absolute alcohol.

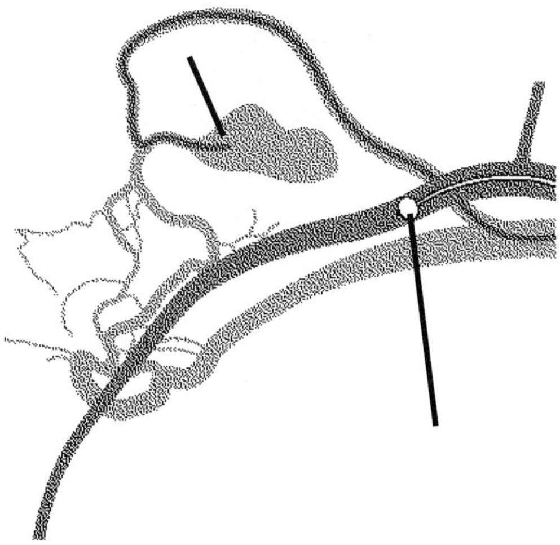

3

4

A follow-up subclavian arteriogram performed 6 months after embolization demonstrates complete obliteration of arteriovenous shunting.

Complications

Complications relating to this technique are rare. Occlusion of arterial branches supplying the arm and hand are extremely unlikely as the embolization is being performed on the venous side of the arteriovenous communications. Complete obliteration of flow through the malformation during inflation of an occlusion balloon within the subclavian artery is not always achievable, and when this is the case there is the risk of passage of embolic material into the draining veins and pulmonary circulation. If this occurs with isobutyl-2-cyanoacrylate then pulmonary artery branch occlusion may result.

Improving profunda femoris flow

Crawford Jamieson

Introduction

The surgical importance of the profunda femoris artery has long been recognized (Morris *et al.*, 1961). Early experience of direct reconstruction of stenosis of the origin of this artery was recorded by Natali in Paris, and direct endarterectomy was popularized by Martin and Cotton. Martin published a large series of patients treated by 'profundaplasty' but 80% of them had a simultaneous proximal endarterectomy or bypass of an iliac arterial stenosis or occlusion (Martin *et al.*, 1968). Cotton favoured an extended approach to the operation, patching the artery well down into the thigh, and claimed that the results were better the longer the reconstruction (Berguer *et al.*, 1973). Martin, however, had preached the opposite, feeling that when disease extended beyond the first perforating artery, reconstruction tended to be unsuccessful owing to the prevalence of disease in distal branches. This dichotomy of opinion has never been resolved but, in the course of time, the operation of extended profundaplasty has fallen from favour and most surgeons now confine their attentions to stenoses localized to the proximal few centimetres of the artery.

This is an operation which is relatively safe and easy to perform, is capable of producing a new limited increase in the circulation of the limb but has excellent long-term patency (Hopkins *et al.*, 1983).

Indications

Profundaplasty is indicated only in the presence of a significant stenosis of the profunda femoris artery. This statement may appear obvious but it has been claimed that limb flow may be improved by widening a totally normal profunda femoris origin in the presence of a superficial femoral arterial occlusion (Berguer *et al.*, 1975). The logic upon which this decision is made remains, however, rather dubious. It appears from the authors' interpretation of their haemodynamic model that a stenosis exists in the arterial tree which consists of the normal profunda femoris origin but the branching arterial tree maintains, by an increase of area at each branch, a standard and even linear resistance. The decrease in resistance of the arterial tree from the heart to the foot achieved by a local profundaplasty of 2–3 cm is only an alteration in resistance compared with the 1.3 m of artery from heart to foot and cannot therefore be expected to be significant and the operation of profundaplasty of an unstenosed vessel has generally been abandoned.

The operation is not indicated in patients with a patent superficial femoral artery, although theoretically they might suffer from intermittent claudication of the thigh with severe disease of the profunda femoris. This does not, however, seem to occur and another cause must be sought for the aetiology of pain in the thigh if the superficial femoral artery is widely patent, even if disease exists in the profunda femoris. The operation is therefore indicated in patients with a stenosis of the origin of the profunda femoris artery and a co-existent superficial femoral arterial occlusion with or without proximal iliac or aortic disease. In the former circumstances proximal reconstruction plus profundaplasty is indicated whereas in the latter and less common situation profundaplasty alone is indicated.

The most important and difficult decision lies in whether a patient with a profunda femoris stenosis and a superficial femoral arterial occlusion should be treated by profundaplasty, femoral popliteal bypass, or a combination of both.

Successful femoral popliteal bypass restores flow in the foot to normal levels which profundaplasty in the presence of an untreated superficial femoral artery occlusion will never do (Jamieson, 1983). Bypass is therefore peferable to profundaplasty where circumstances are favourable and where a major increase in flow is necessary, either to relieve crippling intermittent claudication or to heal extensive ischaemic lesions of the foot. Profundaplasty is indicated in the relatively uncommon but well-defined alternative circumstances, particularly where there is critical ischaemia and where a rise of ankle blood pressure by 20 or 30 mmHg can be expected to relieve rest pain or allow healing of mild trophic lesions (Hill and Jamieson, 1977). Carefully selected profundaplasty in exactly this group of patients can produce excellent results and the general disenchantment with the procedure has, to a great extent, been due to unrealistic hopes for an increase in circulation by relief of such a local stenosis. Bernhard (1979) has pointed out that patients with a significant drop in pressure in the thigh, as opposed to across the knee on segmental thigh pressure, may be predicted to obtain a better result from profundaplasty than the latter group. Published results of the operation uncombined with a proximal reconstruction indicate that the mean increase in ankle pressure lies around 20% of the rise in the ankle brachial pressure index. The long-term patency of profundaplasty is excellent, late occlusion being rare within the lifespan of the patient.

The major indication for a profundaplasty is as an adjunct to aortofemoral grafting or associated with reconstruction of a unilateral iliac arterial stenosis by direct endarterectomy or angioplasty. Profundaplasty may be vital to maintain an adequate flow and protect long-term patency of a proximal reconstruction, in addition to improving the results of the major proximal operation by increasing flow into the muscles of the thigh.

Simultaneous profundaplasty and femoral popliteal bypass

This is tempting when a superficial femoral block with a good run-off is associated with a severe stenosis of the origin of the profunda femoris artery but is probably unnecessary, and may even be unwise, because theoretically it reduces the pressure gradient between the common femoral and the popliteal artery and therefore the flow rate through the femoral popliteal bypass. Although there is only shaky evidence that patency of femoral popliteal bypass is directly in proportion to the flow, there is no doubt that long-term patency is very poor when flow falls below the critical level of around 150 ml/min (Law and Roberts, 1983). It is probably better to perform the femoral popliteal bypass first, keeping profundaplasty in reserve in case of long-term failure of the bypass.

Preoperative preparation

In addition to the general assessment of the patient for fitness for surgery and the degree of ischaemia of his limb, it is important that angiograms be obtained in two planes, particularly an oblique view, as the profunda femoris origin may be obscured by dye in the origin of the superficial femoral artery in the conventional anteroposterior projection of an angiogram (Beales *et al.*, 1971). Intravenous digital subtraction angiography (DSA) is frequently adequate in this preoperative assessment and direct arterial punture may be avoided, although DSA may not give adequate information on the popliteal runoff and patency of calf vessels when the choice lies between a long bypass and profundaplasty, in which case an intravenous DSA to examine the iliac arterial system followed by a direct femoral puncture and conventional angiogram which gives the best view of the distal vessels of the leg is ideal. Bacteria swabs should be taken of necrotic lesions of the foot and appropriate treatment commenced prior to surgery.

The operation may be performed under local anaesthetic when a proximal reconstruction is not required and is therefore highly suitable for the frail patient.

Position of patient

The patient should be positioned supine upon the operating table with the leg slightly abducted. The whole limb should be prepared and exposed and the abdomen prepared to the costal or even subclavian region if there is any doubt over the quality of the inflow through the iliac artery. A patch of vein is required and it is inadvisable to remove this vein from the saphenous vein at the ankle as the wound may not heal well. We prefer to prepare a segment of forearm to harvest a vein patch rather than sacrifice the saphenous vein itself in its more proximal course.

1

Incision

The incision follows a vertical route, slightly convex laterally, over the course of the iliac and femoral vessels to avoid lymphatic damage.

2

Exposure

The excision is deepened to the deep fascia and the common femoral artery exposed. The inguinal ligament is defined and the femoral pulse reassessed. If the femoral pulse is weak, it may be advisable to perform direct intrafemoral arterial pressure measurements with an intra-arterial injection of papaverine to assess the adequacy of iliac inflow. This test may be misleading when the superficial femoral artery is occluded and the profunda femoris artery is severely stenosed, because even following injection of papaverine peripheral resistance may be so high that a good femoral pulse may exist in the presence of a severe iliac stenosis. Inadequate flow may then only be detected when the artery is opened.

The superficial femoral artery is exposed and the common femoral artery and superficial femoral artery are snared and elevated. This exposes the origin of the profunda femoris artery which may be multiple and is

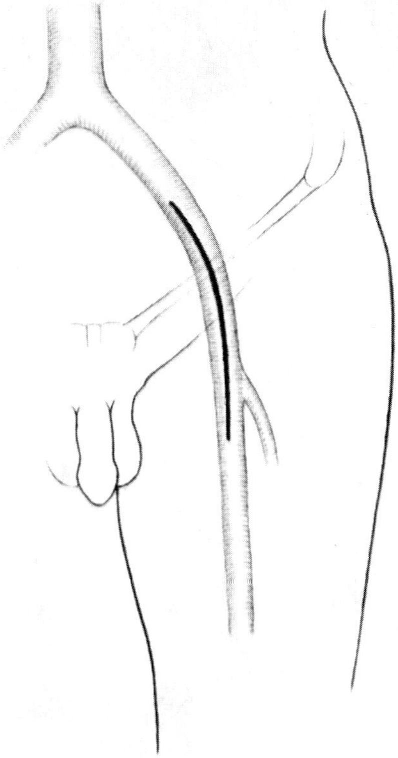

1

crossed approximately 1 cm from its origin by a large vein, the circumflex femoral vein, draining into the termination of the profunda femoris vein. This vein may be up to 1 cm in diameter and must be carefully controlled and divided before the distal artery can be exposed. The exposed course of the vein is very short and it is safer to oversew both ends than ligate them. Distal to this vein, the artery tends to run more parallel to the superficial femoral artery, and as it plunges gradually into the muscles of the thigh, it is crossed by further veins at regular intervals which may require division. The branches of the artery, the circumflex femoral artery and the perforating arteries, tend to arise around the level of these veins and should be controlled individually by snares.

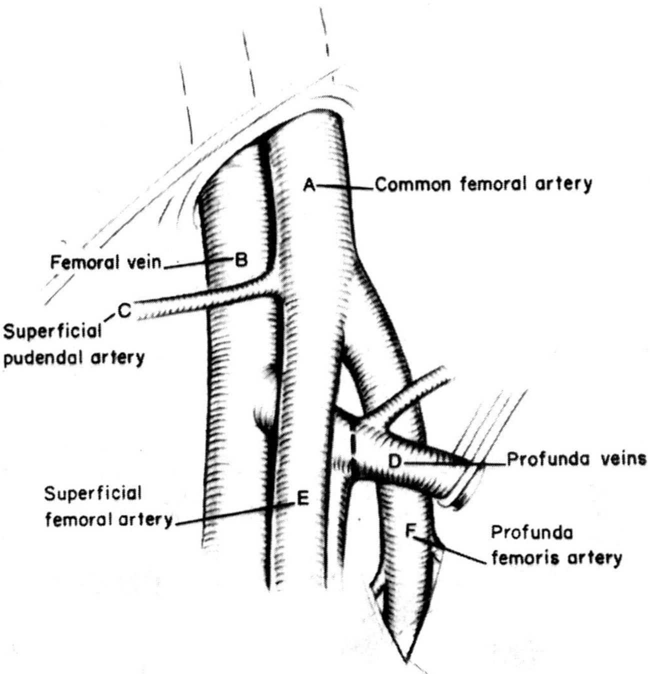

2

3

Reconstruction

The arteries are clamped following intravenous administration of heparin 1.5 mg/kg. The direction and shape of the arteriotomy depends upon which method is selected, but it commences in the distal common femoral artery and is extended down the profunda femoris artery until an adequate lumen is reached. Local endarterectomy may then be performed if necessary, tailing off distally, making quite certain that there is no flap of intima to cause local occlusion. The loose intima should be anchored by a mattress suture inserted in through the endarterectomized segment and out through the unendarterectomized distal intima, to be tied on the exterior surface of the vessel. Avoidance of flaps is best achieved by avoiding endarterectomy where possible as Martin preferred. The adequacy of downflow and backflow are assessed – if downflow is inadequate, proximal reconstruction may

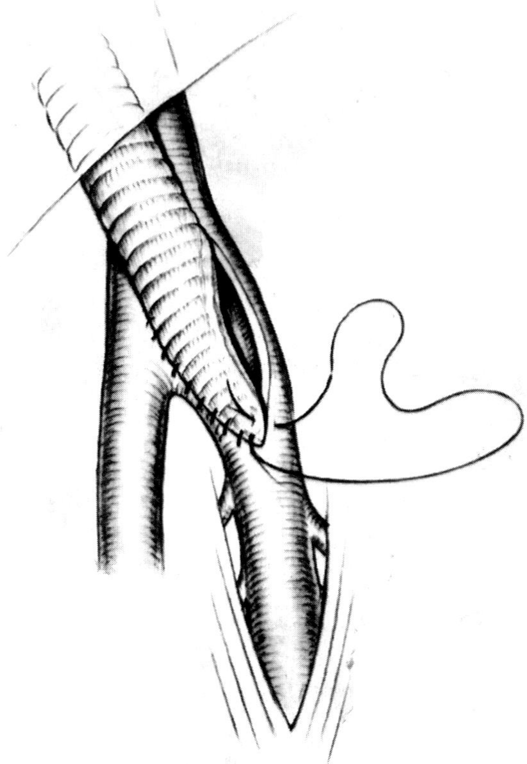

3

be added at this stage, and the profundaplasty is then closed by Dacron end-to-side.

4

If backflow is inadequate, in spite of the gentle passage of Fogarty catheters, it may be necessary to reconsider the decision to perform a femoral distal bypass, but otherwise the arteriotomy is closed with a suitable vein patch. It can be an advantage to cut the vein square-ended as shown. The clamps are removed and anticoagulation is reversed. Operative angiography may be performed to assess the success of the reconstruction. The wound is closed over a suction drain.

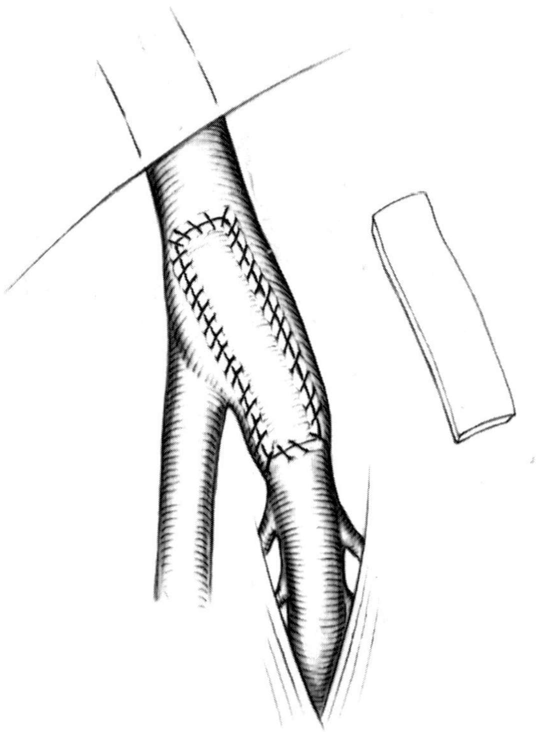

4

5

A variety of permutations exist by which a stenosis of the profunda femoris origin can be relieved. These include use of the segment of endarterectomized occluded superficial femoral artery as a patch, dissected fully free as shown.

6

Alternatively, the endarterectomized superficial femoral artery is left attached and flapped over to widen the profunda origin as a square patch.

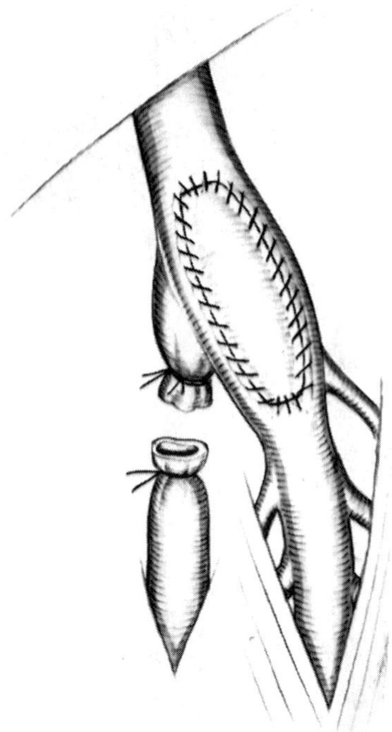

5

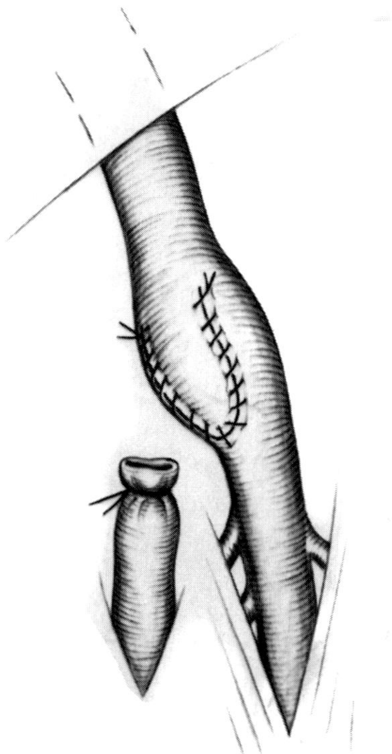

6

7

Widening of the profunda femoris origin can be achieved by suture of a patent or endarterectomized superficial femoral artery to a V-shaped arteriotomy between the superficial femoral artery and the profunda femoris.

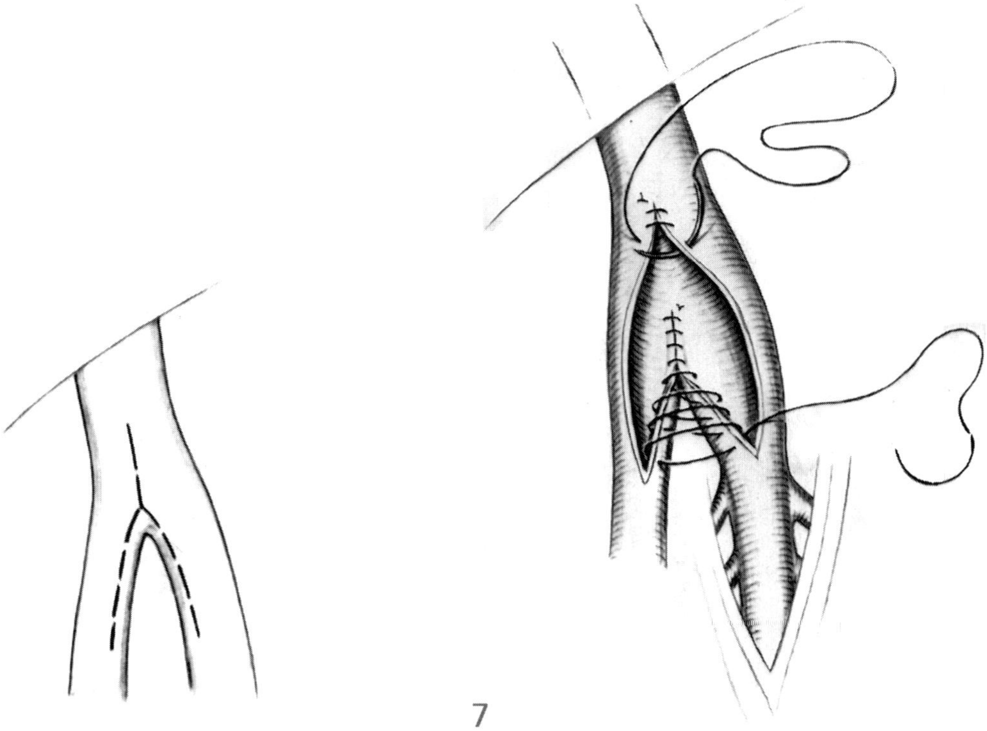

7

a b

Postoperative management

There is little systemic disturbance from this operation and gastrointestinal function is normal. A urinary catheter is not required unless the iliac artery has been exposed, and the patient is allowed up after 24 h, provided there is no excessive lymph leak from the drain. If lymph drainage is considerable it is probably best that the patient be nursed supine until it decreases, as lymph flow is stimulated by exercise of the limb.

Ankle blood pressure is monitored daily for the first few days though early failure of the reconstruction is most unusual. Antibiotic cover is not necessary as autogenous material alone has been used.

Complications

Apart from the general complications of any anaesthetic in a patient with a diffuse vascular disease and wound infection, the only significant complication is a lymphocoele which is unusual and almost always settles with time. It sometimes, however, develops after the suction drain has been removed and if it is large it is best treated by insertion of a further suction drain percutaneously by an oblique route which is left in until the drainage settles. Very rarely, this may take several days.

Profundaplasty combined with proximal reconstruction

The permutations of operation available in profundaplasty plus aortofemoral grafting are covered elsewhere but in spite of the popularity of bypass grafting there is still some place for local endarterectomy of iliac occlusions when the contralateral iliac artery is good. This operation may be performed by an extraperitoneal approach. It is safer, quicker and less traumatic than aortofemoral grafting (Martin *et al.*, 1968) and is associated with less systemic disturbance and ileus. Endarterectomy is technically more demanding than bypass but it is a skill which should be available to every peripheral arterial surgeon and although its detractors state that it only postpones the inevitable, similar operation on the contralateral side, this is not the case, as most patients treated by unilateral iliac endarterectomy do not survive to require an aortobifemoral graft within their limited lifespan.

The preoperative preparation and positioning of the patient are identical to those of pure profundaplasty. The patient lies flat on the operating table.

8

Incision

A thin patient with external iliac occlusion is best treated by an incision carried vertically through the inguinal ligament and muscle layers of the abdominal wall just lateral to the origin of the common femoral artery, and extended proximally along the linear semilunaris. This incision, although apparently traumatic, gives excellent exposure of the external iliac artery and the distal common iliac artery, and is associated with a very low inci-

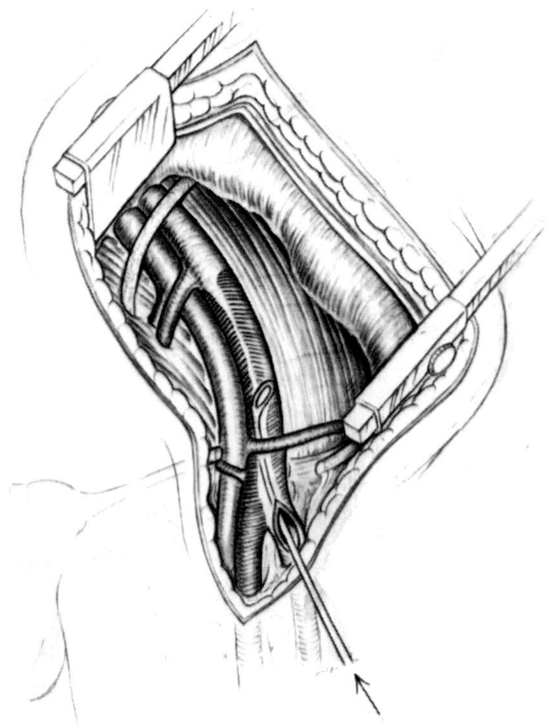

8

dence of incisional hernia provided it is sutured carefully with continuous non-absorbable material of adequate strength. The incision is deepened through the external oblique aponeurosis and the conjoint muscles of internal oblique and transversus. A finger is inserted under the inguinal ligament and the peritoneum gently swept medially, taking great care to avoid damage to the deep circumflex iliac vein which crosses anterior to the distal part of the external iliac artery. The peritoneum becomes more adherent superiorly and medially to the posterior aspect of the rectus sheath and must be mobilized with great care to avoid opening the peritoneal cavity. It is, however, easily separated posteriorly from the anterior aspect of the vessels. The ureter is mobilized anteriorly with the peritoneum until the surgeon's fingers detect the normal pulse proximal to the iliac stenosis.

A Goligher retractor is inserted with a short blade against the iliac crest and a long blade protected by a large swab retracting the peritoneum and viscera. It is most important that this retractor should not exert pressure distally upon the femoral nerve which lies hidden under the fasica just lateral to the termination of the external iliac artery. The blades are opened giving excellent exposure of the external and internal iliac arteries and the common iliac artery. The inferior epigastric artery and deep circumflex iliac artery are controlled by snares as they originate from the distal part of the external iliac artery, and the deep circumflex iliac vein is divided. Lymphatic tissue is cleared from the external iliac artery completely exposing the vessel. The internal iliac artery is snared taking great care to avoid damage to the internal iliac vein which lies deep to it. The distal part of the external common iliac artery is mobilized from the common iliac vein and similarly snared. Venous bleeding at this stage presents the only major hazard of the procedure and the common iliac artery may be so closely tethered to the common iliac vein by periarteritis that snaring is inadvisable, though it is difficult to control it adequately with a clamp unless it is mobilized.

Endarterectomy

The patient is anticoagulated with heparin 1.5mg/kg intravenously. The common iliac artery, internal iliac artery and branch of the common femoral artery are clamped and the distal common femoral artery is then opened in the same manner as for profundaplasty but the arteriotomy is carried proximally to the distal extremity of the external iliac artery. Local endarterectomy is performed upwards from this point using loop or arc strippers to the patent common iliac artery. The arc stripper is extremely valuable for traversing a vessel or varying calibre but has the potential risk of catching in the arterial wall and must not be twisted during its upwards and downwards course in the plane of endarterectomy. It is best located by the surgeon's two fingers on each side of the points of its arc, as it is passed upwards. When the plaque has been loosened by one passage of the ring stripper or four passages of the arc stripper, an arterial clamp is gently closed on the unopened artery at the site of proximal mobilization of the plaque. The gentle closure combined with pressure from the fingers breaks the endarterectomized core, leaving the outer wall intact, and the core may be milked from the endarterectomized vessel.

The manoeuvre is not always successful and excessive force must not be used in attempting to break the plaque as it will result in damage to the external wall. If the plaque does not break open further, arteriotomy must be made at the proximal level of endarterectomy, the plaque divided under direct vision with scissors and the arteriotomy closed with continuous 4/0 polypropylene. Downflow is then assessed and if it is adequate the arteriotomy and the common femoral and profunda femoris arteries are closed with a vein patch as before.

Closure

The abdominal wall is closed with a continuous 2/0 nylon suture in two layers over a suction drain passed along the common femoral artery under the inguinal ligament to lie along the external iliac artery, and the groin wound is closed in layers.

Postoperative course

It is very similar to profundaplasty. Ileus is usually very slight unless the peritoneum has been inadvertently opened.

Combined common iliac endarterectomy and profundaplasty

9

The patient lies with a sandbag to raise the buttock if preferred. The incision described above does not give good exposure of the origin of the common iliac artery without such proximal extension that it risks weakening the muscles of the abdominal wall, and it gives less good exposure in the obese patient. Extensive unilateral iliac arterial occlusion is better treated by a combination of an incision over the common femoral artery and a separate oblique incision in the abdominal wall. The common femoral arterial exposure is extended proximally by division of the inguinal ligament for approximately 1 cm to allow control of the inferior epigastric and deep circumflex iliac arteries.

The abdominal incision is commenced at a point 3 cm above the pubic tubercle over the conjoint tendon and directed upwards and laterally towards the costal margin. It is deepened through the linear semilunaris in its lower part by a combination of splitting the external oblique and cutting the internal oblique and transversus muscles more proximally. The peritoneum is mobilized medially, as in the previous approach, and retracted by a Goligher rectractor as before. This exposure gives much better access to the common iliac artery and even the aortic bifurcation, and division of the inguinal ligament permits control of all the branches in the segment to be endarterectomized.

10

Common iliac endarterectomy requires a separate arteriotomy situated over the distal part of the common iliac artery. The external iliac endarterectomy is performed from a common femoral arteriotomy to the proximal arteriotomy, and common iliac endarterectomy is carried out using loop or preferably arc strippers. The atheromatous plaque in the common iliac artery is ruptured by gentle compression of the origin of the common iliac artery with an arterial clamp. It is obviously vital that this manoeuvre is performed with care, for rupture of the vessel at this point without adequate aortic control might be fatal. The atheroma in the proximal part of the common iliac artery is, however, in unilateral arterial occlusion, frequently soft and virtually non-existent. Frequently, the vessel occludes because of a development of atheroma in its distal part and following a distal occlusion thromboses back to the origin.

In rare circumstances, where external iliac endarterectomy proves to be impossible, it is convenient to insert a Dacron bypass from the common iliac arteriotomy to the common femoral arteriotomy as a unilateral iliofemoral bypass and, in the even rarer circumstance where flow cannot be restored to the common iliac artery, an aortofemoral graft must be used. This last alternative is used to rescue an incorrect clinical decision. These patients are better treated by an aortobifemoral graft if there is extensive distal disease.

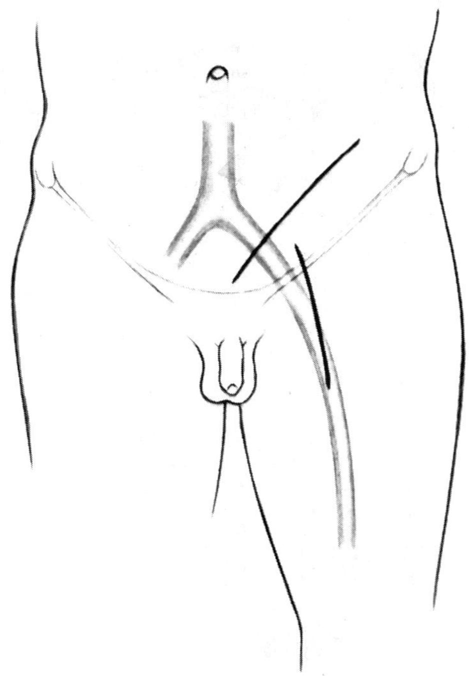

9

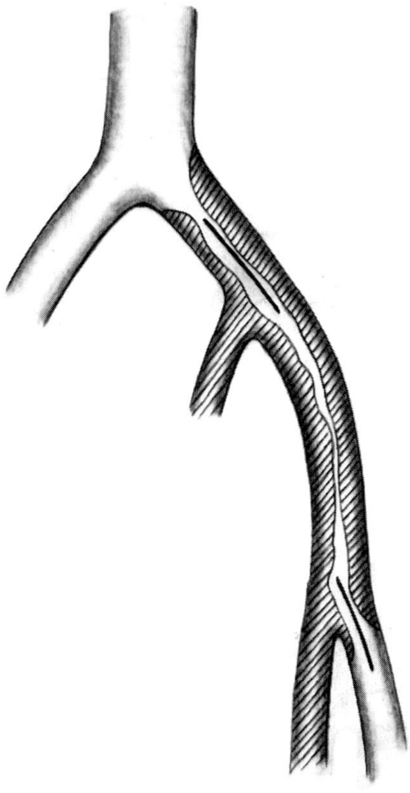

10

The arteriotomy at the lower end of these procedures is always taken into the profunda origin if the superficial femoral artery is occluded and closure is by patch or Dacron graft as for a profundaplasty. Proximal reconstruction of one sort or another is always combined with profundaplasty if the aortoiliac disease significantly limits inflow to the profunda femoris artery.

Acknowledgement
Illustrations by RN Lane.

References

Beales JSM, Adcock FA, Frawley JS *et al.* (1971). The radiological assessment of disease of the profunda femoris artery. *Br J Radiol* **44**: 854.

Berguer R, Cotton LT Sabri S (1973). Extended deep femoral angioplasty. *Br Med J* **1**: 469.

Berguer R, Higgins RF Gotton LT (1975). Geometry blood flow and reconstruction of the deep femoral artery. *Am J Surg* **130**: 68.

Bernhard VM (1979). The role of profundaplasty in revascularisation of the lower extremities. *Surg Clin N Amer* **59**: 681.

Hill DA, Jamieson CW (1977). The results of arterial reconstruction using the profunda femoris artery in rest pain and pre-gangrene. *Br J Surg* **64**: 359.

Hopkins NFG, Polyrakis S, Jamieson CW, Vaughan GMM (1983). Assessment of later patency of profundaplasty. *Surgery* **94**: 814.

Jamieson CW (1983). Profundaplasty: An incomplete alternative to femoro-popliteal bypass. In *Controversies in Surgery* Vol. 2. **Delaney JP, Varcos RL** eds. London/Philadelphia: W B Saunders Co.

Law YF, Roberts, VC (1983). Per-operative haemodynamic assessment of lower limb arterial surgery. *J Biomed Engineering* **5**: 194.

Martin P, Renwick S Stephenson C (1968). On the surgery of the profunda femoris artery. *Br J Surg* **55**: 539.

Morris GC, Edwards W, Cooley DA, *et al.* (1961). Surgical importance of profunda femoris artery. *Arch Surg* **82**: 52.

Reversed saphenous vein for femoropopliteal bypass grafting

K G Burnand, N L Browse

Introduction

Rest pain, pregangrene and frank gangrene of the digits or forefoot in the presence of a good femoral inflow and an adequate run-off via the popliteal artery constitute an absolute indication for the operation. The combination of severe ischaemia and an isolated femoropopliteal occlusion rarely exists. There is almost always some concomitant aortoiliac, profunda or distal vessel disease in limbs with severe ischaemia. Staged or simultaneous aortic reconstruction may then be required and the distal end of the bypass may have to be taken below the popliteal trifurcation if there is a marked stenosis of the popliteal artery or occlusion of the crural vessels.

Intermittent claudication remains a relative indication for the operation: a good early symptomatic improvement must be weighed against the risks of operation and the uncertainty of long-term benefit. Younger, fit and fully employed patients with a unilateral block, a disease-free popliteal segment and a good-calibre saphenous vein are obvious candidates for surgery, although many would claim that such a combination of circumstances is unusual. Patients should ideally have given up smoking for a reasonable period of time and have stable or deteriorating symptoms of several months' duration, which are interfering with their occupation or hobbies to such an extent, that even after a full explanation of the risks and uncertain long-term benefits of procedure, they continue to request operation. Initial enthusiasm for operating in all patients with claudication has now waned in the UK, and more stringent selection criteria are applied to potential candidates for surgery.

Ischaemic leg ulceration, traumatic damage to the superficial femoral artery, cystic change in the popliteal artery, and popliteal aneurysms are alternative indications for vein bypass surgery.

A good-calibre long saphenous vein remains the conduit of first choice for bypassing atherosclerotic obstruction of the femoropopliteal segment. There appears to be little difference in patency between *in situ* and reversed saphenous vein bypasses to the popliteal artery (Harris *et al.*, 1987) and the decision on which method to use appears therefore to be a matter of personal preference. Reversed grafts often lie better when made to the popliteal segment, whereas *in situ* grafts are almost always preferable below the trifurcation.

Assessment

Patients being considered for femoropopliteal bypass should have the basic screening tests outlined in the first chapter: 'Planning the intervention', carried out before proceeding to aortography or digital subtraction angiography. If this shows a satisfactory aortoiliac segment with an isolated femoropopliteal occlusion and satisfactory run-off, we obtain bilateral saphenograms (Senapati *et al.*, 1983) to assess the morphology and diameter of both long saphenous veins before surgery is considered. Duplex Doppler scanning is an alternative method of assessing the calibre and branches of the long saphenous vein. Confirmation of a single lumen saphenous vein of adequate length and diameter in either leg makes recommendation of vein bypass surgery much easier in patients with moderate claudication, whereas a multi-channelled or narrow vein mitigates against surgery in all but the severely handicapped. In patients with rest pain, demonstration of a poor saphenous vein on saphenography may prevent an extensive dissection through poorly vascularized tissue. A prosthetic graft of human umbilical vein, Dacron or polytetrafluoroethylene can then be selected as an alternative bypass.

Preoperative preparation

The affected limb should be fully shaved together with the genitalia and iliac fossa of the same side. Naseptin drops are administered twice a day to the nasal passages for 48 h before operation and the patients have chlorhexidine added to their bath water for the same period. Flucloxacillin 250 mg four times a day is started 24 h before operation and 2 units of blood are cross-matched.

Anaesthesia

The operation is carried out under normotensive general anaesthesia. Good peripheral intravenous access for fluid and blood replacement is essential and an ECG recording and central venous pressure monitoring may be indicated if severe cardiac disease coexists. A Swan–Ganz catheter, an arterial line and continuous bladder drainage are not routinely required, but may be used on certain occasions.

The operation

1, 2

Position of patient

The patient lies supine on the operating table with the end flap of the table lowered to remove the opposite leg from the operating field and provide better access to the popliteal space. The affected leg is supported by a rubber-padded steel strip which is held in place between the metal base of the operating table and the weight of the patient on the antistatic rubber cushion. A large sandbag is placed under the thigh to produce slight knee flexion which aids access to the popliteal space, but excessive knee flexion is avoided because this makes tailoring of graft length difficult. Dissection of the popliteal fossa can then be carried out from the opposite side of the table with the surgeon seated on an adjustable stool. The leg is painted with chlorhexidine or iodine from ankle to mid-abdomen. The unprepared foot is wrapped in a sterile plastic bag, which allows its colour to be inspected and the pulses to be palpated when the reconstruction has been completed. The prepared skin is covered with one or two large plastic drapes.

3

Exposure of the vein

Confirmation of an adequate saphenous vein and avoidance of vein damage are the first two steps of the operation. Our preference is to find the upper end of the vein by a vertical incision placed over the saphenofemoral junction which is then extended up across the front of the inguinal ligament. This incision also allows adequate access to the common femoral artery. Using a combination of blunt and sharp dissection, the vein should be found in the subcutaneous fat as it dips down through the cribriform fascia. The junction of the saphenous with the common femoral vein must be confirmed. If this step is omitted it is possible to trace a large anteromedial or posterolateral thigh vein instead of the main saphenous trunk. Once the vein has been exposed and dissected to its termination, the initial short incision may be extended along the course of the vein by sliding a finger along the perisaphenous space superficial to the vein and carefully incising the skin overlying the surface of the finger with a scalpel. The subcutaneous fat can then be divided with scissors. The finger prevents inadvertent damage to the vein and identifies the direction of its course, so preventing an inaccurate incision and undercutting of the wound edges which predisposes to skin necrosis.

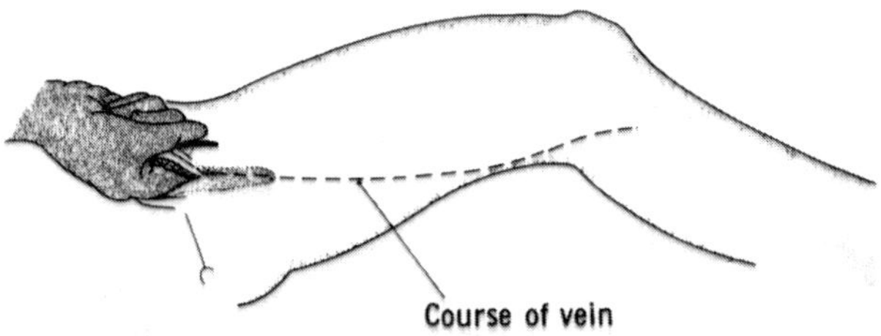

1

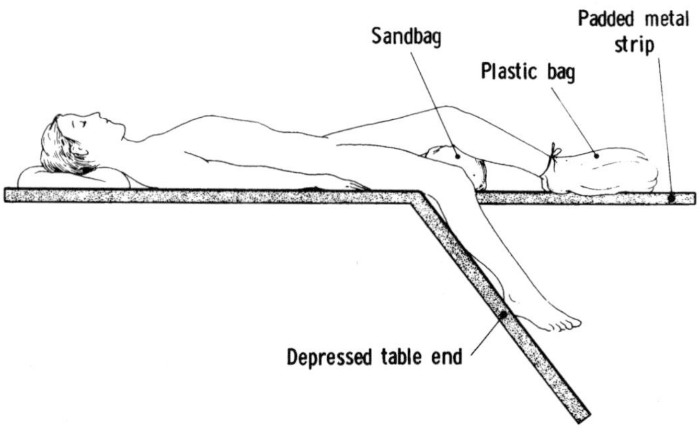

2

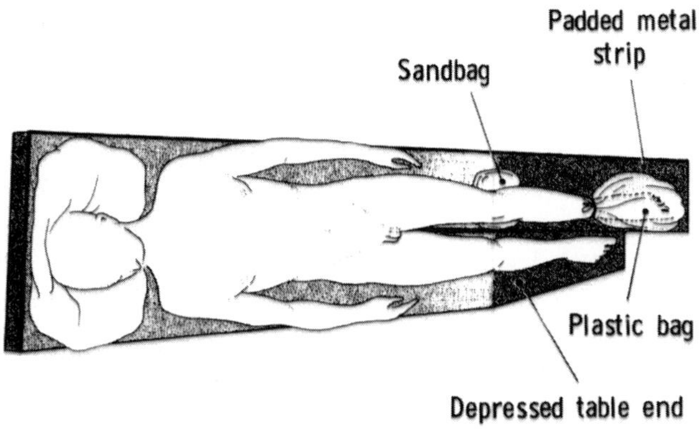

3

4, 5

Dissection of the vein

The skin and subcutaneous tissue over the vein are divided, exposing the appropriate length required for the bypass, using the sliding finger technique already described. It is advisable to overestimate the length of a vein which is required as unused vein may be easily discarded while insufficient length may prejudice successful surgery. The vein becomes more superficial just above the knee and the finger dissection technique may have to be abandoned in favour of blunt tunnelling with scissors under direct vision with scissor division of the overlying skin. Blind tunnelling may perforate and damage the vein. Dabs of patent blue violet are applied to the superficial surface of the vein before it is lifted from its bed. This enables the vein to be carefully aligned without twists when it is later positioned in the tunnel. When the required length of vein is completely exposed two operators working from opposite ends free the vein from the surrounding fat and stringy periadventitia by a combination of sharp and blunt dissection, ligating each small branch of the long saphenous vein with 3/0 silk ties on the vein side and 2/0 chromic catgut or polyglycolic acid at the other end. The ligatures must not be tied too close to the main vein to avoid constriction.

When there is still some doubt over the length of vein that will be required for the bypass, it is better to leave the vein *in situ* (5) and to explore the popliteal artery to determine its suitability (8) before proceeding to harvest the vein (6).

6

Vein distension

When the vein has been lifted from its bed, both attached ends are tied off with 2/0 silk ligatures, before the vein is divided and removed. A cannula is tied into the distal end of the vein. Then, 20 ml of 1 : 400 000 heparin saline solution or heparinized blood are drawn up into a syringe which is attached to the cannula. A bulldog clamp is then placed across the vein and a segment is gently distended by depressing the plunger of the syringe. Side branches that were not ligated when the vein was dissected out are revealed when they emit small jets of perfusate. The stumps of unligated side branches can usually be picked up with accurately placed mosquito forceps and ligated.

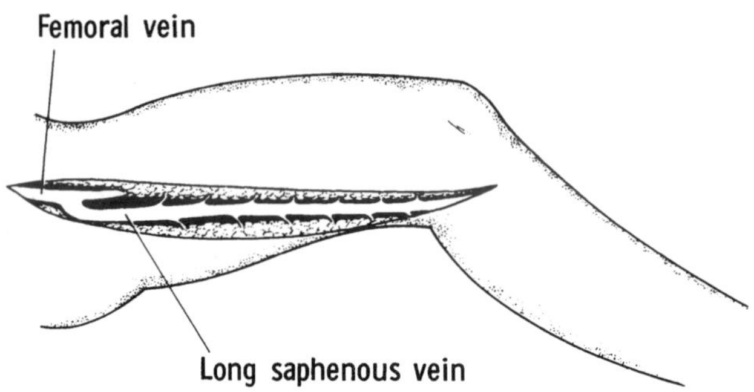

4

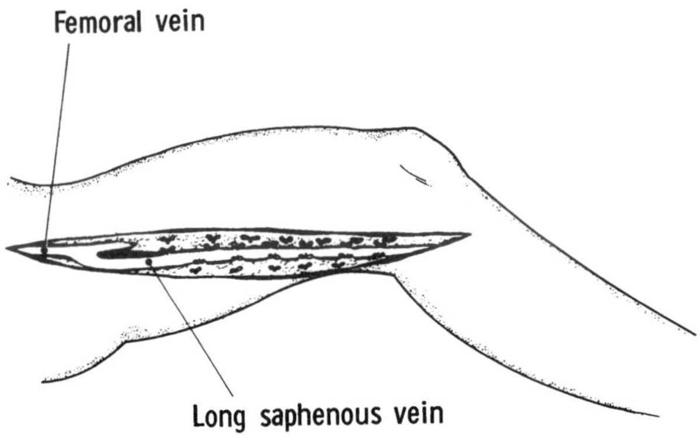

5

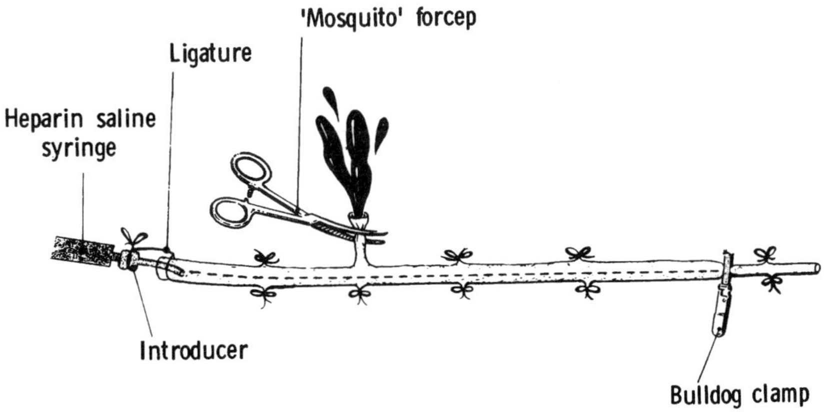

6

A small 6/0 polypropylene stitch is used to close any sideholes in the vein where branches have torn off flush with the main channel. Great care must be taken to avoid narrowing the lumen of the graft when picking up small branches or placing a stitch in the side of the vein wall.

When the entire vein has been distended and rendered watertight, adventitial bands are divided with small curved scissors and the outer layers of adventitia are divided longitudinally to allow maximal venous dilatation. Overdistension of the vein must be avoided, since this has been shown to separate and damage endothelial cells, exposing the underlying collagen, which is known to promote platelet adhesion and thrombosis. Devices to prevent overdistension are now marketed, but we do not use them at present, relying instead on gentle pressure to prevent damage.

7

Femoral artery exposure

The common femoral pulse is palpated through the upper end of the incision which is used to expose the vein. Self-retaining Travers' retractors are inserted to hold the wound edges apart and the subcutaneous fat and deep fascia over the pulse are then divided in the long axis of the limb by sharp dissection until the vasa vasorum on the anterior surface of the artery are clearly seen. The common femoral artery is displayed from the inguinal ligament to its division into the superficial femoral and profunda branches. The three main vessels are dissected free and taped with polythene snares; small branches are ligated and divided or controlled by looped silk sutures.

8

Low popliteal artery exposure

The segment of popliteal artery between the knee joint and the trifurcation is usually the least diseased and this is the segment of vessel usually chosen for the lower anastomosis. The posteromedial border of the tibia is identified by palpation through the lower end of the incision used to expose the saphenous vein. The deep fascia of the calf is then incised vertically about 1 cm behind this bony attachment. This incision is extended upwards, until the tendons of sartorius, gracilis, semimembranosus and semitendinosus are encountered at about the level of the knee joint, and downwards as far as necessary. A finger pushed in front of the medial head of gastrocnemius which lies beneath the deep fascia separates loose areolar tissue between this muscle and the posterior border of the tibia. This space is enlarged by inserting the twin Browse retractors which open up the lower part of the popliteal fossa. These retractors are 'rake-type' paired self-retaining retractors similar to Travers' but with a long and short blade. The short blades sit against the tibia while the long blades 'hold back' the calf muscles. The popliteal vessels lie anteriorly on the posterior surface of the bone with the vein lying on the medial side of the artery and the nerve lying behind. The vein is gently dissected off the artery which is freed at one point and taped with a plastic snare. A reasonable length of artery is then dissected free and a second snare is placed around the artery. Small branches between the snares should be ligated. A Lahey forceps is then passed behind the artery and the vessel is gently palpated against the rigid forceps. This confirms the presence of a satisfactory lumen and allows the extent of the atheroma to be gauged. The

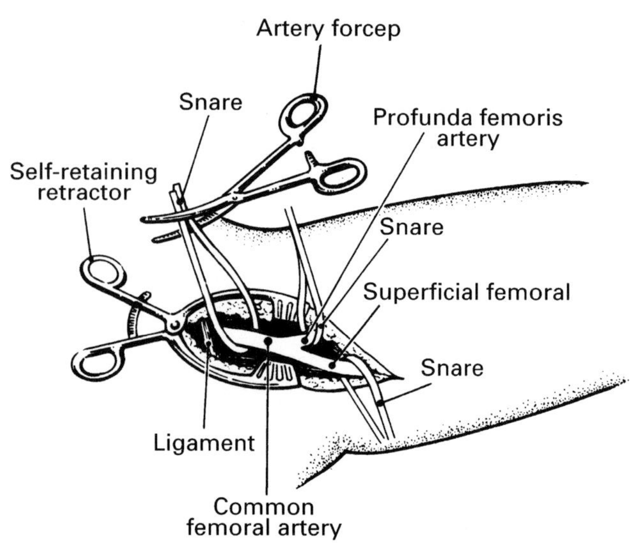

7

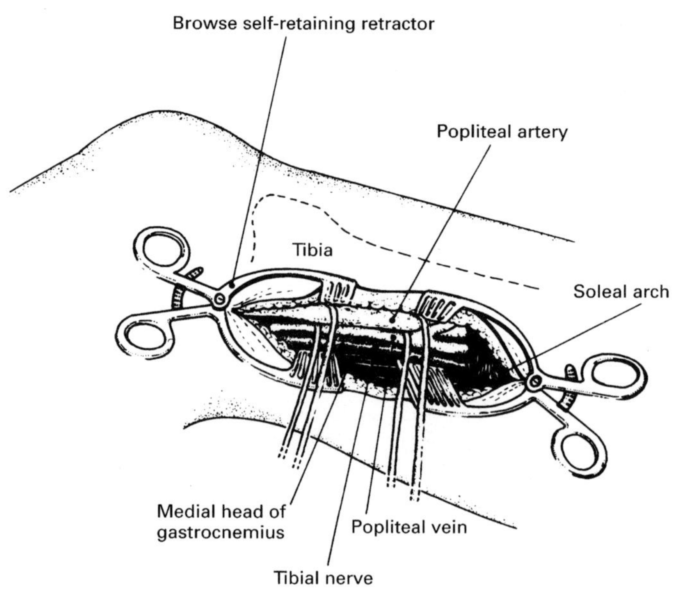

8

optimum site for the lower anastomosis can then be selected. Control of blood flow from the segment of artery to be used for the anastomosis can often be obtained by gently pulling up the snares and holding them taut over the central pinion of the self-retaining retractor. This avoids cluttering the wound with bulldog clamps which are applied if there is continued bleeding. Access to the upper part of the artery is obtained by dividing the medial head of gastrocnemius and the tendons attached to the upper end of the tibia. If exposure of the tibial vessel is required, the origin of soleus and anterior tibial veins can be divided.

High popliteal exposure

Better results are obtained from a short bypass ending above the knee provided the upper popliteal artery is found to have a lumen and is relatively disease-free. The anterior border of sartorius is found and freed above the knee through the incision used to expose the saphenous vein. This muscle is then retracted posteriorly and the upper part of the popliteal fat is exposed. The fat is separated by blunt dissection and the vessels are found lying deeply within the popliteal space. They lie close to the back of the bone and after insertion of the Browse self-retaining retractors are dissected and prepared in an identical manner.

9

The tunnel

A Wilson's or Taylor's tunneller is pushed upward between the heads of gastrocnemius through the apex of the popliteal space, into the thigh medial to the tendon of adductor magnus. The tunneller passes along Hunter's canal deep to sartorius and in front of the superficial femoral artery to emerge in the femoral triangle. The upper end of the saphenous vein is attached to the tunneller or its introducer by a silk suture and pulled back down from the groin to the popliteal space taking great care not to twist the vessel during its passage. This is checked by watching the dye marks previously applied to the surface of the vein, and making sure that they point in the same direction. The proximal end of the vein should lie over the common femoral artery and the distal end should lie over the prepared segment of popliteal artery without tension. The vein should be trimmed at the top end since this is usually its narrowest portion.

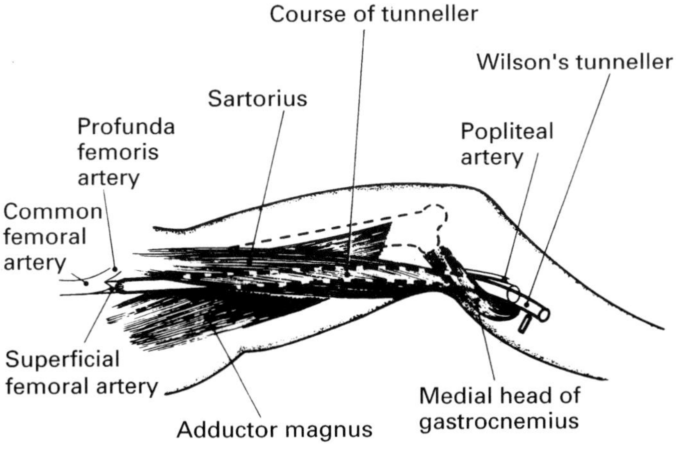

9

The popliteal anastomosis

The upper and lower anastomoses are carried out in an identical manner and may be performed simultaneously if two experienced surgeons are available with adequate assistance. This has the benefit of saving time and reducing the period of distal ischaemia. A dose of 5000 units of heparin is given by the anaesthetist and allowed to circulate. This dose is sufficient to prevent thrombosis during 1 h of arterial occlusion in normal-sized individuals, but it may be increased if the patient is very fat. Further increments of 2000 units are given if the anastomosis takes longer than 1 h.

The surgeon who is seated on a stool on the opposite side of the patient occludes the popliteal artery by tensing the snares over the central pinion of each self-retaining retractor. A small arteriotomy is then made in the centre of the prepared segment of popliteal artery using a No. 15 blade on a long-handled scalpel. A small quantity of blood escapes when the lumen of the vessel is entered. Bulldog clamps are applied if bleeding persists, which may occur in a heavily diseased or calcified vessel. The initial arteriotomy is then enlarged using Potts' scissors, angled on the vertical, until the length of the arteriotomy exceeds the width of the vein (usually 1 cm or more). The arteriotomy should finish well short of both snares. They are then released to assess the volume of back and downbleeding before heparin saline is instilled into the distal and proximal segments via a catheter of appropriate size. The end of the saphenous vein is then tailored to the length of the arteriotomy by cutting it obliquely while ensuring that there is enough vein to reach the distal point of the arteriotomy. The cut end of the vein should be matched for size against the arteriotomy.

10

A double-ended 6/0 polypropylene suture is used for the anastomosis, inserting both needles into the 'heel' of the vein as shown. The needles are then passed out through the proximal end of the arteriotomy on either side of its apex and a knot is tied on the superficial side of the vessel. One needle is then passed back between the attached vein and artery to the far side of the vessel in order to carry out the 'deep side' of the anastomosis.

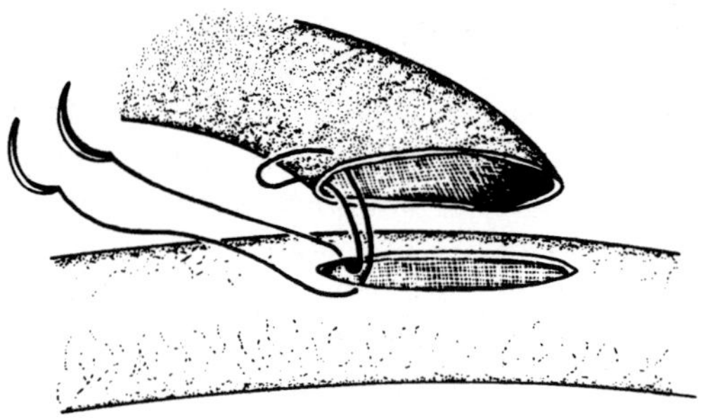

10

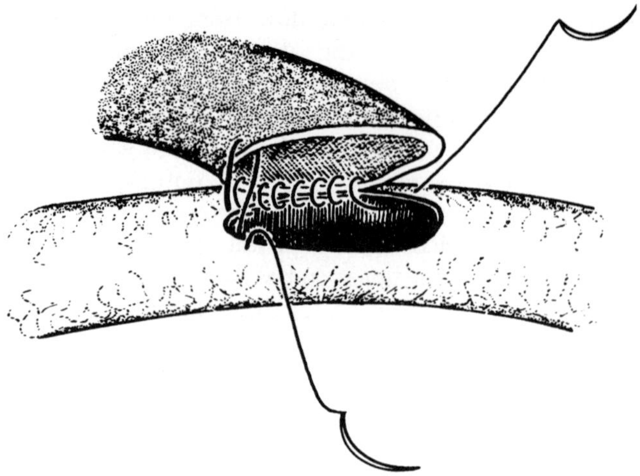

12

11

A standard continuous suture is then begun, entering the vein from out to in and the artery from in to out. Three or four sutures are placed on either side of the 'heel' under direct vision before the backhand side is sutured towards the apex of the graft.

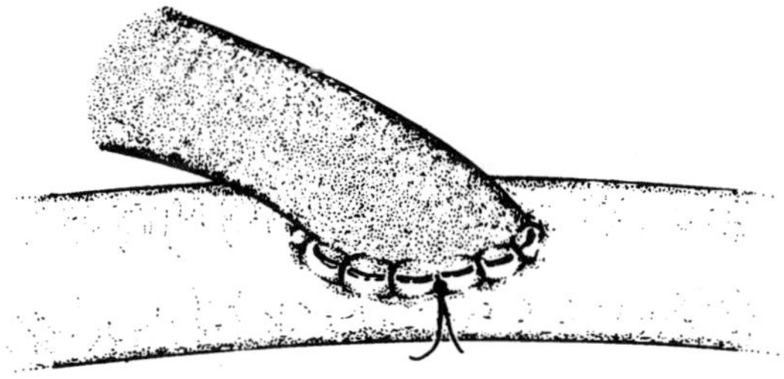

11

12

Carefully placed smaller bites are taken at the apex or 'toe' to ensure that the distal vessel is not narrowed or occluded. This part of the anastomosis must be carefully made to avoid picking up the far side of the vessel and to prevent narrowing.

Alternatively, a number of loops may be inserted under direct vision and pulled tight when the apex has been completed, or the continuous suture may be tied off and a series of carefully placed interrupted sutures put in around the apex.

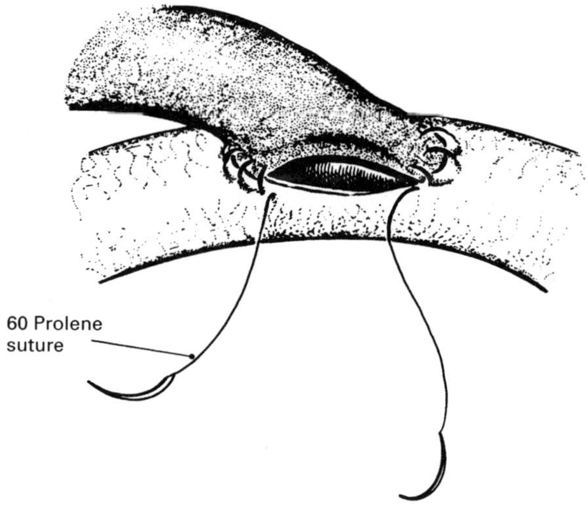

13

13

When the 'toe' has been passed, the over-and-over suture is completed on the near side, tying off both ends in the middle of the forehand side.

A bulldog clamp is then placed on the graft just proximal to the suture line and both snares are relaxed to allow the anastomosis to be checked for leaks and to allow the blood to perfuse the distal vessels again.

14

Alternative anastomosis techniquee

A parachute technique may be used on both the heel and the apex of the anastomosis inserting a number of 'loose' loops on both sides without tying down a knot. After six sutures have been inserted, the vein may be slid down to the artery while gentle traction is applied to the sutures. The central part of the anastomosis can then be completed in the usual manner on both sides.

15

Upper anastomosis

A small, angled Fogarty clamp is placed across the common femoral artery as close to the inguinal ligament as possible. Bulldog clamps are used to occlude the profunda and superficial femoral vessels. An arteriotomy is made in the common femoral artery which may be extended into the profunda femoris artery in the presence

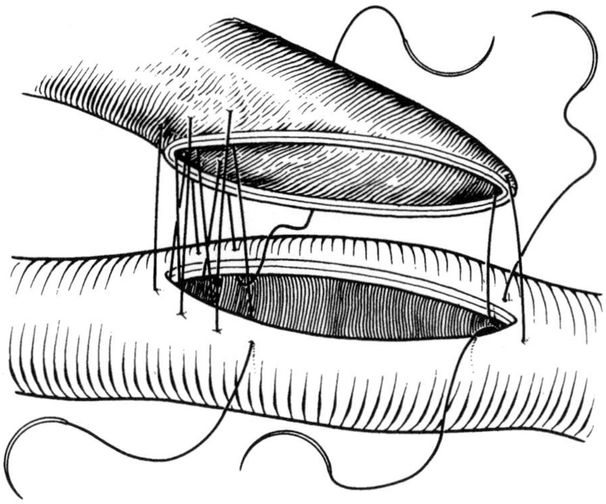

14

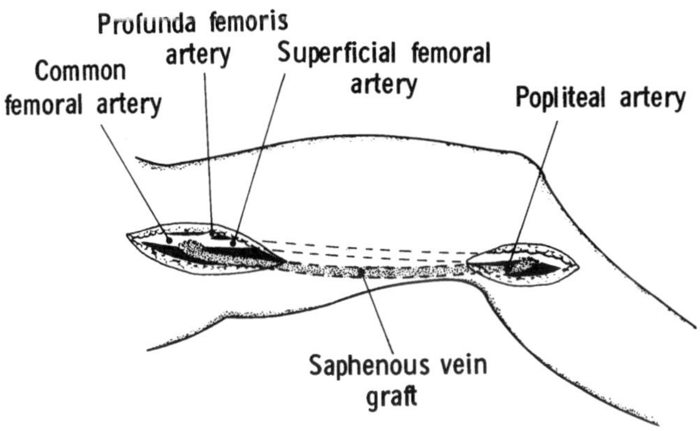

15

of a localized stenosis near its origin. The inflow is checked by releasing the proximal clamp and the back-flow from both superficial and profunda vessels is examined by releasing the bulldog clamps. A few milliliters of heparin saline are instilled into both distal vessels which are then reclamped. The anastomosis is made in an identical manner to that described for the popliteal vessels. When the anastomosis nears completion, the upper clamp is released to expel any thrombus which may have developed in the iliac artery above the clamp, and the final sutures are inserted. The ends are tied together as before. The bulldog clamp is removed from the lower end of the saphenous vein and the clamps on the superficial and profunda vessels are released. The Fogarty clamp is then released and the anastomoses at either end are examined for bleeding. Leaks are occluded by accurately placed single 6/0 polypropylene sutures inserted, if necessary, after the brief reapplication of the upper Fogarty clamp. A reversing dose of protamine 25–50 mg is given by the anaesthetist when it is certain that the vessel will not need to be reclamped again.

Confirmation of patency – operative arteriography

When the anastomoses are dry, the popliteal artery distal to the graft is carefully palpated to confirm the presence of pulsatile flow. The foot pulses are also examined through the sterile plastic bag. A green butterfly needle is inserted into the common femoral artery and an X-ray plate wrapped in a sterile Mayo table cover is placed behind the knee. The common femoral artery is briefly occluded and 20 ml of contrast (Conray or Hexobrix) are injected slowly through the butterfly to outline the graft. A spot film is taken of the popliteal anastomosis and run-off to detect any technical errors which might lead to early occlusion of the graft. We routinely perform operative arteriography after crural bypasses but only perform operative arteriography if in doubt for femoropopliteal bypasses.

Closure

The wound is closed with suction drains inserted near both anastomoses to prevent haematoma formation. The deep fascia and subcutaneous fat are closed with interrupted 2/0 chromic catgut. The skin is closed with 2/0 or 3/0 interrupted nylon mattress sutures or by disposable metal staples if preferred. The wound is covered with sterile adhesive dressings or a thin layer of gauze held in place by zinc oxide tape. Care is taken not to occlude the graft or its outflow by tight circumferential bandaging of the limb.

Postoperative care

The knee is flexed to 10 degrees or 15 degrees by supporting the lower leg on a soft pillow. The ankle is kept free of the bed clothes by a cradle placed over the feet, and the patient is kept in the recovery ward overnight in order that the pulses can be carefully monitored by well-trained staff. Doppler ankle pressures are used if severe distal disease makes the foot pulses impalpable. Some surgeons prefer to use a continuous pulse volume monitor.

The patient returns to the ward the following day provided that the pulses remain palpable and the Doppler pressures are satisfactory. Any disappearance of a previously palpable pulse or a marked deterioration in Doppler pressure is investigated by urgent digital subtraction angiography, conventional arteriography, or re-exploration and operative angiography. Confirmation of graft occlusion is an indication for urgent reoperation unless the run-off is deemed too poor to allow satisfactory graft function to be maintained. The suction drains are removed after 24 or 48 h if the postoperative course is uncomplicated. The patients should begin to walk on the third or fourth day after operation. Our patients can remain in hospital until the sutures or staples are removed on the tenth day, but many now leave hospital on the fifth or seventh day if they have an uncomplicated postoperative course.

Complications

The main complications are early graft occlusion, haemorrhage, infection, skin necrosis from undermining and leg swelling which is common. A careful technique reduces these problems to a minimum.

References

Harris PL, How TV, Jones DP (1987). Prospective randomised clinical trial to complete *in situ* and reversed saphenous vein grafts for femoropopliteal bypass. *Br J Surg* **74**: 252.

Mosley JG, Manhine AR, Raphael M, Marston JAP (1983). An assessment of long saphenous venography to evaluate the saphenous vein for femoropopliteal bypass. *Br J Surg* **70**: 673.

Senapati A, Lea Thomas M, Burnand KG (1983). A trial of saphenous phlebography compared with surgical dissection as a method of assessing suitability of long saphenous veins for use as a bypass graft. *Br J Surg* **70**: 688.

Cephalic and basilic veins as arterial conduits

Peter A Schneider, George Andros,
Robert W Harris, Leopoldo B Dulawa, Robert W Oblath

Introduction

The greater saphenous vein remains the optimal conduit for small-diameter arterial bypass grafts. In the venous circuit, the saphenous vein remains patent at low blood flow rates and it retains this quality when transposed to the arterial system. Its advantages include the highest long-term patency and limb salvage rates, autogenous reconstruction, ease of implantation and low complication rates. We use cephalic and basilic veins as arterial conduits for lower extremity revascularization when ipsilateral or contralateral saphenous vein is unavailable. Long-term follow-up has demonstrated that patency rates are equivalent to that obtained with saphenous vein (Andros *et al.*, 1992).

Decision to use upper extremity veins

Preoperative knowledge of previous saphenous vein excision permits preparation of the patient for alternative vein harvesting in 10% of patients. Intraoperative discovery of an inadequate greater saphenous vein because of phlebitis, varicosities, inadequate size or multiple trunks, occurs in 10–20% of cases. Arm vein can be employed in most clinical situations as a substitute for saphenous vein. Indications include bypass of occlusive disease of the lower limb, upper limb, and the visceral, renal and coronary vessels. Preoperative duplex evaluation of arm veins is beneficial. Past cutdown or phlebitis, usually from intravenous fluid therapy, accounts for the majority of non-usable upper extremity veins. Satisfactory veins can be harvested on the side of permanent pacemaker implantation or previous subclavian catheter insertion.

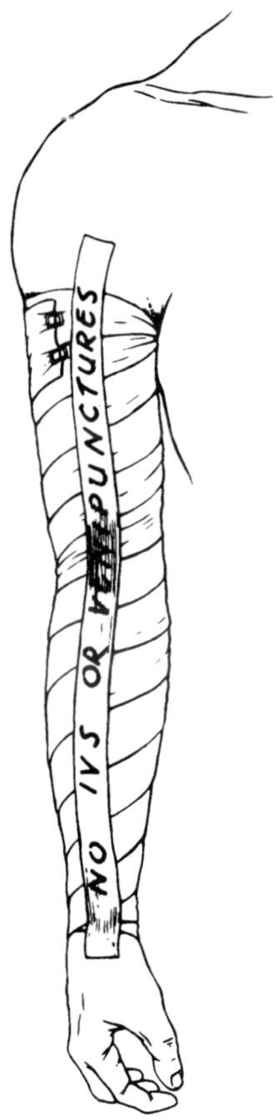

1

Preoperative

1

Preserving a potential graft

The characteristics of size, length and superficial position, which make arm veins desirable arterial conduits also predispose them to potentially damaging venipuncture. Education and protection are needed to prevent vein injury. The patients are shown their own cephalic and basilic veins and instructed to prohibit vein puncture for any reason. Venipuncture is limited to the dorsum of the hand. Signs are placed on the patient's room door, hospital bed, hospital chart and nursing records. The arm is wrapped with gauze upon which is written: NO IVs or VENIPUNCTURE.

2

Arm vein assessment

Arm veins are evaluated preoperatively on physical examination and with non-invasive ultrasonic techniques. The cephalic and basilic veins are examined in a warm room, by inspection and palpation, employing tourniquets, exercise and dependency. Special attention is directed to the antecubital fossa where variations in venous anatomy are often encountered. Inexact preoperative assessment may result from hair, obesity or tattoos. The latter, however, do not produce vein damage. Preoperative arm vein duplex evaluation has proven valuable in identifying useable veins (Salles-Cunha *et al.*, 1986). An arm vein map is constructed for each patient considered for arm vein harvesting. Arm phlebogram and preparatory cephaloradial arteriovenous fistula are not employed, although their use has been described.

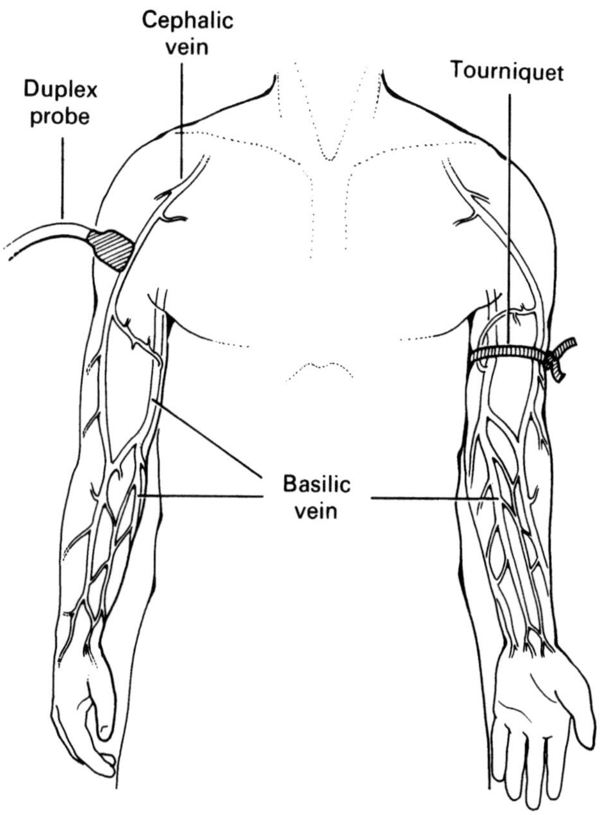

2

3

Upper extremity venous anatomy

The cephalic vein originates distal to the anatomical snuff box on the radial aspect of the wrist. Coursing medially to the antecubital fossa, it joins the median antecubital vein and then continues proximally (centrally), first on the lateral aspect of the biceps brachii and then in the deltopectoral groove, terminating in the axillary vein.

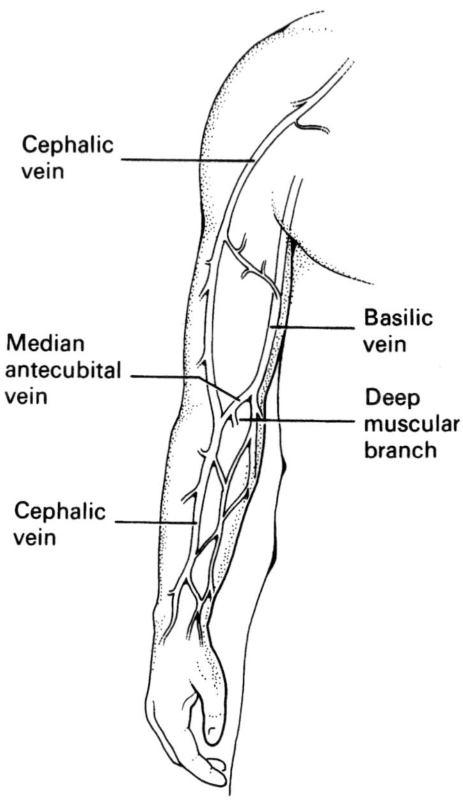

3

The median antecubital vein receives one or more deep muscular tributaries and the forearm tributary of the basilic vein; thereafter it continues as the basilic vein to the axilla. In the forearm the basilic vein diameter is more variable than the forearm portion of the cephalic vein. Males and females appear to have equally usable cephalic veins. Cephalic vein diameter is generally 5–6 mm distally and 6–8 mm proximally. The basilic vein proximally (centrally), is usually 7–10 mm. At the proximal end, both veins are very thin walled. The true cephalic vein from wrist to clavicle is only 15% shorter than the greater saphenous.

Choices of arm vein conduits include; 1) cephalic (forearm and upper arm), 2) forearm cephalic-median antecubital-upper arm basilic, 3) upper arm cephalic-median antecubital-upper arm basilic, 4) forearm basilic-median antecubital-upper arm cephalic (rare).

The operation

4

Operative preparation of the arm

Leg bypasses are generally performed under regional

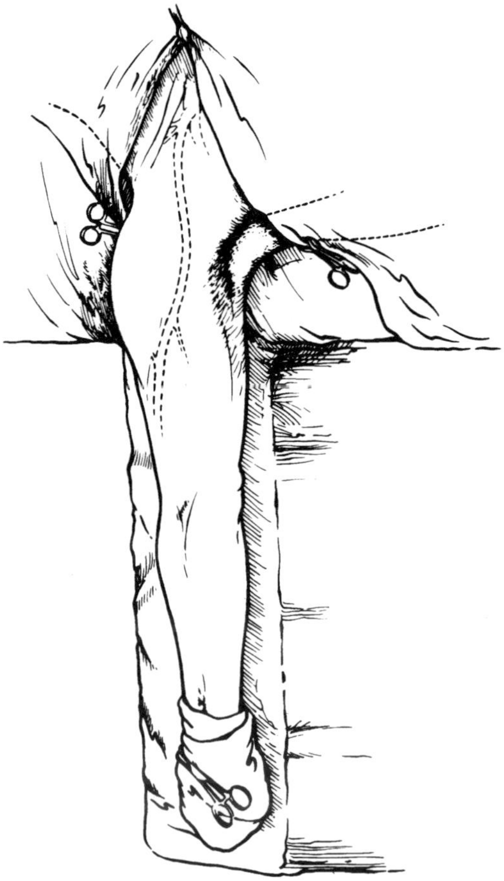

4

anaesthetic. When the decision is made to harvest arm veins, a general anaesthetic is administered. If both arms must be explored for veins, a jugular intravenous line is inserted. The arm is shaved from the wrist to the clavicle, including axilla, and placed on a moveable arm board. The hand is draped out with a towel. If a radial artery cannula is required for blood pressure monitoring, the wrist and hand are excluded from the field and the monitoring extension tubing extends from the towel wrapping the hand. The arm vein duplex map is posted in the operating room.

5 a–d

Unroofing

The antecubital incision is always transverse and is usually made first. Through the antecubital incision, the

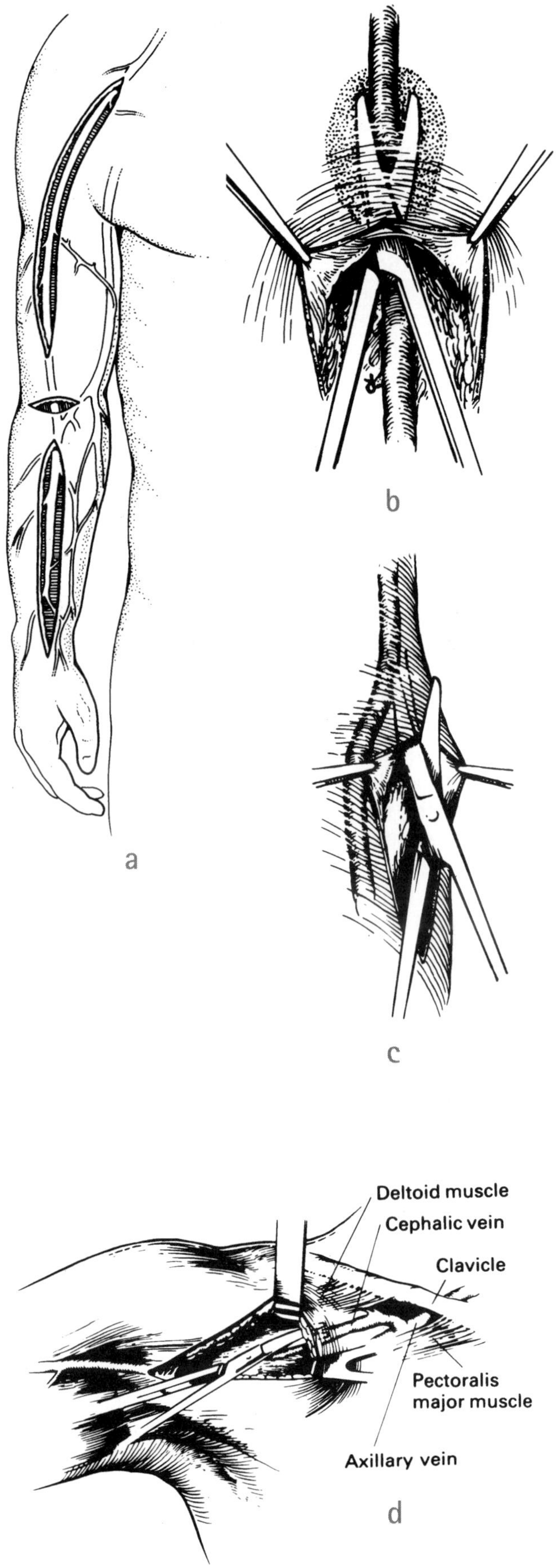

5

upper and lower cephalic and basilic veins can be localized so that longitudinal incisions can be placed directly over the veins. Before excision is undertaken, the entire vein is unroofed. Each incision is started with a scalpel and extended using scissors. Two manoeuvres help to prevent harm to the vein: spreading the scissors between the skin and the vein creates a space (shown as a stippled area) for the scissors' blades when the skin is cut (**5b**); only the body of the scissor blade, and not the tip, is used to cut the skin (**5c**).

Very few branches arise anteriorly and are easily seen as the vein is unroofed. One 2–3 cm skin bridge is generally placed in the proximal forearm and one in the distal upper arm. The proximal cephalic vein is mobilized up to the deltopectoral groove to its junction with the axillary vein (**5d**). The skin is undermined for 5 cm or more to decrease the length of the incision.

6

The antecubital decision

As the cephalic vein is unroofed proximally along the lateral biceps brachii, it may be found to be scarred or small. If so, the vein is usually inadequate all the way to the clavicle. The course of unroofing is then redirected. The transverse antecubital incision is extended medially along the median antecubital vein. The basilic vein is then unroofed through one long incision to the axilla, terminating the incision at the hairline. The upper arm basilic vein is usually free of disease because of difficulty of performing venipuncture in this area.

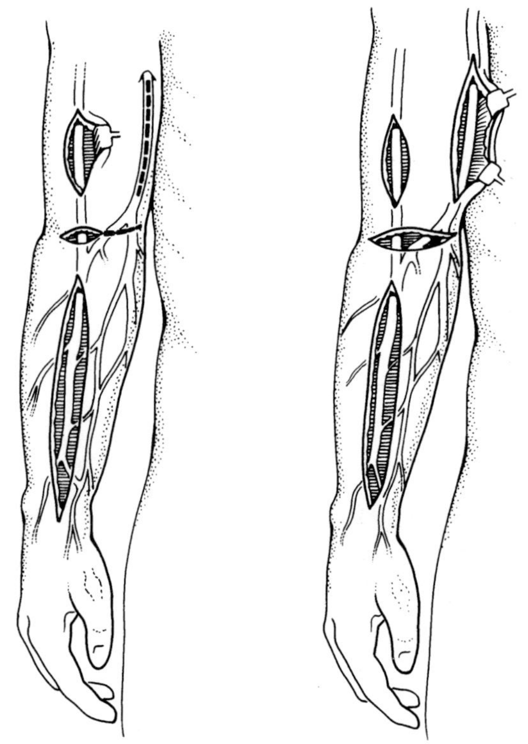

6

7

In situ distension

In situ distension with heparinized saline introduced through a No. 16, 5-cm plastic catheter placed in a side branch is helpful in deciding whether to use the cephalic or the basilic vein. Finger pressure is applied at various sites to permit distension of the segments in question. Some of the vein may be unusable and the decision to use the other arm or alternate graft material can be reached without excising the entire vein or even completely unroofing it.

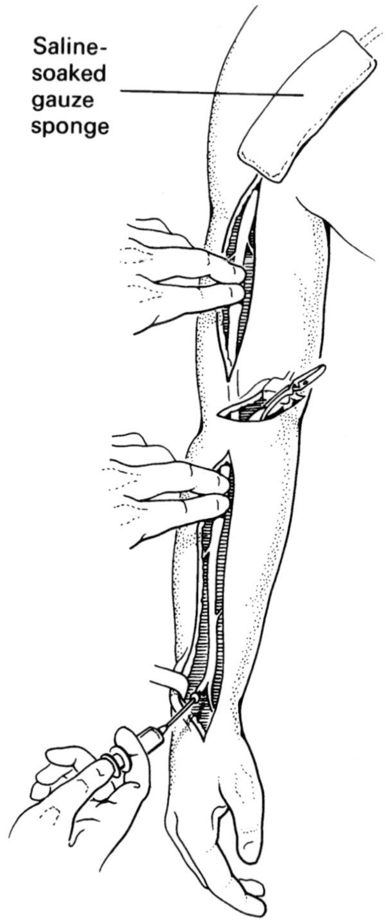

7

8 a, b, c

Excision

Excision of the unroofed vein is begun at the wrist or the most distal site. The vein is tied as distally as possible under the skin to obtain maximum length. It is divided, gently mobilized and rolled on to a wet gauze sponge; the unexcised portion is covered with wet sponges frequently irrigated with saline (**8a**).

The vein and its tributaries are circumferentially dis-

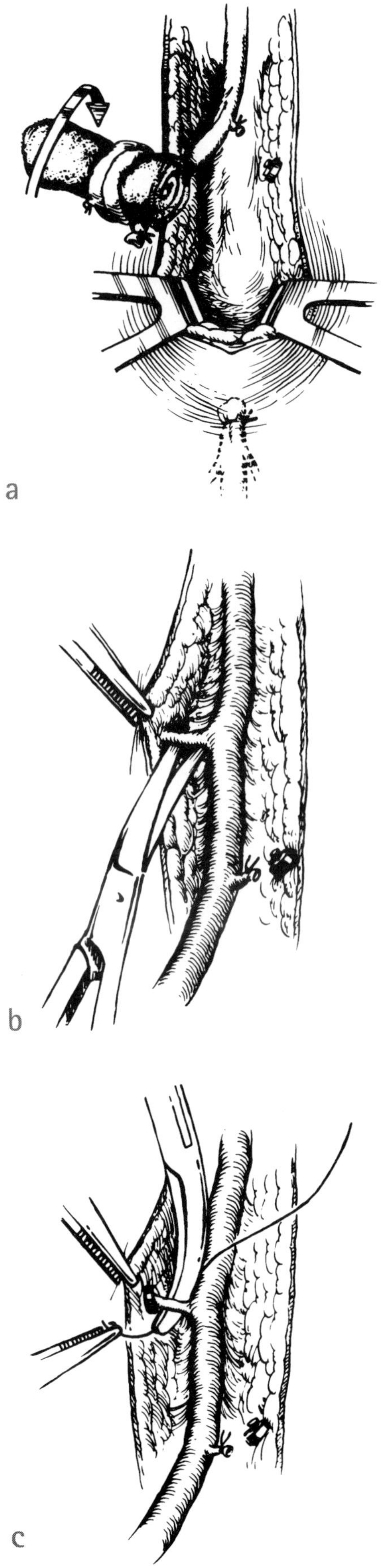

8

sected (8b). It is important to tie branches 1–2 mm from the vein to prevent adventitial gathering; 4–0 silk ligatures are used (8c). The vein is divided so that a 2–3 mm stump extends beyond the tie. Tributaries are haemoclipped distally. The vein is freed under the skin bridges and passed to the next incision. The vein is doubly tied with 2–0 silk at the axillary vein and divided. Venous scarring produced by antecubital venipuncture makes dissection more difficult and risks damage to both the cephalic and basilic veins. If the cephalic vein in the forearm and upper arm are usable, the median antecubital vein is not disturbed. If a segment of vein is diseased, it is excised and a long spatulated venovenous anastomosis is constructed using 7–0 Prolene.

Following excision, reversed venous conduits are filled with heparinized saline. The ease of irrigation is assessed and blood is removed. With a bulldog clamp on the central end, the vein is gently distended to determine length. Easily identified leaking tributaries are ligated with 4–0 silk ties.

9

Implantation

With the vein reversed, the proximal anastomosis is performed using 6–0 Prolene. Whenever possible, prosthetic grafts are avoided for the proximal anastomosis. Lower exremity grafts maintain long-term patency when

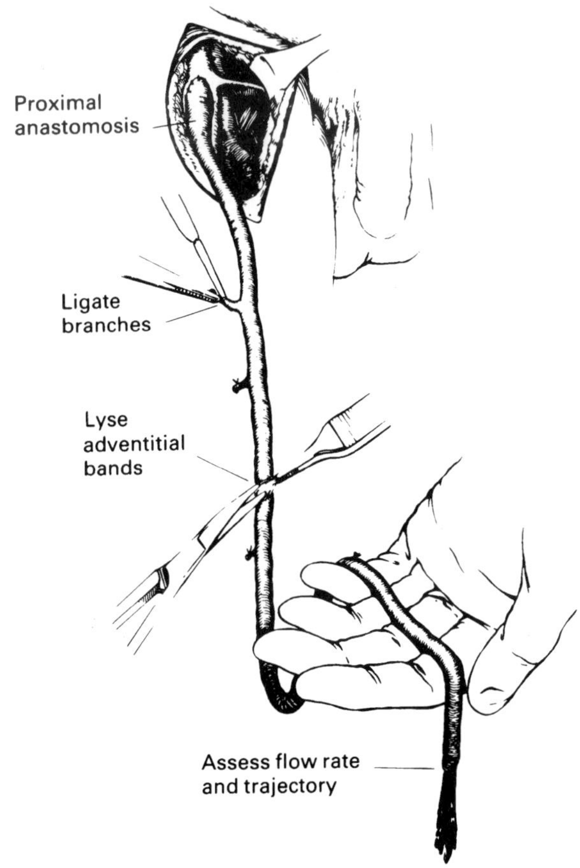

9

originating from the common, superficial or deep femoral arteries and the popliteal artery.

With the proximal anastomosis completed and inspected, the vein graft is allowed to distend with heparinized blood. Constricting adventitial bands are carefully divided. The graft is examined for additional bleeding tributaries. Blood flow from the end of the graft is observed. When a vein segment is placed in non-reversed orientation, valves must be lysed. The valvulotome is placed through the open end of the graft and introduced in retrograde fashion. Valve lysis in arm veins requires greater force than in saphenous veins. Firm counter traction must be held by the assistant. Vein valves can usually be seen through the vein wall. The end of the graft is brought to the distal anastomotic site in a previously formed deep tunnel adjacent to the native artery. By passing the graft when it is distended with blood, the risk of twisting or inappropriate graft length is minimized.

Postoperative anticoagulants are employed in the same way as for saphenous vein conduits begun on the first postoperative day.

10

Wound closure

Subcutaneous tissue is closed with running 3–0 chromic suture and skin is closed with staples. Incisions are covered with povidone-iodine ointment, dry dressings, a gauze wrap and padding over bony prominences. The entire area is wrapped with a 10-cm elastic bandage from the base of the fingers to the axilla. Dressings are removed on the third day and clips removed on the seventh day.

No long-term morbidity has been observed in arms from which veins have been harvested, even when both the cephalic and basilic veins are removed. Surprisingly little postoperative pain or swelling is experienced.

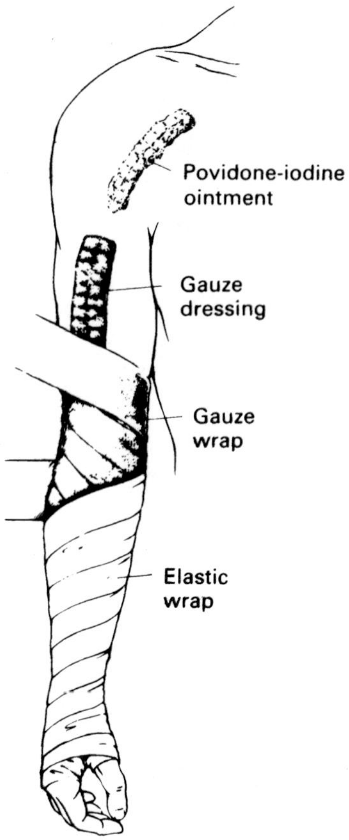

10

Complications

Arm veins are susceptible to all of the early and later complications encountered with saphenous veins. Haemorrhage and infection are infrequent and are treated as with saphenous vein. Thrombectomy within the first day of operation is difficult and should not be performed *in situ*. The vein wall is too thin to withstand catheter thrombectomy. The entire vein is removed, gently stripped of clot, irrigated with heparinized saline and reimplanted. Balloon embolectomy catheters can be hazardous and are best avoided. Late complications of inflow occlusion, neointimal hyperplasia, vein valve hypertrophy, aneurysmal dilatation and progression of outflow occlusive disease have all been observed and are treated as with saphenous veins.

Acknowledgement

We thank Ms Donna Welch for assistance in preparing this chapter.

References

Andros G, Salles-Cunha SX, Harris RW *et al.* (1992). Arm veins for arterial reconstruction surgery: A twenty-three year experience. In *Long Term Results in Vascular Surgery*. **Yao J, Pearce W** eds. Norwalk, CT: Appleton and Lange, pp. 247–258.

Salles-Cunha SX, Andros G, Harris RW *et al.* (1986). Preoperative noninvasive assessment of arm veins to be used as bypass grafts in the lower extremities. *J Vasc Surg* 3: 813.

Semi-closed endarterectomy of the superficial femoral artery

F H W M van der Heijden, T Theodorides, R W H van Reedt Dortland, B C Eikelboom

Introduction

In 1946 the Portuguese surgeon Dos Santos, in attempting a thrombectomy of a brachial artery, not only removed the arterial thrombus but the entire intima and a part of the media as well (Dos Santos, 1947). This was the first endarterectomy ever performed; 35 years later the artery was still patent. Following this first success, endarterectomy found many applications and was the start of a new era in vascular surgery. Dos Santos used the technique for desobstruction of the superficial femoral artery and was the first surgeon to treat arterial occlusive disease. A few years later Kunlin introduced the technique of femoropopliteal reversed venous bypass which has replaced endarterectomy in most hospitals. A number of recent studies have shown that complication rate, mortality and cumulative patency of superficial femoral artery endarterectomy are comparable with those of femoropopliteal reversed venous bypass (Heijden *et al.*, 1993).

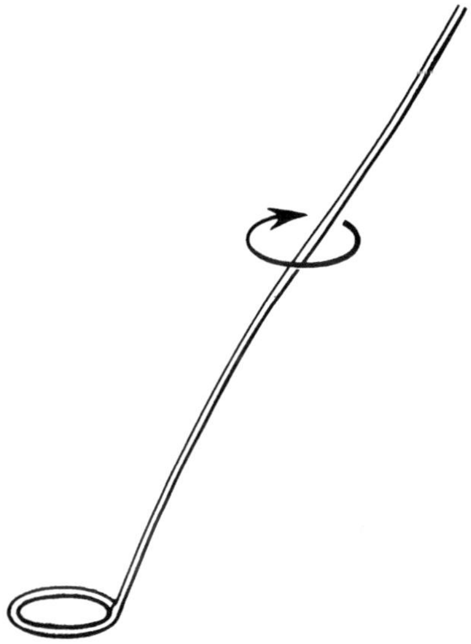

1

1

The technique of superficial femoral artery endarterectomy has since the days of Dos Santos been modified by a number of surgeons. Wylie introduced the technique of open endarterectomy (Wylie, 1952) which was later modified by Edwards (1960) who proposed closure of the entire endarterectomized segment by vein patching. Cannon and Barker (1955) introduced the semi-closed technique with the use of a ringstripper. Many other methods of developing a cleavage plane between intima and media have been used such as gas endarterectomy (Sobel *et al.*, 1966) and saline endarterectomy (Blaisdell *et al.*, 1966). They all proved to be inferior to the ringstripper. The shape of the ringstripper has been altered over the years and a number of devices have been used to replace the ringstripper, like a wire loop or spiral dissector (LeVeen, 1965). From all the techniques described above, the semi-closed endarterectomy with use of a ringstripper with a 45 degree angle is preferred.

2

The operation starts with a groin incision to expose the femoral bifurcation. A curved vertical incision is made over the femoral pulsation below the inguinal ligament. The origin of the superficial and deep femoral arteries are encircled as is the distal part of the common femoral artery.

3

The distal part of the superficial femoral artery and proximal part of the popliteal artery are exposed through a medial supragenual approach. An incision is made in the lower part of the thigh parallel to the long axis of the leg

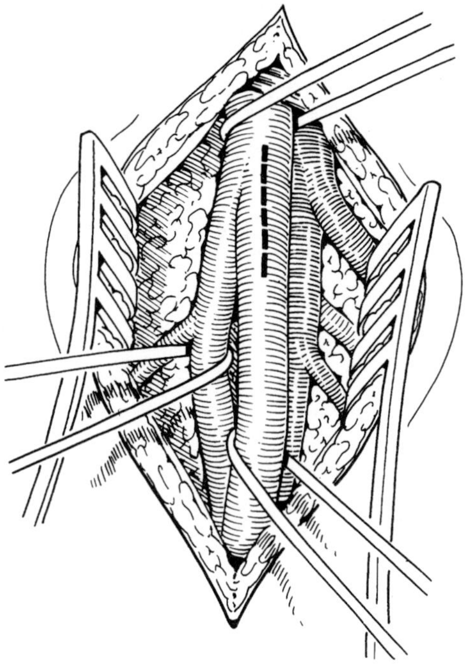

2

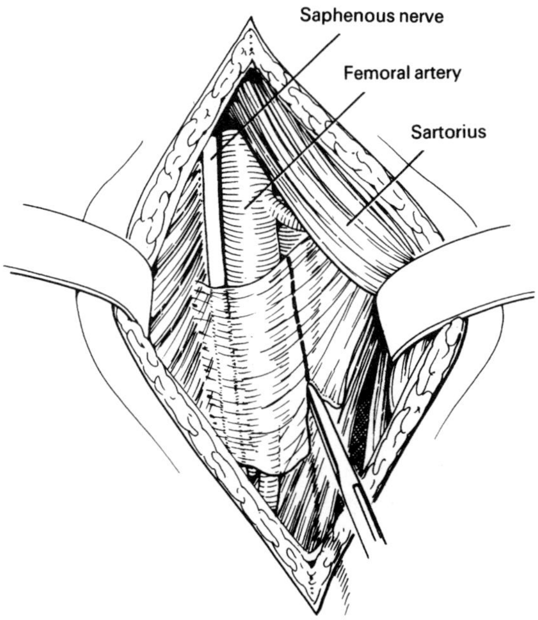

3

in the course of the greater saphenous vein which should be spared. The fascia overlying the sartorius muscle is incised longitudinally. The sartorius muscle is retracted medially and posteriorly. The incision is deepened to the vaso adductor membrane which is bluntly dissected and forms the anterior wall of Hunter's canal. The tendon of the adductor magnus is exposed over its entire length and is resected for better exposure of the artery and to facilitate passage of the ringstripper. Care should be taken not to damage the saphenous nerve.

4

The artery is further exposed and collateral arteries are temporarily encircled with vessel loops. After intravenous administration of 25 mg heparin, the arteries are clamped. The extent of the atheromatous plaque is judged by palpation to determine the site of the arteriotomy. In order to facilitate the arteriotomy the locally clamped arterial segment can be inflated with saline solution. The arteriotomy is placed at the distal end of the atheromatous plaque up into the relatively normal part of the supragenual popliteal artery.

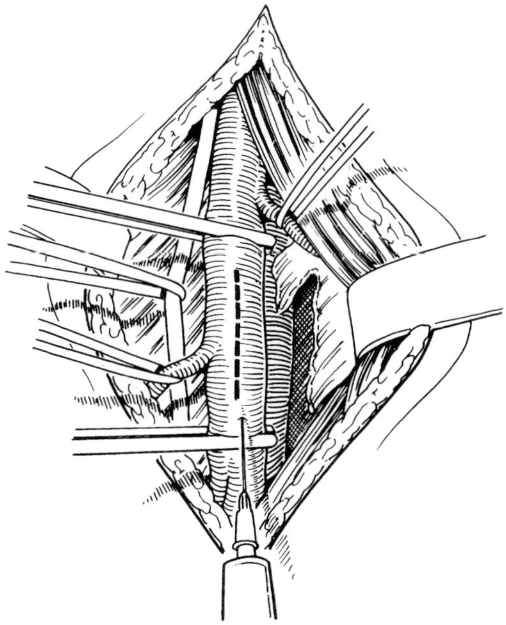

4

5

At this site a local open endarterectomy is performed. One of the most critical technical details of endarterectomy is the selection of the appropriate endarterectomy plane. The optimum plane of dissection lies between the diseased intima and the circular fibres of the media. A dissector is used to open up the cleavage plane between the outer layer of the atheroma and the media. This cleavage plane is easily established partly as a result of the pathological process in the diseased artery.

6

When the local endarterectomy is completed the endarterectomy core is cut. The distal end of the intima is fixed with tacking sutures to prevent dissection by antegrade blood flow. The local open endarterectomy is proximally extended just beyond the arteriotomy.

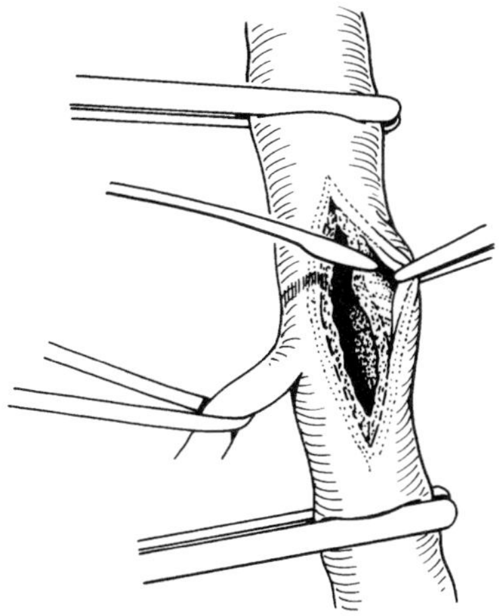

5

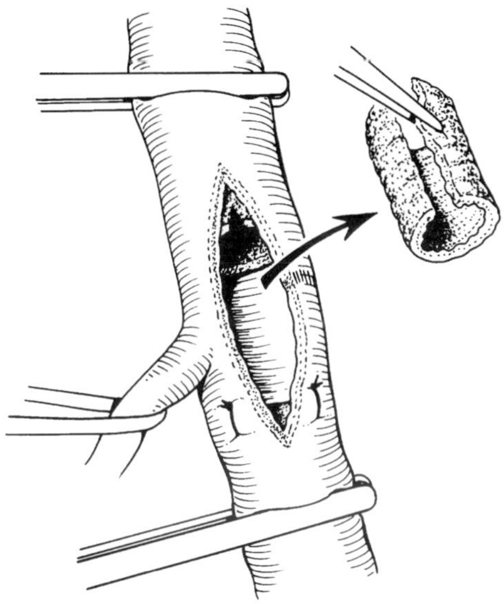

6

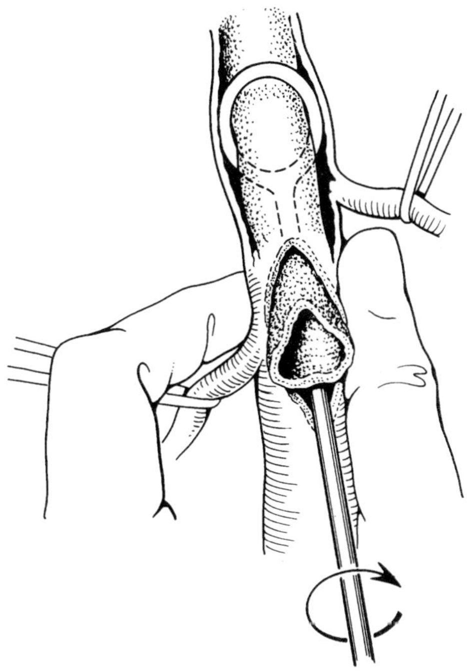

7

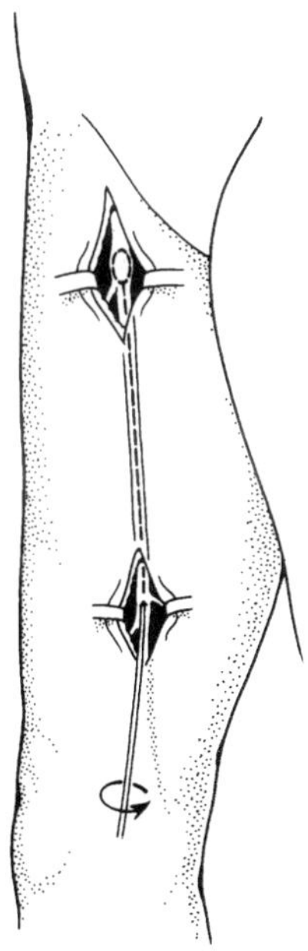

8

7

A ringstripper is selected which just fits inside the artery. The proximal end of the intima is threaded inside the loop of a ringstripper. One hand should hold the arterial wall and intima core fixed together in order to prevent 'roll-up' of the intima, while the other hand operates the ringstripper.

8

With a gentle rotating and thrusting motion the cleavage plane is gradually extended up into the groin. The stripper will usually pass the entire length of the superficial femoral artery without difficulty. If passage of the ringstripper cannot be achieved from this site, the stripper can also be introduced via an arteriotomy at the femoral bifurcation.

9

After palpation of the ringstripper in the groin a longitudinal arteriotomy is made at the femoral bifurcation. The intima core is cut at the origin of the superficial femoral artery. Distally slight traction is given to the intima core and ringstripper, and the entire core can be removed through the distal arteriotomy. The femoral bifurcation is inspected and if necessary an open endarterectomy of the femoral bifurcation is performed. The intima in the deep femoral artery can be fixed with tacking sutures.

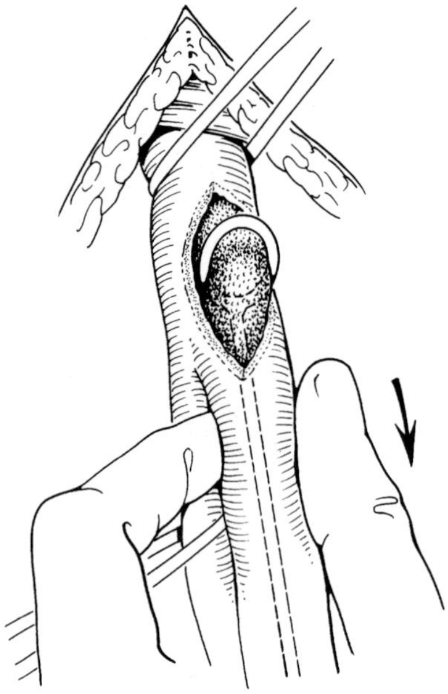

9

10

The superficial femoral artery is then flushed with heparinized saline solution. The diameter of the lumen of the endarterectomized superficial femoral artery is checked by passage of an olive-shaped probe with a diameter of about 6 mm.

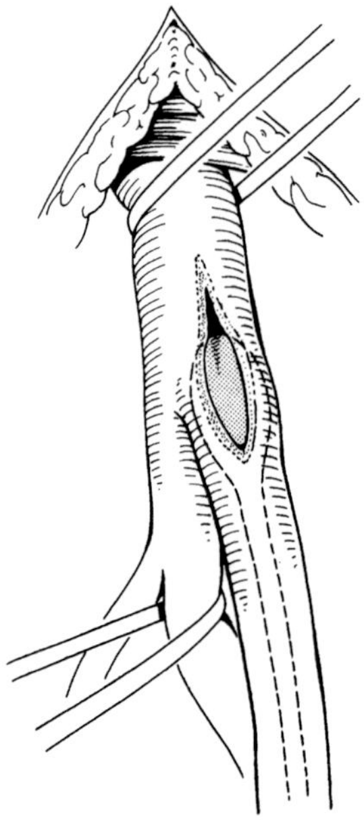

10

11

Both arteriotomies are closed by vein patches taken from the saphenous vein at the level of the ankle. The arteriotomy at the femoral bifurcation is closed first. Pulsations and flow in the distal superficial femoral artery are judged after declamping in the groin. Finally the distal arteriotomy is closed with a vein patch. At this point of the operation it is essential to perform a completion angiogram in order to detect intimal flaps or incomplete removal of the intima resulting in stenosis of the endarterectomized segment. All patients receive coumadines indefinitely.

Endarterectomy is a technically difficult operation with an intraoperative failure rate of 10% (Vollmar *et al.*, 1968). Failure often results from extensive calcification of the arterial wall which makes it impossible to establish a cleavage plane. Therefore if the preoperative angiogram shows extensive calcification of the artery or involvement of the middle or distal segment of the popliteal artery, femoropopliteal venous bypass should be performed.

While performing the endarterectomy special attention should be paid to the distal end of intima. The distal end of the intima should be fixed with tacking sutures to avoid dissection by antegrade blood flow. An arteriotomy at the level of the femoral bifurcation should always be performed. Blind dissection of the proximal end of the intima core will result in incomplete removal of the proximal intima and leads to residual stenosis. To prevent restenosis both longitudinal arteriotomies must be closed with a venous patch. At the end of the operation a completion angiogram should be performed in order to detect incomplete removal of the intima core. Often reopened collateral arteries are seen on the completion angiogram. Loose intimal flaps seen on the com-

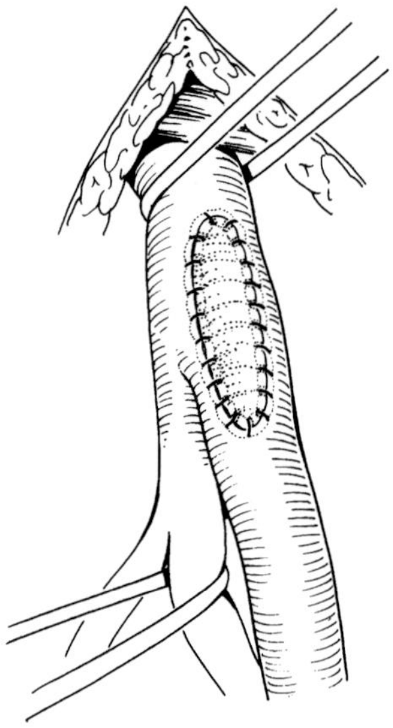

11

pletion angiogram, can be removed with a Fogarty adherent cloth catheter. Although we treat our patients with coumadines following endarterectomy, Schneider showed in a small randomized study that antiplatelet therapy was superior to anticoagulation (Schneider *et al.*, 1979). Therefore postoperative treatment with antiplatelet drugs may be considered as well.

Endarterectomy is a valuable alternative in the treatment of superficial femoral artery occlusive disease. No foreign bodies are being used and the saphenous vein is spared for future use. In case of endarterectomy failure a femoropopliteal above knee venous bypass remains possible. Endarterectomy should be considered as an alternative in patients with superficial femoral artery occlusive disease resulting in claudication. Furthermore the technique can be applied to restore vascular continuity after removal of an infected femoropopliteal bypass.

References

Blaisdell FW, Kall AD, Thomas AN (1966). Surgical treatment of chronic internal carotic artery occlusion by saline endarterectomy. *Annl Surg* **163**: 103.

Cannon JA, Barker WF (1955). Successful management of obstructive femoral arteriosclerosis by endarterectomy. *Surgery* **38**: 48.

Dos Santos JC (1947). Sur la desobstruction des thromboses arterielles anciennes. *Mém Acad Chirurgie* **73**: 409.

Edwards WS (1960). Composite reconstruction of the femoral artery with saphenous vein after endarterectomy. *Surg Gynecol Obstet* **111**: 651.

Heijden FHWM van der, Eikelboom BC, Reedt Dortland RWH van *et al.* (1993). Long term results of semi-closed endarterectomy of the superficial femoral artery and the outcome of failed reconstructions. *J Vasc Surg* **18**: 271.

LeVeen HH (1965). Technical features in endarterectomy. *Surgery* **57**: 22.

Schneidner E, Brunner U, Bollinger A (1979). Medikamentose Rezidivprophylaxe nach femoro-poplitealer Arterienrekonstruktion. *Angio* **2**: 73.

Sobel S, Kaplitt MJ, Reingold M, Sawyer PN (1966). Gas endarterectomy. *Surgery* **59**: 517.

Vollmar J, Trede M, Chir B *et al.* (1968). Principles of reconstructive procedures for chronic femoro-popliteal occlusions: Report on 546 operations. *Annl Surg* **2**: 215.

Wylie EJ (1952). Thromboendarterectomy for arteriosclerotic thrombosis of major arteries. *Surgery* **32**: 275.

Popliteal aneurysm and entrapment

Norman M Rich

Introduction

The popliteal artery is approximately 20 cm in length extending from the adductor hiatus to the lower border of the popliteus muscle. Identification of the many structures in the popliteal area is considerably different from the medial and posterior approaches. The anatomy can be confusing and those with limited experience are frequently at a higher location on the popliteal artery than recognized. An anatomic surface landmark is the head of the fibula, which is usually at the level of the origin of the anterior tibial artery with the continuation of the tibial-peroneal trunk continuing for approximately an additional 3 cm before dividing into the posterior tibial artery and the peroneal artery. Anatomic classification can be confusing because there is frequent description of a popliteal trifurcation which exists in only a very small percentage of patients. There are numerous anatomic variants which should be recognized appropriately. Aneurysms may be difficult to palpate, particularly in the upper third. Aneurysms contain laminated thrombus which can detach an emboli with movement and muscular action. This is an unfortunate complication. Elongation and kinking can accompany dilatation of the popliteal artery and occlusion may occur.

Popliteal aneurysmectomy has been generally abandoned in place of popliteal aneurysmorrhaphy because of the frequent trauma to the popliteal vein which is closely adherent to the wall of the aneurysm. Thrombosis of the popliteal vein with subsequent lower extremity swelling was a frequent complication when aneurysmectomy was performed. A bypass can be used successfully in the majority of cases; however, decompression of a large popliteal aneurysm may be valuable with an incision into the wall of the aneurysm opposite the vein with extraction of the thrombus. Occasionally, there might still be consideration for proximal Hunterian ligation in the very elderly who are at increased risk, especially when the aneurysm is ruptured.

The medial approach for popliteal aneurysmorrhaphy

While general anaesthesia can be used and the patient is monitored as described in the first chapter: 'Planning the intervention', regional anaesthesia may be used, particularly in the elderly who are at high risk. The leg is semiflexed at the knee with support in that position and the foot can be held by a cushion or a heel-ring. The surgeon has the advantage of facing the medial side of the leg.

1

Incision

The incision is usually continuous. It can be placed conveniently over the greater saphenous vein which can be harvested easily. Efforts should be made to prevent undermining skin flaps which may lead to poor healing of the incision. The vein may be obtained at this level or from the groin area and prepared as described in the chapter: 'Reversed saphenous vein for femoropopliteal bypass grafting' (p. 315).

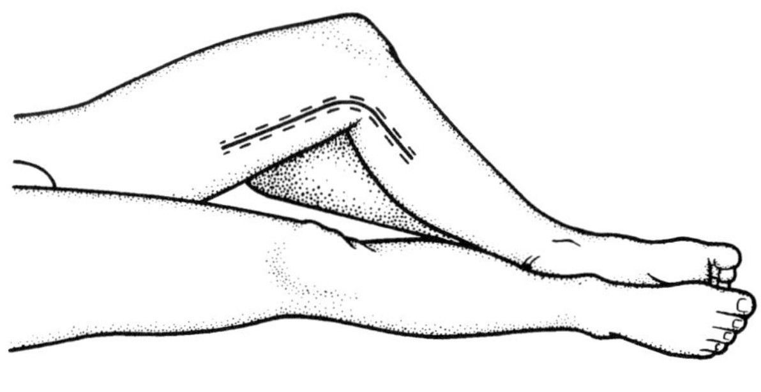

1

2

Approach to the artery

Initially, the popliteal artery is identified as it emerges below the adductor hiatus by separating the sartorius and medialis muscles. Proximal arterial control is obtained by use of a vascular loop (it is also the site of Hunterian ligation which might be considered for a ruptured popliteal aneurysm in the compromised elderly patient). The superficial femoral artery above the adductor hiatus may also be encircled with a vascular tape if this is the intended site of the upper anastomosis.

The popliteal artery distally is approached as described in the chapter: 'Reversed saphenous vein for femoropopliteal bypass grafting' (p. 315). The sartorius, gracilis, semimembranosus and semitendinosus muscles are encountered and usually do not require division. It is usually not necessary to divide the soleus tunnel. The popliteal artery is separated from the popliteal vein and tibial nerve and a vascular loop is placed for distal control. The anterior tibial artery origin is usually easily identified.

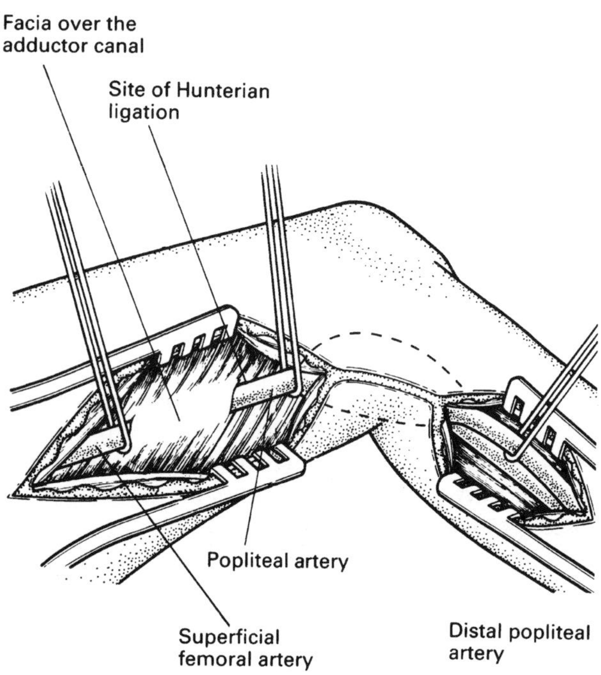

2

3

Anastomosis for the graft

With the patient's blood heparinized, atraumatic vascular clamps can be applied both proximally and distally. At this stage a ligature of strong suture is used to ligate the popliteal artery just proximal to the aneurysm and the distal popliteal artery is ligated as high as possible. An end-to-side proximal anastomosis of the reversed greater saphenous vein bypass is usually accomplished most easily in the distal superficial femoral artery. The distal anastomosis can either be end-to-side or end-to-end using 5/0 vascular suture.

After completion of the proximal anastomosis and near completion of the distal anastomosis, the arterial clamps are removed to fill the vein and to eliminate any air, followed by completion of the anastomosis.

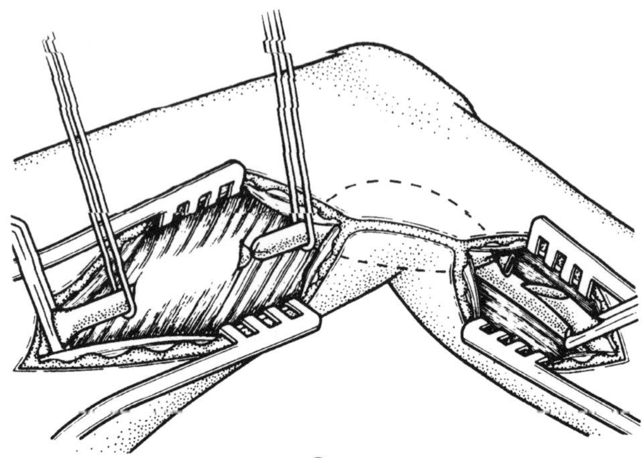

3

4

Tunnelling and the upper anastomosis

There may be variation in the best route for the vein bypass. This may require incision into the aneurysm to evacuate thrombis to prevent tension against the vein. Care must be taken to prevent entrapment of the bypass by the long medial tendons. A subcutaneous route may be elected and satisfactory. The proximal anastomosis may be end-to-end as well as end-to-side. Precise suture techniques are described in the second chapter: 'Techniques of anastomosis' (p. 7).

The incision is closed in layers. The use of suction drains for 12 h is a matter of choice.

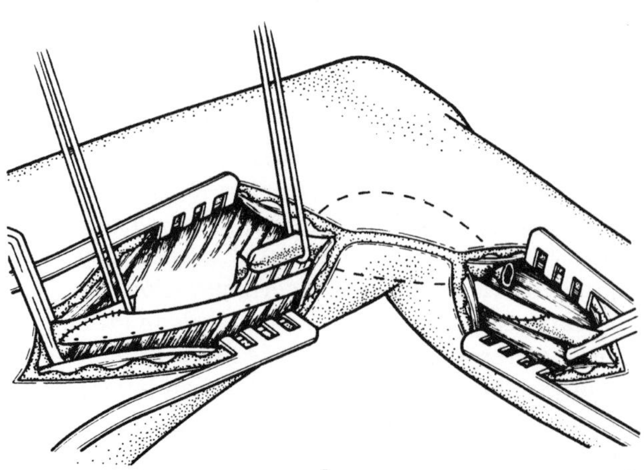

4

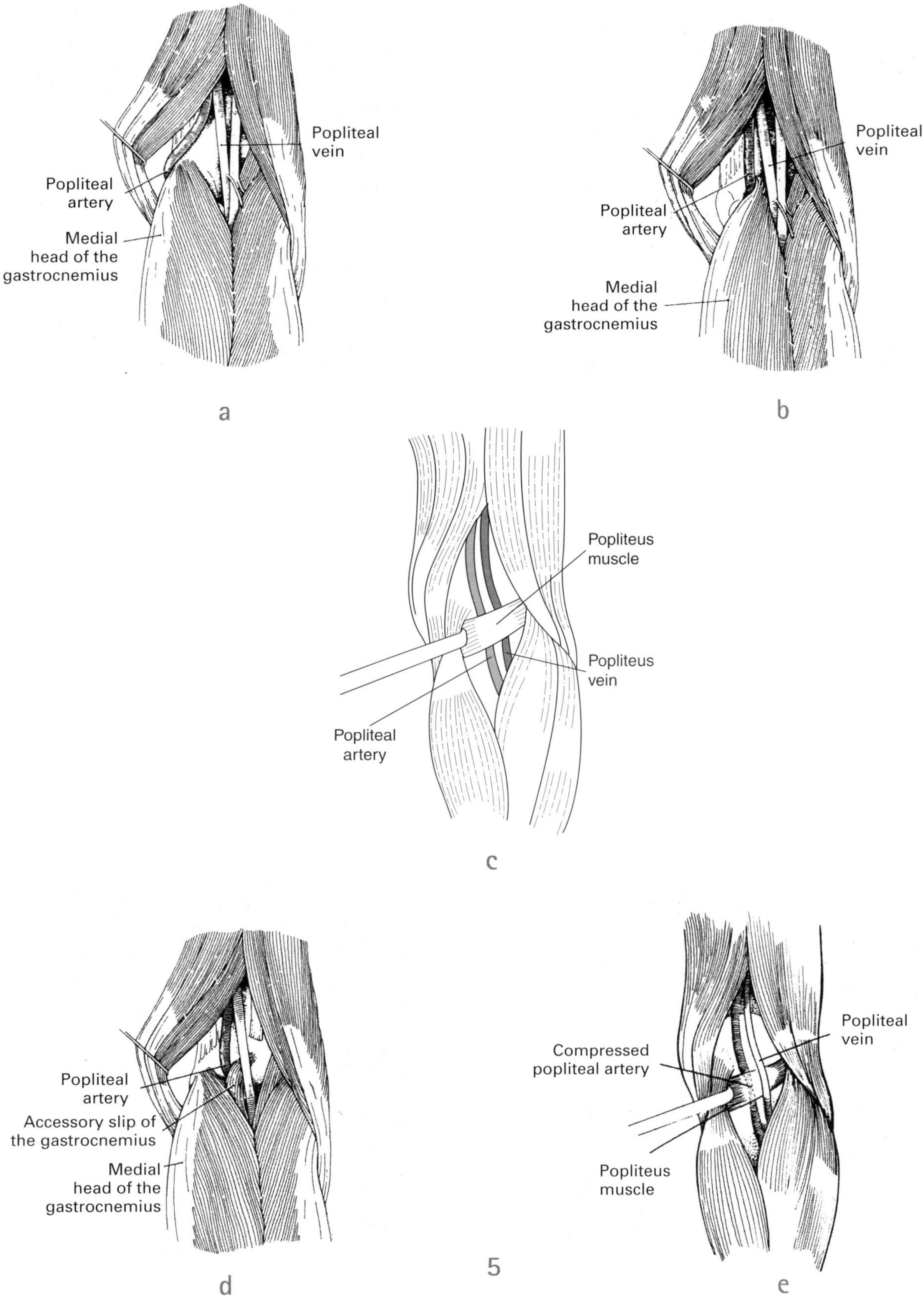

5

5a: Exaggerated medial looping of the popliteal artery around and under normally arising head of the gastrocnemius muscle. Medial hamstring muscles have been retracted.

5b: The course of the popliteal artery is straighter but still medial to and beneath the medial head of the gastrocnemius, which arises more laterally than normal.

5c: Any type where vein follows artery and entrapment follows.

5d: The structure compressing the popliteal artery is an accessory muscle or fascial slip arising more laterally than the medial head of the gastrocnemius muscle.

5e: The popliteal artery is entrapped by the popliteus muscle or a fibrous band in the location. The artery may or may not pass medial to the medial head of the gastrocnemius muscle.

Popliteal entrapment and the posterior approach to the popliteal artery

5 a,b,c,d,e

Since the anomalous course of the popliteal artery was first identified in 1879 by a medical student in Edinburgh, a variety of forms of entrapment of the popliteal artery, and vein, have been identified and one classification includes five separate varieties. Most commonly, however, there is an abnormal lateral insertion of the medial head of the gastrocnemius muscle which can entrap and displace the popliteal artery medially (Rich *et al.*, 1979; Bouhoutsos and Daskalakis, 1981). There can also be accessory slips of the medial head of the gastrocnemius muscle, fibrous bands and an assortment of more unusual anatomic variations.

The posterior approach is preferred to identify the anatomic variants easily, which might be missed when utilizing the medial incision to the popliteal neurovascular bundle. Yet, there might be an associated aneurysm with the entrapment, and the medial approach and bypass might also be selected. For the posterior approach, the patient is prone and the ankle is slightly raised to flex the knee. Colour duplex scanning has been shown to be the ideal diagnostic method for this condition.

6

Incision

The incision is 'S' shaped, being reasonably vertical and midline to follow the course of the artery. At the popliteal fossa the skin crease is included in the incision in an attempt to avoid later skin contracture.

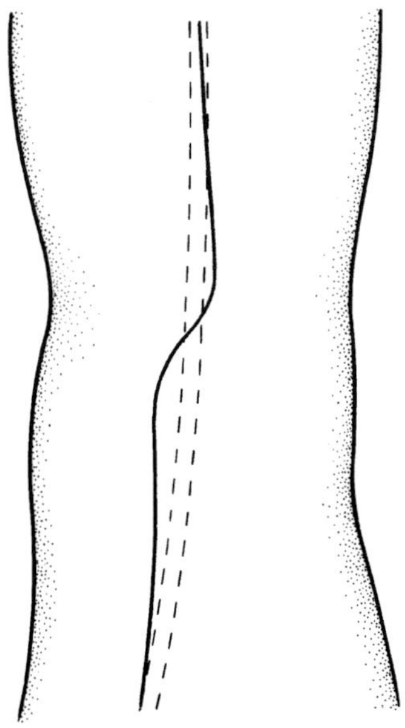

6

7

The incision is extended through the fascia into the popliteal fossa approaching the neurovascular bundle, and then the artery is separated carefully from the vein and the tibial nerve. Vascular loops are placed proximally and distally on the popliteal artery. Usually, it is necessary to divide the small branch of the nerve to the medial head of the gastrocnemius muscle to aid in exposure. Incision through the fibrous portion of the abnormal lateral attachment of the medial head of the gastrocnemius muscle may be all that is required, or similar incision through fibrous bands or accessory muscles may release the popliteal artery, and possibly the vein from the entrapment. If there is poststenotic dilatation which has progressed to aneurysm formation, bypass or replacement with a reversed segment of autogenous greater saphenous vein may be required. If thrombosis of the artery has occurred, an onlay saphenous vein patch graft with thromboendarterectomy may be successful.

The wound is closed in layers. Drainage is not usually required.

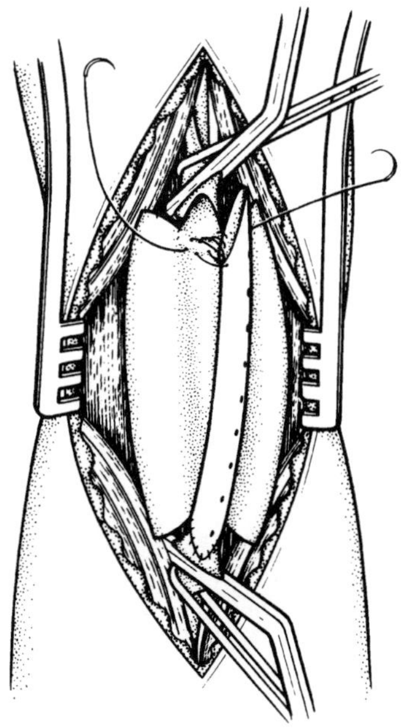

7

Complications

Thrombosis of any arterial reconstruction may be due to technical fault. Re-exploration and removal of the thrombus with a Fogarty catheter is recommended. These problems can be minimized by confirming patency and suture line integrity using on-table angiography at the completion of the reconstruction.

With a popliteal aneurysm care must be taken to see that there is no unnecessary manipulation so as to prevent distal embolization of thrombus from the aneurysm.

Thrombosis of the popliteal vein can occur and this is a reason to avoid unnecessary dissection around the popliteal vein. Elevation of the limb, early inactive calf movements, physiotherapy and compression hose are all adjunctive measures that can be utilized to prevent this complication. If thrombosis occurs, heparin and warfarin therapy should be utilized.

References

Bouhoutsos J, Daskalakis E (1981). Muscular abnormalities affecting the popliteal vessels. *Br J Surg* **68**: 501.

Rich NM, Collins GJ, McDonald PT, *et al.* (1979). Popliteal vascular entrapment *Arch Surg* **114**: 1377.

Sites and approach for tibial anastomoses

Charles N McCollum

Introduction

A feature in the development of vascular surgery in recent years has been the increasing willingness to extend arterial bypass to smaller distal arteries in an attempt to avoid amputation. The posterior tibial artery was first used as the 'run-off' vessel approximately 30 years ago (Palma, 1960; Dale, 1963), but these techniques were not widely accepted until recently. Where an adequate vein is available, and with careful case selection, graft patency rates of 50–70% at 1 year have produced worthwhile limb salvage in these cases (Noon *et al.*, 1969; Davies *et al.*, 1975). However, where the vein is not adequate and a prosthetic substitute has to be used, the results are considerably less encouraging, with graft thrombosis sometimes exceeding 50% within 6 months (Klimach and Charlesworth, 1983). In the absence of a dramatically new material or approach to the bypass of small arterial disease, we can only expect improvement by attention to three main areas. First, the use of saphenous vein could be extended to a greater proportion of patients by one of the techniques for *in situ* vein bypass (Hall and Rostad, 1978; Leather *et al.*, 1979). Second, it may be possible to improve patency by increasing the blood flow within the graft using a distal arteriovenous fistula as suggested by Ibrahim *et al.* (1980) Third, patency may be improved in vascular reconstructions by prescribing platelet inhibitory drugs, although good evidence of their benefit in peripheral reconstruction is only available in patients receiving prosthetic bypasses (Green *et al.*, 1982; Goldman *et al.*, 1983).

The quality of popliteal 'run-off' is important in femoropopliteal bypass with the best results obtained when two to three tibial arteries are patent. It therefore seems logical in bypasses below this level to consider implanting the distal anastomosis to more than one calf artery. This approach has recently been described using both inverted Y vein grafts and sequential anastomoses at and below the knee (Edwards *et al.*, 1976; Piccone *et al.*, 1978). The combination of *in situ* saphenous vein bypass with the use of either a natural or a sutured bifurcation might extend the use of vein, improve total graft flow and increase perfusion to the distal calf and foot. By these means it may be possible to prevent the few frustrating amputations that have to be performed in the presence of a patent femorotibial bypass.

Indications and preoperative assessment

The almost exclusive indication for tibial bypass is ischaemic rest pain or frank tissue necrosis or ulceration of the foot. Occasionally, patients with severely ischaemic feet and lower legs may suffer a minor injury which ulcerates and fails to heal. In these cases reconstruction may have to be considered in the absence of typical rest pain. Reconstruction to the proximal posterior tibial artery may, very rarely, be indicated for severe claudication alone, but the author doubts that reconstruction to the other calf arteries, particularly at the distal sites of anastomosis, should ever be performed for this indication. The peripheral distribution of arterial disease in these patients is such that calf claudication is rarely an important feature in the history. Many of the patients undergoing these procedures will be diabetic and some will have thrombangitis obliterans. These conditions are not contraindications but it is unlikely that a successful outcome will result when none of the calf arteries cross the ankle and communicate with the foot. This does not of course prohibit the use of the peroneal artery where one of the other two arteries is reconstituted at or just below the ankle and may then be filled by collaterals.

Most patients requiring arterial bypass to the distal calf are elderly and usually unfit. The preoperative assessment must obviously include careful evaluation of all the factors already described in the first chapter: 'Planning the intervention'. Angiography is almost always required, not only to assist in the selection of distal anastomotic sites, but to confirm the adequacy of the proximal arterial system. Often with a distal distribution of disease typical in these patients it is possible to site the proximal anastomosis at the superficial femoral artery just above the adductor canal, thereby shortening the length of bypass. The quality of image obtained in the distal calf is often poor, and selective angiography to each limb is essential. It is now well recognized that despite the most carefully performed angiography, patent distal arteries may not opacify. Patency can be detected with greater sensitivity using a standard Doppler flow probe to insonate the three arteries at ankle level which also allows assessment of the pedal arch (Simms, 1988). Angiography detects only a mean of 1.3 patent arteries per leg in patients requiring femorotibial bypass, whereas Doppler insonation will detect a mean of 2.2 arteries per leg. It must of course be recognized that those arteries detected by arteriogram may be more suitable for distal anastomosis and that a higher rate of failure may be associated with Doppler detection alone.

Preoperative preparation

Many patients requiring tibial bypass will already have had either an operative or a chemical lumbar sympathectomy. On the basis that a few patients do improve with sympathectomy alone we usually perform a chemical sympathectomy during the period of evaluation. Although sympathectomy may only increase the flow of blood in arteriovenous shunts in the distal limb this may augment the total graft flow following implantation and theoretically improves the chances of subsequent patency (Terry *et al.*, 1972). Once it has been determined that a femorotibial bypass is possible, the patient is started 2 days preoperatively on the platelet inhibitory combination of aspirin and dipyridamole given orally. At this stage a plan is made as to which arteries should be explored and in what order. Obviously, where two patent calf arteries are known to cross the ankle the selection of distal anastomoses is easy. Finally, on the day before surgery the saphenous vein and, where possible, its natural branches, are marked on the skin to aid the subsequent dissection.

Operative technique

1

Medial incisions and long saphenous vein exposure

The medial incisions are placed over the long saphenous vein to minimize dissection in the subcutaneous fat. The author's preference is for separate incisions with the upper one extending 12 cm below the saphenofemoral junction in order that the first two valves and the upper branches can be seen. Further incisions are made centred 12–15 cm above the knee and 8–10 cm below the knee as these are regions where sizeable branches are usually found. Where there are many branches from the long saphenous vein or where the valve stripper does not pass easily, the incision may be converted to full length without hesitation.

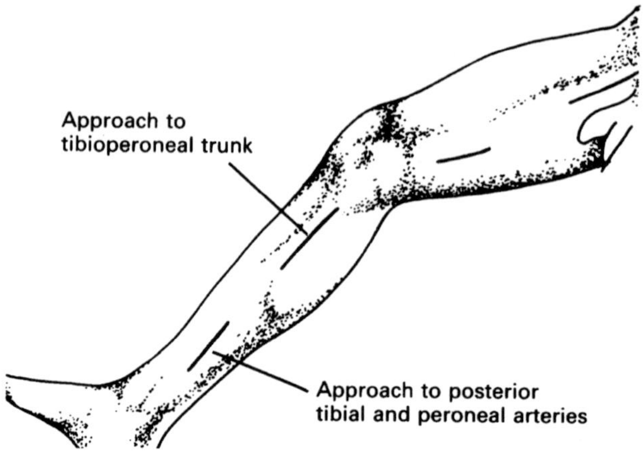

1

2

Exposure of tibioperoneal trunk

The incision used to expose the saphenous vein just below the knee is deepened. The deep fascia is incised 1–2 cm posterior to the upper tibia as shown. The gastrocnemius muscle is retracted posteriorly and in the upper part of the incision the tendons of semitendinosis and gracilis are exposed. Where the distal popliteal artery above the bifurcation of the anterior tibial artery is of adequate quality to receive the graft, these tendons may need to be divided to gain adequate access. The tibioperoneal trunk is found deep to the arch of the soleus which

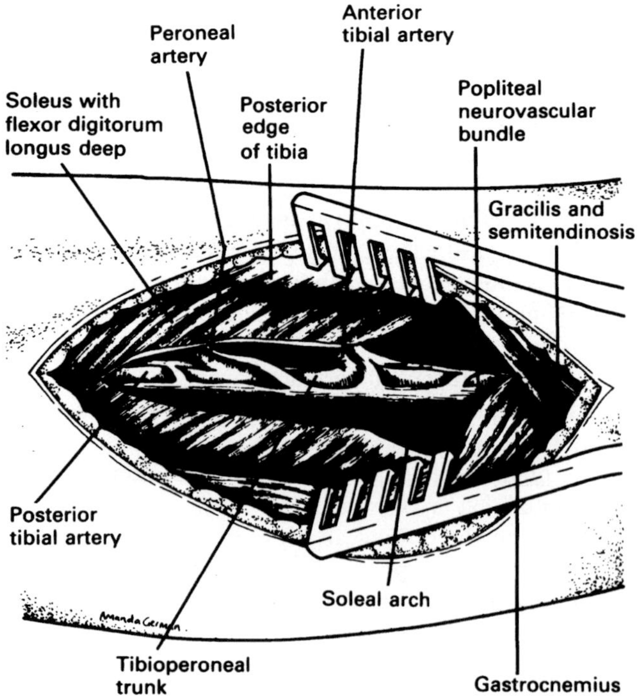

2

is most easily divided 1 cm posterior to its origin on the tibia. A mass of soleal veins usually obscures the anterior tibial artery which must be exposed by gentle dissection with ligation of the venae comitantes that lie superficial to the artery. It is interesting that with severe ischaemia of the distal limb the soleal veins are often found to be thrombosed. Distal anastomosis of a single stem bypass may be placed anywhere along the tibioperoneal trunk, providing its bifurcation into the posterior tibial and peroneal artery is not severely diseased. It may also be placed directly over the peroneal artery to widen the origin, but with disease of the proximal peroneal and posterior tibial artery, bypass to the distal calf seems preferable.

3a, b

Exposure of posterior tibial and peroneal arteries distally

The exposure of the posterior tibia and peroneal artery of the lower calf can best be achieved by placing the incision well distally in the medial calf (see Illustration 1). The lateral approach to the peroneal artery should ideally be avoided and only be used when a bifurcated graft to both the anterior tibial and peroneal arteries is planned. The incision is centred approximately 10 cm above the medial malleolus even if the calf arteries are patent above this level. The deep fascia is incised 0.5–1 cm posterior to the medial border of the tibia and the incision is deepened posterior to flexor digitorum longus (**3a**). The soleus muscle is retracted posteriorly using a self-retaining retractor which engages the posterior tibia. The arteries are still surrounded by the venae comitantes but these are more easily dissected free farther distally. Approximately 5 cm of the healthiest length of artery is mobilized and gently retracted posteriorly. The peroneal artery is exposed by deepening the plane of dissection and incising flexor hallucis longus longitudinally (**3b**). This may be done by finding the peroneal vascular bundle in the upper wound and then dividing the overlying muscle over the jaws of a curved clamp passed in the plane just superficial to the vessels. Dissecting the peroneal artery from its venae comitantes is tedious and demands both good light and magnification.

4a, b, c

Anterior and lateral leg incisions

Exposure of the anterior tibial artery

The anterior tibial artery may be easily exposed throughout its length in the anterior tibial compartment (**4a**). The incision is placed just lateral to the centre of the anterior tibial compartment and is deepened between tibialis anterior and the two extensor muscles (digitorum longus and hallucis longus) (**4b**). In practice, the plane between these muscle groups is not always immediately apparent but it is easy to split the muscles of tibialis anterior. If it is planned to route the graft to the anterior tibial artery from the medial aspect of the leg, a sufficient length should be mobilized and a cruciate incision in the interosseous membrane made 2 cm above the proposed anastomosis (**4c**).

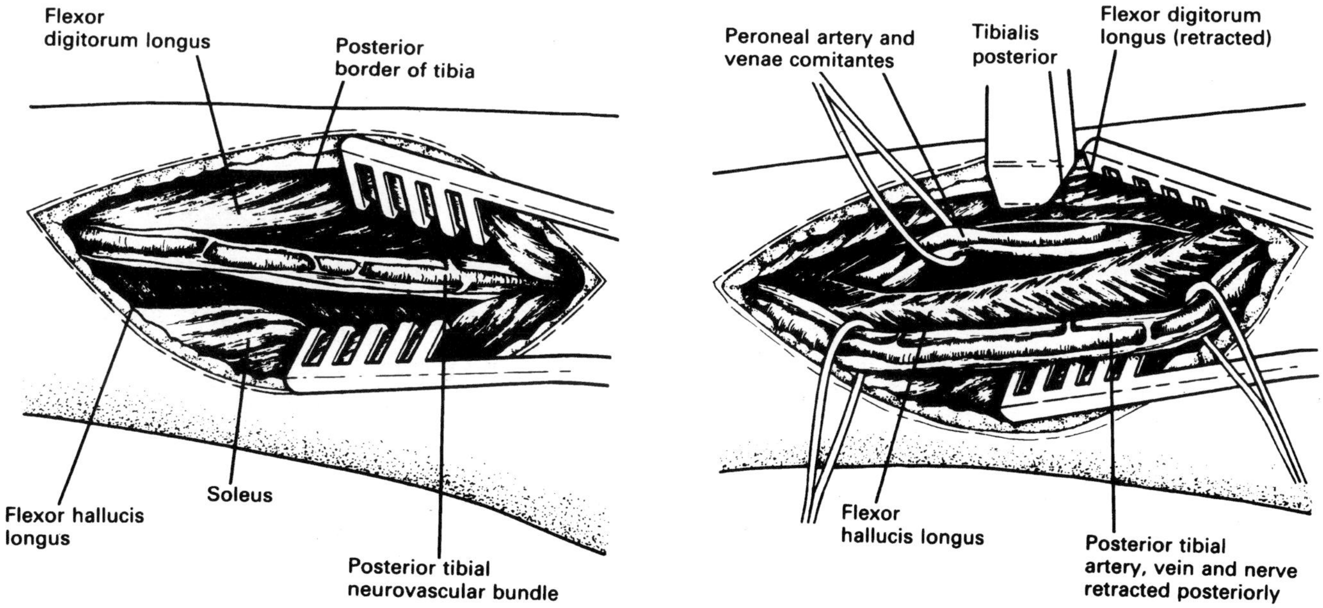

a 3 b

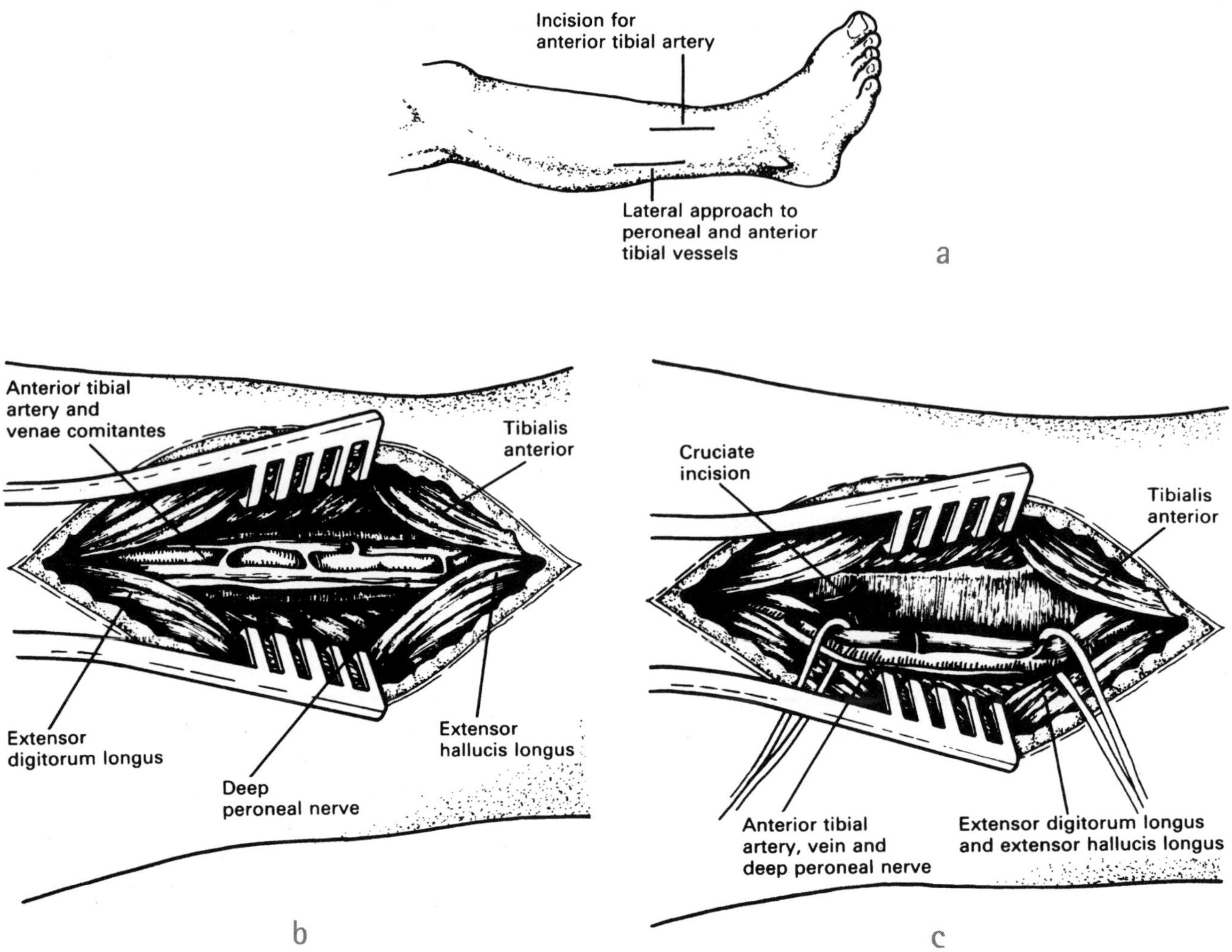
Incision for
anterior tibial artery
Lateral approach to
peroneal and anterior
tibial vessels
a
Anterior tibial
artery and
venae comitantes
Tibialis
anterior
Extensor
digitorum longus
Deep
peroneal nerve
Extensor
hallucis longus
b
Cruciate
incision
Tibialis
anterior
Anterior tibial
artery, vein and
deep peroneal nerve
Extensor digitorum longus
and extensor hallucis longus
c

4

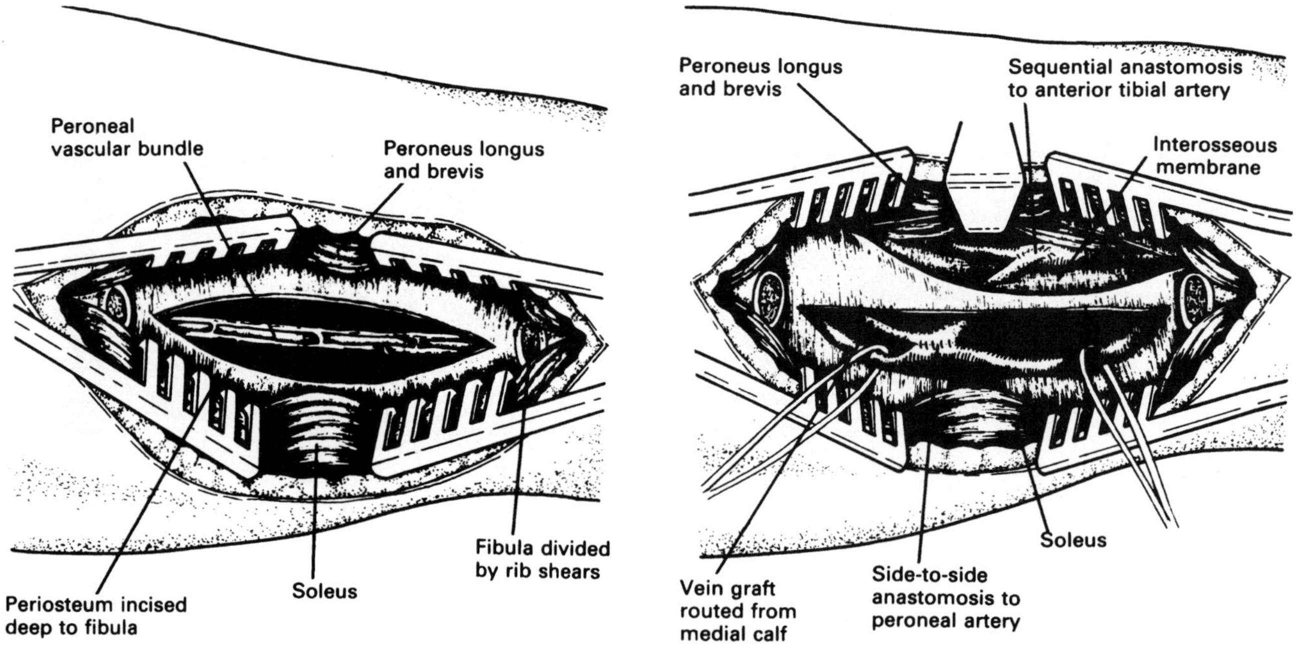
Peroneal
vascular bundle
Peroneus longus
and brevis
Periosteum incised
deep to fibula
Soleus
Fibula divided
by rib shears
Peroneus longus
and brevis
Sequential anastomosis
to anterior tibial artery
Interosseous
membrane
Vein graft
routed from
medial calf
Side-to-side
anastomosis to
peroneal artery
Soleus

a 5 b

5a, b

Lateral approach to both anterior tibial and peroneal arteries

As previously stated, this approach is rarely required. However, where preoperative Doppler evaluation or angiography indicates that the anterior tibial and the peroneal artery are patent, with an occluded posterior tibial artery, then the lateral approach with a view to a bifurcated bypass to these two vessels may be appropriate. The incision is placed directly over the fibula (5a) and deepened between the soleus and the peroneal muscles. The periosteum over the fibula is elevated and a 10–12 cm segment is excised using rib shears. Incision of the periosteum posterior to the interosseous membrane leads to the peroneal vessels and incision anterior leads to the anterior tibial neurovascular bundle. Illustration (5b) depicts a suitable layout for a sequential bypass routed from the medial calf with a side-to-side anastomosis to the peroneal artery and an end-to-side anastomosis to the anterior tibial artery.

6

Routes for bypass

When performing *in situ* saphenous vein bypasses it is undesirable to mobilize the long saphenous vein from its bed. Clearly, the distal and proximal ends have to be dissected free in order to route them to the proposed site of anastomosis, but this dissection should be restricted to the shortest length possible. In effect, this means that the graft should be routed from the medial calf in nearly every case. In bypassing to the upper tibioperoneal trunk or distal popliteal artery it may be necessary to route the distal part of the vein through the popliteal fossa to avoid excessive angulation. However, this is not necessary when bypassing to the distal tibioperoneal trunk or to the posterior tibial artery throughout its length. Routing the vessel to the peroneal artery when exposed through the medial incision is quite simple in that the graft merely lies in the plane of dissection already developed between soleus and flexor digitorum longus. In the majority of cases, we prefer to take the same route for anastomosis to the anterior tibial artery, tunnelling between flexor digitorum longus and flexor hallucis longus and through the interosseous membrane. It is important that the cruciate incision in the interosseous membrane is made at least 2–3 cm above the proposed site of anastomosis, so that the vein can curve laterally around the anterior tibial artery, allowing the anastomosis to be performed on the anterolateral aspect.

Where saphenous vein is being mobilized from its bed, either in a reversed or '*in situ*' orientation, some surgeons prefer to route grafts to the anterior tibial or peroneal artery subcutaneously across the front of the thigh, and

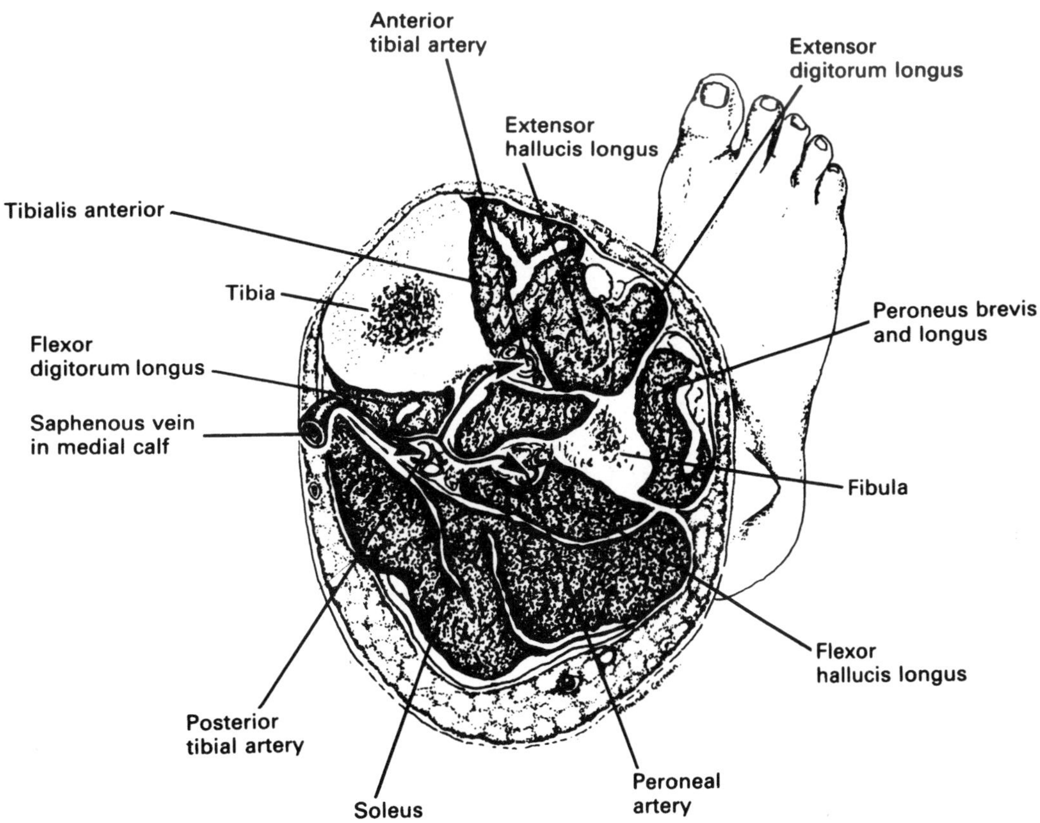

6

then lateral to the knee, passing just anteriorly to the head of the fibula. This route can also be used when a prosthetic graft or human umbilical vein is employed. It is doubtful that it confers any real advantages. However, where the distal anastomosis is to the dorsalis pedis or anterior tibial artery at or just above the ankle, the graft may have to pass from medial to lateral anterior to the tibia. This is far from ideal as necrosis may develop in the overlying skin.

Planning bifurcated grafts

In considering approaches to bifurcated bypass to distal calf arteries it is usually possible to select preoperatively which vessels are most likely to be adequate. In practice there are three possible combinations: posterior tibial and peroneal; posterior tibial and anterior tibial; or peroneal and anterior tibial. Wherever possible the bypass will be routed to anterior or posterior tibial arteries as these cross the ankle but the peroneal artery is available more often as it is relatively spared by atherosclerosis.

Postoperative complications

Patients undergoing femorotibial bypass are usually old, in poor health and may have diabetes. As the major body compartments are not opened, the perioperative mortality should be low, but over the following months and years a substantial number of these patients will die from myocardial or cerebral ischaemia. In contrast, postoperative morbidity often leads to prolonged hospital stay.

Pressure sores are avoided by carefully padding the patient on the operating table and immediately turning the patient and massaging the pressure areas on completion of the procedure. Wound edge necrosis which predominantly affects the distal wounds is related to ischaemia but can be minimized by keeping wound edges moist with saline swabs and releasing the pressure from self-retaining retractors whenever possible. Occasionally, vein grafts may become exposed with the risk of secondary haemorrhage.

Lower leg swelling and oedema occurs in nearly all patients and can be treated symptomatically with leg elevation and gentle elastic compression. Persistent arteriovenous fistulae and anastomotic problems will be reduced to a minimum if intraoperative assessments, including on-table angiography, are used.

Acknowledgement

Illustrations by Amanda Germen.

References

Dale AW (1963). Grafting small arteries. *Arch Surg* **86**: 22.

Davies RC, Davies WT, Mannick J A (1975). Bypass vein grafts in patients with distal popliteal artery occlusion. *Am J Surg* **129**: 421.

Edwards WS, Gerety E, Larkin J *et al.* (1976). Multiple sequential femoral tibial grafting for severe ischaemia. *Surgery* **80**: 722.

Goldman M, Hall C, Dykes J *et al.* (1983). Does indium-platelet deposition predict patency in prosthetic arterial grafts? *Br J Surg* **70**: 635.

Green RM, Roederschecmer RL, De Weese JA (1982). Effects of aspirin and dipyridamole on polytetrafluorethylene graft patency. *Surgery* **92**: 1016.

Hall KV, Rostad H (1978). *In situ* vein bypass in the treatment of femoro-popliteal atherosclerotic disease: a ten year study. *Am J Surg* **136**: 158.

Ibrahim IM, Sussman B, Dardik L *et al.* (1980). Adjunctive arteriovenous fistula with tibial and peroneal reconstruction for limb salvage. *Am J Surg* **140**: 246.

Klimach O, Charlesworth D (1983). Femoro-tibial bypass for limb salvage using human umbilical vein. *Br J Surg* **70**: 1.

Leather RP, Powers SR, Karmody AM (1979). A reappraisal of *in situ* saphenous arterial bypass: its use in limb salvage. *Surgery* **86**: 453.

Noon GP, Diethrich EB, Richardson WP *et al.* (1969). Distal tibial artery bypass – analysis of 91 cases. *Arch Surg* **99**: 770.

Palma EC (1960). Treatment of arteritis of the lower limbs by autogenous vein grafts. *Minerva Cardioangiologica* **1**: 36.

Piccone VA, Moon W, Harry H *et al.* (1978). Limb salvage by inverted Y vein grafts to below-knee arteries. *Arch Surg* **113**: 951.

Simms MH (1988). Is pedal arch patency a pre-requisite for successful reconstruction? In *Limb Salvage and Amputation for Vascular Disease*. Greenhalgh R M, Jamieson C W, Nicolaides A N eds. London and San Diego: W B Saunders Co.

Terry HJ, Allan JS, Taylor GW (1972). The relationship between blood flow and failure of femoro-popliteal reconstructive arterial surgery. *Br J Surg* **59**: 549.

The *in situ* saphenous vein arterial bypass by valve incision

Robert P Leather, Dhiraj M Shah, Benjamin B Chang, R Clement Darling III

Introduction

Technically, the crucial issue in using the greater saphenous vein *in situ*, and the primary reason for its excision and reversal, for femoral to distal arterial bypass, is the elimination of valvular obstruction to arterial flow. All other considerations aside, leaving the saphenous vein *in situ* appears to be the most reliable method of achieving endothelial preservation, provided the valves can be rendered incompetent without injury to this very delicate endothelial cell monolayer. In addition, leaving the vein *in situ* requires interruption of venous side branches, some of which would otherwise become arteriovenous fistulas when the vein is arterialized, and minimal mobilization of its ends for construction of the proximal and distal anastomoses. The objective is to accomplish these manoeuvres with a minimum of operative manipulation of the vein, and especially its endothelial surface with particular avoidance of circumferential longitudinal shear. The simplest, most expedient, and least traumatic method of rendering the bicuspid venous valve incompetent is to cut the leaflets in their major axes, thus bisecting them. This is the essence of the valve incision technique.

The evolution of instruments and constraints of their use to achieve valve incision was guided by an overriding concern toward minimizing the potential for endothelial injury while producing an incompetent valve. Our data show that, particularly with the addition of the intraluminal valve cutter, there was no penalty in performance (Leather *et al.*, 1984) despite the greater potential for circumferential endothelial abrasion, the most devastating form of injury. In concert with this, our technical methodology for performing the *in situ* bypass has been developed with the primary goal of universal application. An *in situ* bypass can be performed by this technique in virtually all cases, regardless of the vagaries of venous anatomy, while minimizing the extent of exposure of the vein necessary for consistently safe and atraumatic valve incision. The high incidence of venous anomalies (up to 30% of double systems) and smaller veins distally 50%, <3.5 mm OD) makes the use of a cylindrical transluminal retrograde valve disrupter such as the Hall, Cartier, or LeMaitre strippers hazardous (Moody *et al.*, 1992; Gruss *et al.*, 1982; Fietze-Fischer *et al.*, 1987; Denton *et al.*, 1983).

For the same reasons, the use of preoperative venous anatomic assessment either by venography or duplex ultrasonography is not only advisable, but mandatory, particularly if a valve cutter is to be used safely. A duplex ultrasonographic venous map provides the relevant information for the careful planning and execution of this procedure. Without this, attempts to define such anatomic variations surgically will result in excessive dissection, increasing the potential not only of injury to the vein, but also of wound complications. Experience with over 2000 duplex mappings has proven its safety, reliability, and utility in the performance of the *in situ* bypass as well as in vein harvesting.

The operation

1

An incision is made in the groin crease and is extended downwards over the saphenous vein. By sharp dissection, 5–10 cm of the proximal of the vein is identified. Its tributaries are ligated with silk or fine Prolene suture ligature and divided, and the vein is dissected from its bed. The saphenofemoral junction lies at the level which commonly corresponds to the bifurcation of the common femoral artery into the superficial and profunda artery. Hence, detachment of the entire saphenous bulb with, if necessary, a small portion of the anterior wall of the common femoral vein will ensure that the upper end of the bypass reaches the common femoral artery.

Alternately unobstructed profunda femoral or superficial femoral arteries can be effectively used as an inflow source without influencing immediate or long-term

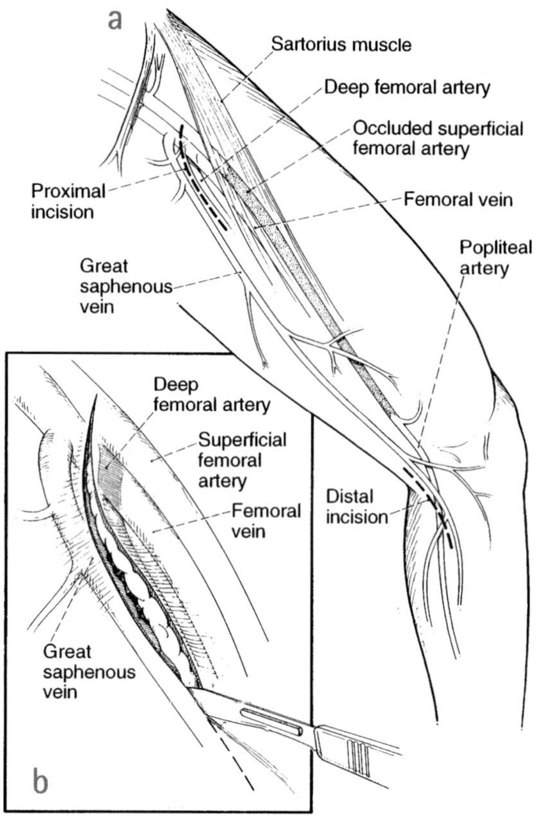

1

patency. It is best approached from the medial aspect (with the surgeon on the opposite side of the table) by incision of the subcutaneous tissue immediately lateral to the saphenous vein and down to the underlying investing myofascia (b). Dissection laterally in this fusion plane to the superficial femoral artery is bloodless. The fascia is incised over the superficial femoral artery and, if it is occluded, a segment of 3–5 cm can be excised, thus facilitating exposure of the deep femoral artery. If patent, a plane is developed between the femoral vein and the superficial femoral artery.

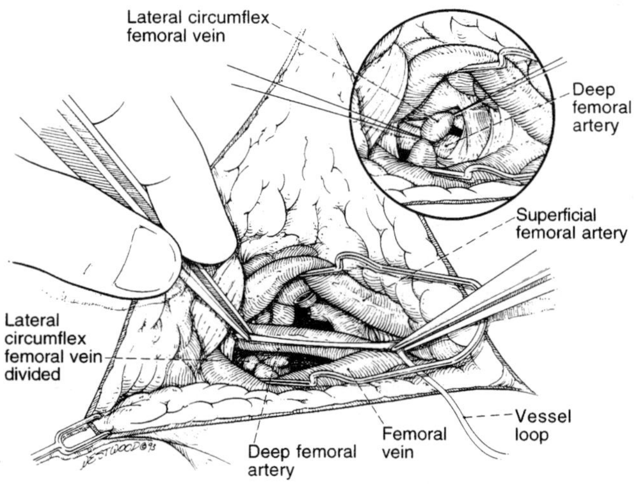

2

2

The lateral circumflex femoral vein is divided, exposing the proximal deep femoral artery which lies immediately deep to it (profundafemoris artery). Having determined the most satisfactory site of proximal anastomosis, the length of the proximal saphenous vein required to reach it is apparent.

3

The most proximal valve at the saphenofemoral junction is excised by lifting each cusp with a fine forceps and excising it through the base of the leaflet (only the transparent part) with a microscissor. For the one to three proximal valves, a valve scissor engages the valve most efficiently when it is in the closed position. The valve can be kept closed by a pressurized column of fluid introduced through a fine catheter at a controlled pressure of 200 mmHg.

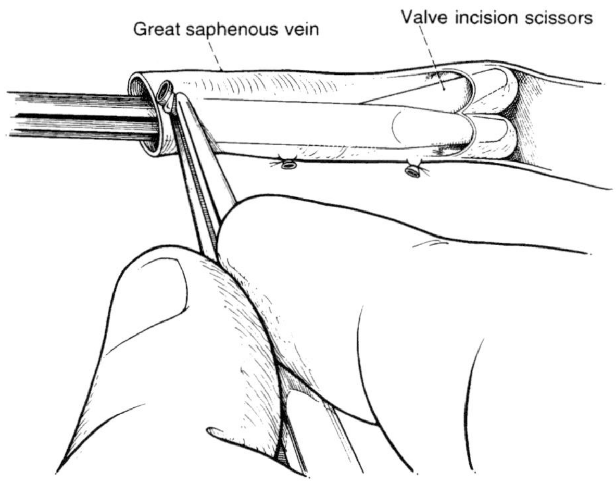

3

4a, b

When the saphenous vein is greater than 3 mm ID (4 mm OD) with a single trunk in its thigh portion, an appropriate size (2 or 3 mm) detachable intraluminal valve cutter is used which divides the cusps up to the level of the knee without the necessity of surgical exposure of the vein (Leather 1984). A small incision is made posterior to the previously marked vein below the level of the knee joint. A branch of suitable size is located and a 3 French Fogarty embolectomy catheter is passed into the saphenous vein and advanced through the detached proximal end with the knee straightened. The catheter is cut obliquely at the 20- or 30-cm mark and the cutter is prepared as shown in **4a**. A 6 or 8 French catheter through which pressurized fluid is delivered into the vein is

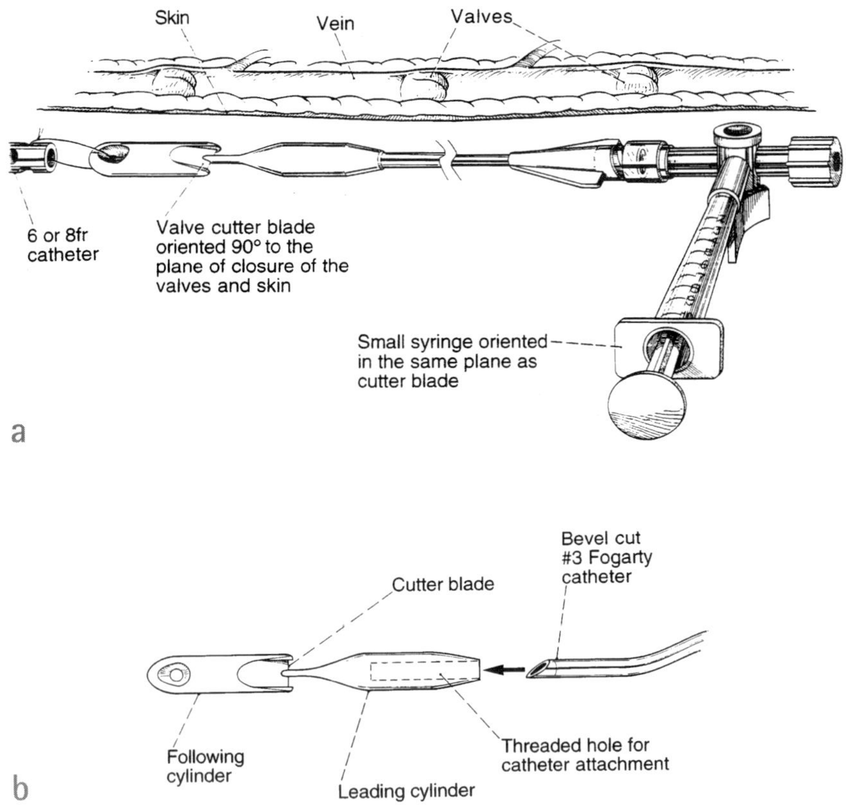

4

attached to the upper end of the cutter ('follower') with a 6/0 monofilament suture. The oblique cut end of the Fogarty catheter is used to firmly screw the self-tapping cutter leader before the pressure catheter is attached. The infusion bag is pressurized to 200–300 torr. The orientation of the cutter within the saphenous vein is shown in **4b** the fluid pressure distends the vein, sealing leakage from the open end of the vein by a 1-mm silastic vessel loop closing the valves so that they will be efficiently engaged by the cutter blades, and provides a fluid interface on which the cutter 'floats' away from the vein wall. The 'leader' centres the device in the saphenous vein and prevents it from engaging any side branches.

The valves are serially cut to the level of the knee joint by one or two passes of the valve cutter. The cutter is then withdrawn with the traction catheter through the proximal end of the vein and dismounted and the catheter is removed from below.

5a, b, c

With clips placed proximally and distally, a deep femoral arteriotomy has been performed at the proposed anastomosis site. The vein is sharply divided from posterior to anterior, and a small tissue bridge will be left connected to a 'handle' for manipulating the vessel (**5a**). All work on the vein is done with a 'no touch' technique using 3.5 × magnification loupes to minimize any potential trauma to the vessel. With traction on the handle, the venotomy on the posterior vessel wall is accurately placed and oriented. Anastomosis of the bypass vein to the deep femoral artery is carried out by the 'open parachute' technique, which allows for accurate and atraumatic placement of each individual suture in the heel portion of the anastomosis. A single, double-needle suture of 6–0 or 7–0 Prolene is used (**5b**). After placement of as many sutures as the length of suture material allows, the vein is drawn down to the artery. The handle will be excised (**5c**). Arterialization of the saphenous vein is completed by continuing the medial suture line clockwise around the arteriotomy to meet the lateral suture line at the midpoint of the arteriotomy.

6

Once arterial pressure has been established down to the knee level, the Mills retrograde valvulotome is used for all subsequent valve incisions. This retrograde valvulotome consists of a 20-cm long, 1 mm flexible shaft, a blade at right angles to the shaft and a ball-tip which protects the vein wall. The instrument is passed either through a side branch or through the open end of the vein after it has been distally detached. Before any intraluminal instrumentation is carried out, the mobilized

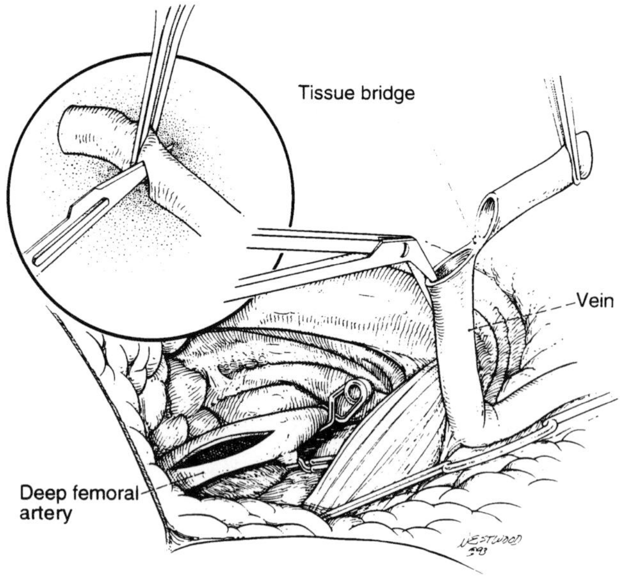

5a

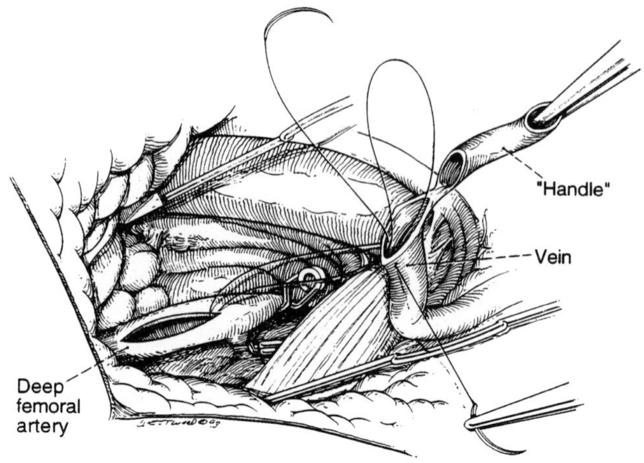

5b

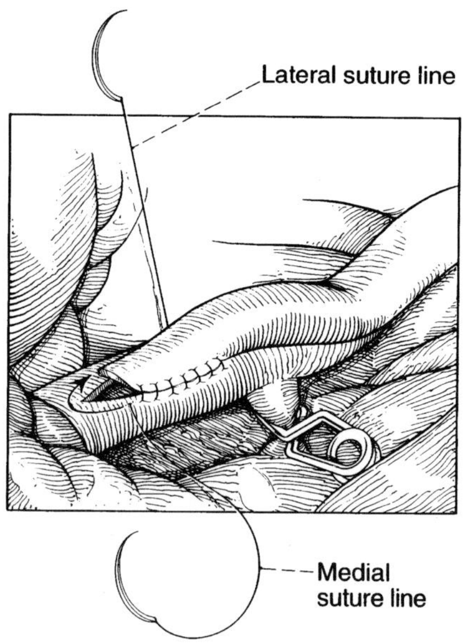

5c

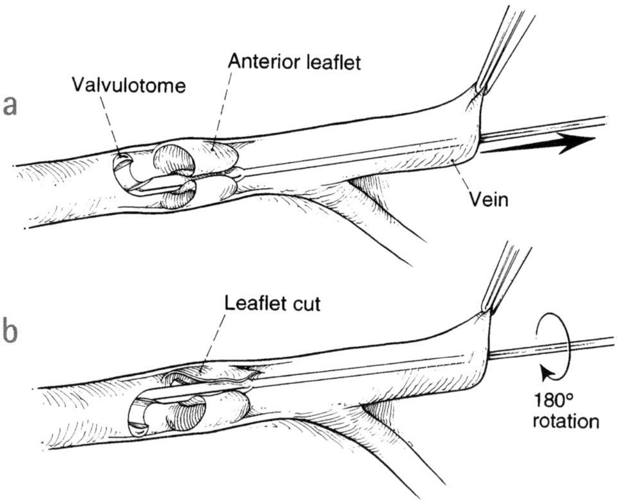

6

segment of vein is dilated with dextran solution at a controlled pressure of 200 mmHg. A retrograde valvulotome is introduced through the distal end of the vein, and as it is with drawn, it cuts one valve leaflet. It is readvanced, rotated 180 degrees, and again withdrawn, cutting the second leaflet.

7

The simple expedient of assessing flow from the distal divided end of the saphenous vein before construction of the distal anastomosis is very reliable in detecting any

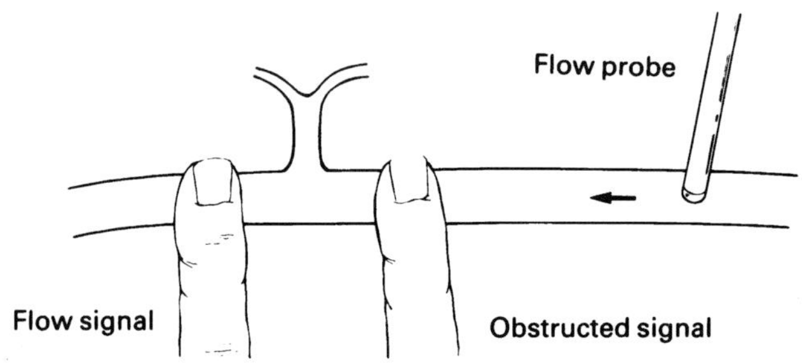

7

proximal haemodynamically significant obstructive lesions. If there is steady, undiminished pulsatile flow, it is unlikely that such a lesion is present proximally with high volume flow in the *in situ* conduit either into a distal fistula or via this distal divided end. A towel is rolled over the entire course of the vein to precipitate closure of any leaflet that has been mechanically placed on the wall and might result in a 'missed valve'. Distal anastomosis is performed using the technique shown in Illustration 5. Elimination of arteriovenous fistulae is not a difficult part of the procedure. The position of most of the branches which will become fistulae will be already identified either from the preoperative venogram or during venous exposure for valve incision as discussed previously. Residual arteriovenous fistulae (usually no more than two) are initially determined by the use of intraoperative Doppler probe as shown here. Sequentially the probe placed in the proximal position provides a flow signal when a fistula is present and an obstructive signal when the vein is compressed proximal to this point. After this, an intraoperative arteriogram (considered to be mandatory) is carried out.

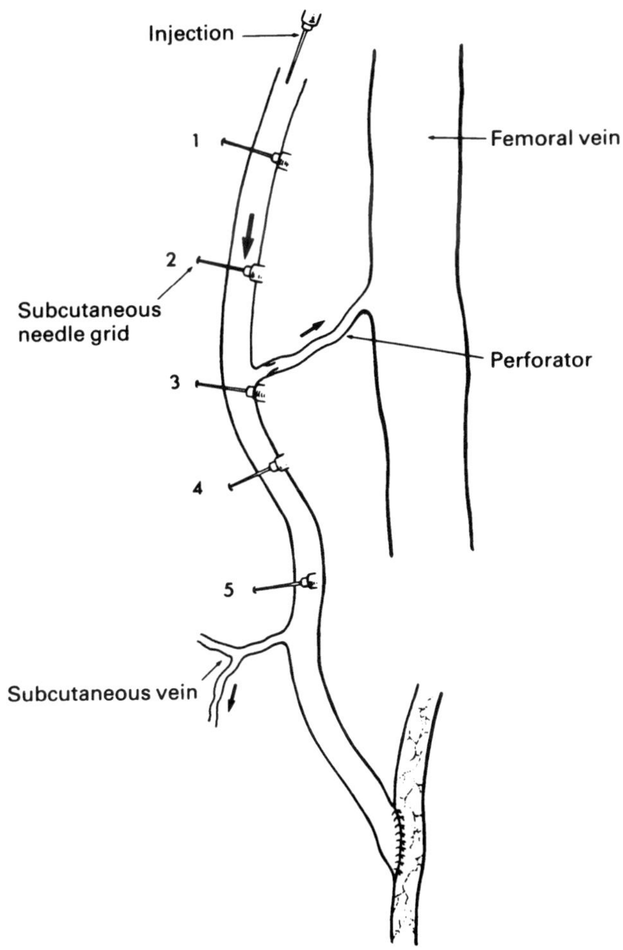

8

8

On the completion arteriogram, remaining fistulae can be readily identified and the technical accuracy of the distal anastomosis can be seen. A 22-gauge plastic sheath is inserted into the proximal part of the vein and contrast is injected. A needle grid shown numerically allows rapid location of the fistulae. The perforating vein which connects directly with the femoral vein is shown at the third needle position. Note that the valve in the vein is directed towards the deep system. A subcutaneous vein which forms a fistula beyond the fifth needle is not of haemodynamic value and can safely be left if desired. Most such fistulae subsequently become occluded because of the formation of true phlebitis within the vein wall.

The distal anastomosis must also be examined on the arteriogram. Its adequacy should be confirmed in this way as well as by Doppler ultrasound of the flow at this point.

Complications

Occasionally, pathological difficulties within the saphenous vein may occur during the operative procedure. These consist of platelet deposition at the site of injured endothelium, unyielding valves because of previous fibrosis, a missed valve cusp, or laceration of the vein wall. Vein wall lacerations are easily identified because of leakage of blood and haematoma formation of the vein wall. When platelet deposition occurs within the vein, this will be seen on the operative angiogram as a foamy filling defect and the Doppler ultrasound will reflect a diminished flow signal. These difficulties, though rare, must be diagnosed and managed intraoperatively if early failure of the bypass is to be avoided.

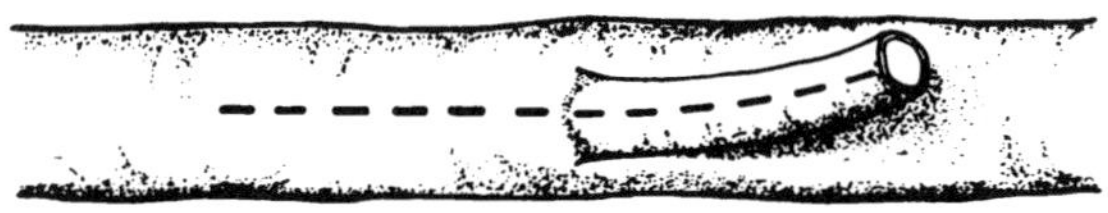

9

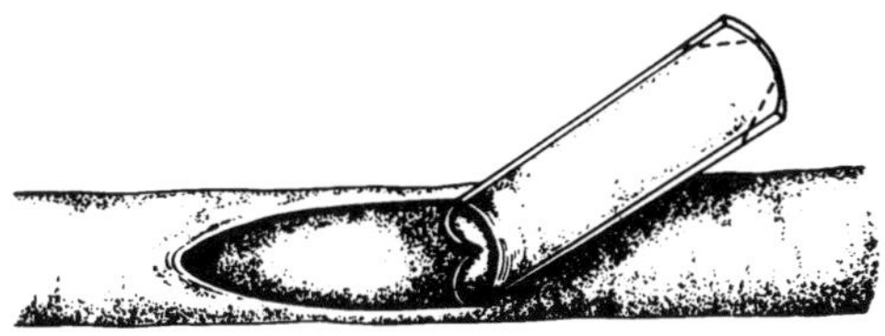

10

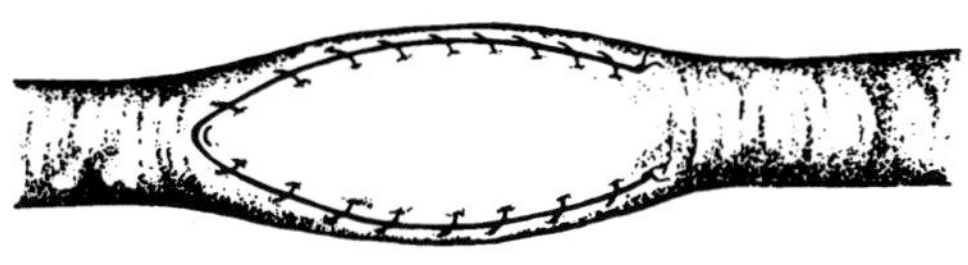

11

9, 10, 11

When such problems occur, they can usually be treated by the technique of vein branch angioplasty. The vein is opened in order to visualize its endothelial surface. Platelets can be removed through the venotomy and/or missed valves dealt with. The venotomy is subsequently closed by patch angioplasty using a venous branch opened in continuity with the diagnostic venotomy.

This technique is in keeping with and preserves the complete *in situ* nature of the entire procedure (Corson *et al.*, 1984). It is stressed that at the termination of the procedure, the predicted physiological criteria resulting from the bypass should be confirmed in the distal limb by non-invasive methods, e.g. Doppler ultrasound, systolic pressures and wave form analysis. In this respect, the intraoperative arteriogram should also be helpful. The patient should not leave the operating suite until the surgeon is satisfied that these criteria have been met.

References

Corson JD, Leather RP, Shah DM, Karmody AM (1984). *In situ* vein branch angioplasty. *Surg Gynecol Obstet* **159**: 283.

Denton MJ, Hill D, Fairgrieve J (1983). *In situ* femoropopliteal and distal vein bypass for limb salvage: Experience of 50 cases. *Br J Surg* **70**: 358.

Fietze-Fischer B, Gruss JD, Bartels D *et al.* (1987). Prostaglandin E1 as an adjuvant therapy in the event of femoropopliteal and crural great saphenous vein *in situ* bypass surgery. *VASA* **17**: 23. (suppl).

Gruss JD, Bartls D, Vargas H *et al.* (1982). Arterial reconstruction for distal disease of the lower extremities by the *in-situ* vein graft technique. *J Cardiovasc Surg*, **23**: 231.

Leather RP (1993a). Overview: history and evolution of techniques. *Semin Vasc Surg* **6**: 3.151.

Leather RP (1993b). The current Albany approach. *Semin Vasc Surg* **6**: 3.159.

Leather RP, Corson JD, Karmody AM (1984). Instrumental evolution of the valve incision method of '*in-situ*' saphenous vein bypass. *F Vasc Surg* **1**: 113.

Moody AP, Edwards PR, Harris PL (1992). *In situ* versus reversed femoropopliteal vein grafts: Long-term follow-up of a prospective, randomized trial. *Br J Surg* **79**: 750.

The use of the vein cuff and polytetrafluoroethylene

Justin H Miller†

Introduction

The cuff (or 'sleeve' as it is often, but less correctly called) is a cylinder of vein interposed between a polytetrafluoroethylene (PTFE) tube and small artery. It was introduced in 1981 (Miller *et al.*, 1984) to facilitate the anastomosis of large (6 mm diameter) stiff PTFE grafts to small (often <2 mm diameter) tibial arteries.

Since 1978 attempts have been made to eliminate this mechanical mismatch problem with variations of the 'Linton patch' (Linton and Wild, 1970), which had the basic problem of accommodating four rows of sutures in a narrow opened vein (6–10 mm wide). In 1979 Siegman suggested linking a Dacron tube to a small artery by a cylinder of vein and this technique was adapted to join PTFE to tibial vessels with encouraging results (Morris *et al.*, 1993).

Its application has now become very widespread, gradually replacing all direct PTFE anastomoses, such as those to the popliteal and profunda femoris arteries. In selected cases, it is also used at the proximal common femoral inflow anastomosis.

Likewise, a recent innovation has been to facilitate the side-to-side anastomosis between the PTFE and an artery, such as sequential ilio-profunda-popliteal reconstructions, or sequential composite PTFE-vein femoro-popliteal-tibial grafts.

While the main advantage of the cuff over direct anastomosis remains its technical facility, evidence is accruing that it leads to improved long-term patency (Tyrrell *et al.*, 1989b). This may well be that it alters the mechanical or elastic mismatch at the distal anastomosis and thereby reduces neointimal hyperplasia (Suggs *et al.*, 1988; Tyrrell *et al.*, 1989a). Another major advantage is that the presence of the cuff facilitates later thrombectomy, thereby extending the life of the graft and limb by reoperation (Morris *et al.*, 1993). The cuff mimics vein at the cuff/artery anastomosis, leading to preservation of the original outflow artery on occlusion of the graft. Moreover, the cuff has less fibrotic reaction than PTFE directly in contact with artery, thereby minimizing the amount of dissection required to control the vessel.

Indications

Femorodistal bypass

It is emphasized that autogenous saphenous vein is still the preferred conduit in all forms of femorodistal grafting. However, PTFE remains a satisfactory alternative when vein (for numerous reasons, not the least of which are multiple previous operations in the same limb) is not available.

The cuff is indicated in all situations where PTFE is to be anastomosed to tibial arteries and is strongly recommended when the anastomosis is to the below-knee popliteal artery, a situation hitherto considered to be a contraindication to the use of any prosthesis. The use of the cuff for the above-knee popliteal artery is not essential but is useful in situations where extensive atheroma makes direct suturing difficult. In the sequential bypass (femoro-popliteal-tibial), the cuff facilitates the side-to-side anastomosis of PTFE (or composite PTFE-vein).

Aortofemoral or crossover bypass surgery

Aortofemoral surgery often requires the distal end of the graft to be anastomosed to the profunda femoris vessel. Mismatch of the graft vessel diameters requires the use of a long tapering graft down the profunda femoris. The cuff is ideal in this situation, reducing the extent of the dissection required and actually reducing the operating time for the anastomosis. The cuff is equally applicable when a crossover femoroprofunda graft is required (Miller *et al.*, 1991). When an inflow operation is combined with a distal bypass (aorto- or ilio-profundapopliteal graft), a cuff applied to the profunda greatly facilitates the side-to-side anastomosis between that vessel and the PTFE graft.

†Justin Miller has died since the third edition of this book was published and we have left his chapter intact. RMG

Special considerations for infrainguinal PTFE grafts with cuff

The total experience in femorodistal bypass grafting has been with 6-mm PTFE, initially with the standard graft, but mostly with thin-walled grafts since 1984. More recently many have found it particularly useful with external supported ringed PTFE. With the profunda femoris as outflow vessel, 8-mm tubing has been used.

Infection

Contrary to accepted belief, the risk of infection (from foot necrosis, nearby wound breakdown after failed surgery or removal of infected graft) has not been a problem. This is provided that the new PTFE graft lies in a new non-devitalized tract, that the suture line of PTFE to cuff is properly buried in living tissue and that the graft remains patent (and this aided by the cuff) (Miller, 1993). Apart from this, prosthetic grafts are at higher risk of infection than vein and the use of preoperative intravenous antibiotics is essential. The agent selected should have good activity against *Staphylococcus aureus* as well as any local cultured organisms, and should be continued for 48 h postoperatively.

Dissection

Anastomosis with prosthesis needs a good blood supply. Local tissue ischaemia should be avoided by minimal and gentle dissection at anastomotic sites. Approaches to arteries should not transect lymph channels and should avoid collaterals. This is especially so in the groin. A less extensive exposure is required for the cuff than a direct anastomosis with PTFE. Often in the presence of difficult atheroma at the inflow common femoral artery anastomosis, deliberate use of the cuff will simplify the operation compared with direct anastomosis.

Graft length

PTFE is more unforgiving than vein and in judging the length of the graft it is better to err on the side of making the graft too black rather than too tight. A rule of thumb is to extend the leg fully, distend to arterial pressure and cut the graft to the exact length plus 1 cm. See Illustration **5b**.

Graft site

Subcutaneous placement of PTFE is preferred to subfascial. However, when the distal anastomosis is to popliteal artery immediately below the knee joint the preference is to run the graft through the popliteal fossa between the heads of gastrocnemius muscle even when using Ringed PTFE. It is possible the cuff allows flexibility of the anastomosis. Because of the narrow popliteal canal PTFE and artery tend to lie parallel just prior to the anastomosis and it is the authors' habit to make a 'double tier' of the distal cuff (see **6a, b**) to avoid the 'cervix' effect of the heel. A minority of surgeons favour running the graft subcutaneously around the medial condyle (even laying it on the anterior shelf) reasoning that this relates to the true centre of movement of the joint. Grafts to the anterior tibial and peroneal arteries are placed on the lateral side of thigh and leg although recently a medial approach to the peroneal artery is favoured even if a segment of fibula has been resected for access.

Clotting

PTFE is intolerant to either stasis of blood within the graft or slow flow, and this must be carefully avoided as follows:

1. Adequate peroperative systemic heparinization is essential. There is little evidence regarding the exact dose to be used but our experience has been to use a bolus of 5000 units of heparin, supplemented by 1000 units/h if the clamp time exceeds 1 h. The advantage of this regime is that it almost never requires reversal with protamine.
2. Heparinized saline (5000 units/1000 ml) is used liberally to irrigate the graft and artery. Once the proximal anastomosis is completed, heparinized saline is forcibly refluxed upstream into the proximal artery of supply prior to clamping of the graft (*see* **5a**). Although there is little evidence of its value in an effort to reduce platelet adherence, I use heparinized rheomacrodex as well as saline.
3. Postoperative systemic heparinization is not used routinely, but it is recommended for at least 48 h or until maximum perfusion is manifest by pulses and reactionary warmth in the foot in redo situations, or when there is poor distal run-off.
4. After thrombectomy, I frequently infuse heparin directly into the graft via a 16-gauge epidural catheter, maintaining moderate therapeutic levels as measured systemically. This has the advantage over intravenous application in that heparin concentrates inside the lower graft and run-off (especially with poor outflow) preventing local thrombus formation before overflowing systemically and risking bleeding from wounds and elsewhere. The dosage needed is much lower than that necessary to achieve the same effect intravenously.

Preliminary clearing of the outflow with fibrinolysis after graft occlusion

1. After occlusion a PTFE graft with vein cuff behaves like vein in that the original outflow tract is retained. Should this not happen (e.g. from progression of disease beyond the graft), it is preferable to clarify outflow with fibrinolysis rather than proceed to a more distal bypass immediately. The original outflow may be restored completely (e.g. retaining an above-knee

segment of artery) or partly (e.g. extending to below-knee popliteal rather than tibial artery). It is also probable that streptokinase augments perfusion by clearing thrombus in the very small vessels in contrast to the Fogarty which can only risk damage to the lining of the larger tibial arteries.

2. A radiological catheter (5 French) is introduced via a sheath by downhill puncture in the ipsilateral common femoral artery (or by traversing the aortic bifurcation by uphill puncture in the opposite femoral artery) and manipulated into the proximal ostium of the graft and down to within 1 or 2 cm of the distal anastomosis. If this is not possible it is better to introduce the catheter through a small incision over the upper graft under local anaesthetic. Repeated attempts at percutaneous puncture directly into the graft are more likely to cause multiple holes which leak. It is important that the entry point is a snug fit in the graft otherwise blood will track back from the outflow artery once connection is established and leak into the tissues. This is best achieved by exposing the surrounding incorporated tissue of the graft but not baring its wall and making the entry point with an 18 G needle.
3. Streptokinase at an hourly rate of 5000 units plus 600 units of heparin is perfused via an intra-arterial pump (e.g. IMED). Alternatively urokinase (120 000 units/h plus heparin), although more expensive causes less allergic reaction, and does not develop resistance. The distal tree is checked via the catheter at 6–8 h intervals and perfusion continues until the run-off is optimal. Systemic monitoring is with usual blood coagulation studies, the most important of which is the fibrinogen level. For optimal benefit the lytic agent must be perfused directly into thrombus before it overflows into the general circulation (if necessary by advancing the catheter into clot in native artery). Overdose in the general circulation declares itself by bleeding from the puncture site and rapidly falling fibrinogen level (>1g/litre). Correction is by fresh frozen plasma or intravenous aminocaproic acid (5 g intravenously). The distal native arterial tree is mostly restored to the original state but usually the distal and almost always the proximal anastomosis will require surgical intervention.

Preparation of the patient: choice of vein for the cuff

The whole limb (or both, if veins are scarce) is prepared in the usual way, and the outflow artery is exposed to establish operability. The vein is chosen from the following sites:

1. Long saphenous vein on the shelf of the medial malleolus, unless as in very critical limb ischaemia the site is unlikely to heal. This can be a problem if there is no boost to the local blood supply by the operation.
2. The lateral saphenous vein in the groin incision. (The main trunk makes an excellent and even better cuff but would be more appropriate in some other capacity, e.g. as a sequential composite graft.) Saphenous vein seems to have the right muscular strength; others such as arm veins can be used but are generally too fragile.
3. The beginning of the short saphenous vein behind the lateral malleolus.
4. In the lower edge of a below-knee approach to the popliteal artery. This segment of long saphenous vein is often spared after coronary artery surgery or previous femoropopliteal bypass. Sometimes an *in situ* vein graft is abandoned at an early stage because the vein is too small at this site; however, it is still adequate for a cuff.

Procedure

The usual order is to suture the cuff on the outflow vessel, then to make the proximal inflow anastomosis, place the graft, cut to length and then join the PTFE to the cuff as the final procedure. Completing the distal anastomosis before the proximal, as is often done with reversed vein graft, is not recommended. PTFE is not as tolerant of stagnant blood as is vein. To shorten operating time it is usually possible for a second operator to execute the proximal anastomosis, while the cuff is being made.

1a, b, c

Cuff and inflow anastomosis

Most consider that a cuff is not necessary at the upper inflow anastomosis, and this is certainly true if it is beyond the takeoff of the profunda femoris. However, a direct anastomosis to the common femoral vessel does constitute a risk to the integrity of the flow of the profunda artery, especially if there is a chance of early graft occlusion and need for removal, e.g. desperate attempts at limb salvage by femorotibial grafting. To minimize this risk the following steps can be taken.

1. Bring a direct anastomosis wholly on to the superficial femoral vessel by enlarging the outlet of the common femoral artery with a vein patch, so that no PTFE intrudes into the main vessel (**1a**). This is most effective.
2. This patch can be varied to resemble that described by Taylor at the outflow end (Taylor *et al.*, 1992) making sure the vein extends up to the common femoral artery and down enough to cover the heel of the PTFE (**1b**). A wide piece of vein is necessary for this manoeuvre to be effective.
3. Sometimes in very complex atheromatous situations it is more expeditious (in the interests of minimal dissection and avoidance of lymph nodes) to simply let in a cuff in any soft spot free from plaque (**1c**). The cuff

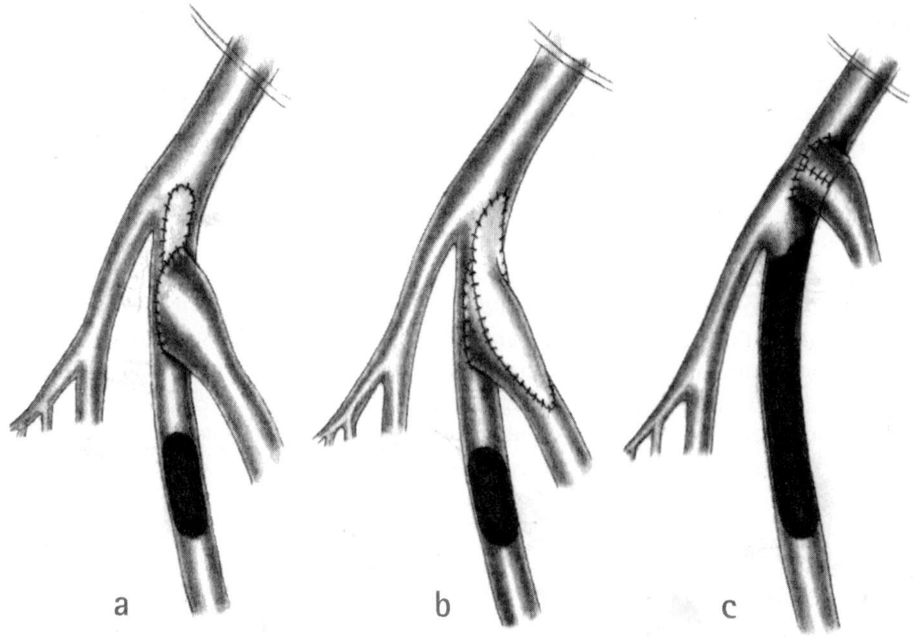

1

helps avoid what experience has shown to be a bad combination (especially in the groin) – endarterectomy and direct suturing of PTFE.

Concomitant profunda disease at the inflow anastomoses

The decision as to whether to combine a profundaplasty with a distal bypass is always difficult. There are times, however, when the need cannot be ignored. With vein, the two procedures combine well by using the hood of the proximal anastomosis as the vein patch for the profundaplasty (Greenhalgh, 1980). The combination of cuff and PTFE can be utilized in a similar and simple manner:

1. Simple orifice stenosis is easily handled by siting the cuff partly on the soft profunda and partly on the common femoral artery without endarterectomy. It is often possible to incorporate the lateral circumflex artery orifice as well.
2. When extensive endarterectomy is necessary (e.g. common femoral orifice coralline atheroma), the combined patch and cuff is useful (see Illustration 6l). Here the cuff can be sited over the junction of endarterectomized profunda and normal intima, so that any tendency to lift will be in the mid-portion of the cuff.

2a–d

Technique of creating the cuff

This is the standard technique for any anastomosis, and despite the many modifications which have been suggested, it remains essentially unchanged since it was first developed in 1981.

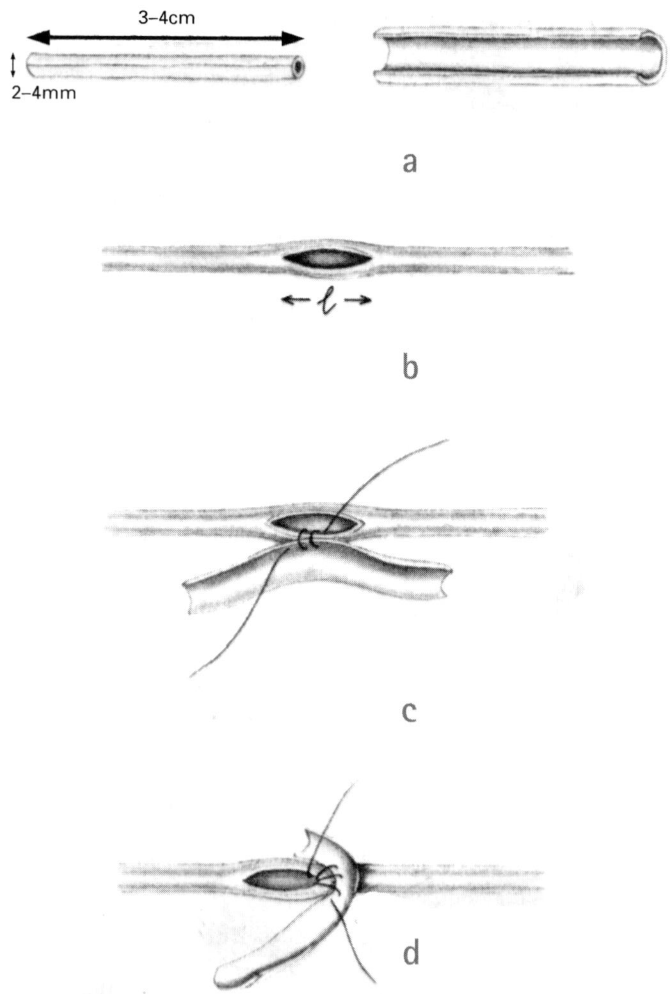

2

A total of 3–4 cm of saphenous vein with a diameter of 2–4 mm is opened up longitudinally (**2a**). A larger diameter makes an even better cuff, but this is an extravagant use of vein. An arteriotomy (**2b**), 1–1.5 cm in length, or approximately twice the diameter of the graft, is made in any soft portion free of plaque. Siting is critical, avoiding 'exploratory arteriotomy' and preferably leaving plaque with potential to lift at the cephalic end. The sleeve is then sutured with continuous Prolene sutures (6/0 for popliteal, 7/0 for tibial) to the inferior edge of the arteriotomy (**2c**). Some surgeons prefer the traditional method of commencing at the distal apex (or 'toe') using the parachute technique to view the lumen first (**2d**). In either case, it is essential to stitch the artery from within out, so that the vein fixes the intima against the medial coat.

3a–d

Suturing the apices

In the middle portion of the arteriotomy, the bite of artery should be larger than that of vein, so as to take the vein well down into the artery to fix the intima (**3a**). As the apex is approached, this bite should be reduced so as to prevent the vein intruding into the lumen. The interval between sutures should be small and they should be left loose to be tightened later (with a nerve hook if necessary) (**3b**). The heel is treated in the same way as the apex. As each suture is placed at both ends, the lumen of the vessel beyond should be clearly visible. This is to preserve outflow in both directions, so that in the event of graft occlusion, artery patency is preserved (**3d**). This is vital at the level of the tibial artery or distal profunda femoris. Suturing is continued on the upper edge until the two separate sutures meet (**3d**), when they are tied together. A sealing corner suture is made by passing one needle out-in through the vein and then in-out through the other edge of the vein, where it is tied to the free length of the suture. Alternatively, if dealing with narrow fragile vein, one might choose to carry on suturing vein to vein. See Illustrations **6a, b**.

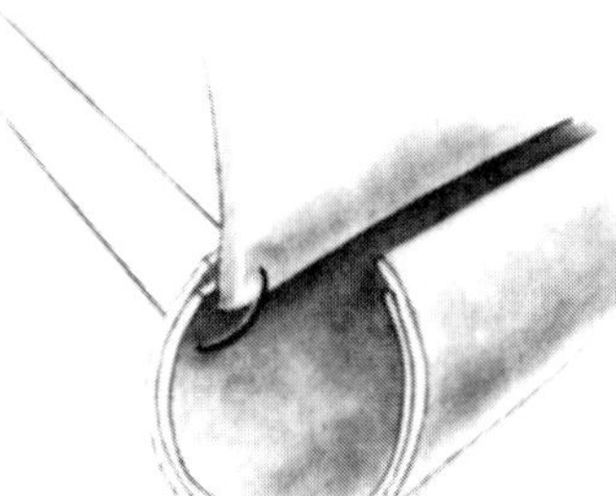

a

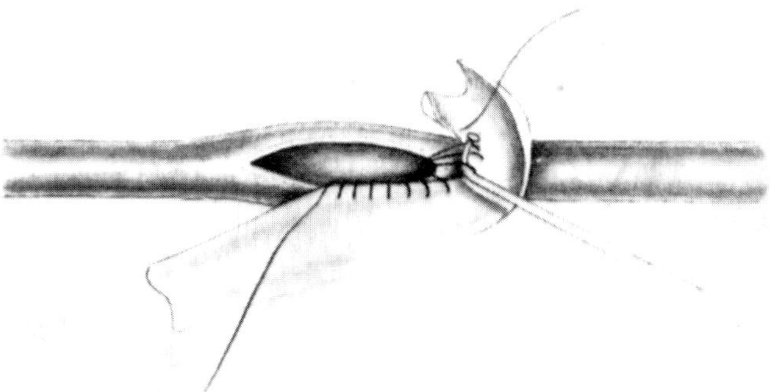

b

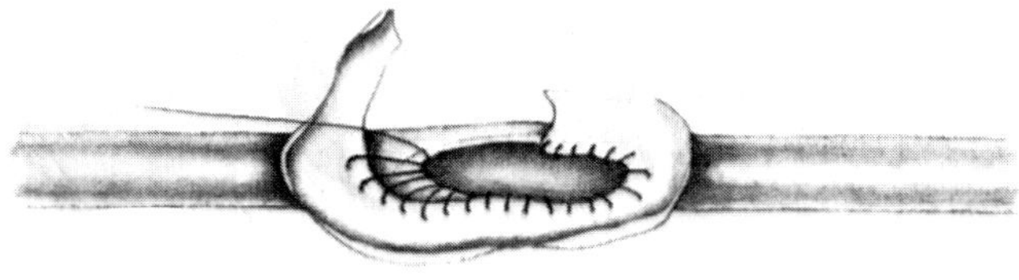

c

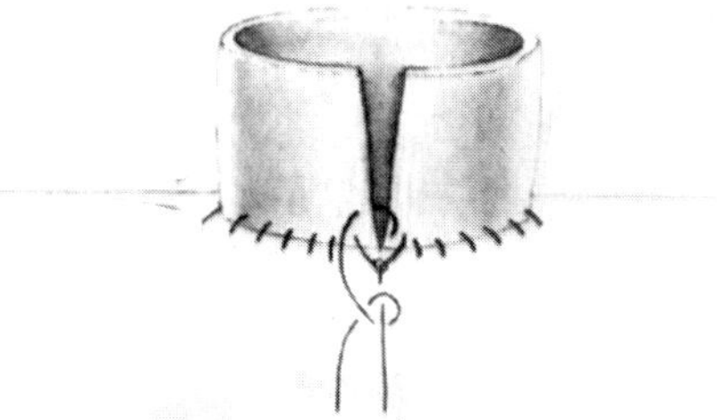

d

3

4a–d

The vein ends are squared off, leaving a little extra for suturing. One thread is cut or used as a stay. The remaining suture is used to approximate the square ends of the vein carefully with frequent bites until the corners meet, where the suture is tied to itself, clipped and used as a stay suture for the next part of the procedure (**4a**). The upper anastomosis is then made and the graft is placed in its appropriate tract. Heparinized saline is forcibly refluxed upstream (see **5a**) and the graft is clamped distally.

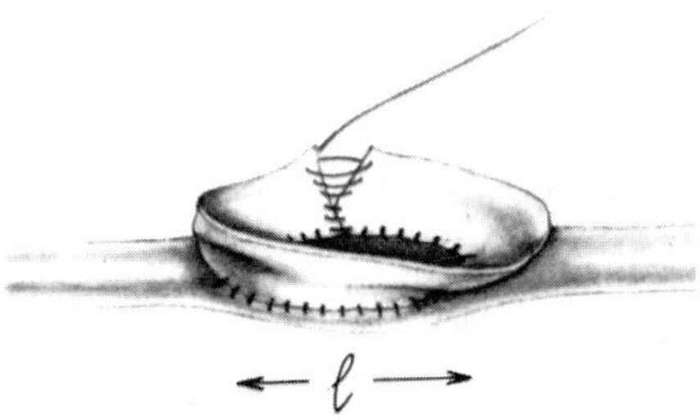

4a

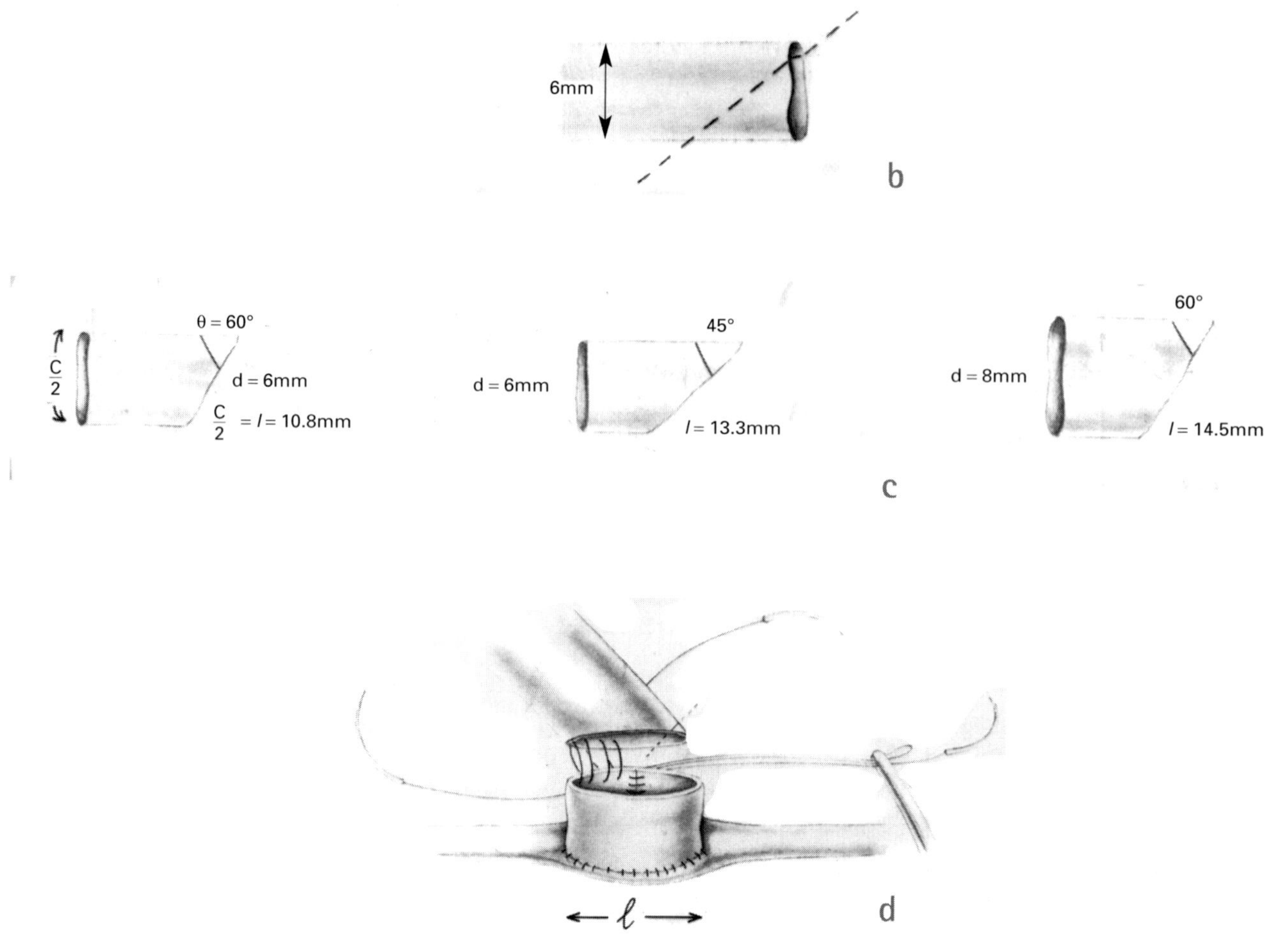

4

The PTFE is cut at the appropriate angle with a blade (conveniently along a clamp). The angle at which it is cut will determine its circumference, which should equal the circumference of the cuff. This in turn should be twice the length of the arteriotomy ($c = 2l$). If half the circumference ($c/2 = \pi d/2$) of a 6-mm tube cut at right angles = 9.4 mm, then $c/2$ cut at an angle of 60 degrees = 10.8 mm (9.4/sin 60), $c/2$ cut at 45 degrees = 13.3 mm, and an 8-mm tube cut at 60 degrees = 14.5 mm (*c*).

The circumference of the cut PTFE should now approximate to that of the sleeve. If there is to be a disparity in length, it is better that the cuff diameter exceed that of the PTFE, so that 'tenting' takes place in the vein rather than the PTFE (this makes extra suturing easier). See **6g, i**. By squaring off the tip of the PTFE with a blade, its circumference can be shortened (**4d**). It is a simple matter to join the PTFE and cuff end-to-end (**4d**). A parachute technique using 6/0 prolene is appropriate.

Prior to the completion of the anastomosis, backbleeding from both directions is checked to flush out any thrombus. After a final irrigation both proximally and distally, the suture line is completed and the clamps released. A peroperative arteriogram is performed through a 21-gauge butterfly needle inserted into the PTFE near the distal anastomosis and facing upstream. This allows the minimum amount of contrast to be used to display the distal anastomosis. This is important with tibial artery outflow, where excessive contrast can be harmful.

5a–d

Care of the graft and prevention of clotting

Considerable care is taken to ensure that the graft is of the correct length and that at no stage is there any stationary blood, either in the graft or the well of the cuff and artery, where blood is inclined to accumulate during the execution of the proximal anastomosis. After the proximal anastomosis is made, the graft is placed in its selected tract by a tunneller or sponge-holding forceps. Heparinized saline is then forcibly refluxed upstream through the graft and inflow artery with a 20-ml syringe and malleable cannula (e.g. Oschner), and the graft is clamped distally (**5a**) This has the effect of ironing out any kinks or malrotation and of ascertaining the optimal length under arterial pressure at the moment the graft is cut (**5b**). It also makes absolutely sure that there is no stagnant blood in the graft.

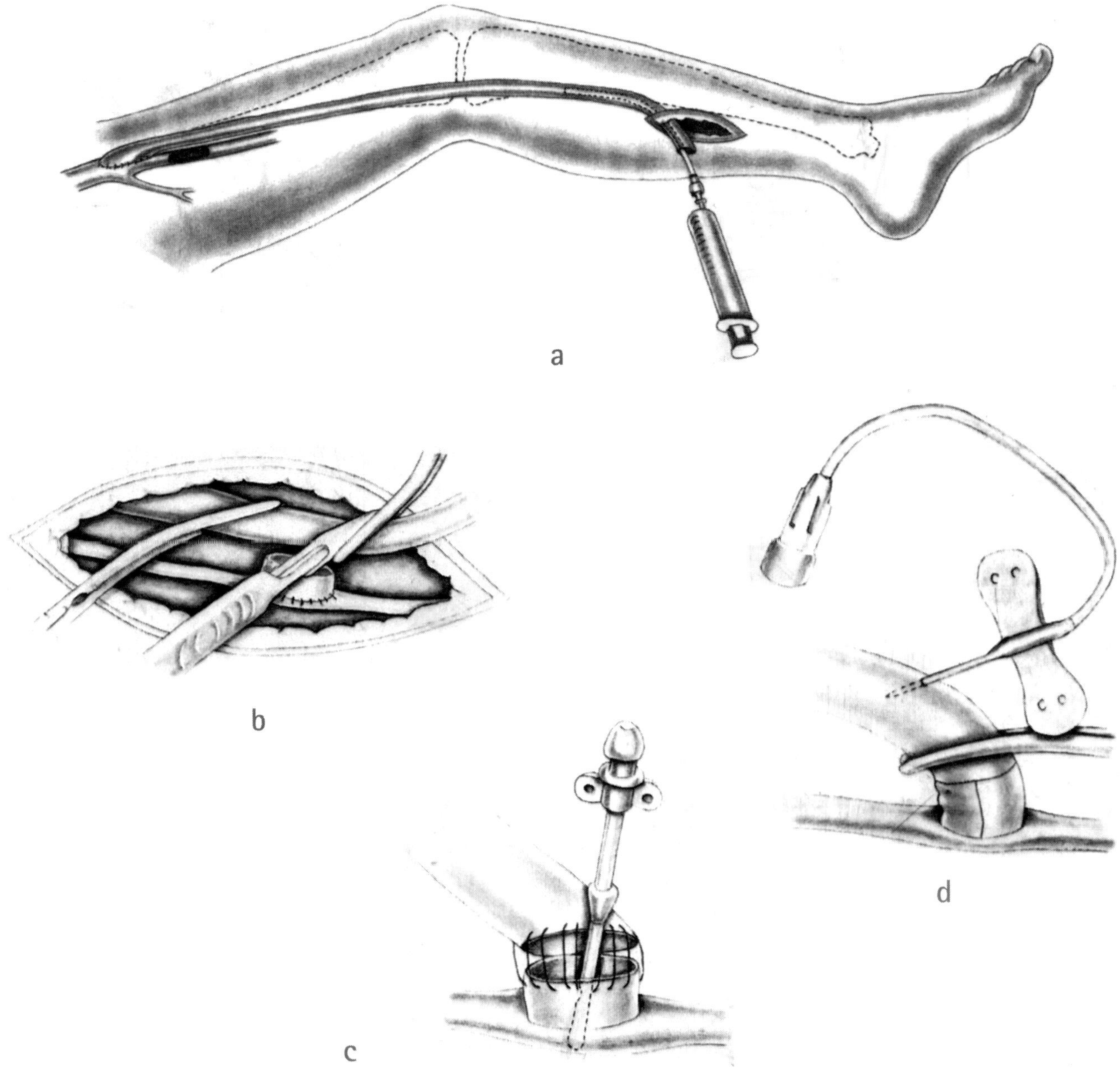

5

Just prior to completion of the anastomosis, the downflow is checked. A cannula is gently inserted between the loose continuous suture and the cavity of the cuff, and then the graft is flushed with heparinized saline with the arterial clamps removed (**5c**). The suture is tightened and the graft clamp is released. This variation in the technique is important with tibial arteries, where backbleeding is often negligible. The perfect tibial clamp is yet to be designed, and therefore clamping and unclamping should be kept to a minimum. Some surgeons make use of the pneumatic tourniquet technique to avoid this clamping (Bernhard *et al.*, 1991).

Most suture line bleeding stops within 5 min with gentle swab pressure. 'Tents' from excess vein to PTFE cause 'spurters', which may require individual suturing with the graft reclamped. At no stage should there ever be stationary blood in the PTFE graft. If clamping longer than 1 min is required for any reason, heparinized saline solution should be refluxed back up the graft (clamped distally) to the proximal anastomosis via the scalp vein needle used for the arteriogram (**5d**).

6a–l

Pitfalls and variations

If the vein is too narrow the sutures to both artery and PTFE get uncomfortably close especially at the vein–vein

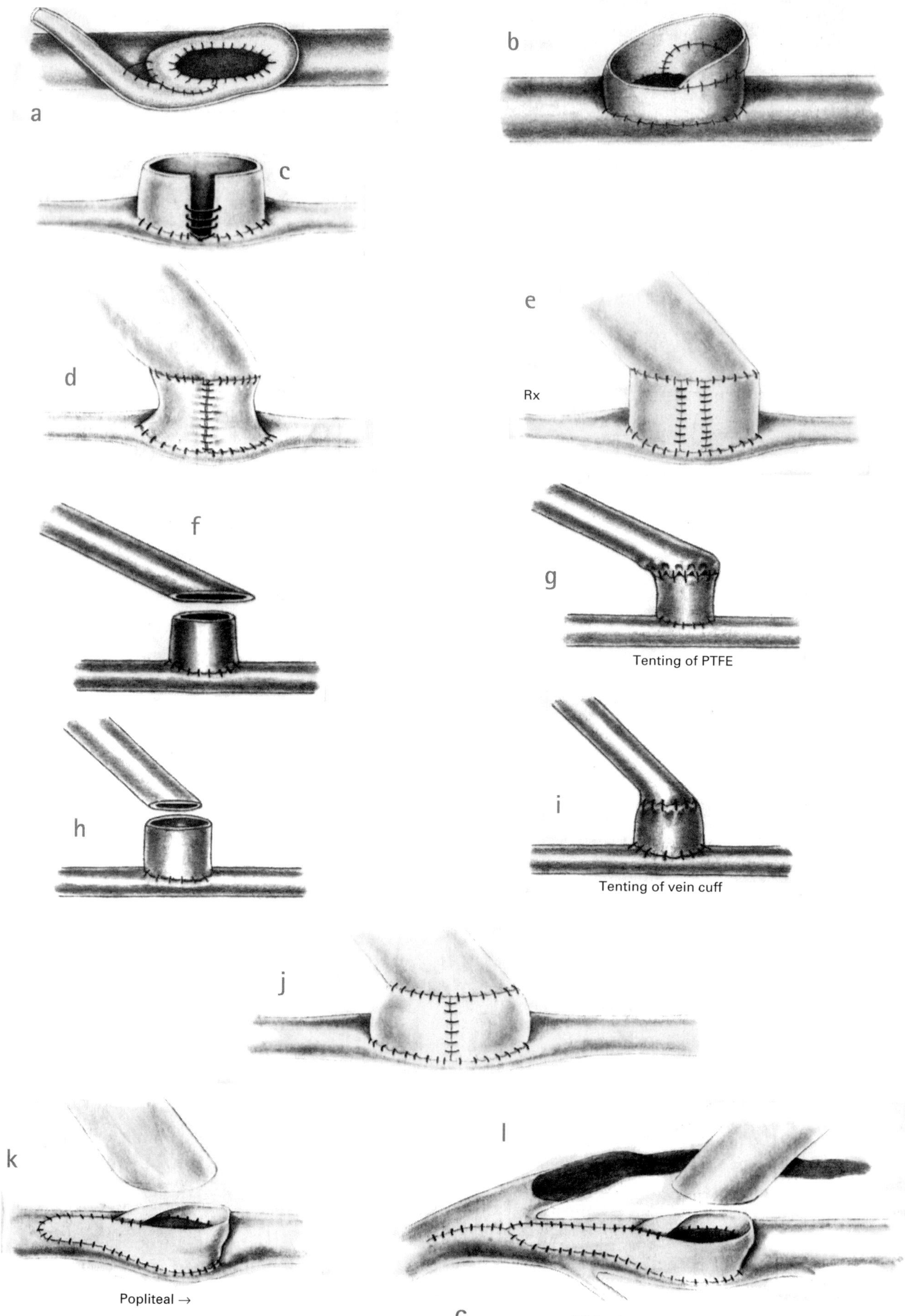
a
b
c
d
e
Rx
f
g
Tenting of PTFE
h
i
Tenting of vein cuff
j
k
Popliteal →
l
Profunda →

6

join. This overcrowding of sutures can be avoided (with suitable length of vein) by continuing suturing to the free edge of the vein initially crossing the apex (**6a**) and finishing on the near side (**6b**) as a 'double tier'. This makes a smoother and more haemodynamic PTFE-cuff join which I often deliberately use when traversing the popliteal fossa to a below-knee popliteal artery insertion.

When the vein is too short, stretching it under tension **6c, d** predisposes to necrosis and bleeding at a later date. It is better to cut another piece of vein and suture this in place, tedious though this might be (**6e**). A common mistake is to cut the PTEE too acutely (e.g. 30 degrees) in an effort to reduce the angle of insertion to cuff-artery complex (**6f**), making the circumference of PTFE longer than cuff. They can then only be matched by 'tenting' the PTFE causing crowding of sutures in more fragile vein (**6g**), risking tearing and bleeding. This is corrected by cutting the PTFE more obtusely (e.g. 45–60 degrees) (**6h**) so that 'tenting' occurs in a vein and tougher PTFE takes the crowding of sutures (**6i**).

If the arteriotomy is too long, the resultant cuff becomes aneurysmal (**6j**). To compensate, part of the vein is sutured in as a patch leaving sufficient as cuff to accommodate the cut PTFE. It is usual to place the cuff component at the downstream end so as to provide for the vital distal outflow lumen (**6k**), unlike Tyrrell and Wolfe (1991), who prefer it as a 'collar' on the upstream end for haemodynamic reasons. The use of this procedure is sometimes made in concomitant profundaplasty. The patch component widens the proximal profunda, and the cuff accommodating the PTFE is placed distally over uninvolved vessel (**6l**).

7a, b, c

Sequential composite femoro-popliteal-tibial graft

The accepted method for composing a femoro-popliteal-tibial graft by making use of a short segment of vein is to

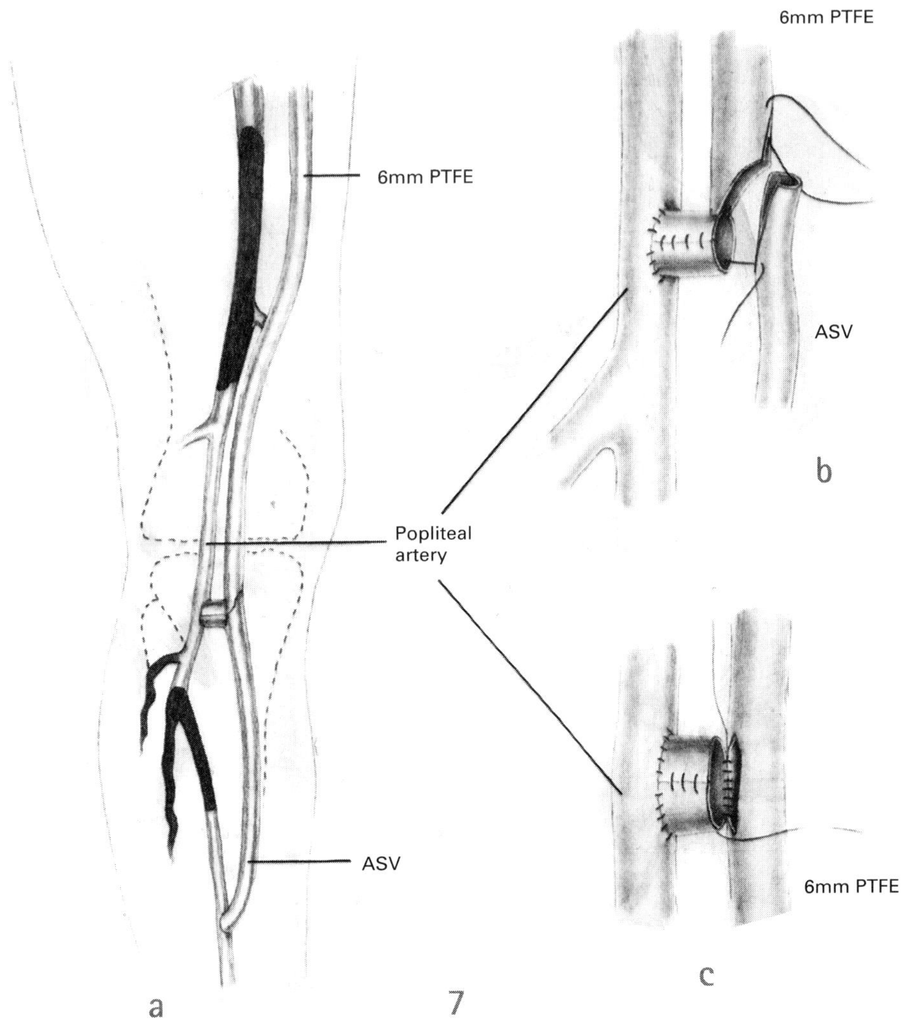

7

make a direct anastomosis of the PTFE to the popliteal artery and run a jump graft from the PTFE to the tibial vessel (Finn *et al.*, 1980), or to join the PTFE distal outflow anastomosis and the vein inflow anastomosis sequentially to the popliteal artery. There are two problems, however. Technically, the proximal portion of the vein is narrow (at the best 4 mm, otherwise it would have been used in its entirety as a complete vein graft) and therefore likely to be narrow immediately at the heel. Second, in the long term, neointimal hyperplasia may develop as a consequence of the compliance mismatch.

By applying a cuff to the intermediate popliteal anastomotic site first (**7a**), the PTFE and the vein can be joined using the sleeve as an intermediary (avoiding the direct vein–PTFE join or the vein to thick-walled artery). The critical heel of the small-diameter vein is first parachuted on to the mid-distal point of the sleeve, and then the wider heel of the PTFE on to the proximal or cephalic side of the sleeve. The apical opened out part of the vein becomes a long patch on the PTFE (**7b**). Alternatively, a single tube of PTFE can be anastomosed side-to-side to the popliteal artery via the cuff (**7c**). A direct side-to-side anastomosis between the PTFE and the artery is very difficult.

8a, b, c

Sequential composite aorto-(ilio)-profunda popliteal graft

An aorto-(or ilio)-profunda popliteal graft is constructed in the same way using a cuff on profunda femoris as an intermediary to link 8 mm PTFE to 6 mm PTFE or the narrow end of reversed saphenous vein. It is possible to use the proximal portion of the reversed vein in continuity as the cuff component. The vein is simply opened as though it were being used for the hood of a conventional proximal anastomosis (**8a**), sutured all the way around the arteriotomy as for the cuff (**8b**), but is continued down the open vein suturing vein to vein, widening the proximal vein as a funnel especially opposite the heel (**8c**) (Vladimirovich, 1985). With more romantic than geographical insight this manoeuvre is known as a 'Hungarian wrap'. It is equally as effective in the femoro-popliteal-tibial situation.

9a, b

Late thrombectomy of occluded PTFE graft and cuff

When a PTFE graft occludes (often years later), the presence of a cuff facilitates the thrombectomy. Usually, the original outflow artery remains open and shows up on the arteriogram. If not, it can sometimes be cleaned out by local infusion of streptokinase via the graft. Failing this, the main body of the graft can be thrombectomized and extended with a fresh piece of PTFE to a new site lower down via a cuff. It is unlikely that simply clearing the graft at its midpoint with a Fogarty catheter will have any lasting outcome. Both ends must be exposed and cleaned under direct vision. Similarly, lysis of the popliteal trifurcation is preferable to Fogarty exploration.

Clearing the distal anastomosis

The junction of the PTFE and cuff is exposed by sharp dissection, as are both the upstream and downstream arteries, sufficient to control backbleeding using straight clamps and without formal taping. It is best not to bare the original vein-to-artery stitching. An arteriotomy is made across the PTFE and cuff (**9a**).

Thrombus is then lifted from within the vein-artery cavity. This results mostly in backbleeding from either end. It is not usually necessary to pass a Fogarty catheter, but this can be decided upon using the arteriogram. Very occasionally, a vessel full of clot can be cleared from here, but it is more likely that the artery lining will be damaged. On rare occasions, neointima may line the junction of the PTFE and vein cuff, possibly extending to the arterial lumen. This will endarterectomize cleanly (it is quite distinct from atheroma), leaving natural endothe-

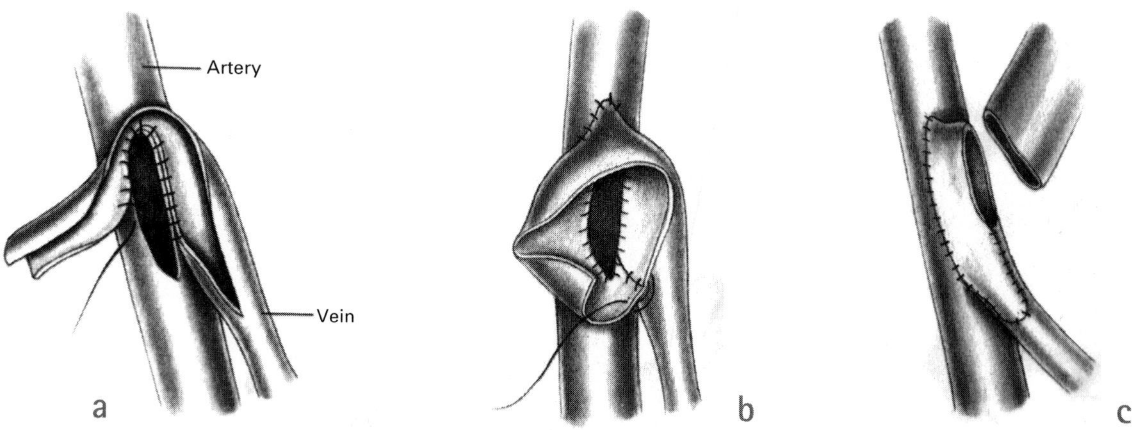

8

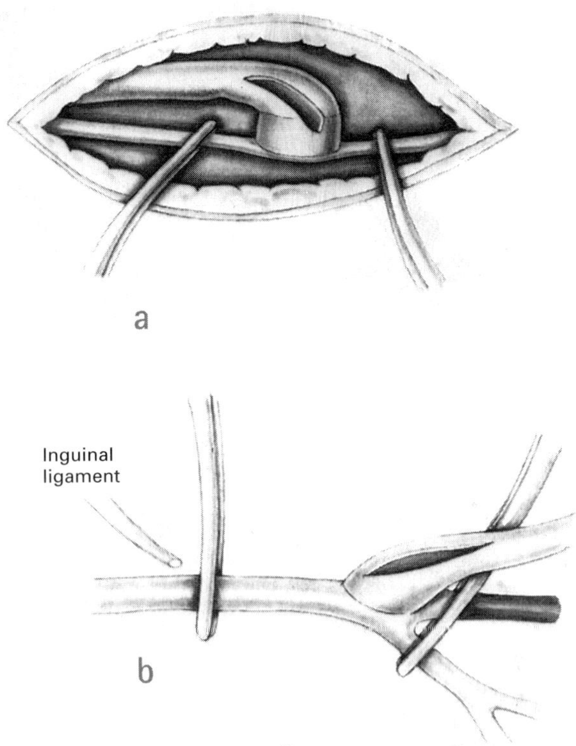

9

lium. No attempt should be made to clear out above with a Fogarty catheter at this stage.

Clearing the upper anastomosis
The upper graft is exposed by sharp dissection and followed up to the anastomosis. It is preferable to avoid laying bare the previous sutures. The common femoral artery is then similarly dissected just under the inguinal ligament, separating the femoral vein to the lateral side and the femoral nerve laterally. This should be virgin territory. Taping, which risks damaging the backwall, is not necessary; a Bainbridge DeBakey clamp directed backwards will suffice. Profunda backbleeding is controlled using a similar clamp across the superficial femoral and profunda artery complex (**9b**). Again it is preferable that the profunda femoris is not taped.

The hood of the PTFE is opened and the cavity is cleared of fibrin. This is facilitated if there has been a previous cuff. The downflow is then checked and, if found to be inadequate, a Fogarty catheter or sound may be gently passed to ascertain the need for a patch above the anastomosis. It may be necessary to have profunda backbleeding during the final stages of cleaning. A view is obtained using a blunt paediatric sucker and irrigation. A common mistake is to shift to a new anastomosis more proximally. Ultimately, this only prejudices the profunda circulation, lengthens the graft and leads to a lower patency rate. It is possible to use the original anastomosis over and over again.

10a–e

The graft is then cleared through both openings. A No. 4 Fogarty catheter is passed from below upward to extract the main thrombus (**10a,b**). Often there is surprisingly little. This procedure should be carried out with care unless a thin layer of fibrin is disturbed. The passage of the catheter from above downward is to make sure there are no kinks. Finally, a large malleable cannula (e.g. Oschner) is introduced from above and the graft is vigorously flushed downwards with heparinized saline (**10c**).

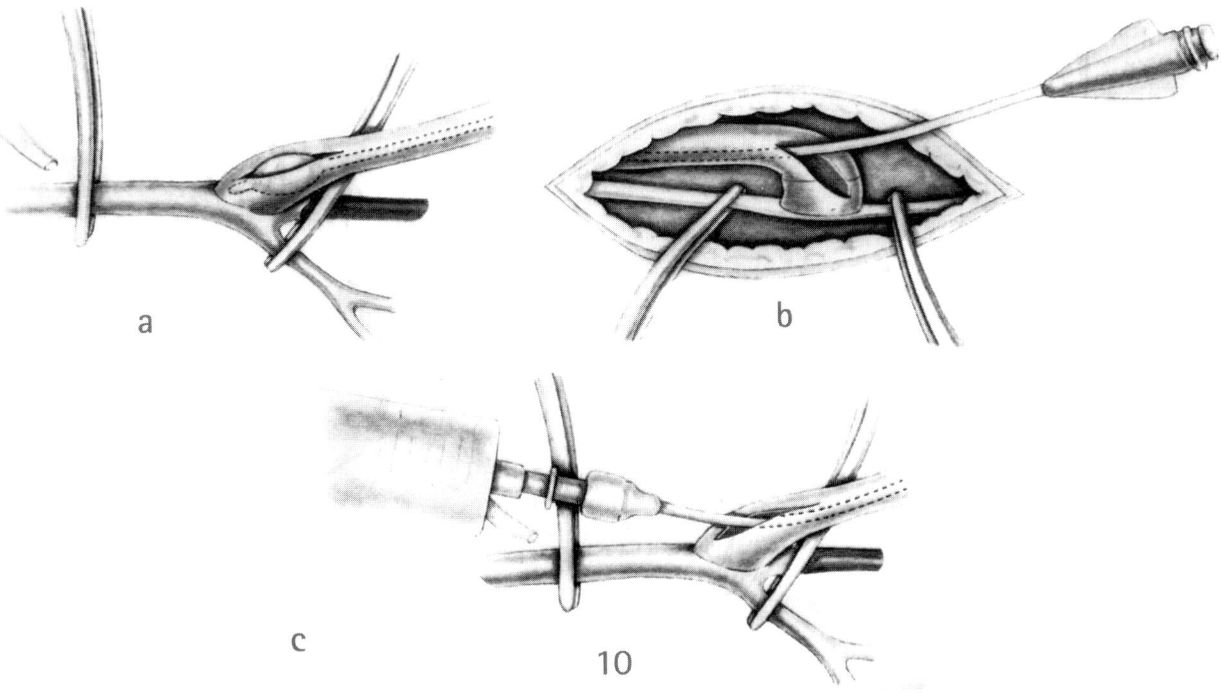

10

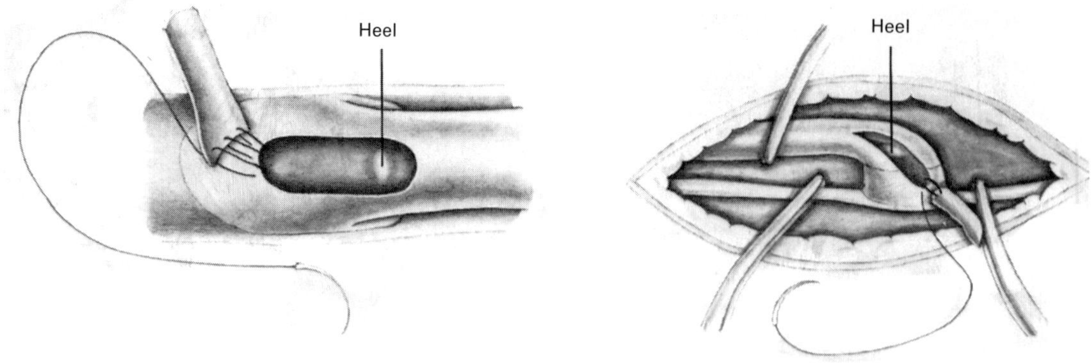

d 10 e

The upper opening is then closed (after checking downflow). Sometimes, a protruding mound ('cervix') presents from the original heel of the PTFE graft. If so, it is preferable to add a patch of PTFE or vein (**10d**). It is best not to clamp just beyond this suturing, in case clot accumulates. Instead, heparinized saline (or rheomacrodex) should be refluxed against the bloodstream as described (see **5a**), and a clamp attached just above the distal opening. This allows any debris to separate and prevents it from going down the outflow vessel. A brisk outflow when the clamp is released ensures the flow is not impeded.

Finally, the bottom opening is closed. Usually, a patch is required (preferably vein), especially if there is a protuberance of the original PTFE heel. The apex of the patch parachutes nicely into the previous cuff (**10e**).

10f

After thrombectomy, it is recommended that immediate full heparinization and long-term anticoagulation be instituted. It is my practice to run heparin (750–1000 u/h) directly into the graft via a 16-gauge epidural catheter introduced through the lower end of the upper wound (**10f**) maintaining a level of 2 × N APPT (50–60 therapeutic > 32) as measured systemically, until distal perfusion is optimal (as manifest by a 'hot foot'), if necessary for several days. The catheter can be used for a distal arteriogram (with digital subtraction angiography) and causes no bleeding on ultimate withdrawal.

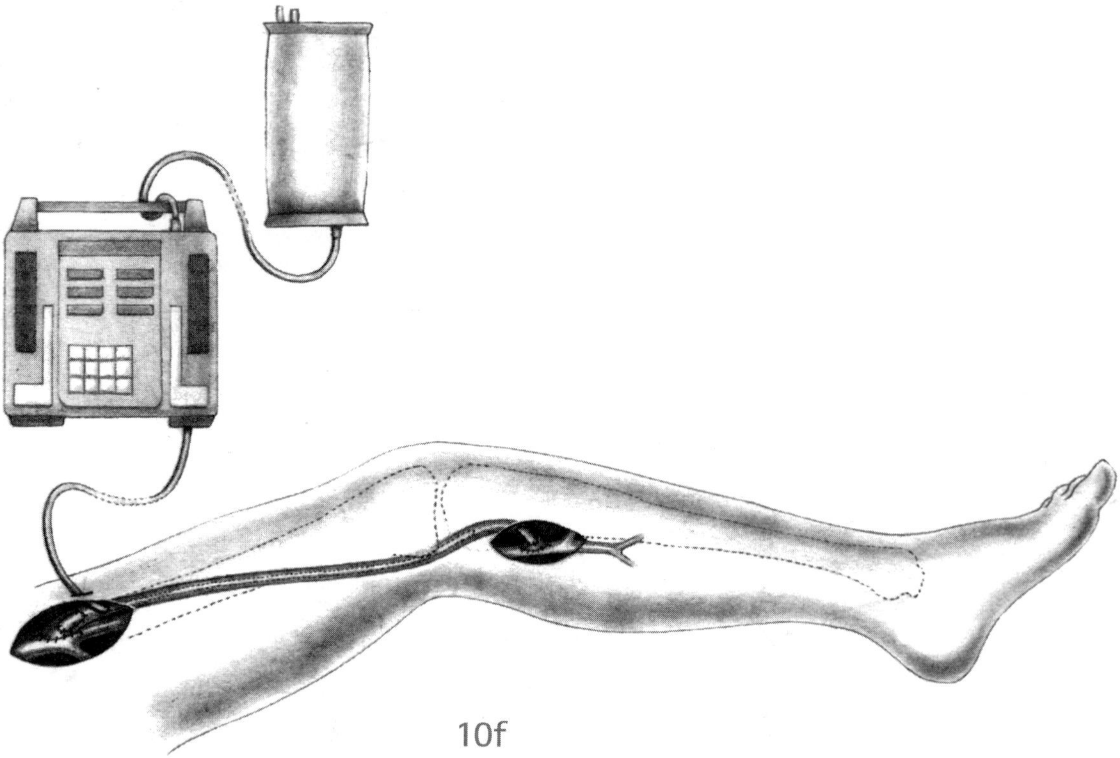

10f

Acknowledgements

Illustrations by Deirdre Cain.

References

Bernhard VM, Parent FN, Hunter GC, McIntyre KE (1991). The pneumatic tourniquet as an alternative to clamps for anastomoses below the knee. *J Cardiovasc Surg* (Suppl.) **32**: 65.

Finn WR, Flanigan DP, Verta M J *et al.* (1980). Sequential femoro-tibial bypass for severe limb ischaemia. *Surgery* **88**: 357.

Greenhalgh RM (1980). Profunda femoris reconstruction with and without distal bypass. In *Operative Techniques in Vascular Surgery* 1st edn. Bergan J J, Yao J S T eds. London/Orlando: Grune and Stratton, p. 189.

Linton RR, Wild WL (1970). *Surgery* **67**: 234.

Miller JH (1993). Partial replacement of an infected arterial graft by a new prosthetic polytetrafluoroethylene segment: A new therapeutic option. *J Vasc Surg* **17**: 546.

Miller JH, Foreman RK, Ferguson L, Faris I (1984). Interposition vein cuff for anastomosis of prosthesis to small artery. *Austral N Z J Surg* **54**: 283.

Miller JH, Allen D, Berce MB, *et al.* (1991). Profunda femoris artery as outflow using PTFE with vein cuff. *J Cardiovasc Surg* (Suppl.) **32**: 96.

Morris GE, Raptis S, Miller JH, Faris IB (1993). *Eur J Vasc Surg* **7**: 329.

Siegman F A (1979). Use of venous cuff for graft anastomosis. *Surg Gynecol Obstet* **148**: 930.

Suggs WD, Henriques HF, DePalma RG (1988). Vein cuff interposition prevents juxta-anastomotic neointimal hyperplasia. *Annl Surg* June, 717.

Taylor RS, Loh A, McFarlane RJ *et al.* (1992). Improved technique for polytetrafluoroethylene bypass grafting: long term results using anastomotic vein patches. *Br J Surg* **79**: 348.

Tyrrell MR, Wolfe JHN (1991). New prosthetic venous collar anastomotic technique: combining the best of other procedures. *Br J Surg* **78**: 1016.

Tyrrell MR, Clark G H, Wolfe JHN (1989a). Consideration of the mechanical properties of the distal anastomosis of PTFE may improve patency rates. *J Cardiovasc Surg* (Suppl.) **30**: 91.

Tyrrell MR, Grigg MJ, Wolfe JHN (1989b). Is arterial reconstruction to the ankle worthwhile in the absence of autogenous vein? *Eur J Vasc Surg* **3**: 429.

Vladimirovich KV (1985). Plasty of proximal anastomosis in femoro-popliteal reconstruction with a small autovenous graft. *International Congress of Angiology, Athens* (Abstracts), 50.

Repair of the failing femorodistal graft

John H N Wolfe, Peter R Taylor

Introduction

In recent years the number of bypass grafts performed to the more distal arteries in the lower limb has increased considerably. Despite experience and improved operative techniques, the failure of these arterial grafts continues to be a problem of considerable magnitude. Reported failure rates of femoropopliteal and femorocrural grafts range between 20 and 50% at 5 years. Brewster and colleagues (1983a) showed that 65% of graft failures occurred within the first postoperative year, and that 79% of grafts occlusions occur within 2 years of operation.

Graft failures can be divided into three groups, based on the postoperative time interval:

1. *Immediate failures.* These occur within 1 month and are almost invariably attributable to errors of surgical technique or judgement. Such failures can be minimized by careful objective intraoperative assessment with Doppler probes and arteriography (Whittemore *et al.*, 1980).
2. *Early failures.* This group accounts for the majority of graft failures and spans the time period from 1 month to 1 year following operation. This group may benefit particularly from graft surveillance techniques (Wolfe and McPherson, 1987).
3. *Late failures.* These occur after 1 year and are usually secondary to progression of the original atherosclerotic disease process. Although graft surveillance may be useful, the failure rate at this stage is only 25% per annum for vein grafts and 7% per annum for prosthetic grafts (Berkowitz *et al.*, 1981).

Techniques of graft surveillance

1. *Serial ankle Doppler pressure measurements.* Initial reports using this technique were encouraging (Taylor and Fox, 1977). However, more recent studies show that if this method is used alone, many graft stenoses are missed (Wolfe *et al.*, 1987; McShane *et al.*, 1987; Moody *et al.*, 1989).
2. *Serial intravenous digital subtraction angiography.* This is a reliable method for detecting graft stenoses, providing that the patient has a good cardiac output. However, patient compliance remains a drawback despite the introduction of non-ionic contrast medium.
3. *Serial duplex Doppler assessment.* This non-invasive method can detect graft stenoses before they become haemodynamically significant. Graft flow measurements are inaccurate (Grigg *et al.*, 1988a), but changes in peak systolic velocity of 50% or more within a 2-cm length of graft suggest the presence of a stenosis (Grigg *et al.*, 1988b).

If patients are monitored regularly for the first year, approximately 20% of grafts will develop stenoses (Wolfe *et al.*, 1987; Cohen *et al.*, 1986). However, not all stenoses will be haemodynamically significant. Our current policy is to monitor their progression. When the change in velocity suggests a 50% reduction in diameter (equivalent to a 75% reduction in cross-sectional area), we intervene, since we believe that the graft is at risk of occlusion from a haemodynamically significant stenosis. Whittemore *et al.* (1980) have shown that the results of thrombectomy are much worse than those of graft repair before occlusion. Not all stenoses progress to become significant, and in approximately half no progression is seen so that intervention is not indicated. Difficulties in imaging may be encountered when the graft is very deep to the skin, such as the area immediately adjacent to a popliteal anastomosis. Distal grafts to the crural vessels are more superficial and reliable recordings can be obtained. Colour flow Doppler imaging may be useful in this regard since the deeper grafts are more easily identified (Buth *et al.*, 1991). This policy of graft surveillance leads to a number of re-operations on arterial bypass grafts. These secondary procedures can be classified into the following three categories: (1) inflow problems, (2) graft problems and (3) outflow problems.

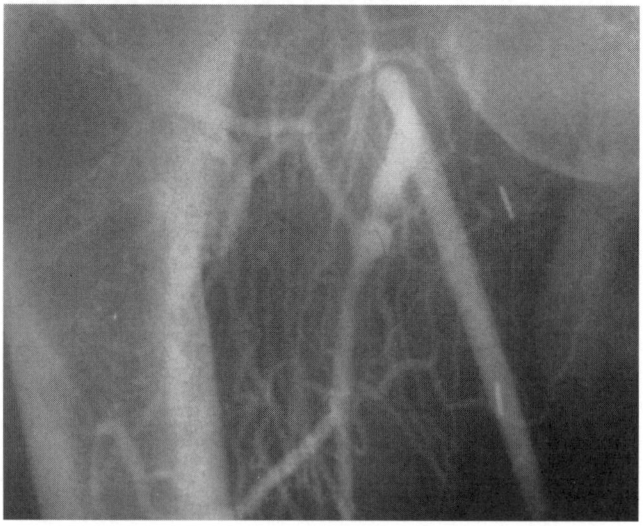

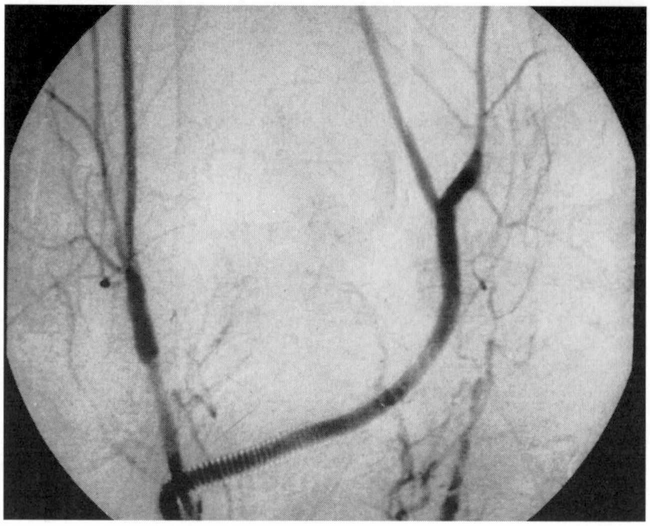

a 1 b

Secondary procedures

Inflow problems

1a, b

In the presence of ipsilateral iliac artery occlusion, vein grafts may remain patent even though clinically they do not pulsate (**1a**). In these patients an appropriate procedure is performed to improve the inflow of the graft. This may include a femorofemoral crossover graft, iliofemoral crossover graft (**1b**), unilateral iliofemoral graft or an aortobifemoral graft. The upper end of the graft is anastomosed, end-to-side, to the new graft using the usual anastomotic technique. There is no purpose in interposing parent artery between the two grafts. Clamp injury may damage the common femoral artery, but in our experience this is rare (Grigg *et al.*, 1988b).

2a, b

A more common problem is aggressive myointimal hyperplasia occurring at the site of femoral endarterectomy performed to facilitate the proximal anastomosis (**2a**). This can be repaired with a vein patch (**2b**) across the stenosed segment.

Graft problems

3, 4

Short fibrotic stenoses occurring in vein grafts are frequently related to valve cusps. These can be treated by either vein patch (taken from either the arm or the short saphenous vein) or percutaneous balloon angioplasty. However, balloon angioplasty is not as successful as surgery (Whittemore *et al.*, 1980; Cohen *et al.*, 1986; Brewster *et al.*, 1983b; Veith *et al.*, 1984), and assessing the discrepancy in results between three centres it became apparent that stenoses >2 cm should be treated surgically (Taylor *et al.*, 1990). The use of a 2.5 mm cardiac balloon may improve results since it is more difficult to disrupt vein grafts with these small, softer balloons. We now rarely perform patches, preferring to interpose a short vein segment (see below).

5a, b

Longer stenoses should be treated operatively by using a 'jump' graft to bypass the stenosed segment. End-to-end venovenous anastomoses give better flow characteristics and the use of a long oblique anastomosis using 7/0 prolene protects against stenosis. When long or multiple segments of graft are affected by a stenotic process, surgery is of little value.

6

The right femoropopliteal graft is older but the left has developed a long segment of stenosis and myointimal hyperplasia. It is unlikely that intervention will assist this graft.

Outflow problems

7a, b, 8a, b

We have had some success with balloon angioplasty in treating 'web' stenoses close to the distal anastomosis, but others are more sceptical. More commonly we perform a bypass 'jump' graft from the graft to a crural vessel distal to the stenosis using arm vein or short

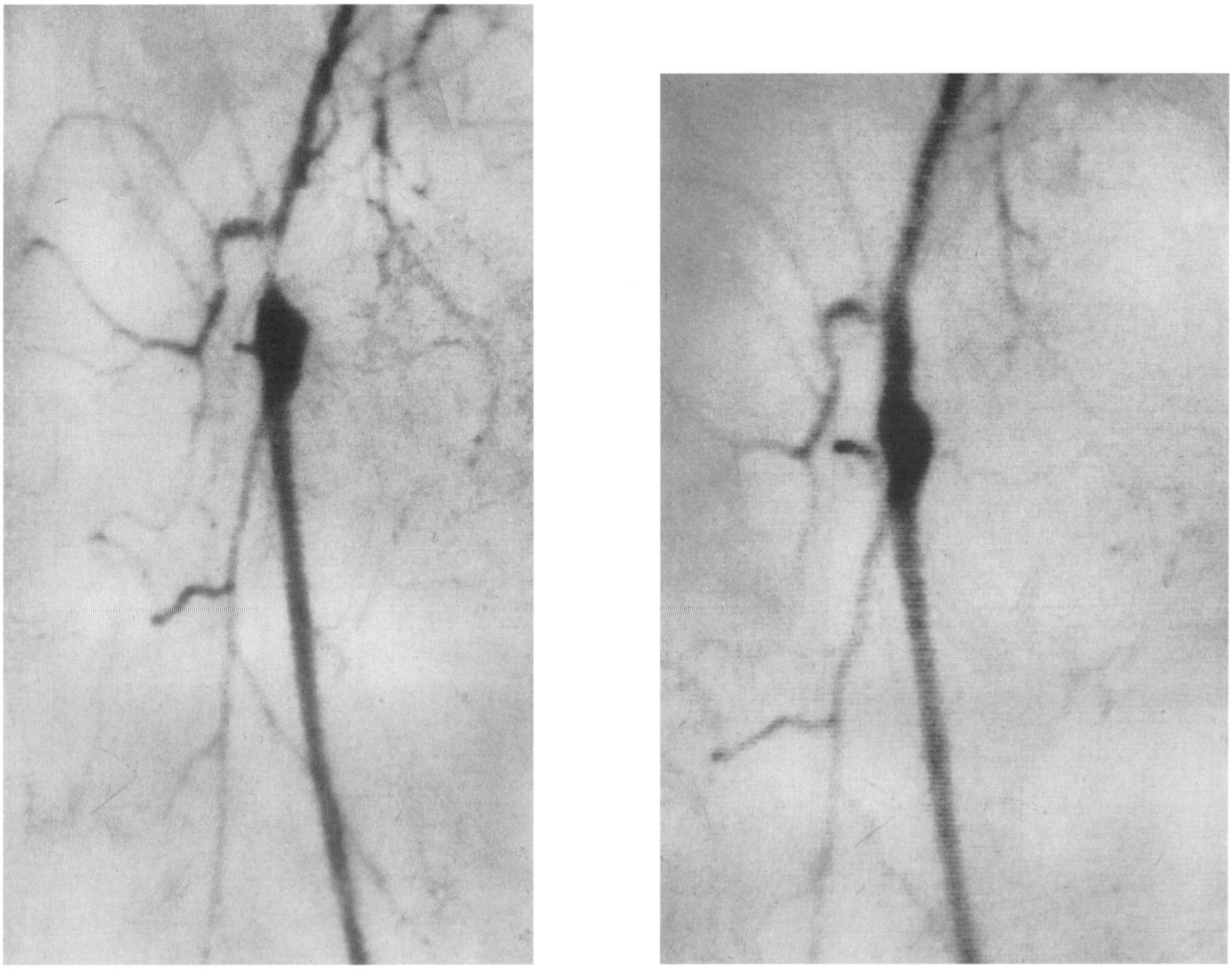

a 2 b

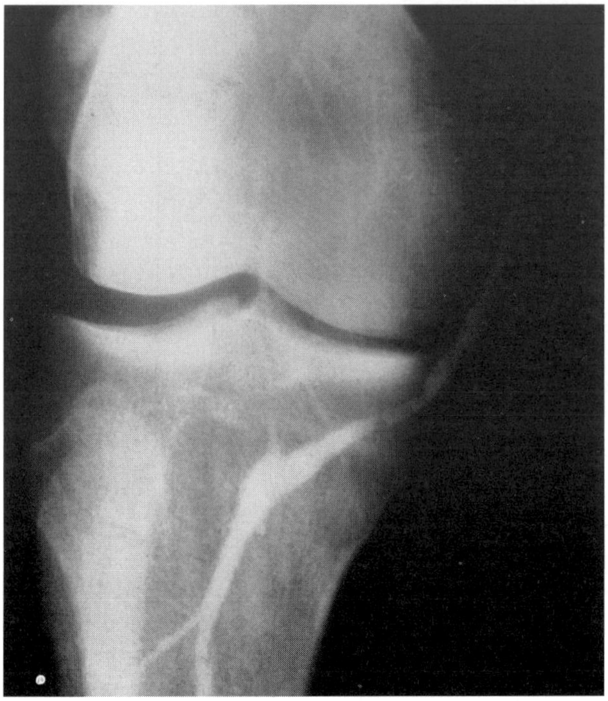

3

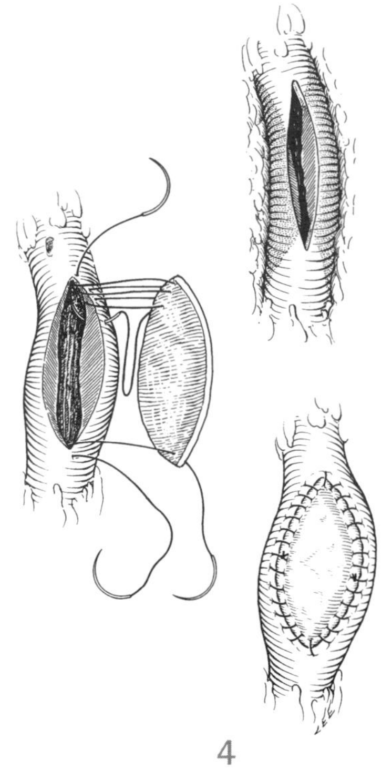

4

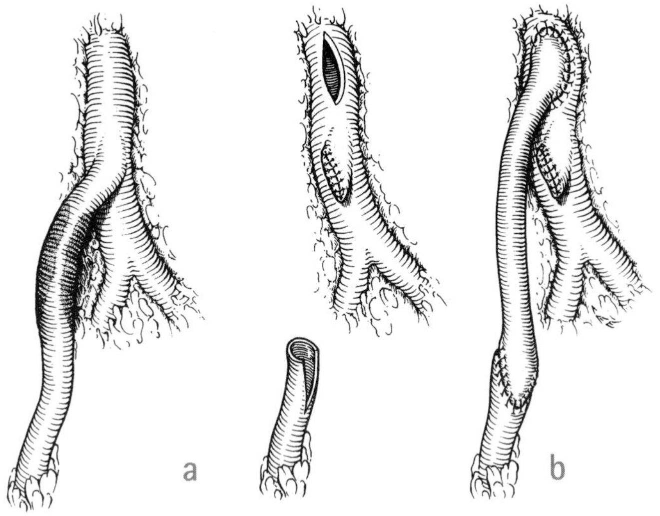

5

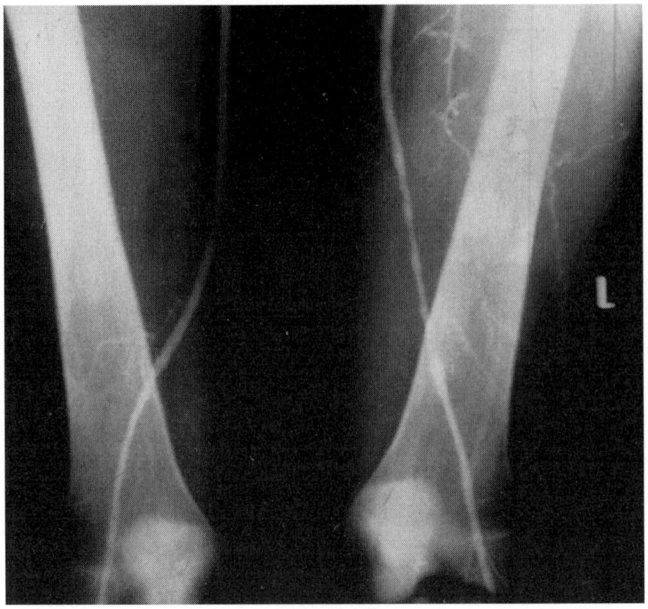

6

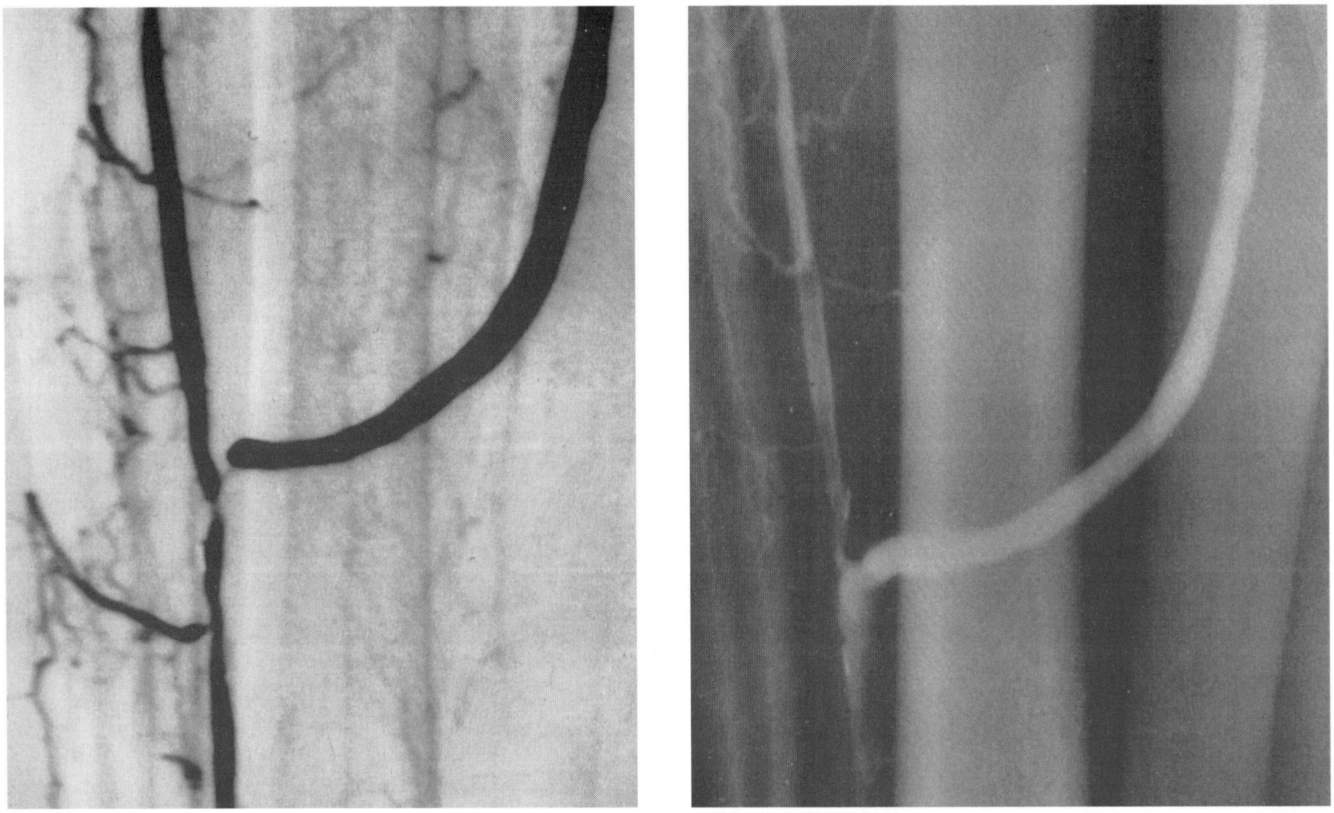

a b

7

saphenous vein. The graft is tunnelled subcutaneously. The dissection of the distal vessel is relatively straightforward providing the previous operating field can be avoided.

9

Except under rare circumstances, no attempt should be made to dissect out the previous anastomosis. The dense scar tissue resulting from the previous operation makes this a procedure fraught with hazard. When it is neces-

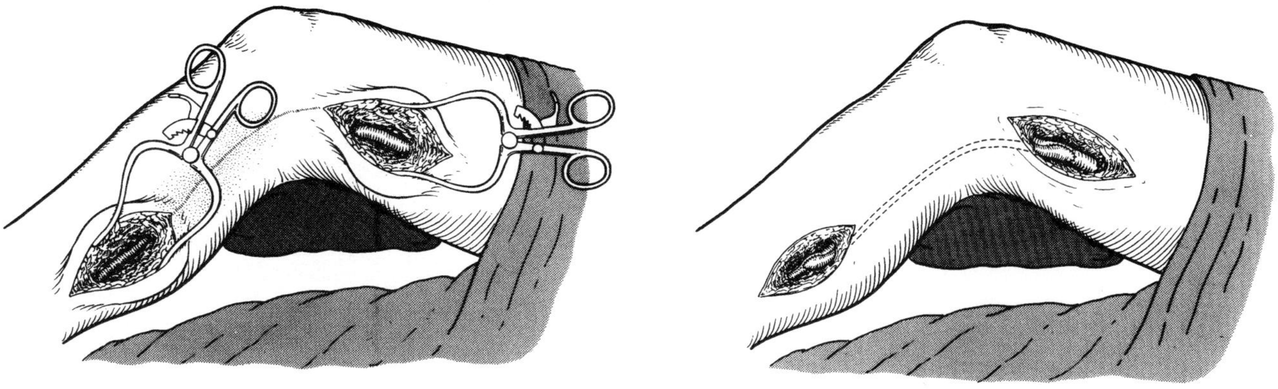

a 8 b

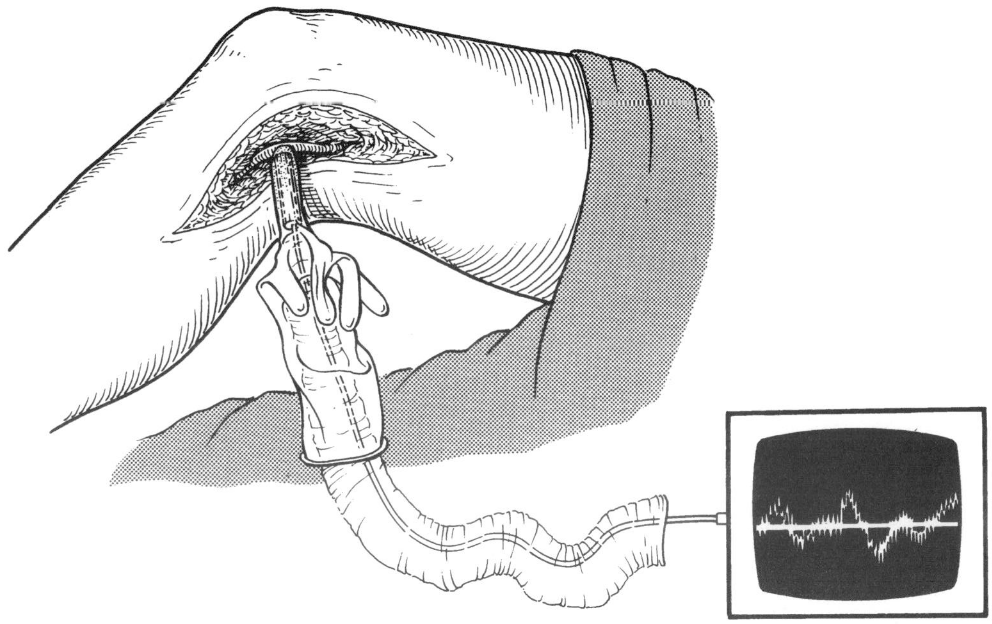

9

sary to dissect a graft from this scar tissue, it can be extremely difficult to visualize or palpate, and a hand-held Doppler probe placed within a sterile operating glove may be invaluable in localizing the graft.

References

Berkowitz HD, Hobbs CL, Roberts B *et al.* (1981). Value of routine vascular laboratory studies to identify vein graft stenoses. *Surgery* **90**: 971.

Brewster DL, La Salle AJ, Robison JC *et al.* (1983a). Factors affecting patency of femoro-popliteal grafts. *Surg Gynecol Obstet* **157**: 437.

Brewster DC, La Salle AJ, Robison JG *et al.* (1983b). Femoro-popliteal graft failures: Clinical consequences and success of secondary reconstructions. *Arch Surg* **118**: 1043.

Buth J, Disselhoff B, Sommerling C *et al.* (1991). Colour flow duplex criteria for grading stenoses in infrainguinal vein grafts. *J Vasc Surg* **14**: 716.

Cohen JR, Mannick JA, Couch NP, Whittemore AD (1986). Recognition and management of impending vein graft failure. *Arch Surg* **121**: 758.

Grigg MJ, Wolfe JHN, Tovan A, Nicolaides AN (1988a). The reliability of duplex haemodynamic measurements in the assessment of femoro-distal grafts. *Euro Vasc Surg* **2**: 171.

Grigg MJ, Nicolaides AN and Wolfe JHN (1988b). Femorodistal bypass graft stenoses. *Br J Surg* **75**: 737.

McShane MD, Gazzard WH, Clifford PC *et al.* (1987). Duplex ultrasound assessment and femoro-distal grafts – correlation with angioplasty. *Eur J Vasc Surg* **1**: 409.

Moody P, DeCossart LM, Douglas HM *et al.* (1989). Asymptomatic strictures in femoropopliteal grafts. *Eur J Vasc Surg* **3**: 389.

Taylor P, Gould D, Harris P *et al.* (1990). Balloon dilatation of graft stenoses – reasons for failure. *Br J Surg* **7**: 371.

Taylor RS, Fox ND (1977). Ultrasonic prediction of graft failure. *J Cardiovasc Surg* **18**: 309.

Veith FJ, Weiser RK, Gupta *et al.* (1984). Diagnosis and management of failing lower extremity arterial reconstructions prior to graft occlusion. *J Cardiovasc Surg* **25**: 381.

Whittemore AD, Clowes AW, Couch NP Mannick JA (1980). Secondary femoro-popliteal reconstruction. *Ann Surg* **193**: 35.

Wolfe JHN, McPherson GAD (1987). The failing femoro-distal graft. *Eur J Vasc Surg* **1**: 295.

Wolfe JHN, Thomas ML, Jamieson CW *et al.* (1987). The early diagnosis of femoro-popliteal graft stenoses, a prospective one year follow up. *Br J Surg* **74**: 268.

Adjuvant arteriovenous fistula at the distal anastomosis of a femorotibial bypass graft

P L Harris

Introduction

An arteriovenous fistula is constructed at the distal anastomosis of a long prosthetic femorotibial graft in order to increase the velocity of blood flow through the graft above the thrombotic threshold level.

Indications

1. Patients with critical ischaemia whose only alternative is a major amputation.
2. Prosthetic grafts inserted into a single tibial vessel.
3. Poor run-off due to disease in the distal tibial or pedal vessels, determined by:
   a. pedal angiography pre- or intraoperatively;
   b. direct observation of vessels at operation;
   c. objective assessment of peripheral resistance or impedance;
   d. failure of the bypass graft despite adequate inflow and perfect operative technique.

Special requirements

1. Some arterial run-off is essential; the procedure is of no value if the venous system alone is perfused.
2. The deep venous system should be patent and free from post-phlebitic damage.
3. The construction of a fistula using superficial veins is associated with a high incidence of impaired wound healing and skin necrosis due to localized venous hypertension and should be avoided.
4. Unrestricted inflow to the graft is essential. Aortoiliac stenosis must be identified by appropriate non-invasive tests or biplanar angiography and must be corrected before or concurrently with the femorodistal bypass procedure.
5. Adjuvant arteriovenous fistula is not advisable for patients with severely impaired myocardial function.
6. The use of loupe magnification (×2.5) is recommended.
7. Heparin anticoagulation is essential during surgery and oral antiplatelet therapy postoperatively.

The operation

Common ostium fistula

1

The selected tibial artery and its largest concomitant vein are approached as described in the chapter by C N McCollum: 'Sites and approach for tibial anastomoses' (p. 341). A suitable length of these vessels is dissected and controlled with narrow latex slings. Clamps must not be applied to these vessels.

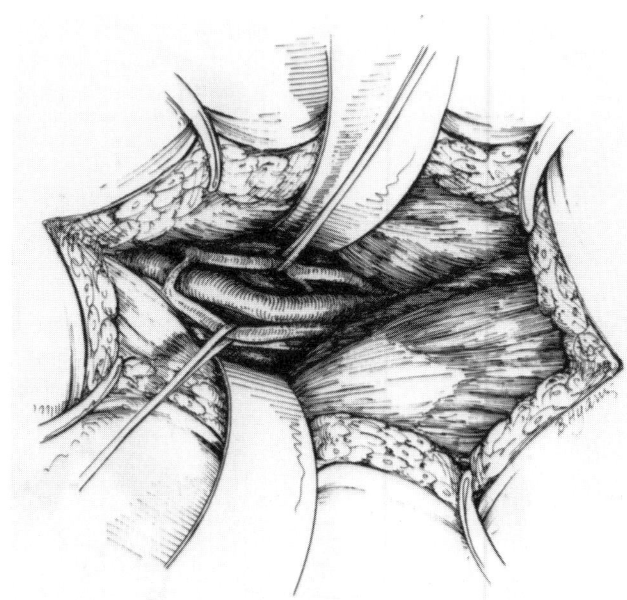

1

2

Longitudinal incisions approximately 15 mm in length are made in the artery and vein. Small catheters (not shown) are inserted into the artery distally and the vein proximally to control bleeding, permit perfusion of heparinized solutions, and to stent the anastomoses during construction. The adjacent walls of the vessels are sutured together using a double-ended 7/0 polypropylene suture.

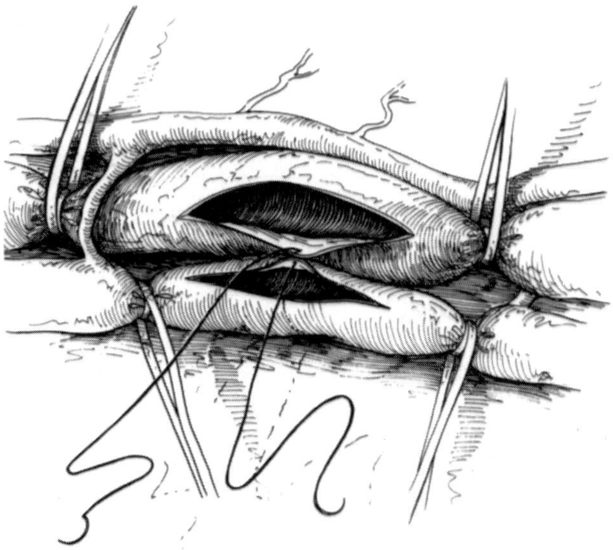

2

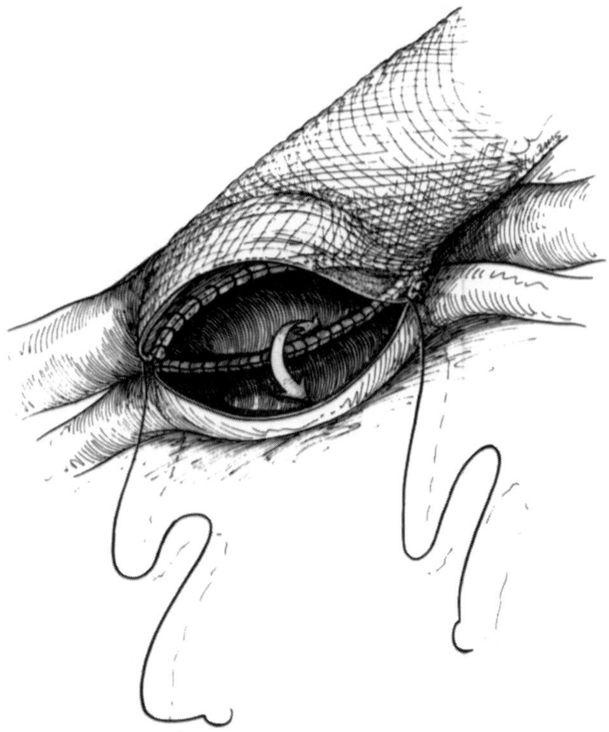

3

3

The distal end of the prosthetic graft is anastomosed to the 'common ostium' using 7/0 polypropylene sutures. Human umbilical vein is shown in the illustration as an example.

4

By reducing the length or the venotomy relative to that of the arteriotomy and constructing the fistula as shown, it is possible to simplify the graft to artery anastomosis at the toe and heel.

This slight modification of technique may help to reduce the risk of technical error at these critical points.

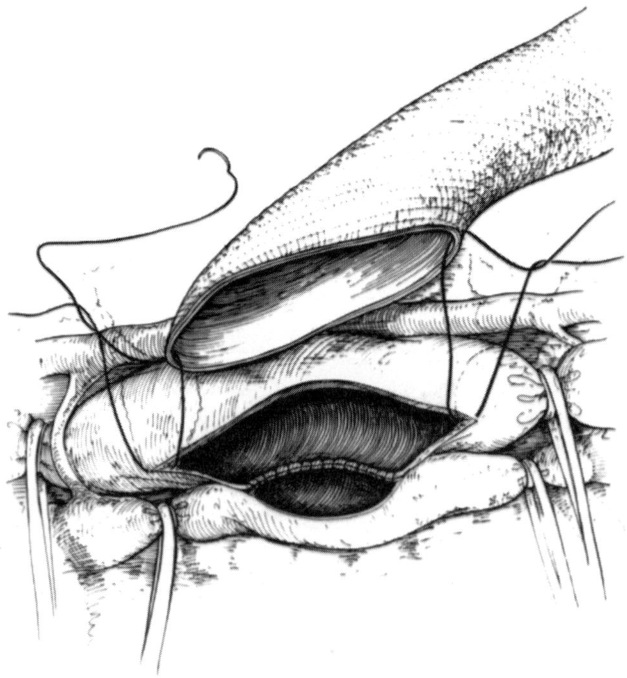

4

5

On completion the presence of a palpable thrill over the anastomosis indicates satisfactory functioning of the arteriovenous fistula. It is helpful to record bloodflow through the graft with an electromagnetic flow probe to assess the effect of the fistula. A mean flow greater than 200 ml per min is to be expected. Experimental studies indicate that less than 20% of the total flow through the graft passes distally into the artery, the remainder being

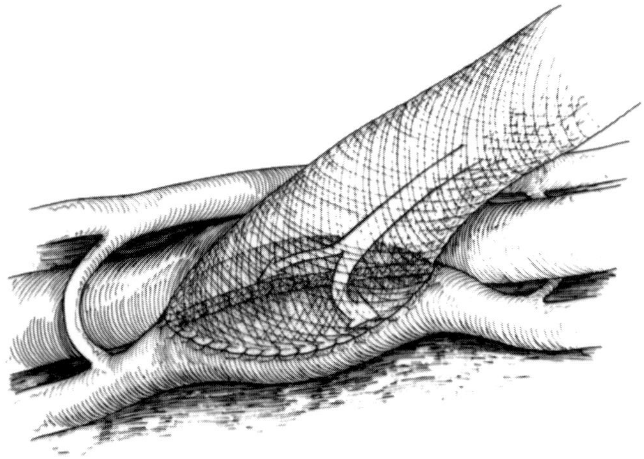

5

shunted into the veins. There is no evidence that a fistula constructed at this site ever results in a 'steal' of blood from the distal arterial circulation in clinical practice.

Alternative method

Pre-anastomotic fistula

6

Construction of a side-to-side arteriovenous fistula at a point 0.5–1 cm upstream of the graft-to-artery anastomosis, as shown, has the following potential advantages:

1. The intervening section of artery acts as a resistance which limits the volume of the shunt. The optimum size of shunt is one which results in a sufficient increase in blood flow through the graft to allow the thrombotic threshold to be exceeded with a small margin of safety. The 'common ostium' type of shunt sometimes results in flows considerably in excess of this with possible detrimental effects.
2. The construction of the graft to artery anastomosis and the fistula separately is less complicated and therefore subject to fewer technical errors.
3. The simpler form of construction may improve the flow characteristics at the graft-to-artery junction with less turbulence.

In practice the patency rates of grafts with common ostium and pre-anastomotic adjuvant fistula are similar.

7

Remote postanastomotic arteriovenous fistula

The construction of an arteriovenous fistula at a point downstream to the graft-to-artery anastomosis carries the advantage of drawing a larger volume of blood flow into the recipient artery than the methods previously described.

However, this disposition can result in a very much reduced perfusion pressure in the arteries distal to the fistula. For this reason a postanastomotic fistula should be sited as remotely as possible in the limb. Another concern regarding this technique is that the fistula may not be of sufficient size to achieve the primary aim of accelerating blood flow in the graft above thrombotic threshold levels.

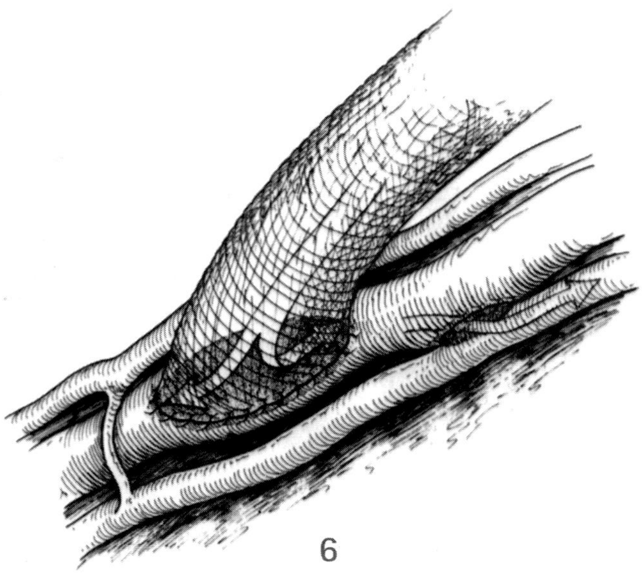

6

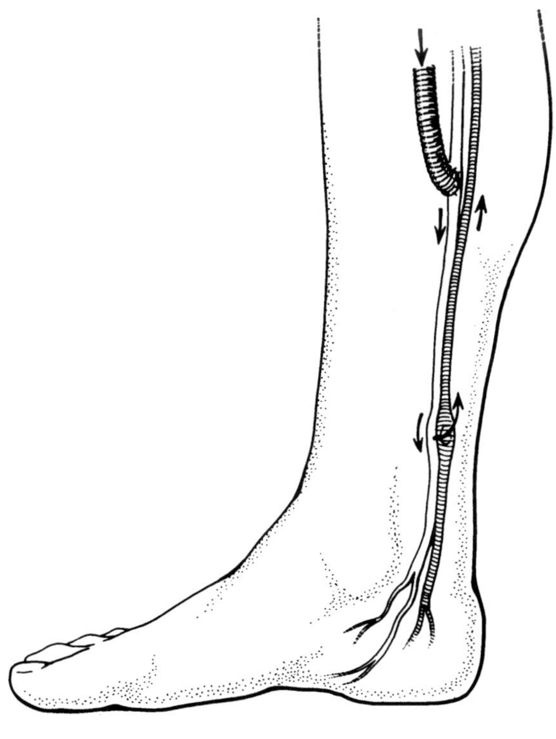

7

Acknowledgement
Illustrations by B Hyam.

References

Harris PL, Campbell H (1983). Adjuvant distal arteriovenous shunt with femoro-tibial bypass for critical ischaemia. *Br J Surg* **70**: 377.

Dardik H, Sussman B, Ibrahmin M *et al.* (1983). Distal artero-venous fistula as an adjunct to maintaining arterial and graft patency for limb salvage. *Surgery* **94**: 478.

Remote endarterectomy using the MollRing Cutter followed by endolining (ENDURING)

Joep AW Teijink, Frans L Moll

Introduction

Treatment of occlusions or multiple stenosed segments in the superficial femoral artery continues to be a challenging field in vascular surgery. Remote endarterectomy is a minimally invasive technique for revascularization that shortens hospital length of stay and reduces patient morbidity and mortality.

Remote endarterectomy with the MollRing Cutter®

With the use of the MollRing Cutter (Vascular Architects Inc., San Jose, CA), a modification of the single ring stripper, the surgeon is able to cut the endoluminal atheroma core remotely. The surgical exposure of the superficial femoral artery can be limited to a small single arteriotomy at the origin in the groin.

The MollRing Cutter consists of two shafts that telescope into each other. Two symmetric single ellipse-shaped rings at a 135-degree angle are attached at the most distal part of each shaft. The ellipse-shaped rings are symmetrical and come in different sizes, ranging from 5 mm to 10 mm inner diameter. Both parallel rings have sharpened inner edges that cut like a pair of scissors when both rings shear along each other. The remote cutting mechanism is activated with a handle at the end of the shafts.

Technique of remote endarterectomy

1

The patient should be prepared according to the institution's practice for open surgical procedures. A small pillow placed beneath the ipsilateral buttock allows for elevation of the incisional area (1) and facilitates the passage of both the ring dissector (Vollmar Dissector, Aesculap®, South San Francisco, CA) and the MollRing Cutter. A radiopaque ruler should be placed alongside the level of the distal superficial femoral artery and proximal popliteal artery.

2

Exposure of the proximal superficial femoral artery should be performed according to standard surgical technique. The dissection should allow for control of the distal common femoral artery, the profunda femoral artery and the proximal segment of the superficial femoral artery. A doubled vessel loop is placed around the distal portion of the superficial femoral artery to control anticipated back bleeding after successful endarterectomy.

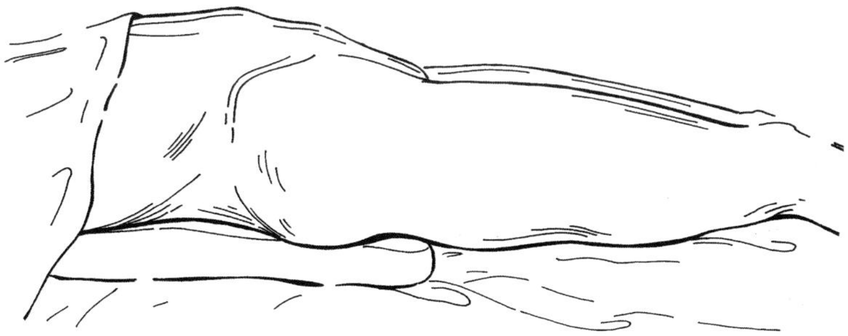

1

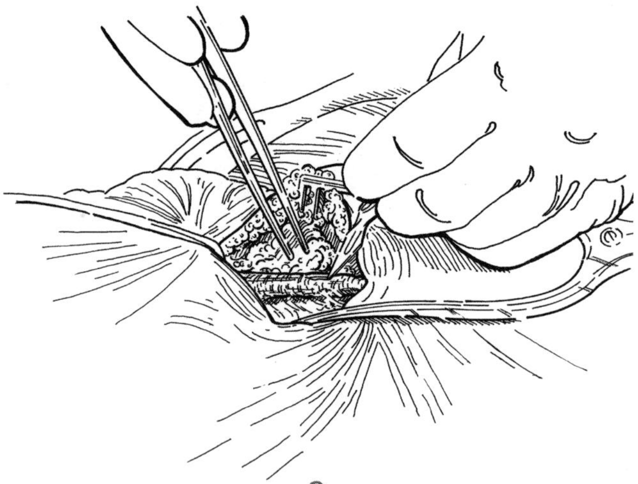

2

Angiography is performed in a retrograde manner into the distal common femoral artery. The distal superficial femoral artery and proximal popliteal artery are visualized. Close attention should be paid to the expected site of transection of the atheroma core, which is the endpoint of the remote endarterectomy. Note the ruler position of this endpoint if applicable.

Administer heparin intravenously according to recommended standards.

Place an angled clamp at the most proximal part of the superficial femoral artery. In case of a complete occlusion, the use of an artery clamp at this point of the procedure is not necessary.

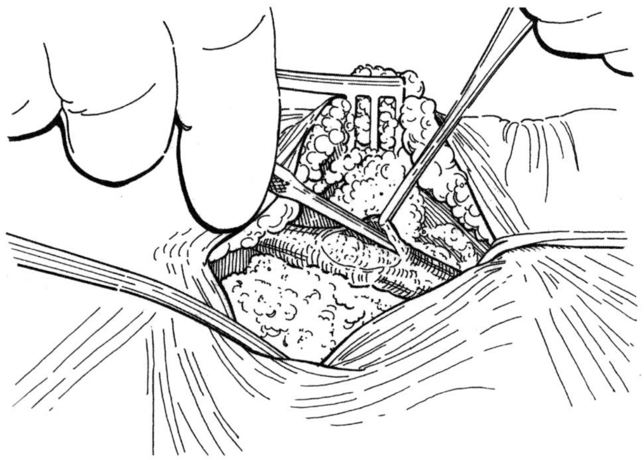

3

3

Use a No. 15 or No. 11 scalpel blade to incise 3–4 cm of the adventitia of the proximal superficial femoral artery in order to enter the subadventitial plane (2). Use of a Halle or Freer elevator facilitates the establishment of a subadventitial dissection plane (3). The vessel wall is dissected away from the core in the arteriotomy and 1–2 cm distally.

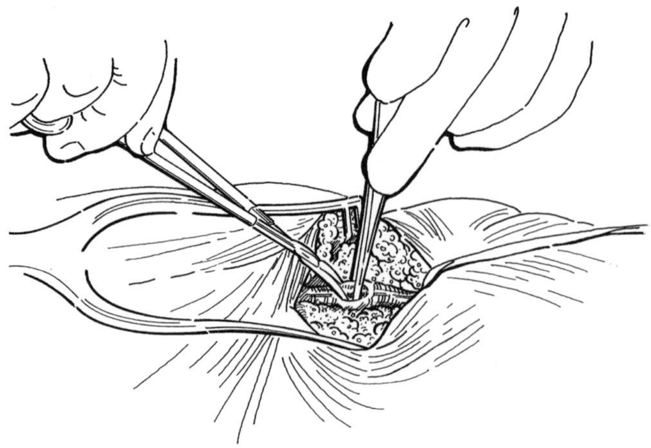

4

4

The core is then transected proximally in the arteriotomy (4). The resulting core should be long enough to be grasped by the assistant during both the ring stripper dissection as well as removal of the core after transection.

5

Determine the appropriate size ring dissector. Assemble the ring dissector and handle according to the manufacturer's instructions. Place the ring dissector over the core (5). Orient the distal tip of the ring posteriorly. The handle of the ring dissector should be positioned close to the groin.

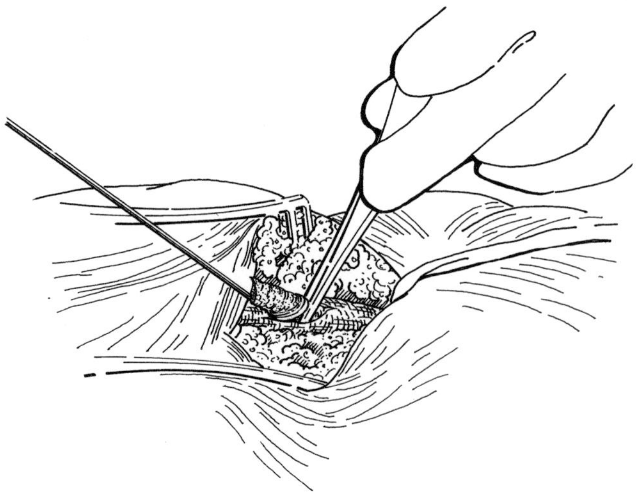

5

Using slow controlled movements the ring dissector is advanced distal to the vessel loop that is then gently retracted to prevent back bleeding. Continue the dissection of the core distally with a slow and controlled to and fro motion of the dissector handle. Rotate the dissector as it moves toward the endpoint but not more than 360 degrees clockwise or counterclockwise to prevent entanglement of the core around the ring dissector. Alternating use of a different size ring dissector can be useful if localized calcification of the core is encountered resulting in different core diameters.

Under fluoroscopy, continue the dissection of the core to the area 1cm above the previously chosen endpoint of the core. Obtain a freeze frame picture to document the position of the dissection endpoint. Gently withdraw the ring dissector, rotating the ring whenever resistance is encountered.

6

Choose the appropriate sized MollRing Cutter based on the size of the ring dissector that has been used. Confirm the cutting motion of the MollRing Cutter prior to passing the rings over the core. The proximal end of the MollRing Cutter consists of a handle and knob that are locked together by a small metal tab. To unlock the handle and knob, pull up on the metal tab. While holding the knob portion firmly, pull the handle portion towards you. The cutting occurs as the rings pass each other. When the handle portion is returned to its original position flush with the knob, the rings return to the original overlapped position. Place the selected MollRing Cutter over the core and advance distally to the endpoint of the previous dissection. Once you have confirmed the initial endpoint, advance the MollRing Cutter 1–2 cm beyond that point. Orient the MollRing Cutter so that the distal angulation is pointing ventrally (**6**). Since most of the residual plaque is usually located on the posterior wall of the vessel, this orientation will allow transection of the least diseased area distally. Transect the plaque. Perform the cutting procedure a second time to confirm that a complete transection of the plaque has occurred.

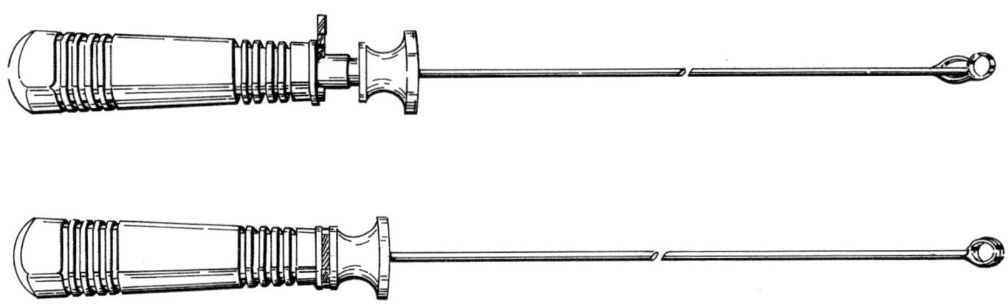

6

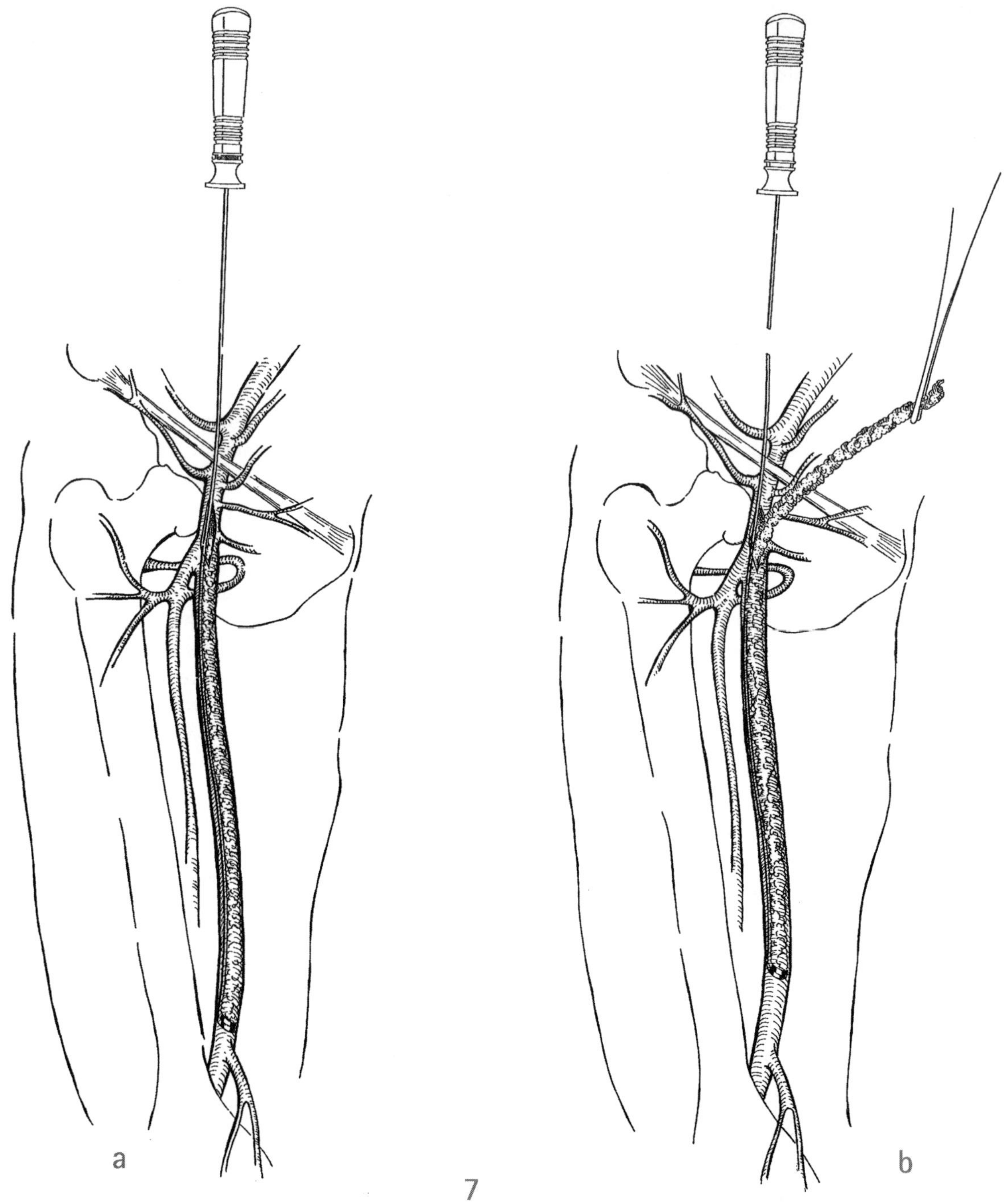

7

7

Return the MollRing Cutter to a position where the rings are one-third deployed. This position will grasp the distal end of the core. Using DeBakey pick-ups or a mosquito clamp, the core is removed (**7a, b**). It is important to maintain equal tension on both and to keep the relative position of MollRing Cutter and core head constant.

After complete extraction of the core, the vessel loop is tightened to control back bleeding. If the core fractures during withdrawal, use a biopsy forceps or a similar instrument to grasp the core and continue the withdrawal. The MollRing Cutter can also be used to grasp any residual core segments. Place an 8F introducer sheath into the superficial femoral artery and obtain an angiogram to view the entire endarterectomized segment. Record a magnified view of the endpoint area.

With the use of an 0.035 inch angled glidewire and a multipurpose angiographic catheter the popliteal artery lumen is catheterized.

Pass a 14 Fr introducer sheath over the guidewire and locate the end of the sheath approximately 2 cm beyond the endarterectomy termination.

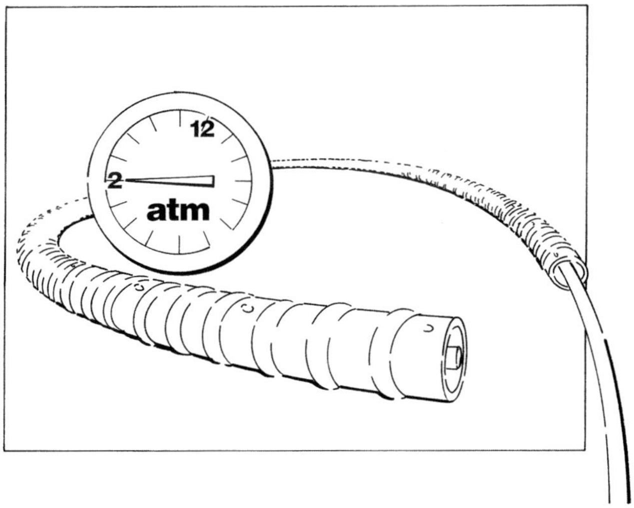

8

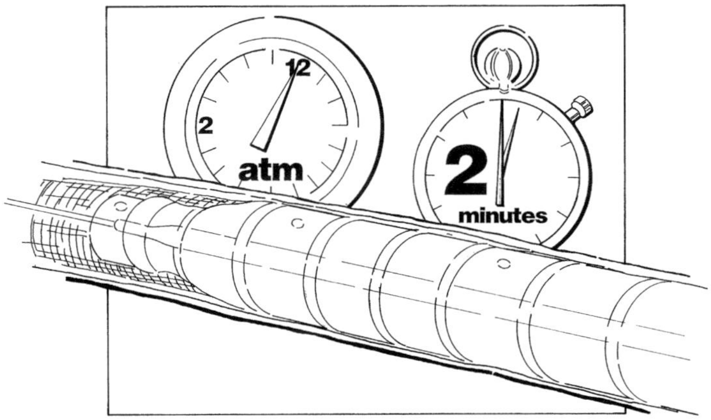

9

8

Select the appropriate balloon size from the sizing table. Load the ENDURING® vascular graft (WL Gore and Associates, Flagstaff, AZ, USA) onto the balloon and align the distal end of the graft (as denoted by the most distal gold marker) with the catheter tip (**8**). Using a high pressure inflation syringe filled with an equal mixture of contrast media and saline, inflate the balloon to approximately 2 atmospheres so the graft is held firmly by the balloon during delivery. The use of lower pressures may result in slippage of the graft on the balloon during delivery. Higher pressures may cause premature distention.

With the gold markers facing anteriorly, place the balloon catheter over the guidewire and deliver the graft through the arteriotomy. Ensure at least 2 cm (three gold markers) of the graft is placed distally past the endarterectomy termination securing any distal flaps and preventing dissection of the media upon perfusion. Ensure proper placement of the graft before initiating high pressure deployment. The graft cannot be repositioned after deployment. Slide the introducer sheath back, thereby exposing graft.

9

Distend the graft by slowly inflating the balloon to 12 atmospheres. Maintain the 12 atmosphere pressure for 2 minutes (**9**). Slowly deflate the balloon.

Under fluoroscopic guidance, carefully reposition the balloon distally so the image of the distal balloon marker just begins to overlap the image of the most distal graft marker. Distend the graft by slowly inflating the balloon to 12 atmospheres. Maintain the 12 atmosphere pressure for 2 minutes. Deflate the balloon.

Sequentially distend the entire length of the graft to beyond the arteriotomy by repositioning the balloon proximally. Ensure there is at least 1 cm balloon overlap of previously distended graft portion and distend graft at 12 atmospheres for 2 minutes. Note: If a tapered graft configuration is desired, insert a larger balloon and sequentially distend the appropriate graft portion. Remove the balloon catheter and guidewire.

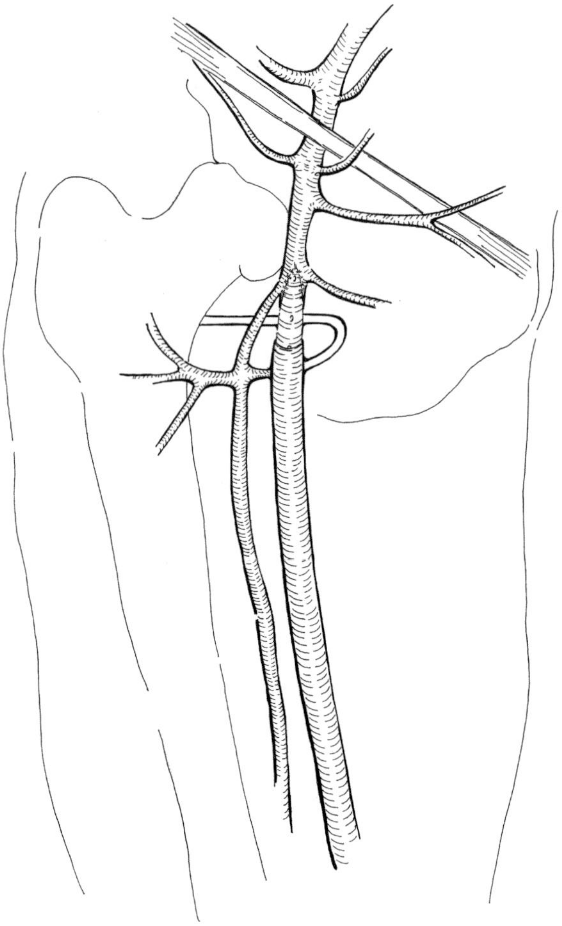

a

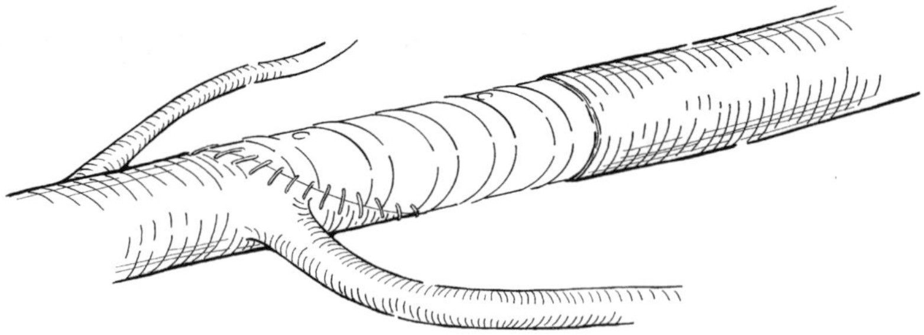

b

10

10a, b

Transect the proximal superficial femoral artery, cut the proximal end of the distended graft to the appropriate length and create a bevelled anastomosis (**10a**, **b**).

Perform a completion angiography to verify that proper flow and a good seal has been obtained at the distal graft end.

Surveillance and medication

The surveillance programme consists of duplex scanning within 6 weeks postoperatively and after 3, 6, 9 and 12 months. Recurrent stenoses developing after 1 year seem to have a different natural history and need intervention only for clinical symptoms (Ho *et al.*, 1999). The authors give all patients an antiplatelet drug (aminosalicylic acid (ASA) 100 mg daily).

Future perspectives

The MollRing Cutter device enables the surgeon to perform a remote endarterectomy of virtually any occluded peripheral artery. Iliac and popliteal arteries have already been successfully treated in our institution, using a retrograde approach for the iliac artery. The results of this procedure may approach those of grafts for femoral supragenicular popliteal bypasses and can be chosen as a first option for treatment of superficial femoral artery occlusive disease. If in the future the occurrence of restenosis after endarterectomies can be reduced, the role of bypass grafting turns into a bailout procedure.

Reference

Ho GH, Buren PA van, Moll FL *et al.* 1999. Incidence, time-of-onset, and anatomical distribution of recurrent stenoses after remote endarterectomy in SFA occlusive disease. *J Vasc Surg* 30: 106–113.

Embolectomy for acute lower limb ischaemia

Hans O Myhre, Ola D Saether

Introduction

In the Scandinavian countries, embolectomies for acute limb ischaemia have increased. Approximately 50% of the procedures are performed by junior staff. The reasons for the increasing incidence of embolism may be due to an increase in the elderly population and the fact that more patients survive major cardiac disease.

In acute limb ischaemia the differential diagnosis between emboli and acute arterial thrombosis is important, because the treatment must be selected accordingly. Thus, an aggressive surgical approach is justified in most cases with emboli, whereas initial conservative treatment may be preferred following acute arterial thrombosis provided the limb is viable (Dale, 1984).

1

The diagnosis of embolism is based on the presence of a potential source and the sudden onset of symptoms. The location of the arterial obstruction may also indicate the source. Thus, an embolus leading to ischaemia of an isolated toe usually arises from atherosclerotic changes in the aorta or the iliac arteries, whereas an embolus in the aortic bifurcation most likely has a cardiac origin. An embolus usually lodges where the artery divides and its calibre reduces.

In arterial thrombosis the onset of symptoms is gradual, often with a previous history of intermittent claudication without signs of cardiac disease. In addition, the pulses may be absent on the contralateral limb.

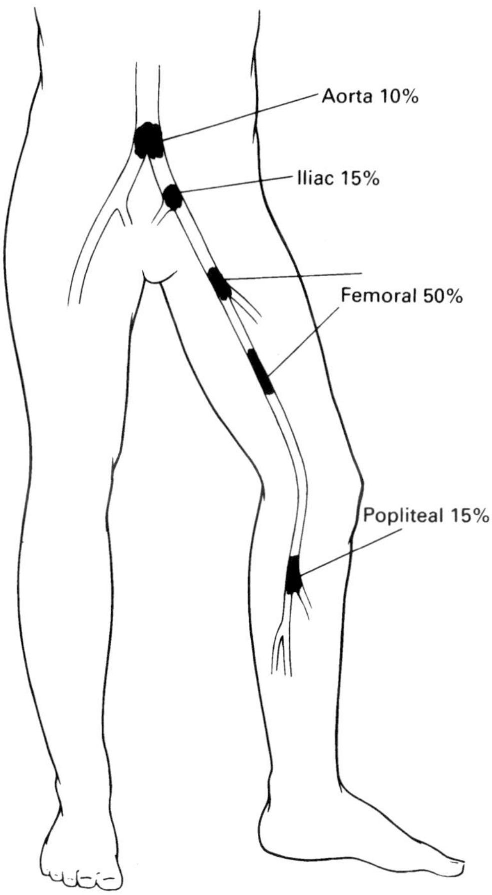

1

Preoperative considerations

Critical ischaemia is indicated by loss of sensitivity, discolouration that blanches with pressure, decreased skin temperature and moderate rigour of the calf muscles. It is generally agreed that embolectomy is indicated even in these patients (Tawes *et al.*, 1985). Although early diagnosis and treatment is important, the time from onset of symptoms to admission is of less importance than the clinical status of the limb. Thus, the time factor does not contraindicate embolectomy by itself.

In irreversible ischaemia there is blotchy cyanotic discolouration which is not influenced by digital pressure.

The calf muscle has a firm consistency and, in addition, there is anaesthesia and paralysis of the extremity. The treatment of choice for patients with irreversible ischaemic changes is primary amputation.

Patients with a clear-cut history of emboli are not referred to preoperative angiography. Angiography should, however, always be done when there is doubt about the diagnosis or when acute arterial thrombosis is suspected.

If present, cardiac insufficiency and dehydration should be corrected preoperatively, but the operation should not be delayed by lengthy evaluations.

Heparin is given intravenously as a bolus of 100–150 international units per kg bodyweight, taking into consideration that heparin may influence the selection of anaesthesia. Blood is typed and cross-matched and the patient is transferred to the operating room.

In general, the patient is prepared from the nipples to the toes of both feet, keeping in mind that more extensive surgery can become necessary and that multiple emboli often occur. For unilateral femoropopliteal embolectomy when the femoral pulse is palpable, some surgeons prepare the groin and limb only.

Anaesthesia technique and monitoring

Local anaesthesia with lidocaine 0.5–1% is recommended when the embolectomy can be completed via the common femoral artery. Local anaesthetics with adrenaline must be used with care in patients with severe coronary heart disease. Should clinical signs or angiography indicate that additional proximal or distal surgery becomes necessary, local anaesthesia may be a disadvantage. Epidural anaesthesia is contraindicated if the patient is already heparinized, but spinal anaesthesia by a thin needle can be used in these patients without risk of intraspinal bleeding. However, most surgeons prefer general anaesthesia when the operation cannot be completed with local anaesthesia.

Since there is a high incidence of concomitant cardiovascular disease, close monitoring is necessary, especially to detect the systemic effects of revascularization. Monitoring of central venous pressure, systemic arterial pressure and urine output is recommended. In patients with advanced ischaemia, monitoring of central haemodynamics by a Swan-Ganz catheter is justified. Prior to re-establishment of blood flow in such patients, a high urinary output should be obtained by volume therapy and osmotic diuretics. The acid-base status should be closely monitored and sodium bicarbonate added in case of acidosis (Tawes *et al.*, 1985).

The operation

Femoropopliteal embolectomy

2

The advantage of the Fogarty balloon catheter is that emboli can be removed from the aorta as well as the leg arteries via a local arterteriotomy in the common femoral artery. Most femoropopliteal embolectomies can be performed by this approach.

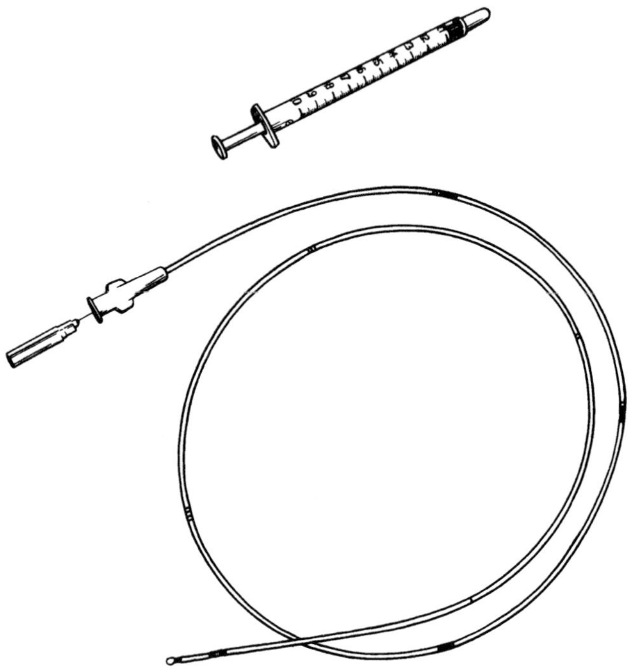

2

3a, b

A vertical incision in the groin is used (**3a**), and the common, superficial and the deep femoral arteries are dissected (**3b**). Elastic vascular tapes are applied to these arteries for vessel occlusion rather than vascular clamps, so as to minimize blood loss during repeated introductions of the embolectomy catheter. Furthermore, vascular clamps may break the embolic material making it more difficult to remove.

A small incision in the common femoral artery is performed using a No. 11 scalpel blade. A longitudinal arteriotomy of about 1.5 cm is made using fine-angled scissors just proximal to the orifice of the profunda femoris artery. Stay-sutures are applied to the edges of the arteriotomy to facilitate repeated introductions of the Fogarty catheter without damaging the artery, which should not be handled by forces (**3b**).

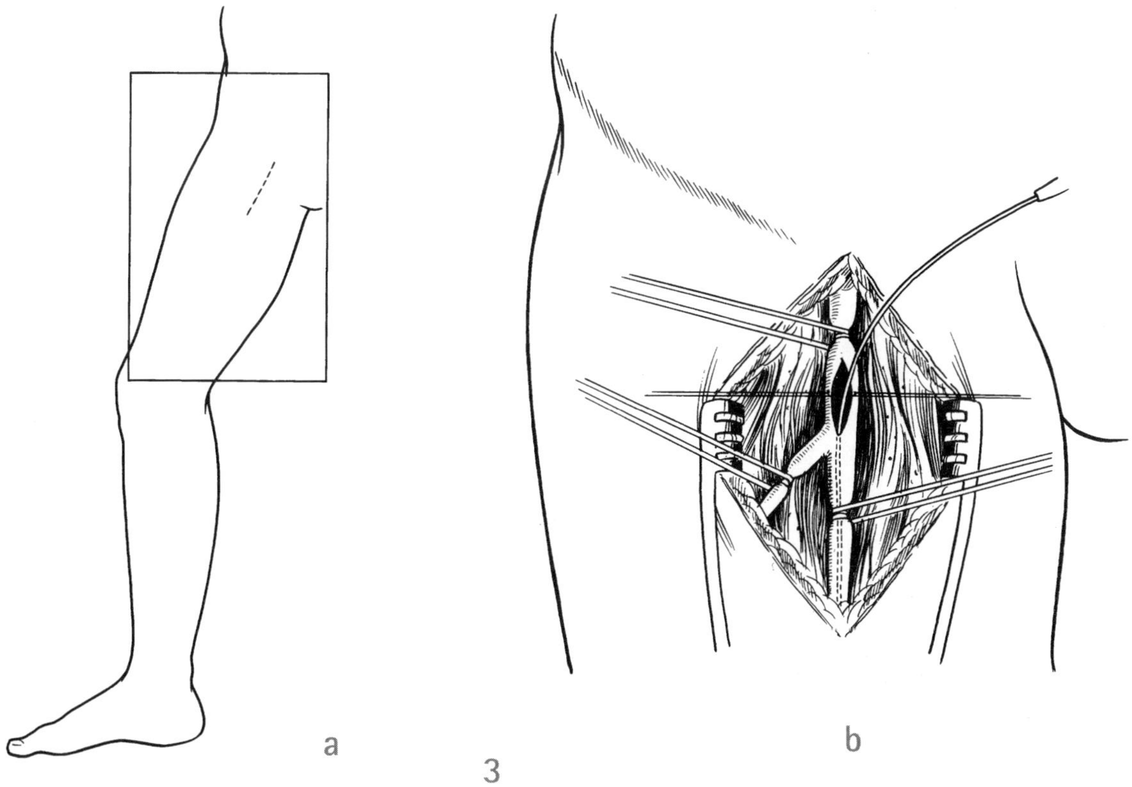

a b

3

The stylet of the embolectomy catheter is removed and the patency of the balloon is tested by inflation of saline as recommended for each catheter size. A 1-ml tuberculine syringe is useful for the inflation of a No. 4 embolectomy catheter. Various modifications of the balloon embolectomy catheter have been presented. A channel at the end of the catheter can be used for intraoperative angiography and for irrigation with heparin saline solution. Side-ports central to the balloon may be advantageous for the removal of adherent embolic material and will probably minimize intimal damage. Resterilized catheters should not be used.

The end of a deflated No. 3 or 4 Fogarty catheter is dipped in heparin saline solution or blood and then introduced into the superficial femoral artery (**3b**). In patients without atherosclerosis, the catheter can usually be advanced to the foot. The catheter is withdrawn 0.5–1 cm and the balloon is then inflated while moving the catheter to prevent excessive shear forces (Dobrin and Jorgensen, 1985). The grade of inflation must be varied according to the calibre of the artery. Extra caution is necessary during embolectomy of small arteries to avoid overdistention of the balloon. The catheter should be inflated and pulled back by the same surgeon.

3c, d, e

The embolic material is now removed through the arteriotomy (**3c**). The procedure is repeated until no residual embolic material is found, keeping in mind that several withdrawals with a high shear force can induce subsequent intimal hyperplasia (Bowles *et al.*, 1988; Schwarcz *et al.*, 1988). Coagulated blood and debris must be cleaned off the catheter between each introduction. Brisk backbleeding from the distal arterial tree can now be expected, but is not synonymous with a complete embolectomy.

Embolectomy of the profunda femoris artery is now performed. It is extremely important that this artery is free of embolic material. The catheter can usually be advanced about 20 cm from the orifice of the artery. The arteries are flushed with heparine saline solution (1000 international units in 100 ml saline) and blood flow from the proximal arteries is tested before the arteriotomy is closed. Provided the artery is unaffected by atherosclerosis and of good calibre, the arteriotomy can be closed by direct suture using 5/0 or 6/0 monofilament suture material (**3d**). A patch graft angioplasty is preferred to avoid stenosis during closure of narrow arteries or when there are atherosclerotic changes in the arterial wall (**3e**). The saphenous vein is harvested at the ankle and used for patch graft material.

Completion angiography is mandatory following femoropopliteal embolectomy, since incomplete embolectomy has been found in 25–40% of the cases when judged by backbleeding only (Bosma and Jorning, 1990).

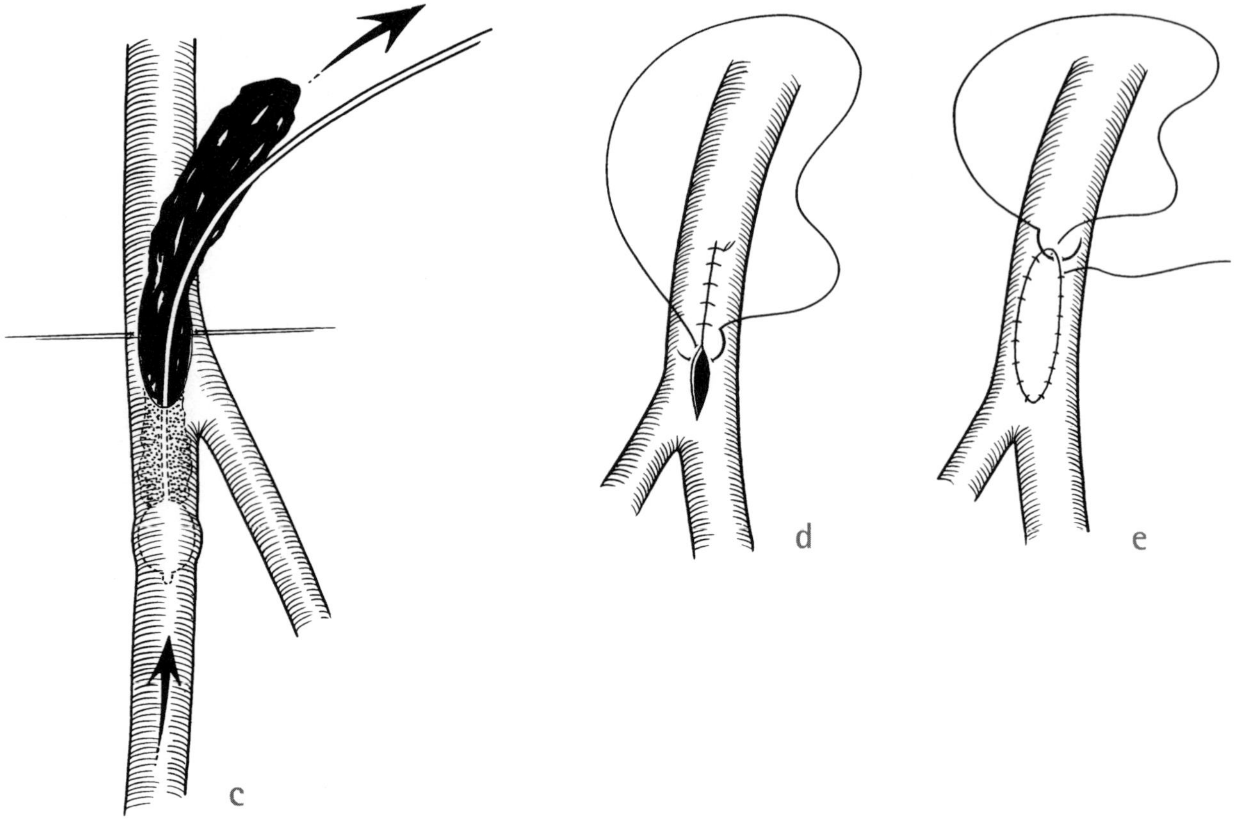

3

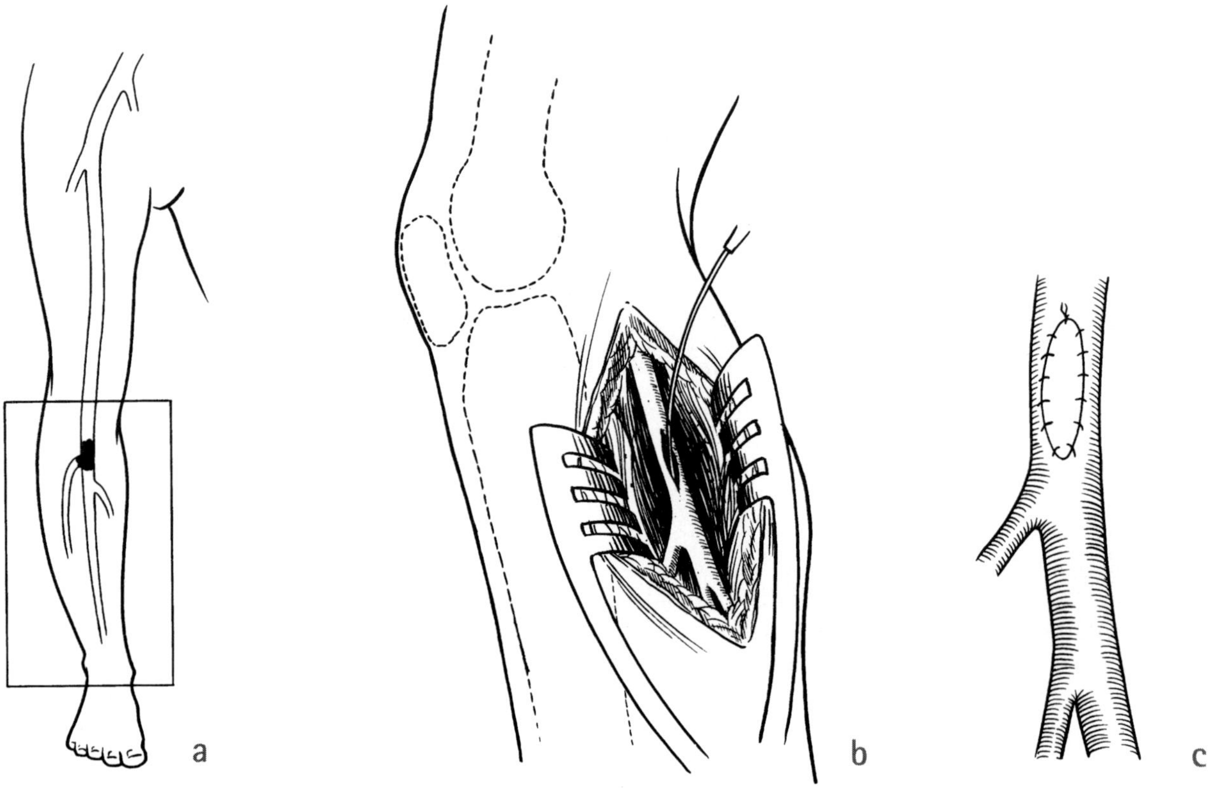

4

4a, b, c

The peroneal and posterial tibial arteries may be embolectomized through the common femoral artery by bending the tip of the catheter. However, not all types of catheters can be manipulated in this way (Gwynn *et al.*, 1987). The anterior tibial artery is not readily accessible by this approach. When the popliteal pulse is palpable preoperatively, we explore the popliteal artery below the knee (**4a, b**). Following arteriotomy, a No. 3 embolectomy catheter can then be introduced into the different leg arteries. The arteriotomy is closed by patch graft angioplasty (**4c**) (Abbott *et al.*, 1984).

In all cases, embolic material should be investigated by microscopy for verification of the aetiology.

5a, b

Aortoiliac 'saddle' embolectomy

Patients with emboli at the aortic bifurcation or the iliac arteries have a more serious prognosis than patients with femoropopliteal embolism (Busuttil *et al.*, 1983). The abdomen and the lower extremities are prepared as previously described. Vertical incisions are made in both groins and the femoral arteries dissected as described for femoropopliteal embolectomy, preferably by two surgeons working simultaneously (**5a**).

A deflated No. 5 or 6 Fogarty catheter is introduced into the aorta through the arteriotomy of the common femoral artery. The balloon is distended and the catheter withdrawn, thereby removing embolic material. The risk of losing embolic material into the contralateral limb can be reduced by compressing the common femoral artery, thereby reducing the blood flow of the contralateral iliac system. When sufficient blood flow from the iliac artery on the embolectomized side is obtained, the embolectomy is repeated on the contralateral side (**5b**).

A No. 3 or 4 catheter is then introduced into the superficial femoral and profunda femoris arteries on both sides to remove possible embolic material. The arteriotomies are closed as previously described. A suction drain is routinely left close to each arteriotomy and can usually be removed on the following day.

A similar approach as described for the removal of saddle embolus is used for iliac embolectomy. It is usually sufficient to expose the arteries of one groin only, but great care is taken not to push embolic material into the opposite leg.

Percutaneous aspiration thromboembolectomy

This is performed through a specially designed catheter-sheath system for clot extraction. The advantage is that it can be used at the time of diagnostic angiography. It is not within the scope of this presentation to describe the technical details of percutaneous aspiration thromboembolectomy, which is preferably used for removal of smaller emboli from the distal arterial tree (Wagner and Starck, 1992).

Handling of special problems

Intraoperative thrombolysis appears to be a safe and effective way of removing a residual embolus (Beard *et al.*, 1993).

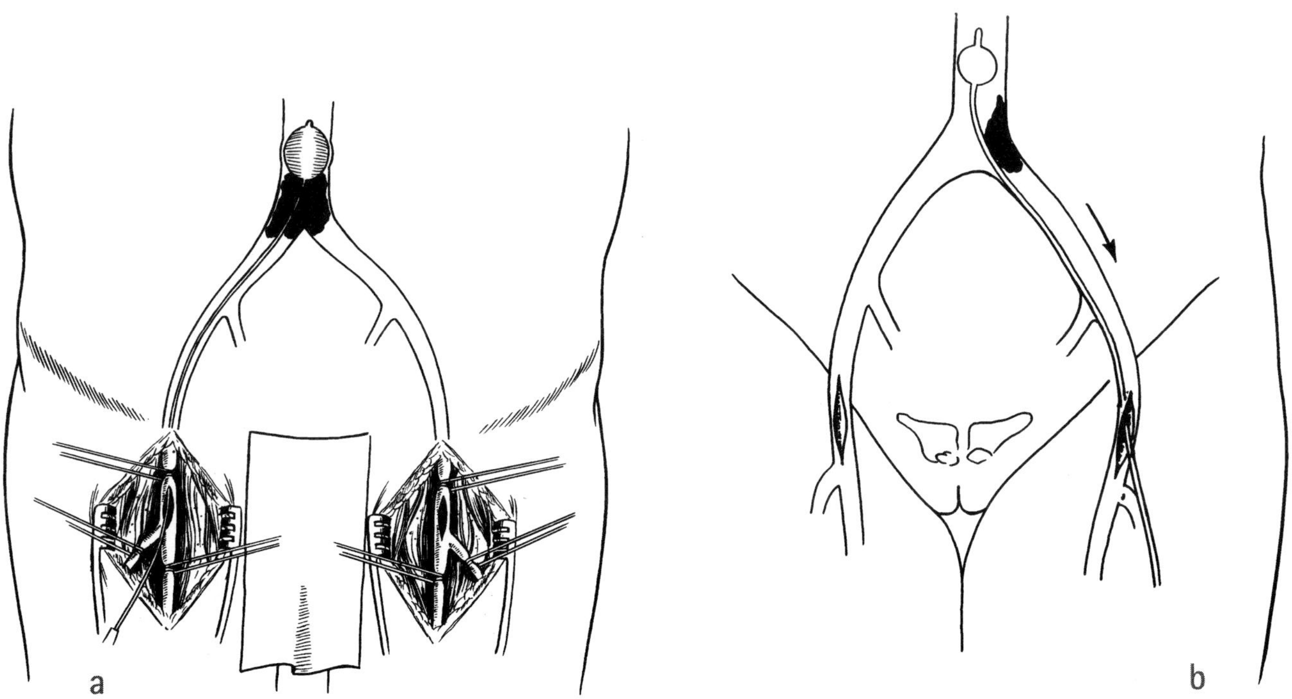

5

During delayed embolectomy a cleavage plane between the embolus and the arterial wall may be difficult to identify. A ringstripper can then be used as a supplement to the balloon catheter, or a bypass graft is applied for revascularization.

Sometimes, the embolus may consist of atherosclerotic material from the proximal arterial tree. Removal of the source of embolus is indicated in most of these patients on an elective basis. If the limb ischaemia is caused by aortic dissection, revascularization of the extremity is performed, the anticoagulation therapy must be reversed and further investigation of the aortic dissection is carried out. When acute arterial thrombosis is found to be the cause of critical ischaemia during operation, the surgeon should be prepared to proceed with arterial reconstruction following angiographic investigation. Thrombosis of a popliteal aneurysm may also be the cause of ischaemia. The aneurysm is excluded from the circulation and arterial reconstruction is performed.

Complications

Complications following use of the balloon catheter include rupture of the balloon, intimal injury, arteriovenous fistula, fragmentation of the clot with distal embolization and inadequate removal of the material. Furthermore, dissection of arterosclerotic plaques may occur. Perforation is indicated by difficulties during withdrawal of the catheter. The balloon should be deflated immediately and the catheter removed.

Fasciotomy is performed in cases with preoperative severe ischaemia when repeated postoperative examinations indicate a closed compartment syndrome.

The post-perfusion syndrome can be suspected in the same group of patients. This syndrome is indicated by a urine specimen with Guajac positive pigments, but without red blood cells on microscopy. Prophylaxis by isolation of the femoral vein followed by withdrawal of 300–500 ml of blood during the first pass of arterial blood has been recommended and may be indicated in selected cases (Tawes *et al.*, 1985).

Postoperative considerations

The patient should be observed in the intensive care unit during the first 24 h following the operation. In addition to general monitoring, the circulation of the first toe should be recorded continuously by a non-invasive technique. The patient can be mobilized on the first postoperative day. Heparin is given postoperatively by continuous infusion according to body weight, sex and age. Warfarin-sodium is started immediately following the operation. When a prothrombin time of 5–10% of normal value is obtained heparin therapy is discontinued. In most patients, including those with cardiac disease, we find lifelong treatment with warfarin-sodium indicates prevention of recurrent emboli.

References

Abbott W M, McCabe C, Maloney R D, Wirthlin L S (1984). Embolism of the popliteal artery. *Surg Gynecol Obstet* **159**: 533.

Beard J D, Nyamekye I, Earnshaw J S *et al.* (1993). Intraoperative streptokinase: a useful adjunct to balloon-catheter embolectomy. *Br J Surg* **80**: 21.

Bosma H W, Jorning P J (1990). Intra-operative arteriography in arterial embolectomy. *Euro J Vasc Surg* **4**: 469.

Bowles C R, Olcott C, Pakter R L *et al.* (1988). Diffuse arterial narrowing as a result of intimal proliferation: A delayed complication of embolectomy with the Fogarty balloon catheter. *J Vasc Surg* **7**: 487.

Busuttil R W, Keehn G, Milliken J *et al.* (1983). Aortic saddle embolus. A twenty-year experience. *Ann Surg* **197**: 698.

Dale W A (1984). Differential management of acute peripheral arterial ischemia. *J Vasc Surg* **1**: 269.

Dobrin P B, Jorgensen R A (1985). Balloon embolectomy catheters in small arteries: A technique to prevent excessive shear forces. *J Vasc Surg* **2**: 692.

Fogarty T J, Cranley J J, Krause R J *et al.* (1963). A method for extraction of arterial emboli and thrombi. *Surg Gynecol Obstet* **116**: 241.

Gwynn B R, Shearman C P, Simms M H (1987). The anatomical basis for the route taken by Fogarty catheters in the lower leg. *Euro J Vasc Surg* **1**: 129.

Schwarcz T H, Dobrin P B, Mrkvicka R *et al.* (1988). Early myointimal hyperplasia after balloon catheter embolectomy. Effect of shear forces and multiple withdrawals. *J Vasc Surg* **7**: 495.

Tawes R L, Harris E J, Brown W H *et al.* (1985). Arterial thromboembolism. A 20-year experience. *Arch Surg* **120**: 595.

Wagner H J, Starck, E E (1992). Acute embolic occlusions of the infrainguinal arteries: percutaneous aspiration embolectomy in 102 patients. *Radiology* **182**: 403.

Initial lysis and catheter clot removal for occlusive disease in critical ischaemia

B Nachbur, F Mahler
Do-Dai-Do, E Schneider

Introduction

Catheter clot lysis (CTL) is gaining increasing acceptance as it becomes evident that not all cases of critical ischaemia are best treated surgically. Our own experience in Berne comprises well over 250 cases with streptokinase, urokinase and tissue plasminogen activator (rt-PA) being used in that order. Although success rates, i.e. patency rates, have risen from 73 to 85%, the differences are statistically not significant, there being no proof that any one fibrinolytic agent is superior to the other as far as efficacy is concerned. If the results with streptokinase are somewhat less favourable it should be borne in mind that this is most likely attributable to a period during which experience with this new form of treatment had to be gained. In the light of this we look back upon our results with streptokinase with satisfaction and are actually using either this drug or urokinase again.

No doubt streptokinase is no less potent than urokinase, but the latter is generally preferred over streptokinase because it is associated with fewer side-effects (slightly less bleeding complications) and because streptokinase cannot be used repeatedly if anaphylactic reactions to antibodies are to be avoided.

Although Hess and others (Hess *et al.*, 1982a, b; Schneider and Largiadèr, 1987) have advocated local clot lysis in the treatment of arterial occlusions with symptoms of complete ischaemia, we feel that it is best indicated for treatment of viable limbs presenting with acute thrombotic occlusion associated with localized or widespread atherosclerotic lesions.

It is agreed that acute thromboembolic occlusion of the iliofemoral segment is best treated by the Fogarty balloon extraction catheter, local thrombolysis is especially suitable for acute thrombotic lesions involving the femoral and/or popliteal arteries including the popliteal trifurcation. Furthermore CTL is indicated in the treatment of early re-occlusions after percutaneous transluminal angioplasty (PTA) and recanalization of acute occlusions of femoropopliteal grafts.

As the clot is gradually being dissolved, underlying stenotic lesions are uncovered and thus become amenable to PTA, which on its own merit must be considered an integral part of catheter clot lysis therapy because it deals with the causative mechanism of thrombotic occlusion. The rate of local thrombolysis can be considerably hastened by aspiration or extraction of loosened clots (CTE) whereby clearance of the vessel is more actively promoted. As a consequence short-term CTL has become the rule, long-term lytic therapy on the other hand the exception.

Method of CTL and CTE

Following preliminary studies by Demski and Zeitler in 1978 the concept of local intrathrombus catheter lysis was developed by Hess and co-workers in 1980. By placing the catheter directly into the thrombus activated plasmin remains where it is needed in high concentration for a lengthy period. Thus smaller doses of fibrolytic agents are needed and the effect greatly enhanced when compared with the regional fibrinolysis applied by Dotter earlier in 1974. If systemic or regional lysis is compared with digestion without chewing, then the combined procedure of CTL and CTE would correspond to digestion *with* chewing (Mahler, 1990).

Methodology

The technical requirements and therapeutic steps are listed as follows:

1. Fluoroscopy.
2. Seldinger technique for introduction of a percutaneous catheter.
3. Percutaneous catheter introducer (PCI kit), for use with a 0.035–0.038 inch diameter guidewire, manufactured by Argon, containing:
   a. 6–9 (=2.8 mm) French radiopaque sheath;
   b. removable haemostasis valve with side-port exten-

sion for injection of heparin or dye and removable stopcock;

c. vessel dilator (Illustrations 1 and 2).

4. Introduction of a French 5 or 6 polyethylene catheter under fluoroscopy.
5. Gradual infusion of fibrinolytic agent.
6. Stepwise advancement of catheter tip.
7. Suction of fresh, loosened thrombi.
8. Percutaneous dilatation of atherosclerotic plaque.

1, 2

For introduction of a percutaneous catheter the Seldinger technique is used with anterograde puncture of the common femoral artery. This can pose problems in obese patients because the puncture site should be below the inguinal ligament in order to avoid retroperitoneal haematoma.

The superficial femoral artery (or graft) is catheterized selectively in local anaesthesia. Primary introduction of a radiopaque sheath (6–9 French) is performed to avoid excessive trauma of the vessel wall during repetitive catheter manipulations. Any bleeding tendency is increased in any case because of the drugs in use (heparin and lytic agents). Usually CTL is performed by introducing an angiography catheter (5 or 6 French) in the vessel dilator shown in Illustrations 1 and 2.

3

The tip of the catheter is placed 3–4 cm into the thrombus without piercing through it. The infusion of a fibrinolytic agent is begun, preferably by using an

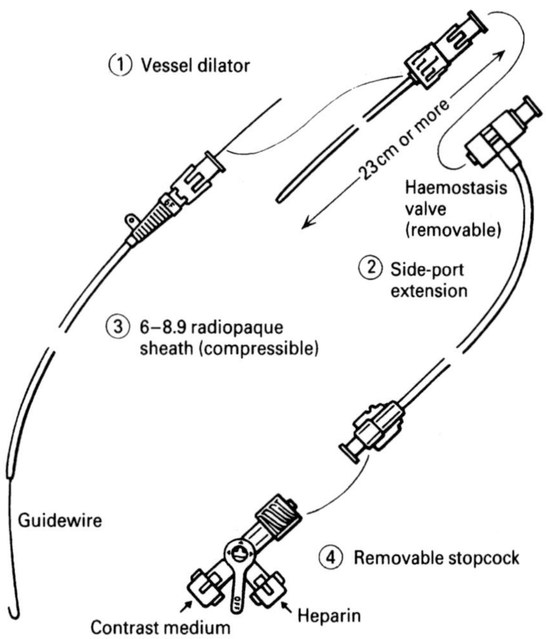

1

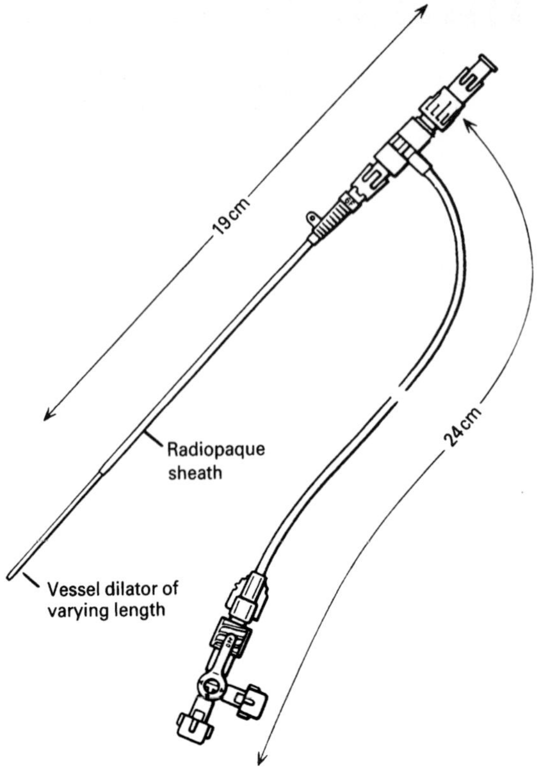

2

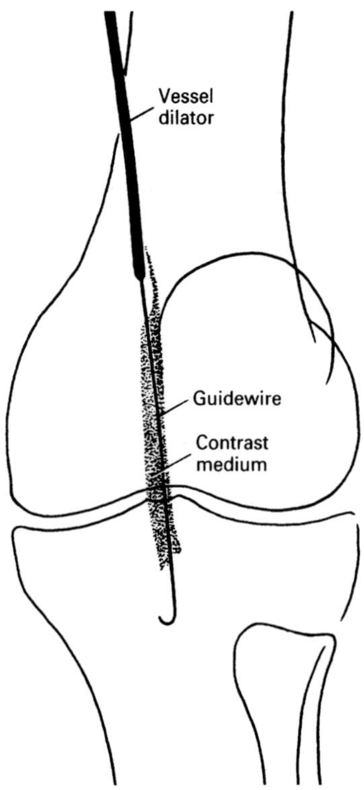

3

infusion pump providing a volume of 20 ml/h. The catheter is advanced stepwise cm by cm every 2–5 min under fluoroscopic control. The result is checked radiologically with diluted contrast medium at least once an hour. As soon as the distal end of the occluding thrombolic mass is reached the lytic agent flows into the distal vasculature. For increased efficacy of lysis a catheter tip with side holes enabling sprinkling is advantageous.

4

For aspiration of loosened thrombi a catheter with an internal diameter of 2 mm is used. It should have a single opening at the end and no side holes – as used for sprinkling – and must be attached to a 20 ml or even 50 ml syringe to achieve the necessary suction force. The thrombus is withdrawn together with the catheter. The mechanism of catheter clot removal by suction is depicted. Laboratory examinations during CTL include the analysis of prothrombin time, thrombin time, coagulation factors II, V, VII and X, reptilase time, an ethanol test and fibrinogen levels. During long-term lysis the thrombin time values are kept from exceeding twice the normal by adjusting the doses of heparin given.

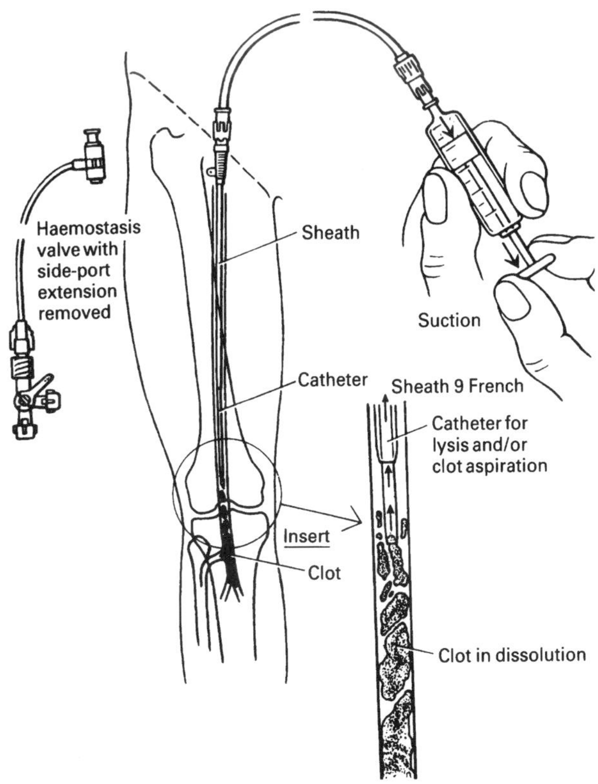

4

Dosage

Streptokinase

In our hands we have used between 2000 and 4000 international units per cm length of clot keeping the catheter in one place for at least 5 minutes. Thus we apply between 40 000 and 100 000 units of streptokinase in one 90-min session. When patency is achieved the procedure is terminated, and 5000 units of heparin are given.

If, after 90 min, the flow through the initially occluded segment is unsatisfactory, the procedure is continued on the ward as a long-term regional thrombolysis after insertion of a 3 French catheter via the introducer sheath. The dose of streptokinase is 4000 units per hour for 8–72 h. Heparin is infused through the side branch of the introducer sheath to prevent pericatheter thrombolysis. Clinical assessment is confirmed by contrast injection through the indwelling catheter at intervals of at least 24 h.

Clinical success is defined by either a return of pedal pulses or a reduction in the arterial ankle pressure deficit of at least 50 mmHg.

Urokinase

If lytic therapy has already been performed once before then thrombolysis will have to be performed using urokinase which is – as opposed to streptokinase – a physiological lytic substance. It is 2–5 times less active than streptokinase per unit. Therefore we use per cm length of clot 5000–10 000 units. For long-term lysis we apply 10 000 units per hour. The total dose should not exceed 500 000 units per day.

Tissue plasminogen activator (rt-PA)

In our own series we have used 10 mg rt-PA per hour successfully. We noted with the doses used by us, with an average of 15 mg rt-PA for an average of 15 cm occlusion, a drop of fibrinonogen levels from 2.7 ± 0.8 g/litre to 2.3 ± 1.0 g/litre which serves to prove that systemic activity is relatively low. Hess has decreased his dosage recently to 2.5 mg rt PA/h.

Table 1. Fibrinogen levels before and after CTL with three fibrinolytic agents; bleeding and complications

	Streptokinase	Urokinase	rt-Pa
Fibrinogen (g/litre)			
before CTL	2.7 ± 0.7	2.6 ± 0.7	2.7 ± 0.8
after CTL	2.0 ± 0.5	2.5 ± 1.2	2.3 ± 1.0
Bleeding complications	8%	4%	4%

5

Illustration **5** shows clot material retrieved by catheter extraction (suction) after initial intrathrombus lysis in a patient successfully treated by combined CTL and CTE.

6a, b, c

Illustration **6a** shows an anteriogram of a long popliteal occlusion of thrombotic origin in a 74-year-old male patient. Clinically, the patient presented in a state of critical ischaemia. The percutaneous catheter shown in Illustrations **1** and **2** is introduced via the common femoral artery into the superficial femoral artery. A vessel dilator, 40–60 cm in length, can be introduced directly into the superficial femoral artery or with the help of a bent guidewire, which in PTA is advanced through the occluded segment down to the patent vessel lumen beyond the occlusion to ensure avoidance of subintimal catheterization. A guidewire is used in this case for better orientation.

In **6b** the guidewire can be seen approximately 3 cm below the knee joint in the same patient as shown schematically in Illustration **3**. The tip of the catheter is recognizable at the level of the upper border of the knee cap. By comparison with **6a**, one can see that the catheter has been unmistakably advanced into the proximal part of the clot. This manoeuvre is performed very slowly and without undue force. Thrombolysis is induced by gradual infusion of streptokinase in doses of 2000–4000 units for each advancement of the catheter tip, allowing about 2–5 min/cm. If urokinase is used, the average dose necessary for each advancement is between 5000 and 10 000 units. For rt-PA, 1 mg is required. From time to time a little contrast medium is injected via the stopcock (see Illustrations **1** and **2**) to ascertain the progress of clot lysis. It is possible to identify some contrast medium within the formerly totally occluded popliteal artery. The important aspects of this are shown.

The completion angiogram for the same patient as in **6a, b** shows the lower level of a formerly occluded popliteal artery 24 h after initiation of CTL. The popliteal trifurcation can now be seen clearly.

Note the well-defined circumscribed atheromatous plaque near the origin of the anterior tibial artery. This lesion might have been the reason for thrombotic occlusion. Once it is uncovered by thrombolysis, it can be dealt with by PTA, which is an integral part of the treatment modality.

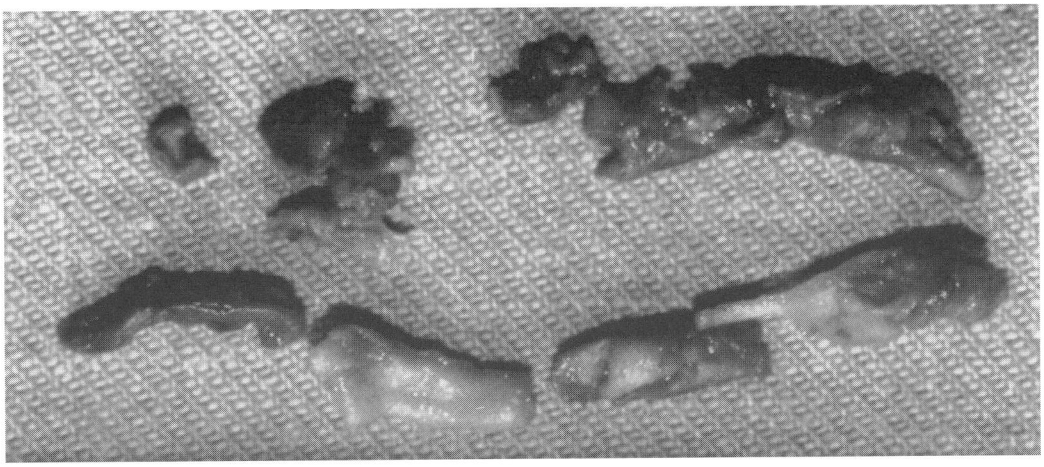

5

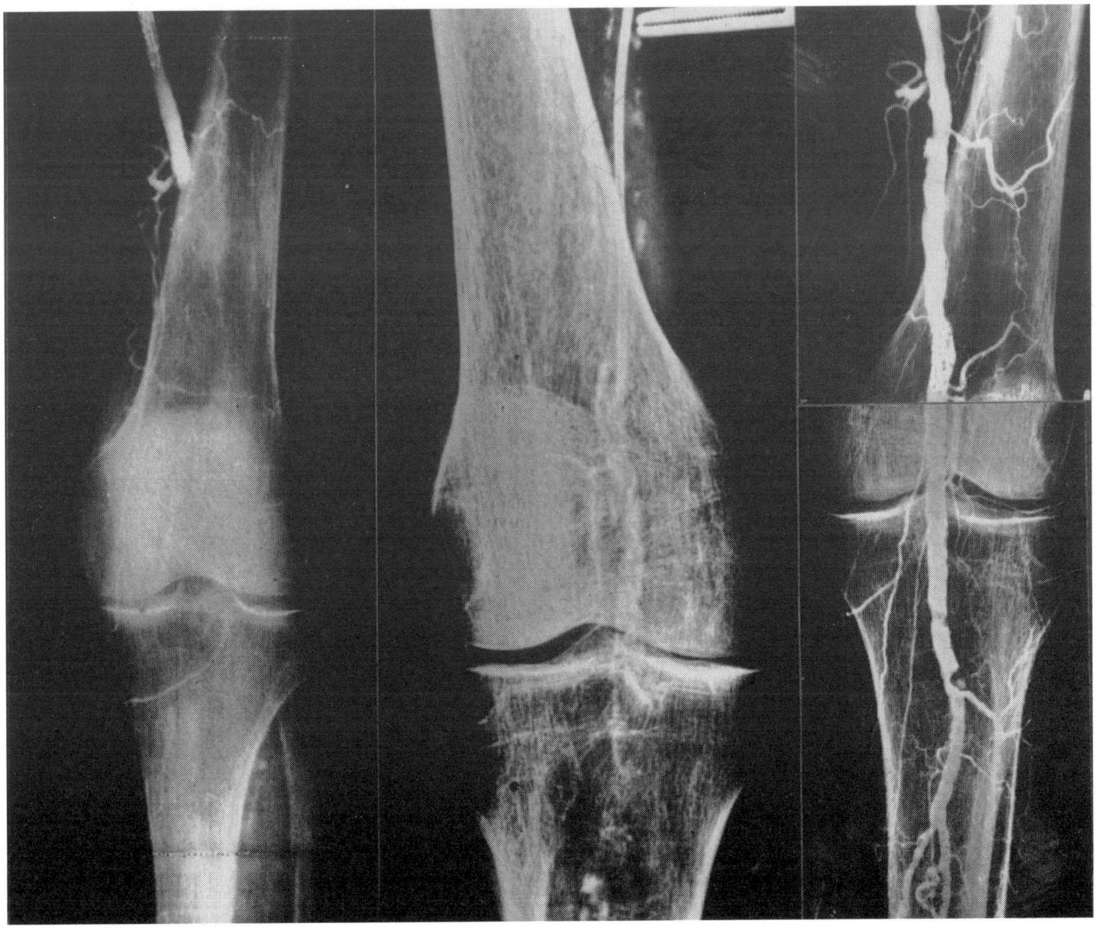

a b c

6

Further examples of initial lysis and catheter clot removal for occlusive disease in critical ischaemia

7a, b, c

Example 1

Illustration **7** shows a sequence of angiograms (**7a**, **b**, **c**) performed before, during and after thrombolysis and catheter clot removal in a 64-year-old female patient presenting with acute arterial occlusion with subtotal ischaemia. Radiologically there is clear evidence of thrombotic occlusion attending extensive atherosclerotic disease. Initial local CTL with streptokinase was followed by CTE and completed with PTA. Repeat angiogram and clinical evaluation 1 year later confirmed patency.

This example illustrates how even long thrombotic occlusions can successfully undergo percutaneous catheter lysis with the added advantage that the underlying cause for thrombotic occlusion (a plaque) can thereafter be localized and flattened by PTA.

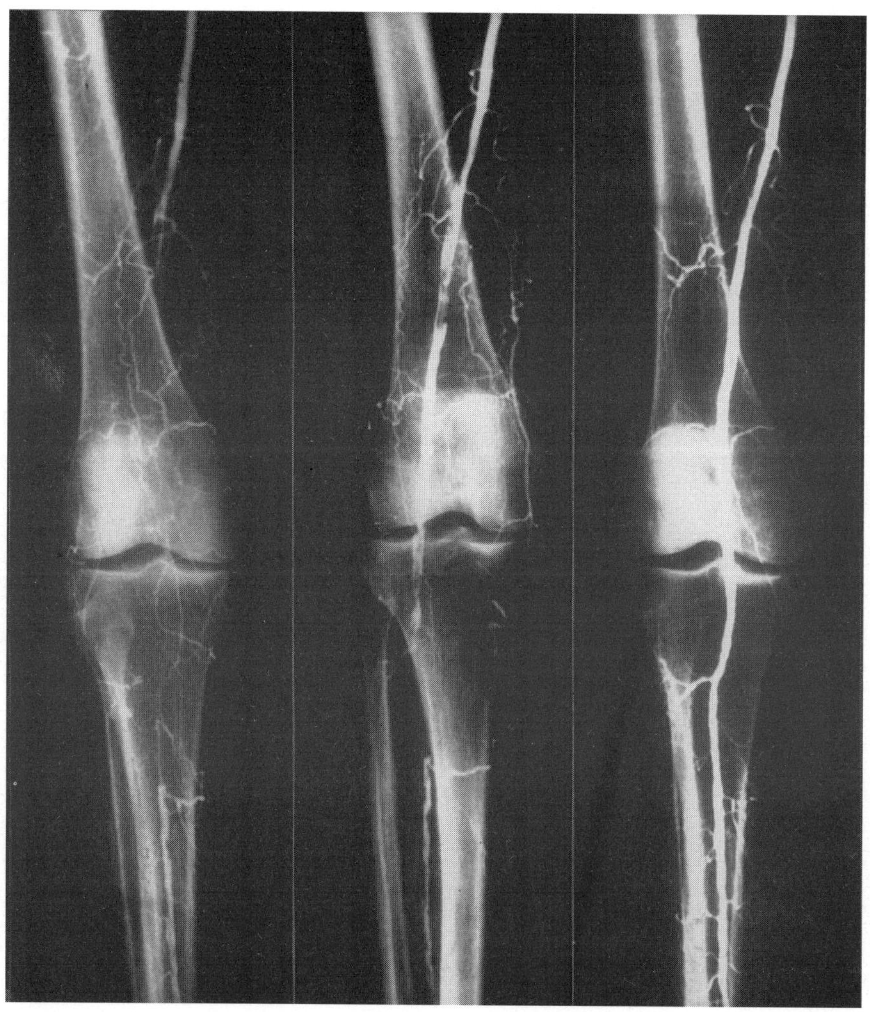

a b c

7

8a, b, c

Example 2

This case involved a 76-year-old female patient with sudden onset of arterial occlusion. Angiograms show (8a) before, (8b) during and (8c) after local thrombolysis and PTA.

Catheter clot lysis was started immediately after performing the initial angiogram on this 76-year-old female patient. Thrombolysis was accelerated by extracting considerable amounts of clot. In this case, an open distal run-off segment can be identified at the upper level of the femur condyles. As soon as complete thrombolysis is achieved, there is suddenly considerable reflux when the haemostasis valve is removed (see Illustrations 1 and 2). Loosened clots can then only be suctioned or extracted if the haemostasis valve is regularly removed and replaced afterwards for further manipulation. In the example presented here, there is residual subtotal occlusion of the proximal popliteal artery and a protruding plaque in the distal part of the superficial femoral artery. Both lesions underwent successful PTA. One year later, a control angiogram showed clear evidence of sustained patency of the femoropopliteal axis.

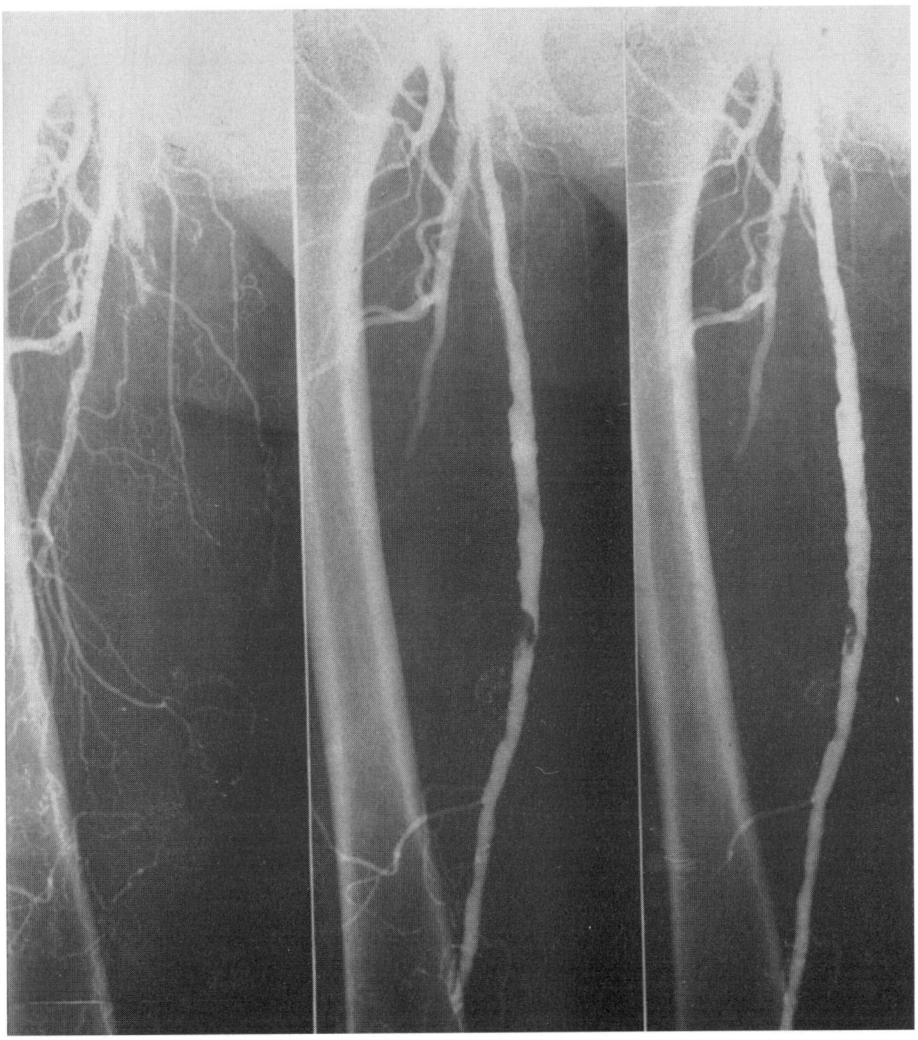

a b c

8

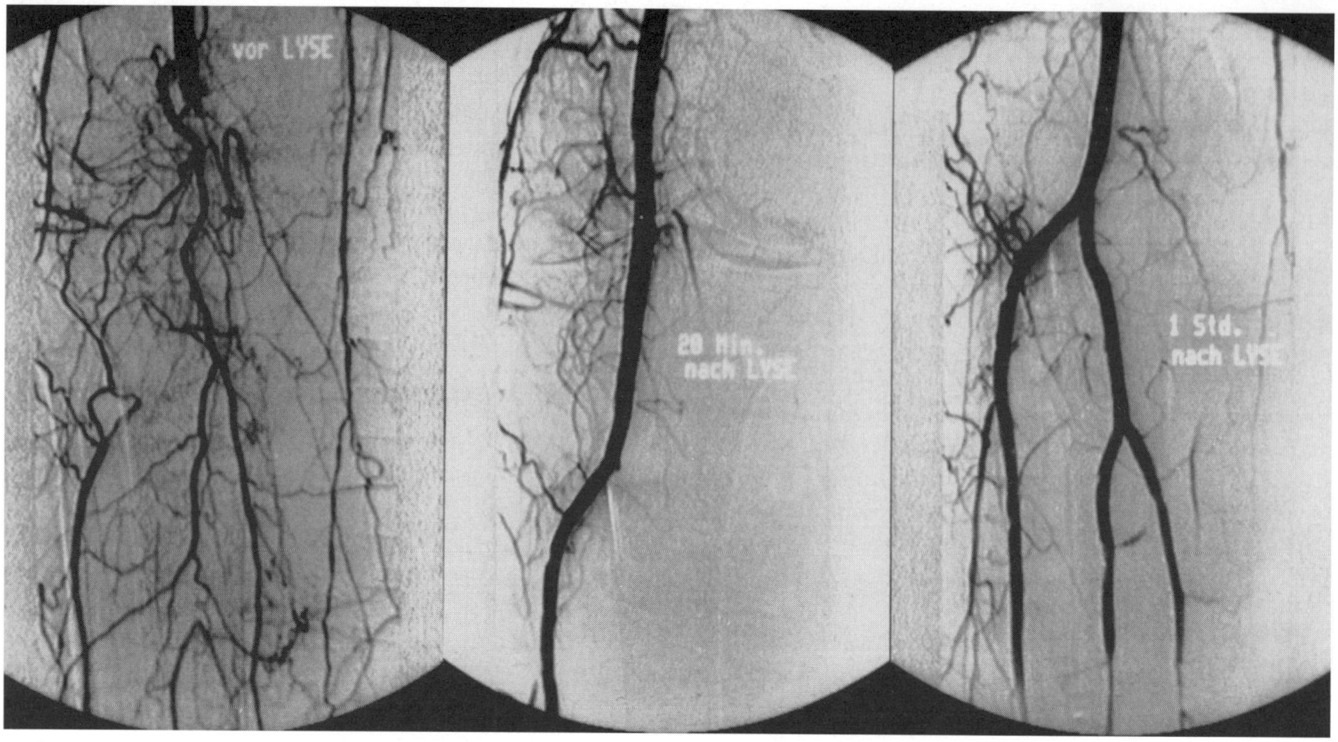

a b c

9

9a, b, c

Example 3

Illustrations **9a, b, c** show how rapidly embolic occlusions of the popliteal trifurcation can be lysed successfully within 1 hour (in this case with 200 000 units of urokinase and without the accessory help of clot suction or extraction). The vascular wall is smooth, slight traces of small atherosclerotic plaques can nevertheless be observed.

References

Do DD, Mahler F, Probst P Nachbur, B (1981). Combination of short and long-term catheter thrombolysis for peripheral arterial occlusion. *Eur Radiol* 1: 235.

Do DD, Mahler F, Triller J (1989). Catheter thrombolysis with streptokinase, urokinase and recombinant tissue plasminogen activator for peripheral arterial occlusion. In *Pros and Cons in PTA and Auxiliary Methods* **Zeitler E** ed. Berlin: Springer, pp. 157–159.

Demski JC, Zeitler E (1978). Selective aterial clot lysis with angiography catheter. In *Percutaneous Vascular Recanalization.* **Zeitler E, Grüntzig A, Schoop W** eds. Berlin: Springer, pp. 157–159.

Dotter CT, Rösch J, Seaman AJ (1974). Selective clot lysis with low-dose streptokinase. *Radiology* **111**: 31.

Hess H, Mietaschk A, Ingrisch H (1982a). Niedrig dosierte thrombolytische Therapie zur Wiederherstellung der Strombahn bei arteriellen Verschlüssen. *Dtsch Med Wschr* **105**: 787.

Hess H, Ingrisch H, Mietaschk A, Roth H (1982b). Local low dose thrombolytc therapy of peripheral arterial occlusions. *New Engl J Med* **307**: 1627.

Mahler F (1990). *Katheterinterventionen in der Angiologie.* Stuttgart: New York: Georg Thieme Verlag, pp. 113–131.

Schneider E, Largiadèr J (1987). Therapiekonzept beim akuten Verschluss von Extremitatenarterien. *Therapeut Umsch* **44**: 653.

Iliac lesions: when to stent, when not

Jean-Pierre Becquemin,
Gian-Luca Smedile

Introduction

Endovascular treatment has become the first choice option for patients with some symptomatic iliac occlusive disease. Results vary according to the type of lesions, whether they are occlusive or stenotic, short or diffuse, calcified or not. Also the site of the lesions influences the results with a better outcome for common iliac disease than external iliac artery lesions. In order to allow a comparison between series, the Committee of the Society of Cardiovascular and Interventional Radiology defined four categories of iliac lesions: category 1 stenoses less than 3 cm, category 2 stenoses between 3 and 5 cm, category 3 stenoses between 5 and 10 cm/or occlusion less than 5 cm, and category 4 stenoses more than 10 cm or occlusions more than 5 cm.

In 1999, we reported our experience of iliac angioplasty (Becquemin *et al.*, 1999). The cumulative patency rates of 260 percutaneous transluminal angioplasty were 92.9% ± 1.5% at 1 month, 86.5% ± 1.7% at 1 year, 81.2% ± 2.3% at 2-years, 78.8% ± 2.9% at 3 years, and 75.4% ± 3.5% at 5 and 6 years.

The category of the lesion as defined above was predictive of long-term patency. The 2-year patency rate was 84% ± 3% for category 1 lesions and 69.7% ± 6.5% for categories 2, 3, and 4 together ($p = 0.02$)

In our series a stent was used selectively for what we thought were unfavorable lesions for angioplasty alone and for failed angioplasty. The patency was the same whether a stent was used or not.

Non-controlled retrospective series have shown excellent results with the use of stent (Sullivan *et al.*, 1997). In a meta-analysis of six percutaneous transluminal angioplasty studies (1300 patients) and eight stent placement studies (816 patients) published in 1990 or later, stent placement and percutaneous transluminal angioplasty yielded similar complication rates, but the technical success rate was higher after stent placement and the risk of long-term failure was reduced (Bosch and Hunink, 1997). However, systematic use of stent is questionable. The Dutch prospective randomized trial comparing systematic and selective stenting concluded that there were no substantial differences in technical results and clinical outcomes of the two treatment strategies both at short-term and long-term follow-up. Since angioplasty followed by selective stent placement is less expensive than direct placement of a stent, the former seems to be the treatment of choice (Tetteroo *et al.*, 1998).

Thus there is evidence for limiting the use of a stent in selected cases. The question remains as to which are those cases.

A stent can be deployed after suboptimal results of balloon angioplasty or on purpose, as a primary procedure. Secondary stenting for suboptimal results is a relatively obvious option. On the contrary, the only justification of primary stenting is the prevention of expected complications related to balloon angioplasty alone.

Stenting for suboptimal results

Suboptimal results are defined by a residual stenosis, due to plague recoil or thrombus formation, and extensive dissection. Restenosis may also be considered for stenting.

Stenting for residual stenosis

1, 2

Following balloon angioplasty the quality control of the revascularization is of paramount importance. There are three ways of controlling the immediate results of balloon angioplasty.

Completion angiogram
To be accurate, both anteroposterior and lateral views are necessary. We consider that there is a residual stenosis when the lumen is narrowed by more than 20%. In these circumstances, we inflate the balloon a second time and place a stent if the results are still unsatisfactory.

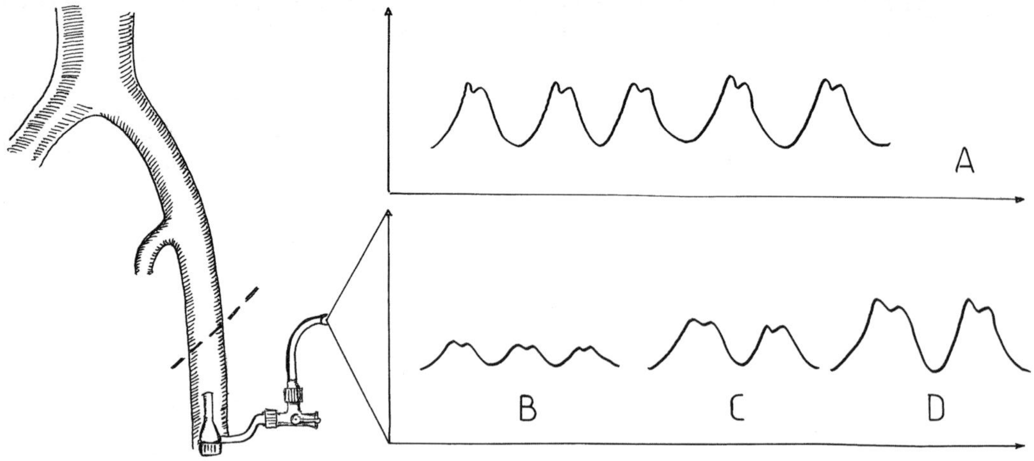

1

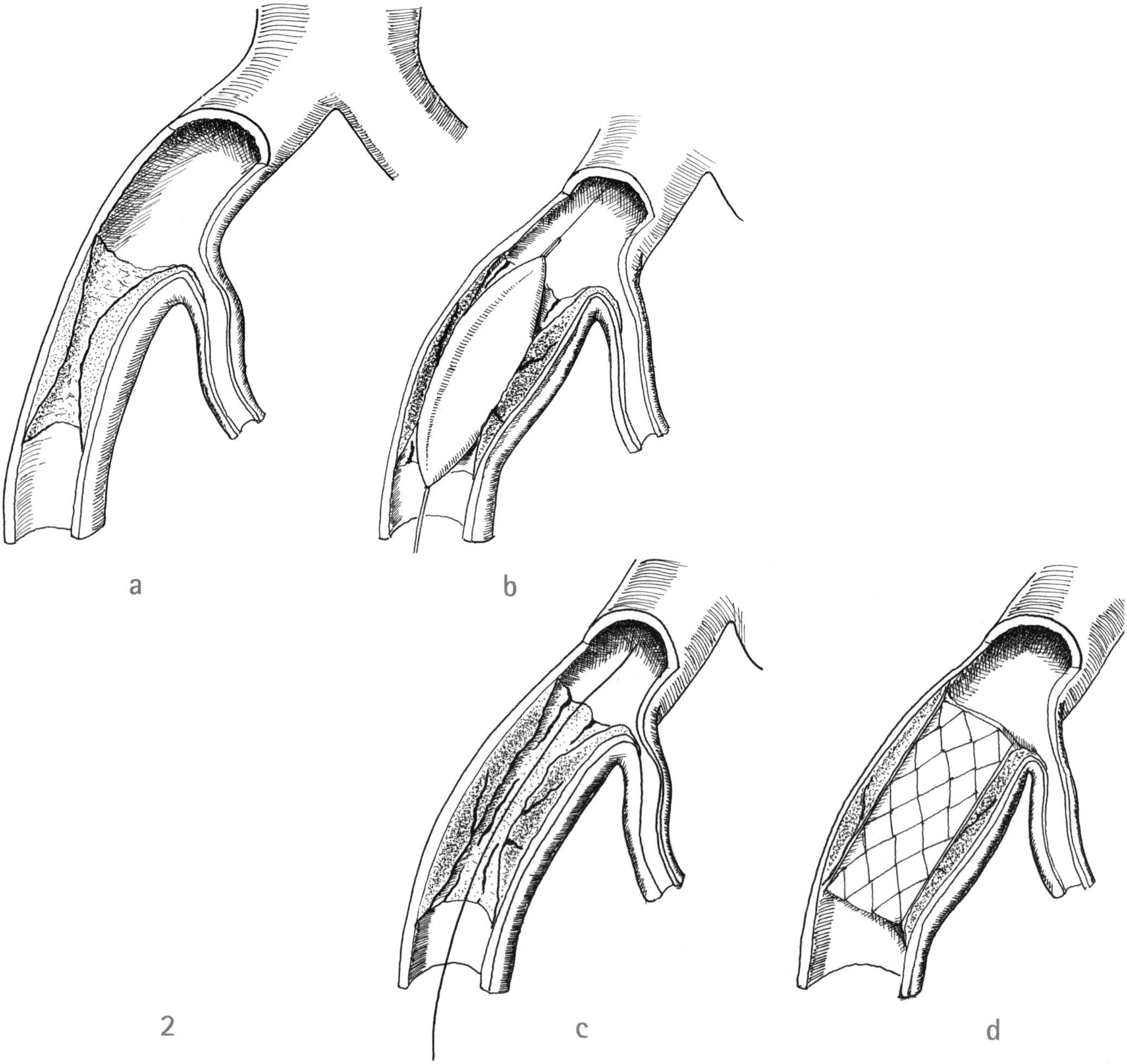

2

Pressure measurement

This gives a haemodynamic assessment, which is more physiological than the angiogram alone. Illustration 1 shows how we proceed. A pressure probe is plugged into the lateral channel of the introducer sheet. Curves are displayed on the same screen as the brachial pressure curves and compared. Curve A is from the brachial artery. Curve B is from the femoral artery, before balloon angioplasty. Curve C shows that after balloon angioplasty the pressure has increased but is still suboptimal. Curve D shows what the final optimal results under baseline condition should be. To be certain that the endovascular treatment will be efficient, we also measure the pressures after intra-arterial injection of 40 mg of papaverine or of Buflomedyl. When the pressure does not drop, the operation is stopped, without any further steps. When there is a 10% gradient of pressure in baseline condition or a drop of 10% or more after the pharmacological test, we inflate the balloon one more time and, if still unsatisfactory, we place a stent. The four steps of the procedure are shown in **2a, b, c, d.**

Intravenous ultrasound evaluation

Intravenous ultrasound has been shown to detect insufficient plague crushing, or incomplete stent apposition (Vogt *et al.*, 1999). However, it is expensive and on a routine basis it has no proven efficiency for improving the overall results of iliac percutaneous transluminal angioplasty. We currently use intravenous ultrasound in a very limited number of cases when there are doubts about the final results of percutaneous transluminal angioplasty or to accurately locate the ostium of the hypogastric artery before stenting.

Stenting for dissections

3

There is no firm evidence that stent is useful for dissection after balloon angioplasty. Balloon angioplasty widens the arterial lumen by fracturing the plaque, and then dissection is almost always present after balloon angioplasty. However, the exposure of the media or of the internal layer of the adventitia to the blood components, is a strong activator of platelet deposition. In the worst cases it induces thrombosis. In a lighter scenario it contributes at least to trigger the biological process leading to intimal hyperplasia. Dissection may also create an intimal flap, which is a potential cause of thrombosis. So there is a general trend to use a stent in the case of a large dissection. Illustration 3 shows an artist's conception of a dissected artery and the beneficial plastic effect of a stent.

Restenosis

Systematic stenting for restenosis is questionable. First, it is difficult to differentiate restenosis occurring at the site of the dilatation, from suboptimal percutaneous transluminal angioplasty left untreated, or from new stenosis which proximal or distal to the angioplastied site.

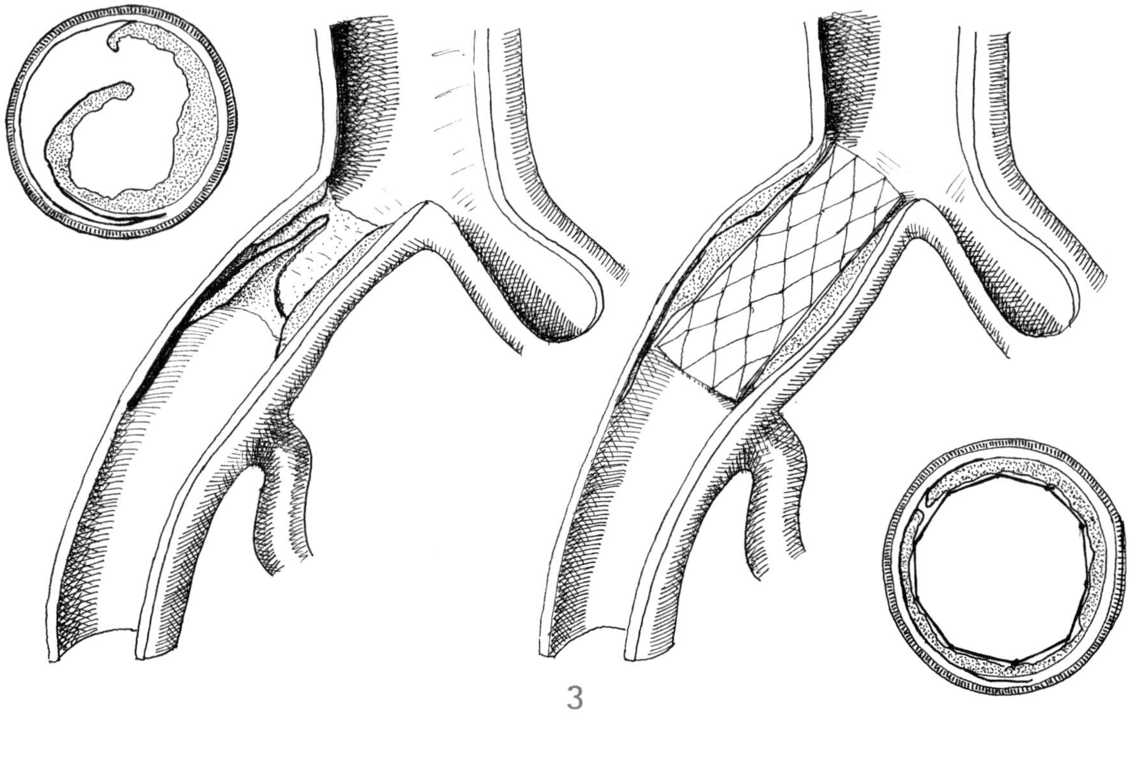

3

Second, we do not know if stenting is a better option than angioplasty alone for those lesions. So we do not currently stent iliac restenosis if the results of a new balloon angioplasty are optimum.

Stenting on purpose

Stenting on purpose may be indicated in the following circumstances.

Totally occluded iliac artery

4

Common iliac occlusions are excellent indications for endovascular treatment. In more than 80% of the cases the guidewire can be pushed within the thrombus up to the lumen of the aorta. The iliac lumen can then be reopened with a balloon. However, old and fresh clots crushed on the arterial wall are unstable materials which may recoil immediately or migrate toward the ipsilateral arteries or into the contralateral arterial tree. Thus it is probably safer to place a stent on purpose. Immediate and long-term results compare favorably when a stent is used (Henry *et al.*, 1998; Reyes *et al.*, 1997) than when it is not (Leu *et al.*, 1999). From a technical point of view, the stent can be deployed as a primary procedure, or after balloon angioplasty. The former option allows the thrombus to be trapped at first; the latter avoids the rather uncomfortable situation of blocking the stent at a wrong place within the iliac artery. When there is no proximal stump, it is of paramount importance to pro-

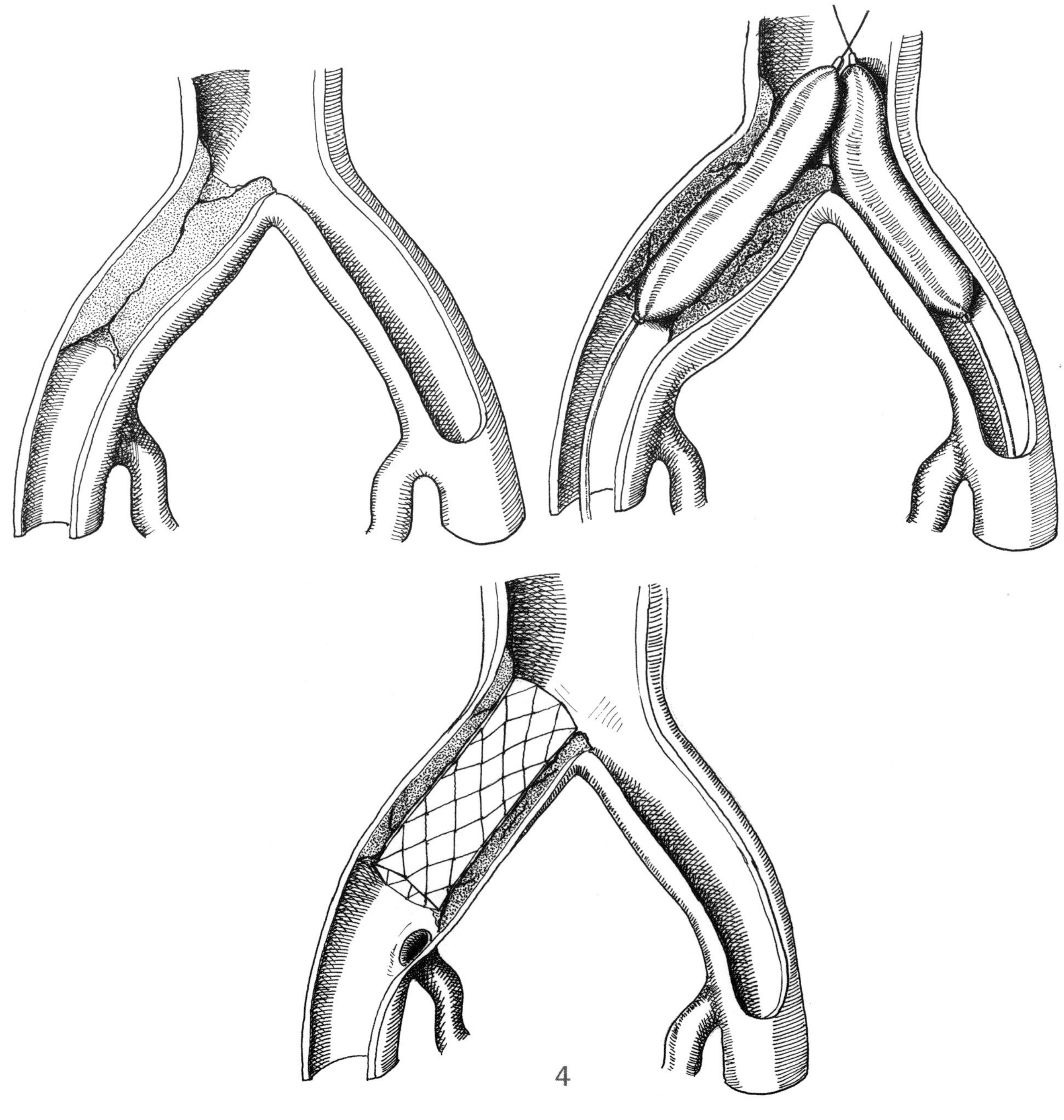

4

ceed with the kissing technique, as shown in **4**. In the drawing, we have shown a single stent. However, to treat lesions involving the aortic bifurcation which is quite frequent, two stents are deployed, one in each of the common iliac arteries. The proximal tips of the stents are placed a few millimetres within the aorta.

Multi-segmented lesions

5

Although an interesting patency rate has been reported with multi-segmented lesions (Powell *et al.*, 2000), results are poorer than those obtained with focal lesions. One way to improve patency would be to systematically stent the entire length of the diseased iliac artery. See **5** for an example of such a long lesion. Spectacular successful cases have been reported. However, in the long term the results remain poor despite the use of unique or multiple stents (Henry *et al.*, 1998). So far we do not know if covered stents such as the Hemobahn® will improve the results for those lesions.

Acute complications
In rare cases rupture occurs after balloon angioplasty. Heavy calcified lesions are prone to such a dramatic complication. Rather than performing surgery, the placement of a covered stent is a smart option (Formichi *et al.*, 1998).

When not to stent

We could schematically say that in all the remaining cases it is probably unnecessary to stent. In our experience and current indications we do not stent 80% of the iliac lesions amenable to endovascular treatment.

Two particular situation are to be discussed:

The covering of the hypogastric artery

6a, b

We are reluctant to cover the ostium of a patent hypogastric artery with a stent, especially when the contralateral hypogastric is occluded. However, when the lesions involve the distal common iliac artery or the proximal external iliac artery, and a stent is indicated based on the previously discussed guidelines, then we go for a stent. In our view, stent is not a firm contraindication since in most cases the hypogastric artery does not occlude by the sole presence of the stent. When occlusion happens, it is more frequently related to plaque protrusion or dislodgement within the hypogastric from the iliac artery. To avoid this potentially hazardous event, we protect the hypogastric using a technique derived from the kissing iliac technique. In this situation the iliac balloon is pushed from the ipsilateral groin and the hypogastric balloon from the contralateral groin, with the crossover technique (**6a, b**).

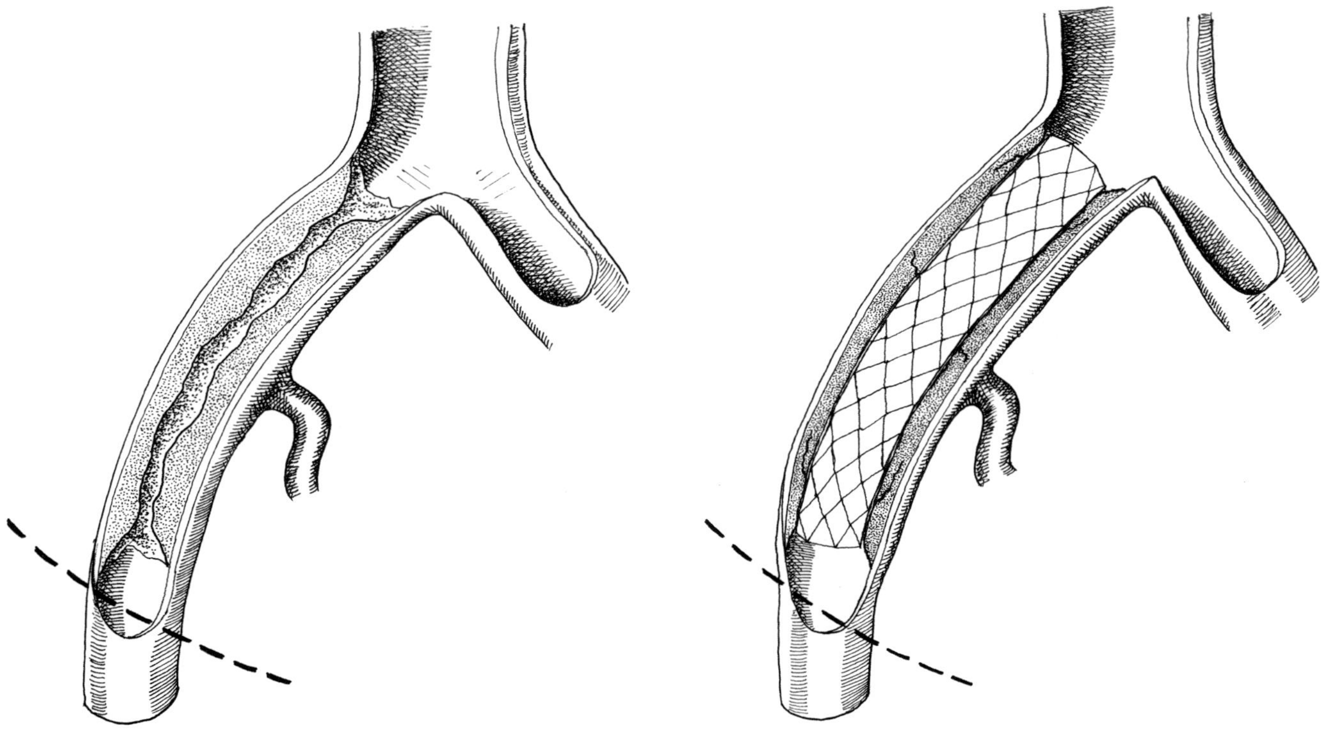

5

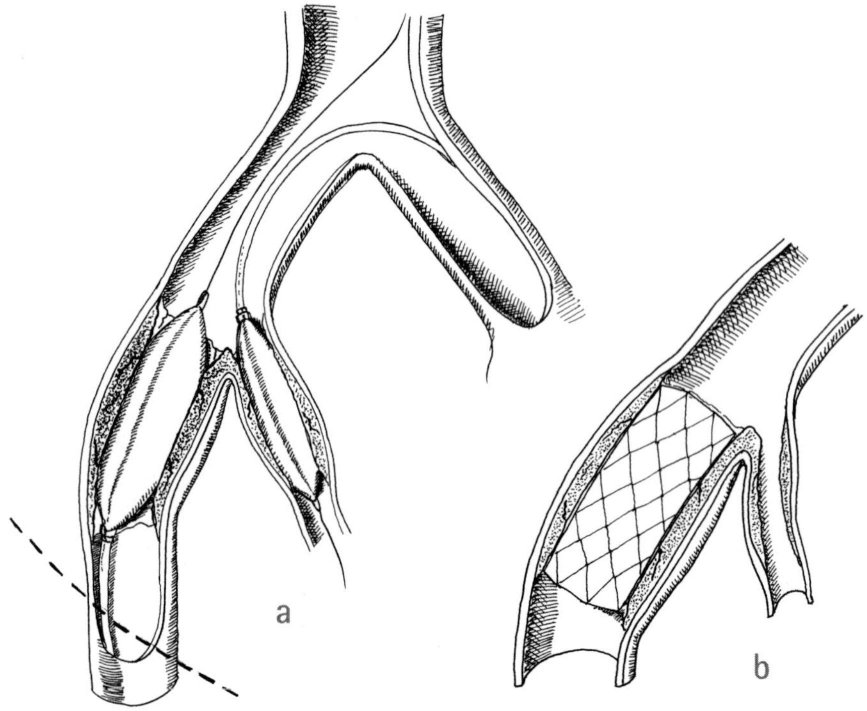

6

The external iliac artery

Diffuse occlusive or stenotic lesions of the external iliac artery, are not well treated by endovascular means (Powell *et al.*, 2000). There are probably several reasons for a poor outcome. The lesions are frequently calcified, the distal part of the iliac artery is mobile under the arcade and finally the atherosclerotic process almost always involves the common femoral artery. In this location, balloon angioplasty does not work well, and the motion of the hip may crush the stent. Thus in our view these patients are best treated surgically.

Acknowledgement

Illustrations by G-L Smedile

References

Becquemin JP, Allaire E, Qvarfordt P *et al.* (1999). Surgical transluminal iliac angioplasty with selective stenting: long-term results assessed by means of duplex scanning. *J Vasc Surg* **29**: 422–429.

Bosch JL, Hunink MG (1997). Meta-analysis of the results of percutaneous transluminal angioplasty and stent placement for aortoiliac occlusive disease [published erratum appears in *Radiology* 1997; **205**: 584]. *Radiology* **204**: 87–96.

Formichi M, Raybaud G, Benichou H, Ciosi G (1998). Rupture of the external iliac artery during balloon angioplasty: endovascular treatment using a covered stent. *J Endovasc Surg* **5**: 37–41.

Henry M, Amor M, Ethevenot G *et al.* (1998). Percutaneous endoluminal treatment of iliac occlusions: long-term follow-up in 105 patients. *J Endovasc Surg* **5**: 228–235.

Leu AJ, Schneider E, Canoval CR, Hoffmann U (1999). Long-term results after recanalisation of chronic iliac artery occlusions by combined catheter therapy without stent placement. *Eur J Vasc Endovasc Surg* **18**: 499–505.

Powell RJ, Fillinger M, Bettmann M *et al.* (2000). The durability of endovascular treatment of multisegment iliac occlusive disease. *J Vasc Surg* **31**: 1178–1184.

Reyes R, Maynar M, Lopera J *et al.* (1997). Treatment of chronic iliac artery occlusions with guide wire recanalization and primary stent placement. *J Vasc Interv Radiol* **8**: 1049–1055.

Sullivan TM, Childs MB, Bacharach JM *et al.* (1997). Percutaneous transluminal angioplasty and primary stenting of the iliac arteries in 288 patients. *J Vasc Surg* **25**: 829–838.

Tetteroo E, van der Graaf Y, Bosch JL *et al.* (1998). Randomised comparison of primary stent placement versus primary angioplasty followed by selective stent placement in patients with iliac-artery occlusive disease. Dutch Iliac Stent Trial Study Group. *Lancet* **351**: 1153–1159.

Vogt KJ, Rasmussen JG, Just S, Schroeder TV (1999). Effect and outcome of balloon angioplasty and stenting of the iliac arteries evaluated by intravascular ultrasound. *Eur J Vasc Endovasc Surg* **17**: 47–55.

Iliac angioplasty and stenting

Tony A Nicholson

Percutaneous transluminal angioplasty, with or without stent, is one of the most commonly performed percutaneous interventional radiological procedures. During the first 6 months of 1999, 3619 iliac angioplasties were performed and 1208 iliac stents inserted under the National Health Service in England and Wales (NCEPOD, 2000). The indications for intervention include lifestyle-limiting intermittent claudication, rest pain/gangrene and to improve inflow prior to infrainguinal surgical or percutaneous revascularization. Prior to percutaneous iliac recanalization due to atheroma, patients require an assessment and modification of risk factors, adjunctive medical therapy and an exercise programme. Patient care also requires the establishment of standards for quality control, and accurate follow-up. Thus, direct access to patients, collaboration with vascular surgeons, physicians and general practitioners, regular interdisciplinary conferences and the collection of clinical information on the outcomes of procedures are mandatory.

Pre-procedural considerations

The iliac system consists of the common, external and internal iliac arteries. Each has a different pattern of stenotic or occlusive disease and each responds differently to intervention. When considering a patient for percutaneous revascularization of the iliac arteries the following should be taken into consideration.

1. Is the disease occlusive or stenotic?
2. Does the disease involve the lower abdominal aorta?
3. Is the disease uni or bilateral?
4. Does the disease extend into the common femoral artery and would stent insertion cross the hip joint?
5. What is the diameter and length of the segment to be treated?
6. Are the internal iliac arteries patent and might they be compromised in any subsequent revascularization?
7. What is the shape of the aortic bifurcation and can it be crossed from a contralateral approach?

Prior to angioplasty, all patients should receive 300 mg of aspirin. If aspirin cannot be used, clopidogrel should be prescribed, 300 mg the day before the procedure and 75 mg per day following the procedure.

Equipment and materials required

1. Modern fluoroscopic unit with road-mapping/tracing facilities and 17–39 cm image intensification. Preferably pulsed fluoroscopy should be available to keep the radiation dose as low as achievable.
2. Preferably a power injector for contrast.
3. Electrocardiogram, pulse oximetry, pulse and blood pressure patient monitoring equipment.
4. Pressure monitoring equipment
5. A full range of protective equipment, including lead coats, glasses and thyroid shields.
6. A full range of torquable femorovisceral catheters and wires, including stiff and hydrophilic coated wires.
7. A full range of angioplasty balloons with diameters ranging from 4 mm to 12 mm.
8. Non-ionic contrast at both 150 and 300 strength.
9. Self-expanding stents with a diameter range from 6 mm to 12 mm and a length range from 4 to 10 cm.
10. Pre-mounted balloon expandable stents with the same diameter and length range.
11. Heparin.

Technique for iliac angioplasty

The femoral approach is used in nearly all patients. The brachial artery or axillary approach can also be used and some have used the popliteal approach for recanalization of iliac disease.

Following diagnostic digital subtraction angiogram to localize the stenosis/occlusion, 3000–5000 international units of heparin are injected. The lesion is traversed using a combination of guidewire and catheter through a sheath inserted at the puncture site. Sheaths are useful as they allow rapid and atraumatic exchange of catheters and wires. Occasionally, especially where the artery is occluded, it may be necessary to try several different shaped catheters or wires but 98% of lesions in the iliac arteries should be crossed in this way. A wire that appears to take on an S-configuration is probably in the subintimal space. If the artery is not calcified it may be possible to re-enter the true lumen and perform a subintimal procedure. If, however, the artery is heavily calcified or the wire does not enter the true lumen at or before the bifurcation, it is best to withdraw the catheter and wire to the origin of the occlusion and try and find a different channel. It is not advisable to try and perform subintimal angioplasty in the external iliac artery as it is more prone to rupture than the common iliac artery, a fact borne out by the relatively high mortality for iliac angioplasty and stenting in NCEPOD.

Stenosis

1, 2, 3, 4

Stenoses should be crossed with curved catheters and torquable wires. The intension should always be to treat stenotic lesions by balloon angioplasty (1 – 3). Illustration 1 shows the left common iliac stenosis at the common iliac origin. In 2 sheaths have been inserted into the common femoral arteries and the stenosis crossed with a combination of steerable wire and catheter. In 3 the arterial diameter has been measured and an appropriate size balloon inserted to dilate stenosis. Pre-angioplasty

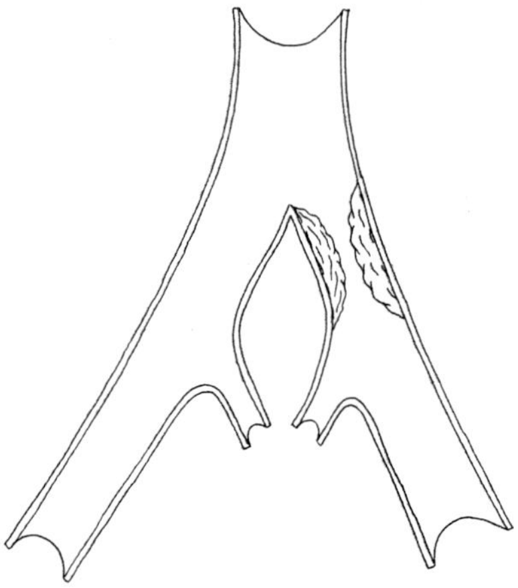

1

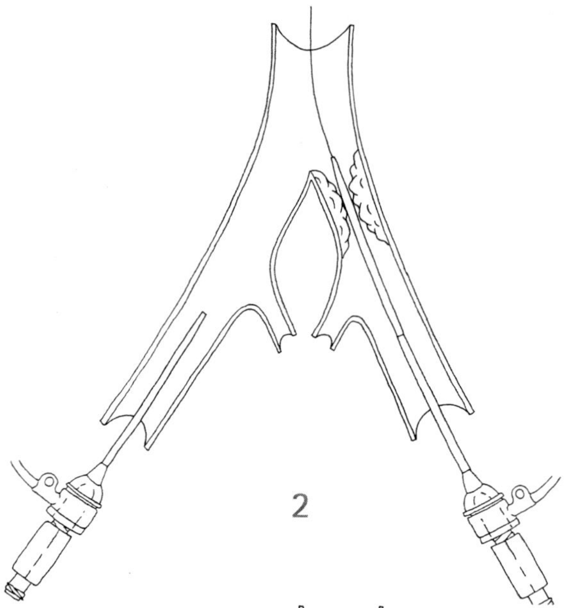

2

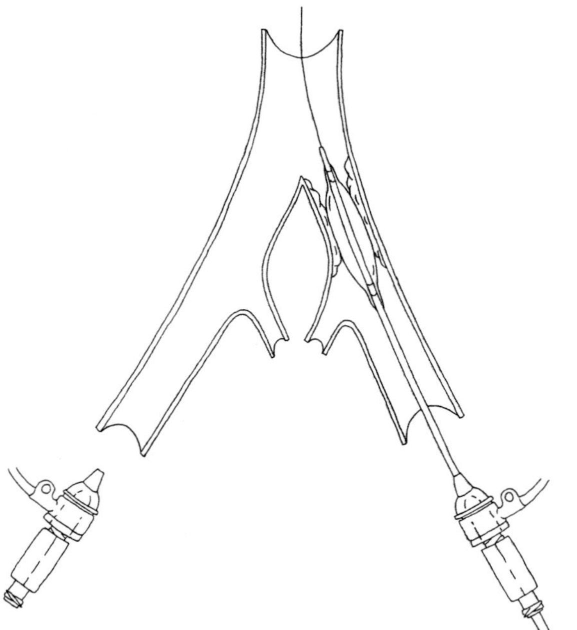

3

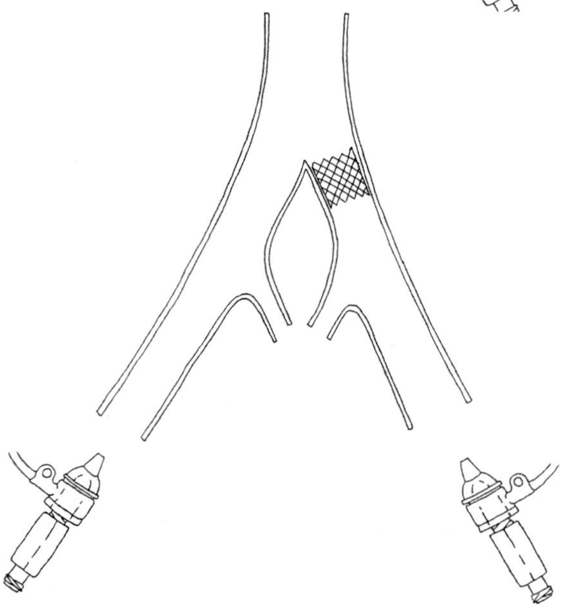

4

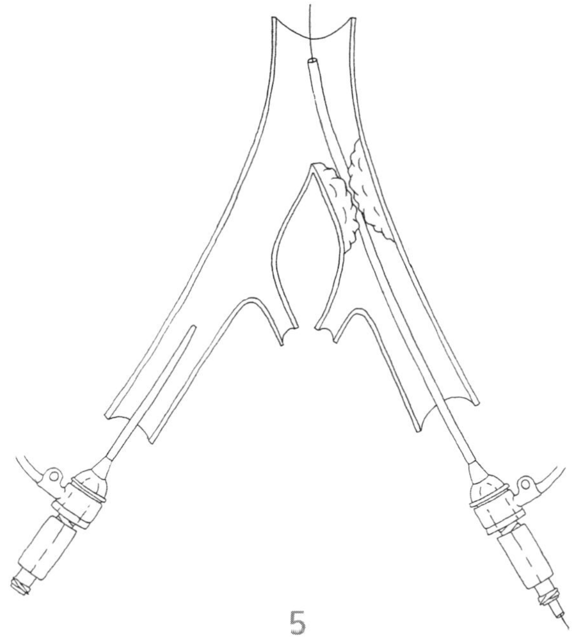

5

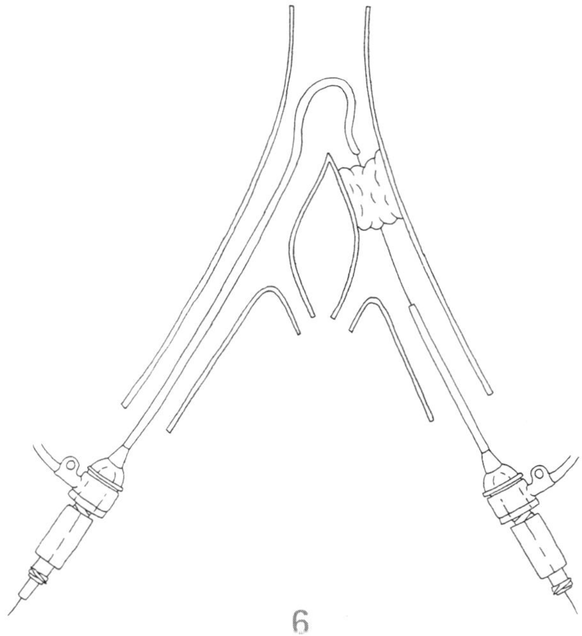

6

vasodilator assisted pressure gradients should be measured as a baseline. In the common and internal iliac arteries the dilatation can match the diameter of the artery. However, the external iliac artery is prone to rupture and it is best to under dilate by a millimeter. The decision to accept the result depends on the angiographic appearance and the pressure gradient. If the final angiographic appearance shows less than 10% residual stenosis/recoil and if there are no potentially occlusive dissections and if the vasodilator assisted gradient is reduced to less than 10 mmHg the result can be accepted. But if these criteria are not met it is reasonable to insert a balloon-mounted stent of appropriate length and diameter (**4**). This approach has been shown to be cost-effective and improves the long-term patency of the recanalized segment (Bosch *et al.*, 1998; Tetteroo *et al.*, 1998; Bosch and Hunink, 1997).

Occlusions

5, 6, 7, 8

Initially attempts should be made to cross iliac occlusions from the ipsilateral side (**5**). In Illustration **5** a completed occlusion of the left common iliac artery has been crossed from the ipsilateral side with a curved catheter and steerable wire. If this approach fails, the contralateral 'crossover' approach invariably works (Roth and Cappius, 1981). Here a 7 French sidewinder catheter is reformed in the aortic arch and turned to face the contralateral side to access the 'Channel' in the occluded segment. It is then pulled into the aortic end of the iliac occlusion, which is then probed with a hydrophilic curved wire (**6**). Once the patent distal artery has been entered the wire is then guided into the previously inserted common femoral sheath and pulled out through the haemostatic valve. A curved hook catheter is then passed up the ipsilateral side into the contralateral iliac artery (**7**). The wire is then turned around so that the floppy end now faces up the aorta, the curved catheter gently withdrawn and turned to face upwards to access the aorta. The wire is then passed up into the aorta (**8**).

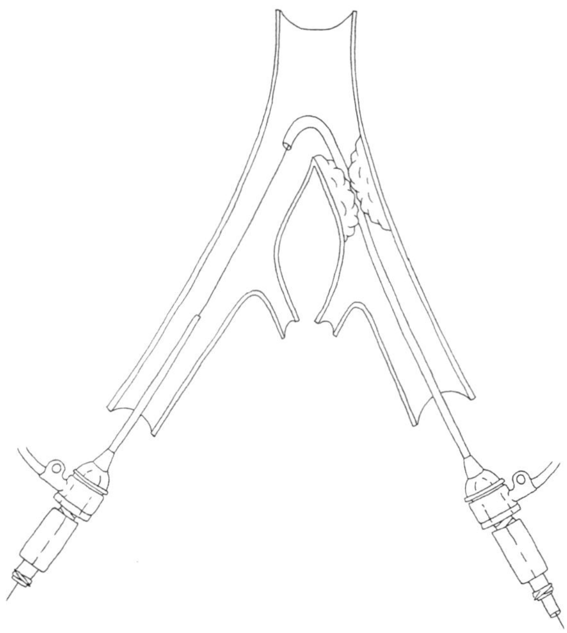

7

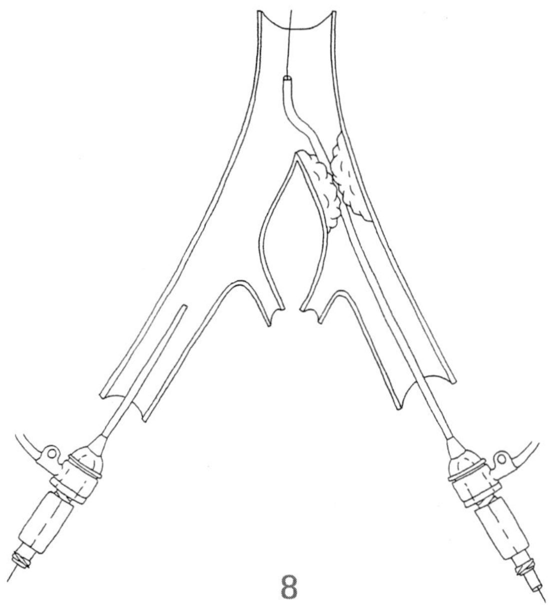

8

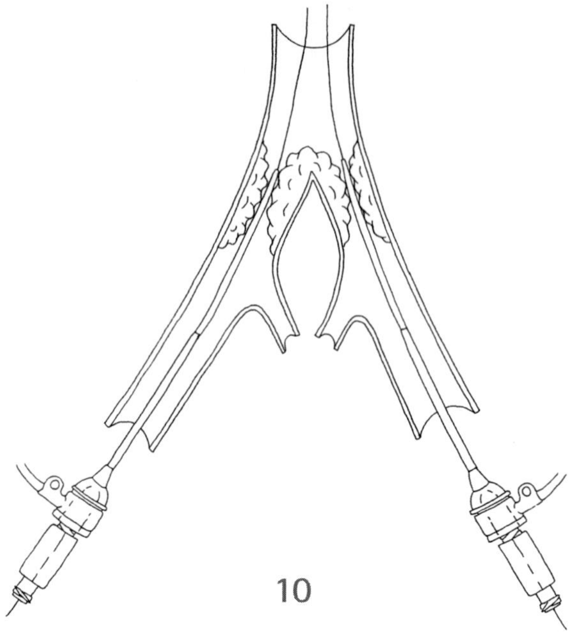

10

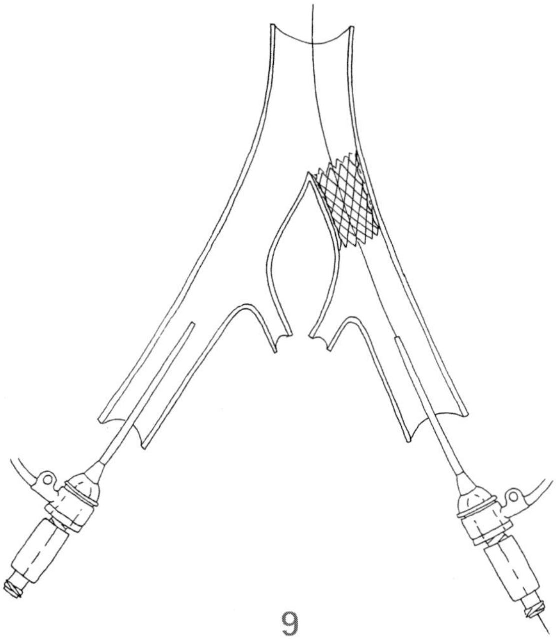

9

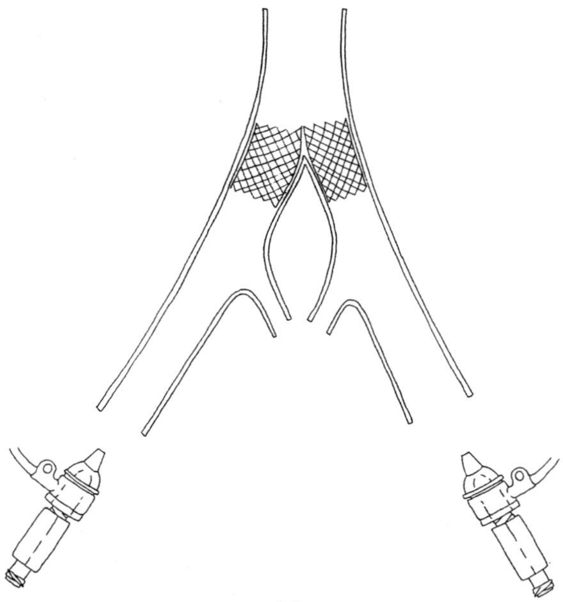

11

9

It is my practice to primary stent all occlusions. There is little literature evidence that iliac stenting is superior to iliac angioplasty for the treatment of iliac occlusions. However, prior to 1990 many centres had abandoned angioplasty of iliac occlusions as the complication rate was high. Embolization rates as high as 40% were recorded. Most of these emboli were large and required surgical removal. In the 10 years since we started stenting we have inserted 1256 stents in 945 patients. We have had only two embolic episodes in that time both in the first 12 months of our experience and at a time when we pre-dilated all occlusions prior to stent insertion (Wijesinghe *et al.*, 1999). It has been our practice for the last 8 years to insert an appropriate sized self-expanding stent across the occlusion without pre-dilatation. Once successfully released the stent is balloon post-dilated to size as for stenosis (9). Pull-back pressure measurements confirm completion of the procedure.

10, 11

Where common iliac occlusions are bilateral it is best to try and position stents at the origins of the arteries

(10,11). If this is not possible or if the distal aorta is also stenotic it may be necessary to place 'kissing stents' effectively reconstructing the aortic bifurcation. Though the literature evidence is not available my own results suggest that patency for the 'kissing stent' technique is not as good as for accurately placed iliac stents (Wijesinghe *et al.*, 1999) Illustration 11 shows stents in place in both common iliac arteries.

Acknowledgement

Illustrations by Rachel Quarenta.

References

Bosch JL, Hunink MG (1997). Meta-analysis of the results of PTA and stent placement in aortoiliac occlusive disease. *Radiology* **204**: 87–96.

Bosch JL, Tetteroo E, Mali W (1998). Iliac arterial disease: Cost effectiveness analysis of stent placement vs PTA. *Radiology* **208**: 641–648.

NCEPOD (2000). Report on Vascular Radiology. *NCEPOD.*

Roth FJ, Cappius G (1981). 'Cross-over' Technik zur Behandlung von Leistenarterien. *VASA* **11**: 22–24.

Tetteroo E, Van der Graf Y, Bosch JL (1998). Randomized comparison of 1ry stent insertion vs primary angioplasty by selective stent insertion in iliac artery occlusive disease. *Lancet* **351**: 1153–1159.

Wijesinghe LD, Nicholson AA, Ettles DF *et al.* (1999). Predictors of outcome after stenting of the common iliac artery for stenotic or occlusive disease. *VSS BSIR* (abstract).

The complications of iliac and subclavian artery stenting

T M Buckenham

Aortoiliac kissing stents

1, 2

The placement of bilateral common iliac stents to create a new bifurcation is controversial particularly if this technique is used to treat unilateral disease. In these cases a non-stenosed iliac artery is stented to prevent impingement of the contralateral stent on the asymptomatic iliac artery. There are a number of complications that can arise from this technique. Illustrations 1 and 2 indicate how mal-positioning and undersizing of the iliac stents can lead to aortic or common iliac artery occlusion. In 1 a kissing stent is shown with compromise of the left common iliac artery. Illustration 2 shows how undersized aorta kissing stents can cause aortic thrombosis.

Some authors have reported good results using self-expanding stents primarily in claudicants but the potential for mal-alignment and the subsequent compromise of an asymptomatic limb has prevented this technique from gaining universal acceptance (Saker *et al.*, 2000; Mendelshon *et al.*, 1998; Houston *et al.*, 1999).

Intramural stent placement

3

Most interventionists believe intraluminal iliac and subclavian stent placement is optimal and the deliberate

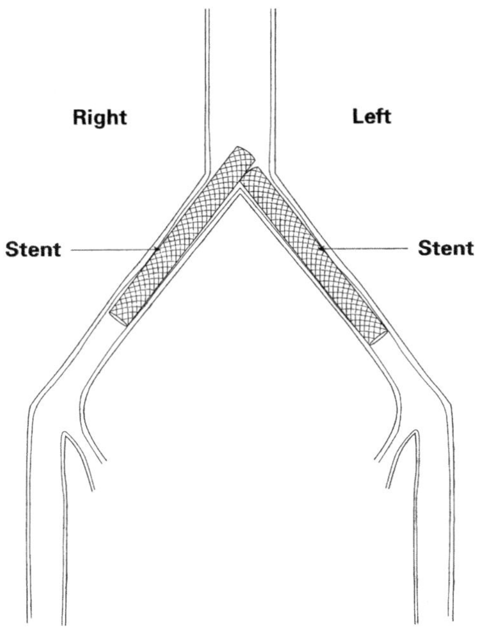

1

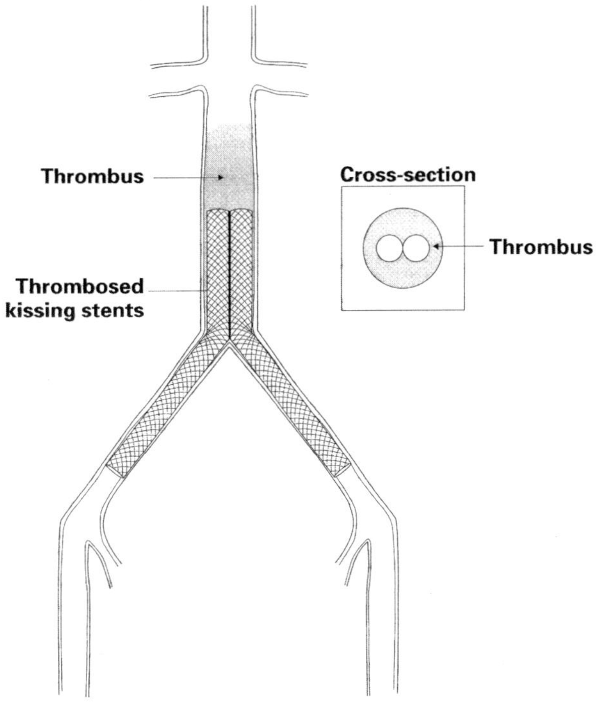

2

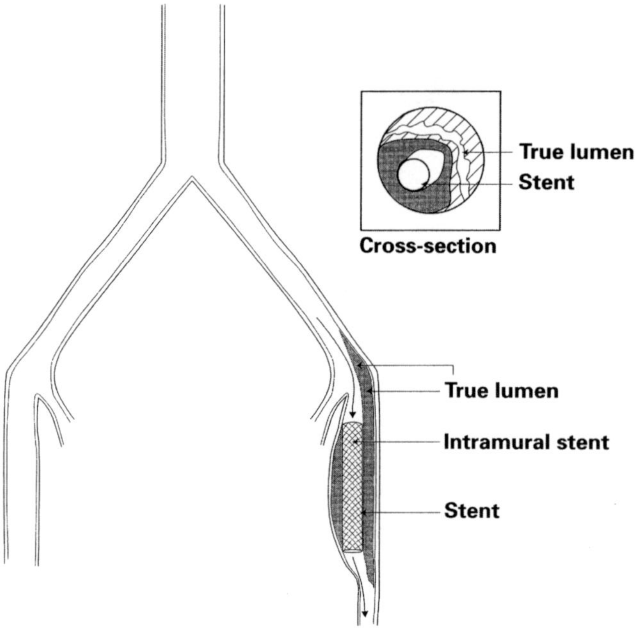

3

intramural neolumin intentionally created in the infrainguinal circulation advocated by some operators is less acceptable above the inguinal ligament. Intramural dilatation and stent placement can predispose to rupture and flow limiting flaps. In the absence of intravascular ultrasound it may be difficult to determine if placement is intraluminal or extraluminal (Navarro *et al.*, 2000).

Stent fracture in the subclavian artery

4

Stents have been used in both the subclavian artery and vein for the management of occlusive disease and venous hypertension. When placed across the first rib these stents are subject to repeated compression between clavicle and first rib on arm abduction and this may lead to stent fracture. The use of self-expanding stents with the ability to reconfigure after distortion has not obviated this problem and there are reports of these stents fracturing (Phipp *et al.*, 1999). Excision of the first rib has been suggested as a routine adjunct to subclavian stenting. Illustration **4** shows mechanical disruption of a subclavian stent in the thoracic outlet.

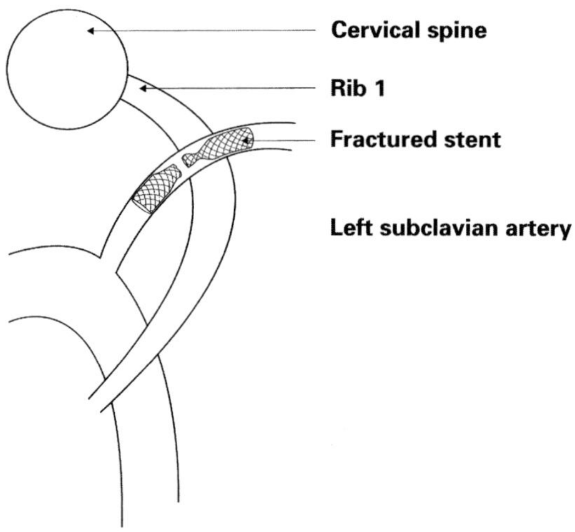

4

Iliac artery rupture

5

The risk factors for iliac rupture are location, (the external iliac artery (**5**) is more prone to rupture than the common) and sex, (the complication is more frequently seen in women). Intramural dilatation is also associated with rupture and the most important indication of impending rupture or intramural dilatation is pain which does not resolve with balloon deflation. Rupture will be apparent on fluoroscopy as the contrast-filled bladder will be displaced away from the site of injury. Most ruptures can be tamponaded with balloon inflation and many can be successfully treated with the percutaneous placement of a covered stent obviating the need for surgery (Joseph *et al.*, 1987). Early recognition and the appropriate equipment to enable percutaneous repair are essential to prevent serious complications or death (Cooper and Sofocleous, 1998).

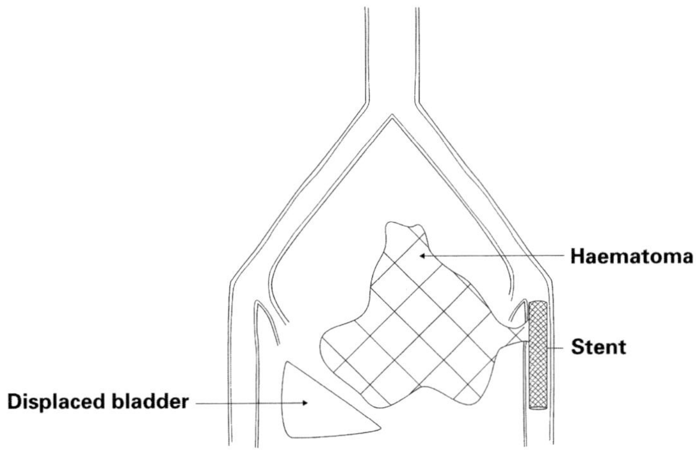

5

Balloon rupture

6

Peripheral angioplasty balloons are designed to rupture longitudinally to reduce the difficulty in withdrawal through a diseased vessel or a stent. Occasionally the balloons may rupture transversely or invert causing entanglement (6) with a partially deployed stent. Some of the self-expanding stents have been reported to cause balloon rupture by puncturing the balloon with sharp stent interfaces. Removal of the ruptured balloon can usually be achieved percutaneously with a large sheath or a vascular snare. The use of a manometer to ensure safe inflation pressures should also reduce the risk of rupture (Ettles and Taylor, 2000; Keelan *et al.*, 1995; Bersin, 1993).

Embolization

7

Peripheral embolization is a serious complication of iliac or subclavian dilation (Rekas *et al.*, 1998; Vorwerk *et al.*, 1995). The rates of distal embolization vary in the

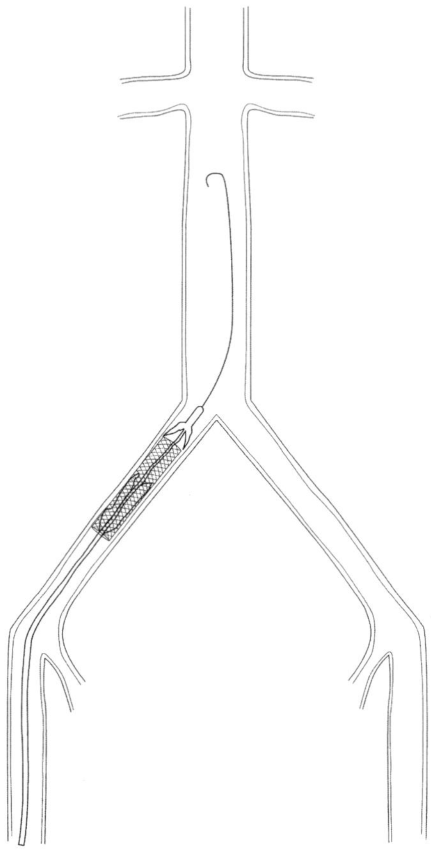

6

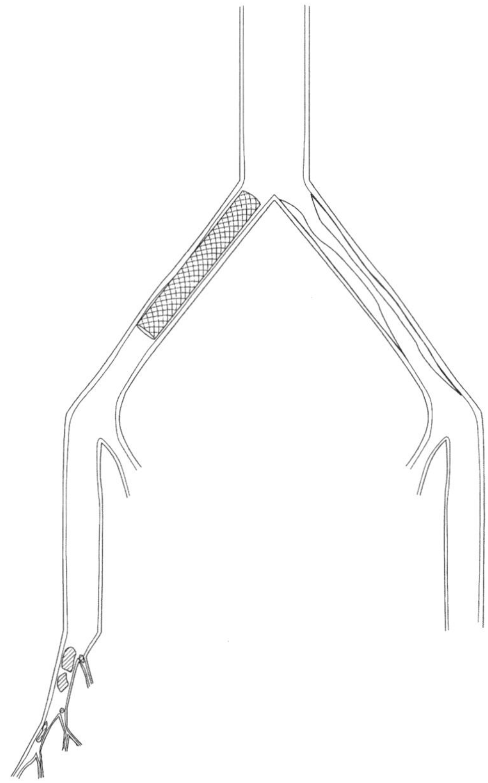

7

literature but simple balloon dilation (without stenting) of iliac occlusions are associated with the highest risk and primary stenting the lowest. On completion of the stenting procedure arteriography of the infrainguinal circulation should be carried out to exclude this complication. The most common site for embolic to impact are the profunda femoris artery (7) (particularly in the presence of superficial femoral artery occlusion) and the popliteal trifurcation. Percutaneous aspiration can be used to treat this complication in the leg at the time of stent placement, this option is more difficult in the arm. Aspiration should be performed with a soft-tip guiding catheter and a detachable hub sheath under fluoroscopic control.

Stent infection

8

Arterial stent infection has been reported in the iliac, subclavian and renal arteries, the causative bacteria is usually *Staphylococcus aureus*. These infections are associated with local pseudoaneurysm formation and in some cases septic emboli. The use of prophylactic antibiotics is unproven. Management is usually surgical removal and bypass grafting (Hassel *et al.*, 1981; Rapoports *et al.*, 1985; Deiparine *et al.*, 1996; Chalmers *et al.*, 1993; Malek *et al.*, 2000). Illustration **8** shows a mycotic false aneurysm associated with stent, and also right common femoral artery access site false aneurysm.

Misplaced arterial stents

9

Balloon-expandable stents either pre-mounted or self-mounted may dislodge from the underlying balloon especially when being advanced through a tight stenosis or occlusion. The stent may then lie over the shaft of the balloon or may be displaced from the balloon entirely. In the former situation the balloon may be remounted by placing a smaller balloon over the wire and inserting it into the undilated stent. The stent then maybe deployed in the appropriate position but will require reinsertion of a larger balloon for full expansion. A stent that has been lost totally from the balloon will only need to be retrieved if it is in a clinically significant location and this may be achieved percutaneously with a vascular snare (Harnell *et al.*, 1995).

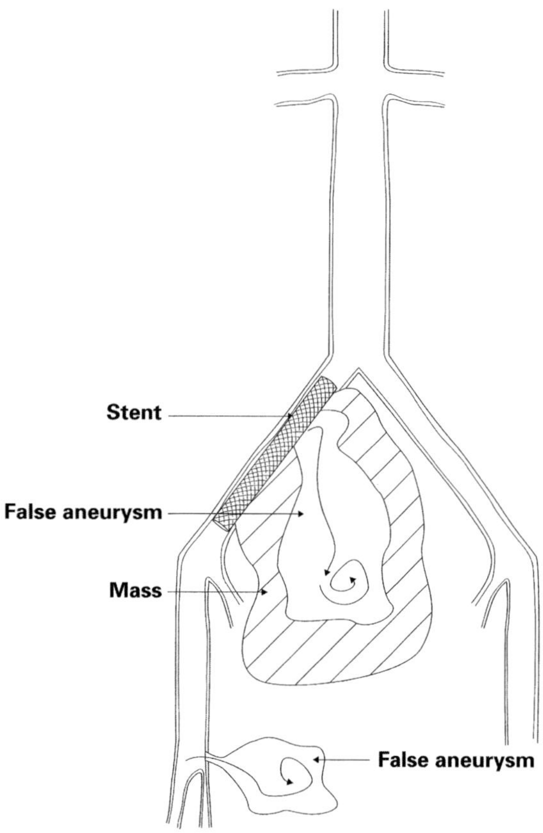

8

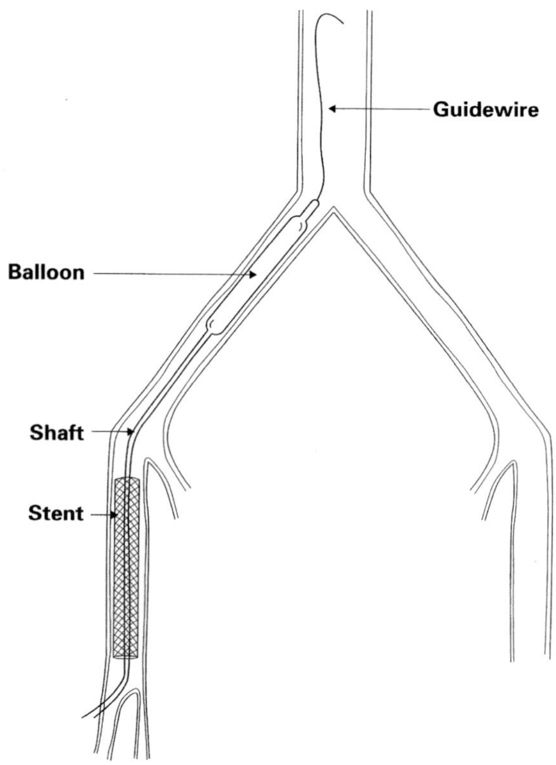

9

References

Bersin RM, Gold RS Jr (1993). Balloon rupture during peripheral stent implantation: a new technique for balloon retrieval. *Cathet Cardiovasc Diagn* **29**: 292–295.

Chalmers N, Eadington DW, Gandanhamo D *et al.* Case report: infected false aneurysm at the site of an iliac stent. *Br J Radiol* **66**:946–948.

Cooper SG, Sofocleous CT (1998). Percutaneous management of angioplasty related iliac artery rupture with preservation of luminal patency. *J Vasc Intervent Radiol* **9**:81–83.

Deiparine MK, Bellard JL, Taylor FC *et al.* (1996). Endovascular stent infection. *J Vasc Surg* **23**:529–533.

Ettles DF and Taylor PR (2000). Complications of endovascular procedures. *Text Book of Endovascular Procedures.* Edinburgh, London: Churchill Livingston, pp. 49–61.

Harnell GG, Jordan SJ (1995). Percutaneous removal of a misplaced Palmaz stent with a coaxial snare technique. *J Vasc Interv Radiol* **6**:799–801.

Hassel SJ, Adams DF, Abrams HL (1981). Complications of angiology. *Radiology* **138**:273–278.

Houston JG, McCollum PT, Stonebridge PA *et al* (1999). Aortic bifurcation reconstruction, use of the memotherm self-expanding nitinol stent for stenosis and occlusions. *Cardiovasc Interven Radiol* **22**:89–95.

Joseph N, Levey E, Lipman S. (1987). Angioplasty related iliac artery rupture: treatment by temporary balloon occlusion. *Cardiovasc Intervent Radiol* **10**:276–279.

Keelan ET, Nunez BD, Berger PB, Holmes DR Jr, Garratt KN (1995). Management of balloon rupture during rigid stent deployment. *Cathet Cardiovasc Diagn* **35**:211–215.

Malek AM, Higashida RT, Reilly LM, Smith WS *et al.* (2000). Subclavian arthritis and pseudoaneurysm formation secondary to stent infection. *Cardiovasc Intervent Radiol* **23**:57–60.

Mendelshon FO, Santos RM, Crowley JJ *et al.* (1998). Kissing stents in the aortic bifurcation. *Interven Radiol* **136**:600–605.

Navarro F, Sullivan TM, Bacharach JM (2000). Intravascular Ultrasound assessment of iliac stent procedures. *J Endovasc Ther* **7**;4 :313–319.

Phipp LH, Scott DJ, Kessel D, Robertson I. Subclavian stents and stentgrafts: cause for concern? *J Endovasc Surg* **6**:223–226.

Rapoport S, Sniderman KW, Morse SS *et al.* (1985). Pseudoaneurysm: a complication of faulty technique in femoral artery puncture. *Radiology* **154**:529–530.

Rekas J (1998) A balloon protection sheath to prevent peripheral embolisation during aorta iliac endovascular procedures. *Cardiovasc Intervent Radiol* **21**:431–438.

Saker MB, Oppat WF, Kent SA *et al.* (2000). Early failure of aortoiliac kissing stents: histopathologic correlation. *J Vasc Interv Radiol* **11**:333–336.

Vorwerk D, Guenther RW, Shurmann K *et al.* (1995). Primary stent placement for chronic iliac artery occlusions. *Radiology* **194**:745–749.

Techniques in subintimal angioplasty

A Bolia

Initiation of a dissection and entry into thc subintimal space by intention

1 [A – B]

The dissection is initiated at the origin of an occlusion by directing the tip of a curved guidewire, usually an angled 0.035 hydrophilic guidewire, towards the wall of the artery in the direction away from any important collaterals. The wire is then pushed into the occlusion, which takes the path of least resistance, which is in the subintimal space. The wire may not advance by itself into the dissection, in which case the support of a 5F Teflon Van Andel catheter is helpful. A combination of a Van Andel catheter and hydrophilic guidewire are usually sufficient to initiate the dissection. The dissection may be initiated by the use of a 'J' wire protruding from the tip of the shaped catheter which is directed towards the wall, away from any collaterals. As shown in the (1), the 'J' wire protruding out of the catheter is pushed together as a unit, into the dissection. Once the catheter is in a dissection, the position can be confirmed by a small amount of contrast which will outline the dissection space. Also, the guidewire will seem to be moving and looping freely into the potential dissection space.

A - B

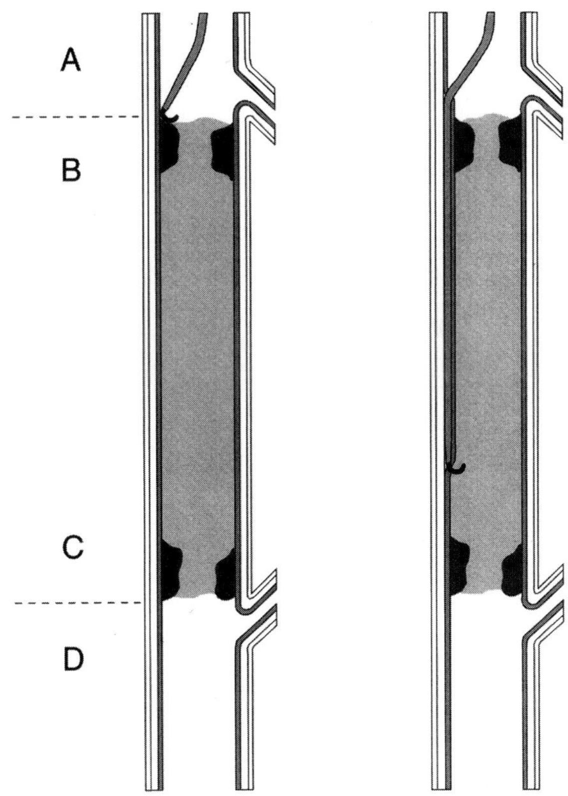

1

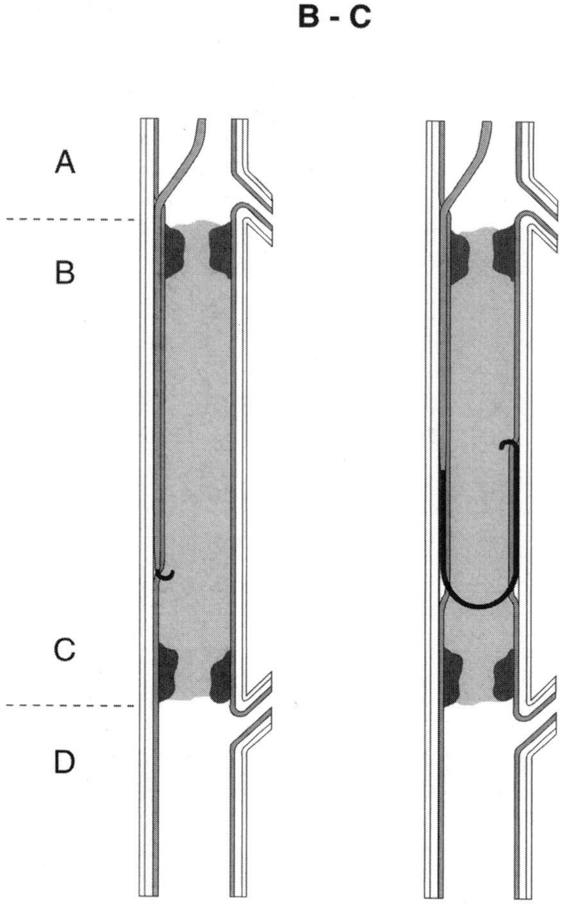

2

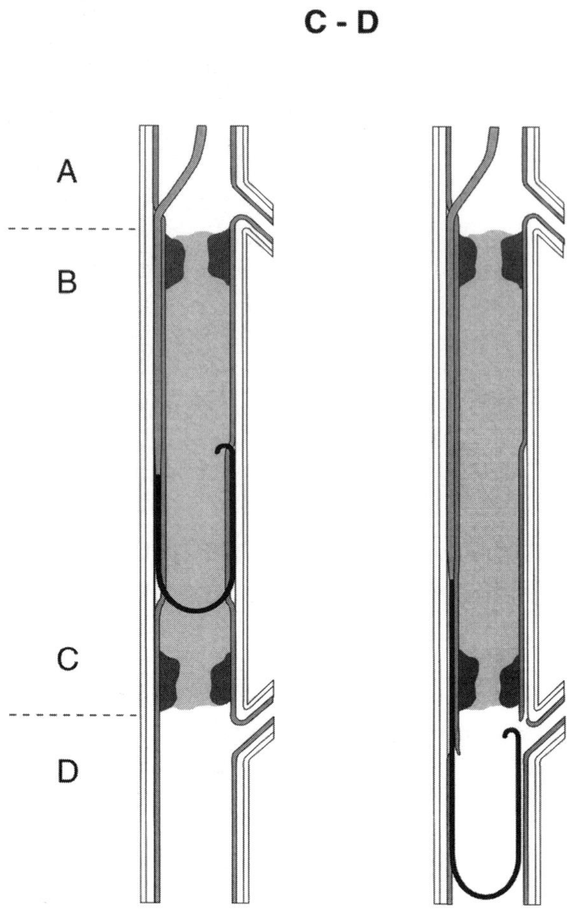

3

Dissecting along the length of the occlusion

2 [B – C]

Once the catheter is in a dissection, a hydrophilic wire passed through it can be advanced through the dissection space. This is achieved by pushing the guidewire and, when necessary, support is provided by the Van Andel catheter which follows the advancing guidewire. The dissection is usually extended with ease by the use of a loop in the hydrophilic guidewire as shown in (2). The loop is advanced through the dissection and when it advances no further, the Van Andel catheter is advanced forward, in order to provide support to one limb of the loop. This allows the loop to be pushed further forward until the length of the occlusion has been traversed but re-entry not achieved.

Re-entry into the lumen from the dissection space

3 [C – D]

Re-entry into the lumen from the dissection space is usually achieved with the help of a large loop in the hydrophilic guidewire. Support is usually necessary from the Van Andel catheter to one limb of the loop in the wire. The leading edge of the loop achieves re-entry back into the lumen spontaneously, particularly when the artery beyond the occlusion is disease free. This phenomenon of the wire loop re-entering into the relatively disease free segment in the distal artery can be likened to the surgical situation whereby the dissecting Cheyne–Watson instrument achieves re-entry back into the lumen of the disease-free distal internal carotid artery during carotid endarectomy.

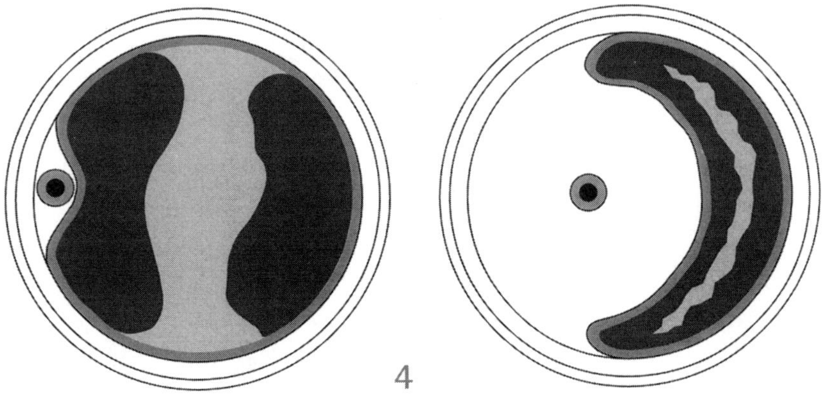

4

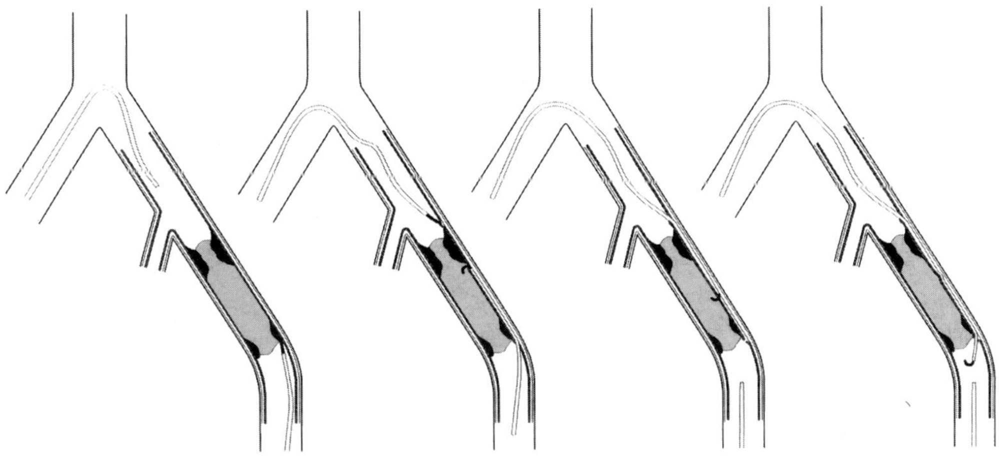

5

Subintimal and intraluminal angioplasty: cross-section

4

During intraluminal angioplasty, the catheter position is in the middle of the artery, surrounded by atheromatous disease. Upon balloon dilatation, the atheroma cracks and the disease is displaced in a concentric fashion.

With subintimal angioplasty, the catheter position is eccentric, between the diseased intima and media. Illustration 4 shows that after balloon dilatation the atheroma and occluding material is displaced eccentrically. A wide crescent-shaped, disease-free channel becomes available for blood flow.

Iliac subintimal angioplasty

5

After an ipsilateral puncture, a dissection is initiated from the distal part of an occlusion using an angled hydrophilic guidewire and the supporting Van Andel catheter. Whilst in some cases, recanalization can be achieved by ipsilateral dissection alone, in the majority of cases, the retrograde dissection has a tendency to extend upwards into the common iliac artery and the aorta. Since the intima becomes thicker as we extend towards the aorta, it becomes difficult to achieve re-entry. Hence, using a contralateral puncture and with a help of a sidewinder catheter, a dissection is initiated in an antegrade manner, using either a 'J' wire or an angled hydrophilic guidewire. The hydrophilic wire appears to work best in initiating a dissection. Have initiated the dissection, the hydrophilic guidewire is extended into the dissection space and manipulated, in order to meet up with the retrograde dissection. Since the two dissections are in the same plane, usually the antegrade crossing is achieved after manipulations. Having crossed the lesion antegradely, a balloon catheter is passed by crossover and the occluding lesion dilated. If the flow is impaired in any way or an inadequate channel is achieved, then the lesion is stented, usually with a self-expanding stent.

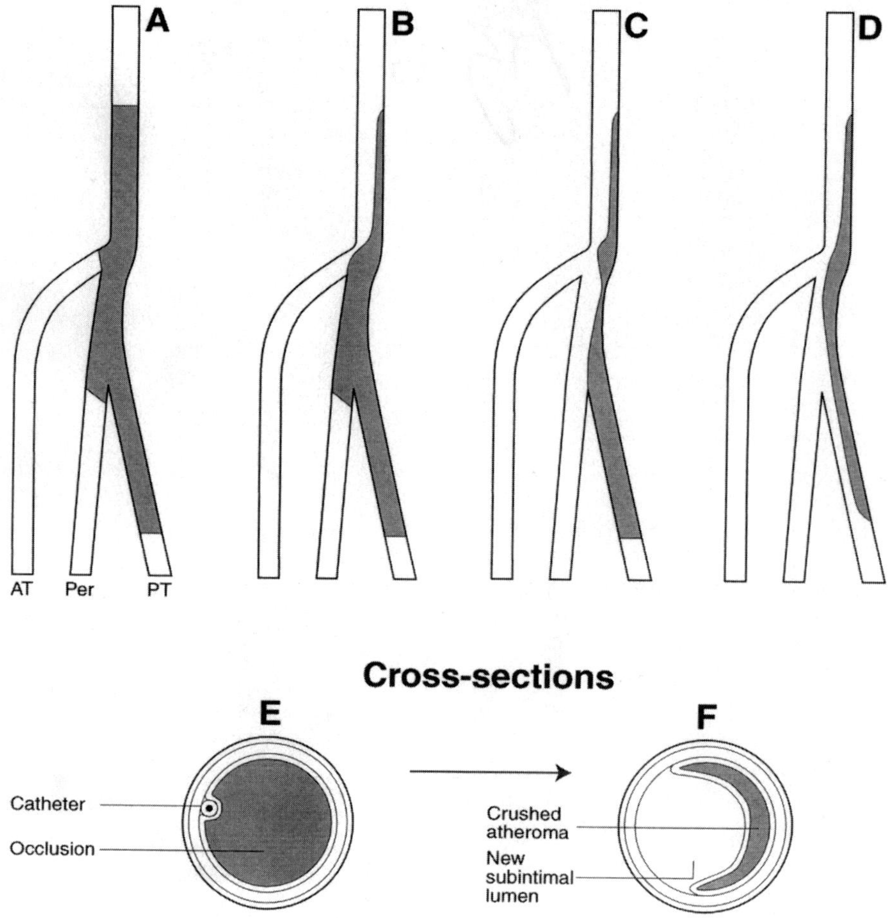

6

Subintimal angioplasty of a popliteal occlusion extending into the trifurcation

6

In patients with critical limb ischaemia, this is not an in frequent situation and would normally require a femorodistal bypass operation. With subintimal angioplasty, one or more of the run-off vessels can be recanalized and quite often, the entire trifurcation can be reconstructed. Dissection is initiated in the manner described for femoropopliteal occlusions. Using a loop in the hydrophilic guidewire, the dissection is extended until the trifurcation is reached. The hydrophilic wire normally moves quite freely in the dissection space but when there is an origin of a vessel, for example the anterior tibial artery, then the tip of the angled hydrophilic guidewire will 'catch' at the origin. At this point, the tip of the wire is persuaded to enter the origin of the artery, usually with the help of a backup catheter until it enters the origin of the anterior tibial artery. As soon as it has entered the origin, the wire is manipulated to form a loop which then allows extension of the dissection into the anterior tibial artery until re-entry is achieved into the patent part of the artery. The anterior tibial artery is dilated with a small balloon, usually 3mm in diameter and then the popliteal artery is dilated with a larger balloon, usually 5mm in diameter. Having established flow into one of the run-off vessels, the procedure is repeated, so that the dissection is then extended into one of the other run-off arteries, for example the peroneal artery. Flow is then established into the peroneal artery. Subsequently the posterior tibial artery is recanalized in the same fashion achieving reconstitution of all three vessels. The advantage of achieving all three run-off vessels is that the recanalized segment of the popliteal artery will have a better chance of a long-term patency because of the three run-off vessels rather than one.

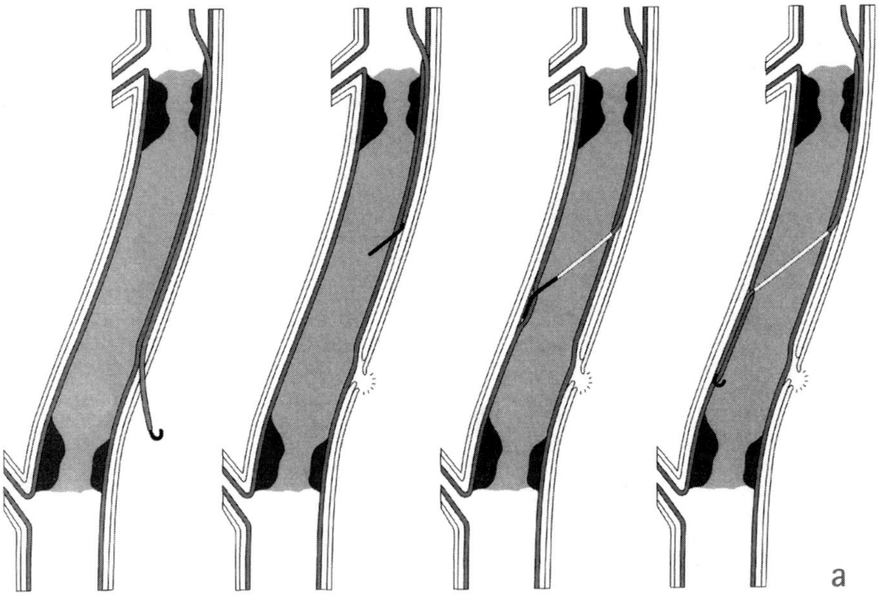

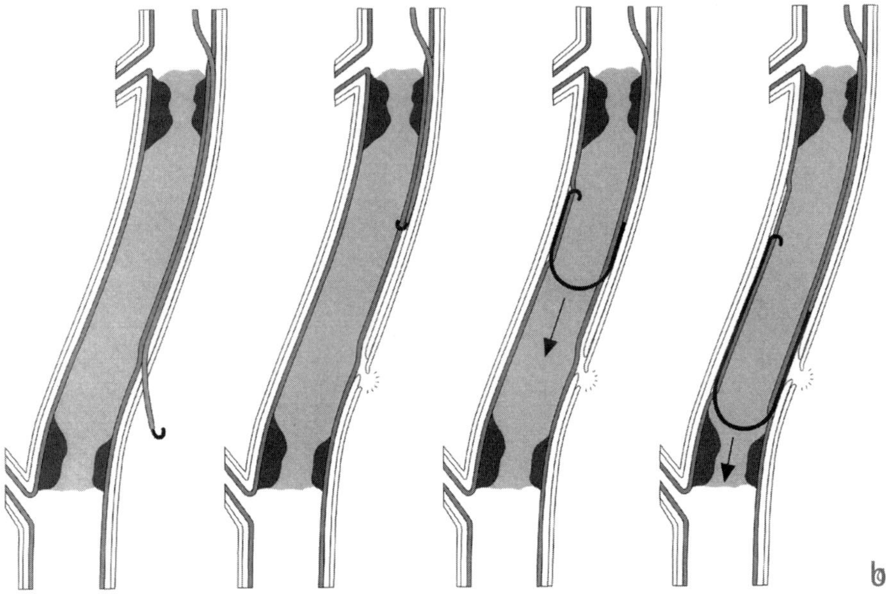

7

Avoidance of a perforated site using subintimal angioplasty

7a, b

When there is a hard and calcified occlusion, sometimes the catheter leaves the artery wall rather than extend through the dissection. In such situations, subintimal angioplasty allows the procedure to be continued, usually with a successful outcome. There are two ways of dealing with this situation: (**7a**) the catheter/guidewire combination is withdrawn from the site of the perforation and with the help of an angled wire and/or catheter, an alternative route of dissection is found and the procedure is continued to completion. (**7b**) Alternatively, having withdrawn the catheter above the site of the perforation, a large loop is formed in the guidewire. The loop is then extended through the length of the dissection. Assuming that the site of the perforation is not larger than the loop, then the loop will have a tendency to overshoot the site of the perforation and go along the dissection beyond the perforation. The procedure can then proceed as normal. The whole length of the dissection space is dilated as normal. The perforation is of no consequence, since the preferential flow is along the main dissection space through the length of the artery.

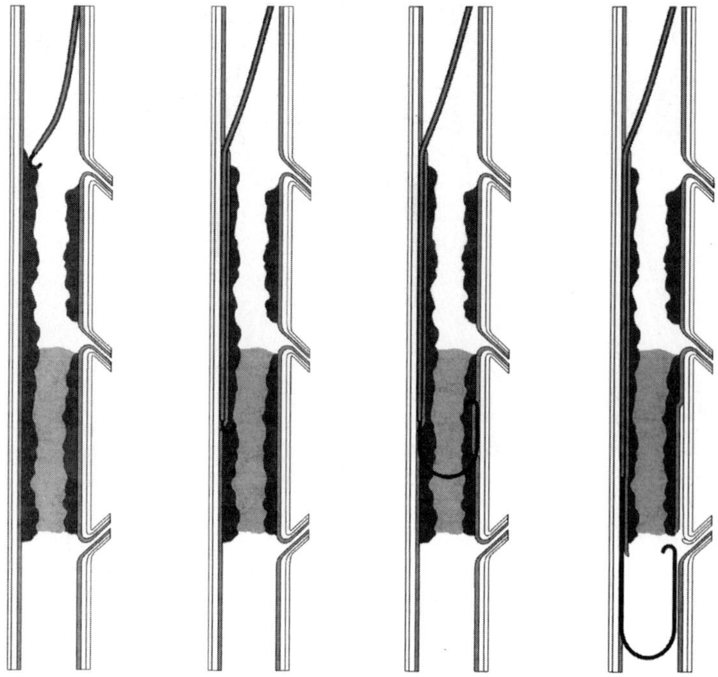

8

Dissecting the entire diseased segment

8

In some situations only part of the total diseased segment of the artery is an occlusion. It is our belief that long-term results are better with a lumen achieved by dissection rather than an intraluminal angioplasty. This being the case, we believe that the entire diseased segment must be excluded from the lumen by dissection rather than just the length of the occlusion. Hence, a dissection is initiated at the level where the diffusely diseased segment starts. Dissection is usually initiated with the help of an angled catheter (cobra shape), pointing towards the wall of the artery away from any collaterals. It may be necessary to use the hard end of an ordinary guidewire which has been angled to allow it to be directed towards the wall. Advancing this hard end of the guidewire into the wall of the artery allows the dissection to be initiated. The catheter is then advanced into the dissection and once the catheter tip is in this position, the hard end of the wire is substituted for an angled hydrophilic guidewire. The dissection is then extended in the usual manner and after re-entry is achieved beyond the occluding lesion, the whole length of the diseased segment is balloon dilated.

Acknowledgement
Illustrations by Kate Radford.

References

Bolia A (1998). Percutaneous intentional extraluminal (subintimal) recanalization of crural arteries. *Eur J Radiol* **28**: 199–204.

Bolia A, Bell PRF (1995). Femoropopliteal and crural artery recanalization using subintimal angioplasty. *Semin Vasc Surg* **3**: 253–264.

Bolia A, Fishwick G (1997). Recanalization of iliac artery occlusion by subintimal dissection using the ipsilateral and the contralateral approach. *Clin Radiol* **52**: 684–687.

Bolia A, Miles KA, Brennan PRF (1990). Percutaneous transluminal angioplasty of occlusions of the femoral and popliteal arteries by subintimal dissection. *Cardiovasc Intervent Radiol* **13**: 357–363.

Bolia A, Sayers RD, Thompson MM, Bell PRF (1994). Subintimal and intraluminal recanalization of occluded crural arteries by percutaneous balloon angioplasty. *Eur J Vasc Surg* **8**: 214–219.

Reekers JA, Bolia A (1998). Percutaneous intentional extraluminal (subintimal) recanalization: How to do it yourself. *Eur J Radiol* **28**: 192–198.

Femoropopliteal angioplasty followed by polytetrafluoroethylene stent-graft

Jacques Bleyn

Introduction

Angioplasty of long (> 7 cm) occlusions in the femoro-popliteal vessels has demonstrated poor long-term patency. Therefore other techniques are being developed including subintimal angioplasty (Bolia), stenting and stent grafting (Cejna *et al.*, 1999; Cikrit and Dalsing, 1998; Conroy *et al.*, 2000; Gray and Olin, 1997; Gray *et al.*, 1997; Karch *et al.*, 2000; Vroegindeweij *et al.*, 1997; Zdanowski *et al.*, 1999).

Long occlusions and a low flow state are typical for the superficial femoral and popliteal axis, as is the absence of important collateral vessels between the profunda and Hunter's canal.

When grafting of the popliteal artery is involved, a very flexible graft is necessary (**6b**).

Initial experience with bare stents and with self-made grafts including two Palmaz stents attached at each end of a polytetrafluoroethylene (PTFE)-graft (Impra® 3 mm) that were expanded after introduction through an incision in the proximal superficial femoral artery have had poor patency rates, mainly because of incontrollable neointimal hyperplasia in the exposed stents.

A new graft (Hemobahn® – Gore®) (**3**) with an expanded PTFE-lining inside a self-expandable nitinol stent with thermal memory makes it possible to create a PTFE in-line graft, a 'thru-pass' that gives patency rates comparable with classical femoropopliteal prosthetic bypass grafts (primary patency rate at 1 year: 79%; secondary: 93%) (Lammer *et al.*, 2000). These better results are because there is no interface between the blood and the stent material. This graft comes in diameters from 6 to 13 mm and in lengths of 5, 10 and 15 cm.

Diagnosis

Vascular diagnosis is made at the first visit of the patient and includes clinical examination, continuous wave Doppler with pressure measurements and a duplex scan ('one stop shop').

An intravenous digital subtraction angiography is performed when the extent of the occlusion or the outflow assessment is not clear after the non-invasive studies.

An appointment is made for treatment in our specialized one-day vascular unit (Antwerp Blood Vessel Centre).

Technique

Preparation of the patient

The patient has to restrain from food but is advised to have a liquid breakfast and to continue drinking the morning of his procedure. Anti-platelet aggregation medication is pursued. No premedication is given. The ipsilateral groin is shaved and an intravenous line installed. A cushion elevates the ipsilateral buttock to lengthen the femoral vessels (**1**).

Anaesthesia

Around the puncture site 10 cc of Xylocaine 1% with adrenaline is given.

Puncture

1

A 2-mm stab wound is made with an 11 blade and an antegrade puncture of the common femoral artery is performed 1–2 cm above the femoral bifurcation (**1**).

A 5 French Introducer is then placed in the origin of the superior femoral artery.

When the superficial femoral artery is occluded from its origin, a subintimal channel is created with a J-Terumo 0.035 inch guidewire loop (**2**).

Intra-arterial digital subtraction angiography of the popliteal artery and the tibial vessels is performed to indicate the site of recanalization of the popliteal artery under Hunter's canal and to document the base-line tibial anatomy. This first angiogram is essential to identify peripheral embolization during the procedure, as most patients have no preoperative angiogram,

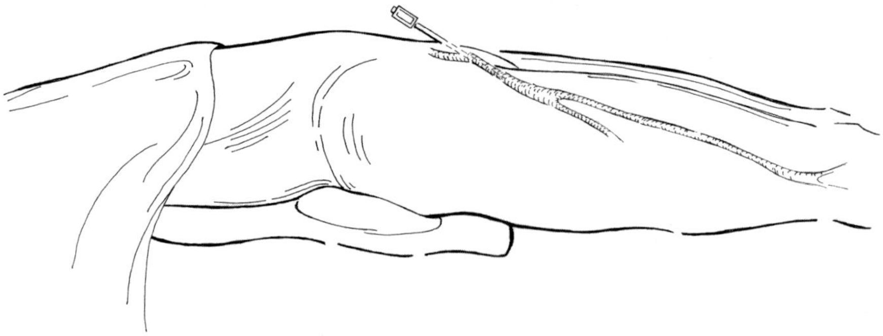

1

Subintimal angioplasty

2

The technique for subintimal angioplasty followed by a balloon dilation described in the previous chapter by Aman Bolia is followed (2). The radiological image of the subintimal channel is often not very reassuring. Therefore the study of the flow after intra-arterial papaverine (50 mg) will help us decide to cover this helicoidally dissected channel (5) with a PTFE stent-graft. In our experience, this will happen in 50% of the cases. When the flow is low, 5000 units of heparin are administered intravenously. Otherwise only 2500 units of heparin per 1000 cc of saline are used as a flushing solution for introducers and angiocatheters without general heparinization.

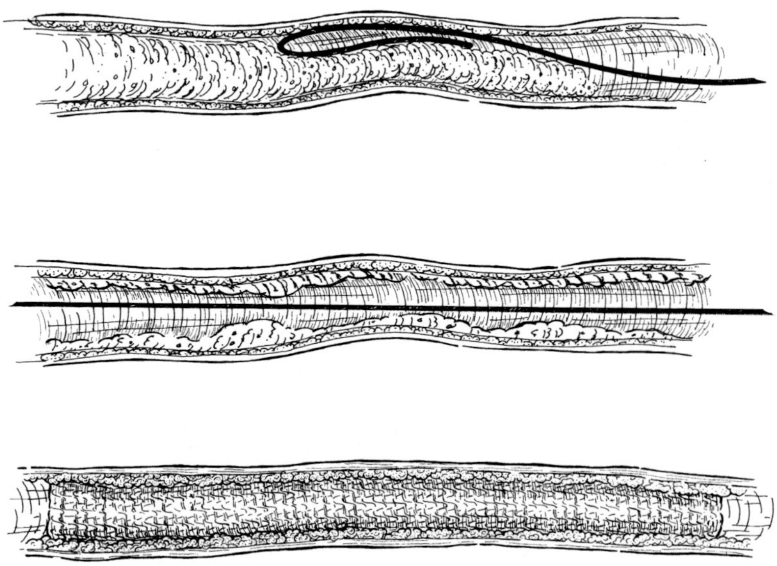

2

Stent-graft insertion and deployment

3

Over the guidewire, the 5 French introducer is exchanged for an 8 or 9 French. Then, the 0.035-inch guidewire is exchanged for one of 0.025 inches. The diameters of the popliteal artery, distal to the recanalized lesion, and of the superficial femoral artery proximal to the lesion are measured as well as the total length of superior femoral artery that we want to cover.

First the distal graft, mostly 6 mm × 15 cm, is positioned at the popliteal level. Deployment is done by an assistent who pulls the laced suture that constrains the graft. Deployment of the stent-graft inside the vessel is shown in 3. The graft deploys from proximal to distal and does not foreshorten (3). A 10-cm long 'touch-up' balloon with a diameter equal to that of the graft takes out eventual wrinkles. A second graft is then introduced proximally into the first one with a minimum overlap of 1 cm. Usually this graft has the same diameter as the distal one but it can be up to 2 mm larger in diameter.

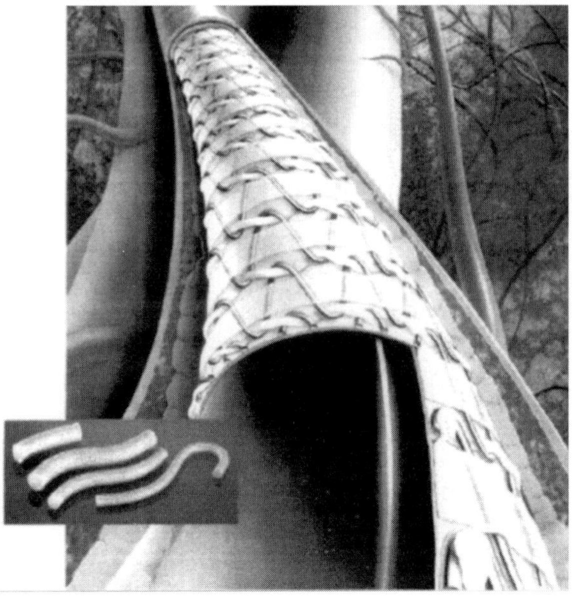

3

When the superficial femoral artery is occluded from its origin, a reference arteriogram is taken with the image intensifier inclined 45 degrees towards the treated side to have a deployment of the proximal graft as close as possible to the origin of the profunda (7). One should not forget to withdraw the introducer into the common femoral artery with such a proximal deployment.

Experience has shown that the proximal 1–2 cm of the superficial femoral artery have a marked tendency to restenose, jeopardizing the distal reconstruction. 'Touch-up' ballooning of the proximal graft and the junction of both grafts is performed with a matched balloon.

A control angiogram is taken after an additional 50 mg of papaverine through the introducer to document a good anatomical reconstruction (6). Special attention is given to the below-knee vessels to identify eventual periferal embolization. This happens in 7% of the cases and can be treated immediately by catheter aspiration or *in situ* thrombolysis with urokinase.

Closure of the puncture site

A percutaneous suturing closure device (Perclose®) (8) is always used because, in our opinion, compression of the groin with impairment of superficial femoral artery flow and even possible obstruction of the proximal part of the stent-graft will have a negative impact on outcome. Because the procedure is done on outpatients, early ambulation is safer with a suture on the groin puncture especially when it is situated above the inguinal ligament.

Postoperative medication

Acetyl salicylic acid is given when there is good flow; clopidogrel is additionally prescribed in low-flow situations or with poor outflow vessel quality.

Patient examples

4, 5, 6, 7, 8

Illustration 4 shows total occlusion of the right superficial femoral artery.

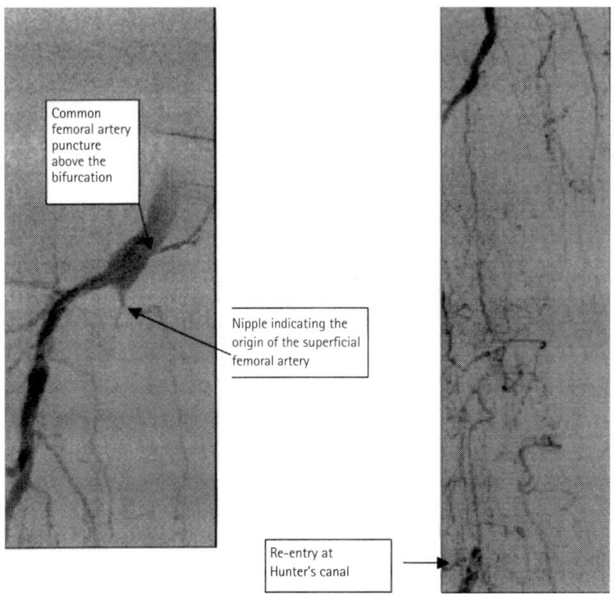

4

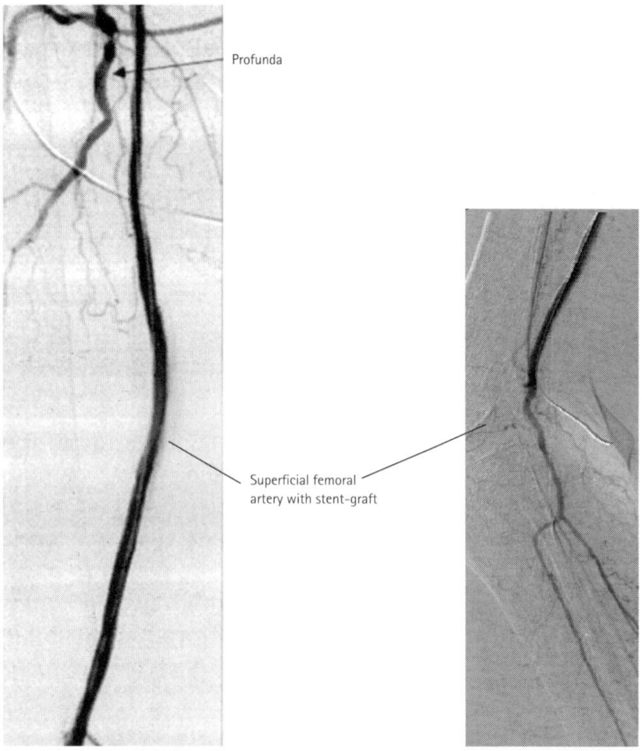

6a 6b

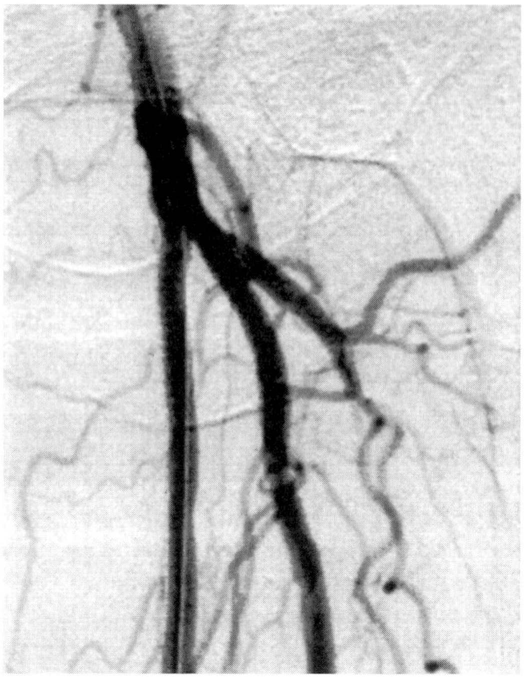

7

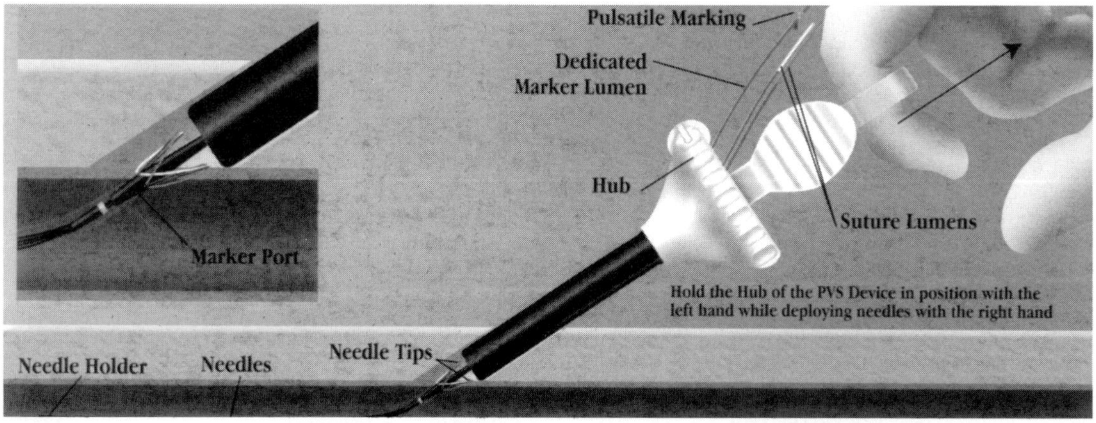

8

Illustration 5 shows helicoidal aspect after subintimal recanalization and percutaneous transluminal angioplasty.

Illustration 6 shows endovascular lining with a PTFE stent-graft: no kinking at the knee joint.

Illustration 7 shows the placement of the stent-graft right at the origin of the superficial femoral artery.

Illustration 8 shows subcutaneous suture placement on the vessel puncture.

Conclusion

When subintimal angioplasty of femoropopliteal occlusions fails to give an acceptable radiological image or a sufficient flow, internal lining with a PTFE-covered 'thru-pass' stent-graft will give in the long run good primary and secondary patency rates that are comparable with those of femoropopliteal synthetic bypass grafts. Experience shows that the whole superficial femoral artery has to be covered because the progression of the atheromatous degeneration of the proximal superficial femoral artery is much faster than anticipated.

Although this procedure is performed under local anaesthesia on outpatients, the cost-benefit analysis has still to be determined.

References

Cejna M, Schoder M, Lammer J (1999). PTA vs stent in femoro-popliteal obstruction. *Radiologe* **39**: 144–150.

Cikrit DF, Dalsing MC (1998). Lower-extremity arterial endovascular stenting. *Surg Clin North Am* **78**: 617–629.

Conroy RM, Gordon IL, Tobis JM *et al.* (2000) Angioplasty and stent placement in chronic occlusion of the superficial femoral artery: technique and results. *J Vasc Intervent Radiol* **11**: 1009–1020.

Gray BH, Olin JW (1997). Limitations of percutaneous transluminal angioplasty with stenting for femoropopliteal arterial occlusive disease. *Semin Vasc Surg* **10**: 8–16.

Gray BH, Sullivan TM, Childs MB *et al.* (1997). High incidence of restenosis/reocclusion of stents in the percutaneous treatment of long-segment superficial femoral artery disease after suboptimal angioplasty. *J Vasc Surg* **25**: 74–83.

Karch LA, Mattos MA, Henretta JP *et al.* (2000). Clinical failure after percutaneous transluminal angioplasty of the superficial femoral and popliteal arteries. *J Vasc Surg* **31**: 880–887.

Lammer J, Dake MD, Bleyn J *et al.* (2000). Peripheral arterial obstruction: prospective study of treatment with a transluminally placed self-expanding stent-graft. International Trial Study Group. *Radiology* **217**: 95–104.

Vroegindeweij D, Vos LD, Tielbeek AV *et al.* (1997). Balloon angioplasty combined with primary stenting versus balloon angioplasty alone in femoropopliteal obstructions: A comparative randomized study. *Cardiovasc Intervent Radiol* **20**: 420–425.

Zdanowski Z, Albrechtsson U, Lundin A *et al.* Percutaneous transluminal angioplasty with or without stenting for femoropopliteal occlusions? A randomized controlled study. *Int Angiol* **18**: 251–255.

Endovascular treatment of popliteal aneurysm

G Deriu, P Frigatti, S Bonvini,
S Lepidi, R Ragazzi, F Grego

1

Initial information on aneurysm size and neck measurements can be obtained by colour coded Duplex scanning.

Digital subtraction angiography is required to evaluate:

- Aneurysm extension.
- Proximal and distal necks.
- Significant collateral vessels originating from the aneurysm.
- Distal outflow.

The choice of stent sizes is based on data from both examinations. Contraindications to endovascular treatment are:

- Distal neck < 1 cm.
- Poor distal runoff.
- Symptoms of nerve and vein compression.

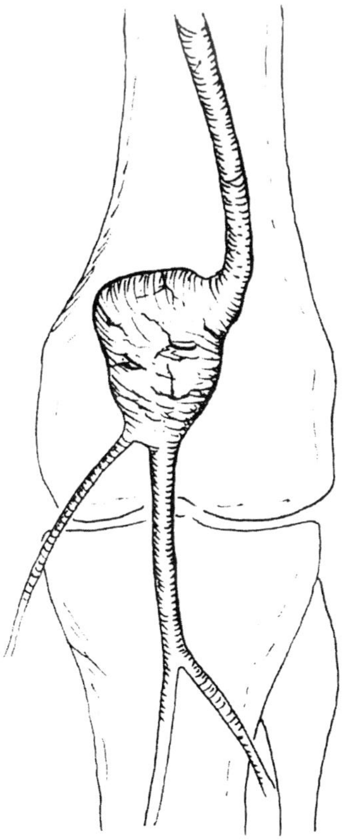

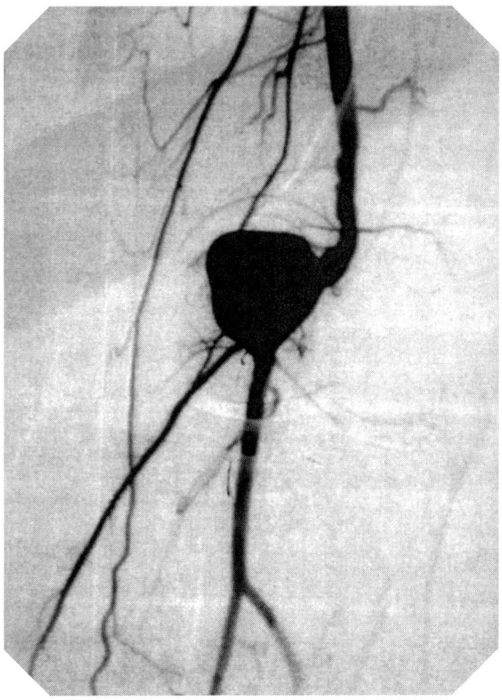

a 7 b

2

The Hemobahn® (Gore, Falstaff, Arizona, USA) endoprosthesis was used for the popliteal aneurysm treatment.

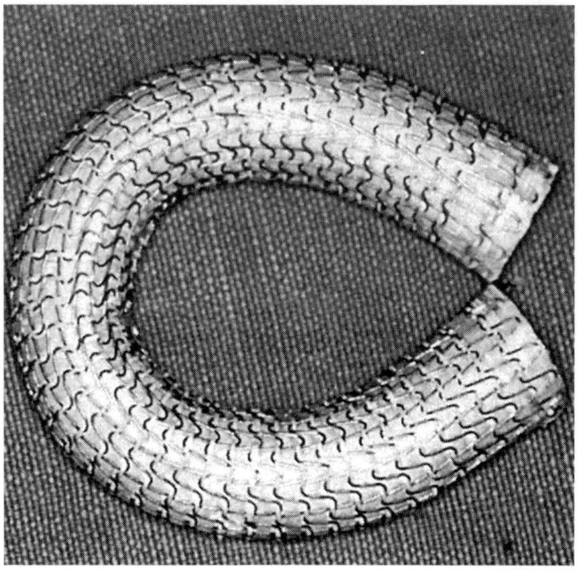

2

Knee joint movements should be taken into account in the endovascular treatment of popliteal aneurysm. The ideal graft should have good flexibility and resistance to external compression, so that occlusion and dislodgement are avoided.

The Hemobhan is a self-expanding nitinol stent, internally covered by an ultra-thin polytetrafluoroethylene (PTFE) graft. Therefore, it is a biocompatible graft with a smooth blood contact surface. Moreover, the special nitinol stent design, reducing the number of net junctions, allows the combination of flexibility and radial stiffness. Kinking risk is reduced.

The Hemobahn graft sizes range from 6 mm to 13 mm in diameter, and from 5 cm to 13 cm in length.

Two clear linear radiopaque markers along the graft allow an easy and exact deployment in the target vessels. The stent graft is released from the catheter as containing lacing fibre is withdrawn.

3a, b, c, d

The anterograde percutaneous transfemoral puncture (18 G needle, 9 F sheath, Terumo guidewire 150 cm, 0.025) (3a) is performed under local anaesthesia.

The final choice of stent sizes is confirmed by the intraoperative angiography. [See the 5 mm rx opaque marker in 3c.]

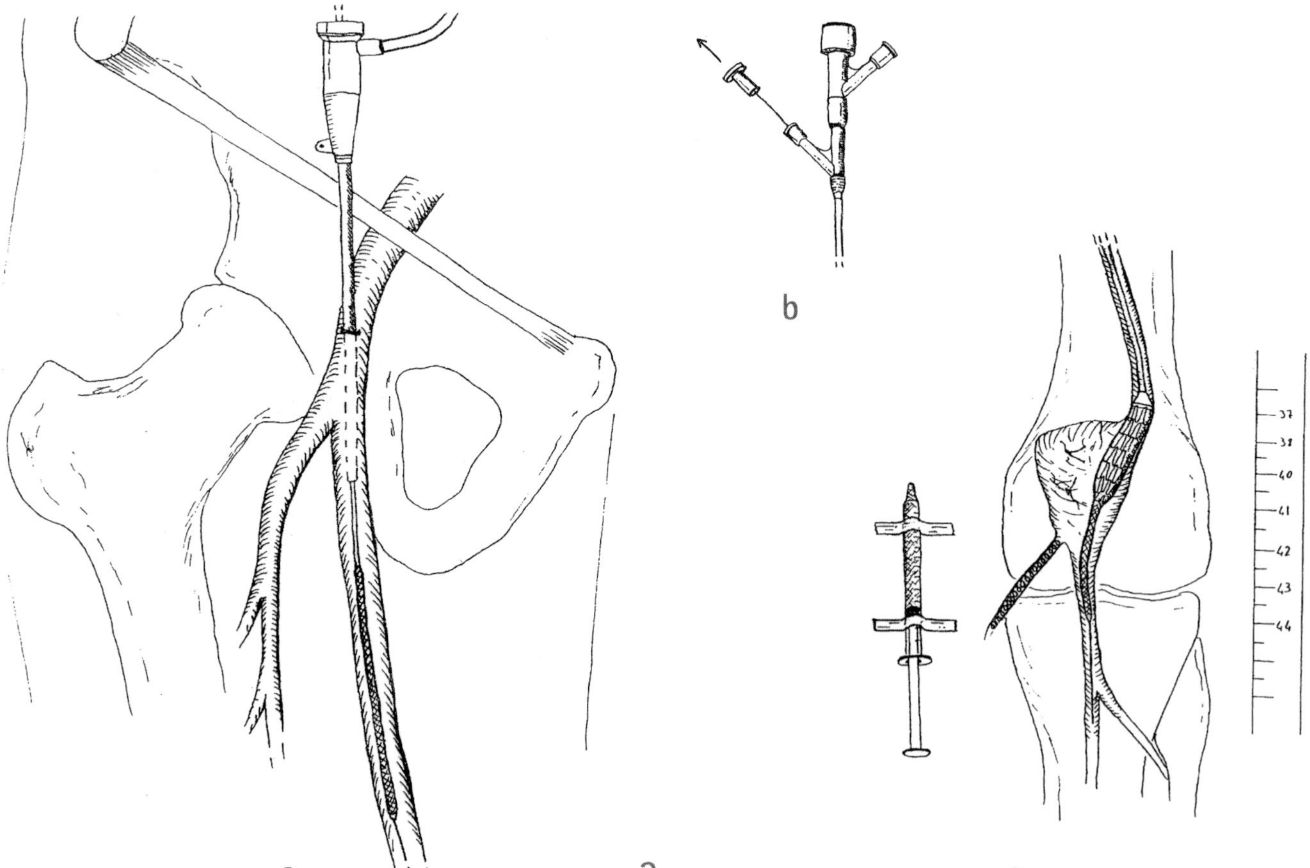

a b c

3

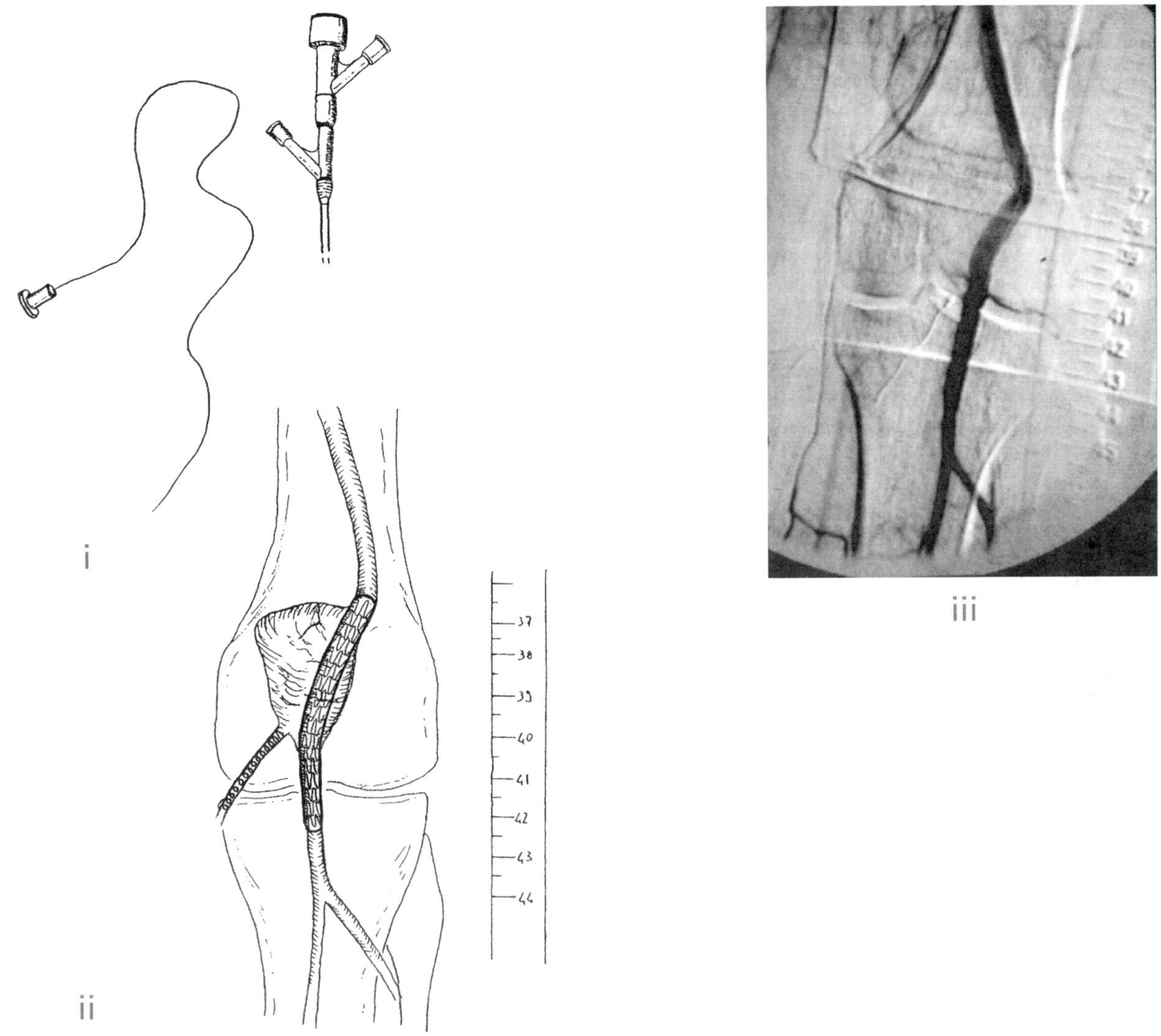

3d

Stent diameters must take into account a 20–25% oversizing.

In choosing the graft length, it is necessary to consider that the stent extremity should not land at the knee joint region or very proximal to it (2–3 cm). Indeed, in this anatomical area, the popliteal artery shows the maximal flexibility.

Deployment begins with a steady, continuous pull of the deployment knob (**3b**).

The stent-graft is released from the catheter as the lacing fibre is withdrawn, beginning from the proximal end (**3c**). Deployment is complete when the expanded ePTFE lacing fibre is fully withdrawn from the catheter (**3d**).

When significant sural branches are present (as in the case presented), coil embolization is required before stent introduction, in order to avoid the possibility of a grade II endoleak. [See angiography **1b** and **3c**.]

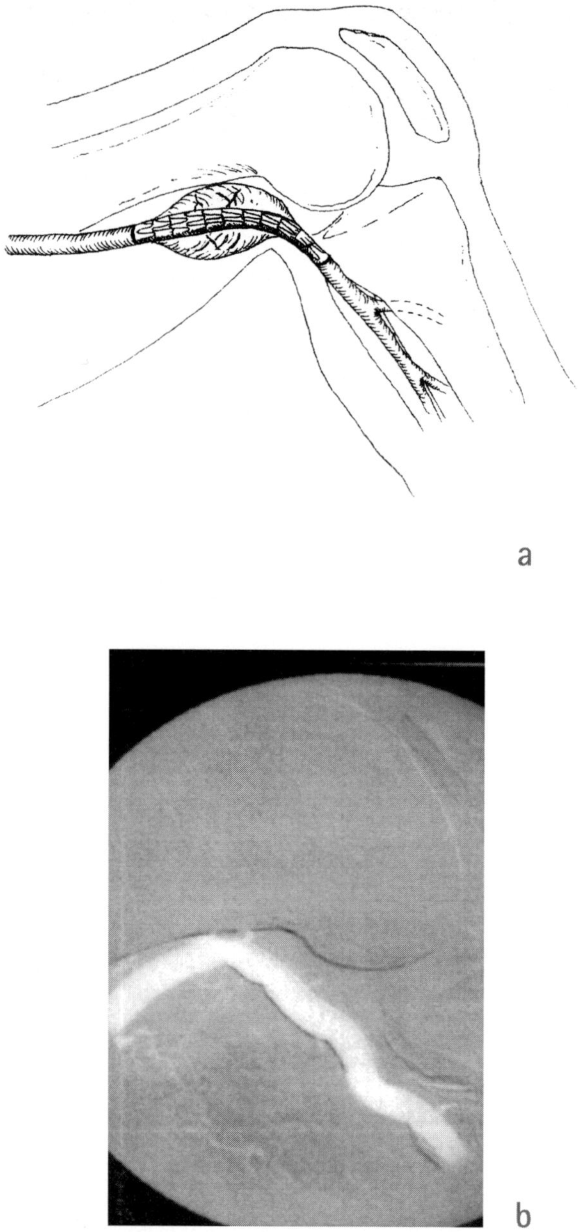

a

b

4

4a, b

The endovascular procedure is considered successful when popliteal aneurysm is completely excluded with no signs of endoleaks. No stent kinking should be detected during forced leg flexion and other knee joint movements.

Above-knee amputation

Hero Van Urk

Introduction

Although the ratio of above-knee amputations to below-knee amputations has changed over the last decades in favour of the latter, the actual number of above-knee amputations has not decreased dramatically.

Whenever possible, an above-knee amputation should be avoided if it is possible to perform either a below-knee or through-knee amputation. The functional results of rehabilitation of patients with a below-knee prosthesis is infinitely better than those with an above-knee prosthesis.

In almost all cases where this operation is indicated, the superficial femoral artery is occluded, leaving the profunda femoral artery (or its remaining branches) as the only remaining blood supply for the thigh muscles. Usually, this arterial supply is further compromised, resulting in insufficient oxygenation of the distal part of the muscles. Hence the principle of preserving as much leg length as possible no longer applies once the decision to perform an above-knee amputation has been taken.

1

Conventional knee mechanisms extend 8–10 cm into the thigh portion of the prosthesis. Therefore, if a thigh amputation is performed too far distally, this may cause problems with prosthetic fitting and unequal knee height. This difficulty has caused some reluctance on the part of surgeons to perform through-knee amputations, but the most recent prosthetic techniques have overcome this. Nevertheless, a too distal diaphyseal amputation may result in an excessively long stump, which is of no benefit to the patient; such a stump end has poor weight-bearing abilities, in contrast to the mid-diaphyseal or through-knee amputation.

On the other hand, an amputation which leaves the limb too short, is equally to be avoided. About 10 cm below the minor trochanter is the upper limit of an amputation. A shorter stump will lead to a flexion-abduction contracture, which poses a problem both cosmetically and functionally. Disarticulation in the hip is preferred in such cases, usually after a high above-knee amputation has failed to heal properly.

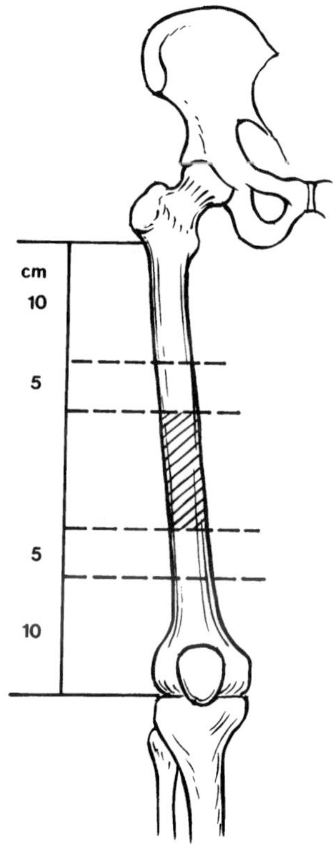

1

The operation

2

The patient is placed in the supine position. Usually, general anaesthesia is preferred, but epidural anaesthesia or a regional block can be given to elderly patients with a critical medical condition.

If gangrene of the foot or lower leg is present, the foot can be packed in a plastic bag. In cases of wet gangrene, the author prefers to administer antibiotics intravenously the evening before the operation. If there is dry necrosis or rest pain only, antibiotics are started just after induction of anaesthesia and continued for 24 h postoperatively.

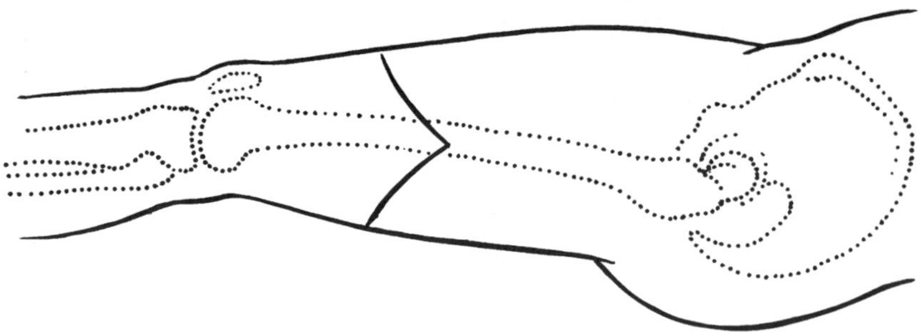

2

After suitable skin preparation and draping, the intended skin incision is marked with a sterile marker pen, having the dorsal flap slightly shorter than the anterior flap. The apex of the angle between the anterior and posterior flaps is approximately at the level of transection of the shaft of the femur. On both sides this point is in the mid-medial and mid-lateral line of the thigh or slightly more to the dorsal side.

3

An incision is made through the subcutaneous tissue and the fascia femoris. If still intact, the greater saphenous vein is transected and ligated. In cases where an *in situ* saphenous vein bypass has previously been performed, this conduit is likely to be thrombosed, but, if not, special care should be taken to avoid blood loss from this source.

After completion of the skin and fascia incisions, the skin usually retracts somewhat on both sides. The muscle incision should be in the same line as the skin incision, because of the tendency of muscles to retract even more than skin.

The anterior and lateral muscles are divided first. When the medial muscles are incised, care should be taken to locate the superficial femoral vessels first. After separate ligation of artery and vein, the deep femoral artery and the sciatic nerve are exposed. In order to minimize neuroma formation, the sciatic nerve is identified anteriorly to the hamstring muscles and is pulled down and divided after ligation of the arteria concomitans. The author prefers not to ligate the sciatic nerve itself, because this is thought to cause more neuroma formation and/or phantom pain.

There seems to be no guaranteed method of avoiding neuroma formation, but the nerve should always be allowed to retract well upwards between the surrounding muscles. It may be of some value for pain relief in the immediate postoperative period to inject the nerve with a local anaesthetic like Marcaine® (bupivacaine).

4

When all muscles have been divided and all bleeding points are clamped and ligated proximally, the periosteum of the femur is incised circumferentially. The periosteum is then pushed upward 3–4 cm. The femoral shaft is divided with a saw, the level of the bony amputation being 4–5 cm more proximal than the musculocutaneous flap.

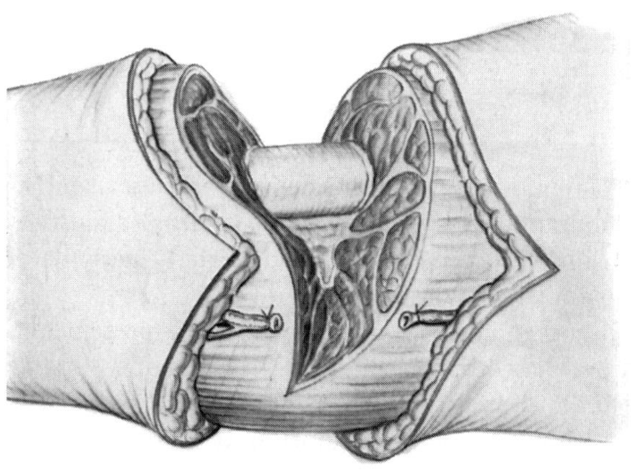

3

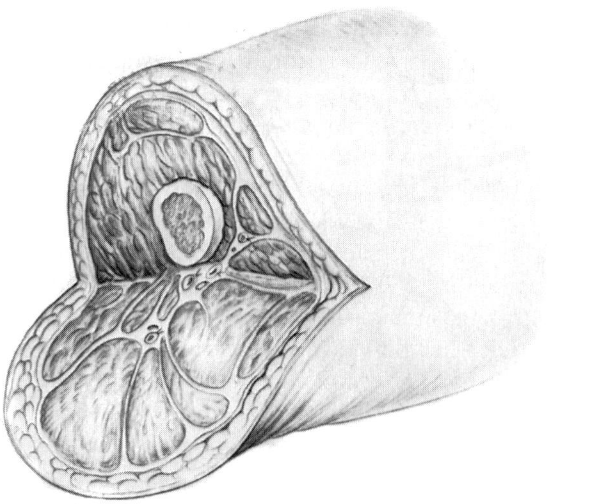

4

After the muscle flaps have been bevelled, accurate haemostasis is obtained. In diabetic patients with calcified small vessels, all bleeding points need to be ligated, preferably with absorbable material, because electrocautery may not be sufficient in such cases.

5

In order to prevent retraction of the muscles causing the overlying skin to press directly against the femoral stump, a myodesis is desirable in most cases and especially when the muscles are hypotrophic. Three to five holes are drilled in the distal femoral cortex with a thin (2–2.5 mm) drill.

Using absorbable sutures, the fascia of the anterior quadriceps flap can be fixed over the top of the femoral stump to the dorsal side of the cortex, together with the dorsal muscles.

The wound is then closed by approximating – with minimal tension – the anterior fascia to the posterior fascia, using interrupted sutures. One or two suction drains are left deep in the wound. No subcutaneous sutures are necessary and the skin is closed in one layer, preferably with interrupted monofilament nylon sutures.

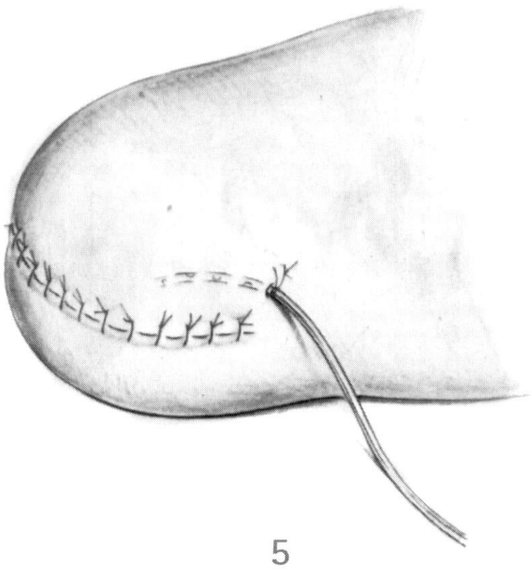

5

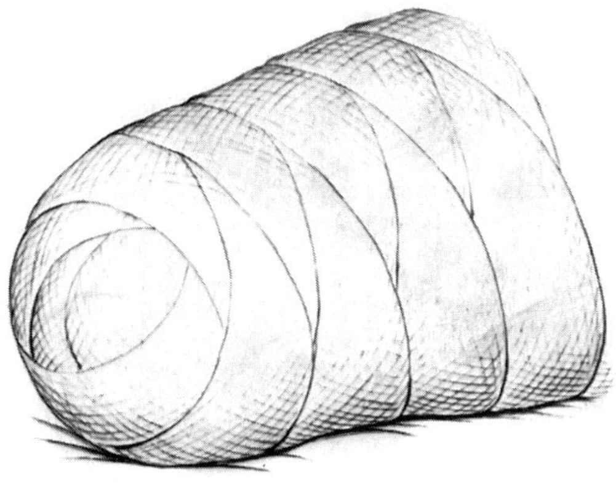

6

Postoperative care

6

Sterile dressings are applied, followed by synthetic orthopaedic padding and, finally, a cotton stretch bandage. This dressing can be left in place for several days unless the patient complains of increasing pain, which may be caused by swelling of the stump.

In some clinics, elevation of the stump on a pillow for the first 24–48 h is advised. The author prefers to keep the stump flat on the bed to prevent a flexion contracture. Exercises can be started after the first few postoperative days. Lying in a prone position for several short periods during the day may be helpful in the prevention of a flexion contracture.

Cotton elastic bandages are applied and regularly changed in order to aid shrinkage of the stump. In contrast with below-knee amputations, no temporary plaster cast is used; instead, a prosthesis is fitted directly when the stump is free of oedema after application of the elastic dressings. Unfortunately, only a small proportion of vascular patients are able to follow a complete rehabilitation programme, and the number of elderly patients who are eventually able to walk again is disappointing.

Acknowledgement

Illustrations by R N Lane.

Through-knee amputation

Kingsley Robinson

Introduction

The through-knee amputation is the quickest major lower limb amputation that can be performed as no bony structure needs to be divided and ligation of the single large popliteal artery and its accompanying veins controls nearly all the bleeding that can be encountered. Only the long saphenous vein usually requires an additional ligature. The large size of the femoral condyles means that ample skin must be provided for adequate and lax skin cover, otherwise skin necrosis can be produced by tension across the edges of the articular surface. It is also important that the patella retains its normal position on the front of the knee rather than being drawn down where it may be subjected to weight-bearing stresses and produce extreme discomfort. The procedure is so atraumatic and speedy that it can be carried out as a debriding procedure prior to a definitive higher amputation. The absence of noise, because no saw is required, is a great asset when operating on patients under regional anaesthesia.

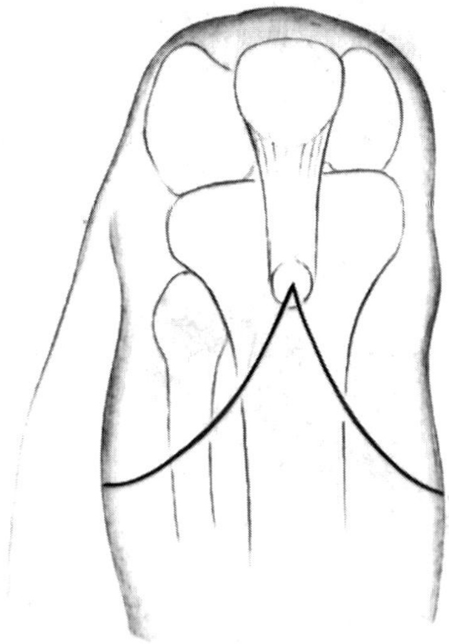

1

1

Lateral and medial sagittal flaps centred on the tibial tubercle anteriorly and the fold at the flexion line in the popliteal fossa constitute the most satisfactory skin flaps. The classical skin flap is a long anterior flap with a transverse scar across the popliteal fossa, and if this incision is used the patient is best placed prone with the distal part of the leg flexed to provide access to the anterior structures. This is an unsatisfactory position for the severely ill patient with vascular disease and a supine position with the hip flexed is entirely satisfactory if sagittal flaps are utilized. The skin incision is cut at one with the subcutaneous fat but the fascia lata and aponeurotic fibres of the lower leg muscles need not be incised.

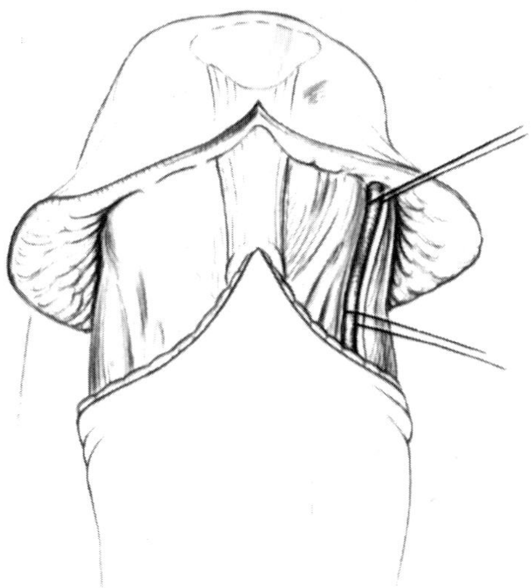

2

2

The skin flaps are elevated by brushing upwards with a wet swab and the patella tendon is defined and its insertion into the tibial tubercle. At this stage the long saphenous vein will be ligated with fine catgut or vicryl, care being taken to avoid inclusion of the saphenous nerve.

3

Retraction on the medial and lateral flap will be necessary to obtain exposure of the tibial plateau. The patella tendon is then divided, erasing it from the patella tubercle to obtain a maximum length and held in a tissue forcep. The patella tendon can be elevated to provide additional retraction and exposure of the fat pad that is anterior to the synovial membrane covering the cruciate ligaments. The joint capsule is incised transversely to each side of the patella tendon exposing the condyles of the femur and if correctly placed the genicular cartilages should be left attached to the tibial plateau. Further flexion of the knee allows clear exposure of the cruciate ligaments. The hamstring tendons and the medial ligament of the knee joint can then be divided as can the lateral ligaments and biceps femoris tendon, allowing further flexion when the cruciate ligaments themselves can be divided leaving as much length as possible attached to the femur.

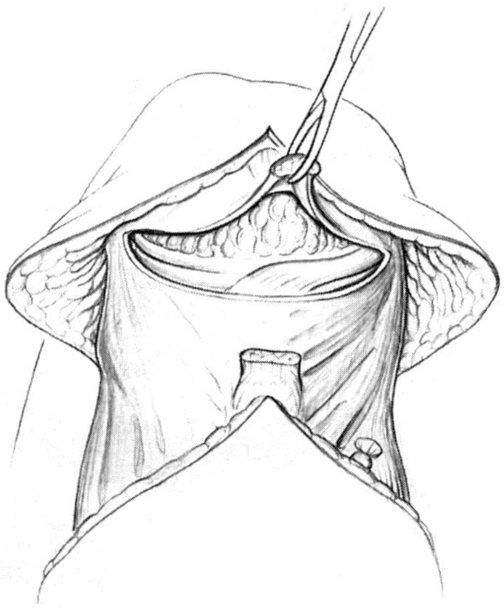

3

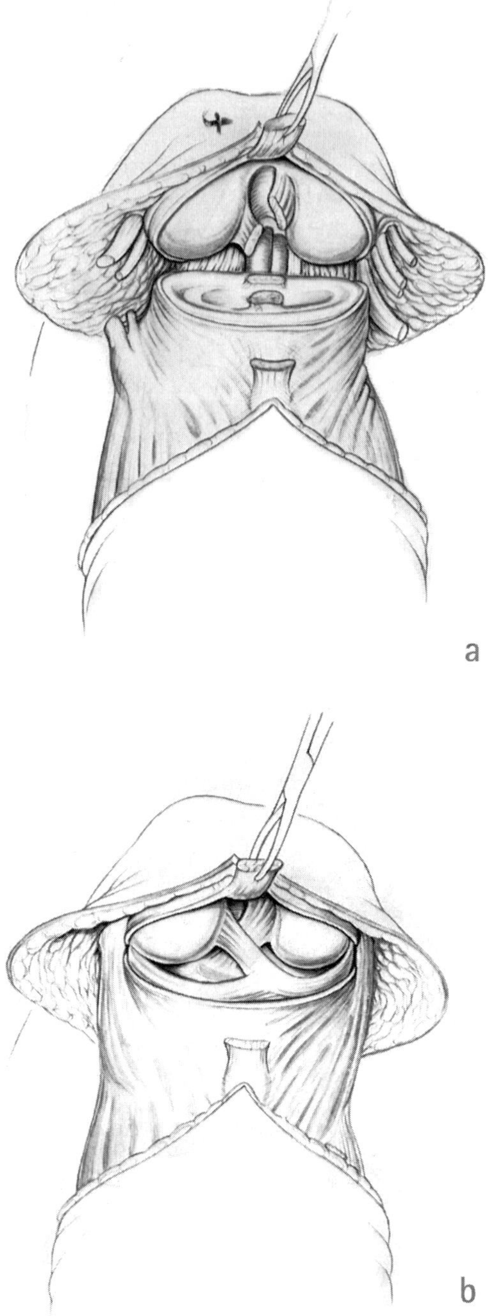

a

b

4

4a, b

The posterior part of the knee joint capsule can then be incised. Access to the popliteal artery and its veni comitans can either be obtained through the back of the knee joint capsule with some traction on the tibia or, alternatively, a finger can be hooked around the medial head of the gastrocnemius which can then be erased from the point of origin above the femoral condyle when the popliteal artery has been ligated and divided. The two elements of the sciatic nerve can also be transected under tension with the proximal end allowed to retract as far as possible. The lateral head of the gastrocnemius can also be divided.

5, 6a, b

When all these structures are completely divided the specimen is freed. The hamstring tendons and biceps tendons are marked with artery forceps and preserved and haemostasis secured. Myoplasty is effected by anchoring the biceps femoris tendon and the semimembranosis gracivis and semitendonosis tendons being attached to

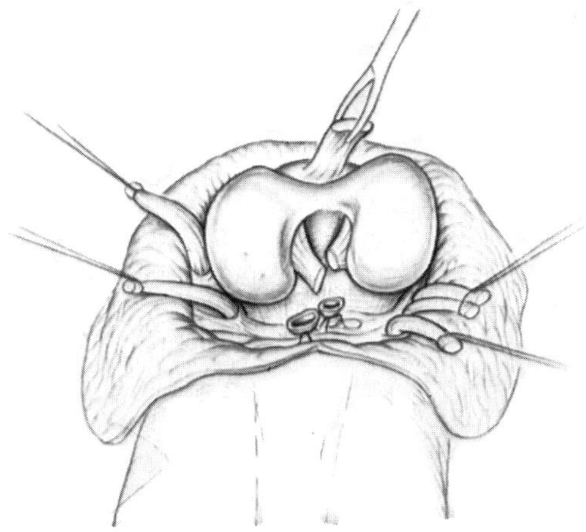

5

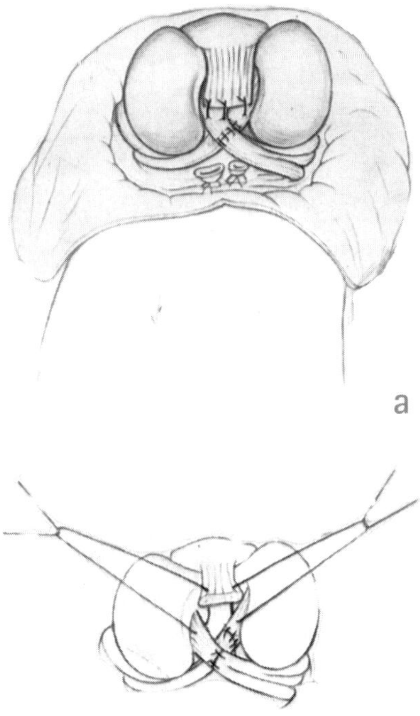

a

b

6

the residue of the cruciate ligaments. These sutures have to hold the tendons against considerable tension when the muscles are active and must be at least 1 chromicatgut or 0 vicryl. At this stage the patellar tendon is also sutured into the intercondylar notch securely attached to the residue of the cruciate ligaments, and care must be taken not to pull the patellar tendon down too far and to allow it to remain in its anatomical position in relation to the anterior surface of the femoral condyles. At this stage

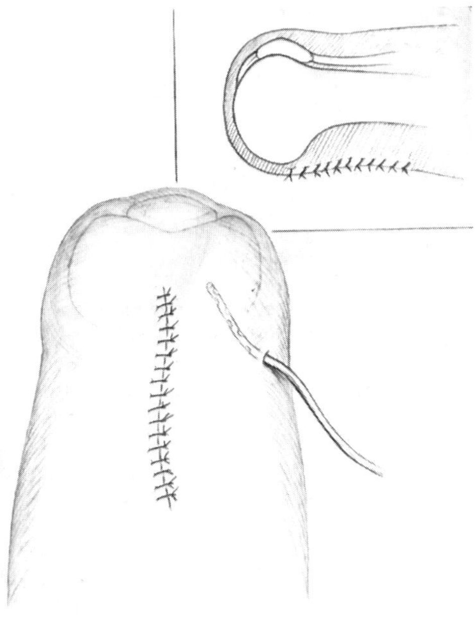

7

there should be an appreciable excess of skin in the flaps and the skin can usually be closed in a single layer. In case of continuing synovial fluid production a Redivac drain is best placed across the condyles and, leaving the stump well above the condylar area, the skin is closed as a single layer of subcutaneous fat using vertical interrupted mattress sutures.

7

When the suture line is complete it will be found that the scar lies entirely within and above the femoral intercondylar notch and the skin area related to the inferior surface of the femoral condyles is free of any sutures or scar tissue. This allows the stump to be used for terminal weight-bearing, a great advantage in prosthetic design as ischial weight-bearing can be avoided. Many patients with bilateral through-knee amputations learn to crawl on the stump ends and may be mobile without any prosthesis at all. If the patient finds this mode of progression satisfactory, provision of knee bootees can be of some value.

Acknowledgement

Illustrations by R N Lane.

Posterior-flap below-knee amputation

Charles N McCollum

Introduction

In modern practice, over 80% of all lower limb amputations are for peripheral vascular disease with the majority performed by vascular surgeons. These amputations are usually necessary because the severity of distal disease prevents arterial reconstruction, acute or severe ischaemia is prolonged, or our reconstructions fail. Nevertheless, the purpose is to relieve pain and to restore mobility to a patient who would otherwise have been immobilized either by pain or by developing gangrene. Amputation surgery therefore requires to be of the highest standard with gentle handling of ischaemic tissues to achieve primary healing. The type of amputation will be tailored to the individual needs of the patient and to their ability to regain full mobility. The surgeon must work in close cooperation with his limb-fitting service, as there is little point in achieving excellent primary healing rates if the resulting stump will only accommodate a difficult or clumsy prosthesis.

In major lower limb amputation, below-knee amputation has substantial advantages for rehabilitation over both through-knee and above-knee amputation. Only 20 years ago it was rarely performed in arterial disease because the anterior flap suffered necrosis and the amputation had to be revised to above-knee. The use of a longer posterior flap was advocated by Kendrick in 1956, but the modern posterior flap technique was popularized a decade later by Burgess (1968; Burgess *et al.*, 1971). Although the proportion of below-knee to above-knee amputations was 6 : 1 in Kendrick's series, the tragedy of vascular surgery over the following 20 years was that this ratio was progressively reversed, with many vascular surgeons rarely performing below-knee amputation.

Selection for below-knee amputation

Where an amputation is essential, or arterial reconstruction is not possible or has failed, it requires to be performed in such a way as to ensure the greatest chance of the patient returning to full mobility and independence and with the objective of achieving primary healing. Perhaps one reason that above-knee amputation became so frequent was that primary healing could almost be guaranteed. In below-knee amputation, particularly when operating in an ischaemic calf, the technique is critical to achieve primary healing. On our vascular surgical service, above-knee amputation is now reserved for those patients with crippling disability, such as hemiplegia, where mobilization is impossible. As a result, we have only performed 24 such procedures over the last 5 years, with 6 of these being revisions of below-knee amputations. Over the same interval, we have performed 61 below-knee amputations with an in-hospital mortality of 6.5% and revision to above-knee in just under 10%. These results can be achieved even where there is no recordable arterial pressure at the ankle by Doppler as the long posterior flap is based on the collateral blood supply to the calf.

Blood supply to the posterior flap

1

In the majority of patients for amputation, the popliteal artery and the posterior calf arteries are completely occluded, otherwise arterial reconstruction would be possible. An example of a typical arteriogram in a patient where distal reconstruction may not be possible is shown (1) where the superficial femoral artery is patent down to the mid-popliteal with complete occlusion of the distal popliteal and all calf arteries. An almost invariable feature of such cases is a fan of collaterals, including the sural artery, arising with its apex in the suprageniculate vessels. These collaterals fill either from thigh collaterals if the sugrageniculate popliteal is occluded or from the suprageniculate arteries themselves. They then ramify distally, posterior to the gastrocnemius with branches entering the gastrocnemius. These vessels may represent the main source of supply of the lower limb as there are very few collaterals passing down in the tissues anterior to the knee. Clearly collateralization to the anterior skin

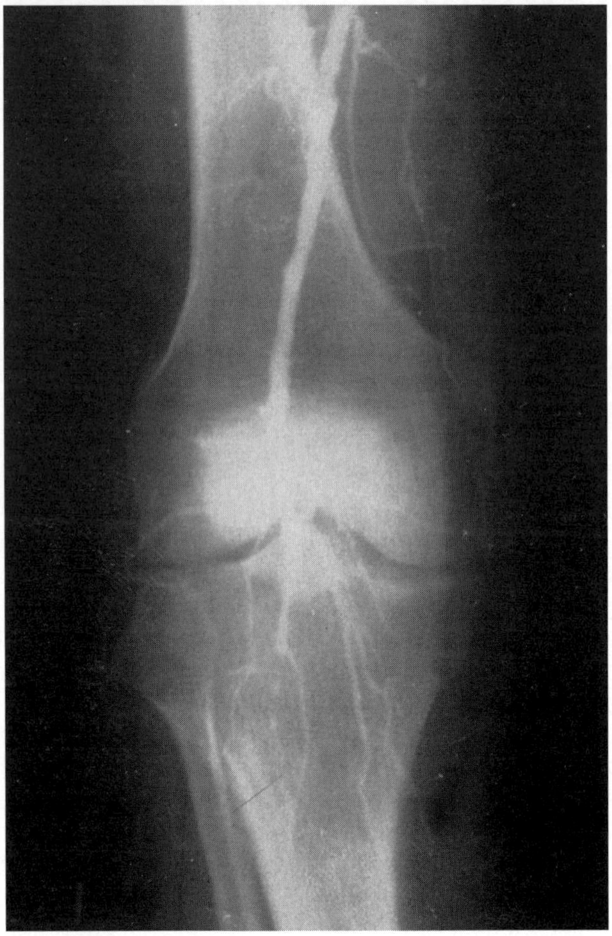

1

will be poor, as there is no easy communication between the posterior compartment of the calf and the peroneal or anterior compartments, other than in collaterals within the skin itself.

As these posterior calf collaterals may also be the main source of supply for the lower leg, including the soleus muscle and the anterior and peroneal compartments, there may be considerable 'steal' of blood from the posterior calf compartment. The available blood supply to the posterior flap is, therefore, improved on amputation of the lower leg, providing all tissue anterior to the gastrocnemius is removed. It is for this reason that I emphasize that the soleus muscle should be completely removed up to a level just above the division of the bone.

Preoperative preparation

As the mean age of these patients is over 70 and the early postoperative mortality in the range of 7–14%, these patients require careful assessment for anaesthesia and close postoperative supervision (Hayes and Middleton, 1981; Harrison *et al.*, 1987; Sethia *et al.*, 1986; Robinson *et al.*, 1982). Associated cardiovascular or respiratory disease and diabetes add to the risks. Often, these patients have become debilitated and malnourished through prolonged opiate therapy for rest pain, or may have already undergone arterial reconstruction or previous attempts at conservative amputation. Despite this, amputation should not be delayed, because the patients will usually continue to deteriorate with pain, spreading infection or gangrene.

Once the decision to amputate has been made the leg should be elevated to reduce tissue oedema and antibiotics started if there is evidence of infection or gangrene. Diabetes should be carefully controlled by soluble insulin infusion and the patient rehydrated. Where malnutrition is a problem, fine bore gastric feeding may be started, even though amputation should be scheduled within 24 h. The level of amputation is carefully explained and consent obtained for below-knee amputation only, unless there is spreading gangrene and the viability of the calf muscles is in doubt.

Selecting amputation level

Much has been written about methods of assessing tissue perfusion for the selection of the most distal amputation site likely to heal. This is critical, as the more distal the amputation the greater the proportion of patients who achieve complete rehabilitation, whereas the more proximal the amputation the higher the chances of primary healing. Methods described to measure them objectively include Doppler segmental pressures, pulse volume recording, zenon-133 clearance studies, photoplethysmography, muscle pH measurements, thermography and transcutaneous oxygen tension measurement ($TCPO_2$). Of these, the latter appears to be the most promising, with the potential that laser Doppler may be equally valuable in the future. Planning is still difficult, as healing may occur in the face of low $TCPO_2$ levels unless skin heating to overcome vasospasm or high inhaled oxygen concentrations are administered (Spence and McCollum, 1985; Franzech *et al.*, 1982; Rattiff *et al.*, 1984). Furthermore, in below-knee amputation, it is impossible to predict how much the $TCPO_2$ of the skin flap will improve once the distal tissue dependent on the same collaterals has been removed, although some improvement in the flap has been acknowledged (Katsamouris *et al.*, 1984). For most vascular surgeons, there is still no clear indication as to which technique should be used routinely because development has not yet reached the standard that they can be applied generally. From our own results, clinical judgement alone may be used, because reamputation at a higher level was required in less than 10% of patients despite performing below-knee amputations on all patients with viable posterior calf skin. When an adequate posterior flap cannot be fashioned due to ulceration or gangrene, the 'skin flap' technique may be appropriate, but in my opinion requires a better blood supply (Robinson *et al.*, 1982).

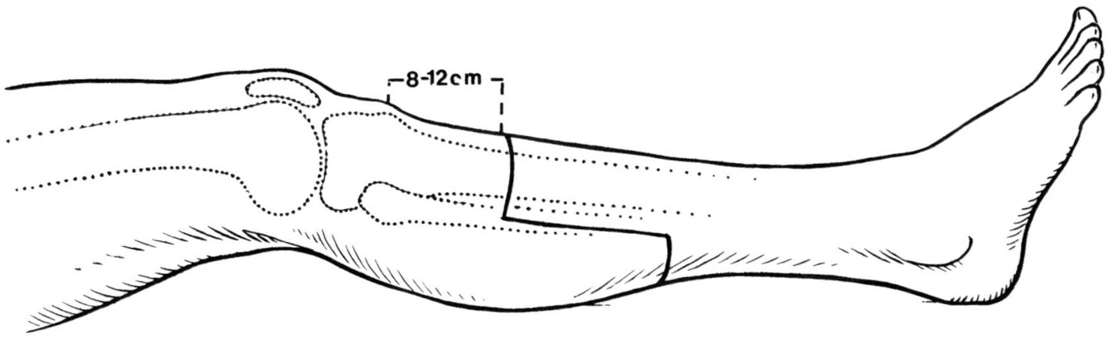

2

The operation

In most cases, general anaesthesia is used, although epidural or spinal local anaesthesia may be appropriate for individual cases. Prophylactic antibiotics are given before incision, or earlier for spreading infection.

2

The skin is marked 8–12 cm below the tibial tuberosity where the anterior skin incision is made and the bone divided. The medial and lateral limits of the anterior incision are then marked, as this will form the base of the posterior flap. This base should be more medially placed by only extending the anterior incision medially 1–2 cm posterior to the border of the tibia, but the lateral incision should extend just posterior to the line of the fibula. The posterior flap will be cut to size later in the procedure.

3

The anterior skin incision is made down to the tibia and through the anterior tibial compartment to the neurovascular bundle. Once this has been ligated the fibula can easily be cleaned of its periosteum and divided using rib shears 3–4 cm above the proposed level of tibial division.

4

Using minimal retraction, so as not to disturb the precarious blood supply to the anterior skin, the periosteum on the tibia is then divided and elevated on its anterior surface, only far enough for the anterior bevel on the tibia to be cut. The tibia is then divided transversely and grasped firmly so that it can be pulled gently forward and the cut end of the fibula brought forward from the bulk of the muscle.

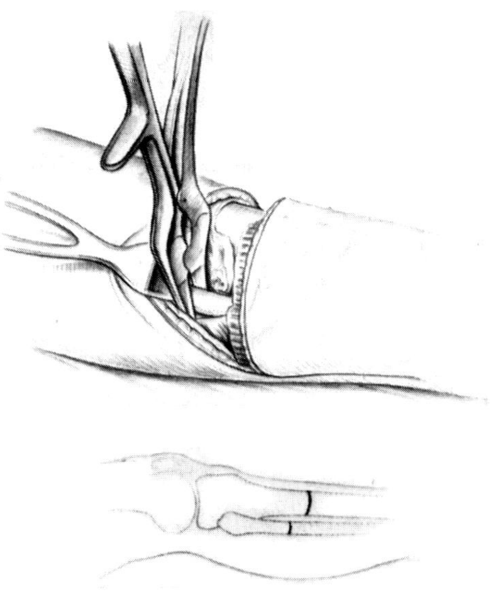

3

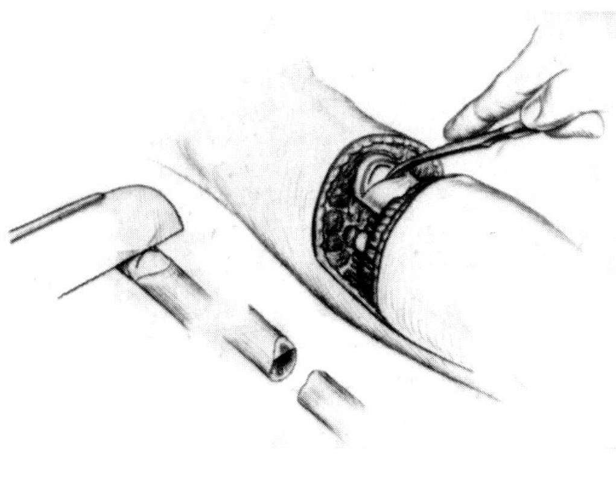

4

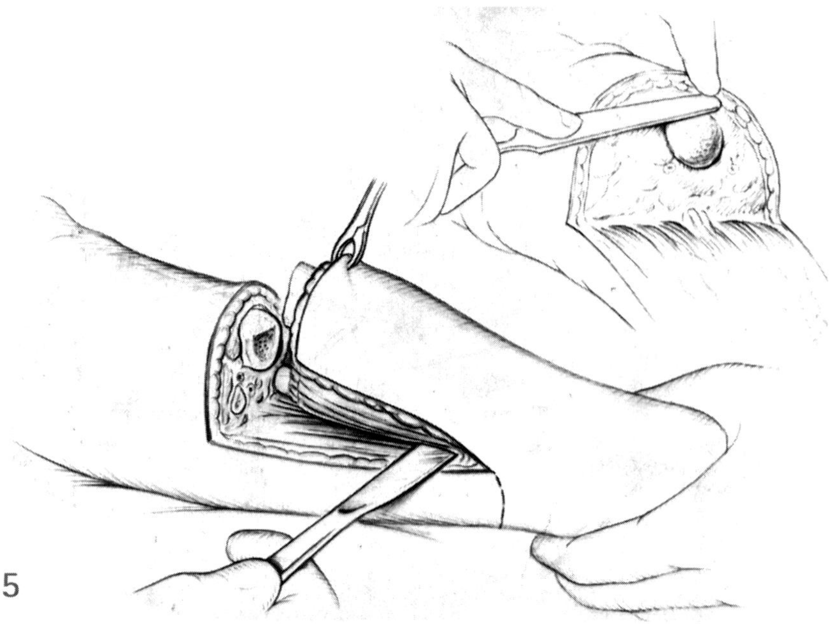

5

5

The posterior flap is cut with long medial and lateral incisions and rapid separation of the calf muscles from the posterior surface of the tibia and fibula. The posterior flap is divided distally to provide excessive length so that it may subsequently be trimmed to fit with absolutely no tension. The cut end of the tibia is rounded by filing and all sawdust and filings rinsed away with saline.

6

The plane between the gastrocnemius and the soleus is easily identified on the medial aspect of the flap and can simply be developed by blunt dissection. This plane is virtually avascular, demonstrating that the posterior flap is supplied by the sural arterial and not from the tibial vessels. The soleus is firmly adherent to the tendon of the gastrocnemius in the lateral part of the flap, but this may easily be divided leaving no soleus on the flap.

7

Once fully mobilized, the soleus is pulled distally and divided transversely at the level of the tibia, ligating the posterior tibial vessels and securing haemostasis at this stage. This procedure greatly reduces the bulk of the posterior flap so that the flap may be shortened without undue tension, improving the shape of the stump, preventing 'dog ears' and reducing the disproportion in thickness between the anterior and posterior tissues.

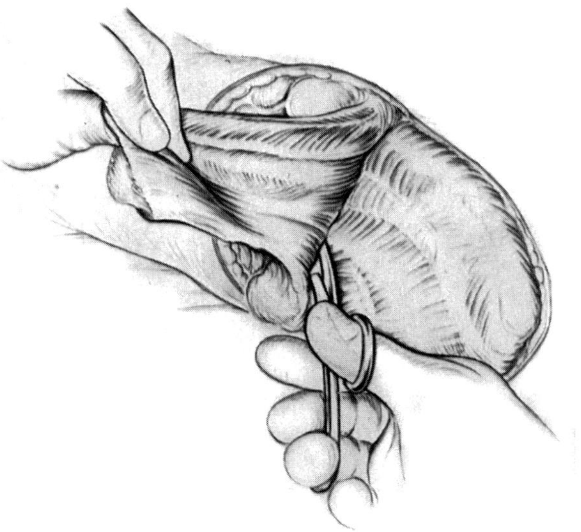

6

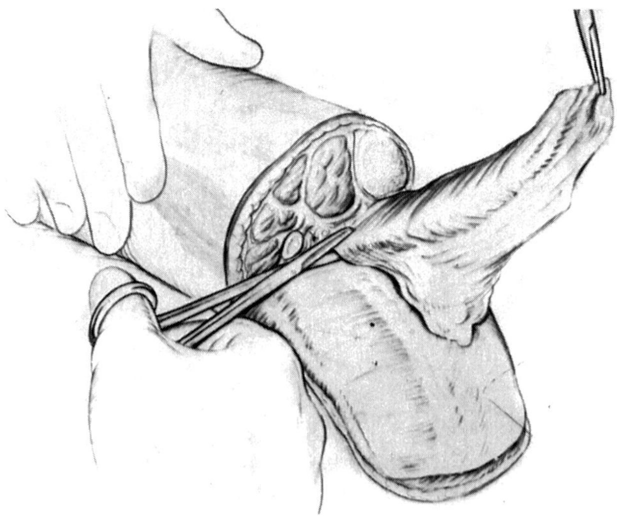

7

8a, b

The gastrocnemius tendon and deep fascia are divided first and sutured anteriorly, ensuring complete muscular cover of the bone end. Only then is the skin folded up and divided to an exact fit with no tension.

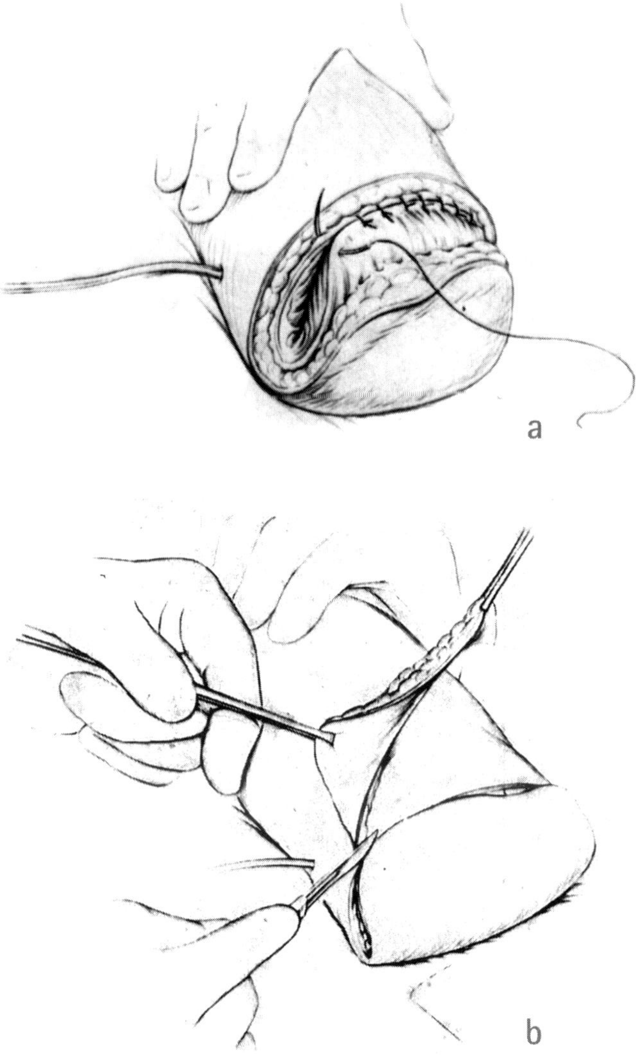

8

9

Three or four 4/0 Prolene sutures are loosely placed, but the main skin aposition is achieved with 0.5-inch wide steri- or suture-strips. I routinely use a Redivac drain and the stump is then wrapped in a generous layer of wool, held in place by a gentle crêpe bandage applied to exert as little pressure as possible on the stump.

Postoperative care and rehabilitation

The patient is encouraged to mobilize the knee from the first postoperative day, with elevation initially and vig-

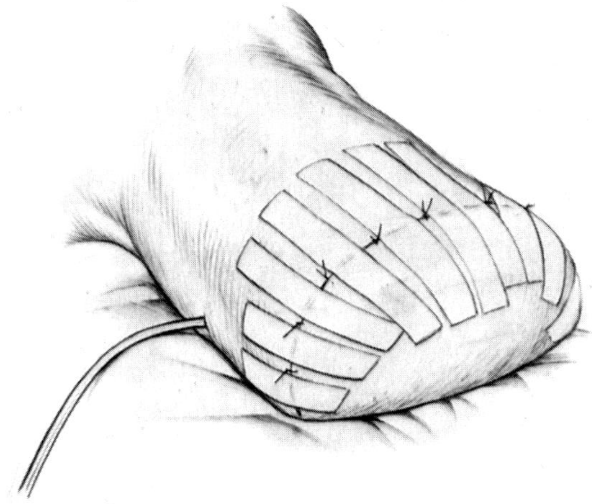

9

orous physiotherapy to ensure complete extension of the knee joint. As the suture strips maintain skin aposition the skin sutures may be removed after 5 or 6 days. The suture-strips are left until wound healing is adequate, which may be anything between 8 and 20 days. Physiotherapy ideally starts prior to amputation and is designed to relieve any contractures that may be developing as a result of rest ischaemia. The emphasis is on the rapid recovery of a full range of movement in the knee joint so that the patient can 'drive' a patella tendon-bearing prosthesis. In this respect, knee extension must be complete so that mobilization with a pneumatic limb starts in the second week and a temporary prosthesis may then be fitted within 3–4 weeks.

Acknowledgement

Illustrations by R N Lane.

References

Burgess E M (1968). The below knee amputation. *Bull Pros Res BRP* **10**: 9.

Burgess E M, Romano R L, Zett J H, Schrock R D Jr (1971). Amputations of the leg for peripheral vascular insufficiency. *J Bone J Surg* **53A**: 874.

Franzech U K, Talke P, Bernstein E F *et al.* (1982). Transcutaneous PO_2 measurements in health and peripheral arterial disease. *Surgery* **91**: 156.

Harrison J D, Southworth S, Callum K G (1987). Experience with 'skew-flap' below knee amputation. *Br J Surg* **74**: 930.

Hayes I G, Middleton M D (1981). Amputation for peripheral vascular disease. Experience of a district general hospital. *Ann Surg* **63**: 342.

Katsamouris A, Brewster D C, Megerman J, (1984). Transcutaneous oxygen tension in selection of amputation level. *Am J Surg* **147**: 510.

Kendrick R R (1956). Below knee amputation for arteriosclerotic gangrene. *Br J Surg* **44**: 13.

Malone J M, Godstone J (1986). Lower extremity amputation. In *Vascular Surgery: A Comprehensive Review*, 2nd edn. Moore W ed. London/San Diego: Grune and Stratton.

Rattiff D A, Clyne C A C, Chant A D B *et al.* (1984). Prediction of amputation wound healing: The role of transcutaneous PO_2 assessment. *Br J Surg* **71**: 219.

Robinson K P, Hoile R, Coddington T (1982). Skew flap myopastic below-knee amputation: A preliminary report. *Br J Surg* **69**: 554.

Sethia K K, Berry A R, Morison J D *et al.* (1986). Changing pattern of lower limb amputation for vascular disease. *Br J Surg* **73**: 701.

Spence V A, McCollum P T (1985). Evaluation of the ischaemic limb by transcutaneous oxymetry. In *Diagnostic Techniques and Assessment Procedures in Vascular Surgery*. Greenhalgh R M ed. London/San Diego: Grune and Stratton.

Skew-flap below-knee amputation

Kingsley Robinson

Introduction

This technique is designed to make the best use of the blood supply to the below-knee skin in patients with peripheral vascular disease to form a stump which is shaped to be suitable for prosthetic use at the conclusion of the surgical operation, and which has a standardized technique that is reproducible in the hands of different surgeons, so that a stump with the same characteristics can be consistently produced.

1

The length of the stump is determined by the line of bone section which is measured from the articular surface of the tibial plateau and according to the patient's build is between 10 and 14 cm below this level. The level should be judged to be just above the maximum convexity of the calf muscle mass and not shorter than a point that allows 4 cm of stump to protrude beyond the hamstring tendons when the knee is flexed to 90 degrees. The line of bone section is drawn on the skin overlying the tibia and a circumferential equator line is extended around the limb at this point. It is important to use a fully waterproof marking device, and if the skin marking is performed in the anaesthetic room, a waterproof fibre-tip cartridge writer is ideal and the skin can be subsequently prepared with a spirit-based antiseptic without removing the marks. A point 2 cm lateral to the subcutaneous tibial crest is marked on the equator line and a vertical mark parallel to the axis of the limb is extended upwards for 2 cm. This point represents the junction of the anteromedial and posterolateral skin flap. To identify the diametrically opposite point on the back of the limb a tape is passed around the equator line and cut to that length. This tape folded in half will then indicate the posterior junction of the flaps. If the same tape is then folded to obtain a quarter length, this will indicate the midpoints of each flap along the equator line from which the quarter circumference length can be drawn on the skin to indicate the length of the skin flap at its maximum extent. A semicircular line then connects the three marks to form the skew flaps. The skin is incised together with the subcutaneous fat, the periosteum over the tibia and the anterior tibial compartment and peroneal compartment fascia.

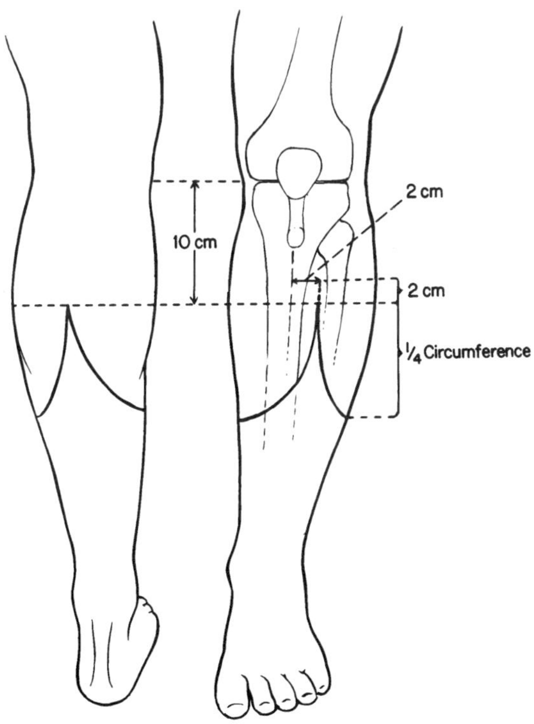

1

2

When the skin incision has been completed and the skin retracted, the long saphenous vein and the short saphenous vein need to be secured with artery forceps and ligated with fine catgut or vicryl 3/0, while the saphenous nerve and sural nerve are separately divided under some tension to allow the ends to retract. Very few bleeding points require attention at this stage and the skin flaps can be elevated to expose the anterior aspect of the tibia

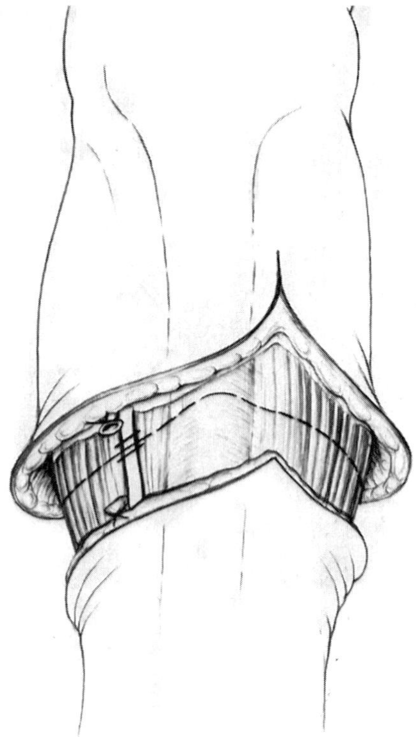

2

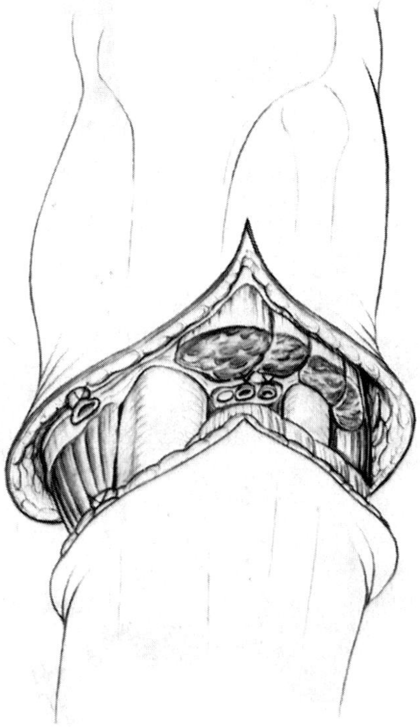

3

and the peroneal and anterior tibial muscle compartments. The tibial periosteum and the anterior tibial muscles are divided along the line of the equator mark on the skin, the upward extension of the skin incision providing access to the anterior tibial compartment with moderate retraction.

3

The dissection is carried through the anterior tibial peroneal muscles, a few muscle fibres at a time, either with a scalpel or diathermy point, until the anterior tibial nerve and the musculocutaneous nerve are revealed in each compartment, allowing them to be drawn down under tension and cut transversely with a scalpel so that they can retract clear of the area of the stump end. The anterior tibial artery and its venae comitans are revealed close to the interosseous membrane and can be divided between haemostats and ligated with a fine vicryl or catgut suture. The anterior surface of the fibula and the lateral surface of the tibia are now exposed together with the interosseous membrane. The latter is divided in the line of the dissection and a periosteal elevator is used to clear all surfaces of the tibia at this same level. The fibula can similarly be cleared and retraction will expose an adequate length to allow the fibula to be divided 2 cm proximal to the line of bone section marked on the skin.

4

The fibula is divided first. Bone forceps should not be used for this purpose because the fibula will fragment into sharp pieces and may split along its whole length. A Gigli saw is convenient for dividing the bone, although a cantilever power-saw is much easier to manage. Sometimes the nutrient vessels of both the fibula and tibia are encountered at this level and may produce some

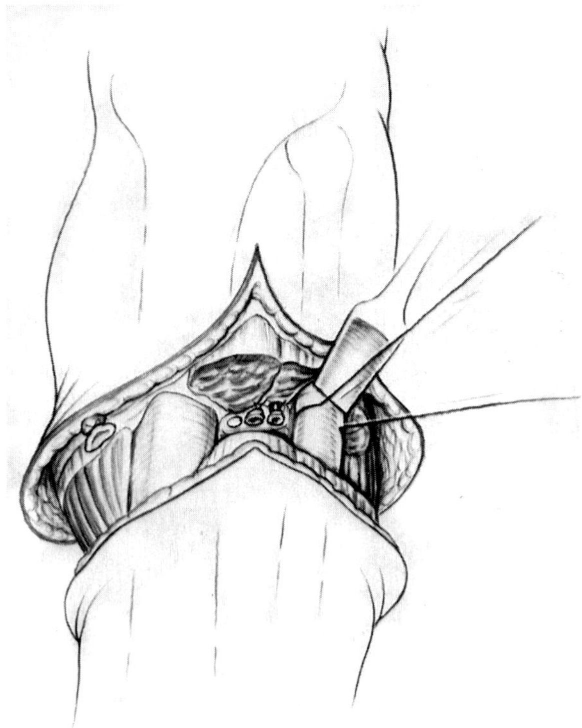

4

bleeding that has to be controlled with a pack until better access is obtained after the bones are divided. Once the fibula is divided, the tibia can be transected.

5

The tibia is most conveniently cut with a cantilever power-saw while copious irrigation is maintained to avoid any heat damage to the bone ends and to remove the bone dust and fragments. The cantilever power-saw will permit a gentle anterior curve to be described as the bone is transected, but if a hand-saw is used, a sloping cut is made through the anterior half of the bone and then a transverse cut through the remaining half to produce a partial bevel which can then be rounded by subsequent filing. Once the tibia is completely divided, the distal fragment is stabilized by inserting a sharp bone hook into the medullary cavity and applying some traction.

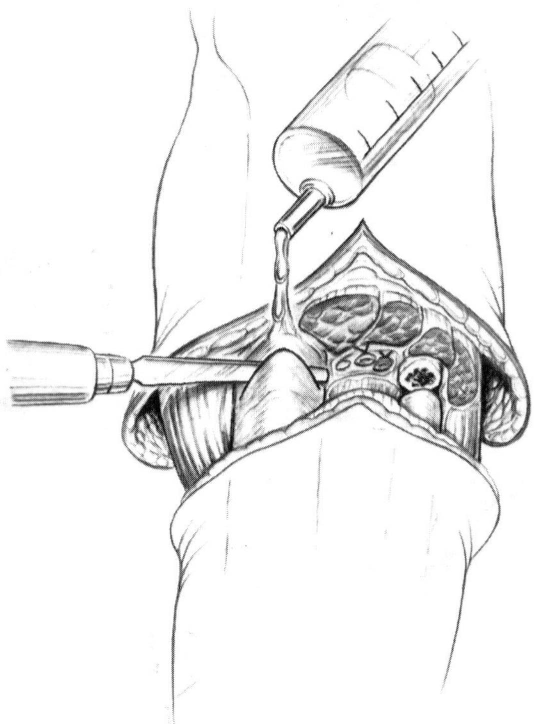

5

6

While downward traction is maintained on the distal fragment of the tibia, the tibialis posterior muscle is clearly visible and can be divided a few fibres at a time until the neurovascular bundles and the posterior tibial nerve are revealed beneath it. The most convenient technique to handle the neurovascular bundles is the application of a large artery forcep of the Robert's type with enough length being allowed for a second forcep to be applied behind the first so that the posterior tibial nerve can be extricated, and both the peroneal and posterior tibial arteries and their venae comitans can then be separately secured and the temporary proximal forcep removed. The posterior tibial nerve, the largest encountered in the dissection, is drawn down strongly and cut across with the scalpel and allowed to retract well away. Some bleeding from its concomitant artery may be encountered and this is never a problem. The skin flaps are separated from the distal part of the limb by a blunt dissection and drawn down to allow access to the full thickness of the gastrocnemius soleus muscle mass which is extricated from the distal portion of the limb, the very distance at least equal to the vertical thickness of the formed stump. If the assistant presses firmly across the upper part of the calf muscles, a degree of control of the remaining vessels is obtained and the gastrocnemius muscle mass can be transected at the chosen distal level with a minimum of blood loss.

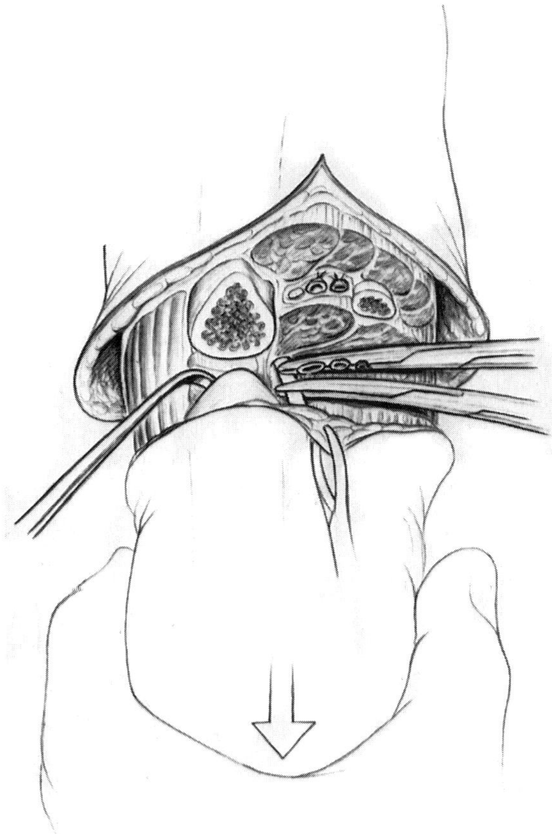

6

7

At this point the myoplastic flap to be formed from the gastrocnemius soleus mass is formed. The muscle tongue is pulled out with tissue forceps and a slope is cut from

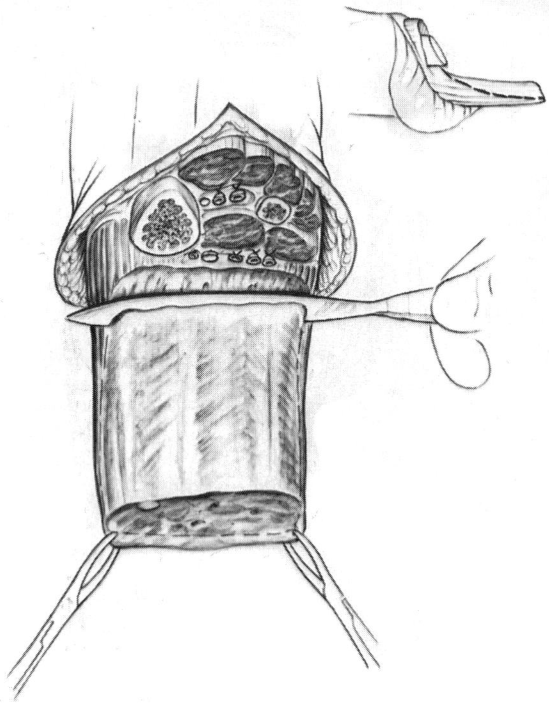

7

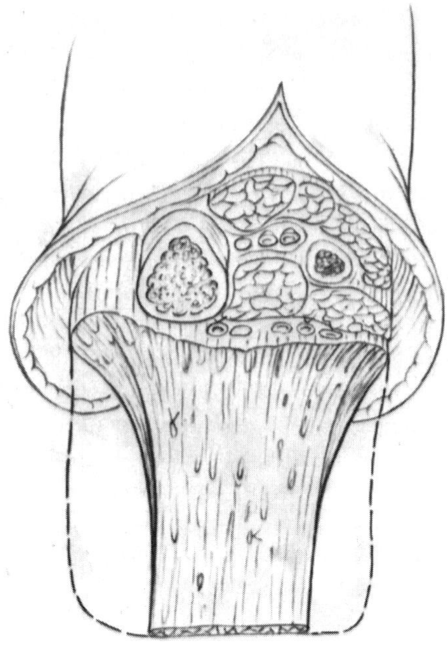

8

the line of bone section to the distal end of the flap leaving only aponeurosis for the last few millimeters. This will transect the soleal venous sinuses and numerous small arteries which will require individual transfixion and underrunning with sutures to obtain full haemostasis. The use of diathermy ligaclips and simple ligatures is rarely successful and an underrunning suture will save a considerable amount of time.

8

Once haemostasis is obtained and the tapering flap has been constructed, the dimensions of this are then checked by folding it forward to approximate its distal end to the anterior tibial periosteum and the anterior tibial fascia. This will demonstrate how much bulk the folded muscle mass will produce at the medial and lateral aspects and, following accurate trimming of the distal end of the flap, the sides of the muscle mass must then be reduced to make sure that there is no widening when the muscle flap is folded over.

9, 10

A large scalpel is used to trim away the excess muscle tissue and the trimming process may have to be extended above the line of bone section into the peroneal muscle group and on the medial side of the gastrocnemius. Some further venous sinuses may require underrunning and ligation. At this stage attention is paid to the bone ends

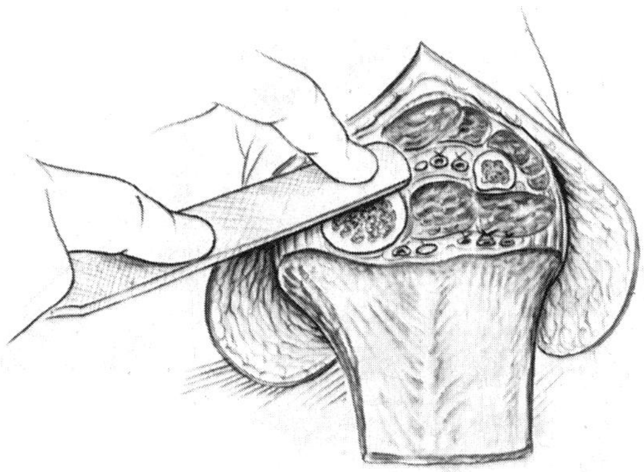

9

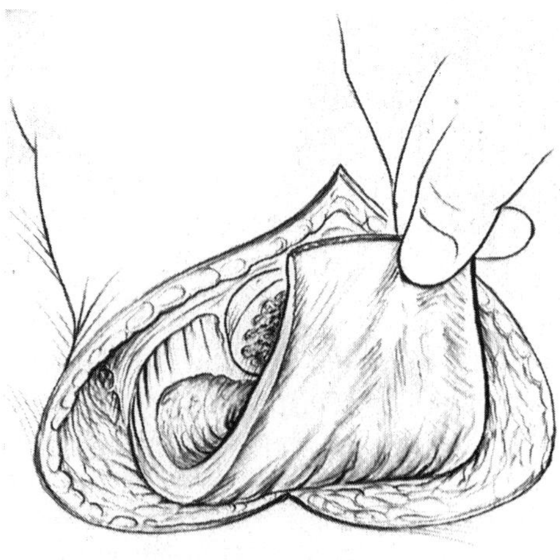

10

which are then carefully shaped with a coarse rasp and then a fine bone file to produce a rounded corner with a smooth surface in all dimensions. Similar attention must also be paid to the fibula end so that there is no excess scar tissue formed by trauma due to movement of bone fragments in the muscle tissue. A careful wash out is required to remove all the calcium fragments and a suction drain is placed in relation to the bone ends and passed through the skin laterally and secured with a stitch. The myoplastic flap is now finally folded over.

11

The folded flap is carefully opposed to the anterior tibial fascia and the anterior tibial periosteum. A continuous suture of '1' chromic catgut or '0' vicryl is used to run along the whole anterior aspect of the stump and to complete the myoplasty. The skin flaps remain partially attached to the gastrocnemius soleus mass and a small degree of separation may be required to allow them to come into comfortable apposition and the skin and subcutaneous fat are sutured with interrupted stitches – usually vertical mattress sutures of 3/0 nylon – to approximate the skin edges along the line of the skew flaps. It is recommended that the anterior and posterior sutures are inserted first and then a central stay stitch to

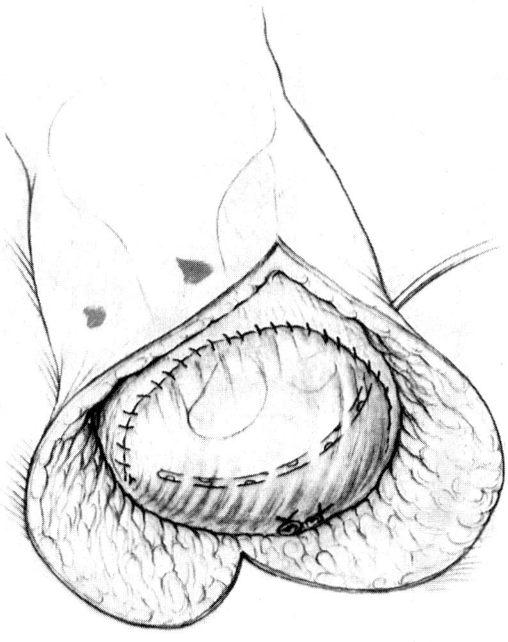

11

allow any fine adjustment in the alignment of the flaps to be obtained before closure is complete. The application of steri-strips to the skin between each interrupted suture may relieve tension loading on the sutures.

12

At completion, the stump is usually well-rounded, parallel-sided and symmetrical, with the suture line just clear of the anterior tibial crest and the tibia and fibula bone ends. The soft tissues are not excessive or redundant and the patient may be allowed to apply stress to the stump between 2 and 4 days from the completion of the operation. Definitive stump bandaging is not recommended and our current practice is to use finely fluffed cotton

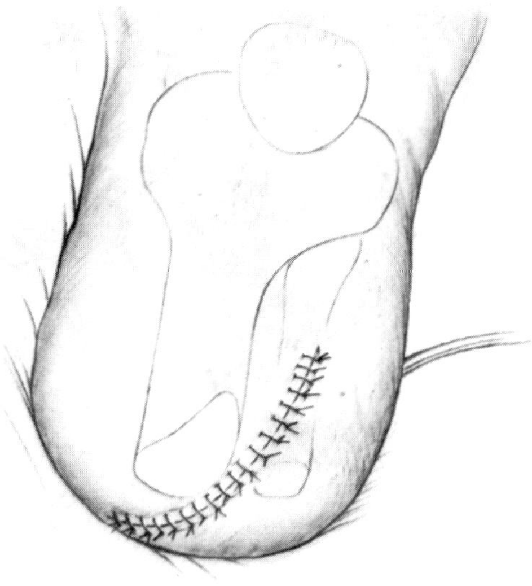

12

gauze without any cotton wool or padding applied to the stump, and a spiral of 4″ crêpe bandage keeps the fluffed gauze in place without applying any pressure or constriction to the stump itself. At the first dressing change, a netalast elastic net is used to retain the dressing, and as soon as possible the dressing is discarded altogether.

Acknowledgement

Illustrations by R N Lane.

Toe and foot amputations

Frank J Veith, Sushil K Gupta, Enrico Ascer, Kurt R Wengerter

Introduction

Performance of successful toe or partial foot amputation can be a critical part of limb salvage surgery in many patients who have gangrene and/or infection with or without ischaemia from arterial occlusive disease. These amputations within the foot include ablation of one or more toes, toe amputation with a portion of the adjacent metatarsal bone, partial (medial or lateral) transmetatarsal amputation, complete transmetatarsal amputation and a variety of unnamed or free-style partial foot amputations or debridements designed to remove necrotic or infected tissue and allow healing of enough of the foot to permit functional weight-bearing on the residual part of the extremity.

General principles

Before considering the specific techniques for these amputations within the foot, several principles must be emphasized. The first is that with normal or near-normal arterial circulation to the foot and adequate debridement or excision of infected and necrotic tissue, remarkable healing of the residual foot can be obtained. Moreover, even a small remnant of the foot can be effectively used for bipedal ambulation in sick, old patients, with one or more other disabilities. Salvage of less than half the foot with its plantar skin intact will permit more effective ambulation than a below-knee amputation if the patient has had a contralateral major amputation or a stroke. In this regard, we have found it possible to remove a major portion of the heel, including the Achilles tendon and the weight-bearing part of the os calcis, and still have the patient use the foot effectively in walking. Similarly, loss of the toes, metatarsals and most of the tarsal bones, leaving a foot remnant one-third the length of normal, does not preclude effective bipedal ambulation, which is not achieved in more than 30% of our patients undergoing below-knee amputation because of their frequent intercurrent disabilities.

A second principle relates to the importance of confirming adequate arterial circulation to permit successful performance of amputations within the foot. Simple toe amputations will occasionally heal with somewhat diminished ankle brachial pressure indices and pulse volume recordings, but they almost never will when the ankle brachial index is less than 0.6 and forefoot waves are flat or less than 5 mm in amplitude. Moreover, complex partial foot amputations and particularly some of the free-style transtarsal amputations to be described require near-normal arterial circulation to the foot. If a normal pedal pulse is not palpable or non-invasive tests do not indicate direct or straight-line arterial flow to the foot, the amputation within the foot should not be undertaken until arteriography and successful revascularization of the foot have been performed.

A third set of principles relate to the decision to close the skin primarily or leave the wound open. Although this decision requires careful judgement, there are certain guidelines which the surgeon should follow. If infection is evident or tissue viability is in question, the wound must be left open. Skin closure should never be under tension. Any wound that is closed must be reopened if wound edges become dusky or tension develops because of oedema. Open wounds are best kept moist with saline. This can be accomplished effectively by incorporating impermeable plastic within the saline-soaked dressing.

Fourthly, control of infection and normal or near-normal circulation are necessary for successful healing by secondary intention. Adequate debridement of infected and necrotic tissue is also essential and may require several trips to the operating room. Split thickness skin grafting can hasten healing once a clean granulating wound is obtained. Even on weight-bearing surfaces, such skin grafts can help to save feet.

Fifthly, there are no absolute barriers to debridement. Infected or necrotic tissue must be removed even if it requires exposure of joint interiors between the tarsal bones or even the ankle. With good circulation, adequate debridement and postoperative care healing can be achieved. A rongeur is a most useful instrument to perform adequate debridement of infected or necrotic tissues within the foot. This includes soft tissue, tendons, cartilage and bone.

A sixth and final principle is adherence to the use of minimally traumatic technique to handle all remaining tissue. Crushing of tissue and grasping of the skin with forceps must be avoided. Haemostasis should be complete but no adjacent tissue should be ligated or coagulated with blood vessels.

Specific amputations within the foot

1

Simple toe amputation

This is performed by making a circular incision in the skin of the toe as close to the proximal interphalangeal joint as possible, thereby assuring adequate skin length to permit closure by primary or secondary intention. The actual position of the skin incision is determined by the amount of remaining viable skin left on the toe. Care is taken to make the incision in viable skin. The soft tissues are then sharply divided down to the proximal phalanx. A flap of soft tissue is raised to provide access to the base of the proximal phalanx and the bone is divided using a bone-cutting forceps or rongeur without entering the metatarsal–phalangeal joint. If the skin is clearly viable and uninfected and closure without tension can be performed, a few monofilament sutures are placed in the skin to close the wound in a transverse plane. If any of these conditions cannot be fulfilled, the wound is left open to heal by secondary intention. If the metatarsal–phalangeal joint is entered, all of the cartilage, the entire proximal phalanx and much of the head of the metatarsal bone should be removed with a rongeur. Care is taken to remove all bone spicules and tissue fragments using the same instrument.

2

Removal of one or more toes with a portion of the corresponding metatarsal bone

If all the phalanges and all of the associated metatarsal bone are amputated, the procedure is often described as a 'ray' amputation. The 'ray' amputation is frequently required for quite severe osteomyelitis in association with diabetic gangrene. However, more frequently, the degree of infection dictates only that the head of the metatarsal needs to be excised with the toe, as is described here.

The skin incision is performed at the distal-most limit of viability. This incision is deepened to bone. The formation of flaps with so-called racquet handle incisions is kept to a minimum, but proximal extension of the incision is acceptable to provide proximal exposure of the metatarsal shafts. A periosteal elevator is used to expose the metatarsal–phalangeal joint and the distal portions of the metatarsal bones. These are transected in their midshaft with bone-cutting forceps or a vibrating saw. Sharp

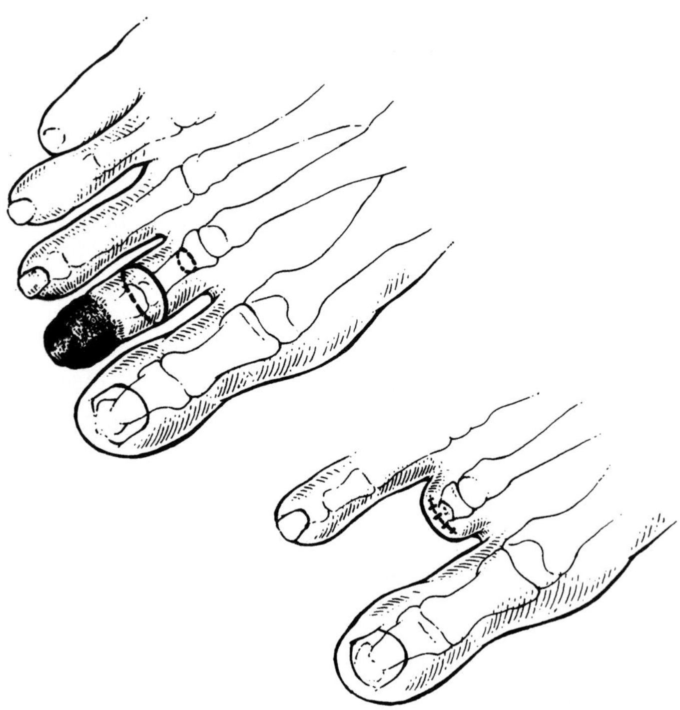

1

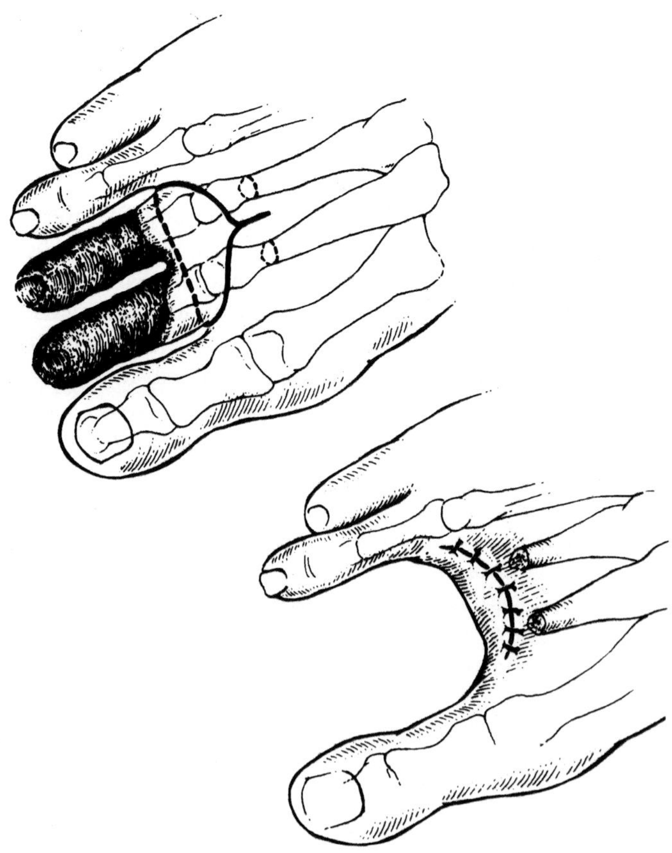

2

or projecting bone fragments are smoothed with a rongeur, and the same instrument is used to facilitate excision of deep soft tissue that may be non-viable or infected. The presence of dark thrombosed small blood vessels in the soft tissues indicates both infection and non-viability, and all such tissue must be excised. Haemostasis is obtained, and the wound edges are then loosely approximated or left open according to the principles already outlined.

3

Partial (medial or lateral) transmetatarsal amputation

These procedures are useful when gangrene involves the proximal portions of one or two toes medially or laterally with or without involvement of the adjacent webspace or webspaces. Again the skin incision is made to preserve as much viable skin and soft tissue as possible. The incision is deepened to bone and the thickest possible flaps are raised using sharp dissection with a scalpel supplemented by a periosteal elevator. The metatarsal bone or bones are then transected through their shaft with bone-cutting forceps or a vibrating saw as far proximally as is necessary to permit the skin and soft tissue to fall together over the bone ends without tension. The interior of the wound is carefully inspected for bone spicules and tissues of questionable viability. These include remnants of divided tendon and joint capsule. All these elements which require debridement are sharply excised by grasping them with a rongeur and transecting them with this instrument or cutting them with a scalpel while they are held in tension by the rongeur. This particular technique with a rongeur is useful in all debridements and excisions of necrotic tissue within the foot. It is the most effective way to assure smooth bone ends and minimally traumatic removal of all tendonous and ligamentous remnants which tend to have a poor blood supply.

4

Transmetatarsal amputation

This operation is indicated when gangrene involves all the toes including one or more webspaces. It produces a very functional foot without the need for a prosthesis or special shoe. If only the distal portion of four or five toes are necrotic, several simple toe amputations are performed in preference to a transmetatarsal amputation. Although the resulting foot remnant after multiple toe amputations may be less pleasing aesthetically, it has the advantage of preserving the important weight-bearing and step-off functions of the metatarsal heads. In addition, leaving the webspaces intact preserves important collateral circulation to skin edges and maintains skin bridges which minimize tension on the suture line.

Transmetatarsal amputation is performed by making an incision through the distal-most viable skin. Because of its greater thickness and tolerance to weight-bearing, preservation of plantar skin is particularly important. Accordingly, if possible, the end of the foot remnant should be covered with a relatively longer plantar flap.

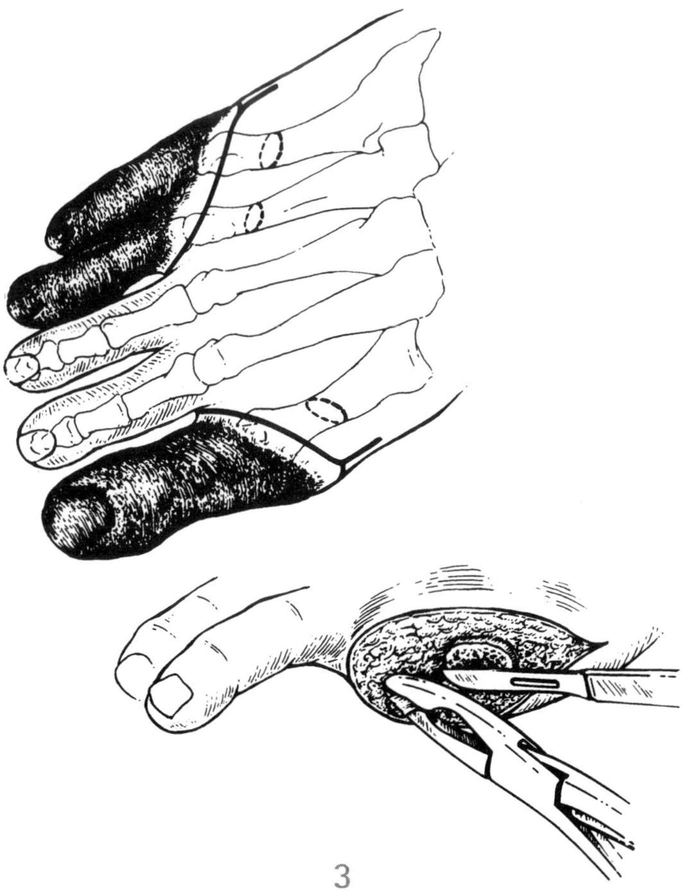

3

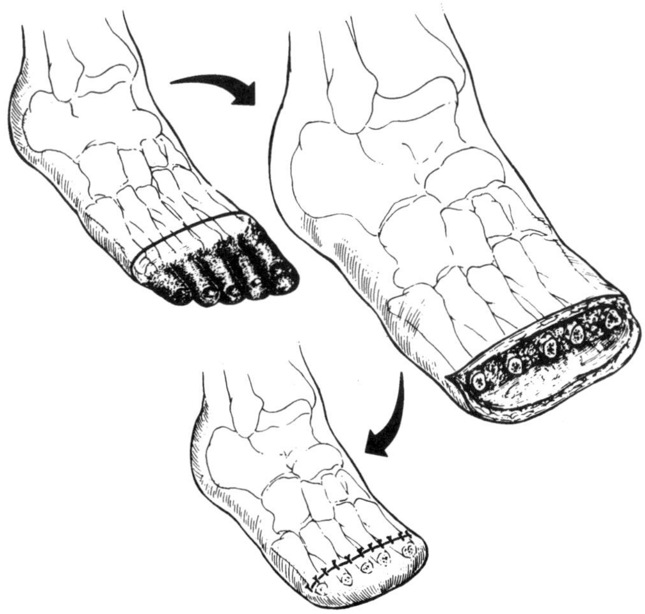

4

However, if viable plantar skin is limited, closure can be achieved by leaving more of the dorsal skin. If closure of viable skin without tension or residual infection is not possible, the wound may be left open to heal by secondary intention with or without skin grafting. Although this may require a protracted hospital stay, the resulting foot remnant can provide excellent function. Occasionally, if a portion of the wound is questionable, the rest of it may be closed loosely by adhesive strips and the questionable part left open and treated with wet dressings.

After the plantar flap is developed superficial to the tendons of the toe flexors to the level of bone transection, the forefoot is plantar flexed and the dorsal incision is carried down to the metatarsal heads. With continued plantar flexion, all tendons are incised as far proximally as possible. The forefoot is then dorsiflexed and the plantar tendons divided as far proximally as possible. The metatarsal shafts are then transected by already described techniques that will permit approximation of wound edges without tension. The rongeur-scalpel techniques described above are then used to provide smooth bone ends and to debride devitalized tissue and tendon ends. Haemostasis is secured and the wound approximated completely or partially, or left open depending on the pathology and principles already discussed.

5

Freestyle foot amputations (transtarsal amputations, heel amputations, excision of metatarsal–phalangeal joint and excision of toe bones)

The first two of these procedures facilitate removal of necrotic or infected tissues that are more extensive than those treated by the standard procedures already described. The other two procedures preserve the soft tissue of the toes and permit excision of bones that are involved with osteomyelitis, thereby facilitating healing of toe or foot lesions. In all four instances excision of involved bone and soft tissue is accomplished by the rongeur-scalpel techniques already described and

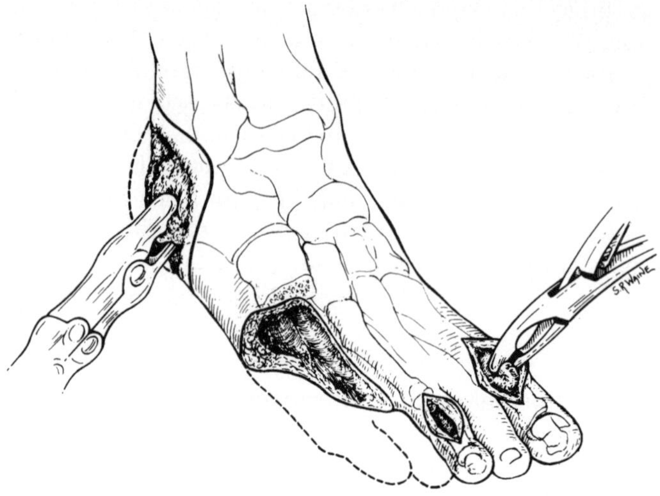

5

wounds are left open to heal by secondary intention with or without skin grafting. If transtarsal amputation is performed the Achilles tendon should be divided by dorsiflexing the foot remnant and cutting the stretched taught tendon with a No. 11 blade inserted alongside the tendon via a 3-mm skin incision.

Conclusions

All of these foot amputations can be valuable in preserving bipedal gait in patients with extensive gangrene and/or infection. In general, as much viable foot as possible should be preserved. Although multiple operations may be required and normal or near-normal arterial circulation is usually a prerequisite, the foot has a remarkable ability to heal and, by using the techniques described in this chapter, functional remnants of foot can be preserved despite the presence of surprisingly extensive gangrene and infection.

Acknowledgements

This work was supported in part by the Manning Foundation, The Anna S Brown Foundation and the New York Institute for Vascular Studies.

Basic principles in the surgical management of vascular trauma

John V Robbs

Introduction

Trauma to the major arteries and veins may present the most taxing technical problems encountered by the operating surgeon. This entails not only access to the major vessels in certain areas, but also control of haemorrhage and the sometimes exacting exercise of accurately restoring continuity of the involved vessels. There are few areas in surgery less forgiving of imperfect technique. The major thrust of this chapter will be towards management of arterial injury.

Mechanisms and pathology of arterial injury

1a, b, c

An understanding of the mechanisms of injury and pathology encountered is essential in order to treat these injuries rationally. In Table 1, mechanisms of injury, each of which results in a specific type of pathology, are summarized. The pathology encountered is illustrated below (1a–f). Following penetration by a sharp instrument or a low-velocity missile (for example, from a small-calibre hand gun) the tissue damage is essentially confined to the track of the penetrating agent. Low-velocity missiles may, however, compound the injury by fragmentation of soft-nosed bullets or fragments of bone; ricochet may also be responsible for more extensive damage.

High-velocity missiles are defined as those in which the muzzle velocity exceeds approximately 600 m/s (2000 ft/s). Under these circumstances, there is a highly significant energy release during passage through the tissues which causes a cavitation effect resulting in a great deal of soft tissue damage around the track. In addition, extraneous material such as clothing is drawn into the wound.

Penetrating trauma may result in a lateral perforation of the artery with formation of a false aneurysm. Total transection with or without loss of substance of the vessel may also occur and the artery frequently develops spasm at its severed ends (1b) with resultant thrombosis. Simultaneous lateral perforation of artery and adjacent vein may result in the formation of an acute arteriovenous fistula, with or without an associated false aneurysm (1c).

1d, e

Direct blunt trauma is exemplified by a direct localized blow to the vessel against a rigid bony structure. Indirect injuries are caused by distraction which may occur with joint dislocation or acceleration–deceleration trauma with its associated shearing forces at areas of fixity of the artery. An example of the latter is the aortic disruption

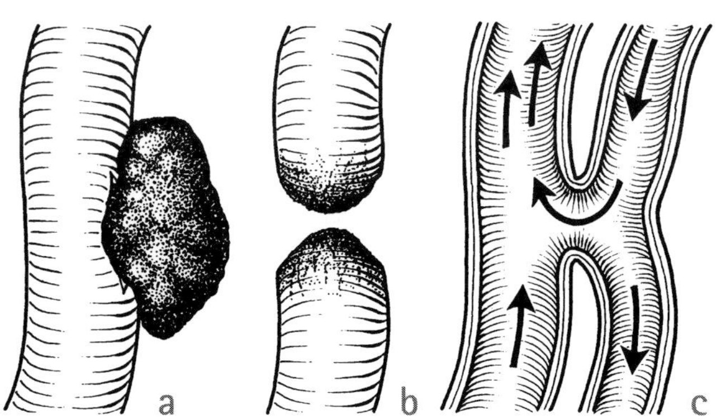

1

Table 1. Mechanisms of vascular injury	
Penetrating	Stab
	Missile
	high-velocity (600 m/s or 2000ft/s)
	low-velocity
Blunt	Direct
	Indirect
Blast	Shotgun
	Bomb
Iatrogenic	

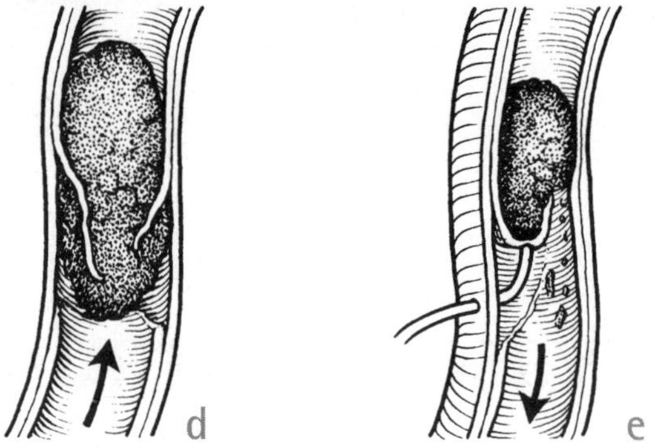

1

found at the isthmus or aortic valve ring in road traffic accident victims. The intima and media of the vessel wall are less elastic than the overlying adventitia and when the vessel is subjected to the type of forces described, it tends to disrupt from the less elastic layers on the inside towards the adventitia in proportion to the degree of violence. If the adventitia remains intact with an intimomedial tear in the smaller calibre vessels, superimposed thrombosis occurs due to a combination of exposure of blood to the thrombogenic raw surface and the elevation of a distally based flap (**1d**). In larger vessels such as the aorta, thrombosis does not occur to any great extent but an aneurysm tends to form at that site. Obviously with this type of trauma, if the forces are great enough all layers disrupt through part or all of the circumference, with perforation of the artery.

Shotgun blast injuries result in extensive soft tissue destruction which is contaminated by multiple small pellets which remain firmly embedded in the tissues. This is particularly noticeable when birdshot has been used. In addition, there are frequently multiple sites of perforation within the neurovascular bundle.

Bomb explosions may produce similar multiple penetrating wounds and soft tissue trauma but, in victims close to the explosion, high-velocity fragments may result in extensive cavitating injury and the situation may be compounded by surface flash burns.

Istrogenic vascular injuries warrant separate consideration. The most frequently encountered is catheter trauma associated with diagnostic radiological procedures. Laceration at the arterial puncture site may occur with the formation of false aneurysm or free haemorrhage. However, in smaller vessels (as in children), or the brachial artery in adults, thrombosis may occur at the site of the puncture due to the associated intimal damage. In atherosclerotic vessels, dislodgement of plaque and the formation of a flap with subsequent thrombosis or even distal embolization of atheromatous debris may occur (**1e**). Passage of the catheter between the layers of a diseased vessel with subintimal injection of contrast resulting in superimposed thrombosis is also occasionally seen following diagnostic radiological procedures.

Excessive inflation of the balloon of an embolectomy catheter may result in significant arterial injury. This applies particularly when the balloon is filled with fluid, thus creating a hydraulic system which is capable of transmitting extremely high pressures. The types of lesions caused range from intimomedial tears or stripping with subsequent thrombosis to transmural rupture with perforation. It is strongly recommended that air be used to inflate the catheter balloon during its use.

Intra-arterial injection of lipid-soluble substances may be responsible for injury to the arterioles by fixing in the intimal tissues with superimposed intense spasm and thrombosis. In clinical practice this is occasionally seen following inadvertent injection of sodium pentothal or diazepam which are both widely used for premedication purposes during anaesthesia or invasive diagnostic procedures. A similar spectrum of pathologies is seen in drug abusers following intra-arterial injection of a variety of agents. These lesions are not amenable to direct arterial reconstructive surgery.

1f

Arterial spasm

This is always associated with trauma to an artery whatever mechanism may have been responsible and whatever the underlying pathology may be. In addition, the lack of intraluminal pressure in the arterial tree distal to the site of injury results in marked diminution in calibre of these vessels due to the unopposed sympathetic tone which further aggravates distal ischaemia. Spasm occurring in isolation as a cause of distal ischaemia is exceptionally rare and in our own series, which numbers well in excess of 1000 cases of arterial trauma, it has been found to be the sole cause of the problem in less than 1%. Spasm as a cause of distal ischaemia is therefore a retrospective diagnosis made at the time of surgical exploration.

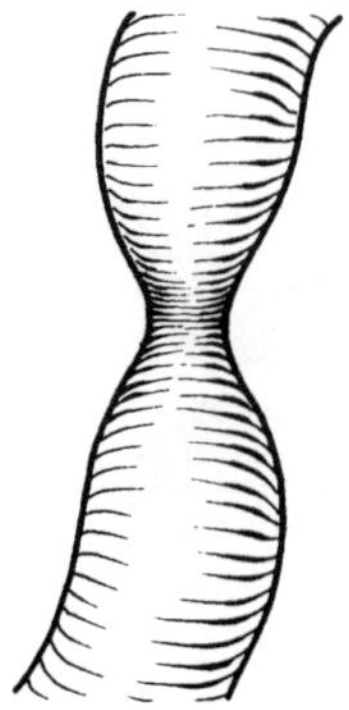

1f

Preoperative evaluation and diagnosis

Diagnosis rests upon a high index of clinical suspicion, and vascular injury should be entertained in every patient who has a penetrating wound of the neck and extremities and in every long-bone fracture or joint dislocation. In patients with multiple injuries, once ventilatory and haemodynamic deficits have been stabilized, every injury must be considered on its particular merit and remote injuries should not be allowed to distract from the possibility of an arterial injury, particularly in the extremities. An accurate assessment of peripheral perfusion cannot be made in a hypovolaemic peripherally vasoconstricted patient and it is important to reserve final clinical assessment of peripheral perfusion until the patient has been adequately volume resuscitated.

Arterial injuries *per se* present in principle with either occlusion, haemorrhage or arteriovenous fistulation. Occlusion invariably results in a pulse deficit with or without significant signs of ischaemia. It must be re-emphasized that in isolation, arterial spasm will never cause significant peripheral ischaemia. Another important pitfall which must be avoided in patients who have sustained blunt trauma is the entity of delayed thrombosis, as it may take several hours of occlusive thrombus to develop on an area of intimal disruption and patients with high-risk injuries such as knee dislocation or lower third femoral fractures must be continually reassessed during the first 24 h following injury.

Haemorrhage may be overt with obvious arterial or venous bleeding occurring through a wound; contained haemorrhage may manifest as a false aneurysm. Bleeding may also be concealed and occur into the pleural or peritoneal cavity or the retroperitoneum. A fairly frequent occurrence, particularly in patients with penetrating wounds, is the finding of unexplained shock or a low haematocrit with no obvious site of haemorrhage, which is encountered in patients who have sustained transection of a major vessel which has ultimately thrombosed. Arteriovenous fistulae are always associated with a machinery-type murmur. However, this may be subtle, and unless specifically sought will be missed. This is the most common pathology found in patients with arterial trauma who present late.

Place of preoperative angiography

While Doppler ultrasound is an extremely useful screening test when there is doubt, angiography provides the definitive diagnosis. In addition, angiography is essential for the localization of, and hence operative planning in, inaccessible areas such as the superior mediastinum, the base of the skull and the abdominal vasculature. In general, in the presence of focal trauma to the mid-cervical region or the extremities, the performance of angiography is time-wasting, as the injury is easily located on clinical grounds. However, in an ischaemic limb which has multiple fractures, it is essential to image the vascular tree at every fracture site as it is not uncommon to find arterial disruption in more than one area. It is best under these circumstances to perform the investigation on the operating table before embarking upon exploration. It must be emphasized that the patient must be volume resuscitated and haemodynamically stable before angiography is performed. In our own experience, the retrograde femoral route is usually preferable utilizing the digital subtraction technique. In young healthy adults, the complication rate is negligible. In children, as far as possible, digital subtraction angiography via the intravenous injection technique has been found adequate. An overview of the indications for preoperative angiography in our practice is summarized in Table 2.

Table 2. Indications for arteriography in trauma

Suspected cervicomediastinal injury
Pulse deficit
False aneurysm
Haemorrhage
Overt
Unexplained shock
Low haematocrit/haemoglobin value
Bruit
Injury to anatomically related nerves
First rib fracture
Widened mediastinum on chest radiograph
Suspected renal artery injury
Upper quadrant/loin pain
Proteinura
Non-function on intravenous pyelography
Suspected intraperitoneal haemorrhage
Pelvic fracture
Ongoing haemorrhage
Pulsating or expanding retroperitoneal haematoma
Ischaemic extremity
Severe soft tissue injury
Multiple fractures

Indications for operation and prioritization

The urgency for the operative procedure ranges from the 'crash' exploration in the 'clinically dead' patient, to the stabilized patient in whom a planned urgent procedure can be conducted, to the individual who presents months or years later with the long-term complications of a misdiagnosed or conservatively treated lesion. The question often arises in the stable patient without distal ischaemia or any other significant manifestations of arterial disruption other than an abnormal arteriogram, whether repair should be undertaken. While the precise incidence of complications in injuries that have been misdiagnosed or treated non-operatively is not known, when they do occur they may be life-threatening and indeed cause considerable morbidity. With penetrating wounds, secondary haemorrhage may occur between 5 days and 3 weeks after injury. This is probably due to low-grade sepsis with clot lysis resulting in active haemorrhage, or the acute onset of a false aneurysm which compresses surrounding structures. This most frequently applies to nerves and, in particular, to the brachial plexus. The prognosis for nerve recovery under these circumstances is guarded and when it does occur it may take anything up to 1 year for full function to be restored. Similarly, neglected false aneurysms or haematomas are susceptible to infection. Arteriovenous fistulae with a significant shunt may return with cardiac problems, due to the hyperdynamic circulation and when situated in the extremities with associated distal ischaemia and venous hypertension. Claudication or growth disparity in children are important long-term considerations with occluded arteries in the extremities.

Contraindications to reconstruction

Limb salvagability in the presence of extensive trauma may be an extremely difficult decision to make and should certainly not be left to the junior staff. In general terms, it is probably better to give the patient the benefit of the doubt and to proceed with revascularization under most circumstances. However, in the presence of extensive crush trauma associated with bone comminution and neurological dysfunction, the outlook is generally poor.

Similarly, the decision whether an extremity is irreversibly ischaemic or not may considerably exercise clinical judgement. Fixed skin staining and muscle rigidity in all compartments obviously preclude vascular reconstruction. However, in the presence of localized muscle compartment rigidity, such as the extensor compartment in the lower extremity, for example, a good functional result can still be obtained.

The general approach to the patient with a vascular injury should comprise concerted combined effort on the part of the involved disciplines with rapid resuscitation and definitive therapy as soon as possible. In virtually all instances we believe that the vascular injury should take priority over orthopaedic or plastic surgical intervention. The proviso, however, is that the vascular surgeons remain in attendance, until the procedures are concluded. In our experience, it is exceptionally uncommon for orthopaedic manipulations to disrupt the vascular repair. We believe that this approach is preferable to the use of temporary shunts which serves to prolong the operative procedure considerably.

Operative procedure

Access and positioning

2

Besides meticulous surgical technique the basis for successful surgery is to be on the alert for the unexpected and to provide wide access to the area of injury. It is certainly preferable to overexpose than the converse and there is no place for 'keyhole' or cosmetic surgery. In principle, the aim should be to plan operative exposure to the major vessels in a definitive way in order to obtain control of the vessels proximal and distal to the site of injury. It is ill-advised to attempt to approach the injury by enlarging pre-existing stab wounds, particularly in the root of the neck, because the bony confines of the superior mediastinum make rapid access difficult if torrential haemorrhage from a superior mediastinal vessel is initiated by manipulation through an inadequate incision. The most difficult anatomical areas to deal with from the access point of view are injuries near the base of the skull, the root of the neck and superior mediastinum and the major abdominal vessels, particularly the aorta and its branches above the level of the renal artery. The optimum utility incisions for injuries in these various areas are shown (2).

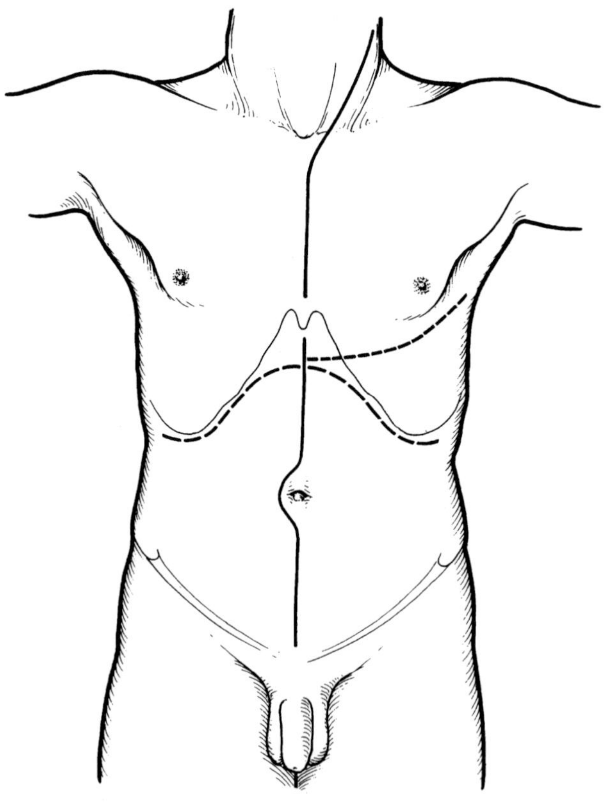

2

In principle, for cervicomediastinal injuries, the entire neck, sternum and left thoracic cage down to the posterior axillary line should be prepared and draped with the neck in extension and a bolster placed between the scapulae in order to brace the shoulders and thrust the aortic arch and mediastinal vessels forward. An oblique incision placed along the anterior border of the sternomastoid muscle, and extending from the mastoid process to the suprasternal notch is the best utility approach to neck wounds. To expose the distal internal carotid, the sternomastoid muscle can be divided close to its origin from the mastoid process. The incision can be readily extended into a median sternotomy which provides the best access to the superior mediastinum and heart. Left thoracotomy via the fourth or fifth intercostal space provides good exposure of the descending thoracic aorta and structures in the pulmonary hilum. Under certain circumstances the proximal subclavian artery is best approached in this manner.

Similarly, when intra-abdominal vascular injuries are suspected, the entire abdomen and thoracic cage should be prepared and draped and both lower limbs should be free-draped and prepared down to the level of the knee. The initial utility incision is a mid-line from xiphisternum to pubis. There should be no hesitation to extend this incision either by subcostal incisions into the flanks or into the lower thoracic cavity via one of the lower intercostal spaces should this become necessary. The proximal abdominal aorta and its branches are exposed by mobilization of the left colon, spleen and pancreas towards the right side of the patient. The suprarenal inferior vena cava is exposed by mobilization of the right colon to the left, together with Kocher's manoeuvre to the duodenum. For access to the retrohepatic inferior vena cava, the right lobe of liver must be mobilized in addition by division of the right triangular ligament.

3a, b

When the injuries are confined to the extremities the entire limb should be prepared and free-draped and there should always be access to the groins in order to obtain a long saphenous vein graft should this be necessary. In every case, arrangements should be made for the ready availability of on-table angiographic facilities. The upper limb should be abducted to 90 degrees and we find it most convenient to place it on a narrow arm board rather than to use a conventional arm table (3a). It is also helpful to place a bolster behind the shoulder which serves to thrust the axillary vessels forward. The major access problem is provided by vessels in the vicinity of the shoulder girdle and it is usually necessary to divide the insertions of both pectoralis minor and major muscles in order to obtain adequate exposure and control of the proximal axillary vessels. This applies particularly if the anatomy is distorted by the presence of a large aneurysm which fills the axilla, a frequent accompaniment of pen-

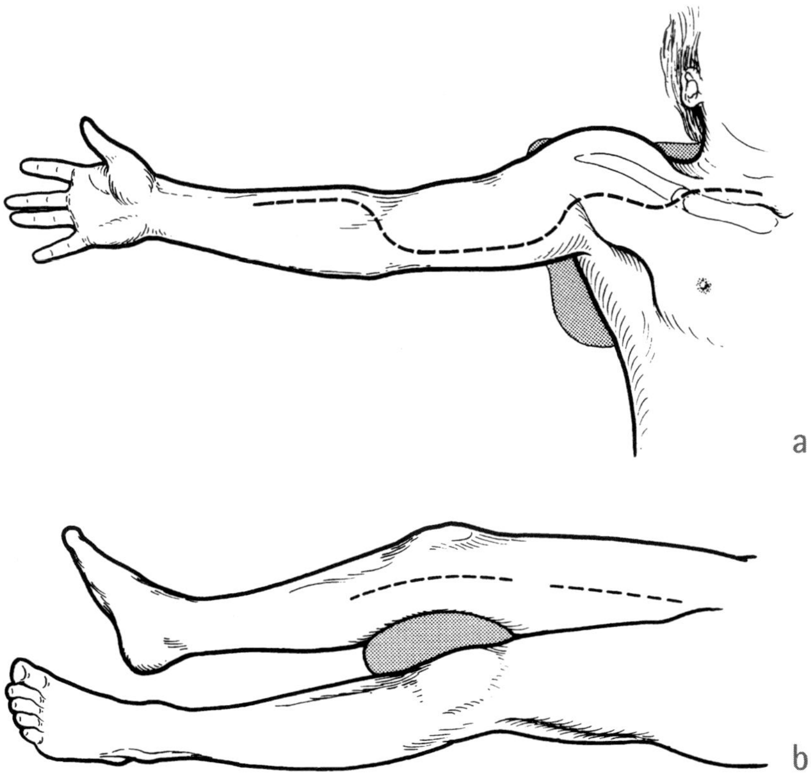

a

b

3

etrating injury. Adequate exposure of the distal subclavian vessels usually requires division of the clavicle midshaft. We have never found resection of the clavicle, in part or whole, necessary. The brachial is easily approached directly as illustrated.

The lower limb should be positioned with the knee slightly flexed on a bolster (**3b**). The femoral vessels can be directly exposed via an overlying incision. The optimum approach to the popliteal vasculature is via a medially placed incision. When the injury is situated in the artery behind the knee the hamstrings should be detached as a unit from their insertion on the tibia, together with a cuff of periosteum which can be stapled back into position.

Control of active haemorrhage

Should active bleeding be initiated during dissection it is essential to avoid the blind application of clamps as this will frequently cause unnecessary associated injuries to surrounding nerves or veins. It is usually possible to control bleeding by judicious application of pressure using a finger or sponge stick while resuscitation proceeds, and definitive proximal and distal control can be obtained by dissecting out the relevant vessels and applying atraumatic vascular clamps. Under certain circumstances it may be possible or even desirable to pass intraluminal balloon catheters and to control haemorrhage in this way until more definitive control is obtained.

Principles of repair

Once the pathology has been identified and the vessel controlled the options for repair include lateral suture, patch angioplasty, end-to-end reconstruction and interposition grafting. Under certain circumstances, arterial ligation may be necessary. In order to fully appreciate the significance of the various manoeuvres involved in the techniques or repair, it is important to understand the common reasons for early failure of arterial reconstruction. These may be summarized as follows:

1. Narrowing at the suture lines.
2. Inadequate calibre graft.
3. Anastomotic tension.
4. Failure of intimal apposition with the formation of a distal flap.
5. Adventitial incorporation into the lumen.
6. Inadequate distal run-off due either to underectected thrombosis or additional distal injury.
7. Infection causing thrombosis or disruption of the suture lines.

4

Assessment of inflow and the distal arterial tree

Backbleeding is not a reliable sign of distal patency, as a short collateral network may result in considerable back-

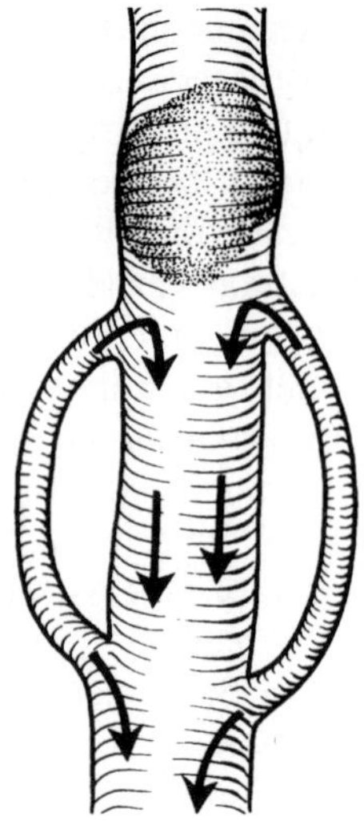

4

bleeding even in the presence of propogated thrombus distal to the collateral network. A small (size 3) balloon embolectomy catheter should be routinely passed into the distal vessel, gently inflated with air and withdrawn. This serves to extract any distal thrombus and to break gently co-existing arterial spasm. We do not believe that there is any place for the use of topical vasodilators such as papaverine or local anaesthetic agents. Should the catheter fail to pass the full length of the extremity, an intraoperative angiogram should be obtained. It is also advisable to pass the embolectomy catheter into the proximal artery and ensure that any proximal propagated thrombus is removed and that good pulsatile inflow is obtained. Both proximal and distal segments should be copiously irrigated with dilute heparin solution (10 000 units/litre normal saline); systemic heparin is not recommended in the trauma context.

5a, b, c

Preparation of artery for repair

The edges of the artery at the site of injury should be debrided back to healthy intima. The adventitia should be trimmed sufficiently by sharp dissection to prevent incorporation into the suture line; however, care must be taken to avoid excessive adventitial stripping which may result in the sutures cutting out. Thrombosed segments should be excised back to healthy non-oedematous arterial wall; this usually comprises 2–3 cm of vessel wall.

6, 7

Lateral suture

This can only be performed when closure will not result in narrowing at the site of the suture line. It is important to pick up all layers of the vessel wall and the sutures should be spaced approximately 2 mm apart and about

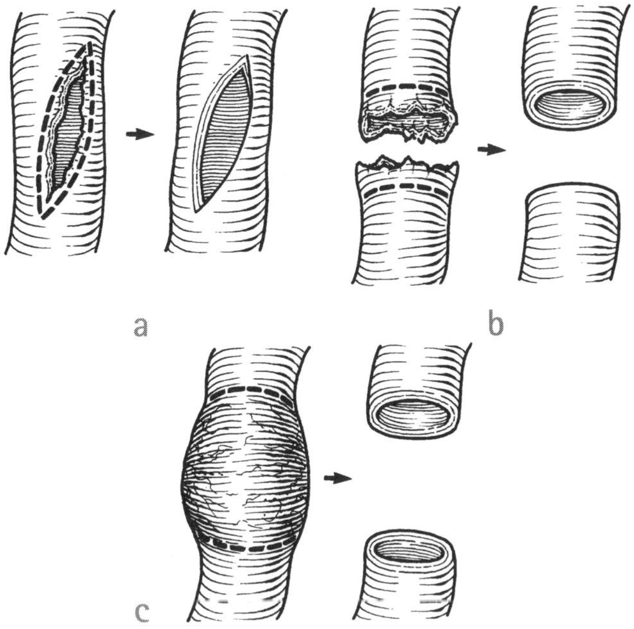

5

the same distance from the edges. In this way, blocks of tissue are opposed and intimal apposition is secured. The principle applies to any vascular suture line.

Puncture wounds in the aorta compatible with survival are usually relatively small. Illustration **7** illustrates a useful technique. Bleeding is controlled by digital pressure and the laceration is closed by means of interrupted mattress sutures placed deep to the finger. This technique is, however, not applicable to smaller calibre vessels as it would result in significant narrowing.

8a, b, c

Patch angioplasty

This should be used whenever simple lateral suture will result in narrowing. Any regional subcutaneous vein may be used and cut to size. Prosthetic material should be avoided in view of the danger of infection. The initial corner suture is of the mattress type in order to evert the suture line and ensure intimal apposition (**8a**). The suture line is then completed by an over-and-over technique at approximately 2-mm intervals using the principles described for lateral suture (**8b, c**).

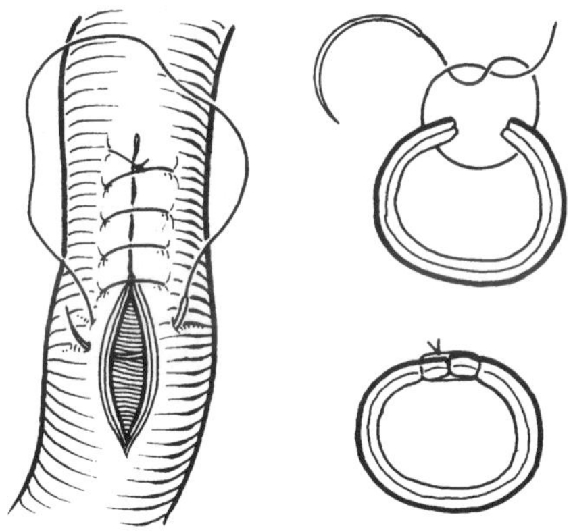
6

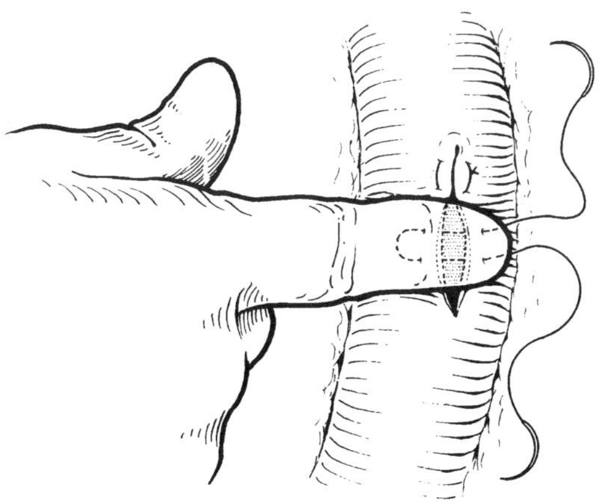
7

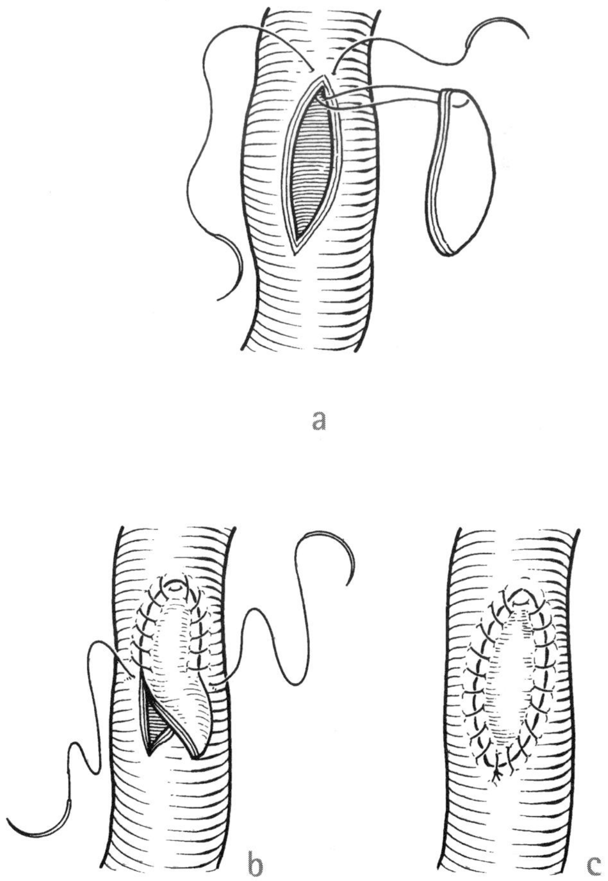

8

9a–d

End-to-end anastomosis

This can only be performed when apposition between the vessel ends can be maintained without tension. The best parameter to use in this regard is whether the single corner tethering stitch can maintain apposition of the ends with the limb in full extension. If tearing out results under these circumstances it is preferable to insert an interposition graft. After adequate debridement the ends of the vessel are fish-mouthed at opposite ends to prevent narrowing (**9a**). It is best to commence the suture line at the posterior corner with a mattress tethering suture (**9b**), and it is preferable not to simultaneously tether the opposite corner so that the intimal surface of the suture line can be inspected at all times while the artery is being sutured. In general, interrupted sutures are preferable, placed approximately 2 mm apart as described for lateral suture (**9c**). In larger vessels a continuous over-and-over suturing technique may be used. In deeply situated vessels in which ready access to the posterior wall is difficult, e.g. the great vessels in the superior mediastinum, it is possible to suture the posterior third of the anastomosis intraluminally (**9d**). The initial suture is placed posterolaterally at approximately the 4 o'clock point on the circumference and knotted outside the lumen. The lumen is re-entered and a full thickness over-and-over suture placed from within the lumen. Once the posterior part of the suture line is complete (approximately one-third of the circumference) this can be knotted on the adventitial surface at about the 7 o'clock point on the circumference and the anastomosis completed in the conventional manner, preferably with interrupted sutures. Whatever technique is used, it is important that the ends be accurately approximated without obliquity of the suture line, the sutures should be evenly spaced, and should always lie at right-angles to the cut ends of the artery.

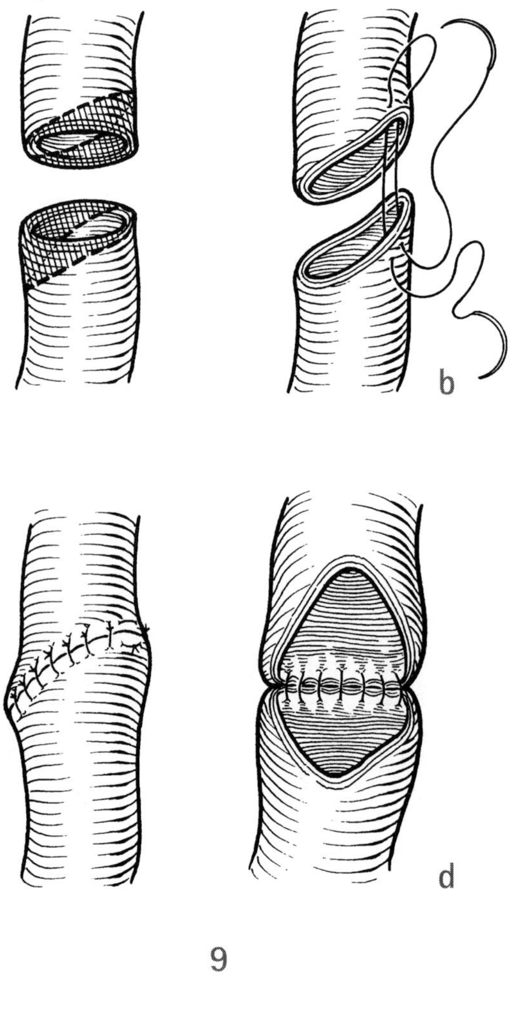

a b c d

9

Interposition graft

10

The long saphenous vein taken from the groin area provides the most suitable graft in terms of calibre and ease of handling. We have used the cephalic and internal jugular veins on occasion, but found these to be too thin-walled and, in the case of the cephalic vein, too small under most circumstances. Regarded as being of adequate calibre for reconstruction in the extremities is a vein which measures 4–6 cm in diameter in its native state. It is possible on occasion to fashion a larger calibre vein graft by suturing a panel taken from another vein into the circumference. In most instances, the graft is short and can be seen in its entirety at completion of the procedure, so that in preparation it is not necessary to distend it with saline but preferable to allow arterial blood pressure to distend the graft once the clamps have been released, thus avoiding excessive trauma to the

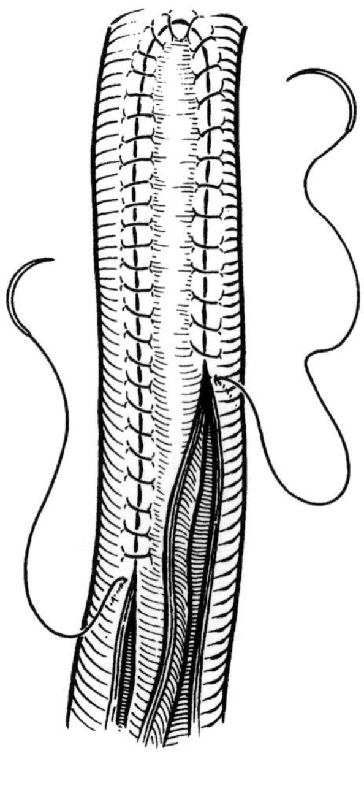

10

graft. It is also unnecessary to totally denude the graft of adventitia and just sufficient should be dissected free from the anastomotic areas to allow suture without adventitial incorporation into the lumen. The principles of anastomosis are identical to those described for end-to-end reconstruction.

11a, b

As a general rule, prosthetic grafts should be avoided in view of the hazards of infection, particularly following penetrating wounds. An exception to this rule is to be found with injuries to the great vessels close to the aortic arch, particularly when a through-and-through perforation of both anterior and posterior walls has occurred (**11a**). Attempts to restore in line continuity invariably results in difficulty in closing the posterior wall as the aorta tends to slip out of the clamp as the medial layer retracts. It is therefore preferable to obtain initial control by means of a side-biting clamp and to oversew the origin of the vessel. Continuity is then restored by means of a Dacron graft which takes origin from the intrapericardial ascending aorta (**11b**). Should a prosthetic graft be required elsewhere as a last resort, we have found polytetrafluoroethylene (PTFE) to be the most satisfactory substitute.

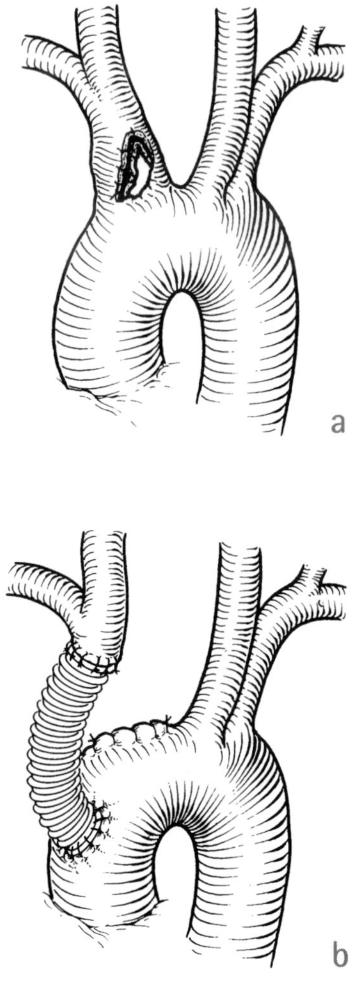

11

Ligation

Arterial ligation should be limited to 'non-essential' vessels, e.g. branches of the external carotid, or an intercostal vessel. An additional consideration is the situation in which prolonged reconstructive operation is inappropriate to the general clinical condition of the patient ('life or limb').

In a grossly contaminated operative field, attempts at in-line reconstruction are ill-advised. A fairly common example would be the combination of colonic and iliac vessel disruption with gross faecal soiling. When this situation pertains, the injured artery should be ligated and flow to the lower limb restored by means of an extra-anatomical bypass, such as an axillofemoral graft. Once the infection has settled the latter may be taken down and anatomical continuity restored, which may be many months later. The same principles apply in any grossly contaminated operative field and ingenuity may be sorely taxed in finding an extra-anatomical route.

Venous reconstruction

In general, repair in the venous system does not yield equivalent results to arterial construction. This is due mainly to the slower blood flow velocity which makes any technical errors such as stenosis, adventitial invagination or intimal irregularity assume far greater significance in terms of subsequent thrombosis. In addition, the thin-walled delicate structure of the venous system makes it far more susceptible to trauma from clamps or rough handling. There is also a tendency for these vessels to collapse because of their low intraluminal pressure which makes localization and hence control of the bleeding area more difficult. Bleeding from large veins should in most cases be controlled by the use of proximal and distal pressure using sponge sticks or intraluminal balloons in order to avoid tearing collaterals and small branches which aggravate the bleeding and make localization still more hazardous by attempts to encircle and mobilize the vein proximal and distal to the injury. An additional important consideration in dealing with injuries to the neck, mediastinum and abdomen is the danger of significant air embolism. Definitive repair of venous lacerations follows the principles outlined for arterial trauma and entails debridement of the edges and closure by means of lateral suture, patch angioplasty or reanastomosis. Suture technique must be fine and meticulous with close attention to detail. Complex injuries present a great problem and if an interposition graft is required the long saphenous or jugular system make the best grafts. We have found prosthetic grafts in the venous system to be uniformly unsatisfactory and thrombosis is the inevitable result. However, the use of temporary arteriovenous fistulae to improve flow has been shown to be effective in improving patency rates. An example of this technique is the anastomosis of the long saphenous vein to the superficial femoral artery to maintain patency in the iliac system or inferior vena cava. Haemodynamic problems may, however, result if these fistulae exceed 5 mm in diameter and they should be closed within 4–8 weeks. Prolonged reconstructive manoeuvres for complex venous injuries are seldom indicated, as these patients frequently have associated arterial and other injuries that mandate reconstruction and, under most circumstances, ligation of the major veins may be performed without immediate adverse effects. For example, in the superior mediastinum, an extensive analysis of our own experience has shown that any major veins cephalad to the azygous confluence may be ligated with safety, with minimal, if any, postoperative sequelae with regard to oedema. An additional problem in treating inferior vena caval and iliac venous injuries is that a thrombosed repair might theoretically result in pulmonary embolism. The morbidity from chronic venous insufficiency in the lower extremity following failure to repair femoral and distal venous injuries is well established, and every attempt should be made to repair these. On the other hand, more recent reports on long-term follow-up of these patients in civilian practice has indicated a more benign course in those in whom veins have been ligated as this level. Following venous repair to the great veins, in view of the theoretical possibility of pulmonary embolism, it is probably advisable to heparinize these patients until they are fully mobile.

Arteriovenous fistula

In our own experience, these have always occurred as a complication of penetrating trauma and the usual pathology is a lateral perforation of adjacent artery and vein with or without an interposed false aneurysm. Perforations are usually relatively small and the most frequent area involved is the neck and mediastinum. In most instances, the diagnosis is made soon after injury, but in a significant proportion in whom arterial haemorrhage is not a major presenting feature due to immediate decompression into the vein, the fistula only becomes evident some time later with the emergence of haemodynamic complications or the detection of a bruit. Patients frequently notice the latter themselves. The sooner repair is effected after injury, the easier it is technically. Once fibrosis has become established, it adds greatly to the difficulty of control and repair of the component vessels and the concept of waiting for a fistula to mature is historical. Ideally, control of both afferent and efferent arterial and venous components should be obtained and can usually be performed without difficulty in the recently acquired lesion. However, when extensive fibrosis has occurred, this may prove hazardous or, indeed, impossible. Under these circumstances, the venous components can usually be readily identified and isolated by palpation of the thrill as they lie on a more superficial plane to the artery. In addition, in the extremities and cervicomediastinal areas, no vital structures cross the major veins. The thrill pinpoints the situation of the fistula which can then in most cases be occluded by direct transvenous pressure using a finger. Arterial control may then be obtained by sharp dissection proximal and distal to this site. Distal control may on occasion prove difficult, especially when the vessels involved are close to the base of the skull. Under these circumstances, once arterial inflow has been isolated and controlled, and proximal and distal venous control obtained, the fistula should be exposed transvenously and arterial backbleeding controlled digitally. More definitive distal control may then be obtained by means of an intraluminally placed inflated balloon embolectomy catheter. Arterial and venous injuries should be repaired on their respective merits as described in some detail earlier.

While recurrent fistulae undoubtedly occur, in our own experience we have found this to be usually due to a second fistula which remained undetected at the original operation. These have more frequently been a consequence of gunshot or, in particular, shotgun wounds. It is therefore important to study and trace the trajectory of the penetrating agent and ensure that the machinery bruit has disappeared at the conclusion of the operation. While the classically held concept is that soft tissue should be interposed between the arterial and venous repairs, we have not made this standard practice as this proves difficult on occasion unless considerable tissue mobilization is performed.

Interventional radiology

Occlusion of fistulae by embolization using thrombin pellets, detachable balloons or various coil devices via transarterial catheters are well adapted to the treatment of surgically inaccessible post-traumatic arteriovenous fistulae involving smaller vessels. Particular application is found in the kidney, smaller intra-abdominal vessels such as the pancreaticoduodenal, and the vertebral and carotid near the skull base. In the latter instance, virtually all afferent flow enters the fistula with very little distal flow into the brain, which makes occlusion safe from the point of view of cerebral blood supply.

These embolization techniques have also proved invaluable in arresting haemorrhage arising from branches of the internal iliac artery as a complication of pelvic fracture or penetrating wounds in the buttock or perineal area.

There has been some success with the use of covered stents in the treatment of arteriovenous fistulae. This pertains mainly to lesions involving the subclavian and proximal axillary vessels. This procedure is not advised for arteriovenous fistulae involving the carotids as thrombus frequently forms in proximity to the fistula and there have been incidences of embolization.

Wound management

Primary closure of a contaminated wound invites septic complications. The most serious of these is disruption of suture lines with massive exsanguinating secondary haemorrhage. In the presence of a compound wound with false aneurysm formation, significant associates blunt tissue injury, multiple foreign bodies (e.g. shotgun wound), and patients with penetrating trauma presenting more than 8–12 h after injury, primarily suture of the wound is inadvisable. Under these circumstances, the deep fascia and skin should be left unsutured and the wound covered with an absorbent, non-adherent dressing. Copious irrigation with antiseptic or antibiotic solution should be performed. Vascular repairs must not be left exposed in the wound but should be covered with muscle or, under certain circumstances, a split skin graft.

The wound should be inspected under sterile conditions 48 h later and further debridement performed if necessary. This should be repeated at regular intervals until the wound is healthy, at which stage formal closure is effected. This regimen significantly reduces the infection rate and hence secondary haemorrhage from the repair site in our own experience.

Postoperative management and complications

Careful monitoring of peripheral pulse status and for evidence of excessive haemorrhage is essential during the postoperative period as a routine. Early complications occur within 5–10 days of operation and may be local or systemic. Local complications are thrombosis, haemorrhage, compartment syndrome, infection and recurrent arteriovenous fistula. Graft thrombosis usually has a mechanical cause and occurs within 24–48 h of operation. Haemorrhage may result from inadequate haemostasis due often to reperfusion of traumatized tissues, but may also occur 5–7 days later due to infection with disruption of the anastomosis. Compartment syndrome may become manifest within the following 6–24 h and must be anticipated, particularly if there has been prolonged preoperative ischaemia or extensive soft tissue injury; its development demands urgent fasciotomy. Compound injuries are contaminated by their very nature and significant infection usually supervenes in the presence of non-viable tissue. Open wound management and frequent inspections with a view to debridement are important. Recurrent arteriovenous fistula as such is rare and persistence of the physical signs usually indicates failure to detect additional fistulae which are not uncommon after missile wounds.

Systemic complications such as adult respiratory distress syndrome and disseminated intravascular coagulation are complications of severe multiple trauma and massive blood transfusion must be anticipated in these patients. The myonephropathic syndrome (crush syndrome) accompanies severe crush trauma or revascularization of necrotic tissue. The major issue is acute renal failure due to the deposition of myoglobin crystals in the renal tubules. In addition, at the time of allowing reperfusion to occur, the patient undergoes a severe metabolic insult in that a bolus of 'metabolic debris' including potassium and lactic acid which in turn may cause diffuse vasodilatation and myocardial depression with hypotension. It is therefore vital to anticipate this complication in the severely traumatized patient in the appropriate clinical setting. Prior to release of the clamp with reperfusion of the limb, the patient should be well volume resuscitated, should be rendered alkalotic by means of bicarbonate infusion and an osmotic diuresis initiated by means of mannitol infusion. The clamp should then be gradually released and reapplied should the blood pressure fall. At this stage the metabolic acidosis should also be carefully monitored. During the postoperative period, diuresis must be maintained at a level of at least 150–200 ml/h by means of adequate crystalloid volume replacement and, if necessary, mannitol administration. The urine should also be carefully monitored for the presence of myoglobin which has a characteristic brown discolouration. Renal failure can be largely eliminated by this regimen.

References

Costa M, Robbs J V (1988). Nonpenetrating subclavian artery trauma. *J Vasc Surg* **8**: 71.

Hirshberg A, Thomson S R, Robbs J V (1988). Vascular complications of diagnostic angiography via limb arteries. *J R Col Surg Edinb* **33**: 196.

Meek A C, Robbs J V (1984). Vascular injury with associated bone and joint trauma. *Br J Surg* **71**: 341.

Robbs J V, Baker L W (1979). Late revascularisation of the lower limb following acute arterial occlusion. *Br J Surg* **66**: 129.

Robbs J V, Baker L W (1984). Cardiovascular trauma. *Curr Prob Surg* **XXI**(4).

Robbs J V, Costa M (1984). Injuries to the great veins of the abdomen. *S Afr J Surg* **22**: 223.

Robbs J V, Naidoo K S (1984). Nerve compression injuries due to traumatic false aneurysm. *Ann Surg* **200**: 80.

Robbs J V, Reddy E (1987). Management options for penetrating injuries to the great veins of the neck and superior mediastinum. *Surg Gynecol Obstet* **165**: 323.

Robbs J V *et al.* (1981). Cervicomediastinal arterial injuries: A surgical challenge. *Arch Surg* **116**: 663.

Cervical trauma

Malcolm O Perry, M Kathleen Reilly

Introduction

Most cervical injuries are caused by penetrating trauma, usually from knives or low-velocity bullets and the damage therefore is usually confined to the wound tract. High-velocity weapons are capable of causing considerable damage because of the blast effect. Vascular injuries caused by blunt trauma are more difficult to manage and can be easily overlooked because often there is no superficial evidence of injury to the neck. Moreover, patients sustaining blunt trauma sometimes have associated closed head injuries and other wounds that require an array of diagnostic tests.

Most patients sustaining penetrating cervical trauma are males. In the authors' series, 14% of the vascular wounds were in the cervical region, but there is a trend seen in recent publications suggesting that the incidence of penetrating cervical trauma may be as high as 38% (Fry and Fry, 1987; McCormack and Burch, 1979).

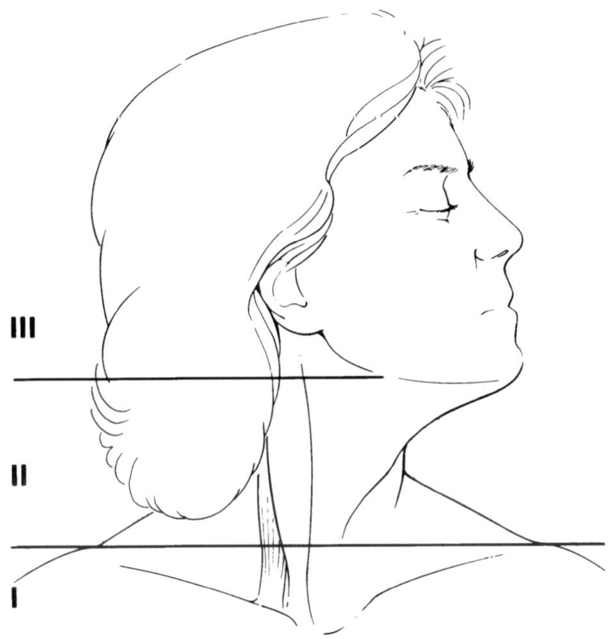

1

1

In evaluating patients with penetrating cervical trauma it is useful to divide the neck into three zones as described by Monson *et al.* (1969). Zone I extends from 1 cm above the clavicle down to include the base of the neck and the thoracic outlet. Zone II is from 1 cm above the clavicle to the angle of the mandible and Zone III extends from the angle of the mandible to the base of the skull.

It is the authors' practice to explore all penetrating wounds of the anterior triangle of the neck that pierce the platysma muscle (Perry, 1981). This is controversial, and if the patient does not have an obvious injury, some surgeons prefer to observe the patient and perform various diagnostic manoeuvres. Patients with injuries of the oesophagus or trachea may have subcutaneous air or drainage; surgical exploration is mandatory. In patients who do not have clear evidence of injury to the aerodigestive tract, endoscopy and contrast studies have been used to exclude injury. These tests have an incidence of false-negative results and cannot be relied upon to exclude damage, particularly to the hypopharynx.

A thorough neurological examination is mandatory in all patients because of the anatomic relationships of the major nerves and vessels. It is important to identify injuries to the cranial nerves or brachial plexis preoperatively, not only to assess the extent of injury, but to document pre-existing damage prior to an operative procedure.

Arteriography may be used to exclude the need for an operation in patients with no obvious injuries. In others, an arteriogram may be helpful in planning the operation, or perhaps will identify a clinically unsuspected injury (Perry *et al.*, 1980). It is the authors' practice to obtain four vessel arteriography in all patients is stable condition who have penetrating trauma to the neck in Zones I and III, as well as in patients with neurological deficits from injuries in Zone II. Patients with penetrating injuries in Zone II, but who have no neurological deficit, can safely undergo operative exploration without arteriography.

Because the main concern in these patients is the possibility of a carotid artery injury, it is useful in planning treatment to divide them into three neurological groups (That *et al.*, 1974) (Table 1). The majority of patients fall into the first group – those who have no neurological deficit. Their prognosis is good and one can anticipate a successful surgical repair. The second group contains those patients with a moderate neurological deficit, generally manifested by hemiparesis or monoparesis, or transient episodes of cerebral ischaemia. Repair of carotid injuries in these patients is also expected to be successful. Group 3 consists of patients who have severe neurological deficits, and often have carotid artery occlusion. In this group the eventual outcome is directly related to the severity of the neurological deficit before surgical treatment. It is the authors' practice to repair all carotid injuries in patients in Groups 1 and 2. We recommend repair of carotid injuries in Group 3 if prograde arterial flow is preserved and if the patient does not have an acute severe stroke with coma.

Most injuries of the vertebral artery are treated by ligation, but if the injured artery is a large dominant vessel it should be repaired. Those methods described for the carotid artery are used in this situation as well (Fry and Fry, 1987).

Jugular vein wounds are also usually treated by simple ligation. If both veins are damaged, it is prudent to repair the larger of the two. The vessel is often of a size that will permit lateral venography, but vein patch venoplasty may be needed.

2

A standard oblique neck incision is made along the anterior border of the sternocleidomastoid muscle. The dissection continues through the plastysma muscle, reflecting the sternocleidomastoid muscle posteriorly, thus exposing the carotid sheath. The exposure of the carotid artery is begun at the base of the neck. If haematoma is identified in the sheath or in the periadventitial tissue surrounding the carotid artery at this level, the incision may be extended as a median sternotomy as demonstrated by the dotted lines. This will enable the surgeon to obtain proximal control of the great vessels in the thoracic outlet.

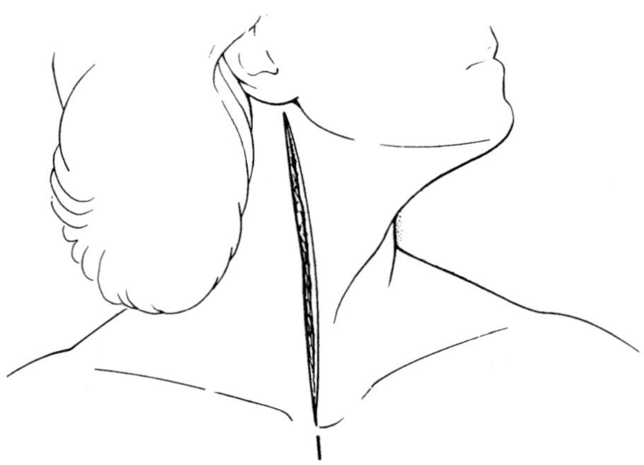

2

3

As the bifurcation of the carotid artery is approached, the jugular vein and sternomastoid muscles are retracted laterally. Beginning the dissection of the common carotid artery first enables the surgeon to establish proximal control. This step also centres the dissection at the proper depth (deep to the visceral fascia) to identify and protect the vagus and hypoglossal nerves, and their branches. The superior laryngeal nerve is hidden by the carotid bifurcation, and if the artery must be freed from its bed, that nerve is protected – it passes forward and medially adjacent and behind the bulb.

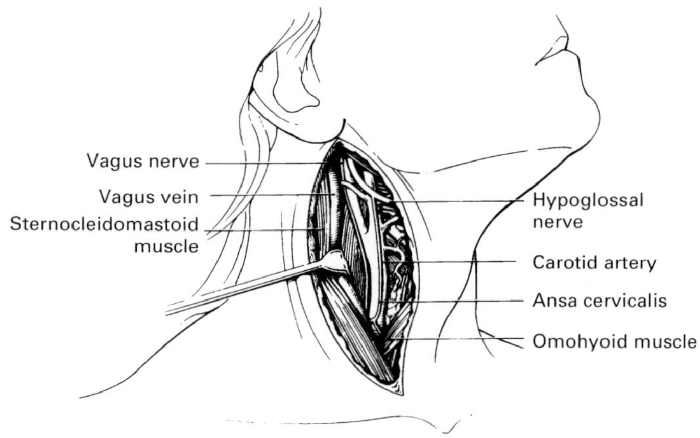

3

4a, b

This demonstrates the exposure obtained by anterior subluxation of the mandible. This manoeuvre is useful when arteriograms show injuries to the internal carotid above the level of the angle of the mandible. With the mandible in the normal anatomic position (**4a**), the dissection enters a progressively smaller area at the apex of the triangle near the base of the skull. If the mandible is moved anteriorly (**4b**), this narrow apex of the triangle can be expanded by 1.5–2 cm, thus facilitating exposure up to the base of the skull. This eliminates the need for mandibular osteotomies. It is usually helpful to divide the digastric muscle and perhaps excise the styloid process.

There are several methods of obtaining and holding mandibular subluxation. The maxillary wires shown eliminate the need for continuous traction that is required when only mandibular wires are placed at the mentum.

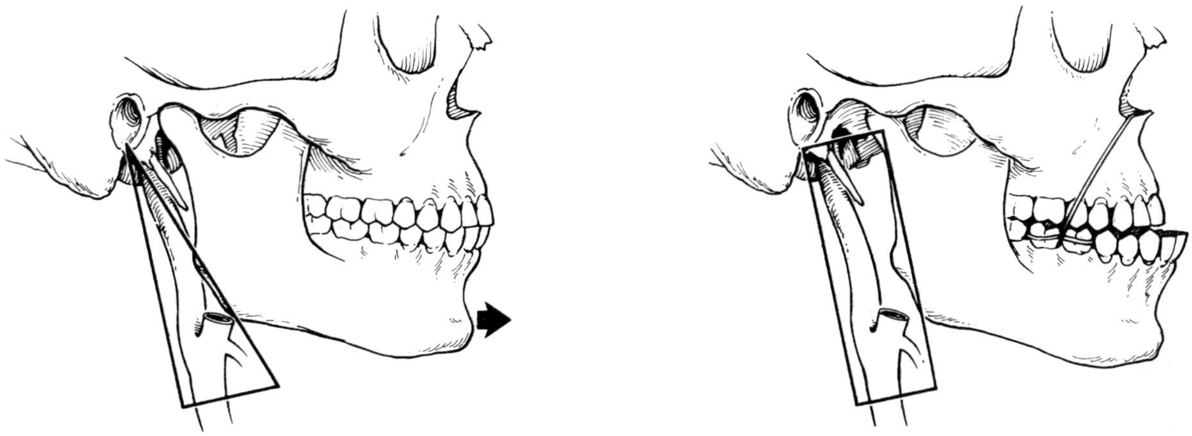

a 4 b

The mandible should be brought directly and evenly forward, and not permitted to assume an angled position because this may compress the opposite carotid artery. Little disability has been seen in these patients after subluxation, although the procedure is rarely needed.

5

Simple oblique lacerations – the kind often seen from a knife injury – are best repaired by simple suture repair after debridement of devitalized wound edges. Intimal coaptation is particularly important in the carotid artery because of the damage to the brain from microemboli.

Most surgeons prefer small monofilament sutures. Often these lacerations are best managed by interrupted suture techniques.

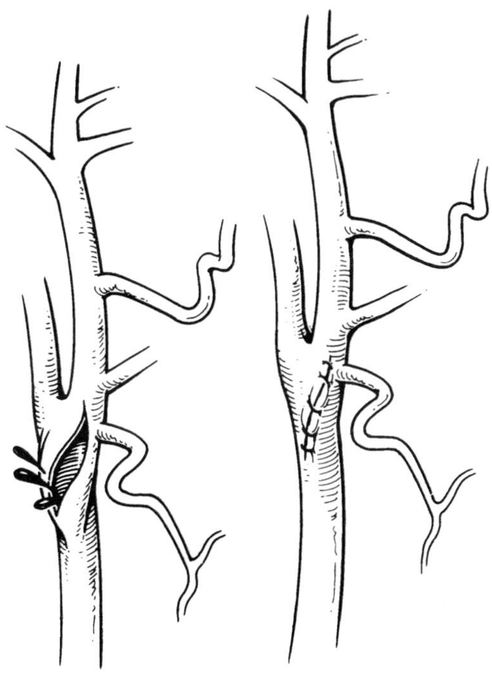

5

6a, b, c

An extensive injury involving the carotid bifurcation, with loss of most of the circumference of the vessel, generally results from a bullet wound. It is most easily treated by resection of the involved segment as shown in **6b**, and then a simple end-to-end anastomosis is performed (**6c**). Injuries to the internal carotid artery involving extensive loss of vessel may be treated by similar technique.

If the artery has a small diameter (4 mm), interrupted sutures are preferred but, alternatively, a spatulated, running suture anastomosis may be chosen.

7a, b

When the internal carotid artery cannot be repaired directly, continuity may be obtained by substituting the external carotid artery. A standard end-to-end anastomosis is constructed between the proximal external carotid and the undamaged distal part of the internal carotid artery. In patients who have multifocal arterial occlusive disease, the external carotid may be an important collateral pathway, and should be preserved. In this situation, an interposition saphenous vein graft is preferred.

8a, b, c

When the internal carotid artery is severely damaged, direct repair or vein patch graft angioplasty may not be possible. An interposition saphenous vein graft is obtained from the groin (these areas should be prepared in all of these cases, since vein grafts may be needed in several situations).

If there is scanty backflow from the internal carotid artery, rather than bright red, brisk, pulsatile flow, a temporary inlying shunt is threaded through the prepared vein graft and put in place to support cerebral blood

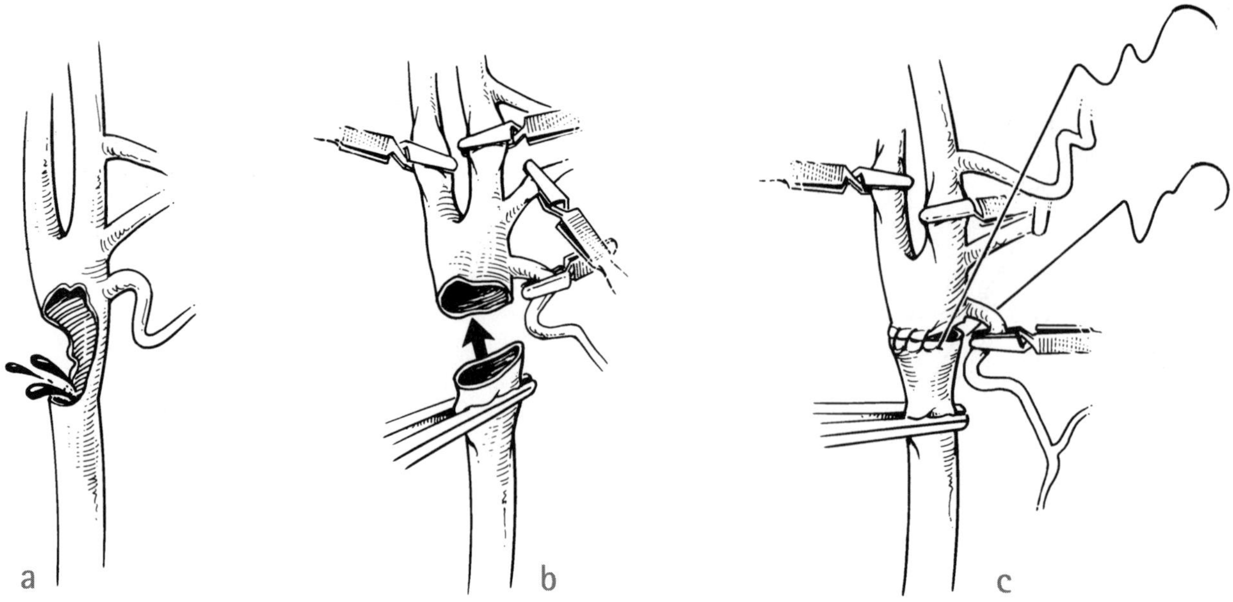

6

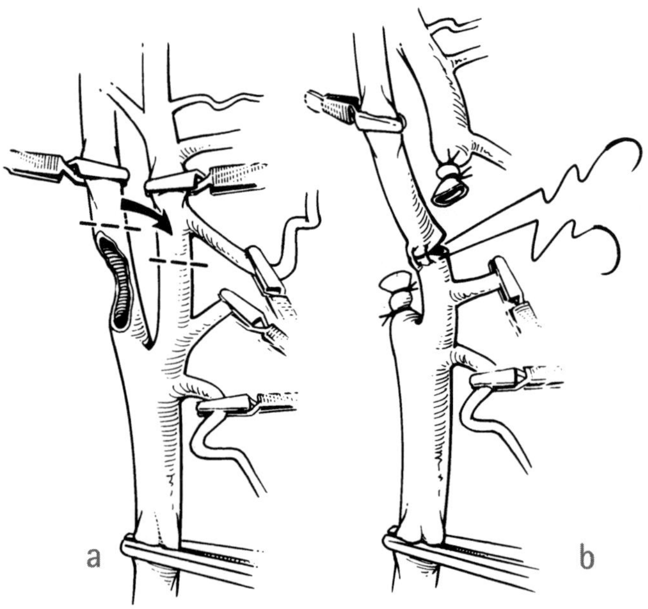

7

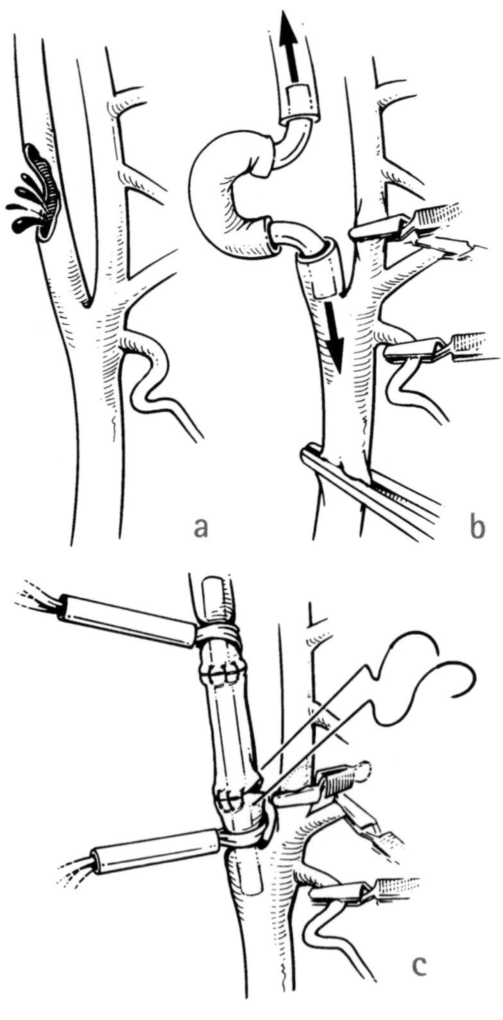

8

flow. Alternatively, the surgeon can measure the back pressure in the internal carotid artery. If it is greater than 70 torr, it is thought to be safe to proceed without a shunt. Some surgeons do not employ a shunt in any of these situations.

During these operations a dilute heparin-saline solution (1 : 10) is used to prevent local thrombosis. Since many of these patients have multiple injuries, full systemic doses of heparin my be contraindicated. If there is only the isolated carotid artery wound, 5000 units of heparin are administered intravenously as soon as control of the bleeding is obtained.

Summary

Although thromboembolic events following the repair of carotid artery injuries are unusual they may cause serious neurological problems on rare occasions if frequent evaluation of the haemodynamic and neurological status of these patients is mandatory. Any alteration in the neurological findings is a clear indication for further studies, usually arteriograms. If a build-up of thrombus in the arteries is suspected, some of the non-invasive tests may be helpful, but often an arteriogram would be required to be certain. If a patient has a frank stroke it is best not to delay for confirmatory studies, but return the patient to the operating room for exploration and restoration of cerebral blood flow as rapidly as possible. The problem is most likely a clot at the site of the repair, and if this is treated before cerebral infarction supervenes, the outcome is usually satisfactory.

Long-term results of repairing carotid artery injuries are quite good (Table 2). In the absence of infection and if the patient does not have a neurological deficit prior to operation, a majority of the patients recover without incident. As seen in Table 2 carotid injuries caused by penetrating trauma have a more favourable outlook than those caused by blunt trauma (Table 3). As indicated in the preliminary remarks of this section, if the patients can be successfully operated upon prior to the development of a neurological deficit, the prognosis is usually favourable. Once the patient has a cerebral infarction then the amount of recovery will depend on the extent of brain damage.

Table 1. Carotid injuries

Group	Degree of neurological deficit	n
1	None	49
2	Mild	8
3	Severe	15

Table 2. Carotid injuries: penetrating trauma

Group	Mortality	
	n	%
1	0	0.0
2	1	1.3
3	5	6.9

Table 3. Carotid injuries: blunt trauma

Group	Mortality	
	n	%
All cases	4/17	23
Carotid operations	2/14	14
Successful repair	0/7	0

References

Fry W J, Fry R E (1987). Management of carotid artery injury. In *Vascular Surgical Emergencies*. Bergan J J Yao, J S T eds. New York: Grune and Stratton.

McCormack T M, Burch B H (1979). Routine angiographic evaluation of neck and extremity injuries. *J Trauma* 19: 384.

Monson D O, Saletta J D, Freeark R J (1969). Carotid-vertebral trauma. *J Trauma* 9: 987.

Perry M O (1981). *The Management of Acute Vascular Injuries*. Baltimore: Williams and Wilkins.

Perry M O, Snyder W H, Thal E R (1980). Carotid artery injuries caused by blunt trauma. *Ann Surg* 192: 74.

Thal E R, Snyder W H, Hays R J, Perry M O (1974). Management of carotid artery injuries. *Surgery* 76: 955.

Upper and lower limb vascular trauma

Aires A B Barros D'Sa

Introduction

Vascular injuries of the limbs which once occurred almost exclusively in wartime, are now observed not only on the field of battle and following criminal violence so typical of large conurbations, but also as a consequence of road traffic and industrial accidents. Blood vessel injuries of the extremities represent approximately two-thirds of all vascular trauma. Confronted with these undoubtedly challenging injuries, the vascular surgeon must swiftly control life-endangering haemorrhage and initiate resuscitation which proceeds in concert with definitive operative treatment. The objective of surgery is to preserve the viability of a limb by precise repair of damaged arteries and veins using accepted principles in the knowledge that failure may lead to crippling disability, amputation and sometimes to death.

The scenario within which penetrating vascular injury of the extremities takes place, i.e. the nature of the wounding agent, the mode of injury and the lapse of time before admission, will strongly influence operative management. Knives, splinters of glass, shards of metal, bullets, shrapnel and fragments from a variety of explosive devices, account for injuries ranging from mere contusion or puncture to complete transection of a vessel. Stab wounds, usually sustained by the upper limb, may sever major vessels quite cleanly with minimal soft tissue injury. In contrast, a missile has a considerable wounding capacity which is proportional to its mass, muzzle velocity and distance before impact. Whereas a low-velocity missile usually only disrupts a vessel segment lying in its path, the temporary cavitational effect of a high-velocity missile will cause traumatic displacement and destruction of tissues sufficient to stretch and tear neighbouring arteries. If bone is struck, dissipating most of the energy of such a missile, the resulting fragments of bone, now behaving as secondary missiles, will wreak havoc on the soft tissues. A shotgun fired at close range can inflict massive damage to a limb, particularly to soft tissues, including blood vessels. Survivors of bomb explosions sustain a multiplicity of injuries with widespread destruction of all body tissues caused not only by the blast wave, initially faster than the speed of sound, but also by flying fragments, secondary missiles, and falling masonry. A few of the thousands of transfemoral and transaxillary diagnostic procedures undertaken by cardiologists and radiologists in modern hospital practice, represent a further iatrogenic source of penetrating limb vascular trauma.

In road traffic accidents, a sharp bony fragment may directly lacerate a vessel, but more frequently indirect damage may ensue as a result of the intense shearing forces generated by the sudden fracture of long bones. Particularly vulnerable arterial segments are those which lie adjacent to a long bone or at points of relative fixity, especially in close proximity to joints. Sudden violent angulation of the shaft of a long bone or the traction associated with fracture dislocations at the knee, progressively disrupts the layers of the vessel wall beginning with the intima. Crush injuries caused by falling masonry after air raids and bomb explosions are observed in peacetime following industrial, mining and train accidents, and earthquakes. The ischaemia consequent upon injury, whether in the form of extrinsic compression and contusion or division of a vessel, will accelerate the progression of a 'crush syndrome' and renal failure.

Limb vascular trauma may result in blood loss, and hypovolaemic hypotension which compounds the ischaemia of arterial injury. These effects and the impaired drainage due to concomitant vein injury are rapidly overtaken by complex and interdependent pathophysiological events (Barros D'Sa, 1980, 1988). If resuscitatory measures and vascular repair are not forthcoming, the protracted hypoxia will increase capillary permeability, causing a rise in intracompartmental pressure, which may herald a disastrous outcome either in the form of Volkmann's ischaemic contracture or amputation.

Preoperative measures

A firm pad and pressure bandage is preferable to a clamp which, when blindly applied, may add to the injury. The principal resuscitative measure must be the re-expansion of the circulating volume. Prophylactic tetanus toxoid and broad-spectrum antibiotics are prescribed. If the patient is not hypotensive a narcotic analgesic will decrease vasospasm and assist peripheral perfusion.

The surgeon runs through a mental checklist of clinical signs of limb vascular injury: a tense and expanding haematoma in blunt closed injuries, persistent arterial or venous bleeding in penetrating injuries, the presence of a thrill or bruit suggestive of incomplete occlusion or an acute arteriovenous fistula. It should be remembered that pulses may still be palpable beyond an injured artery which on exploration almost invariably reveals intimal damage and mural thrombosis. Doppler ultrasound assessment of pulse waveform and ankle systolic pressure is helpful. Evidence of concomitant bone and nerve injury should be documented.

In the shocked patient, delay in the radiology department may endanger life but in most instances plane films which define the bony injury and identify foreign bodies are of value in planning the best incisional approach. Preoperative angiography wastes valuable time in situations of impending loss of life or limb, whereas a policy of selective angiography based on clinical judgement will rule out arterial injury and prevent unnecessary surgery. In these times the medicolegal implications of not having obtained an arteriogram when the ultimate outcome turns out to be less than ideal, should be emphasized. In institutions unaccustomed to a round-the-clock emergency angiography service, the simple alternative of one-shot percutaneous angiography represents a fast, efficient and effective way of using resources. In certain circumstances such as delayed admission, persistent ischaemia after fracture reduction or doubt as to the trajectory of the wounding agent, a negative angiogram supports the surgeon's decision not to explore the wound and, by the same token, a positive angiogram makes operation mandatory. Biplane arteriograms of good quality will define the site and type of injury, and a lateral projection is of particular value in demonstrating a potentially, sinister popliteal injury such as an intimal tear, often missed in an anteroposterior view.

The operation

The operation must be undertaken with the least possible delay, the objectives being control of bleeding, wound toilet, restoration of circulation and prevention of complications. Delay in diagnosis or improper management may result in amputation or lasting functional disability. All wounds in anatomical proximity to a major vessel should be explored.

Emergency amputation

If tissue death and gangrene have supervened due to delayed admission, amputation at the appropriate level must be carried out expeditiously. Following massive destruction and irreparable mutilation of a limb, for example following a bomb explosion, it may be prudent, after careful deliberation, to proceed to immediate amputation so avoiding gas gangrene, sepsis, haemorrhage and renal failure. In such cases, amputation should include vigorous wound toilet and excision of all devitalized tissue, doubly ligating the vessels within viable boundaries and leaving the stump to drain. After inspection, delayed closure, no earlier than 5 days later, is undertaken, using whatever tissue has been preserved to fashion definitive flaps in order to create a functioning rather than cosmetic stump.

Incisions and exposure

1

In upper limb injuries, peripheral and central venous lines should not be inserted on the injured side. The patient lies supine, the upper limb is abducted and extended palm-upwards at right-angles to the body and the draping should provide an operative field with access to the chest, neck and arm if needed. One lower limb should also be prepared and draped in case donor vein is required. The incisional approaches are illustrated.

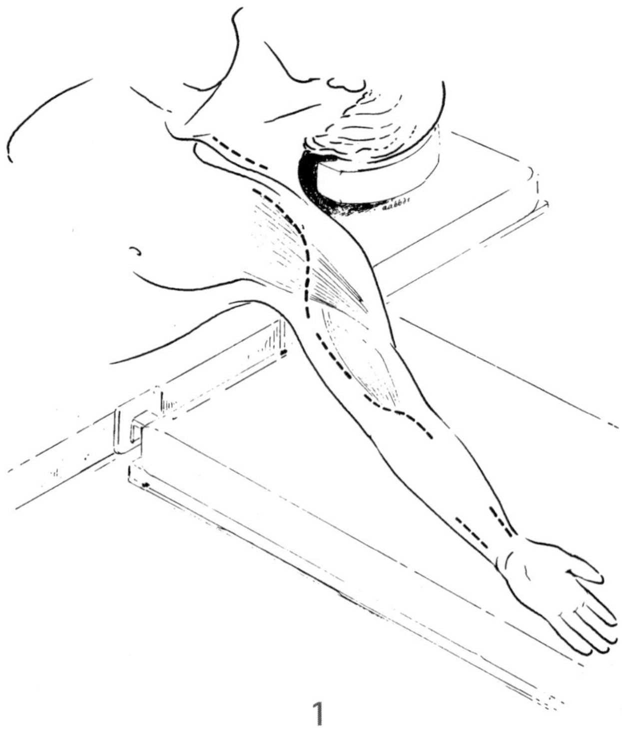

1

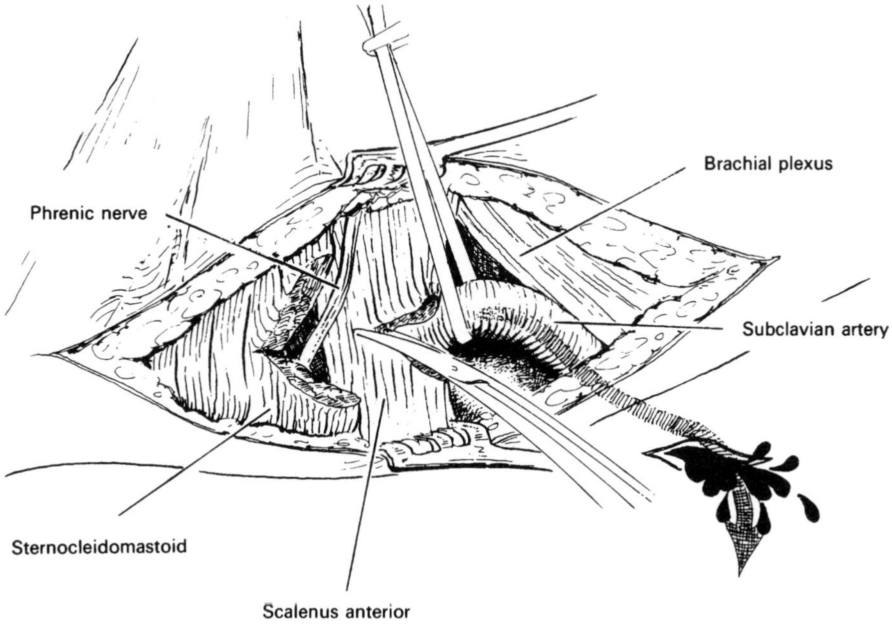

2

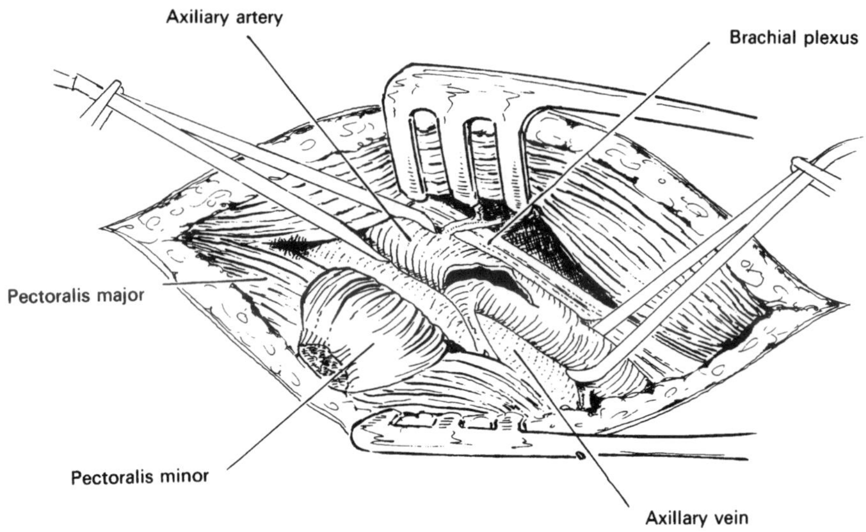

3

2

In injuries such as stab wounds of the first part of the axillary artery it is wise to secure proximal supraclavicular control of the subclavian artery. Partial division of the clavicular head of the sternocleidomastoid, and identification and delicate retraction of the phrenic nerve medially before careful division of the scalenus anterior will reveal the subclavian artery which can be encircled.

3

The incision to approach the axillary artery commences below the clavicle and is extended laterally down the deltopectoral groove and continued distally if required along the course of the brachial artery. This means that the axillary artery can be approached either above or below the margins of the pectoralis major or by separating the fibres of this muscle, as shown. The pectoralis minor tendon has been divided. For rapid access in occasional exsanguinating situations the pectoralis major tendon may be divided at its insertion. Dissection in this area should be meticulous in view of the intimate proximity of nerves and collateral vessels.

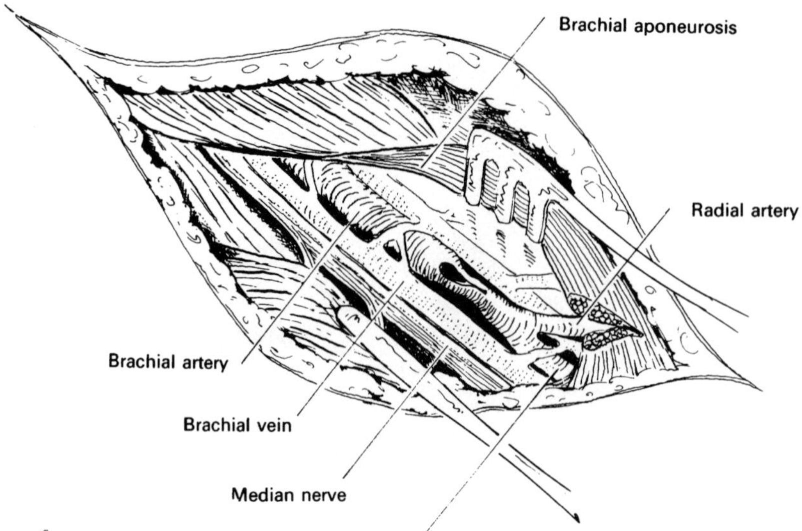

4

4

The brachial artery in the upper arm or at the elbow is exposed via a standard longitudinal incision of sufficient length to expose the injured segment and to establish control. Diagnostic cannulation of this vessel may cause intimal fracture, dissection and thrombosis. Short longitudinal incisions over radial and ulnar arteries are usually quite adequate.

5

In most instances of lower limb vascular injury the patient lies supine and both lower limbs are prepared and draped to permit proximal and distal extension of longitudinal incisions in the injured leg and to enable the procurement of a donor vein from the contralateral leg.

6

Of particular importance are vascular injuries of the groin associated with torrential bleeding, where control of the external iliac artery may have to be established through an oblique muscle-splitting incision affording retroperitoneal access above the inguinal ligament. While this is in progress, digital pressure over the bleeding artery is maintained and only after the external iliac artery has been clamped can the groin incision be made.

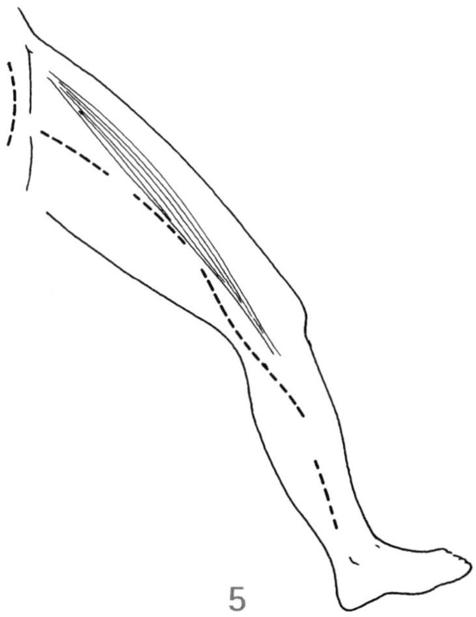

5

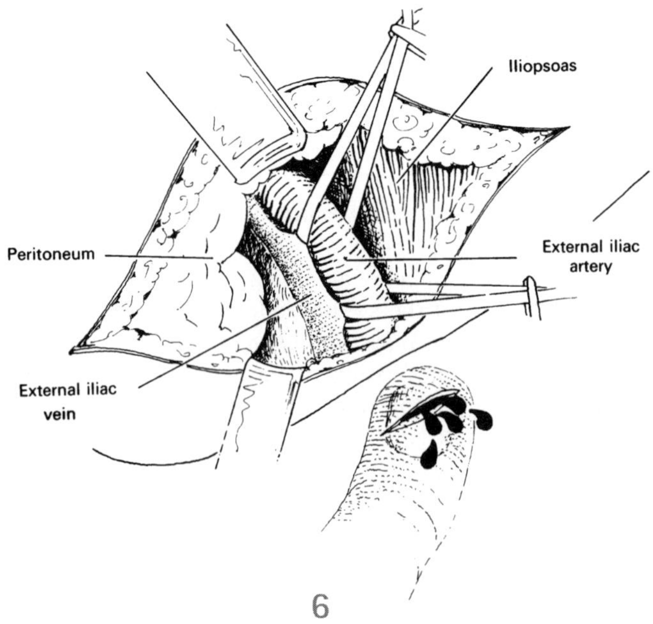

6

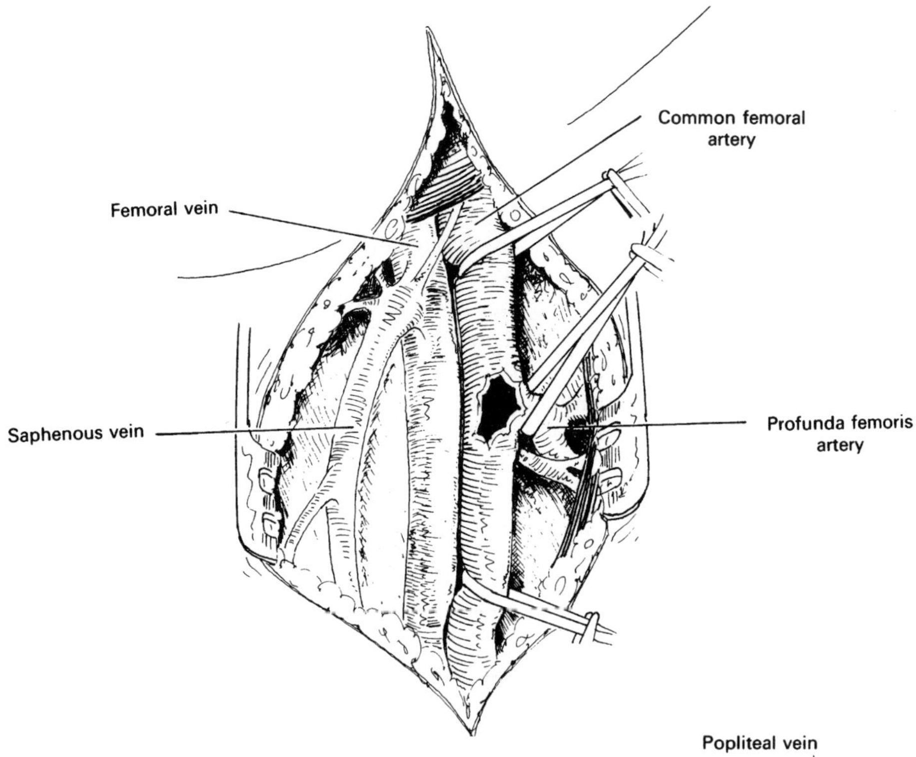

7

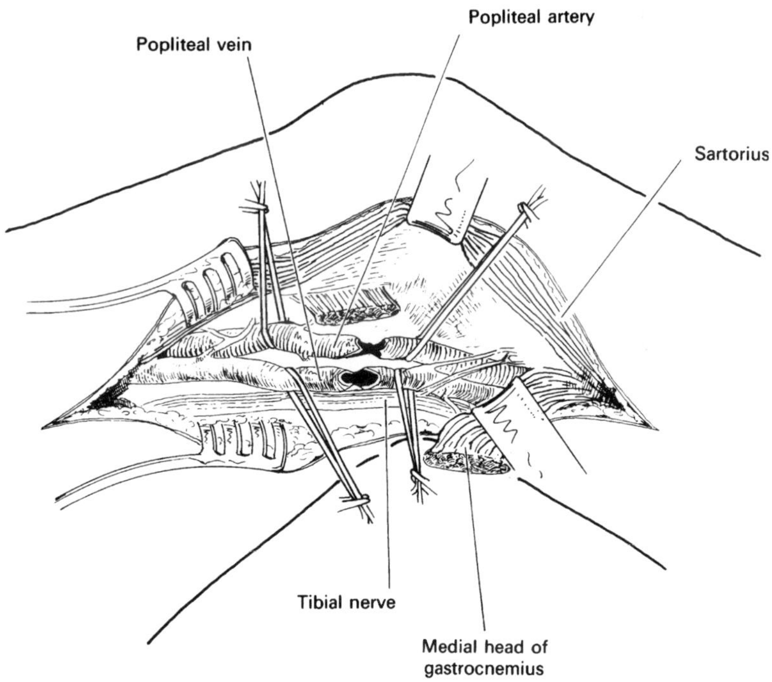

8

7

Classical longitudinal incisions are employed in the approach to vessels of the lower limb. The common femoral artery and adjacent vein are exposed. Injuries at the common femoral artery bifurcation will also require encirclement and control of the superficial and deep femoral arteries.

8

The medial approach parallel to and preserving the long saphenous vein will expose the entire length of the popliteal vessels. External rotation of the thigh and 50 degrees knee flexion using a pack of two sterile gowns for lateral support at the hip, is the ideal position. This exposure usually necessitates division of the medial head of the gastrocnemius.

9

A posterior approach with the patient lying prone is convenient for localized mid-popliteal artery injuries. A gentle 'S'-shaped incision in an oblique axis, commencing medially above and proceeding laterally downwards provides adequate exposure. In these instances, both legs are routinely prepared enabling a segment of distal long saphenous vein to be removed with moderate ease from the opposite leg when it is flexed at the knee. Alternatively, with the patient supine, the upper long saphenous vein is harvested and the incision closed before turning the patient over for a posterior approach to the popliteal artery. The deep fascia is incised, watching for the short saphenous vein which may be ligated as it enters the popliteal vein. The tibial nerve should be handled gently as it crosses the vessels in the distal fossa. The popliteal vessels lie on the floor of the fossa, the vein superficial to the artery and united to it by dense areolar tissue, which may be carefully snipped to facilitate encirclement.

Control and preparation of vessels

10

The damaged vessels in a wound are quickly exposed and bleeding controlled initially by digital pressure. Using sharp dissecting scissors the segments of an artery above and below are dissected free before encircling them with silastic loops of suitable thickness before clamping. Care is taken to preserve significant branches, which in turn are doubly encircled for control. A sufficient length of artery on either side of the injury is exposed so that it can be trimmed back if necessary to a point where the wall is intact. Minor venous tributaries can be ligated.

11

If ischaemia has been prolonged, release of the upper clamp may wash out a plug of clot but a balloon catheter may also be required. Distal balloon exploration, delicately employed, will often recover clot, especially when backbleeding is poor or absent. Lack of backbleeding is ominous, and in these circumstances vigorous upward milking of the limb musculature distal to the injury may express recent propagated clot. In the young patient

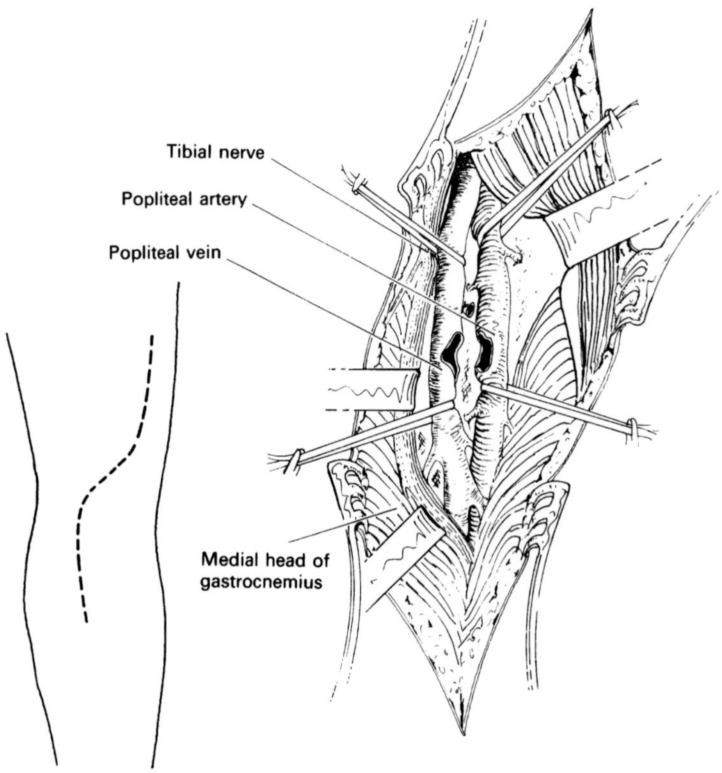

9

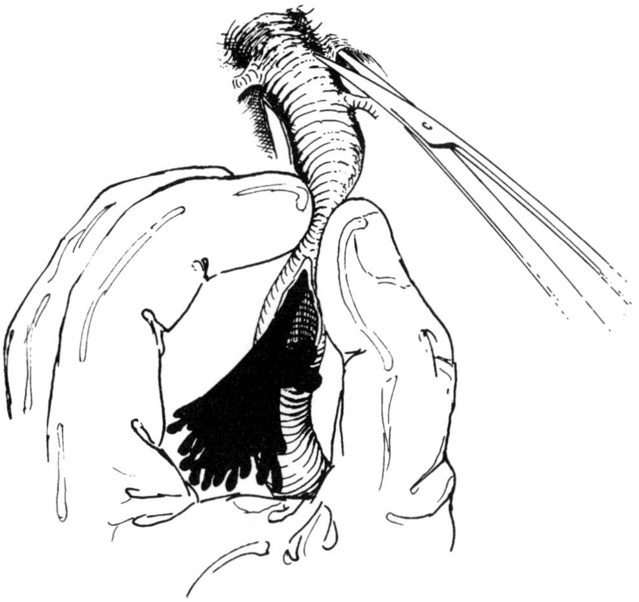

10

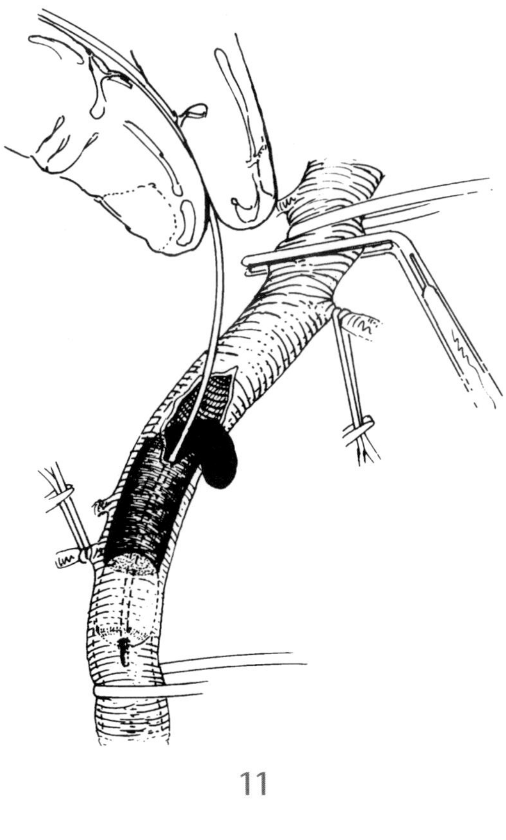

11

lacking an established collateral network, backbleeding will be limited making arterial repair even more essential if the limb is to be salvaged. The distal arteries are then perfused with heparinized saline in a ratio of 5000 units of heparin to 250 ml saline. In the absence of other injury, systemic heparinization is both reliable and easily reversible.

Shunting

When flow through an artery or vein has been interrupted, a policy of routine intraluminal shunting has contributed to improved operative technique, a reduction in complications and enhanced viability (Barros D'Sa, 1982, 1988). Intraluminal shunts of the Brener, Sundt and Javid type of appropriate size, employed in carotid artery surgery, are reasonably effective and a new purpose-built shunt system for vascular trauma has been designed (Barros D'Sa, 1989). When shunts are used, demarcation between viable and dead muscle is more clearly apparent, facilitating accurate debridement and ensuring better haemostasis. In the event of a patient being admitted with multiple injuries, limb-threatening vascular trauma can be safely ignored after shunt insertion, so buying valuable time to complete life-endangering surgery first.

12

A Brener shunt inserted in a torn popliteal artery revitalizes the distal limb and a Javid shunt placed in a severed vein prevents the inevitable rise in intracompartmental pressure, thereby limiting tissue damage and in consequence significantly reducing the need for fasciotomy. The side arm of a Brener shunt forms a convenient port for the delivery of heparinized saline and antibiotics and also for blood sampling, pressure monitoring and on-table angiography if distal injury is suspected.

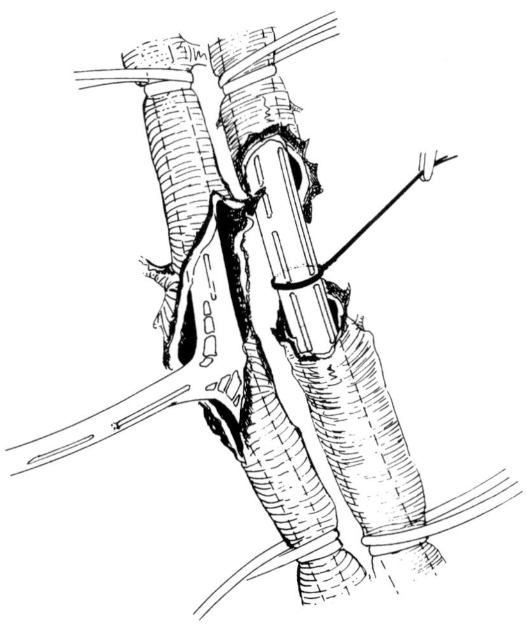

12

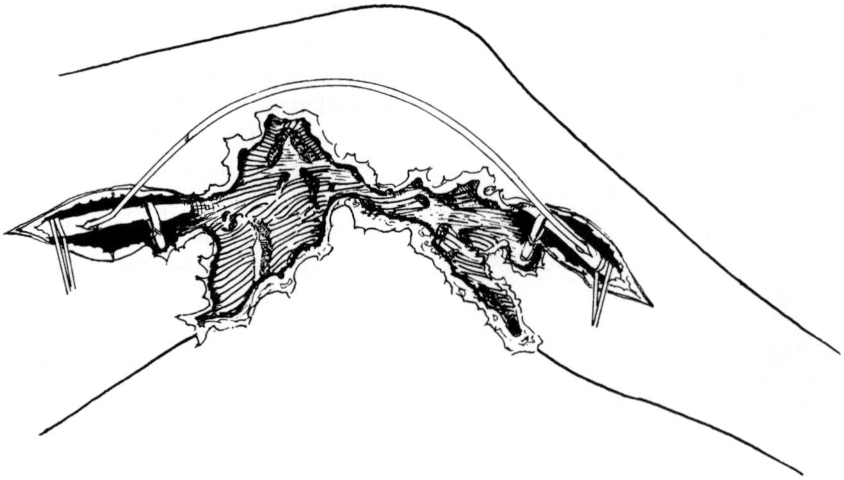

13

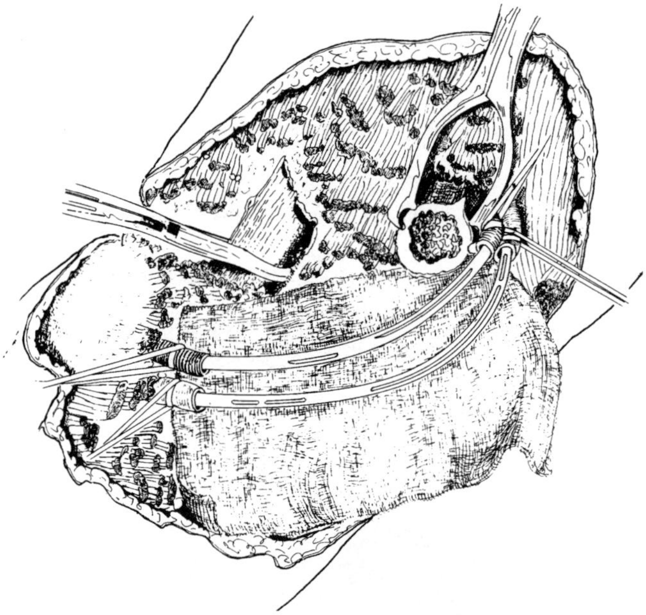

14

13

When a long arterial segment in either upper or lower limb is associated with extensive soft tissue trauma, much time may elapse before restoration of flow. In such cases, a long outlying Pudenz shunt, picking up flow proximal to the injured segment and inserted beyond the injury, will revitalize the limb, and if bleeding through damaged veins is excessive the shunt may be clamped intermittently.

14

When skeletal and vascular injuries co-exist a logical policy formulated around the use of inlying shunts streamlines and co-ordinates operative management. After an agreed incisional approach, if necessary by extending an open wound as when confronted with a case of virtual dismemberment just below mid-thigh level, the vascular surgeon re-establishes flow through artery and vein by means of shunts. He is then relieved by the orthopaedic surgeon who can proceed methodically without undue haste approximating the bone ends and using the most suitable method of fracture stabilization, which in penetrating trauma is usually by external fixation.

15

The vascular surgeon then returns to execute the vascular repair using long vein grafts to bridge the gaps in the confident knowledge that they will not be disturbed. A great deal of debate still takes place about the order of repair when artery and vein are injured concomitantly, but such controversy is dispelled if both vessels are shunted. In the past an understandable desire to restore limb flow speedily led to exhortations to repair the artery before bony fixation, but this policy was attended by the real fears of suture line disruption of a delicate vessel repair during the robust manipulations necessary to achieve alignment of bone fragments. Shunts render this approach almost obsolete.

Care of the wound

Excision of knife wounds is usually unnecessary and only a small margin of devitalized tissue around the edge of a low-velocity bullet wound is removed. Debridement of high-velocity wounds must be adequate if infection is to be averted, and therefore a liberal longitudinal incision dividing the investing fascia is required. All devitalized muscle, recognized by its deep purplish colour and failure to bleed and contract, is trimmed back to a point

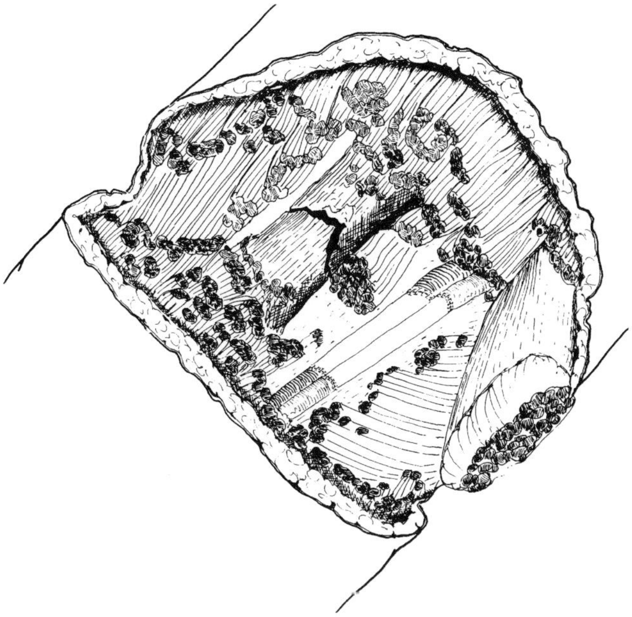

15

plete disruption by avulsive forces. In practice, various permutations of these morphologically simple subdivisions may be present in a single vascular injury. The diagnosis of 'spasm' is both presumptive and dangerous if it leads to inactivity in the presence of limb-threatening arterial injury.

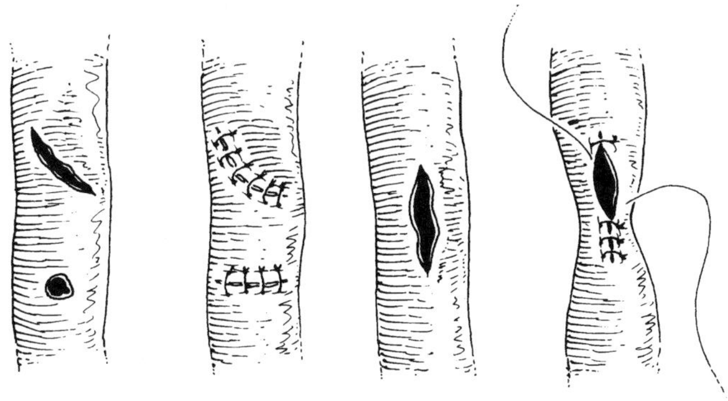

16

16

Lateral suture

Lateral suture is acceptable in a small puncture wound, especially if it can be performed transversely using interrupted sutures. Transverse and short oblique lacerations with sharp edges may be repaired similarly. When the laceration is longitudinal and particularly if it is contused, adequate excision followed by lateral suture will narrow the lumen and could endanger the extremity, notably in critical vessels such as the brachial and popliteal.

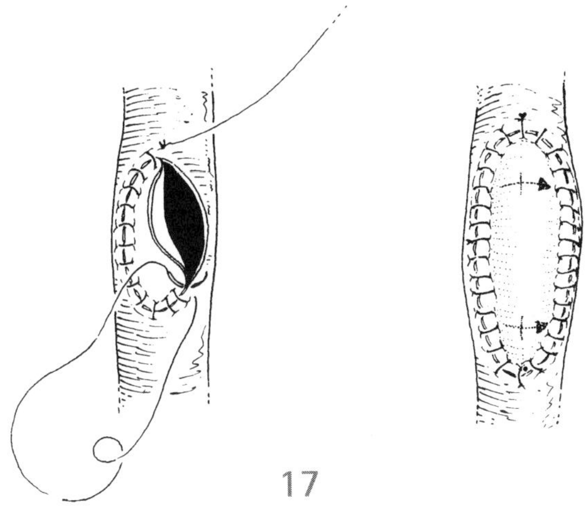

17

17

Patch angioplasty

In order to preserve the calibre of the artery an angioplasty using a vein patch is preferable to lateral suture. In a closed

where it does. Bone fragments are detached from periosteum and foreign bodies, missiles and contaminants are meticulously removed, aided by copious and if possible pulsatile irrigation. A contused nerve is simply left alone, but if transected in a clean wound accurate primary repair is advisable. If damage is extensive following severe blunt injuries and gunshot wounds, the sheath of each nerve end is simply tagged so that delayed secondary repair can be undertaken as an elective procedure.

Arterial repair

While it may be reasonable to ligate minor arteries and veins, in principle all damaged vessels should be repaired, a precept which is particularly applicable to the small calibre brachial or femoral artery of a child whose limbs require sufficient blood flow for proper growth and development. Tibial arteries should be reconstructed, especially if two of them are known to be damaged. The presumption that axillary or brachial artery ligation will not lead to upper limb amputation due to the protective presence of adequate collateral blood flow should be diminished. Brachial artery injuries should not be regarded as innocuous and left to be repaired by a novice, as opportunities to obtain a good result diminish with each repeated attempt. The Allen test should be used in determining the importance of repairing injured radical and ulnar arteries. The choice of vascular repair indicated will obviously depend on the nature of the injury. The morphological types of injury (Barros D'Sa, 1988) include varying degrees of intimal fracture and dissection with thrombic occlusion, laceration or a lateral defect sometimes complicated by false aneurysm and arteriovenous fistula formation, transection and com-

or uncontaminated injury to a large vessel such as the iliac or common femoral artery, it would be quite acceptable to employ a suitable prosthetic patch graft in the knowledge that it will heal with an endothelialized flow surface in a matter of a few weeks (Barros D'Sa *et al.*, 1980).

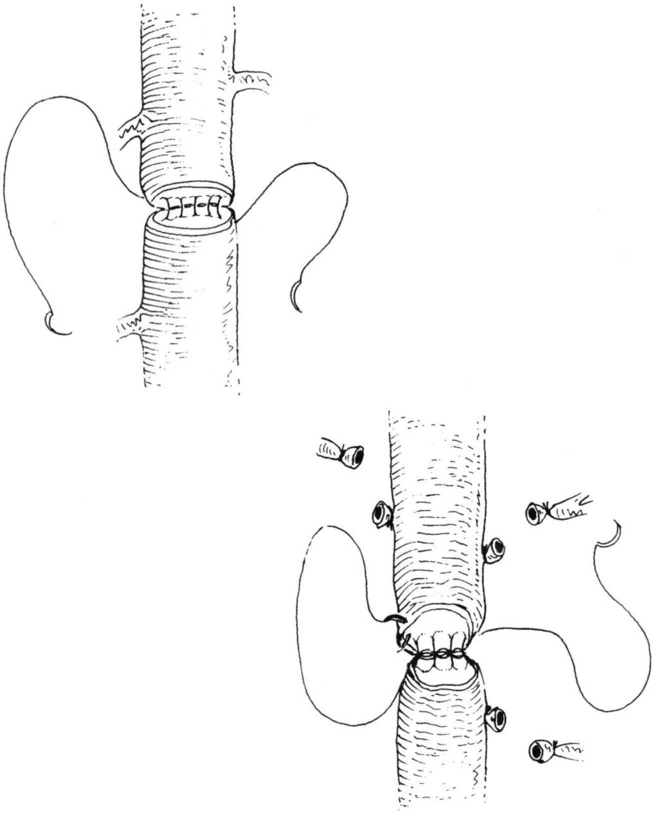

18

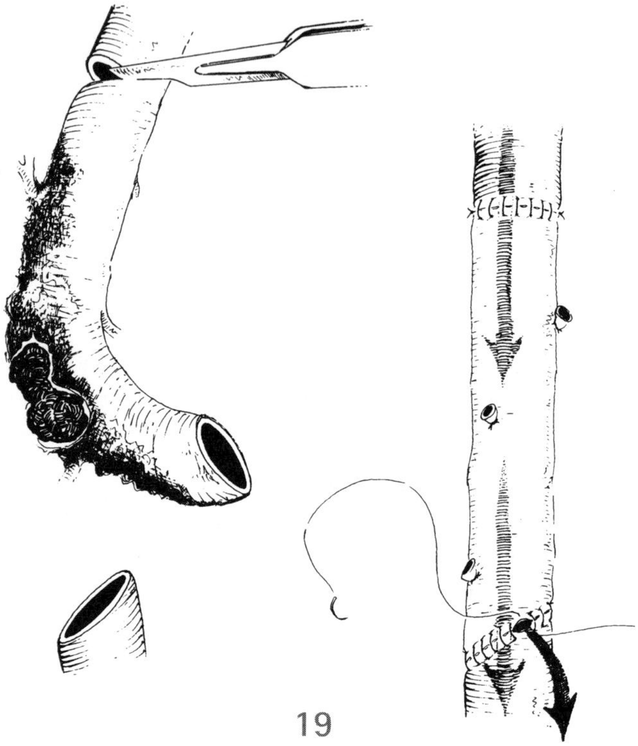

19

18

Direct anastomosis

Direct end-to-end anastomosis is possible after stab wounds or after excising the edges with limited loss of length. The presence of excessive anastomotic tension may well lead to disruption or thrombotic failure. If a joint has to be flexed and if major collateral channels, particularly in an atherosclerotic artery, have to be sacrificed to permit approximation, then excision and vein grafting is indicated. These limitations are once again particularly applicable to the popliteal artery.

Vein grafts

Autogenous tissue is durable, resistant to infection and can develop nutrient flow from surrounding viable tissue. Long-term promise of patency makes vein the most desirable graft, especially as vascular trauma largely afflicts the young. The indiscriminate use of prosthetic arterial grafts in combat wounds predisposes to infection, secondary haemorrhage and a high amputation rate, and has been avoided with beneficial results (Barros D'Sa, 1980, 1982; Barros D'Sa *et al.*, 1980). An institutional policy of using substitute arterial conduits in the form of polytetrafluoroethylene (PTFE) prostheses in gunshot wounds has shown early promise (Feliciano *et al.*, 1984), but should not lead to complacency.

19

The excision of only a centimetre of apparently normal vessel with a No. 15 scalpel blade on either side of an obvious vascular injury may be inadequate, particularly in high-velocity bullet trauma or the complex traction injury of the popliteal vessels in a motor-cycle accident. The external appearances of an injured artery often belie the extent of damage to the intima, and therefore the arterial wall may have to be trimmed back further with sharp scissors to a point where it is visibly intact. The practice of interposing a reversed vein graft which is easily available encourages adequate excision of a damaged artery. The long saphenous vein of the opposite leg is the usual source for donor graft, the ipsilateral vein representing a precious drainage channel in circumstances where the deep vein may be injured. The vein graft is reversed and is usually used at once but may be stored temporarily in cold Hank's solution or heparinized saline.

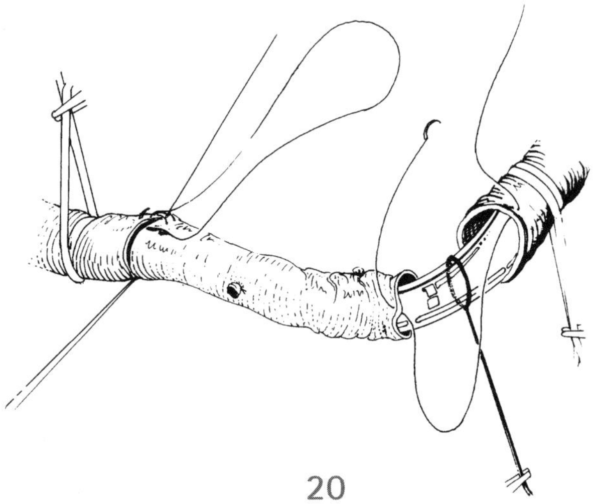

20

20

In larger vessels such as the axillary and femoral, a polypropylene everting suture commenced at diametrically opposite points is continued along the suture line, access to which is gained by a measure of rotation on the axis of the vessel. If a shunt is in place, the vein graft can be drawn over it. The shunt then acts conveniently as a stent, permits a more disciplined suture technique and prevents purse-stringing of the anastomosis.

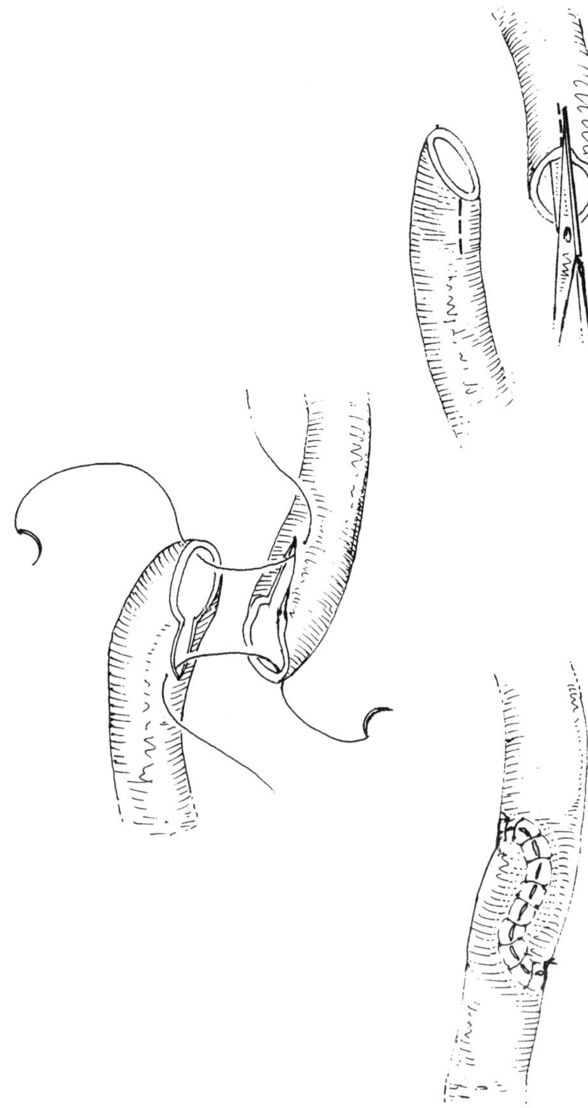

21

21

If the arterial diameter is less than 4 mm, careful thrombectomy using a size 2 balloon catheter is essential. Meticulous attention is paid to technique in executing the anastomosis using loupes and fine instruments. Small arteries of children are prone to vasospasm which may be abolished by judicious inflation with a fine rounded catheter. The ends of the vein graft and host vessel are cut obliquely and spatulated, a necessary step which will accommodate increasing vessel diameter without stenosis as the child grows. Repair is then undertaken by interrupted 6/0 to 8/0 polypropylene sutures carefully placed without tension so as to prevent constriction at the suture line. Accurate coaptation of intimal surfaces while everting the edges will prevent inward protrusion of adventitial strands.

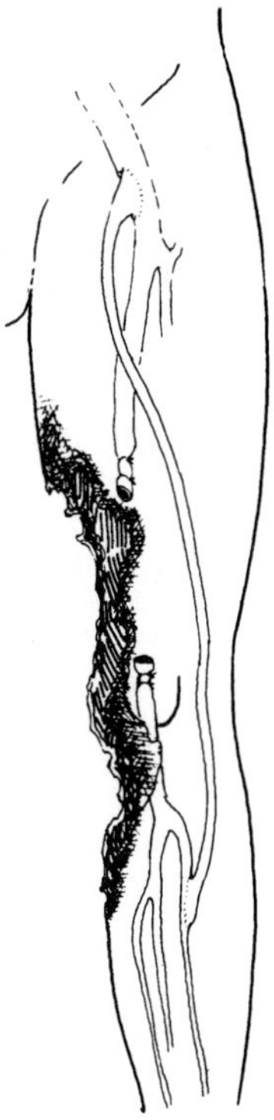

22

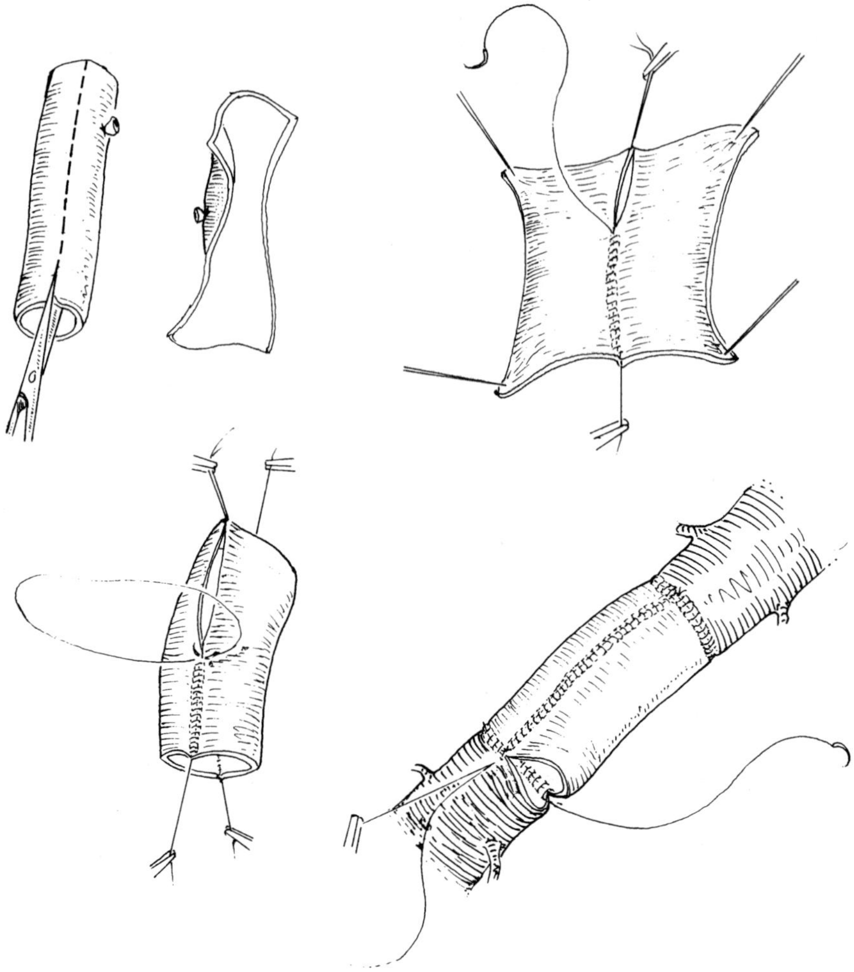

23

22

If a lengthy segment of atheroscierotic artery is damaged, emergency bypass surgery may be necessary. If soft tissue loss is extensive and if contamination is extreme, then an extra-anatomic vein bypass through clean tissues should be considered. If, for example, a lengthy femoropopliteal segment has been destroyed in a large contaminated wound, the trimmed ends are ligated and an extra-anatomic vein graft, unreversed but with its valves disrupted, is inserted subcutaneously from the common femoral to, for example, the anterior tibial artery.

23

When the calibre of the donor vein is much smaller than that of the host vessel – often a vein – the graft will fail unless a panel compound graft of larger diameter can be constructed to ensure laminar flow. It is fashioned 'on the bench' by taking two segments of vein opened longitudinally to form panels and these are sewn together side by side with 6/0 polypropylene to achieve proportions comparable with the host vessel (Livingston and Wilson, 1975). These grafts have to be made slightly longer than the gap to be bridged.

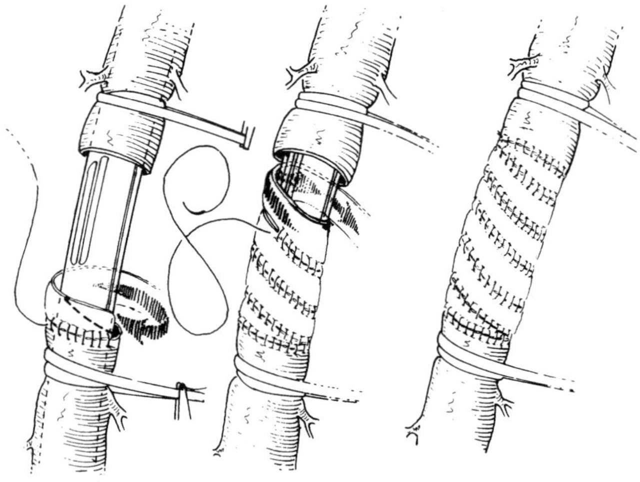

24

24

For larger vessels such as the femoral vein, three rather than two panels may be required. Alternatively, a technique used to replace a segment of the vena cava can be employed and it may have particular value in contaminated wounds. A length of vein is slit open longitudinally and wrapped spirally over a shunt of sufficiently wide bore to act as a stent and then the adjoining margins of vein are sewn together using a continuous 6/0 polypropylene suture.

25

False aneurysms

A false aneurysm may develop in a partially penetrating injury which has been missed usually because distal flow did not appear to be compromised. Most frequently, false aneurysms follow diagnostic transfemoral cardiac catheterization. For obvious reasons, these patients may not be fit for general anaesthesia and regional or local anaesthesia may have to be used. After establishing proximal and distal control, the aneurysm is opened and the profunda femoris which could not be exposed initially is now clamped. The thrombus is removed and the aneurysm excised. The vessel lumen is inspected for intimal damage, if necessary by transverse extension of the opening. If a loose atheromatous flap is present on the posterior wall, it is tacked down with a 5/0 or 6/0 polypropylene suture. The laceration is repaired transversely with interrupted 5/0 double-ended sutures, picking upper and lower edges from within outwards. In the case of a chronic larger fusiform aneurysm, patch angioplasty or segmental excision and replacement with an interposed vein graft or prosthetic conduit is preferred.

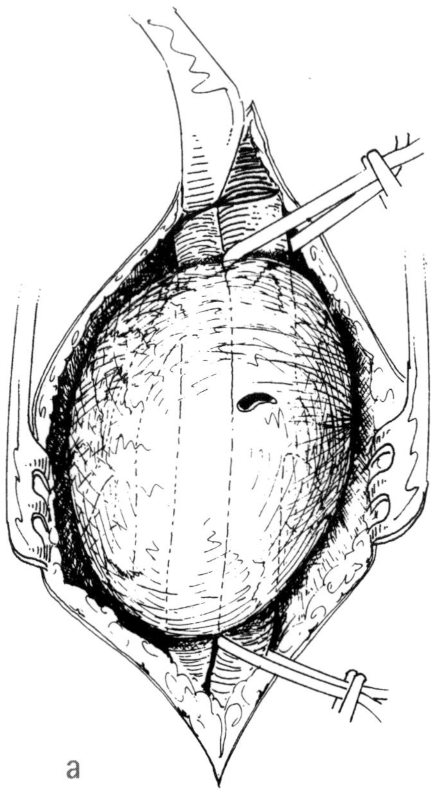

a

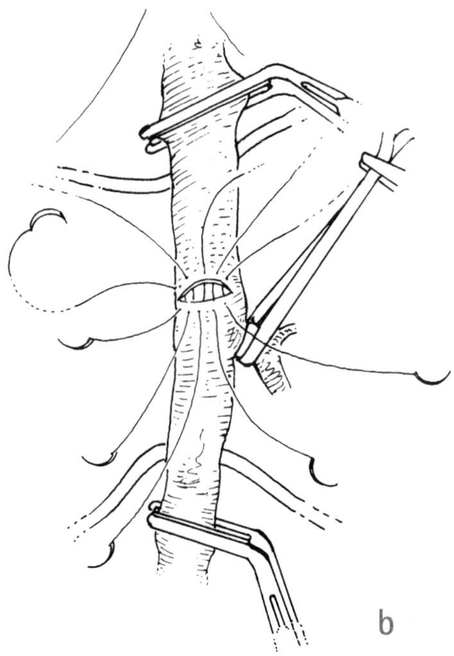

b

25

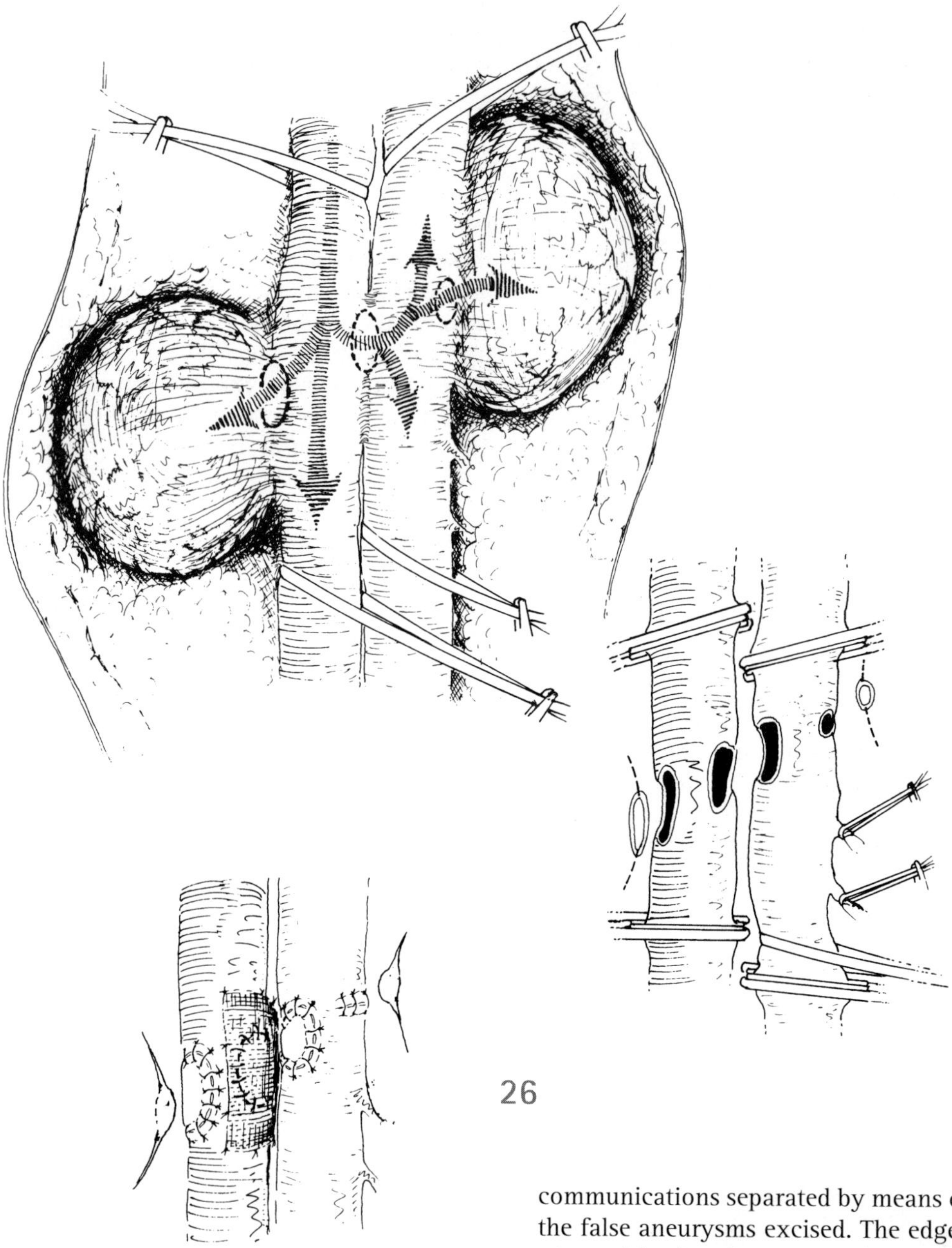

26

26

Arteriovenous fistulae
Arteriovenous fistulae may be missed both clinically and at operation due to inadequate exploration and will present much later, usually accompanied by one or two false aneurysms. The intraoperative use of a sterile stethoscope may have some value, especially in cases of shotgun wounds, to ensure closure of all fistulae. The artery and vein are exposed, brought under control, the fistulous communications separated by means of a fine scalpel and the false aneurysms excised. The edges of the defects are trimmed back to intact vessel wall. The openings in the artery are best repaired by vein patches and, if required, by excision of a segment and vein graft replacement. The vein is usually repaired successfully either by lateral suture or by insertion of a vein patch. Finally, a flap of fascia may be interposed between adjacent suture lines to prevent recurrence.

On-table angiography
Clinical evaluation of the quality of arterial repair in a severely injured and hypotensive patient whose core temperature has fallen may be difficult simply because distal pulses are weak or absent, and even Doppler ultrasound cannot be relied upon. The only way of excluding technical error or distal thrombotic obstruction is by on-table angiography which takes a few minutes and provides visual evidence of the adequacy of surgery.

Venous repair

The mistaken attitude that ligation of a damaged vein, while not helpful, would do no harm, or that venous repair is possibly less important than arterial repair, should not be perpetuated. When both vessels are injured, vein ligation may result in amputation even after successful arterial reconstruction. Conversely, venous repair will enhance arterial patency. Ligation of a main vein causes venous hypertension and can result in acute massive oedema, in some cases leading to gangrene and amputation and in others to deep vein thrombosis and pulmonary embolism or to disabling chronic odema and postphlebitic changes. Every effort must be made to secure at least one good venous channel at axillary, femoral or popliteal level. A vein tolerates lateral suturing much better than an artery, but loss of diameter must still be guarded against. Repair of a major vein is quite valuable when tissue loss is massive and lymph damage is compromised.

27

If both artery and vein are injured and each is shunted, the order of repair of these two vessels is immaterial, but if neither vessel has been shunted then preliminary vein repair will prevent a serious rise in venous pressure when arterial flow is eventually re-established. With shunts in place in this wound, a simple vein graft has been reversed and interposed perfectly adequately to replace a damaged arterial segment of similar calibre, but it would have been too narrow for the adjacent vein of much larger diameter. As time is not of crucial importance, a panel compound vein graft is constructed to match the host vein, drawn over the shunt and sutured in position.

Fasciotomy

Restoration of arterial flow, especially if delayed, increases intracompartmental pressure, which in turn aggravates peripheral ischaemia. These considerations are of particular importance in brachial and popliteal artery injury, and in the latter case the anterior compartment which lies within rigid confines is most vulnerable. Adequate pedal pulses, good skin flow and satisfactory Doppler signals may be observed, although the muscle within the compartments is dying. Fasciotomy, if carried out early and effectively, is an invaluable adjunctive measure aimed at forestalling the serious complications of muscle ischaemia. The early use of intraluminal shunts in both artery and vein diminishes the need for fasciotomy. If shunts have not been employed, fasciotomy should be considered if any one of the following several factors is present: sustained hypotension, an interval of more than 4 h between injury and surgical intervention, evident oedema or patchy muscle necrosis, concurrent injury to a main vein, marked injury of distal soft tissue, subfascial haematoma and bleeding, muscle paralysis and fixed flexion deformity after initial vascular repair or a compartment pressure in excess of 40 mmHg.

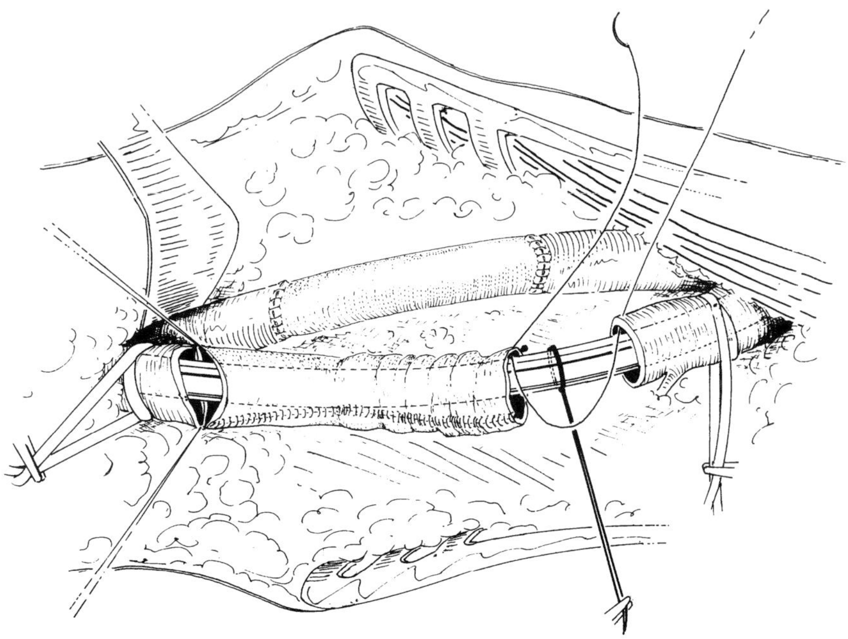

27

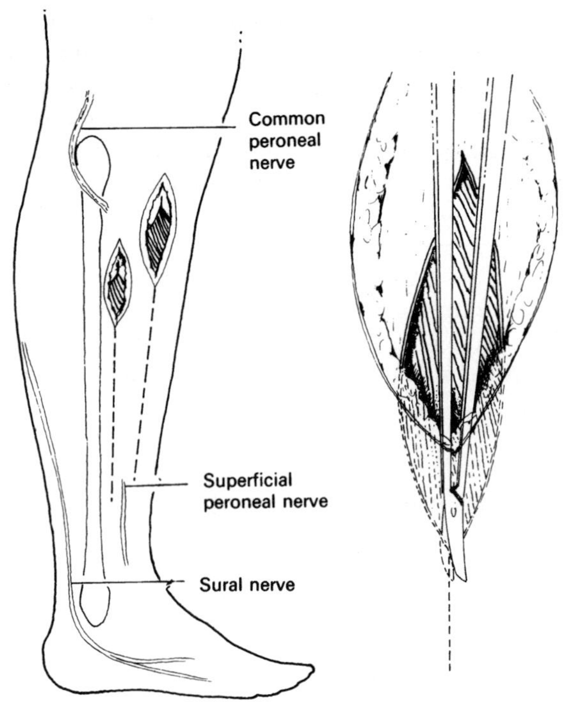

28

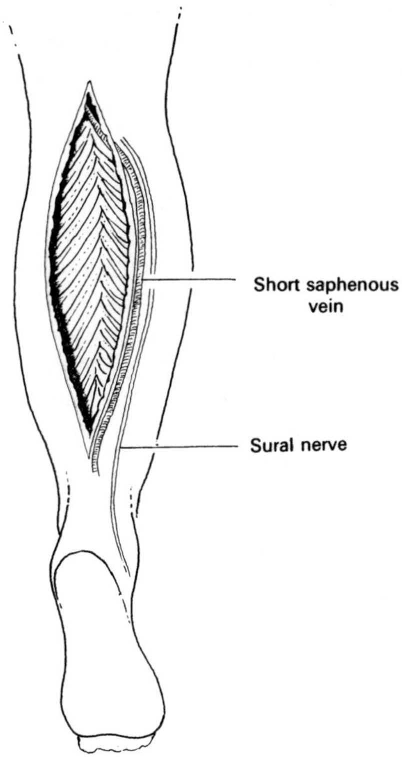

29

28

The classical percutaneous or closed fasciotomy is employed as a rule by using 5-cm vertical incisions into the deep fascia through which muscle tends to bulge. These incisions are made in the centre of the upper anterior compartment, further laterally in the middle of the upper lateral compartment and, finally, medial to the short saphenous vein over the upper posterior compartment. A pair of long curved blunt-tipped scissors is held slightly open to grasp the lower corner of the divided fascia and advanced, slitting it down the length of each compartment. Care is taken to avoid damaging the common peroneal nerve at the neck of the fibula as well as the distal superficial peroneal and sural nerves.

29

If the muscle is pale, grey and firm, or if obvious compartmental tension is still present, the skin and subcutaneous tissues are incised converting it to an open fasciotomy. As tension decreases, these transcutaneous fasciotomy incisions will gradually approximate, but during this period utmost care must be taken to prevent infection within relatively ischaemic tissues.

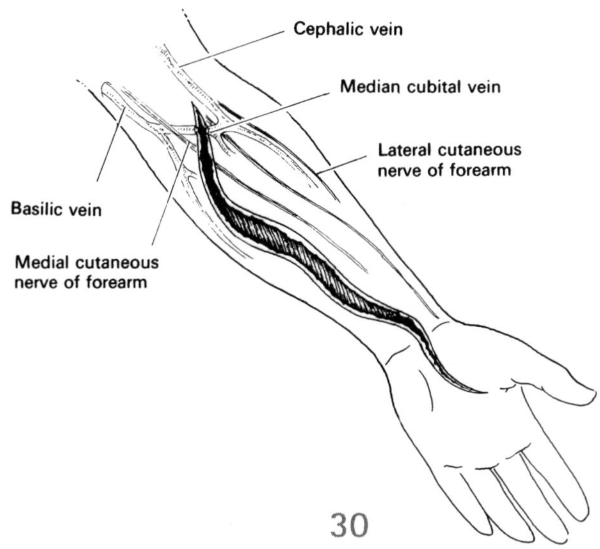

30

30

Open fasciotomy is the technique of choice is severe compression of the muscles of the forearm. The extensor compartment is released by a longitudinal centrally placed incision, while the flexor compartment is decompressed by a long curvilinear incision commencing in the antecubital fossa and crossing the wrist onto the palm along the thenar crease.

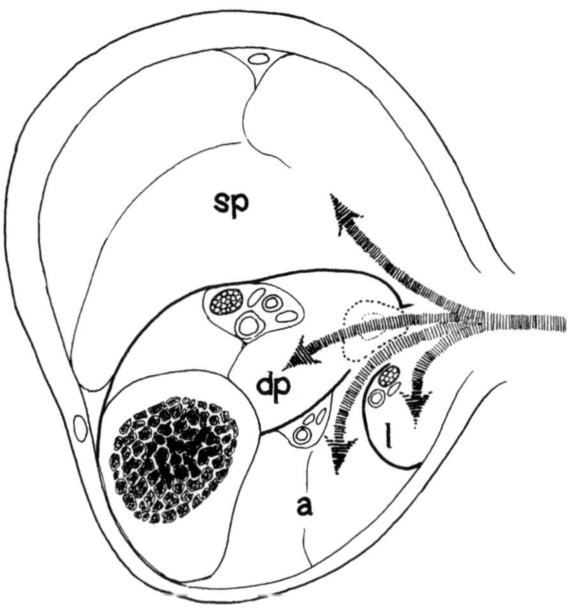

31

31

It should be remembered that a fourth deep posterior compartment is present in the lower leg in addition to the other three, and all four can be decompressed simultaneously after first resecting the mid-third of the shaft of the fibula subperiosteally (Patman and Thompson, 1970). The relationship of the superficial posterior (sp), deep posterior (dp), anterior (a) and lateral (l) compartments to the fibula when imagined in transverse section show how this route of entry can achieve the desired result.

Wound closure and vessel cover

It is important to ensure adequate cover of repaired vessels by adjacent tissues. In closed injuries primary suture of the wound is acceptable, leaving a vacuum suction drain *in situ* for a short period. In contaminated wounds the wisdom of a policy of delayed primary suture 5–7 days later has been borne out by experience (Barros D'Sa, 1980), but that should not be an excuse for slipshod wound excision and toilet.

In situations of extensive loss of skin and soft tissue over a site of arterial repair, the wall of a vein graft or adjacent artery may conceivably undergo ischaemia, desiccation and degeneration followed by catastrophic haemorrhage. While prosthetic grafts are immune to these influences they still represent alien material and if the field is contaminated then infection, thrombosis and suture line dehiscence could follow. This observation has a special bearing on the management of large dirty wounds which have to be left open to drain, making graft cover difficult. Biological dressings, such as porcine heterografts and amniotic membrane, have been tried but the alternative of a vascularized muscle flap requiring the skills of a plastic surgeon is preferable. Many of these difficulties will, of course, have been countered by the employment of the extra-anatomic vein bypass described.

Postoperative management

Ordinarily, following arterial repair, a limb is nursed in a horizontal position, but when the adjacent vein has been repaired, some degree of elevation is justified. As the patient rewarms, a deficiency in fluid replacement, evident from general observation and vital signs, must be corrected to ensure adequate flow through the reconstructed vessels. Anticoagulation with low-dose heparin (5000 units every 6 h subcutaneously) will aid graft patency and prevent deep vein thrombosis.

Failure of repair

Utmost vigilance must be exercised in monitoring flow by checking pulses, skin circulation and Doppler signals. Their absence may be a prelude to amputation unless urgent angiography and further reconstruction are undertaken. In such cases, classical weaknesses of technique are observed, namely, constriction caused by lateral suture, tension at the suture line of a direct anastomosis, insufficient excision of damaged artery, too narrow or too long vein grafts, 'purse-string' effect of a continuous anastomotic suture and poor intimal coaptation. In dealing with graft failure the most reliable sequence of measures is as follows: excise the segment concerned liberally, confirm the quality of the freshly trimmed vessel, perform an adequate balloon thrombectomy, reperfuse the distal artery with heparinized saline and very precisely revise the repair with a fresh vein graft of suitable calibre and length. Systemic heparinization and close observation will avert an unfavourable outcome.

In summary, a number of factors play a role in minimizing the complication rate and incidence of limb loss: routine use of intraluminal shunts in both injured artery and vein, vascular repair after skeletal fixation, early and definitive repair of both artery and vein injury, avoidance of lateral suture and direct anastomosis, use of vein grafts and of panel compound grafts of appropriate diameter when required, immediate fasciotomy when indicated, postoperative vigilance and, in cases of graft failure, expeditious re-exploration and fresh repair.

References

Barros D'Sa A A B (1980). Missile-induced vascular trauma. *Injury* **12**: 13.

Barros D'Sa A A B (1982). A decade of missile-induced vascular trauma. *Ann R Coll Surg Engl* **64**: 37.

Barros D'Sa A A B (1988). How should we manage acute ischaemia associated with trauma? In *Limb Salvage and Amputation for Vascular Disease*. Greenhalgh R M, Jamieson C W, Nicolaides, A N eds. London Philadelphia: W B Saunders Co.

Barros D'Sa A A B (1989). The rationale for arterial and venous shunting in the management of limb vascular injuries. *Eur J Vasc Surg* **3**: 471.

Barros D'Sa A A B, Berger K, DiBenedetto G *et al.* (1980). A healable filamentous Dacron surgical fabric. *Annl Surg* **192**: 645.

Feliciano D V, Camel G, Bitondo P A C *et al.* (1984). Civilian trauma in the 1980s. A 1-year experience with 456 vascular and cardiac injuries. *Annl Surg* **199**: 717.

Livingston R H, Wilson R I (1975). Gunshot wounds to the limbs. *Br Med J* **1**: 667.

Patman R D, Thompson J E (1970). Fasciotomy in peripheral arterial injury. *Arch Surg* **101**: 633.

Surgical techniques in the treatment of varicose veins

Sidney S Rose

Introduction

The surgical treatment of varicose veins has in the past even in experienced hands, produced notoriously bad results. This is due to a number of factors among the commonest of which is the inexperience of the surgeon and the natural prevalence of recurrence. It is felt that it is also attributable in part to the unquestioning acceptance of the hitherto established aetiological concept of primary valvular incompetence and the influence this has on surgical technique. In particular this has led to concentration of operative techniques on proximal ligation of main stem superficial veins and/or ligation of incompetent deep perforators. It is obvious that proximal ligation is necessary in the case of irreversible incompetence at the confluence of the main deep and superficial veins but the necessity for ligation of the deep perforator has been called into question. Full-length stripping has had its advocates and been found wanting because of failure to remove varicose bunches. Routine stripping often removes a saphenous vein which is largely normal and deprives the patient of a possible future bypass conduit.

Our concept of the aetiology based on a series of examinations of the vein wall by transmission electron microscopy is somewhat different and has led us to adopt our present techniques. We believe that the primary lesion is in the muscle cell of the vein wall where a degenerative fibrosis develops, producing first of all loss of tone and then dilatation not only of the vein wall in between the valves but of the valve ring itself. Dilatation at this point leads to secondary valvular incompetence because the valve cusps can no longer meet and eventually undergo disuse atrophy. This applies to both the superficial veins and the deep perforators. The surgical treatment is therefore based on removal of the varicose veins themselves combined if necessary with proximal ligation at the main saphenofemoral or saphenopopliteal junction if incompetence exists at these points. We maintain that meticulous removal of the superficial varices renders it unnecessary to ligate deep perforators as most of the connections to the superficial veins will be interrupted by this procedure, and the veins into which they feed will be eliminated surgically.

The modern technique has been variously described in the centres where it has been developed *viz* 'winkling', multiple excision, ligation-excision, but has now become known for convenience as stab-avulsion although micro-incision would be more descriptive in many circumstances.

Preoperative

Indications for surgery

Relief of symptoms
Varicose veins are often asymptomatic but the sensation of heaviness of the legs and chronic aching in the calves may be so severe as to require treatment. The other symptoms which cause patients to seek advice are night cramps, 'restless' legs, localized pain and tenderness over localized blow-outs, even in the absence of phlebitis. Itching and irritation of the overlying skin may occur. Any of these symptoms may be severe enough to require treatment by surgery.

To treat complications
The common complications of varicose veins are haematoma, possible even after slight trauma, haemorrhage which may be spontaneous or traumatic, eczema which may be local or generalized, recurrent superficial phlebitis, the development of subcutaneous and intradermal induration and varicose ulceration. Deep venous thrombosis may occur although the relationship to varicose veins is not as clear-cut as might be expected. Pulmonary embolism has also been recorded although this may be considered to be related to a subclinical deep venous thrombosis. A history of any of the above complications is an indication for surgery, although an interval of 3 months should be allowed after an attack of

superficial thrombophlebitis before surgery is undertaken.

Cosmetic considerations

There is no doubt that varicose veins can be extremely ugly, both from a subjective and objective point of view. The development of a cosmetic procedure which also provides efficient and long-lasting relief justifies operating for cosmetic reasons. It must be noted here that a purely cosmetic complaint has difficulty in finding a place on a hospital waiting list and some health insurance companies specifically exclude such complaints from benefit.

Contraindications

1. Age and general condition. General condition is more important than age in this respect but it is obviously unwise and unnecessary to carry out operative procedures requiring long anaesthetics in the aged. Removal of symptomatic bunches under local anaesthetic may be carried out in the elderly if otherwise quite fit.
2. Obesity. This increases the hazards of any surgical procedure, and may produce special difficulties in removing varicose veins. This should be corrected if feasible before proceeding.
3. Active superficial thrombophlebitis. This must always be controlled before embarking upon surgery for varicose veins.
4. Subcutaneous induration (lipodermatosclerosis). It is often impossible to remove veins from these areas. The local condition may be improved by support (firm bandaging or pressure-graded elastic stockings), elevation of the legs at night, calf muscle and ankle exercises, and stanozolol in acute cases. The feeding veins may then be dealt with by ligation, sclerotherapy, or a combination of the two.
5. Infected ulceration. The presence of an ulcer alone is not a contraindication to surgery provided it is clean, but infection must be treated first.
6. Pregnancy. It is inadvisable to operate during pregnancy and in any event many of the veins regress within 3 months of parturition.
7. Arterial insufficiency. Peripheral pulses must always be recorded and the state of the peripheral circulation must be identified in patients at risk.
8. The presence of a large intra-abdominal tumour which may be the cause of venous back pressure and will require primary treatment.

Both the latter conditions will have been excluded by the preliminary examination.

Preoperative preparation

A pubic shave is only necessary where the groin is to be explored. The leg must be shaved, especially in men, and the patients are instructed to do this themselves before admission.

The veins are marked with the patient standing using a black or blue fine-point felt pen, the sites of maximum discomfort being marked with a circle, so that special attention may be given to the underlying vein. If the veins are extensive in one leg, both legs are not operated on unless the contralateral limb is only slightly involved. This is because an extensive procedure on both sides will hinder the postoperative walking ability, necessary to minimize phlebitis, and will involve an unjustifiably long anaesthetic.

Anatomy

1

Normal distribution of main superficial veins of the lower limb with common sites of deep perforators (after *Gray's Anatomy*). A similar chart is used to record the distribution of the varicosities at the first examination.

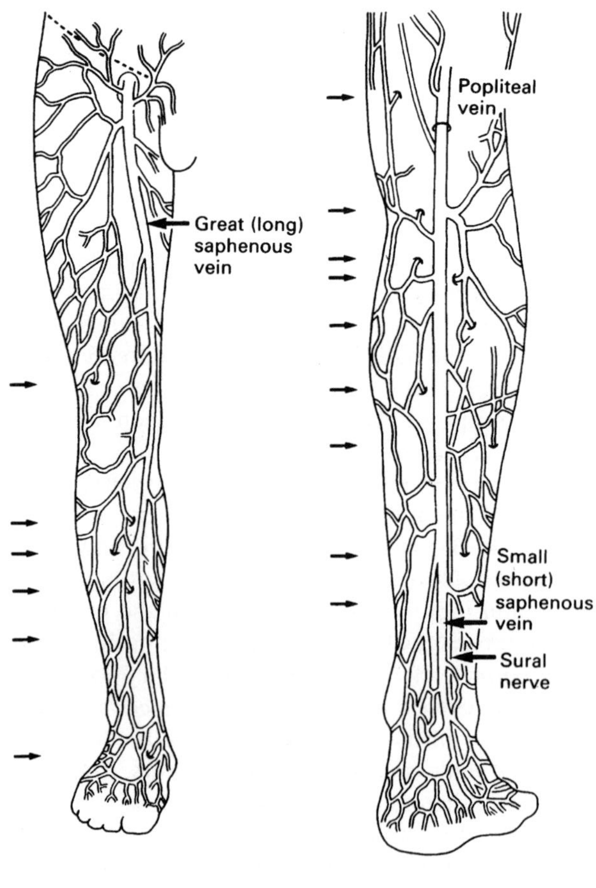

1

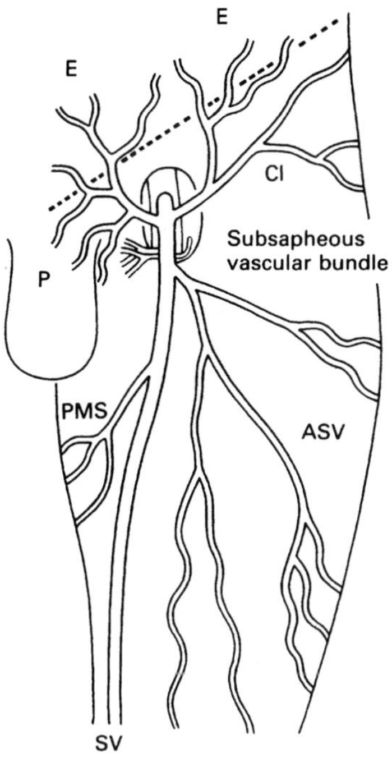

SV = long saphenous vein; ASV = anterior saphenous veins; PMS = posterior medial saphenous veins; P = superficial internal pudendal veins; E = superficial epigastric veins; CI = superficial circumflex iliac veins; L = lateral saphenous veins.

2

2

Normal anatomy of the saphenofemoral junction (after *Gray's Anatomy*). The position of the inguinal ligament is shown dotted, but this is not synonymous with the groin crease. This is usually lower than the inguinal ligament, the distance increasing with obesity.

The operation

Position of patient

The patient is positioned on the table with a sandbag under the contralateral buttock to rotate the affected limb outwards to improve access to the groin, and this is further improved by having the knee moderately flexed.

Most aspects of the limb can be reached by judicious rotation but exploration of the saphenopopliteal junction and veins at the back of the thigh must be carried out with the patient in the prone position. If this is necessary, this part of the procedure is carried out first. It must be remembered that pressure on the abdomen in the prone position causes some obstruction to the vena cava and will increase venous bleeding unless the chest and pelvis are raised off the operating table.

The groin incision

Exploration of the groin is indicated where there is a pronounced cough impulse at the groin on palpation. Reflex may be confirmed by Doppler examination. This may be confined to the immediate vicinity of the saphenofemoral junction or propagated down the leg in more advanced cases. The incision must be placed so that an adequate exposure of the saphenofemoral junction is obtained. Its position and length will be governed by the degree of obesity of the patient since the groin fold only approximates to the inguinal ligament when there is a minimum of subcutaneous fat. It will be appreciably lower in obese patients, in whom the incision needs to be above the groin crease. In any event, the incision is parallel to the inguinal ligament, using the femoral pulse as the lateral landmark, and will be on average 3.5–7 cm long.

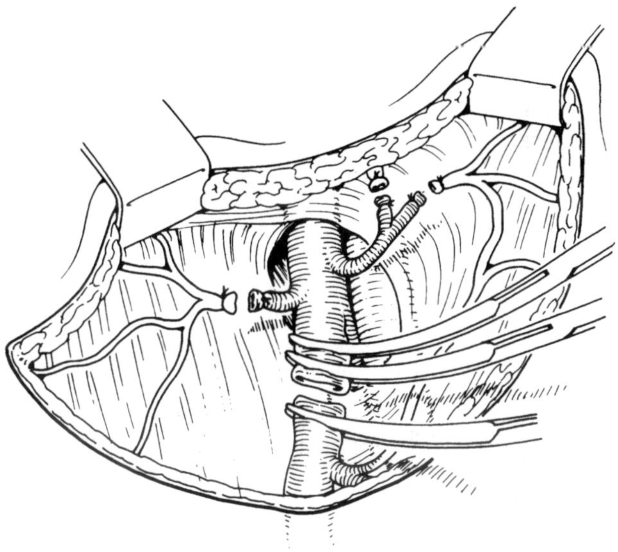

3

3

The saphenous vein and its tributaries are identified by blunt dissection, remembering that it lies much more superficially in the male. The saphenofemoral junction must be clearly visualized before the clamps are applied, since considerable anatomical variation may occur. Two clamps are applied proximally and one distally and the vein is divided between them. It is safer to leave a small proximal stump than to carry out a flush ligation, because if a clamp slips it can be picked up without difficulty. The term flush ligation should be abandoned as it can be misleading for the uninitiated. A short stump cannot be the site of significant thrombus formation. The tributaries are divided and ligated as gentle traction brings them into view.

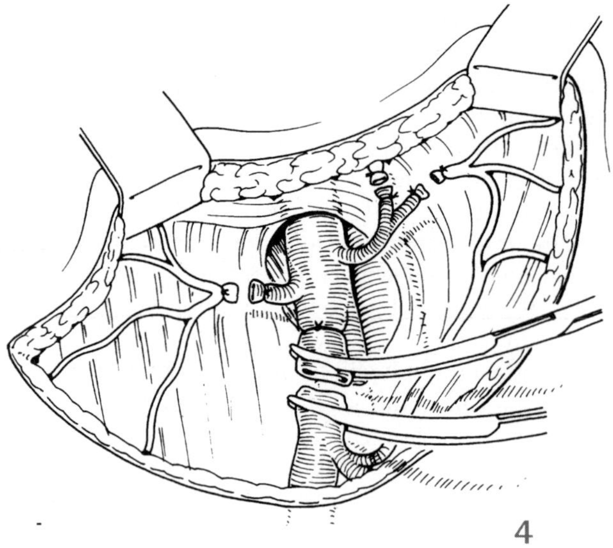

4

4

The saphenous vein is ligated with No. 1 linen thread and the most proximal clamp is removed.

A second ligature of 2/0 linen thread is placed above the second proximal clamp which is then removed.

In cases where there is no downward propagation of the cough impulse, ligation of the distal end with 2/0 linen thread completes the groin operation. The rest of the operation is then completed by multiple removal of the varicosities by the technique described below (see Illustrations 11–16).

Where the impulse is propagated down the leg, limited stripping of the long saphenous vein is indicated and is carried out as follows.

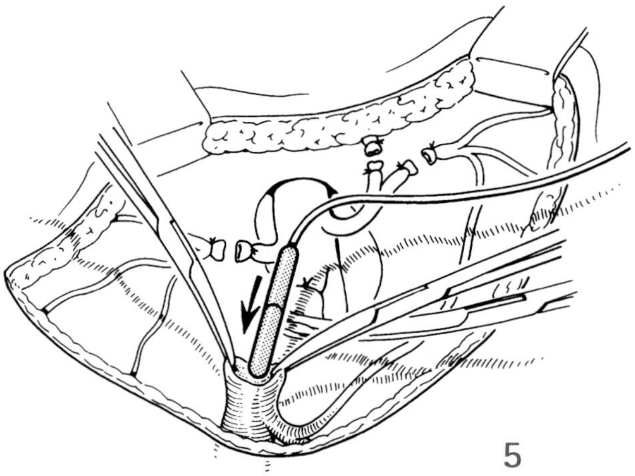

5

Limited stripping of long saphenous vein

5

The stripper is inserted into the upper cut end of the saphenous vein. Mosquito forceps are applied as shown to make this easier.

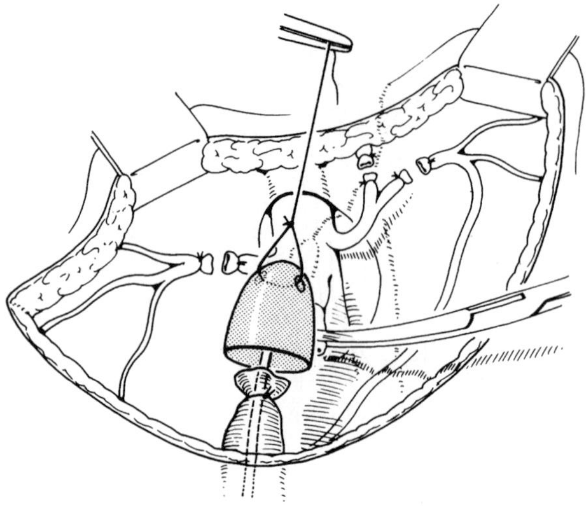

6

6

The vein is tied round the stripper head with 1/0 linen thread leaving one end of the thread long enough to follow the stripper all the way down to the lowest point of the strip. Preferably, the acorn of the stripper is drilled as shown and the long end of the thread is tied through the hole. This prevents the stripper angling at the junction with the acorn when it is drawn upwards. The end of the thread is secured with an arterial clamp.

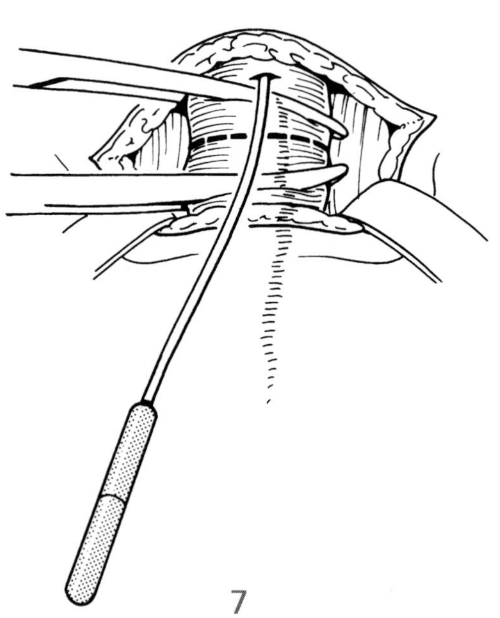

7

7

The lower end of the stripper is identified by palpation and the vein is dissected out through a small transverse incision using curved mosquito forceps. The vein is doubly clamped and the tip of the stripper is drawn out through a small incision in the vein just above the proximal clamp.

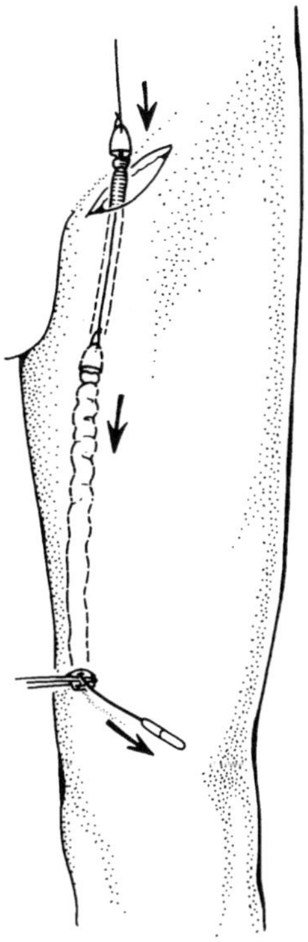

8

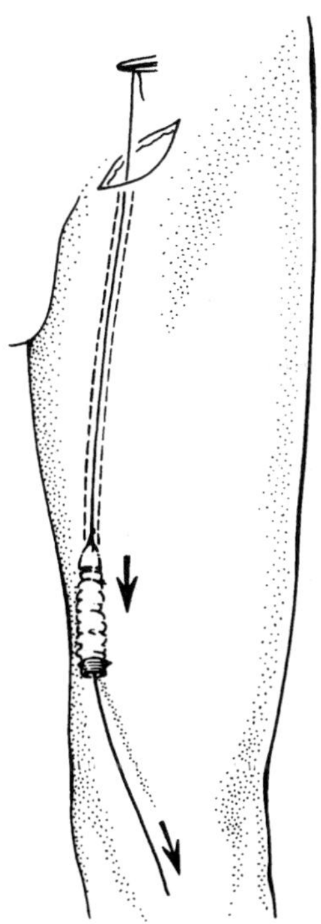

9

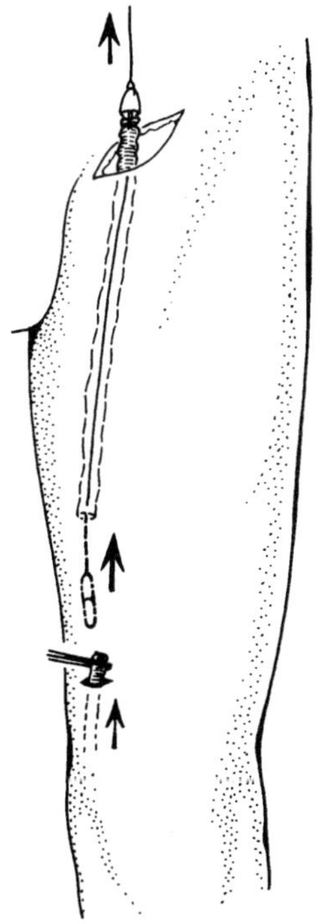

10

8, 9

The vein is divided between the clamps and the stripper is now pulled gently downwards keeping the proximal retaining thread taut until the head of the stripper is just above the lower incision. The end of the vein is freed by traction on the retaining forceps which is now removed.

10

The vein is then removed by upward traction on the retaining thread so that the head of the stripper is removed through the groin incision, thus avoiding enlarging the incision at the lower end to pull the head through.

Firm pressure is applied over the whole length of the stripped channel for a few minutes to prevent haematoma formation. This part of the operation is now completed by removing the lower end of the saphenous vein by firm traction until it breaks in the manner shown in **14**. Haemostasis is again secured by firm pressure.

This method of stripping ensures that only the incompetent saphenous vein is removed and incidentally avoids endangering the saphenous nerve at the ankle – a frequent cause of lingering postoperative discomfort.

Routine orthograde stripping has been abandoned in favour of this technique, since not only does that method endanger the saphenous nerve but it often removes long lengths of normal saphenous vein which should be preserved whenever possible.

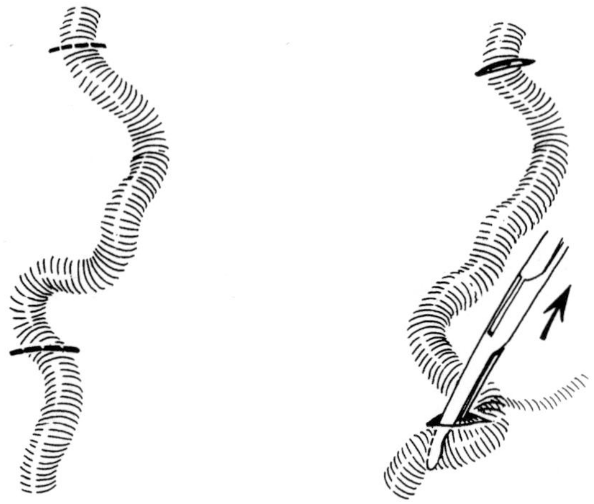

11

Multiple excision of varicose veins

11

Multiple tiny (2–3 mm) transverse incisions are made over the previously marked veins, at such intervals that the maximum length of vein can be removed through the minimum number of incisions. The number will be dictated by the size and the fragility of the veins and by familiarity with the technique. A No. 65 Beaver blade and handle have made extremely small incisions possible. It is often possible to make a tiny stab incision which should go right through the dermis, but if there is any underlying fibrosis or previous scars or a blow out lying very close to the surface it is necessary to make a careful microincision which can be almost as small. Once all the incisions are made, the marking ink is rubbed off with spirit to avoid tatooing of the scars. The incision is opened up using sharp mosquito forceps which are then laid aside in favour of a blunter instrument which is less liable to perforate the vein.

12

Using the blunt curved mosquito forceps, a loop of vein is drawn out through the incision.

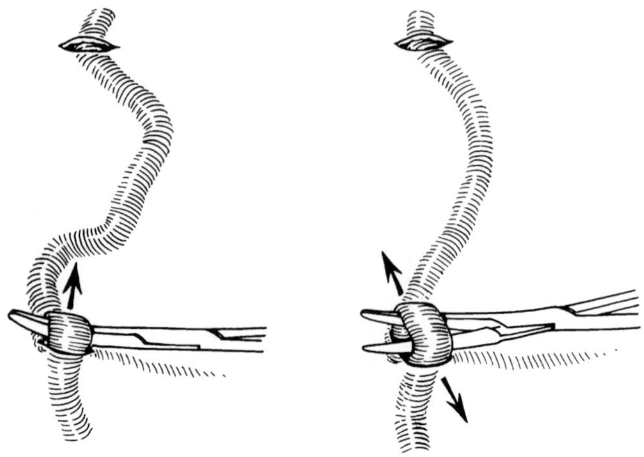

12

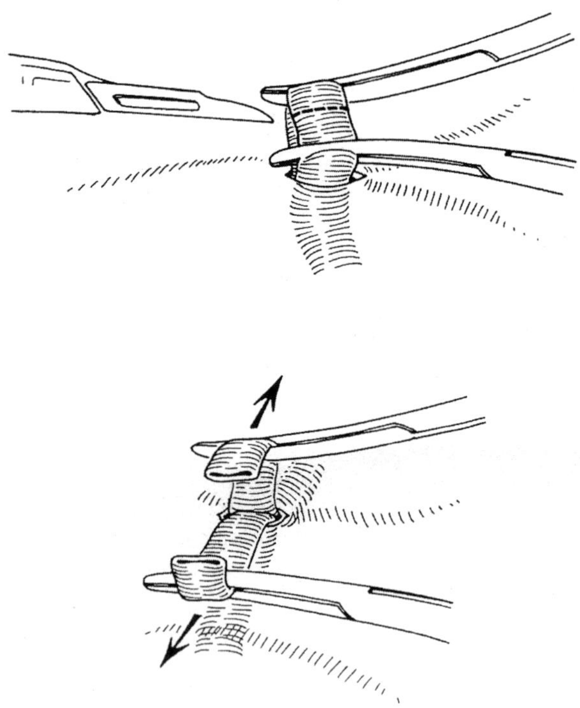

13

13

The vein is now divided between the forceps and each end is 'winkled out' in turn by firm but gentle traction.

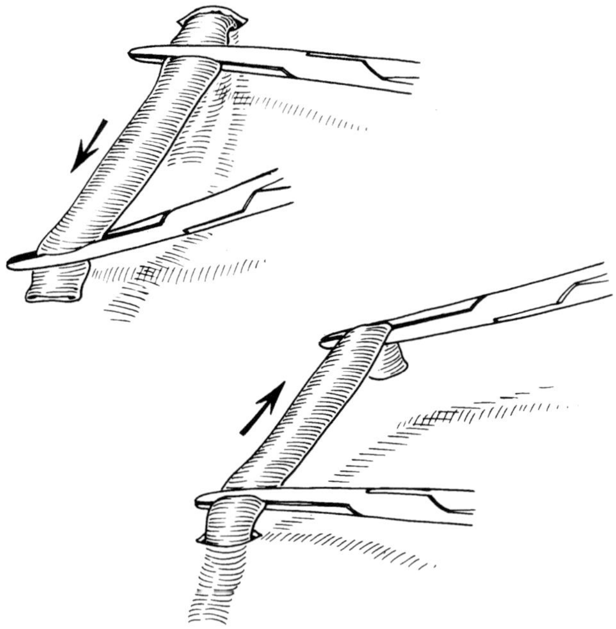

14

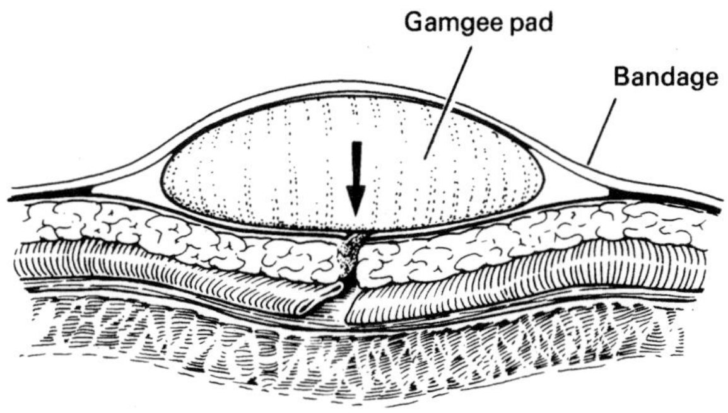

15

14

The vein is always pulled in the direction shown and never across the incision, which would otherwise become enlarged. Heavier curved forceps (Cairns) should be used to apply traction as the broader grip will prevent the vein from breaking prematurely. Sometimes a deep perforator will come into view if traction continues, and it may be grasped and broken by traction in the usual way. No ligatures are required.

15

Haemostatis is secured by firm pressure over each incision as before while the next incision is being explored.

Skin sutures are not necessary and the incisions, when dry, are sealed with steri-strips, applied in the line of the incision without tension and reinforced by a plastic spray. This minimizes blister formation. A gauze roll is applied with the limb elevated.

Firm pressure is maintained by the application of Gamgee pads to include all the operated areas. The limb is firmly bandaged from foot to groin using 15-cm crêpe bandages.

In patients over 50 years of age, 1 unit of Rheomacrodex 40 is given intravenously at the end of the operation to minimize the possibility of postoperative venous thrombosis. The incidence of this complication has been cut to less than 1% since the introduction of this technique.

Postoperative care

The limb is elevated for 8 h postoperatively and this is followed by immediate brisk ambulation. The patient may be treated as a day case or as an outpatient but if the procedure has been extensive an overnight stay is advisable. The limb is rebandaged firmly before discharge after the Gamgee pads are removed. This encourages freer movement of the leg and allows the patient to undertake brisk walking exercise. Patients are advised to do this for 10 min at a time, at least six times a day, for the first 2 postoperative weeks. This is preferable to time-consuming walks of 5–8 km (3–5 miles) and is more likely to be adhered to.

The patient takes a bath on the 7th postoperative day and the strips are allowed to come off with each succeeding bath. A firm tubular bandage support should be worn for a further 4 weeks. Continued pressure helps to accelerate healing. A postoperative instruction sheet is given to the patient as an *aide-mémoire*. The multiple avulsion technique may be carried out under a local anaesthetic as an outpatient procedure. The average patient is able to tolerate as many as 15–20 incisions without difficulty and follows the same postoperative regime. The patient should be kept under observation for about half an hour postoperatively with the leg elevated. In the event of bleeding a firm pressure bandage is applied over the dressings. If bleeding occurs later the patient should be instructed to lie down with the limb elevated while a firm bandage is applied.

Operative treatment of varicose veins with tourniquet

John P Royle

Introduction

1a, b

The initial preoperative assessment of a patient with varicose veins should include Doppler evaluation of the saphenofemoral and saphenopopliteal junctions. These should not be ligated as a routine, but their ligation is required when reflux is present. Clinical examination, particularly in obese patients, often fails to reveal any abnormality at these sites, but such abnormality is revealed with ease by a Doppler (Chan *et al.*, 1983).

After a decision to operate is made, a full duplex ultrasound evaluation should be undertaken before operation. Incompetent perforating veins are frequently missed on clinical examination and examination with a simple Doppler. If short saphenous reflux or perforator reflux is detected, then the sites of these should be marked with the assistance of a duplex ultrasound scan immediately before operation. (It may be convenient to simply do one full duplex ultrasound examination shortly before surgery.)

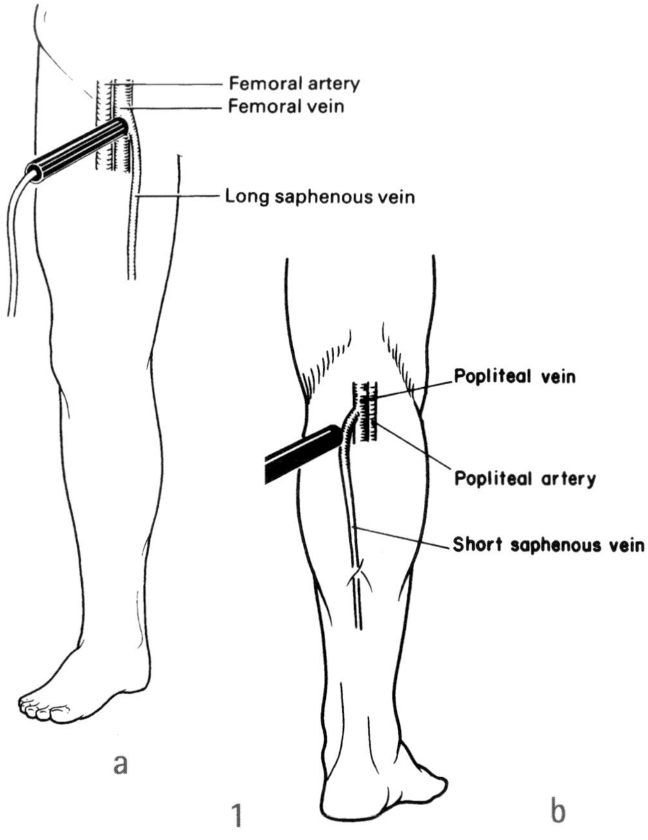

1

2a, b

Marking the veins

Very careful preoperative marking of the varices is performed with the patient in a standing position in a good light. All visible varices are marked and in particular the most superficial portions of the varices are marked clearly (these will be the sites for subsequent stab avulsion). The obvious normal veins on the dorsum of the foot are not marked for removal, but genuine varices on the dorsum of the foot are so marked. The site of an abnormal short saphenous vein or abnormal perforating veins will have been marked with the assistance of a duplex ultrasound scan.

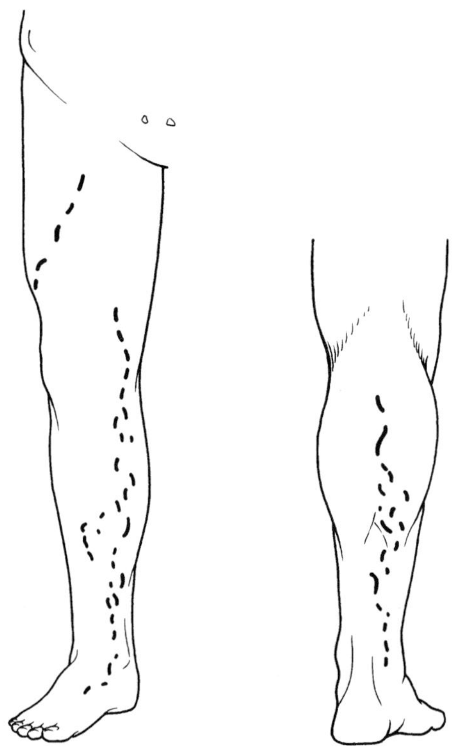

a 2 b

Long saphenous vein

3

Skin incision

The groin incision should be made directly over the saphenofemoral junction, i.e. *above* the groin skin crease. The incision is made in a line parallel to the skin crease centred over a point 1 cm medial to the femoral pulse and 1 cm distal to the line of the pubic tubercle. Except in obese patients, the incision does not need to exceed 4 cm. A small self-retaining retractor is inserted to spread the skin edges apart. The fat separates easily, revealing Scarpa's fascia.

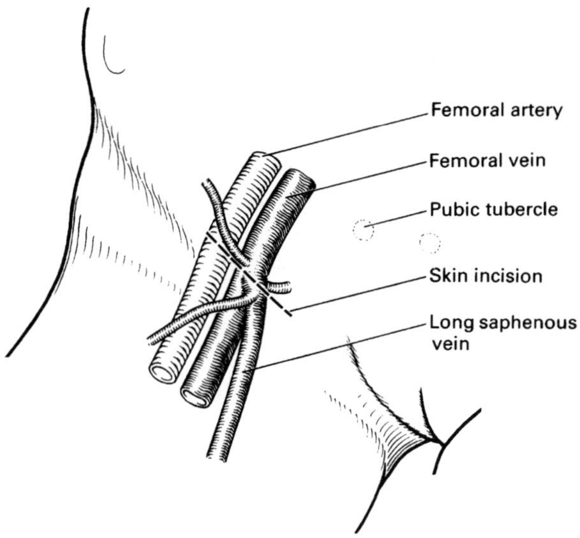

3

4

Scarpa's fascia

The incision is deepened through Scarpa's fascia and the self-retaining retractor is placed in a deeper plane to spread this layer. At this stage the long saphenous vein is usually visible. The vein is grasped with forceps and gently pulled outwards.

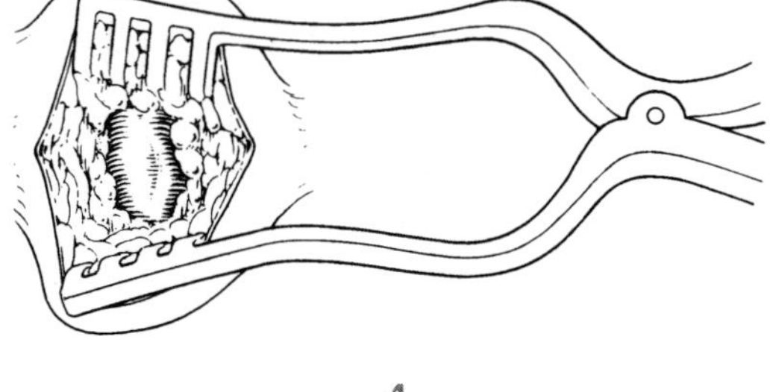

4

5

Division of tributaries

Thereafter dissection takes place in the immediate perivenous plane. The plane immediately alongside the vein is avascular and consists only of loose areolar tissue. The tributaries of the terminal portion of the long saphenous vein are all identified at the site where they drain into the long saphenous vein and pass across this loose areolar tissue. They are ligated and divided.

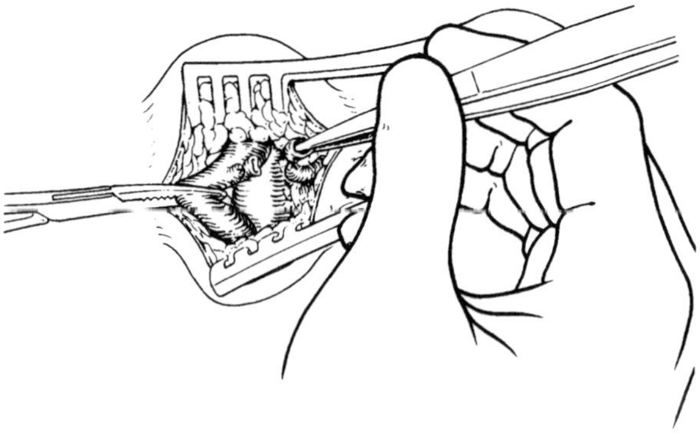

5

6

Saphenofemoral junction

The junction of the long saphenous vein with the femoral vein must be clearly identified before the saphenous vein is divided. The junction on the medial side must be carefully inspected, along with the medial aspect of the femoral vein at this point to check for the point of entry of the deep external pudendal vein. This may enter the long saphenous vein itself, the junction of the long saphenous vein and the femoral vein, or the femoral vein itself (as illustrated). It should be ligated and divided (Royle *et al.*, 1981).

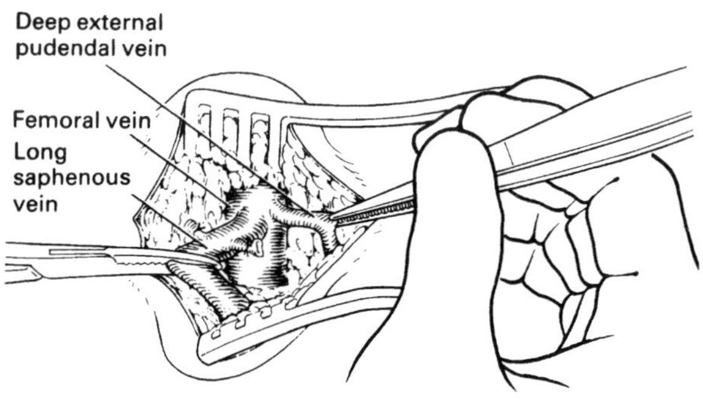

6

7

Flush ligation

The long saphenous vein is divided some 2 cm from the junction, and is then transfixed and tied. To provide a flush ligation, the needle of the transfixion suture enters the long saphenous vein one-half of the diameter of the long saphenous vein away from the saphenofemoral junction. The ligature is then tied, looped around the vein and tied again. The transfixion suture will then lie flush with the femoral vein, and constriction of the femoral vein by the suture is avoided.

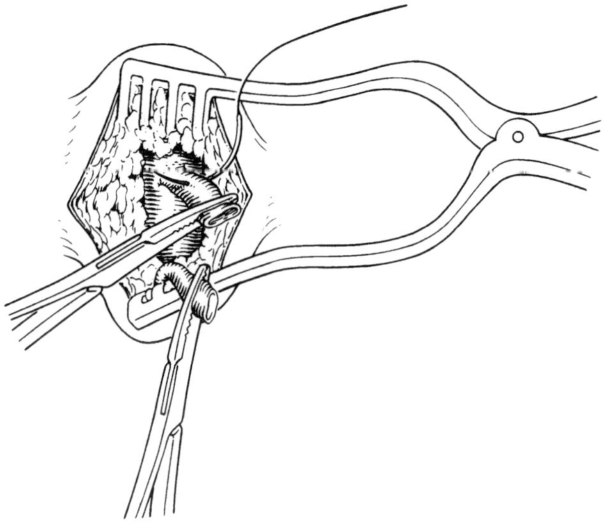

7

8

Long saphenous vein removal

A Codman's stripper is placed into the open cut upper end of the long saphenous vein and passed down to the below-knee level. The stripper is extracted through a small stab incision at that site. The stripper is then pulled distally until the very small knob at the upper end of the stripper enters the upper end of the long saphenous vein. It is then ligated with a long (one metre) length of No 2 thread, firmly anchoring the stripper head inside the vein lumen. The long length of thread is left intact so that when the stripper passes through and extracts the long saphenous vein, the thread will remain along the track of the long saphenous vein.

After extraction of the long saphenous vein, it is checked to see that the full length of vein has been removed. If there is a residual segment remaining, traction on the No 2 thread from each end simultaneously produces a tenting of the skin and enables a stab incision to be made over the residual segment of long saphenous vein which can then be readily grasped with its contained thread.

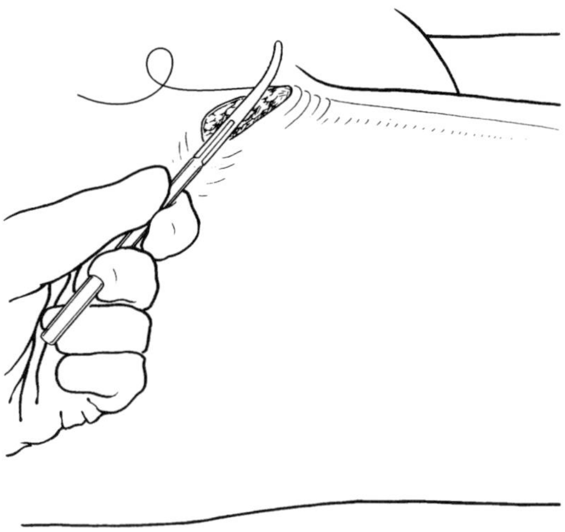

8

To the end of thread protruding from the groin wound, a piece of nylon tape, pre-soaked in 0.5% Bupivacaine HCl and 1:200 000 adrenaline, is tied and then pulled through until it just disappears in the groin wound. This tape is then left along the length of the long saphenous vein extraction track, protruding from the lower end only until the end of the operation when the dressings are being applied, when it is removed. This assists postoperative analgesia and haemostatsis.

If the Codman's stripper does not pass the full way from the groin to below knee but is held up in the thigh by a varix, it can be extracted at that site through a small stab incision and then reintroduced into the vein to once again pass distally. In this way the whole of the long saphenous vein from groin to below-knee level, can be successfully removed.

Groin wound closure

The orifice left by the removal of the long saphenous vein is closed over. This prevents any haematoma from passing up to the groin wound. The subcutaneous tissue in the groin is approximated with an absorbable deep suture. The skin is closed with a subcuticular absorbable suture. The wound edges are infiltrated with 0.5% Bupivacaine HCl local anaesthetic solution. There is then little discomfort in the leg for some hours even when multiple varicose tributaries are also removed through stab incisions (**9–16**).

Varicose tributaries

Thigh veins are approached in the following manner.

9

A small stab incision 3 mm long is made directly over the vein in the long axis of the limb and passing through the dermis only. A pair of toothed mosquito forceps (shown magnified) is passed through the incision and the underlying vein grasped. Mueller hooks can also be used for this purpose, particularly with smaller varicosities. A smaller incision can be used with the Mueller hooks but with large varicosities, a large varix will just not pull through a tiny incision.

Whether toothed mosquito forceps or Mueller hooks are used, the technique described susbsequently (illustrations 10–14) is the same.

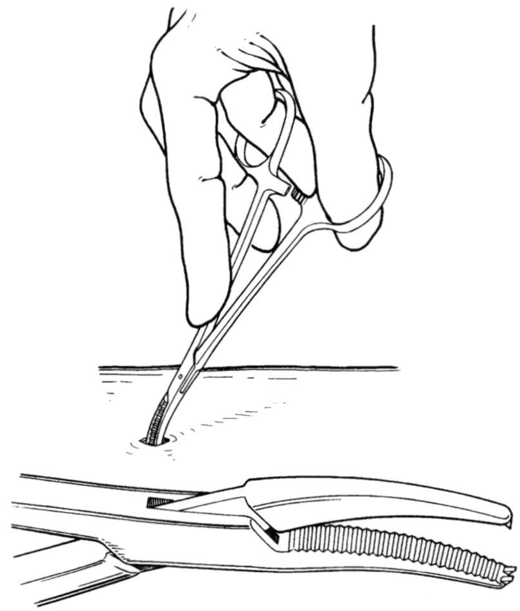

9

10

The grasped vein is pulled to the surface and the toothed forceps are replaced by stronger artery forceps.

11

The vein is pulled further until it emerges as a loop. A pair of forceps is placed on each limb of the loop.

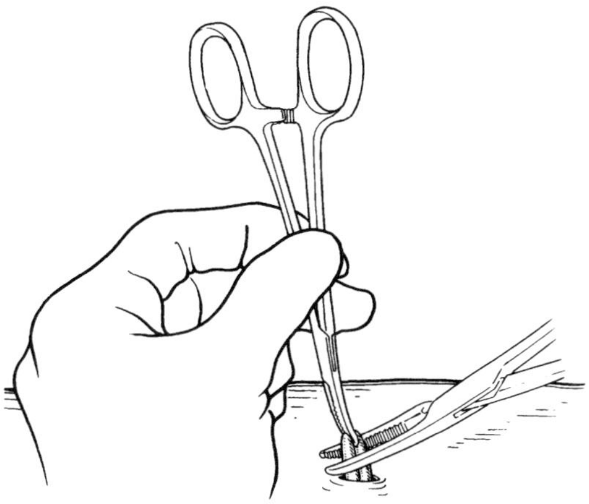

10

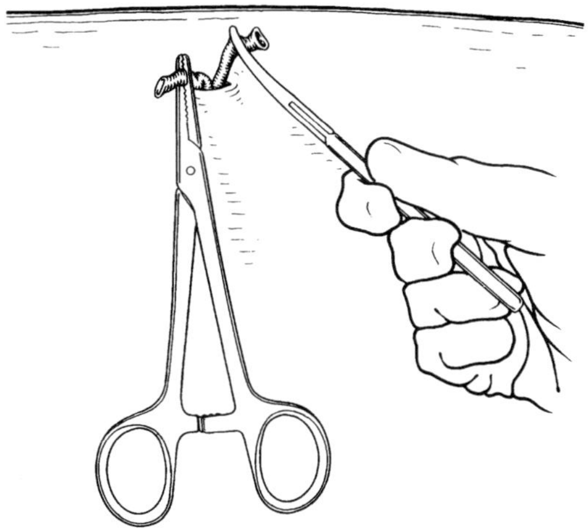

12

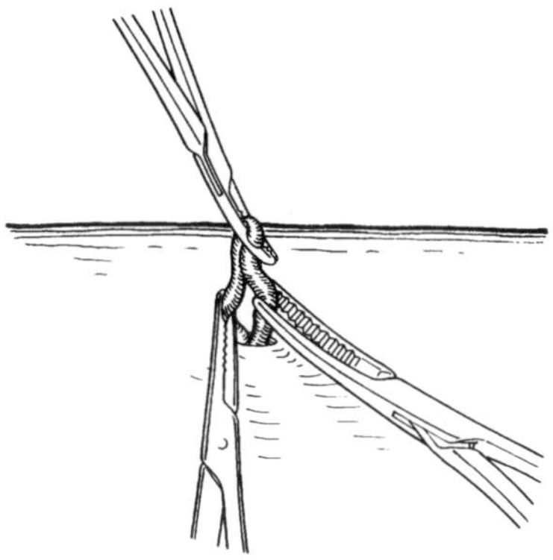

11

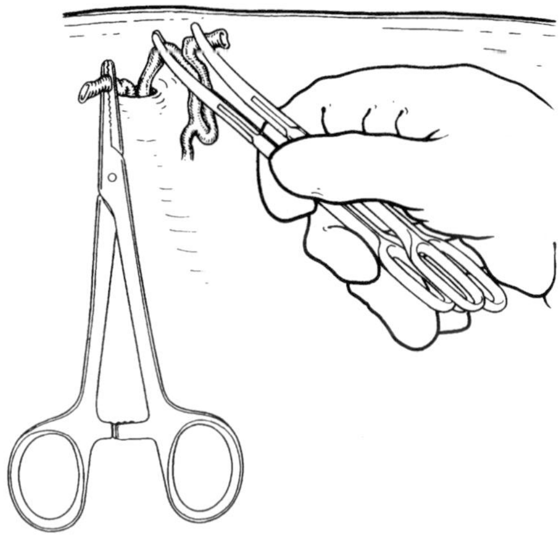

13

12

Taking one limb of the loop at a time, the vein is pulled gently.

13

As it emerges through the skin, the vein is grasped with another pair of forceps near the skin and pulled farther, a new pair of forceps being placed on nearer the skin as every 2 cm or so is extracted.

14

This process is continued until the vein breaks off. A new incision is then made farther down the marked vein to pick up vein again. In this manner the whole of the superficial varicosity is removed.

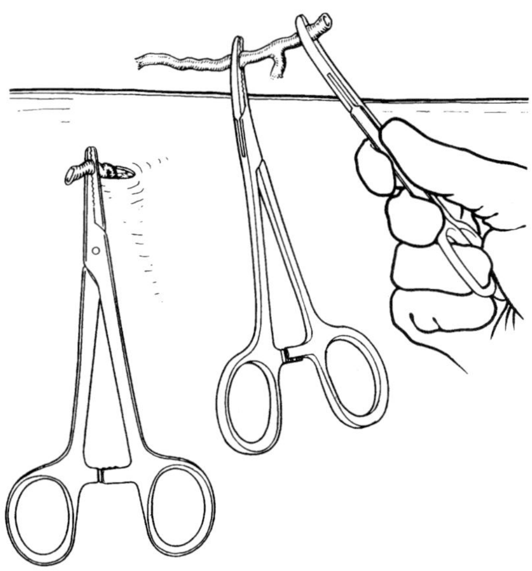

14

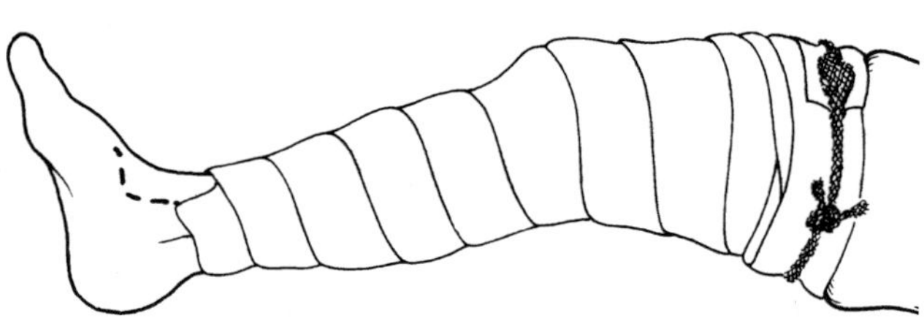

15

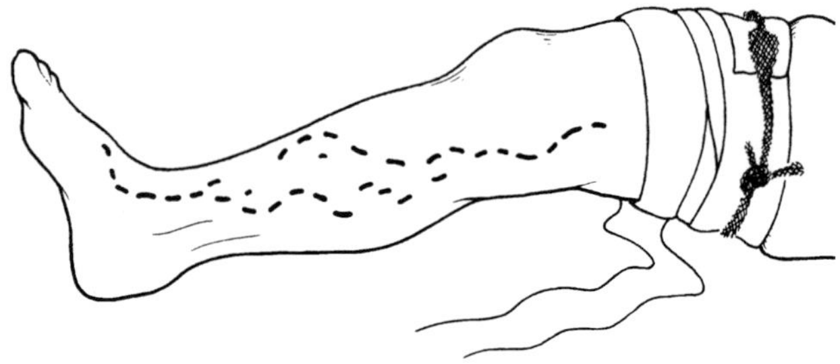

16

15, 16

Tourniquet

When sufficient thigh veins have been dealt with so that a tourniquet can be positioned higher than all the remaining veins, an Esmarch's bandage is applied from medial malleolus to thigh. The upper turns are used on the thigh as a tourniquet and the lower turns are then removed. After application of the tourniquet, the remainder of the varices in the leg are removed from the now avascular field through multiple small stab incisions as described above (**9–14**).

17

Wound dressings

The incisions are *not sutured*; they are dressed with tulle gras, gauze, cotton wool and a crêpe bandage. The bandage must be firm enough to occlude the surface veins, as no venous connections have been ligated except in the groin incision. The wounds distal to the tourniquet are dressed and bandaged while the tourniquet is still in place. The tourniquet is removed and any thigh wounds are then dressed and bandaged. If any bloody ooze comes through the bandages after removal of the tourniquet, an extra, firmer crêpe bandage is applied over the top of the original bandage.

Finally, a TED elastic stocking is placed over the top of the bandages. This keeps the bandages in good position and prevents them from slipping. There is less thigh bruising when such a stocking is used.

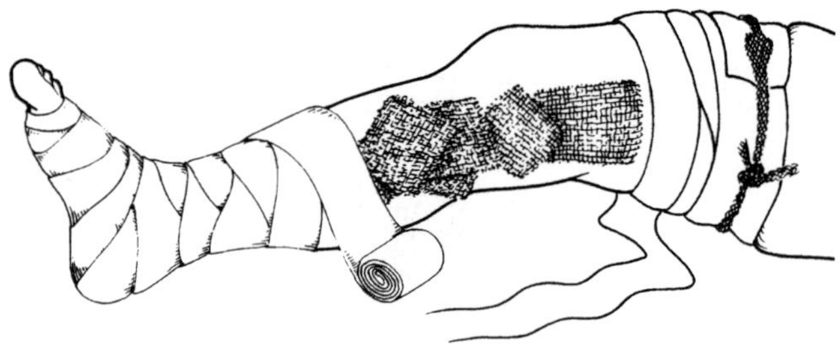

17

Short saphenous vein

18

Duplex scan

The preoperative duplex scan will have enabled accurate preoperative marking of the level of the saphenopopliteal junction. It will also have enabled multiple sources of reflux (e.g. gastrocnemius veins) to be identified.

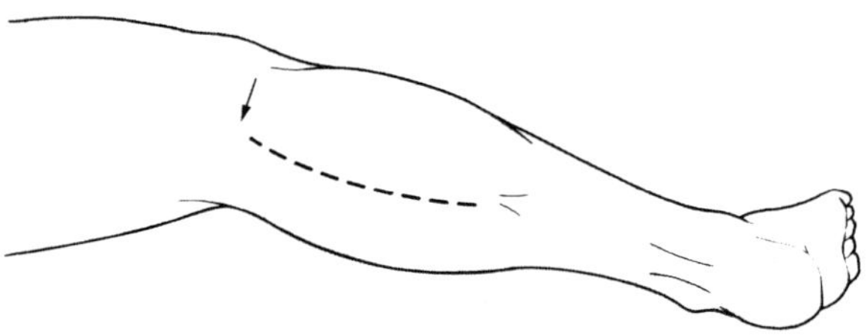

18

Saphenopopliteal ligation

When only the short saphenous vein is abnormal, the patient may be placed in the prone position and an Esmarch's tourniquet applied. When the saphenopopliteal junction is being ligated as part of a more generalized operation on other veins, the flush ligation of the saphenopopliteal junction is usually delayed until after the tourniquet has been applied and all the superficial varices have been removed by stab avulsions as described above (**9–14**). In these circumstances the patient is turned on his side.

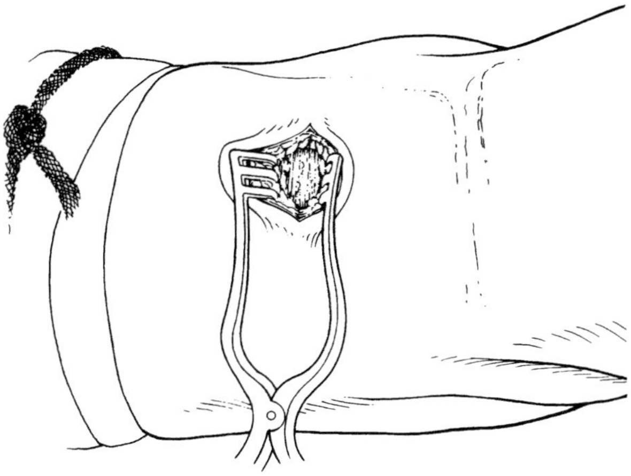

19

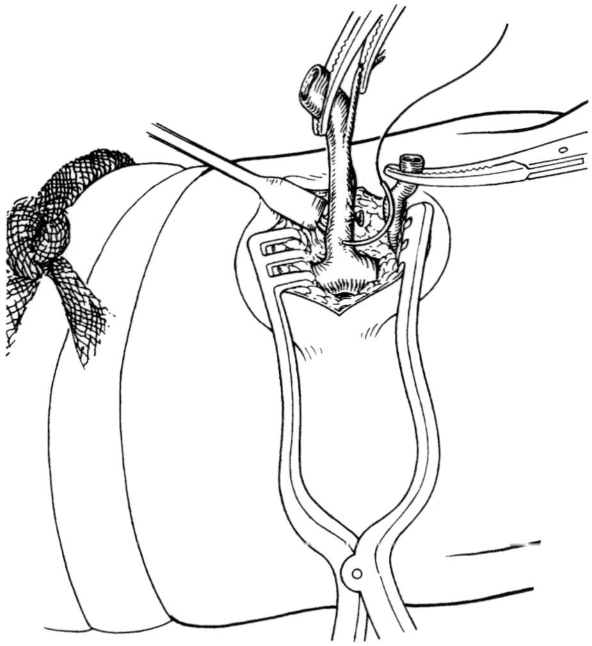

21

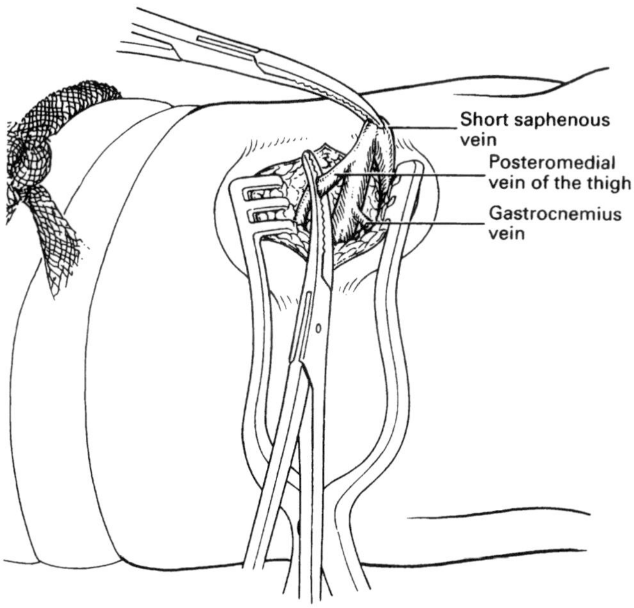

20

19

The skin incision is made transversely 1 cm distal to the level indicated by duplex scanning and a small self-retaining retractor is inserted to separate the skin. The fat usually parts to reveal the deep fascia.

The skin incision is made just distal to the level of the saphenopopliteal junction as described so that it is at a site where the short saphenous vein is still relatively superficial and easily identified. At the saphenopopliteal junction, the short saphenous vein is at quite a deep level.

20

The deep fascia is opened transversely in the line of its fibres. The short saphenous vein can then usually be seen easily.

The short saphenous vein is grasped with forceps and dissection is conducted in the immediate perivenous avascular plane. Care is taken to avoid damage to the sural nerve. All patients undergoing short saphenous vein surgery should be warned of the possibility of post-operative numbness over the sural nerve distribution as this is quite common.

The vein that passes upwards from the short saphenous vein to form the posteromedial vein of the thigh is ligated and divided. Gastrocnemius veins joining the incompetent short saphenous vein are ligated and divided. The dissection of the short saphenous vein is continued down to the saphenopopliteal junction.

21

Flush ligation

A transfixion flush ligation is performed as described for the saphenofemoral junction, with the needle passing through the saphenous vein one-half of the diameter away from the popliteal vein in order to produce a flush ligation without constriction. Any incompetent gastrocnemius vein or popliteal area vein separately draining into the popliteal vein, is divided and ligated adjacent to the popliteal vein.

Short saphenous vein removal

As described for stripping of the long saphenous vein, a Codman's stripper is passed distally down the short saphenous vein to the lower calf level. It is extracted there through an incision large enough to enable clear visualization of the short saphenous vein with its contained stripper. The clear visualization avoids inadvertent grasping of the adjacent sural nerve with forceps which, of course, would leave postoperative numbness and/or pain. The Codman's stripper is secured to the upper end of the short saphenous vein by No. 2 thread and pulled distally, removing the vein by inversion stripping. The stripper is followed by the No. 2 thread, followed by the nylon tape soaked in Bupivacaine and adrenaline, as for the long saphenous vein stripping. The fascia is closed with an absorbable deep suture. The subcutaneous fat is closed with another absorbable deep suture. The skin is closed with a subcuticular absorbable suture. The wound edges are infiltrated with 0.5% Bupivacaine HCl local anaesthetic solution as for a groin wound.

Perforating veins

Any incompetent perforating veins will have been identified by a duplex scan. These are treated as follows:

A vertical incision is made over the site of the marked perforating vein (usually 2–3cm long). The perforating vein is identified and traced to the site where it emerges through the deep fascia. It is ligated and divided at the level of of the deep fascia. It is essential to dissect the perforating vein right to the deep fascia as there are often tributaries at a deep level adjacent to the fascia. If these are left behind, recurrence will occur.

The subcutaneous tissue and skin are all closed with either two or three large nylon sutures. The use of subcutaneous absorbable sutures for the underlying fat tends to produce greater induration beneath the scar than if the fat is approximated by the nylon skin suture.

Postoperative management

The sutures used in closure of perforating vein ligation wounds can usually be removed at about 7 days, although sometimes they may need to stay longer. After removal of the sutures, steristrip dressings are used across the wound to provide support until the wound closure is strong.

Endovenous vein closure

Andrew N Nicolaides, Maura B Griffin, Andrew F Lennox, Zak A Zarka, Gerald Stansby

Introduction

This chapter aims to introduce a method of controlled endovenous heating to obliterate reflux in the long saphenous vein *in situ*, in lieu of surgical stripping, using the Closure© System (VNUS Medical Technologies, Inc., Sunnyvale, CA). This therapy works on the principal of heating precisely, controlled by monitoring vein wall temperature and impedance, which is sufficient to cause collagen contraction without destroying vessel-wall integrity. The aims of this new treatment are to abolish saphenous vein reflux and maintain a long-term clinical and haemodynamic effect. A major advantage would be the ability to achieve this without a groin incision or long saphenous stripping.

Animal studies have determined the temperature needed to cause sufficient vein-wall collagen denaturation with vein-wall contraction and vessel obliteration (Chen *et al.*, 1998).

Thermal effects are confined locally by using bipolar electrodes, which concentrate current density along minimal impedance paths between the poles (Pearce, 1986) and by excluding blood flow from the treatment area by compression during energy application. Withdrawal of the activated electrodes results in complete lumen closure. Effective treatment leaves behind a small thrombus plug in a contracted vessel with de-endothelialized wall and obliterated lumen.

Equipment

1a, b

The equipment consists of a dedicated, computer controlled, bipolar generator and 5F (**1a**) and 8F (**1b**) catheters with sheathable electrodes. The two sizes differ in design in that electrical polarity is exchanged between a single tuft of collapsible electrodes and a central ball tip in the smaller catheter and between two sets of collapsible electrodes, with the ball tip being neutral, in the larger catheter. The two sizes allow for obliteration of veins from 2 to 12 mm in diameter, effectively providing a ring of resistive vein-wall heating 6 to 8 mm long. Both catheters incorporate a central lumen for fluid infusion and the option of passage over a guidewire (Chandler *et al.*, 2000).

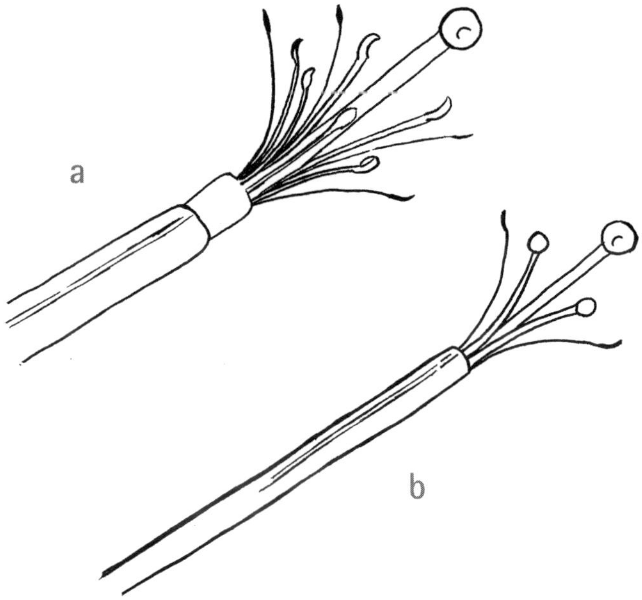

1

2

Each catheter is automatically recognized by the system's generator, which then in turn selects the appropriate algorithm for that catheter's use. Before the start of any treatment the unit delivers a minute, instantaneous current for temperature and impedance measurements via the generator's test button. The latter measurements are used to confirm adequate electrode-vein-wall contact before the treatment circuit is activated. Good wall

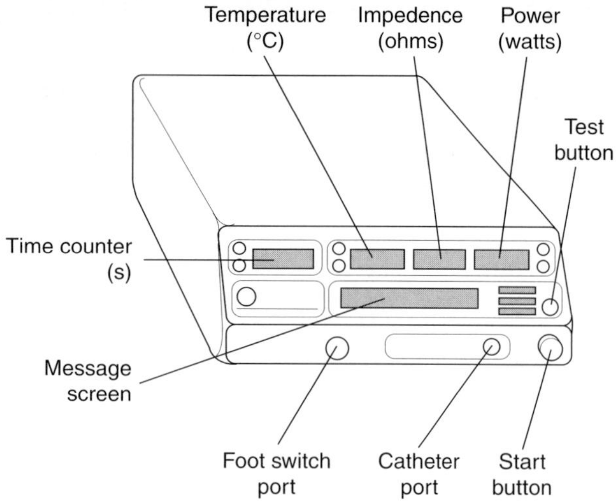

2

contact is defined by a sudden increase in impedance over that displayed when the electrodes are surrounded by blood. Typically a treatment temperature of 85 degrees C is selected, which the generator then attempts to maintain using as little wattage as possible, capped by a pre-set maximum of 6 watts. The generator will cut out at any time during the course of the treatment if impedance or temperature exceeds the upper or lower limits of the controlling algorithm. This can occur if contact with the vein wall is lost or if thrombus forms around the catheter's electrodes. The latter is easily remedied by removal and cleaning of the electrodes.

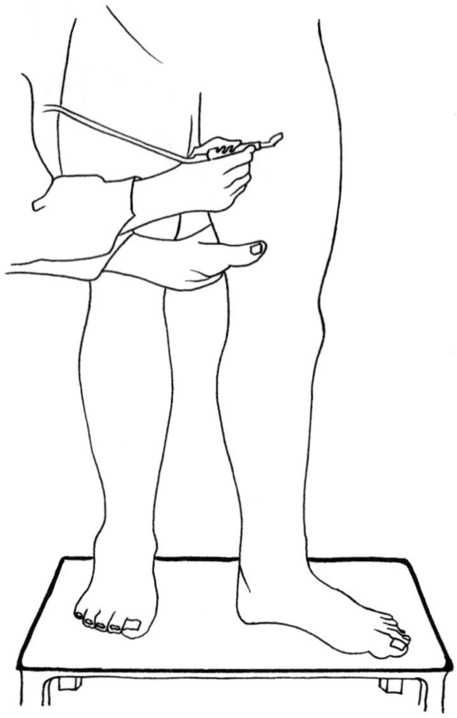

3

Patient assessment and selection

3

Patients suitable for the closure procedure should be symptomatic, and have demonstrable saphenous-vein reflux as determined by colour duplex ultrasound during calf compression with sudden release whilst standing and a vein diameter of 12 mm or less. Patients with a tortuous long saphenous were excluded. Patients undergoing anticoagulation therapy, previous history of deep vein thrombosis, peripheral arterial disease, pacemakers or pregnancy were also excluded.

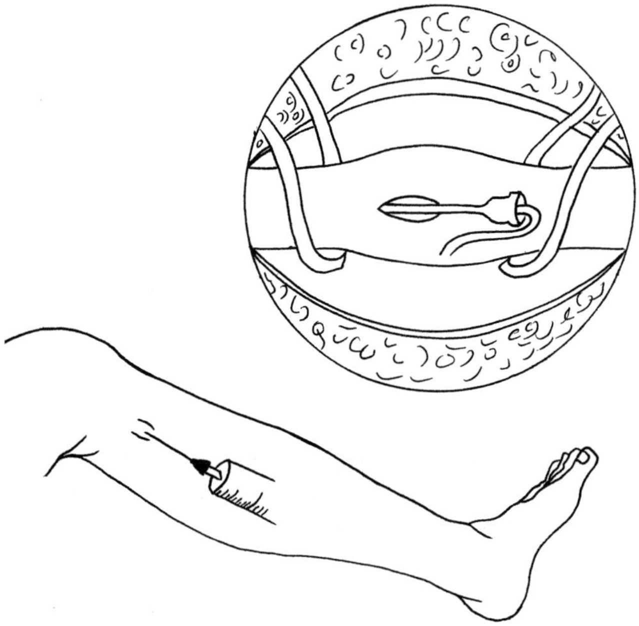

4

Procedure

4

In the majority of cases the long saphenous is accessed percutaneously, employing the Seldinger technique, under ultrasound guidance and palpation (**4a**), but in some cases a small cut-down may be required (**4b**).

5

The catheter with sheathed electrodes is then passed proximally and positioned at the saphenofemoral junction under ultrasound control.

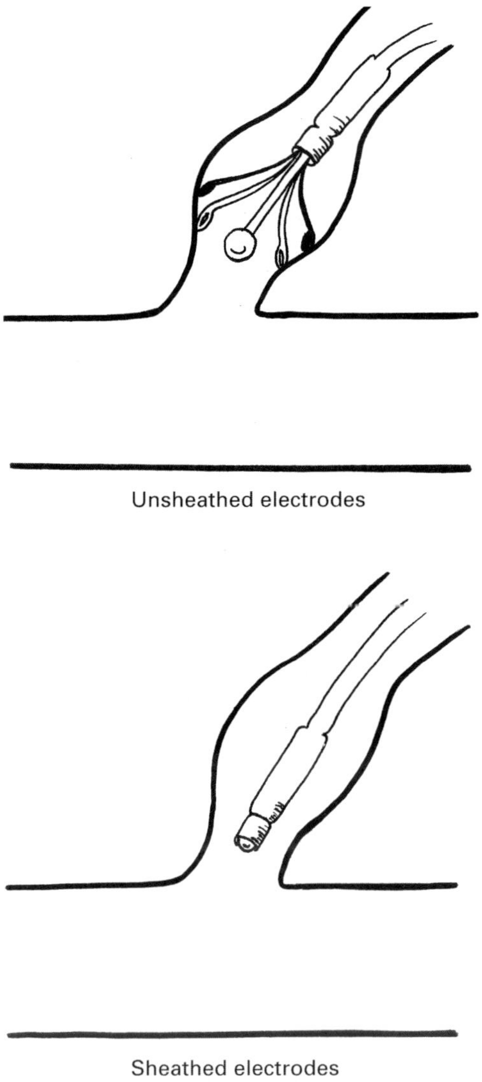

5

6

In order to exclude flow in the superficial veins, of the limb being treated, the leg is wrapped in an Esmarch bandage from toes to groin with the patient in a 15° Trendelenburg position. Care is taken not to disturb the catheter at the level of the knee.

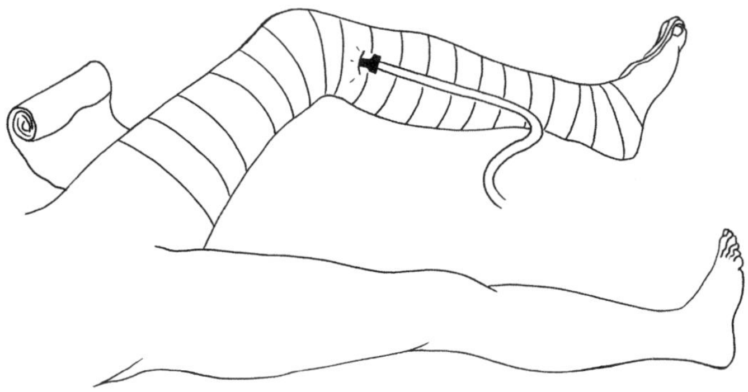

6

7

Manual compression is applied at the saphenofemoral junction which cannot be effectively compressed by the bandage, to clear blood away during the early stages of the treatment.

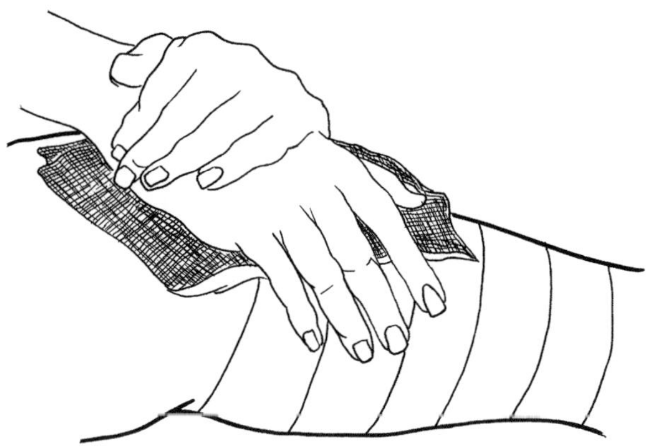

7

8a, b, c, d

An infusion of heparinized saline is given through the central lumen to minimize thrombus formation on the electrodes. The treatment circuit is then activated and once the vein wall temperature reaches the required level the catheter is withdrawn slowly, 2–3 cm/minute, keeping the wall temperature within ± 3 degrees of the set temperature (85 degrees) and the wattage display below 4 watts to ensure the 12–16 second exposure needed for greatest wall contraction.

Illustration **8a**. Shows the end of the catheter with the electrodes within the sheath; **(8b)** the electrodes released; **(8c)** the activated electrodes during withdrawal and **(8d)** the end result of the occluded vein

At the end of the procedure, treated segment is routinely scanned to ensure absence of flow and also non-compressibility of the treated vein. Where necessary, distal avulsions of varicosities are also performed.

Patients and study sites

Our centre was one of several European sites that participated in these clinical trials as well as centres from the United States of America – and Australia, and it is these combined study sites that comprise the VNUS Closure Treatment Study Group. In total 186 limbs were treated in 130 women and 42 men with a mean CEAP Clinical class (Porter *et al.*, 1995) of 2.5±0.9. Closure treatment was combined with high ligation in 60 limbs (32%). High ligation was not performed in the remaining 126 (68%) of limbs. Calf phlebectomies were performed when necessary. Of all the treated veins, the majority comprised

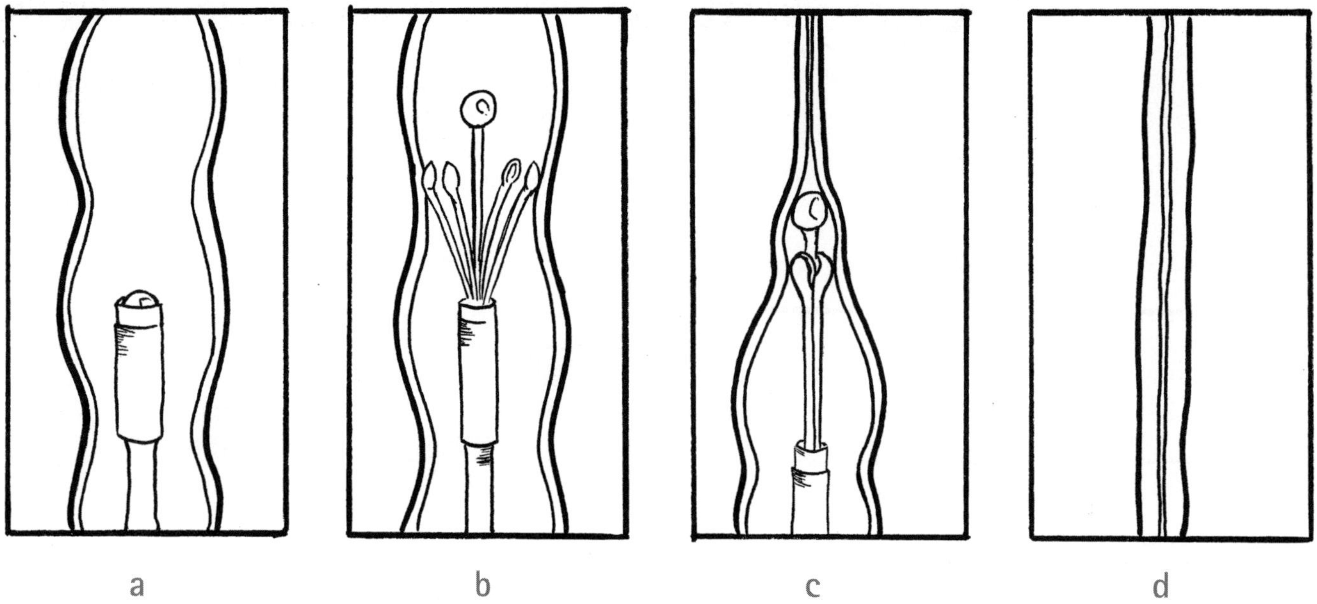

8

treatment of the long saphenous in the thigh (72%). Treatment of the entire long saphemous vein was performed in 22%.

Successful occlusion was obtained in 96% with eight failures, three from a single study site. Three of these failures were recognized before the end of the procedure and were surgically stripped. One of these involved only the below-knee segment of an entire long saphenous vein treatment; the below-knee segment was stripped, and the above-knee portion continues to be evaluated. The remaining five failed cases became evident 1 week after treatment and these were scheduled to undergo stripping or a repeat closure procedure.

Follow-up

Forty-nine successfully treated limbs, from 47 patients, have been followed for 6 months or longer, or to recanalization. To date, eight of 180 veins have recanalized (4.4%). Three veins completely re-opened, two at 6 weeks and one at 3 months. Four other veins showed partial recanalization by 6 weeks, involving 5 to 15 cm segments in the mid thigh or just above the knee. A fifth case of a 5-cm segment that had re-opened was associated with a still unaddressed Dodd's perforating vein. The remainder of the treated vein was not affected, demonstrating the vein lumen to be sufficiently contracted and fibrosed to resist the transmitted deep vein muscle pump pressure.

Of forty-one patients monitored for 6 months or more, 95%, including two with partial recanalization, rated themselves as being symptom-free or substantially improved. At each follow-up interval collective, progressive symptomatic improvement was observed in all patients.

Conclusion

The closure procedure was conceived to exploit the strong contractile forces of collagen denaturation to cause vein wall contraction and permanent obliteration of refluxing superficial veins. Its early therapeutic efficacy is now proven and appears equivalent to saphenous vein stripping. Since closure treatment can be done without high ligation and consequent interference with the normal prograde drainage of superficial abdominal and pudendal veins, it may eventually prove less prone than saphenectomy to thigh neovascularity and recurrent truncal-vein reflux (Edmunds *et al.*, 1988, Nyamekye *et al.*, 1998). Results for 3 and 5 years are now needed.

References

Chandler JG, Pichot O, Sessa C *et al.* (2000). Treatment of primary venous insufficiency by endovenous saphenous vein obliteration. *Vasc Surg* **34**:201–214.

Chen SS, Wright NT, Humphrey JD (1998). Heat induced changes in the mechanics of a collagenous tissue: isothermal, isotonic shrinkage. *J Biomech Eng* **120**:382–388.

Edmunds LH Jr, Clark RE, Cohn LH *et al.* (1988). Guidelines for reporting morbidity and mortality after cardiac valvular operations. *J Thorac Cardiovasc Surg* **96**:351–353.

Nyamekye I, Shephard NA, Davies B *et al.* (1998) Clinicopathological evidence that neovascularization is a cause of recurrent varicose veins. *Eur J Vasc Endovasc Surg* **15**:412–415.

Pearce JA (1986). *Electrosurgery.* New York: John Wiley & Sons. pp. 62–65.

Porter JM, Moneta GL and an International Concensus Committee on Chronic Venous Disease (1995). Reporting standards in venous disease: an update. *J Vasc Surg* **21**:635–645.

Ligation of perforating veins

F B Cockett

Introduction

The perforating veins referred to here are the so-called 'direct' perforators – defined as those veins which perforate the *deep fascia* of the limb to enter directly into a main deep vein (such as the femoral or posterior tibial). These veins are few in number and in definite regular anatomical sites. The termination of the long saphenous vein at the groin and of the short saphenous vein in the popliteal vein behind the knee are the two most well-known perforator sites. There is also the 'Hunterian' or mid-thigh perforator.

This chapter deals with the important direct perforators in the lower half of the leg, which normally drain the venous blood from the subcutaneous tissue and skin of the ankle directly into the posterior tibial and peroneal veins.

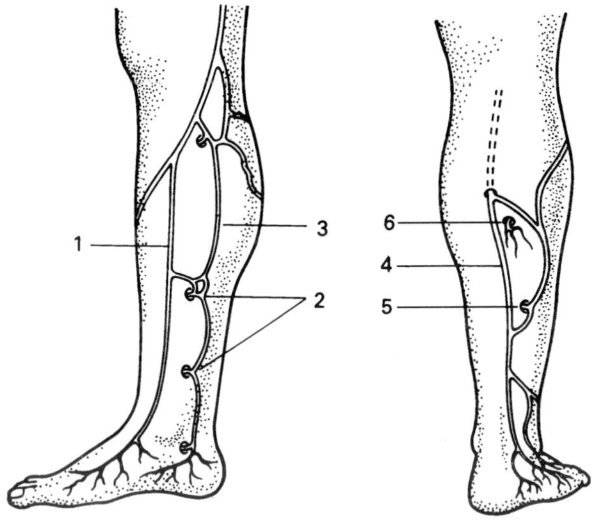

1

1

On the inner side of the limb there are two main direct perforating veins (2) emerging from holes in the deep fascia. They are situated behind the long saphenous vein (1). The upper one is approximately halfway up the leg. The lower one is four fingers' breadth above the medial malleolus. Note that the perforating veins communicate by fine venous arches, and with the long saphenous vein by a large constant posterior arch vein (3) arising at knee level.

On the outer side of the limb there is only one constant large perforator (5) which communicates directly with the short saphenous vein (4). Much less constant is the so-called midcalf perforating vein (6) emerging close to the insertion of the gastrocnemius into the soleus tendon. When present, however, it is often large and important.

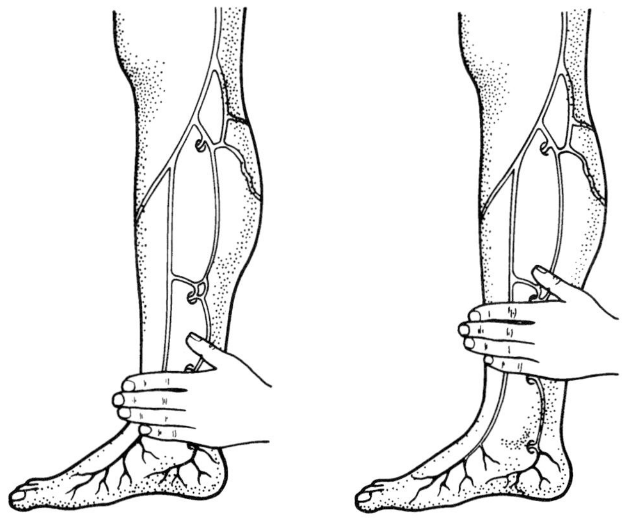

2

2

Clinically, these perforators are easily located by the 'hand's breadth' rule. In other words, the perforating veins on the medial aspect are separated by approximately the breadth of a hand as shown.

3

In the normal erect exercising limb, very high pressure (about 100 mmHg) develops in the deep calf veins during the contraction phase of the calf muscles. Blood is normally prevented from leaking out into the skin and subcutaneous tissue by the valve in the perforating vein, but when this valve is destroyed or becomes incompetent for any reason, the high pressure is exerted directly on to the fine mesh veins on the inner side of the ankle. These veins dilate rapidly, giving rise to the typical and important sign called 'ankle flare'. This process eventually leads to sclerosis and skin destruction – the lesion we know as a venous ulcer.

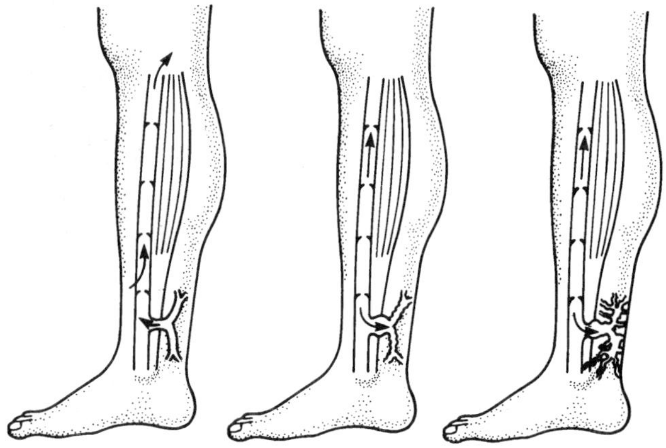

Normal

Perforator leak established

3

Essential diagnostic points

There are three distinct groups of cases in which incompetent ankle perforators occur. In the first two groups, they are the main cause of the steady deterioration of the ankle skin and subcutaneous tissues which leads eventually to venous ulceration.

4

Group 1: Incompetent ankle perforators occurring as a late complication of primary varicose veins

In many longstanding cases of primary hereditary long saphenous incompetence, as the varicose veins of the posterior arch branch become bigger and more prominent, they connect with and drain into a competent medial ankle perforator. This competent perforator 'drains off into the deep veins', the high pressure coming down the long saphenous system, and thus protects the ankle skin. However, in many cases, as time goes on, the

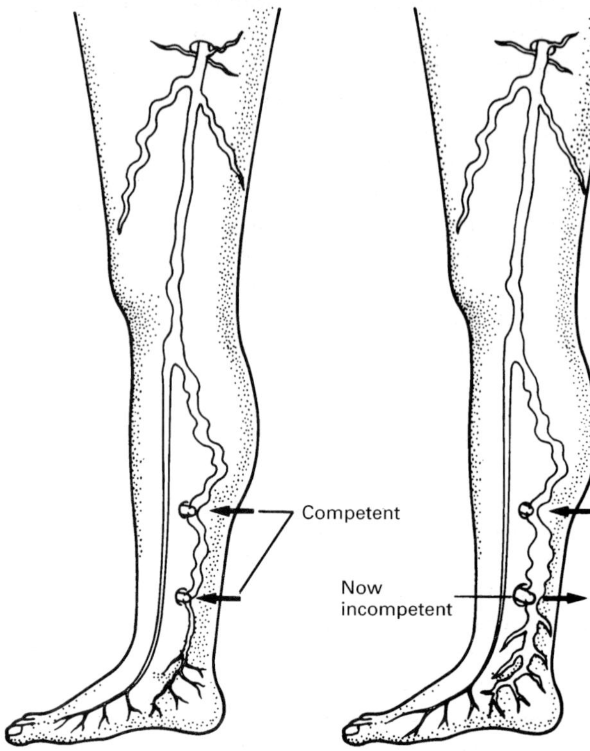

4

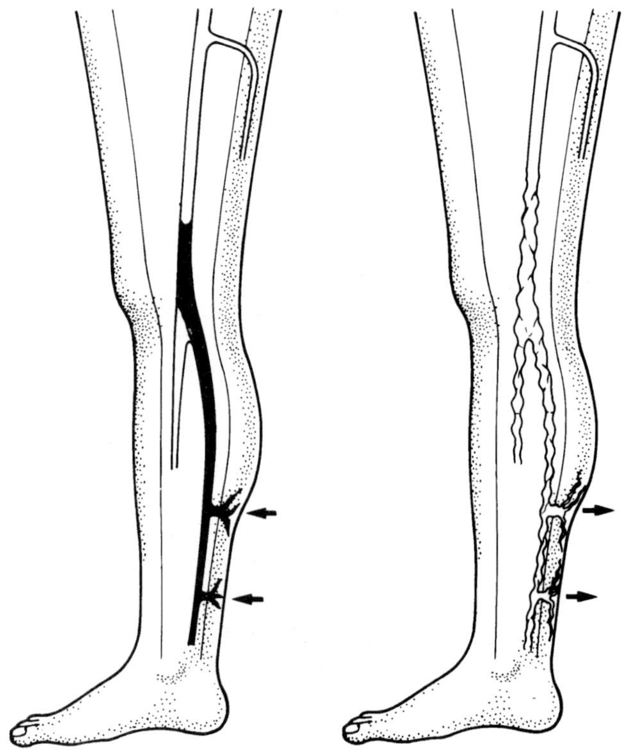

Acute

Post-thrombotic phase (2–5 years later)

5

ankle perforator enlarges and its valve is either destroyed or becomes inefficient. When this occurs a massive venous hypertension from the perforator is added to that coming down the saphenous system, and rapid deterioration of the ankle occurs, leading to ulcer (hence the old name, 'varicose ulcer').

These cases are fairly common, and give the best results after long saphenous ligation and stripping, combined with ankle perforator exposure and ligation. In this group, associated varicose veins will be seen and should be marked as they must be dealt with when the perforating veins are tied.

5

Group 2: Incompetent ankle perforators occurring late (2–5 years) after an acute venous thrombosis of the peripheral type

In this type, the thrombosis starts deep in the calf, either in the calf sinusoids or in the posterior tibial or peroneal veins. It spreads upwards into popliteal or femoral veins, but rarely higher. Usually, the clot spreads into the perforator up to its valve. During the recanalization phase the valve is destroyed and a 'perforator leak' is established. This causes swelling, venular dilatation, sclerosis and pigmentation of the ankle (the classic post-thrombotic syndrome), eventually leading to ulcer.

Often, in these cases, there is a remarkable degree of recanalization of the main deep veins in the post-thrombic phase. Also in the profunda vein and its branches there is usually an efficient collateral channel from the lower leg, so that there is often very minimal deep vein obstruction after a peripheral type of thrombosis, leaving the incompetent perforator as the main lesion responsible for the ankle ulcer. It is essential to discover any past history of possible deep vein thrombosis in order to recognize this state of affairs, because it implies that the only surgery required is ligation of these perforating veins.

6

Group 3: Incompetent ankle perforators occurring after a patient has had a proximal or iliofemoral type of thrombosis

In these cases the thrombosis starts in the iliac vein segment; usually, patients are young and have the developmental anomaly known as the 'iliac compression syndrome'. The left iliac vein is partly (or sometimes wholly) obstructed by the right common artery passing over it and compressing it against the promontory of the sacrum. When this partly obstructed left iliac vein thromboses, the thrombosis usually spreads down to the groin. After this resolves and attempts recanalization, the patient is left with an obstructed iliac vein, but a *normal* calf pump and perforators.

Occasionally, the thrombus extends peripherally right back into the calf, producing a very severe clinical picture (phlegmasia caerulae dolens). When this resolves and recanalizes, there may be extensive deep vein obstruction *plus* incompetent ankle perforators. These patients develop the worst and most intractable ulcers and even though incompetent perforating veins are detected, ligation in this situation gives poor results, because the venous hypertension due to obstructed deep veins is unrelieved. More frequently, venous reconstructive surgery is required.

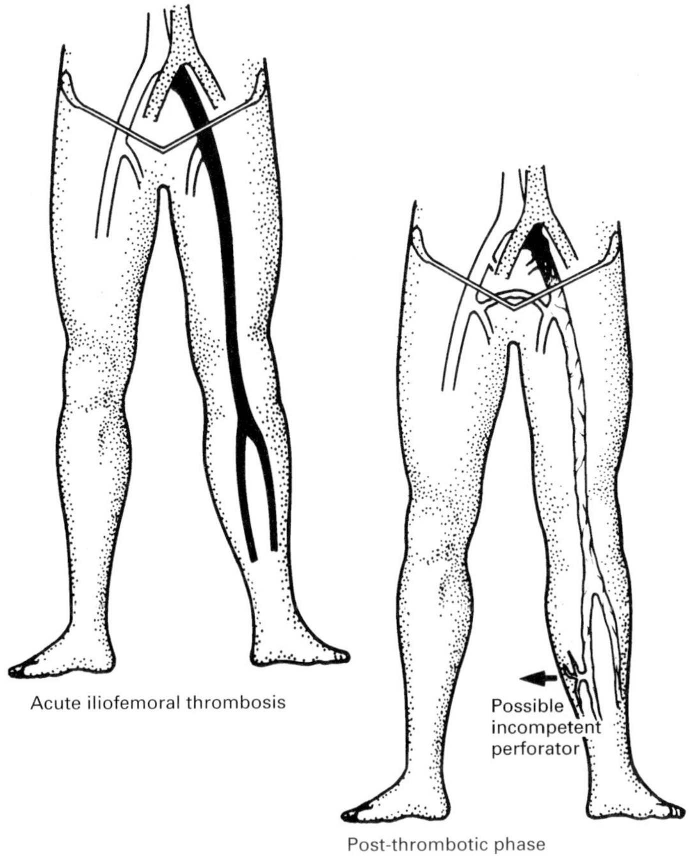

6

Editorial note

Preoperative management and the operative procedure

At present venous ulceration healing is usually achieved by firm compression and ambulation. The four-layer bandage technique requires change of bandages weekly or sometimes twice-weekly. Colour duplex scanning pinpoints the underlying abnormality and surgery relates to this. Perforating veins are usually located by colour duplex scan and the incision is placed just over the perforation. The long incision for extrafascial ligation or subfacial ligation (Linton) or stocking incision (Dodd) is seldom required. The great contribution of these pioneers, however, was to recognize the relative constant situation of the perforating veins. The ligation of perforating veins is now usually performed in conjunction with surgery for primary varicose veins as described by Royle or Rose in the two previous chapters. The patient is usually admitted on the day of operation and stays in hospital at most for one night postoperatively. Compression bandaging continues in the postoperative period for patients with unhealed ulcers.

Acknowledgement
Illustrations by A George.

References

Cockett FB (1955). Surgery of venous ulcers. *Br J Surg* **43**: 179.

Cockett FB, Jones DE (1953). Ankle blow-out syndrome. *Lancet* **1**: 17.

Cockett FB, Lea Thomas M, Negus D (1967). Iliac vein compression – its relation to iliofemoral thrombosis and the post-thrombotic syndrome. *Br Med J* **2**: 14.

Dodd H, Cockett FB (1976). *Pathology and Surgery of the Veins of the Lower Limb*, 2nd ed. Edinburgh: Churchill-Livingstone.

Edwards JM (1976). Sherry operation for incompetent perforating veins. *Br J Surg* **63**: 885.

Moffatt CJ, Franks PJ, Oldroyd M *et al.* (1992). Community clinics for leg ulcers and impact of healing. *Br Med J* **305**: 1389.

Negus D, Friedgood A (1983). Effective management of venous ulceration. *Br J Surg* **70**: 623.

The technique of endoscopic subfascial perforator surgery

Ralf Kolvenbach

Introduction

Before the introduction of subfascial endoscopic perforator surgery, subfascial ligation using multiple stab incisions or the classical Linton procedure were preferred to treat patients with incompetent perforating veins and chronic venous disease (CVD). One of the major drawbacks of these surgical techniques was the high incidence of wound healing problems causing a prolonged hospital stay and increased costs. Subfascial perforator surgery was finally introduced as an alternative because of the possibility of ligating perforator veins by making an incision in a non-diseased skin area (Tawes *et al.*, 1996; Glovitzk *et al.*, 1996; Bergan *et al.*, 1996). The ultimate goal of a subfascial perforator surgery procedure is the reduction of reflux in perforator veins mostly combined with surgery directed at the superficial venous system (Kolvenbach *et al.*, 1999).

1

Saphenous vein stripping as the only procedure does not necessarily suffice to treat incompetent perforating veins. A substantial number of perforators communicates with the posterior arch vein which remains intact after saphenous vein surgery.

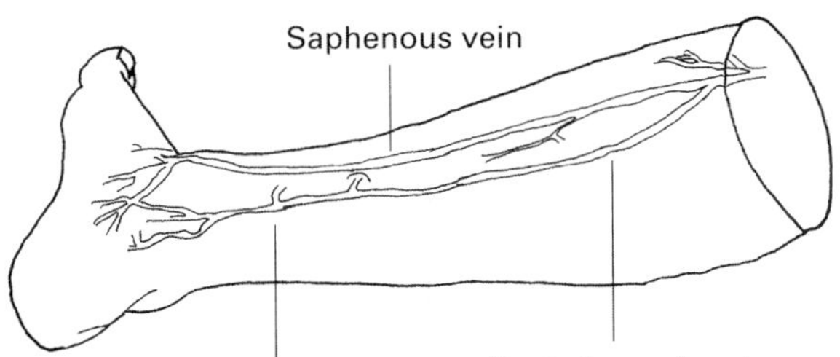

1

Procedure

Patients considered for subfascial perforator surgery are in class IV, V or VI of the CEAP (Clinical status – Etiology – Anatomical distribution – Pathophysiology) classification of the American Venous Forum. Class IV describes patients with pre-ulcerative venous disease states (lipodermatosclerosis, pain, pigmentation), Class V are those cases with healed yet recurrent ulcers and class VI summarizes patients with still an active ulcer that does not respond to compression therapy. The preoperative evaluation consists mainly of a colour duplex examination. The measurements are made using a linear array transducer with a 7.5 MHz pulsed wave Doppler colour flow duplex system with the patient in a near-upright standing position. The criterion for insufficiency is reverse venous flow demonstrated on the Doppler spectral display during the relaxation phase after active dorsiflexion or manual calf compression. Insufficiency is diagnosed if reversed flow persists longer than 0.5 seconds.

Surgical instruments

Most instruments are already available in the operating room for laparoscopic procedures. These include an insufflator to insufflate the subfascial space with carbon dioxide to maintain the working space; a rigid 10-mm endoscope; a three-chip video camera with xenon light source plus and a monitor.

2, 3

Additional instruments are: a balloon dissector (Spacemaker Tyco) [which helps to create a large bloodless operative working space] consisting of a 300-cc

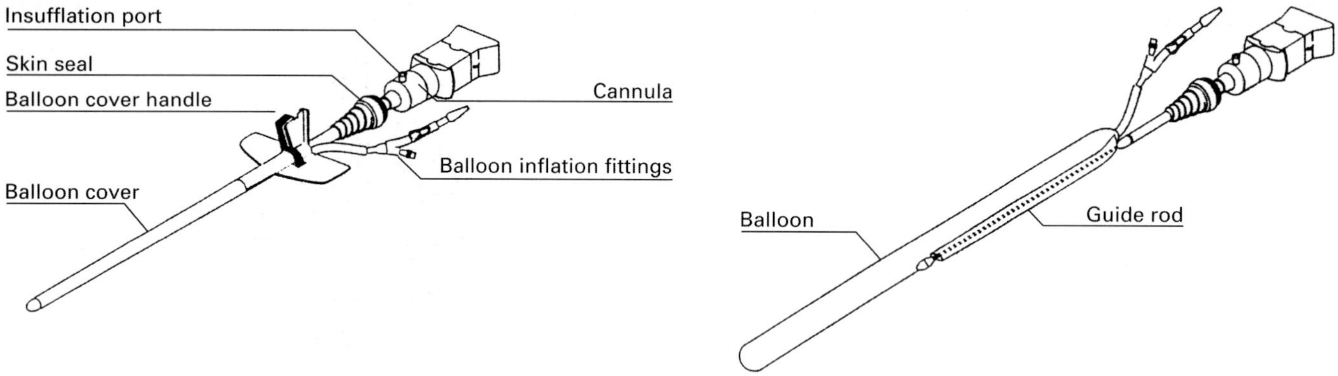

2

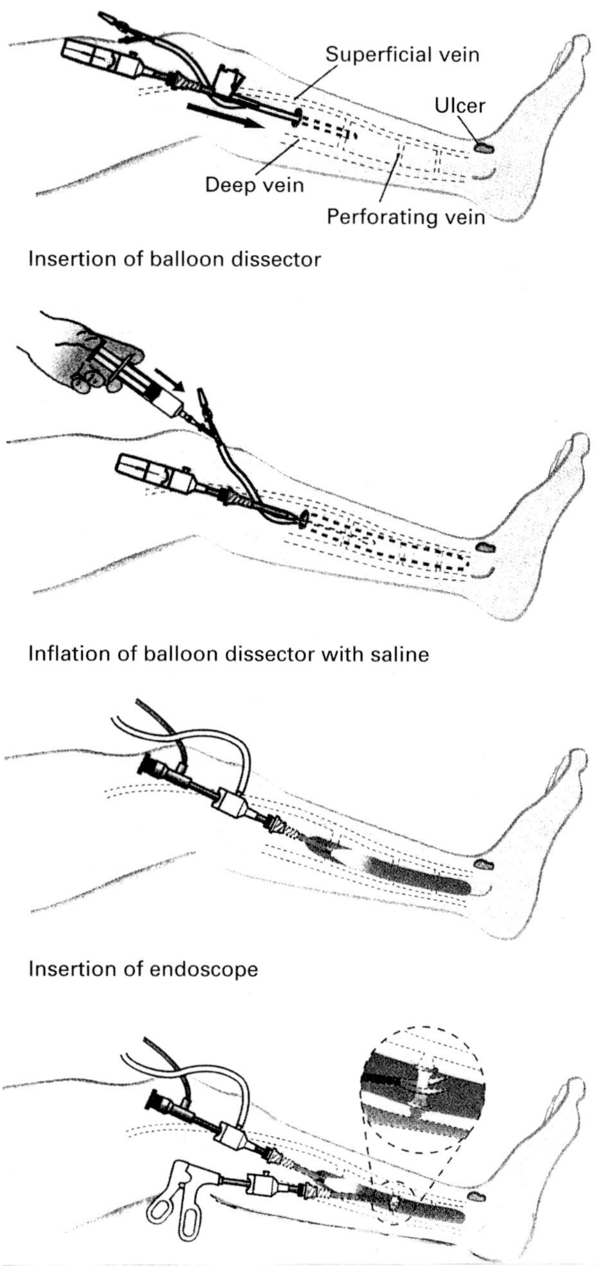

3

capacity balloon with a protective removable cover; a guide rod and a 10-mm laparoscopy canula with a skin seal. When using a 5-mm working port, a 5-mm disposable clip applier is necessary; in a 10-mm working port a reusable clip applier can be introduced.

The procedure is performed with the patient under general or spinal anaesthesia. We do not use any tourniquets. Instead the patient is operated in a Trendelenburg position with the knee slightly flexed and elevated. A 10-mm incision is made through the skin 4 cm medial to the tibia and 10–12 cm below the popliteal crease. After dissecting the subcutaneous tissue an incision is made into the fascia to open the superficial posterior compartment. The balloon retractor is introduced into this space and directed torward the medial malleolus. The balloon is inflated to a volume of 200–300 cc. The balloon is constructed in such a way that radial expansion occurs initially, followed by distal propagation to the malleolus. After deflation of the balloon, carbon dioxide is inflated at a pressure of 15 mmHg. The zero-degree 10-mm rigid laparoscope is inserted and a 5-mm working place is inserted in the mid-calf under direct endoscopic vision. It is important to place this trocar as posteriorly as possible to make a wide working axis and to prevent fencing of the instruments. The working port must not be placed through the gastrocnemius muscle to prevent compromising the subfascial space. All perforators accessible in the posterior superficial compartment are clipped. Division is only necessary when otherwise inspection of more distal areas cannot be performed. We do not use any electrocautery during the procedure to prevent nerve damage. Even with bipolar electrocautery damage of the tibial nerve can occur. Once identified, each perforating vein is double-clipped with the 8-mm titanium clips from the 5-mm clip applier. Regardless of the preoperative duplex findings we try to clip all perforators that are accessible.

4

In the more distal part of the calf there can be a septum intermusculare which is basically a duplicature formed

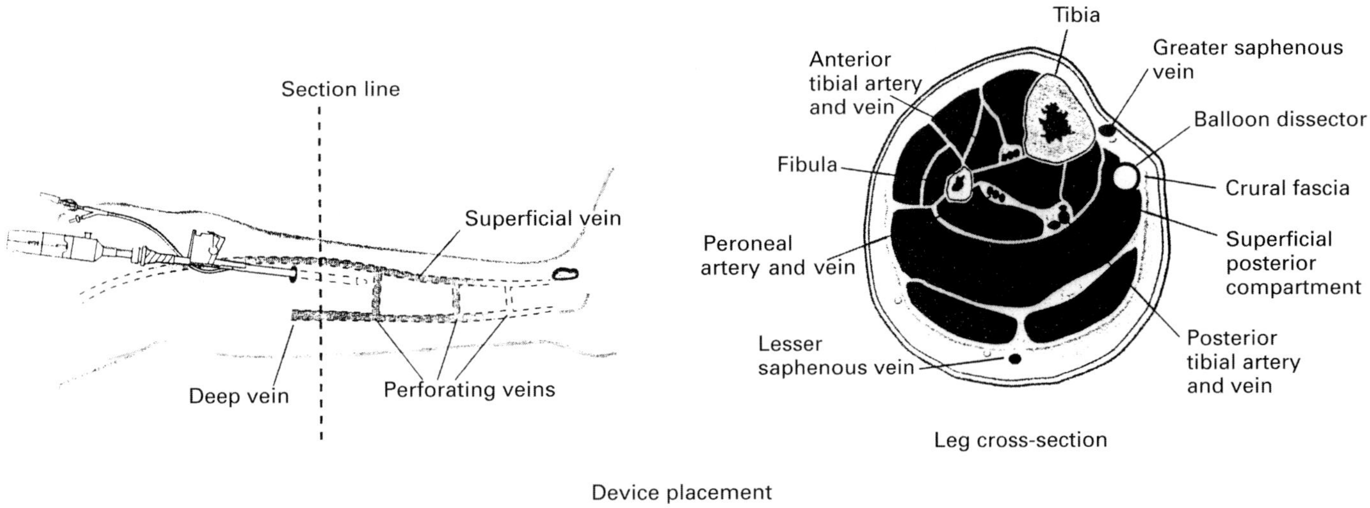

4

by the superficial posterior fascia and the deep posterior fascia (lamina profunda). There still can be e.g. Cockett II perforators in this septum which are missed when it is not taken down. For the same reason the deep posterior fascia has to be identified, and incised. This allows us substantial number of patients in a to identify Cockett perforators and to clip them. When incising the deep posterior fascia, special care must be taken to identify the structures posterior to the fascia such as the posterior tibial artery and the tibial nerve. The deep posterior fascia must be incised down to the level of the medial malleolus. Cockett I perforators dorsal to the malleolus can not usually be reached endoscopically. When they can be identified they can be marked percutaneously and clipped through a small stab incision.

In some cases an optimal degree of freedom to work through the instrument port cannot be achieved. In these cases where we want to reach the Cockett II perforators near the medial malleolus a second 5-mm instrument port is inserted percutaneously which permits dissection of the distal parts of the deep fascia.

Any bleeding e.g. from dislodged clips is controlled by external compression and elevation of the leg. At the end of the procedure the skin incisions are closed and short stretched compression bandages are applied. Superficial varicose vein surgery is performed in the standard fashion including stripping of the saphenous vein using an inversion technique or flush ligation. All patients are encouraged to start ambulation on the day of the operation.

References

Bergan JJ, Murray J, Greason K (1996). Subfascial endoscopic perforator vein surgery: a preliminary report. *Ann Vasc Surg* **10**: 211–219.

Glovitzki P, Cambria RA, Rhee RY *et al.* (1996). Surgical technique and preliminary results of endoscopic subfascial division of perforating veins. *J Vasc Surg* **23**: 517–523.

Kolvenbach R, Ramadan H, Schwierz E (1999). Redone endoscopic perforator surgery: Feasibility and failure analysis. *J Vasc Surg* **30**: 720–726.

Tawes RL, Wetter A, Fogarty TJ (1996) Endoscopic technique for subfascial perforating vein interruption. *J Endovasc Surg* **3**: 414–420.

Venous reconstructive surgery

John J Bergan, James S T Yao

Introduction

Direct surgery of veins has lagged behind direct arterialization of the extremities and viscera partly because surgeons have been more fascinated with the drama of cardiac and arterial surgery and partly because of the genuine difficulties which attend venous reconstruction and anastomosis. The standard operations with expected good results are bypasses of venous obstruction. Kistner has been successful with valveplasty (Ferris and Kistner, 1982), but others have found it to be a technically difficult procedure (Sottiurai, 1988). Kistner's technique of segment transfer is less demanding and enables venous flow to be directed through competent valves; unfortunately, it is applicable to a very small number of patients. The procedure championed by Taheri *et al.* (1982) of transplantation of valve-containing venous segments must await long-term evaluation before it is considered acceptable. Free-segment venous transfer must also be regarded as experimental. This chapter presents our current techniques of direct venous reconstruction.

Femorofemoral crossover grafts

1, 2

In this procedure, the saphenous vein is used as a conduit to bypass contralateral common and external iliac venous occlusion. Exposure is gained through vertical

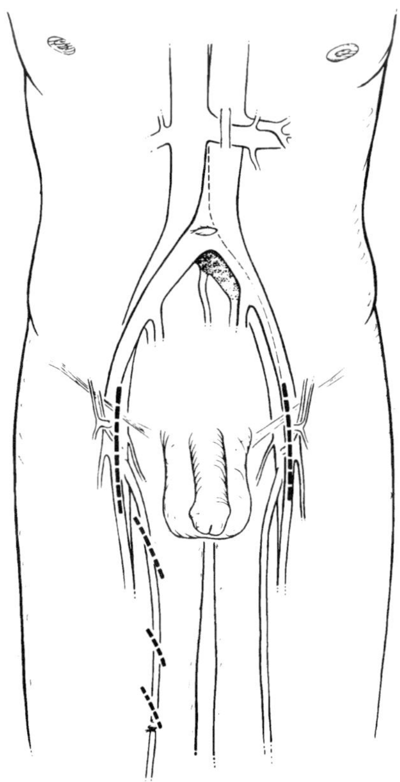

1

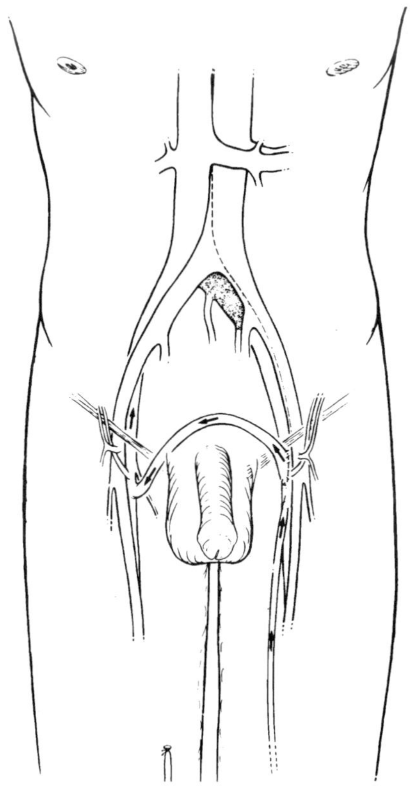

2

incisions over the femoral veins; one-third of the incision extends above the inguinal ligament. The saphenous vein is removed from the thigh under direct vision, through multiple, discontinuous incisions. Preparation of the graft must be meticulous to avoid venous trauma. As much adventitia as possible is carefully removed to allow maximum venous dilation. All tributary veins are ligated and divided at least 2 mm from the main trunk, in order to avoid constriction of the trunk during dilation. The graft is gently distended with heparinized saline solution to check for inadvertent tears or leaks. Localized varicosities, if present, must be dealt with either by resection or external support using normal vein tissue as recommended by Palma (1976).

The junction of the saphenous vein with the femoral vein is left intact. The superficial epigastric and external pudendal tributaries must be maintained so that angulation of the saphenofemoral junction is prevented.

The tunnel is made deeply, but subcutaneously, in the suprapubic region by digital dissection. The saphenous vein is passed through the tunnel using a long vascular clamp. Twisting of the vessel must be avoided. If possible, the graft should gradually curve into Scarpa's triangle on the affected side, and if necessary the vein can be stitched to the deep fascia using adventitial stitches.

The anastomosis should be 2–3 cm in length. It can be made to the saphenous vein on the affected side, but is best made to the common femoral vein, if possible. The venous intima should not be traumatized.

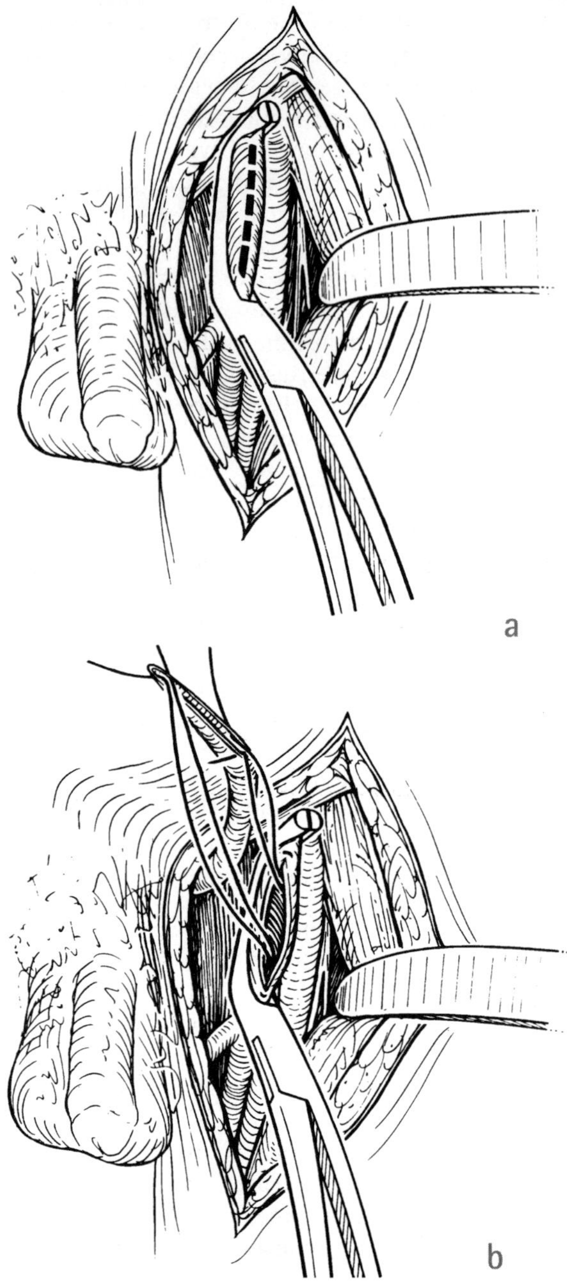

3

3a, b

Illustration **3a** shows the orientation of the structures after mobilization. Atraumatic clamps, as shown here, or siliconized rubber slings can be used for venous occlusion. Illustration **3b** indicates the anastomotic technique, with careful atraumatic eversion of the venous edges and approximation with 6/0 or 7/0 monofilament suture.

The wounds are closed in several layers to obliterate dead space. On our service, the arteriovenous fistula has been abandoned; instead, intermittent calf compression boots are applied using a 15-second on-cycle and 45-second off-cycle. Anticoagulants are not used.

Late results of the procedure are comparatively good. Harris *et al.* (1988), reporting from Sydney, Australia, described a 17-year experience, ending in 1982, involving 40 cross-saphenous bypasses. The crossover bypass graft managed symptoms in all patients, except two who required some distal reconstructive or ablative surgery. There were five late deaths, all unrelated to venous disease; three patients were lost to follow-up. The 5-year cumulative patency rate was 83%, but this was based on clinical judgement only. It is known that eight of the 41 grafts have occluded. In this study, 11 patients had surgical interruption of perforating veins or removal of distal varicosities, either concomitantly (eight) or following the bypass (three). The remaining 28 patients constituted a follow-up group: 11 have normal legs, nine confirmed by photoplethysmography (PPG), and nine have residual calf symptoms controlled with stocking support. Only one patient has had recurrent ulcerations. The eight patients with occluded grafts continue to have swelling, pigmentation and ulceration of the affected limb.

Saphenopopliteal bypass

When deep venous thrombosis of the superficial femoral vein is poorly recanalized, severe distal venous stasis may appear. When wearing of supportive bandages or well-fitted elastic stockings does not relieve stasis symptoms, direct surgical bypass of the obstruction is required. The calf muscle pump is relatively ineffective when working below an obstruction, and the long saphenous vein is inefficient because it is not connected to the muscle pump mechanism. Therefore, the objective of the operation is to provide a conduit to connect the deep venous system of the calf with a patent proximal venous pool.

In the USA, first Warren and Thayer (1954), and then Husni (1970) performed saphenopopliteal bypass. May (1979), in Innsbruck, also advocated this procedure. In 50% of Warren's patients, the saphenous vein was transplanted deep to the sartorius muscle.

As time has passed, we have become increasingly disappointed with this procedure.

For this procedure the poorly recanalized venous segment must be confined to the superficial femoral vein, the iliac system being spared, and the saphenous vein must be of good calibre preferably with functioning valves and no varicosities.

Careful ascending venography should show at least the distal half of the popliteal vein to be completely patent. There should be no evidence of smouldering, subacute venous thrombosis, as this will cause the procedure to fail.

Operative procedure

4

The patient lies supine on the operating table, with the leg slightly externally rotated and the knee moderately flexed. An incision is made parallel to the tibia, distal to its crest. The vein is marked prior to the operation, so that the skin incision can be made directly over it. The saphenous vein is mobilized and transected 2–3 cm distal to the distal end of the operative incision. The deep fasica is divided. The medial head of the gastrocnemius muscle is retracted medially. The soleus is exposed. The popliteal vein may be doubled, but the larger portion will lie posterior to the artery, with the anterior tibial veins crossing that structure.

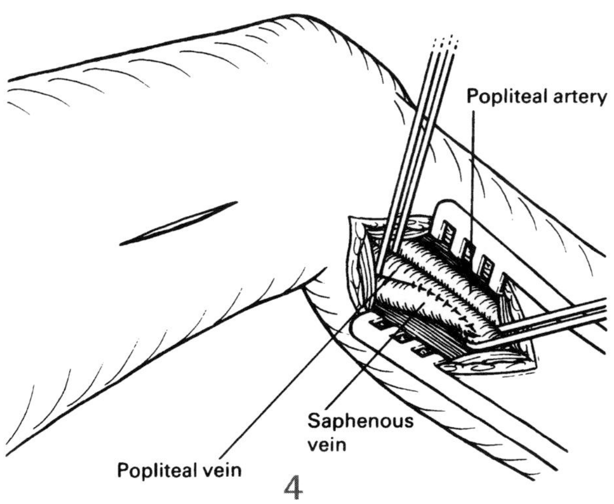

4

Additional exposure can be gained by cutting the semitendinosus and semimembranosus muscles. These do not have to be repaired.

Once an adequate segment of vein for anastomosis has been mobilized, attention is turned to the anteromedial aspect of the thigh. A 6-cm incision is made at the junction of the middle and distal thirds of the thigh and is carried through the deep fascia, displacing the sartorius posteriorly and incising the fascia over the popliteal space. A tunnel is made between the thigh and calf wounds, so that the mobilized saphenous vein can be inserted parallel to the popliteal vessels from above downward and thus lie in a gentle curve in the thigh, without tension behind the knee joint.

The leg is extended to make sure that the saphenous vein is of adequate length, and a site is chosen for the distal anastomosis. Thin, siliconized vessel loops are used to encircle the popliteal vein. A venotomy is created, and the venotomy and the distal end of the saphenous vein are irrigated with heparinized saline solution. The distal end of the saphenous vein is fishmouthed to conform exactly to the venotomy in the popliteal vein. A long anastomosis, 1.5 cm in length, is then made using 6/0 or 7/0 monofilament polypropylene suture.

Following the attainment of haemostasis, the wounds are closed, leaving the fascia open, both in the calf and in the thigh. The skin is approximated with synthetic, adsorbable intradermal suture. Suction drainage may be used, but an arteriovenous fistula is not created.

Postoperatively, the patient is not anticoagulated but may receive 500 ml of 10% Rheomacrodex each day for the first 5 days. An intermittent compression pump is applied to the calf, with a cycle of 15 seconds on, 45 seconds off.

The patency of the anastomosis is monitored by the transcutaneous Doppler technique.

Prostheses in venous reconstruction

Anecdotal reports have been received about the use of polytetrafluoroethylene (PTFE) grafts in the crossover femorofemoral position. None of these has been successful below the femoral vein.

Investigators using prosthetic grafts have been encouraged by experimental models which have used short-segment venous interposition grafts in the portal and vena caval systems, yet the clinical application of PTFE has been limited. There are reports of successful crossover grafts (Clowes, 1980), but these are few, and the operation should be applied with great caution.

As externally reinforced grafts have become available, they have been used clinically although, admittedly, in situations of great difficulty. A 1983 report from Japan (Takaba *et al.*, 1983) included a follow-up of 3–15 months in five patients requiring such femorofemoral crossover grafts. The grafts used were 16, 12, 8 and 6 mm, the last two being externally reinforced.

Direct venous valve surgery

Operations to correct valvular incompetence include direct valvuloplasty, transposition of the venous stream through a competent valve system, and valve transplantation.

Valvuloplasty, as invented by Kistner (Ferris and Kistner, 1982), can be a technically difficult operation. It is performed under magnification, using a 7/0 to 9/0 sutures. It is used in patients who have demonstrated a grossly incompetent superficial femoral valve, through which retrograde flow is visualized on descending venography.

5a, b, c

The femoral vein is exposed through a linear incision extending from the inguinal ligament. After complete mobilization of the superficial femoral vein, the anterior aspect is studied carefully, so that the incision in the vein can be made from below upward exactly through the valve commissure. It is very easy to carry the incision through a valve cusp and destroy the valvuloplasty operation.

6a, b, c

It is essential not to tear the valve cusp while sutures are being placed, and the reefing sutures must be placed precisely, in order to shorten the valve cusp but not excessively.

The venotomy may be closed from above downward to test the competence of the valve under direct vision. A dental mirror may be inserted into the venotomy to check the status of the reconstruction further or, alternatively, as the venotomy is being created from below upward, to assist in placing the venotomy precisely through the valve commissure (Samuels P, 1983, personal communication).

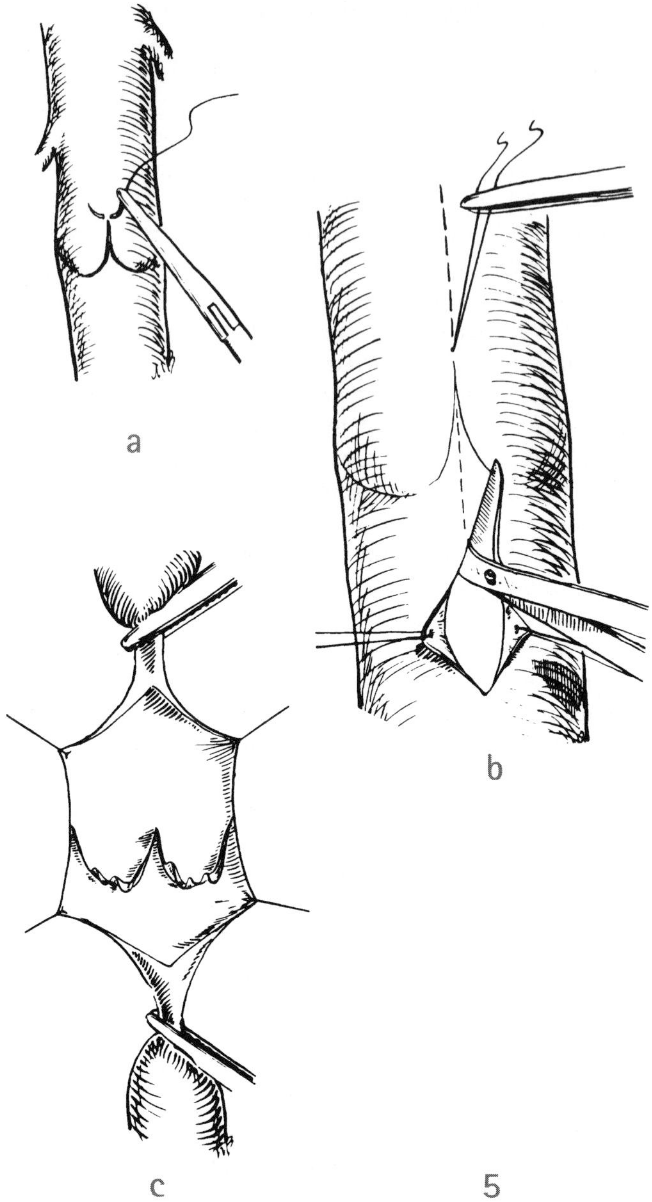

5

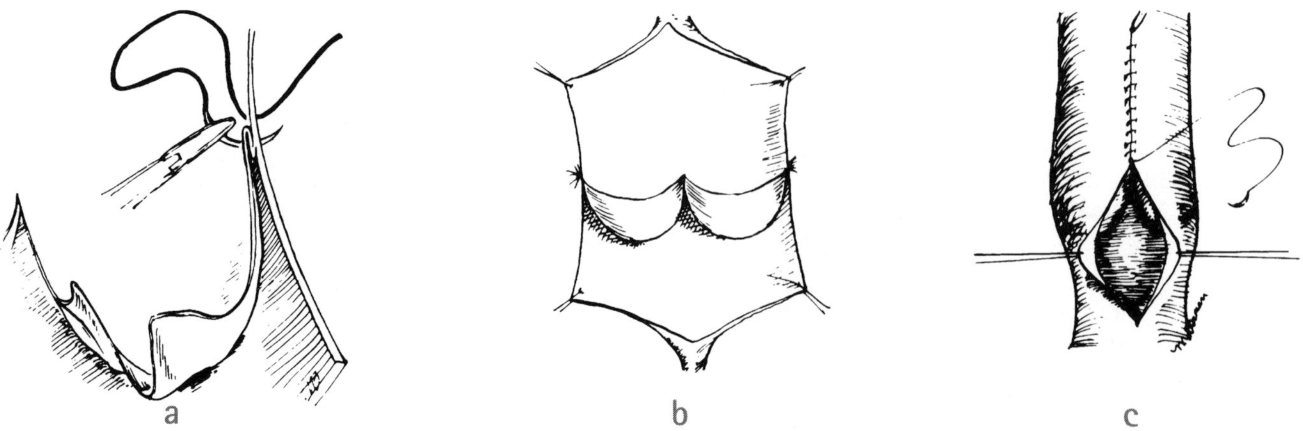

6

Transposition of the venous stream

7a, b, c

Kistner made a second major contribution to direct venous surgery by inventing the procedure of transposition of the venous stream through a demonstrably competent valve. He has called this redirection of venous flow through competent proximal valves the 'segment transfer operation'.

In this procedure, competent valves are identified in the profunda femoris vein, the saphenous vein or the superficial femoral vein by means of descending phlebography. After a competent valve is identified, an adjacent deep vein is transected and anastomosed to the venous segment containing the competent valve. An example of this is transection of the superficial femoral vein, which contains only incompetent valves, and anastomosis of this to the saphenous vein, which contains a competent saphenofemoral valve (**7a**). Another example is anastomosis of the divided superficial femoral vein to a profunda femoris vein which contains a competent valve (**7b**). Otherwise, the superficial femoral vein can be ligated and the saphenous vein anastomosed end-to-side below the ligature (**7c**).

The femoral venous confluence is approached through a linear incision made directly over the veins. One-third of the incision should be above the inguinal ligament, and two-thirds below. The saphenous vein and its tributaries are isolated, the common vein is skeletonized, and the profunda and superficial femoral veins are mobilized for a distance of 3–6 cm. The patient is systematically heparinized prior to the application of atraumatic clamps or occlusion of the major veins with siliconized rubber slings. Anastomosis is done with 7/0 polypropylene suture, ensuring that there is no tension between the structures to be anastomosed. Continuous stitching is utilized.

Competence of the valve is checked by emptying the distal vein through the valve and observing the distal vein for refilling. Wound closure is done in layers to avoid dead space. The skin edges are approximated using intradermal sutures of synthetic absorbable material, such as polyglycolic acid. Suction drainage may be used, but anticoagulants have been abandoned on our service.

Intermittent calf compression can be applied to maintain venous velocity through the reconstructed segment.

Kistner's late 1982 report (Ferris and Kistner, 1982) included 53 venous reconstructions in 46 patients, performed over a 14-year period. Seven of these reconstructions were excluded from evaluation. In two of these, superficial femoral vein ligation was required because of haemorrhage. In two others, superficial femoral vein ligation was required because of valve injury during repair or irreparable valve due to postphlebitic state. In another case, external plication rather than valve repair was done. Two patients had lymphoedema but underwent

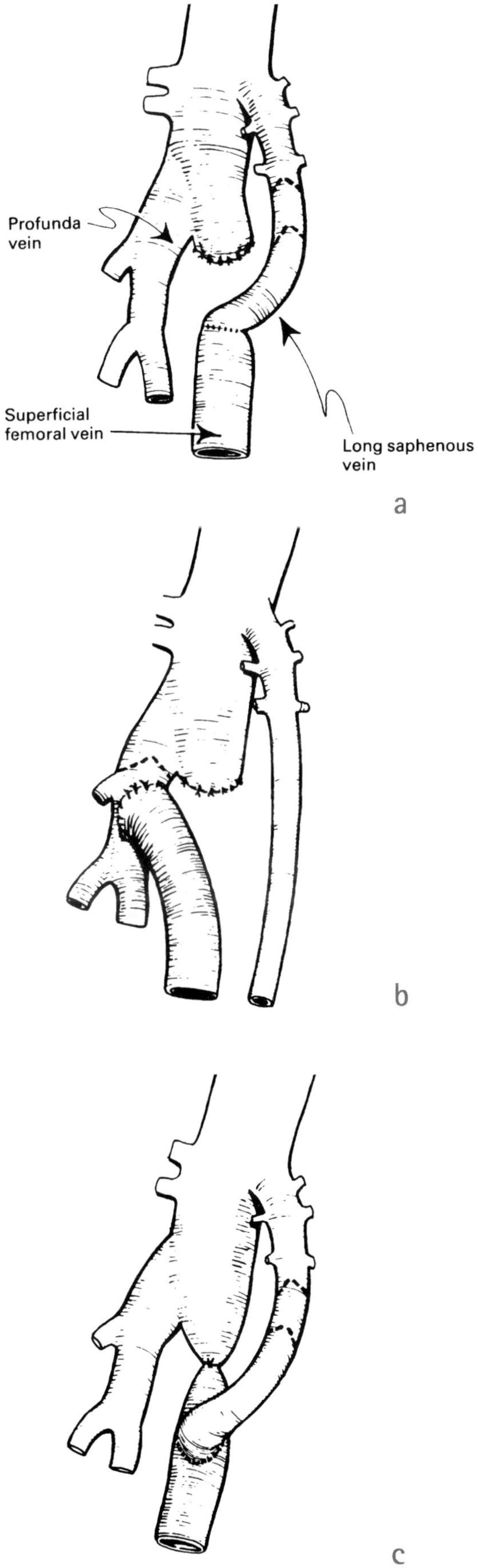

7

repair of a leaking superficial femoral vein valve; their symptoms of lymphoedema persisted.

In the remaining 46 extremities, there were 32 valve repairs and 14 venous segment transpositions. The results were good-to-excellent in 80% of both groups. Patients with stasis and ulceration had better results than those with pain and oedema. Interestingly, descending postoperative venography was performed in 41 of 46 cases, and thrombosis of the reconstructed segment has not occurred in any patient. Improvement of venous competence was demonstrated in 39 of the 41 cases.

It should be noted that incompetent perforators have been treated in conjunction with femoral vein reconstruction in this series. In another series (Queral *et al.*, 1980), in which incompetent perforators were not treated, good results were only achieved in 11 of 16 patients, and excellent results in only one patient. This experience is similar to ours.

Valve transplantation

Taheri has had the greatest experience with valve transplantation. In the original procedure described by him the superficial femoral vein was exposed through a longitudinal incision below the inguinal ligament. Later, he implanted the new segment in the above-knee popliteal vein. The brachial vein is approached through a longitudinal incision 5 cm below the axilla. A 2-cm segment of brachial vein, including valve, is tested for competence and removed. A segment of popliteal vein is excised, and the brachial vein, including the valve, is sutured to the popliteal vein with 7/0 or 8/0 polypropylene suture, using a continuous, everting or interrupted technique.

Taheri uses continuous heparin administration and suction drainage of both the arm and the thigh wound. Oral anticoagulation is used for 3 months.

Taheri, *et al.* (1982) described 38 patients having valve transplantation. Postoperative venography (16 ascending, 12 descending) showed 13 patients with normal venous systems and three patients with thrombosis of the superficial femoral system.

The only other large experience with valve transplantation is that of Raju (1983), who reported 20 valvuloplasties, 22 vein valve transplantations and three Kistner segment transfer operations. Thrombosis of a valve repair was only found in one of 17 patients who had venographic examination of the repair after operation. The valve transplant operation seemed quite satisfactory, with resolution of the primary symptom in 13 limbs (nine ulcers, two oedema, two chronic pain). Of this group, ten limbs showed improvement in the venous haemodynam-

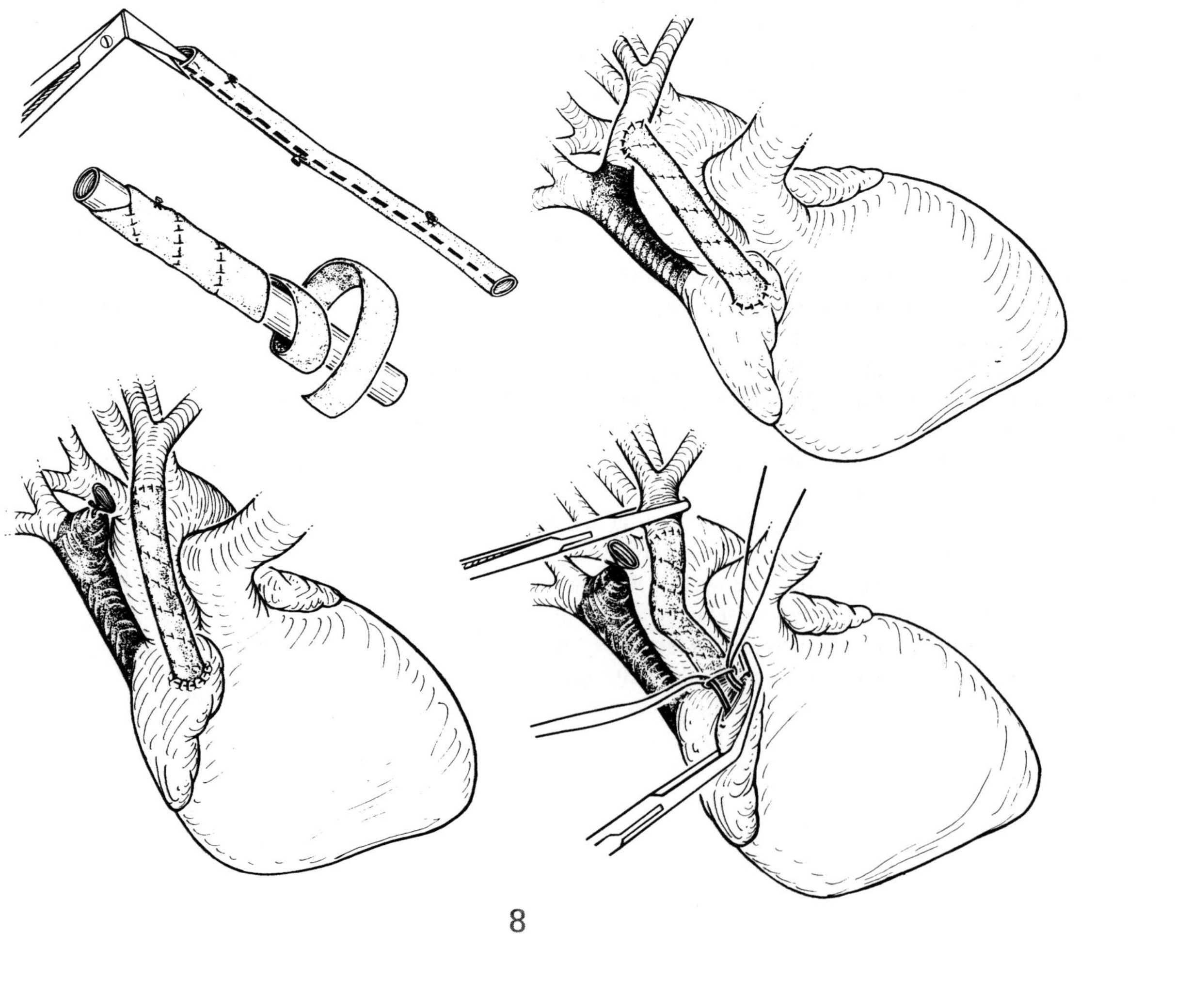

8

ics, as measured in the laboratory, and in three limbs, despite subjective improvement, the laboratory parameters remained unchanged. Eight patients were surgical failures: there was a technical problem in one small axillary vein; in the other seven patients there was recurrence of reflux through the transplanted axillary vein segment, proved by venography venous testing.

Superior vena cava bypass

8

Superior vena cava obstruction may have a variety of causes, including granulomatous mediastinitis, tuberculosis and malignant tumour. When cerebral insufficiency syndromes occur, consideration may be given to the performance of a bypass of the superior vena cava (Chiu *et al.*, 1974; Wright and Doty, 1980). A suitable graft for such bypass may be obtained by removing the long saphenous vein, ligating all of its branches, distending the vein with heparinized saline solution under gentle hydrostatic pressure, and splitting the vein longitudinally throughout its length. The open vein is then wrapped around a previously chosen stent of appropriate size (No. 40 chest tube). The continuous anastomosis can be made utilizing 6/0 or 7/0 polypropylene suture.

A median sternotomy incision is made, and the innominate vein exposed and mobilized throughout its length. The pericardium is then opened through a vertical incision, retracted laterally and held in place with stay sutures. Biopsy of the upper mediastinum can be obtained at this time. The distance between the innominate vein and atrial appendage is measured. The distal anastomosis can be made end-to-end, as preferred by Doty and Wright, or end-of-graft to side-of-innominate vein. Meticulous performance of the anastomosis is eased by use of loop magnification. The suture material is 6/0 polypropylene.

The anastomosis to the right atrial appendage can be done using a partial occlusion clamp. The trabeculated portion of the atrial appendage is excised and the anastomosis constructed with 6/0 polypropylene. The clamps are removed, and the blood flow through the graft is checked. As in all venous surgery, meticulous technique must be utilized for construction of the spiral graft and both of the anastomoses. Fibrous adventitial strings must not be allowed to cross the suture lines; neither should purse-stringing of either anastomosis be allowed to occur.

The pericardium is not closed, but the median sternotomy is closed by peristernal wire, in order to immobilize the sternum entirely. Drainage tubes are left in the mediastinum, but anticoagulation is unnecessary.

Acknowledgements

Supported in part by the Conrad Jobst Foundation, the Seabury Foundation and the Northwestern Vascular Research Foundation.

Illustrations 5 and 6 are from Kistner and Ferris (1980, pp. 293 and 295) Illustration is from Queral (1980, p. 304).

References

Chiu CJ, Terzis J, MacRae ML (1974). Replacement of superior vena cava with the spiral composite vein graft. *Ann Thorac Surg* **17**: 555.

Clowes AW (1980). Extra-anatomical bypass of iliac vein obstruction. *Arch Surg* **115**: 767.

Ferris EB, Kistner RL (1982). Femoral vein reconstruction in management of chronic venous insufficiency. *Arch Surg* **117**: 1571.

Harris JP, Kidd J, Burnett A, Halliday P (1988). Patency of femorofemoral venous crossover grafts assessed by duplex scanning and phlebography. *J Vasc Surg* **8**: 679.

Husni EA (1970). *In situ* sapheno-popliteal bypass grafts for incompetence of femoral and popliteal veins. *Surg Gynecol Obstet* **130**: 279.

Kistner RL, Ferris EB (1980). Technique of surgical reconstruction of femoral vein valves. In *Operative Techniques in Vascular Surgery*. Bergan JJ, Yao JST eds. London/San Diego: Grune and Stratton.

May R (1979). *Surgery of the Veins of the Leg and Pelvis*. London Philadelphia: WB Saunders Co., p. 150.

Palma EC (1976). Vein grafts for treatment of post-phlebitic syndrome. In *Vascular Surgery: Principles and Techniques*. Haimovici H ed. New York: McGraw Hill, p. 857.

Queral LA (1980). Correction of deep venous insufficiency by valvular transposition. In *Operative Techniques in Vascular Surgery*. Bergan JJ, Yao JST eds. London/San Diego: Grune and Stratton.

Queral LA, Whitehouse WM Jr, Flinn WR *et al.* (1980). Surgical correction of chronic deep venous insufficiency by valvular transposition. *Surgery* **87**: 688.

Raju S (1983). Venous insufficiency of the lower limb and stasis ulceration. *Ann Surg* **197**: 688.

Sottiurai VS (1988). Techniques in venous valvuloplasty. *J Vasc Surg* **8**: 646.

Taheri SA, Lazar L, Alias S (1982). Status of vein valve transplant after 12 months. *Arch Surg* **117**: 1313.

Takaba T, Yamamoto N, Fumami M *et al.* (1983). Reconstruction with expanded polytetrafluoroethylene (EPTFE) for iliac venous obstruction (abstract). *J Cardiovasc Surg* **24**: 422.

Warren CB, Thayer TP (1954). Transplantation of the saphenous vein for post-phlebitic stasis. *Surgery* **35**: 867.

Wright CB, Doty DB (1980). Spiral vein grafting: the technique. In *Operative Techniques in Vascular Surgery*. Bergan JJ, Yao JST eds. London/San Diego: Grune and Stratton, pp. 307–310.

Repair of venous valves using silicone cuffs

Rodney J Lane

Introduction

The present indications for the use of silicone valve cuffs are to correct chronic deep venous insufficiency usually associated with ulceration unresponsive to other forms of therapy. Similar silicone cuffs may be used for varicose veins. The underlying aetiology of lower limb venous insufficiency is first determined using non-invasive testing. If deep venous incompetence is thought to be the problem it is confirmed by venography. Grades of III or IV (Kistner) of reflux must be demonstrated and the best results are obtained when the whole venous system is uniformly dilated with multiple valves. These must be clearly demonstrated by venography, particularly by descending venography. Both cusps must be seen to be present and the attachment of the cusps on to the wall must be symmetrical. Radio-opaque markers are essential during all forms of venography in order to allow accurate location of the valves at the time of operation.

There are reservations about this technique in patients with extensive deep venous thrombosis and associated inflammatory changes with destruction of valve cusps. However, patients who have venographically intact valve cusps either above or below a previous thrombosis do not necessarily have to be excluded. At present, at least three valves in more than one area (i.e. popliteal or femoral level) should be corrected. The distal repairs are always performed initially, because one of the operative tests for valve function requires maximal hydrostatic pressure with anaesthetic-induced valsalva. Additional back pressure is created by elevating the head as much as possible and clearly this is best achieved without having interposing competent valves. Main axial valves are selected in order to minimize distal alternate retrograde flow. In patients where the function of a particular valve cannot be totally corrected (but a good pressure gradient can be maintained), additional valves should be repaired. It is essential that all valves are tested at operation usually via the 'milking' and the 'proximal occlusion' techniques to check competence visually. Typically, complete competence is obtained with reduction of the lumen by apparently one-third

Preoperative precautions

Microbiological examination of swabs from the ulcer is used to determine the presence of pathogens and patients are covered with the appropriate antibiotics during the anaesthetic induction. Heparin is also given. Our practice is to give 5000 units subcutaneously and 2000 units intravenously. The level of the valve is marked on the skin with an indelible pencil based on preoperative venogram with magnification taken into account.

The operation

1

The popliteal fossa or thigh is prepared and draped in the usual manner and the skin covered with a suitable plastic drape. The incision is curved to minimize contracture at the skin fold.

2

The incision is carried through the deep fascia and the vein is located adjacent to the artery. Minimal dissection is required in order to obviate or minimize lymphatic interruption. The segment of vein above and below the valve is isolated and minor tributaries are ligated and divided. If there are major tributaries then these are slung.

3

During the dissection the valve is located and appears as an oblique curvilinear line of attachment joining in a proximal apex. There is commonly a bulge just proximal

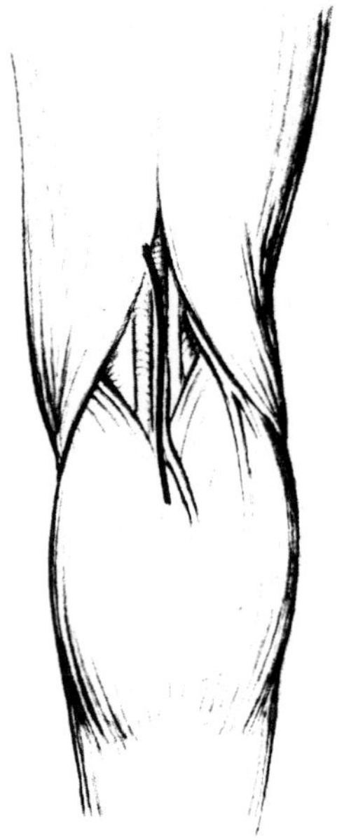

1

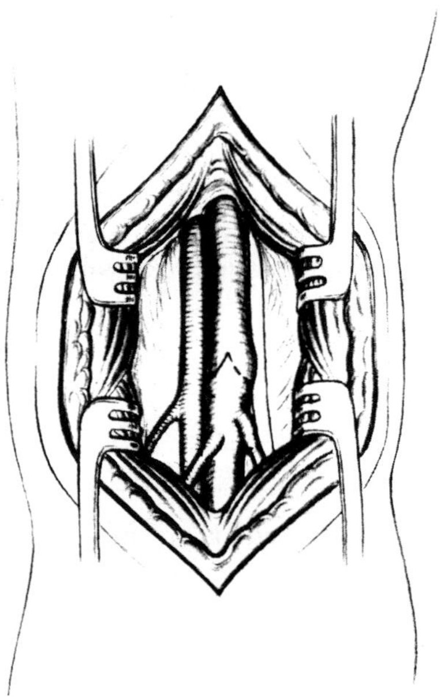

2

to the valve cusp and it may be necessary to refer to the venogram and remeasure the actual site of the valve from a bony prominence.

If the valve cannot be identified by these means, intraoperative B-mode imaging may be used. Occasionally, to decide finally on the presence or absence of a valve, the vein is narrowed to see if competence is achieved. Very gentle dissection is essential as spasm of the valve may occur and cause temporary competence interfering with testing. This can always be overcome, however, by proximal occlusion and digital pressure between the occlusive loop and the valve.

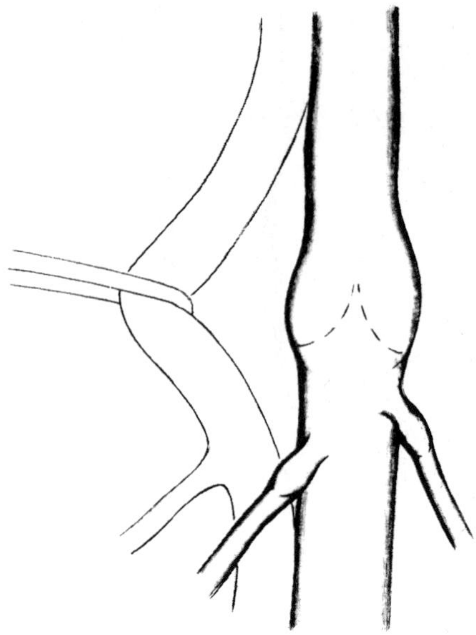

3

4

Having identified the valve and dissected at least 3 cm distally and 1 cm proximally, silastic vessel loops are placed around the vein in order to control inflow and outflow.

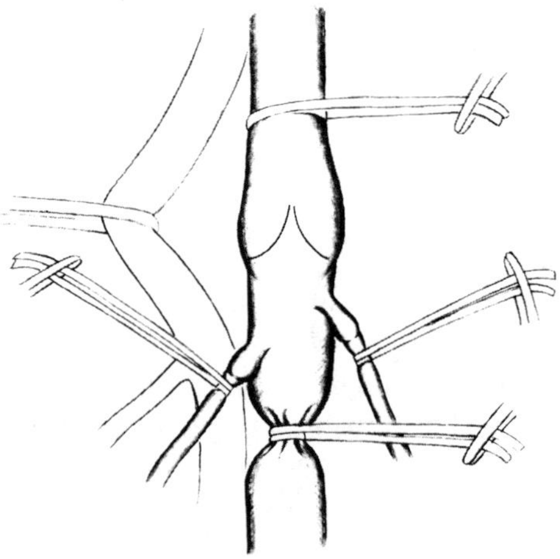

4

5

The silicone cuff used is called the 'Venocuff'. A right-angle forceps is used to pass one end of the Venocuff around the vein. The other end of the Venocuff is already attached to its applicator. Sometimes the end of the Venocuff may impinge upon the vein wall and great care should be taken.

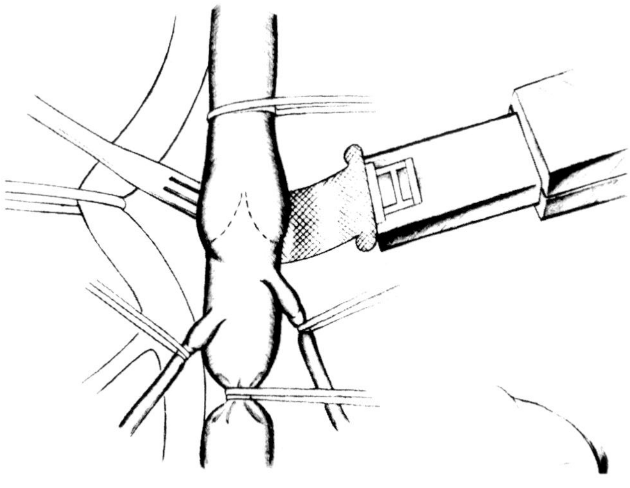

5

7

The applicator tensioning bar is then activated to decrease the valve ring circumference and so bring valve cusps closer together to produce competence. This is checked frequently during the tightening using the 'milking technique'. The inflow is first occluded with the distal silastic slings and the segment up to the valve ring is milked free of blood with the finger and thumb. Maximum 'head up' of the patient on the operating table is required during this testing. A valsalva manoeuvre is performed by the anaesthetist to obstruct venous return and further stress the valve being tested. It becomes clear if the valve withstands the downward force of venous pressure if the distal vein segment stays collapsed. The distal silastic loop is now released to fill the distal segment and again the test is repeated.

6

The free end of the Venocuff is engaged into the applicator Venocuff slot. The Venocuff is now wrapped around the vein and is positioned at the valve site. The buckle action is similar to a car seat belt. At this stage, irrigation solution containing antibiotics in saline is used to irrigate the wound to maintain asepsis. The Venocuff should not be allowed to touch the patient's skin.

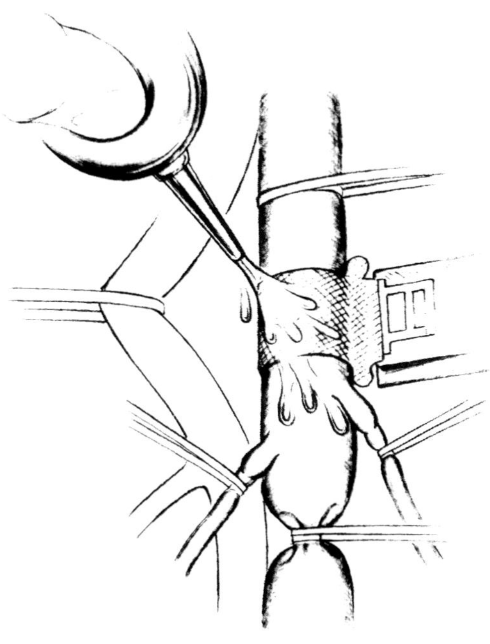

6

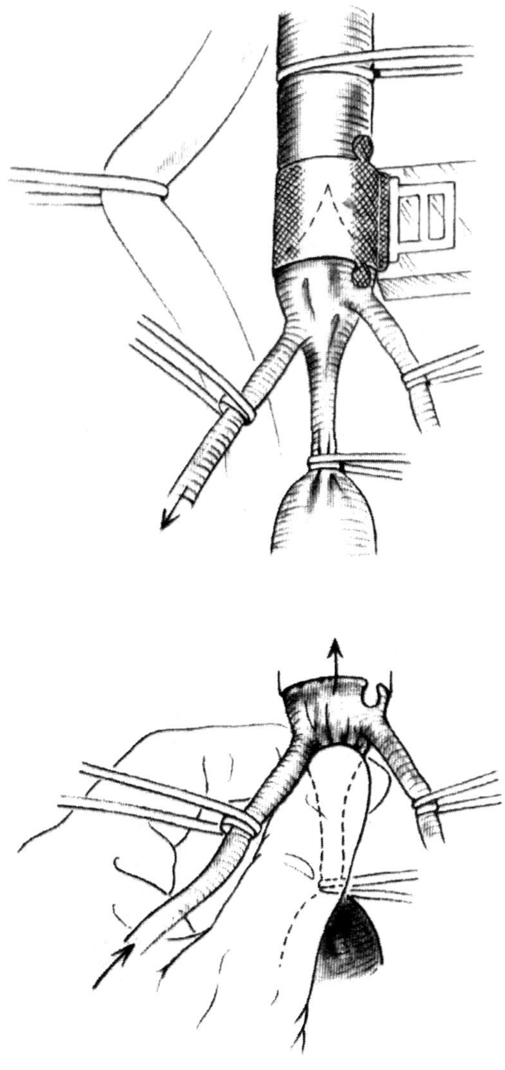

7

8

The proximal compression test or close segment compression test is then performed by obstructing the proximal sling, cranial to the valve being tested and allowing the segment between to fill. Digital pressure then compresses this segment and a competent valve generates a high pressure. This can be compared with the pressure in the distal vein. This test is useful when access to the more distal parts of the vein are not possible because of tributaries or inadequate dissection. If a valve seems to be incompetent following Venocuff application on repeated testing, an unsighted tributary should be sought. In many cases, competence is demonstrated when this hidden tributary is controlled. If the valve is not completely competent under high pressure but clearly maintains a gradient, the Venocuff is left in place.

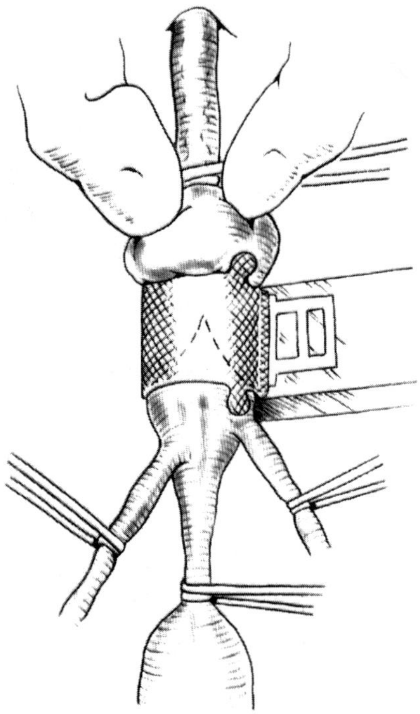

8

9

When valve function has been corrected or, at least, improved, the staple trigger on the applicator is fired and the staple automatically fastens the Venocuff at the appropriate diameter and cuts off excess strapping. Occasionally, the operator may place excessive downward pressure on the actual vein, so that when the applicator has been removed, the valve subsequently becomes incompetent again. Therefore, both testing manoeuvres should be repeated after fastening the Venocuff. The diameter of the Venocuff should always be noted using

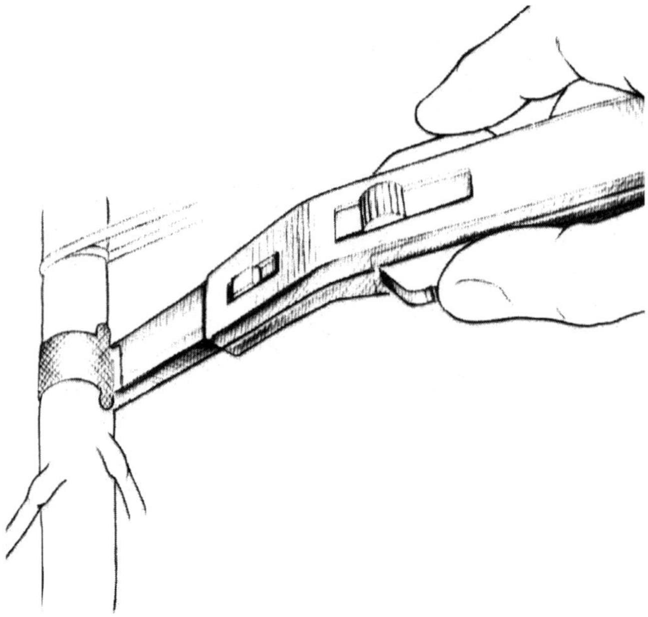

9

the graduations on the applicator. Hence, if incompetence occurs, a new Venocuff is applied and the diameter is further decreased, which usually imparts competence.

10

Occasionally, the ends of the Venocuff require a metal vessel clip at the join of the two straps. These may be inserted at either end above or below.

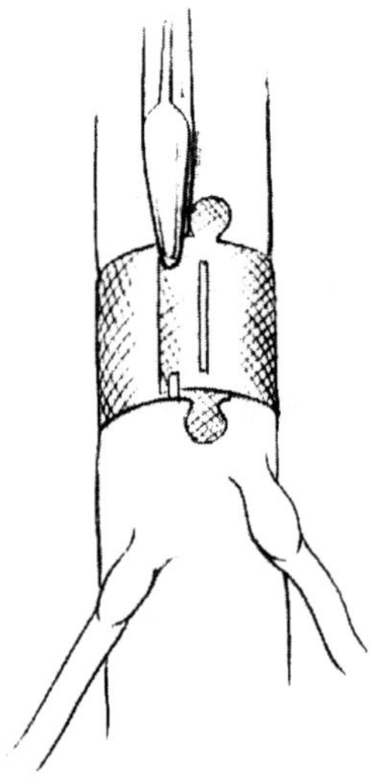

10

11

There are two fixation tags on the Venocuff which are then used to suture the Venocuff to surrounding tissue. A 5/0 polypropylene suture is used to do this. Two further sutures are used to fasten the Venocuff directly to the adventitia of the vein as shown. Sometimes when checking for competence it becomes necessary to cut the distal fixation tag off, and this direct extra suturing to the vein is then mandatory.

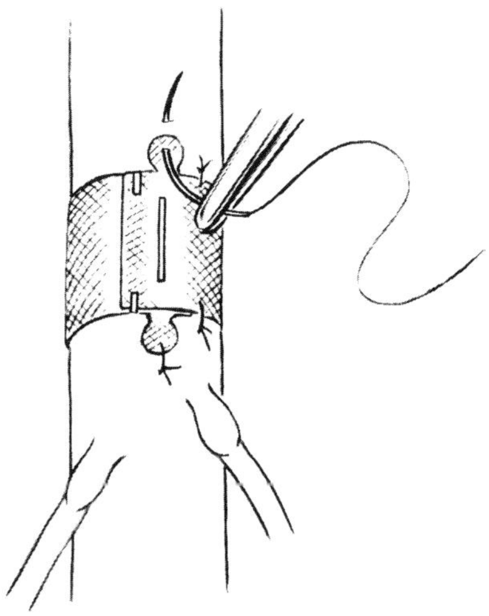

11

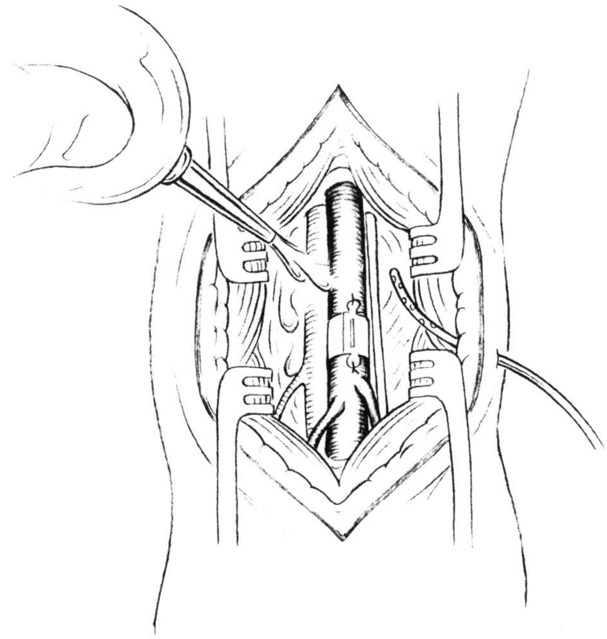

13

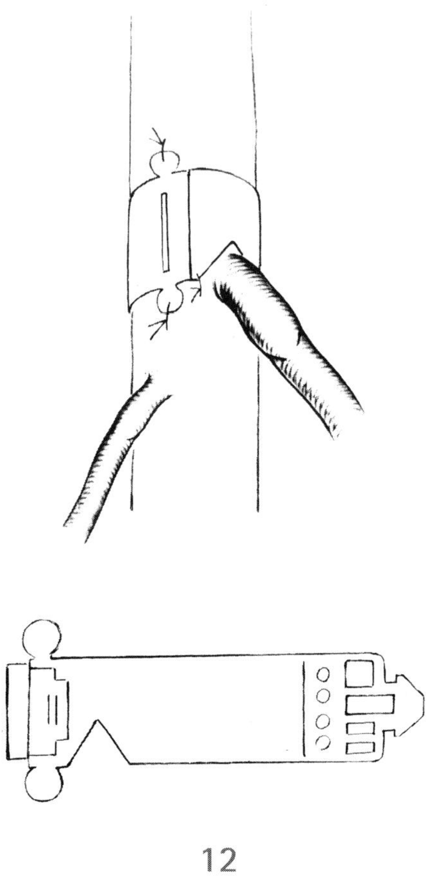

12

12

In cases of a valve being very close to a tributary, a Venocuff with a V-notch (Venocuff S) can be chosen to allow adequate and suitable reduction of the circumference of the valve. There are two notched Venocuffs, the left and right (Venocuff SL and SR), to suit the situation.

It should be emphasized that the corners of the notch must be sutured directly to the adventitia, preferably anteriorly and posteriorly in order to maintain the diameter and tension of the Venocuff.

13

Closure is completed in layers and sterility maintained by again irrigating with an antibiotic solution. A suction drain is used routinely and careful haemostasis is essential. Mobilization should begin as soon as possible, preferably the next day, and subcutaneous heparin is administered until ambulation is complete. Intravenous antibiotics are continued for 24h. The patient is usually discharged at 4 days and ulcer care is continued.

Acknowledgement

Illustrations by R N Lane.

Deep venous thrombectomy

O Wagner

Introduction

Intervention for the removal of acute thrombosis of the iliac and femoral veins consists of thrombolysis or venous thrombectomy. The aim of these procedures is the prevention of lethal pulmonary embolism as well as the immediate restoration of venous blood-flow, thereby also preserving the valvular system and preventing a post-thrombotic syndrome. The advantages of these procedures over elevation and heparin therapy are the immediate relief of the compromised venous drainage, lowered and shortened morbidity, venous valve preservation and prevention of the postphlebitic syndrome in a large percentage of these patients. Success of surgical thrombectomy can only be expected in cases of very recent thrombosis, which means that surgery should be performed within the first few days of occurrence. If thrombectomy is performed after a longer interval, adherence of the thrombus to the vessel wall makes removal of the clot increasingly more difficult and enhances the chance of rethrombosis. Surgery performed later than 6 days after the onset of symptoms shows no better results than conservative treatment; thrombolysis, however, may be successful up to 15 days (Minar *et al.*, 1983).

Preoperative

Indications

Surgery is indicated for thrombosis of the deep femoral and iliac veins with a history of onset up to 5 days. However, floating thrombus or segmental femoral or iliac thrombosis can be operated on successfully up to 4 weeks.

Contraindications

Surgery is contraindicated in patients with a short life expectancy (such as those with inoperable tumour) or when postoperative heparin or anticoagulant therapy is inadvisable.

Preoperative assessment

The clinical course with sudden onset of swelling and pain is characteristic. A reliable diagnosis depends on clinical findings only and can be supplemented by ultrasound examinations. Venography is not obligatory but provides helpful information on the extent of the thrombosis. The blood group should be determined and 2 units of blood prepared in case of extensive blood loss.

The operation

This operation was first described in 1937 by Läwen, Professor of Surgery in Königsberg, Germany and followed up by Mahorner *et al.* in 1957.

The operation is performed under general anaesthesia. In slim patients thrombectomy from the common femoral vein is also feasible in local anaesthesia. Systemic heparinization is attained by administration of 5000 international units of heparin intravenously.

1, 2

A transverse inguinal incision is made just above the groin crease, and the femoral vein, saphenous vein, deep femoral vein and superficial femoral vein are controlled by Silastic slings.

After heparinization a longitudinal incision of 2–3 cm is made at the entrance of the saphenous vein. First the local thrombus is removed; then each orifice is explored for clots which are removed by forceps and Fogarty catheters. The same procedure is performed on the deep femoral veins. The veins are then controlled by bulldog clamps (Fogarty and Kreppoehne, 1965). Proximal clots are removed by passing Fogarty catheters into the iliac venous system. During this procedure the pressure in the intra-abdominal vena cava is increased by hyperbaric respiration to prevent pulmonary embolism. (A blocking catheter from the collateral side should not be used since this would constitute an added trauma to the normal

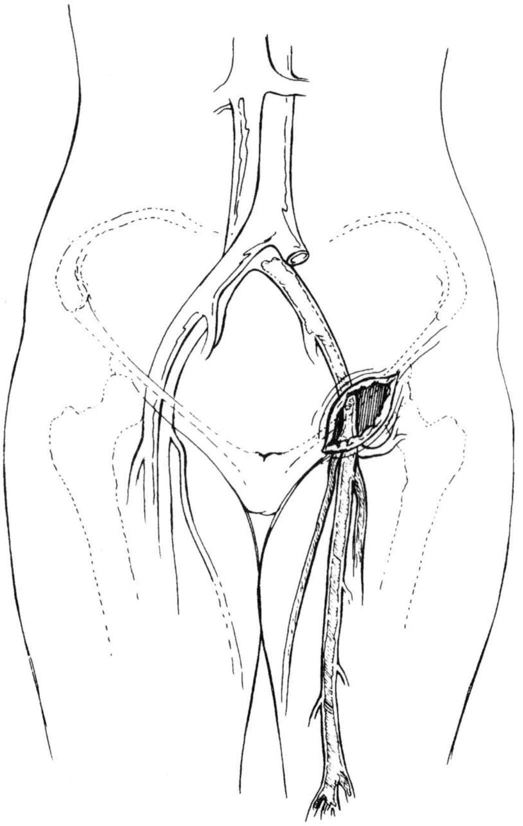

1

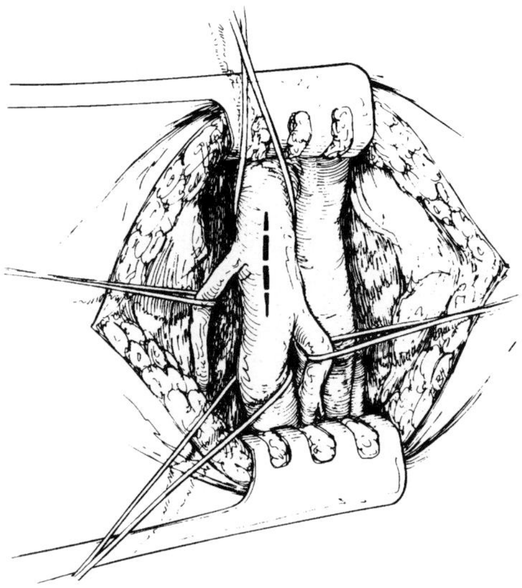

2

collateral vein without providing absolute security against embolization.)

Intraoperative phlebography of the iliac veins is helpful when additional information on the completeness of thrombectomy is necessary. In some patients repeated attempts at thrombectomy are necessary before normal venograms can be obtained.

Intraoperative endoscopy is another possibility for checking completeness of clot removal and to demonstrate residual disease in the iliac veins (Loeprecht *et al.* 1985).

3

If a chronic thrombus in the iliac vein cannot be removed with the Fogarty catheter despite successful catheterization, the Fogarty catheter can be guided through the hole of a ringstripper and used to block the entrance of the common iliac vein. Following this procedure, the ringstripper can be used to remove the thrombotic material with gentle force from the vessel wall. When the clots are loosened they can then be removed by retracting the Fogarty catheter.

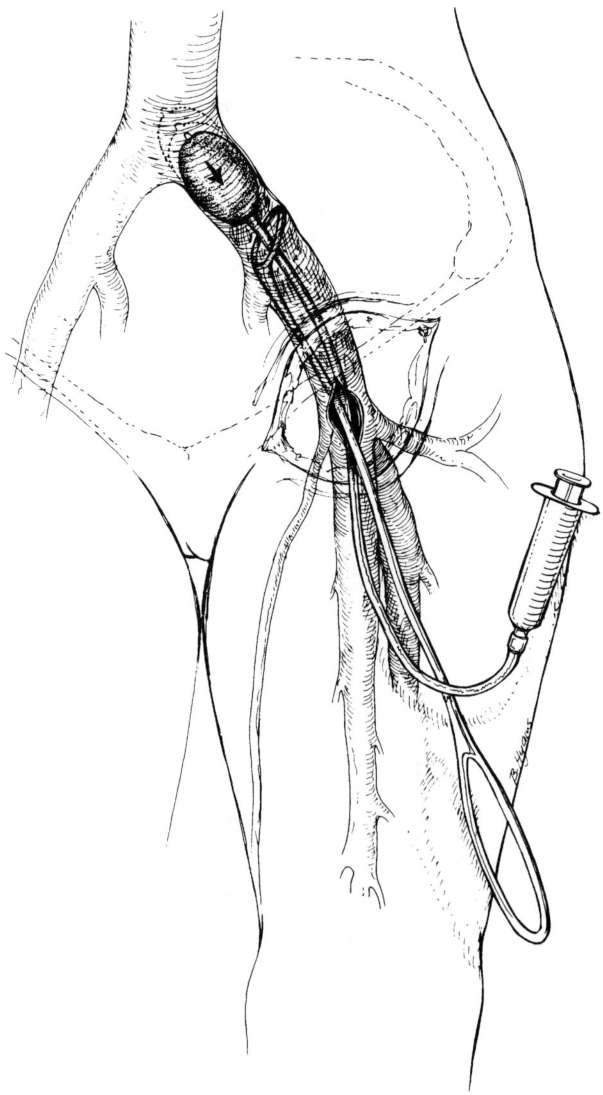

3

4

Finally, the distal clot is removed. When the thrombus is of recent origin and not yet firmly attached to the vessel wall, it can be removed by circumferential manual pressure which is exerted at the calf and gradually advanced upward. In cases of fresh thrombosis, sudden compression of the calf and thigh muscles by hand or with an Esimarch bandage results in complete removal of a thrombus throughout the whole deep venous system. The thrombus is then flushed out *in toto* by the bloodstream.

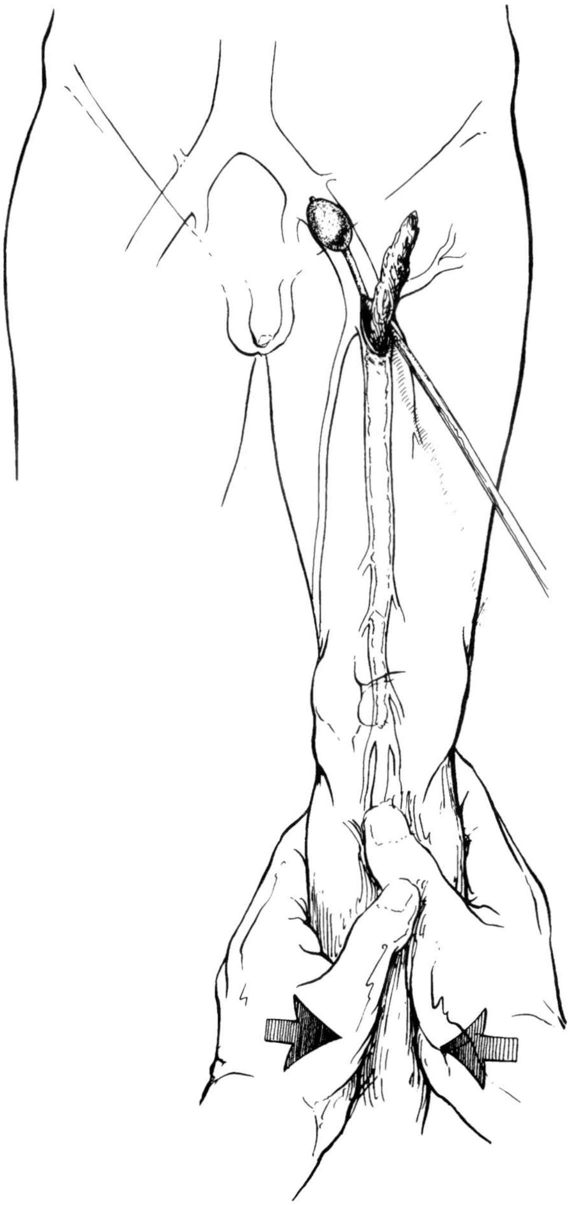

4

5

When the thrombus is adherent and compression does not work, a Fogarty catheter is used. In most cases introduction of this catheter is not possible over a longer distance because of competent valves. In such cases the catheter is attached to a small ringstripper and guided downward through the superficial femoral vein. If this procedure is not successful, because of patent venous valves, an additional incision at the proximal or distal popliteal vein might be helpful. A soft catheter can be brought up from the distal incision, the Fogarty catheter inserted into the lumen of the catheter, moved distally without problems, and the thrombus material can then be removed without interference from the valves.

After satisfactory thrombectomy, the incision(s) is (are) closed with a continuous 6/0 polypropylene suture, a suction drain is inserted and the wound is closed in layers. Postoperative continuous heparin therapy is administered (1000 international units/h intravenously).

The patient is mobilized on the third postoperative day and anticoagulation with warfarin is started as a longer-term therapy. Anticoagulation treatment should be continued lifelong, because the rate of recurrent thrombosis in the diseased leg is very high (50%) among those patients who stopped anticoagulation even some years after their operation (Polterauer *et al.*, 1988).

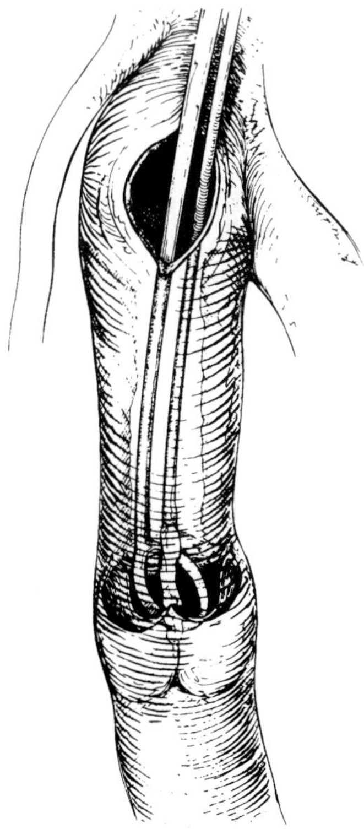

5

Ligation of veins is never performed. If the thrombus cannot be removed during the operation because of its adherence, there is also no danger of pulmonary embolism.

Even if the procedure is not successful because of an unfavourable local situation, the chances of developing a post-phlebitic syndrome are the same as in non-operated cases. The recanalization in the coming months or years is probably not adversely influenced by the surgical exploration (Wagner, 1986).

Problems

6

Venous spur

In 20–25% of cases a circumscribed stenosis at the entrance of the common iliac vein into the vena cava is found which in many of these cases might be the major cause of thrombosis. This stenosis was described by May and Thurner (1957) and is probably caused by the pulsating irritation of the crossing right iliac artery. It is nearly always possible to pass the stenosis with the balloon catheter and to dilate the spur by balloon dilatation and, if available, a stent might be inserted. Direct exploration of this area and surgical resection of the spur is not advisable as this results in a rather extensive operation. The danger of postoperative haematoma or haemorrhage as a consequence of vigorous interference and heparin therapy is high.

7

Impaction in an ascending lumbar vein

Occasionally, the Fogarty catheter, in spite of careful manipulation, repeatedly enters the lumbar ascending vein. In this case the tip of the catheter should be curved (inset). This catheter is introduced for the first few centimeters with the curve backwards and then with the curve towards the medial side of the vein in order to enter the vena cava.

Thrombus of longer duration

Even with a history of recent thrombosis, organized clots may be found during the operation, because old thrombi in the major deep veins are sometimes silent. However, acute symptoms follow sudden propagation, and occlusion of small segments (particularly the common femoral vein) as well as of small collateral branches with obstruction of venous drainage may occur. Therefore, even though the indication for venous thrombectomy is restricted to patients with a history of onset up to 5 days, an old thrombosis may be found unexpectedly during operation in the iliac and/or femoral veins in up to 50% of patients. Since the success of clot removal is directly related to intraoperatively determined thrombus age (which may not necessarily correspond to the patient's history), there are definitely two groups of patients with

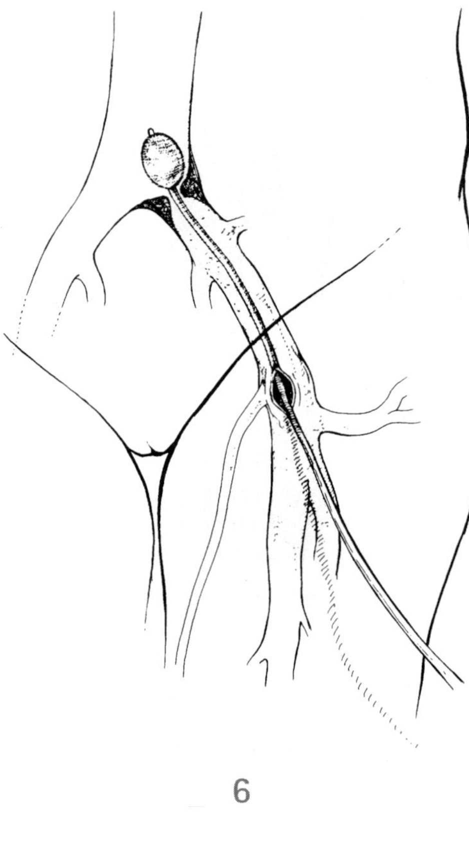

6

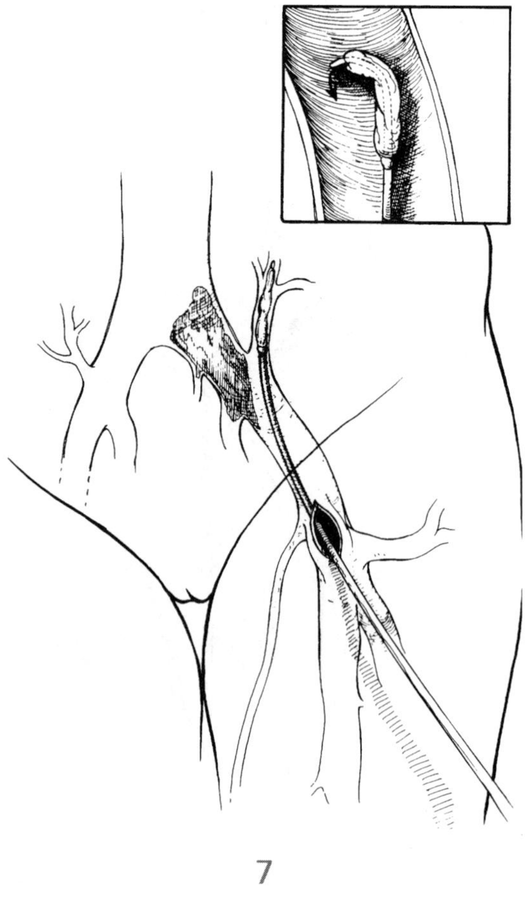

7

an entirely different prognosis. The most favourable prognosis can be made for patients with a short history of thrombosis and when recent thrombosis is found intraoperatively. The success rate is much lower in patients with a history of over a week or when a chronic thrombosis is found during surgery.

Surgical possibilities

Chronic thrombosis of the superficial femoral vein in combination with fresh iliac vein thrombosis Thrombectomy of the acute thrombus is performed on the iliac vein, thus returning the patient to the preoperative asymptomatic condition. Partial thrombectomy is also beneficial if the venous drainage from the deep femoral veins in iliac veins and vena cava can be preserved.

8

Chronic thrombosis of the iliac vein combined with acute thrombosis of the superficial femoral vein In addition to thrombectomy of the acute thrombosis of the superficial femoral vein, thrombectomy of a chronic thrombosis of the iliac vein is often possible. In many of these cases the iliac vein stays patent. If the inflow from the femoral vein is poor, the formation of an arteriovenous fistula at the inguinal level is advisable. This arteriovenous fistula is also indicated when only the deep vein circulation can be obtained. The technique recommended is to mobilize a suitable branch of the long saphenous vein as shown and anastomose its end to the side of the femoral artery.

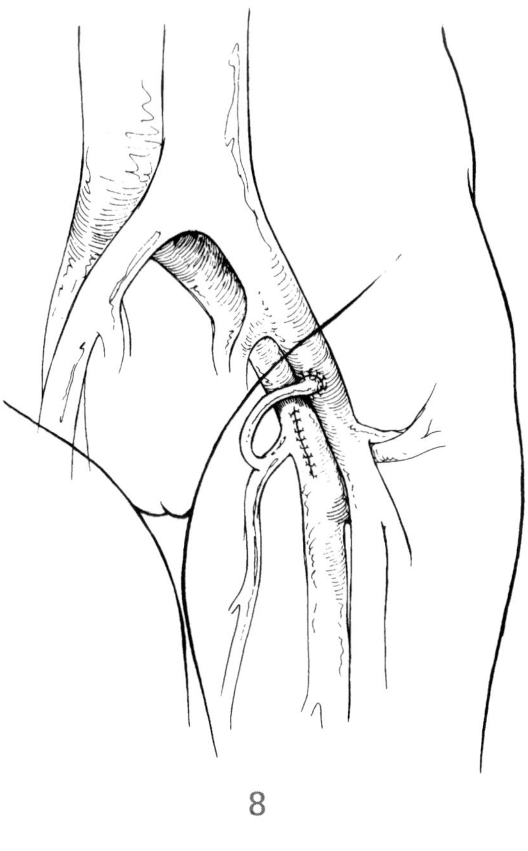

8

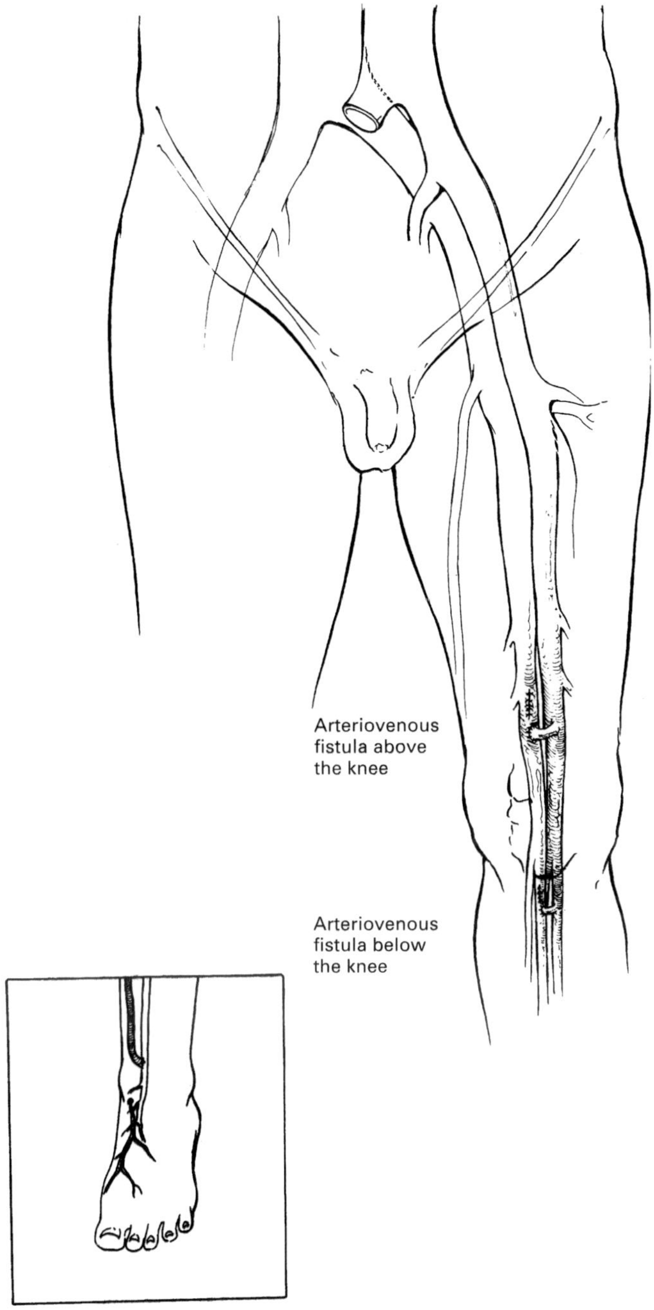

9

Additional technical factors

An obstruction in the thigh caused by a doubled superficial femoral vein makes the removal even of a recent thrombus difficult In these cases distal incisions in the proximal or distal popliteal vein are sometimes helpful. The decision can depend on the preoperatively obtained venogram.

9

A still discussed question is, whether thrombectomy should be combined with a temporary arteriovenous fistula (Swedenborg, 1991). If the thrombus is adherent but removable, a distal arteriovenous fistula on a branch of the artery or the vein keeps the thrombectomized vein open in a sufficient number of cases. These fistulae might be located at the level of the proximal or distal popliteal artery, or even at the ankle (between the long saphenous vein and the posterior tibial artery). Arteriovenous fistulae are marked with a silk suture and should be closed after 2–3 months, if they do not close spontaneously. Closure by an operation often presents a difficult technical problem, while occlusion by placing a detachable balloon under radiographic control might be achieved with a very low complication rate (Neglen *et al.*, 1991). During the function of the fistula percutaneous interventions (dilatation, stent implantation) in the arterialized venous system are feasible.

Obstruction of the iliac veins by tumour, pregnancy or chronic fibrosis of the thrombus When a thrombectomy of the femoral vein can be performed but the iliac vein cannot be cleared of thrombosis, distal thrombectomy should be combined with a femoral crossover saphenous vein bypass (Palma and Esperon, 1960). This procedure was successful in a series of cases of primary undiagnosed pelvic tumour and in cases where pregnancy was the cause of the iliac vein thrombosis (Wagner *et al.*, 1973).

Complications

Intraoperative lethal pulmonary embolism is rare (around 0.5%) when appropriate caution is taken. There are some deaths in the postoperative period in patients where peripheral pulmonary embolisms of longer duration are found, but it is difficult to decide whether this embolization occurred before, during or after surgery. It is well established, however, that the pulmonary embolism rate in patients with iliac vein thrombosis is around 75%. The older patient group also shows an additional low mortality in myocardial infarctions. A rare complication is the loss of a transplanted kidney when the unsuspected intubation of the renal vein with the Fogarty catheter and the subsequent inflation results in an arteriovenous fistula and an untreatable haematuria leading to the removal of the otherwise well-functioning kidney transplant.

Rethrombosis is observed in a variable number of cases. In a few of those, restoration of blood flow can be obtained with a second operation and repeated thrombectomy with and without an arteriovenous fistula. In many cases it is advisable to accept the spontaneous course with rethrombosis and not insist on repeated and sophisticated operations.

References

Fogarty T J, Kreppoehne W W (1965). Catheter technique for venous thrombectomy. *Surg Gynecol Obstet* **121**: 362.

Läwen A (1937). Über Thrombektomie bei Venethrombose und Arteriospasmus. *Zentralbl Chirurg* **64**: 961.

Loeprecht H, Weber H, Monnig J (1985). Vascular endoscopy. In *Diagnostic Techniques and Assessment Procedures in Vascular Surgery.* **Greenhalgh R M**, ed. London/San Diego: Grune and Stratton.

Mahorner H, Castleberry S W, Coleman W O (1957). Attempts to restore functions in major veins which are the site of massive thrombosis. *Ann Surg* **146**: 510.

May R, Thurner J (1957). The cause of the predominantly sinstral occurrence of thrombosis of the pelvic veins. *Angiology* **8**: 419.

Minar E, Ehringer H, Marosi L *et al.* (1983). Klinische, funktionelle und morphologische Spätergebnisse nach venöser Thrombektomie. *VASA* **12**: 346.

Neglen P, Al-Hassan H K, Endrys J *et al.* (1991). Iliofemoral venous thrombectomy followed by percutaneous closure of the temporary arteriovenous fistula. *Surgery* **110**: 493.

Palma E, Esperon R (1960). Vein transplants and grafts in the surgical treatment of the postphlebitic syndrome. *J Cardiovasc Surg* **1**: 94.

Polterauer P, Holzenbein T, Huk I *et al.* (1988). Die akute tiefe Bëin-Beckenvenenthrombose: Retrospektive Analyse chirurgischen Therapie ergebuisse. *Chirurg.*

Swedenborg J (1991). Surgical thrombectomy for ilio-femoral venous thromosis. *Eur J Vasc Surg* **5**: 365.

Wagner O (1986). Chirurgischen Thrombektomie. In *Angiologie 86.* **Widmer L K, Zemp E** eds. Bern: Hans Huber.

Wagner O, Piza F, Müller-Harburg W (1973). Zur chirurgischen Therapie der Beckenvenenthrombose in der Schwangerschaft. *Wien Klin Wochenschr* **85**: 17.

Iliofemoral venous thrombolysis and stenting

Syed A Babar,
AD Platts, A Watkinson

Deep vein thrombosis is amongst the most common postoperative complication. In patients over 40 years old, those undergoing pelvic or abdominal surgery for malignant disease and those having lower limb orthopaedic surgery, the incidence of peripheral venous thrombosis is reported as between 40 and 80% with propagation to involve proximal veins in 10–30% and embolism to produce a symptomatic pulmonary embolism in 0.3–3%. (Mewissen *et al.*, 1999). Post-thrombotic syndrome occurs in up to 60%. Iliofemoral venous thrombosis needs to be differentiated into isolated iliofemoral thrombosis usually due to local causes in that region and thrombosis, which propagates from the calf veins or inferior vena cava retrogradely to involve the iliofemoral segment. This differentiation is important, as the approach to treatment is different in both cases.

Lower limb thrombosis is treated as:

1. Acute (< 10 days after onset of symptoms).
2. Chronic (> 10 days after onset of symptoms).
3. Phlegmasia caerula dolens – malignant compression/occlusion.

The site of the thrombus also influences the treatment options. For iliofemoral thrombosis, May Thurner syndrome and phlegmasia caerula dulens the initial treatment includes aggressive anticoagulation and elevation. If this does not work thrombolysis is the next step.
Thombolysis regimens include

1. Systemic infusion (historical).
2. Catheter directed thrombolysis
   pulse spray technique,
   bolus plus infusion,
   continuous infusion,
   urokinase or rt-PA.
3. Concurrent heparin therapy.

Thrombolysis may reveal underlying stenosis in the venous segments, which can be dealt with by balloon dilatation or stents.

Technique for catheter directed thrombolysis

Indications

1. Limb salvage in phlegmasia caerula dolens
2. Acute iliofemoral thrombosis open parens (persistent swollen symptomatic limb despite adequate anticoagulation with low molecular weight heparin and leg elevation).
3. Chronic inferior vena cava; iliofemoral thrombosis; debilitating lower extremity pain and swelling and venous stasis ulceration.

Potential benefits

1. Rapid clot dissolution.
2. Preservation of valve function.
3. Prevention of post-thrombotic syndrome.

Potential disadvantages

Increased bleeding complications and expensive.

Approach

1, 2

Retrograde – internal jugular vein, brachial and crossover femoral. For isolated iliac vein thrombosis only. Antegrade – femoral, popliteal or posterior tibial vein.

1. The puncture is usually performed using ultrasound guidance, preferably using an echogenic needle because of the close proximity of the popliteal artery and vein in the knee and internal jugular vein and carotid artery in the neck (Illustration 1 Seldinger technique).
2. A 5 F sheath is most commonly used as an access through which subsequent wire and catheter exchanges are performed.

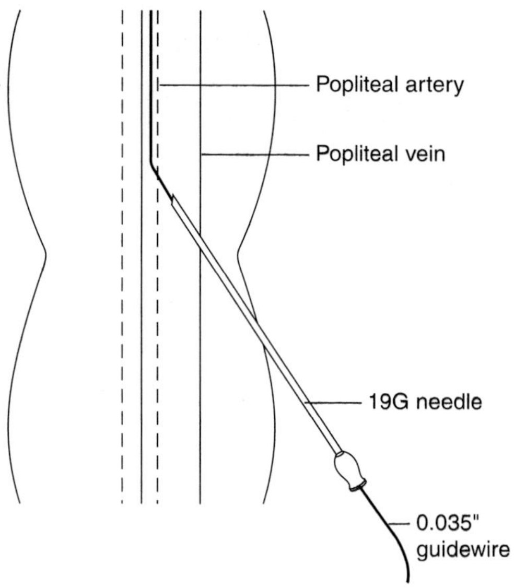

1

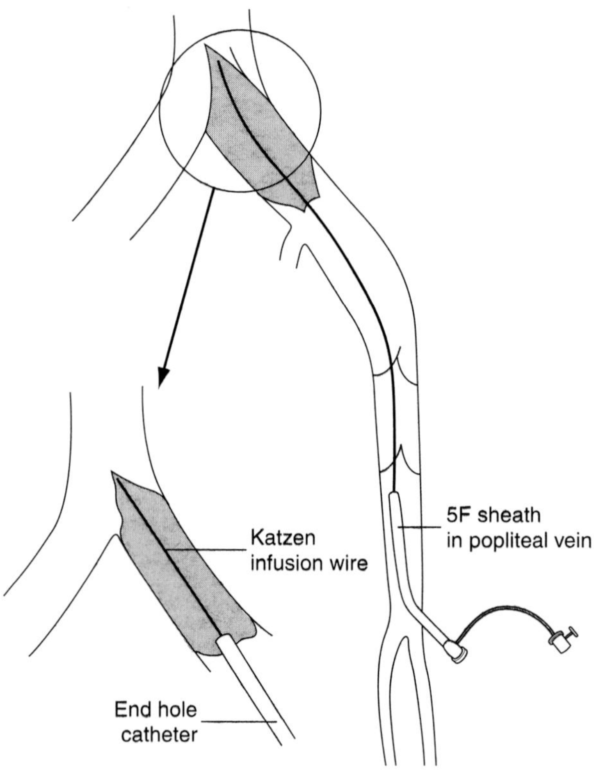

2

3. A 5 F straight catheter is used. Infusions can be performed using a coaxial catheter and guidewire and/or a double lumen multiple side-hole system. With the coaxial technique the tip of the infusion wire is placed at the distal edge of the thrombus while the end-hole catheter is positioned near the proximal puncture end. The infusion wire is about 145 cm in length and 0.035 inch in diameter (2).
4. Urokinase has been more widely used in the USA. Dose range is 0.5–44 million international units (mean 7.8 million international units). Infusion time is 2–147 hours (mean 53.4 hours).
   Altepase (rt-PA). Infusion rate is 3 mg/h and the mean duration is 29.7 h (Verhaege *et al.*, 1997).

Contraindications

1. Recent stroke.
2. Recent surgery.
3. Haemorrhagic retinopathy.
4. Recent major trauma.
5. Pregnancy
6. Intracranial malignancy

Complications

1. Active bleeding-10%.
2. Symptomatic pulmonary embolism-1%.
3. Groin haematoma.
4. Stroke.
5. Peri-catheter thrombosis.
6. Death.

Balloon angioplasty

1. Adjuvant therapy with thrombolysis to dilate stenosis.
2. Has been advocated as a primary treatment for lower limb venous thrombosis in chronic occlusions.
3. Temporary filters are commonly placed in the inferior vena cava to reduce the risk of pulmonary embolism. However research is still inconclusive.

Technique

3

1. For angioplasty in the region of common iliac/external iliac vein stenosis/thrombus, an appropriately sized sheath is used to allow the balloon catheter to pass into the vein.
2. Guidewire is used to cross the thrombus/stenosis. The guidewire tip is placed in the inferior vena cava. An appropriate size balloon is used. The balloon is placed across the stenosis. A slow and long inflation technique is considered more beneficial. A good result should see any waist of the balloon disappear on inflation (3).
3. If there is residual pressure gradient of > 10mm or collateral vessel flow after PTA, then stent insertion is advocated.

Stenting

Results of thrombolysis can be improved by adjuvant therapies namely angioplasty and stenting.

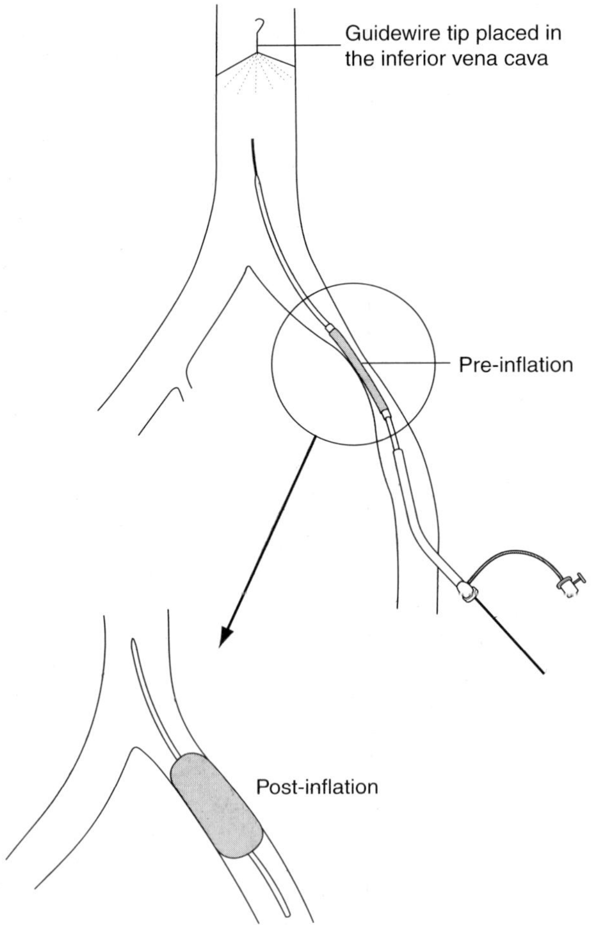

3

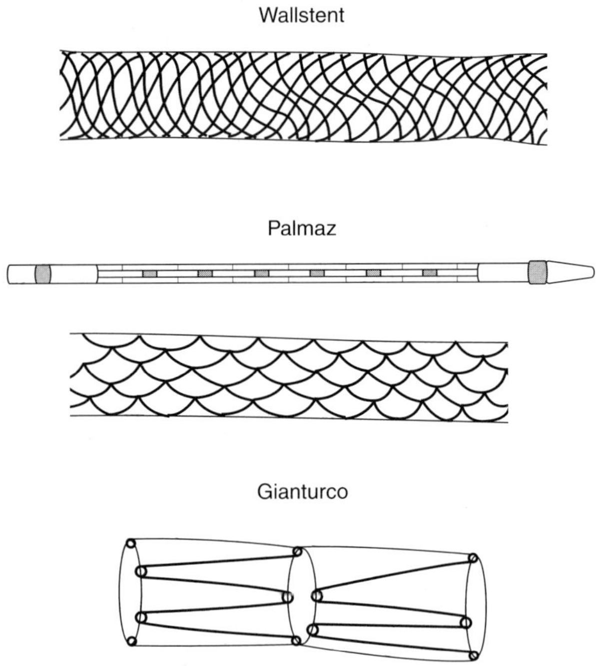

4

Indications

Stent insertion has been described for:

1. Post-thrombotic stenoses.
2. May Thurner syndrome.
3. Malignancy.
4. Radiotherapy or previous surgery.

Types of stents

4

These have been traditionally classified into expandable and self-expanding balloons (**4**).

1. Wallstents
   Commonest to be used.
   Stainless steel.
   Self-expanding.
   Flexible.
   Deployed with removable sheath delivery system.
2. Gianturco Z stent
   Self-expanding.
   Two or three stents can be joined by welding or tying to produce double or triple stents.
3. Palmaz stent
   Balloon expandable.
   Rigid.
   Preloaded on balloon.

Steps

1. Proximal and distal limits of stenosis need to be defined.
2. An appropriately sized sheath with haemostatic valve should be used.
3. Pass a 0.035-inch guidewire through the stenosis.
4. Perform balloon angioplasty prior to stent insertion using dilating balloon of 10% less than wall stent diameter. Leave guidewire across the stenosis.
5. Choose correct size of the stent depending on the size of the native vessel (**5**).
6. Pass the stent catheter over the guidewire and place it across the stenosis with the help of radio-opaque markers.
7. Deploy stent by sliding the sliding T-connector tube over the stainless steel tube.
8. Perform post-procedure angiogram through the sheath.

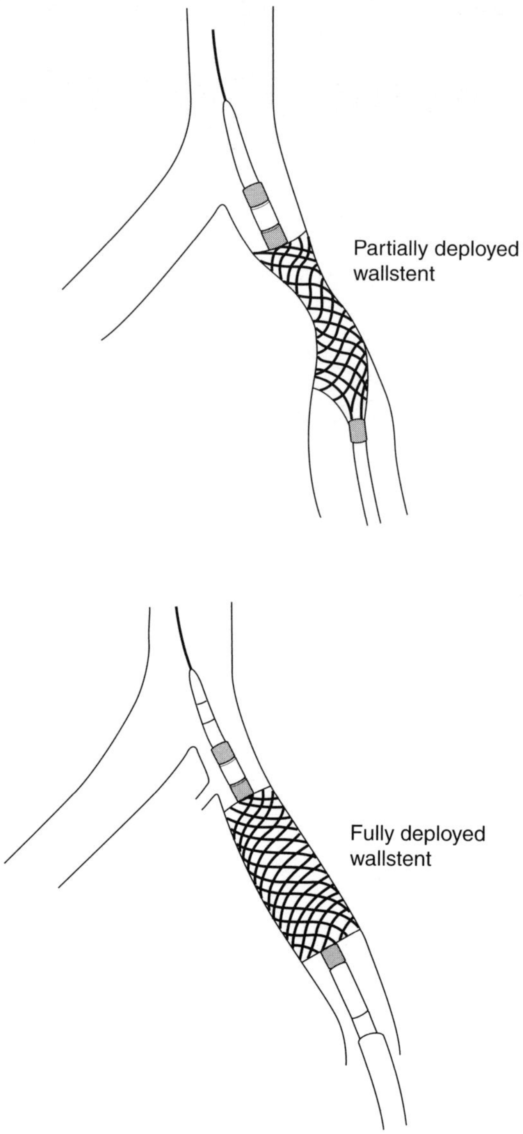

5

Complications

1. Seen in 6–8% of patients (Nazarian *et al.*, 1996).
2. Peri/post procedure haemorrhage.
3. Sepsis.
4. Fractured stents.
5. Slippage.
6. Spasm of the vessel.
7. Emboli.
8. Intimal flap.
9. Dissection.

Patency

Primary and secondary 2-year patency rates for implanted left iliac vein stents are 73% and 82% respectively. Overall primary patency for all venous stents is 50% at 1 year, while secondary patency over the same period is 80%.

Phlegmasia caerula dolens

1. Often related to underlying malignancy.
2. Pallid painful swollen cyanotic limb.
3. Current management is usually a combination of elevation, rehydration and anticoagulation, thrombolysis (both intravenous and intra-arterial), thrombectomy and amputation. If resuscitating the patient with intravenous fluids, anticoagulation and elevation of the limb does not work, proceed to thrombolysis (0.5–1.0 mg rt-PA) (Wlodarczyk *et al.*, 1994).

Summary

Indications for iliofemoral thrombolysis and stenting are:

1. Limb salvage in phlegmasia cearula dolens.
2. Acute iliofemoral thrombosis.
   Persistent swollen symptomatic limb despite adequate anticoagulation with low molecular weight heparin and aggressive elevation.
3. Chronic inferior vena cava – iliofemoral thrombosis.

Debilitating lower extremity pain and swelling and venous stasis ulceration.

References

Mewissen MW, Seabrook GR, Meissner MH *et al.* (1999). Catheter thrombolysis for lower extremity DVT: report of a national multicentre registry. *Radiology* **211**: 39–49.

Nazarian GK, Bjarnason H, Dietz C, Hunter D (1996) Iliofemoral venous stenosis: effectiveness of treatment with metallic endovascular stents. *Radiology* **200**: 193–199.

Verhaege R, Stockx L, Lacroix H *et al.* (1997). Catheter directed lysis of iliofemoral vein thrombosis with use of rt-PA. *Eur Radiol* **7**: 996–1001.

Wlodarczyk ZK, Gibson M, Dick R, Hamilton G (1994). Low dose intra-arterial thrombolysis in the treatment of Phlegmasia caerulea dolens. *Br J Surg* **81**: 370–372.

Transvenous insertion of the inferior vena caval filter

Lazar J Greenfield,
Mary C Proctor

Introduction

Most patients with thromboembolic disease can be effectively managed with anticoagulation; however, there are several situations which require mechanical protection with a vena caval filter. Through the years, the indications for filter placement have remained relatively consistent and address both failures of anticoagulation and individual patient characteristics (Brenner *et al.*, 1992; Greenfield, 1984, 1987). Those who are at risk for bleeding due to injury, physical condition or surgical procedures, those who develop a complication while receiving anticoagulants, or suffer recurrent embolism while therapeutically anticoagulated have a primary indication for filter placement. In addition, those who have undergone pulmonary embolectomy, are noted to have a propagating tail on a thrombus in a major vessel or sustain recurrent embolism after placement of another vena caval device are appropriate candidates for further mechanical protection. A final group of patients to be considered for filter placement include high risk patients with serious, underlying cardiac or pulmonary disease who may not tolerate even small pulmonary embolism. These patients may warrant prophylaxis with both anticoagulant and vena caval filter placement.

Methods

Prior to placement of a vena caval filter, patients should undergo an inferior vena cavagram to determine the level of placement and to identify any anatomical abnormalities of the cava which may affect filter placement such as megacava or extra-anatomic tributaries. Greenfield filters can be safely placed if the diameter of the cava is 28 mm or less in diameter after correction for radiographic magnification.

Multiple factors determine the appropriate level for filter placement. Routinely, the filter is positioned within the inferior vena cava at the level of the L3 vertebral body. If there is thrombus extending to or involving the renal vein or if there is pelvic or ovarian vein thrombosis, the filter should be positioned above the level of the renal veins at T12–L1. This suprarenal location is also appropriate for pregnant patients or young women of child bearing potential. This prevents compression of the filter from the pressure of the gravid uterus. Placement above the renal veins has proved safe and efficacious in long-term studies (Brenner *et al.*, 1992; Stewart *et al.*, 1982; Orsini and Jarrell, 1984; Greenfield *et al.*, 1992). On rare occasions, the filter has been inserted in the superior vena cava in an inverted position when subclavian vein thrombosis has been considered to represent a risk for pulmonary embolism (Owen *et al.*, 1992).

1

The standard Greenfield filter is fashioned from stainless steel and designed to be inserted operatively from either the right jugular or femoral vein. Alternative sites include the left jugular or left axillary vein as well as intraoperative insertion via the right atrium. Interventional radiologists have reported their experience

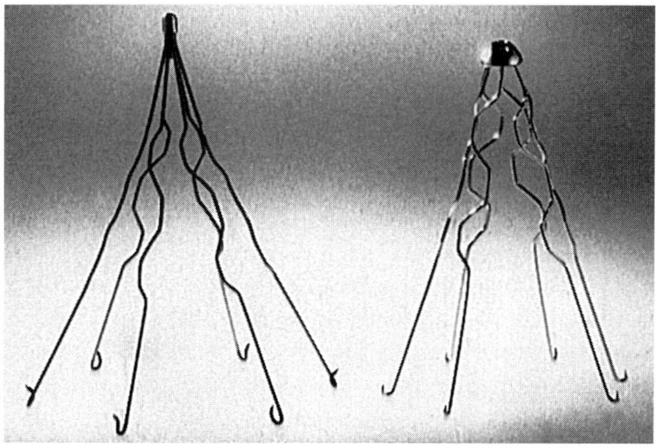

1

with percutaneous insertion of the standard Greenfield filter using the Seldinger technique for progressive dilatation to accommodate a 26 French sheath. This has been associated with a 40% incidence of insertion site thrombosis leading to the introduction of reduced profile vena caval filters designed for percutaneous placement (Kantor *et al.*, 1987; Hye *et al.*, 1990; Rose *et al.*, 1987; Pais *et al.*, 1987).

2

The smaller titanium Greenfield filter (TGF-MH) is designed to be inserted via a 12 French carrier system, is safer for percutaneous insertion and also allows intraoperative insertion directly into the inferior vena cava.

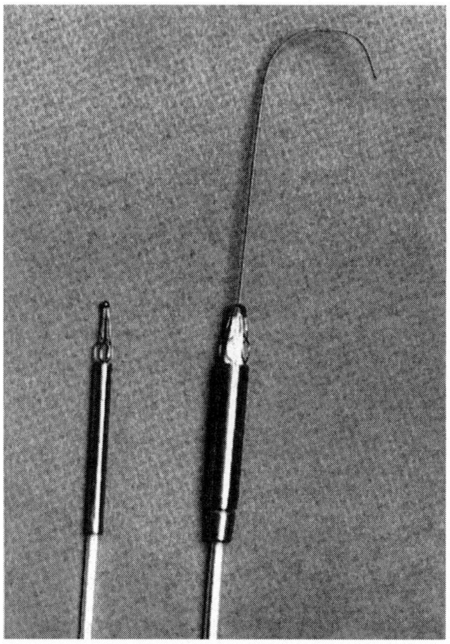

2

Operative technique

The technique of operative insertion of the standard Greenfield filter via the jugular vein will be described, then the technique of percutaneous insertion of the TGF-MH via the femoral vein. The open procedure is usually performed in the operating room on a table which allows portable fluoroscopy. Local anaesthesia is preferred, but general anaesthesia may be necessary to prevent air embolism if the patient is not cooperative.

With the head of the table slightly elevated, the patient is placed in the supine position. In order to facilitate exposure of the base of the neck, a small roll is placed under the shoulders and the head is turned to the left. To prevent wound haematoma, heparin should be discontinued 6 h prior to the procedure and may be resumed during the postoperative period.

3

A transverse incision is made one finger breadth above the clavicle overlying the sternal and clavicular heads of the sternocleidomastoid muscle. Separation of the heads of the muscle allows ready access to the internal jugular vein which is freed for a distance of at least 3 cm. After loops are passed around the vein, a vascular clamp is applied distally, taking care to avoid injury to the vagus nerve. Twill tape is preferred for proximal control to allow repeated clamping by a haemostat.

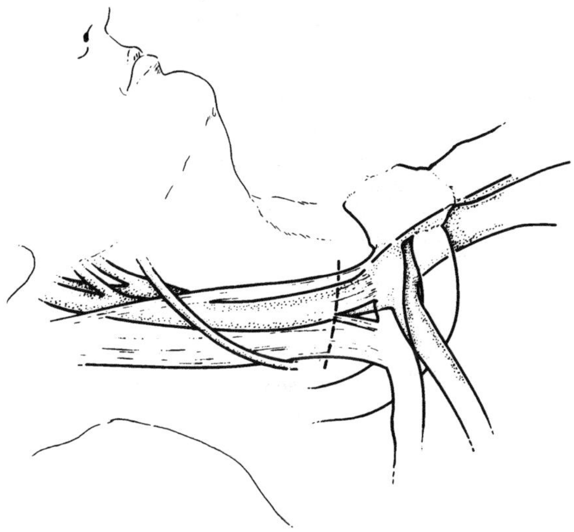

3

4

A 0.035-inch flexible tip Teflon-coated guidewire is passed through a No. 14 plastic sheath needle puncture of the jugular vein and threaded under fluoroscopy to the level of the bifurcation of the inferior vena cava. Torque manipulation is usually required in order to pass the eustachian valve at the atriocaval junction. Once the guidewire is in position, the external end is threaded retrograde through the carrier system of the standard Greenfield filter and a clamp applied to it when it emerges from the proximal catheter. The venotomy is enlarged at the point of guidewire entry by incision and clamp dilation after which the carrier is threaded over the guidewire to the desired level of filter discharge. This would be the L3 level for infrarenal discharge and the T12-L1 level for suprarenal discharge.

5

The locking hub is unscrewed to release the stylet and the main catheter is drawn backward. The filter is uncovered, springs open, and attaches to the wall of the inferior vena cava.

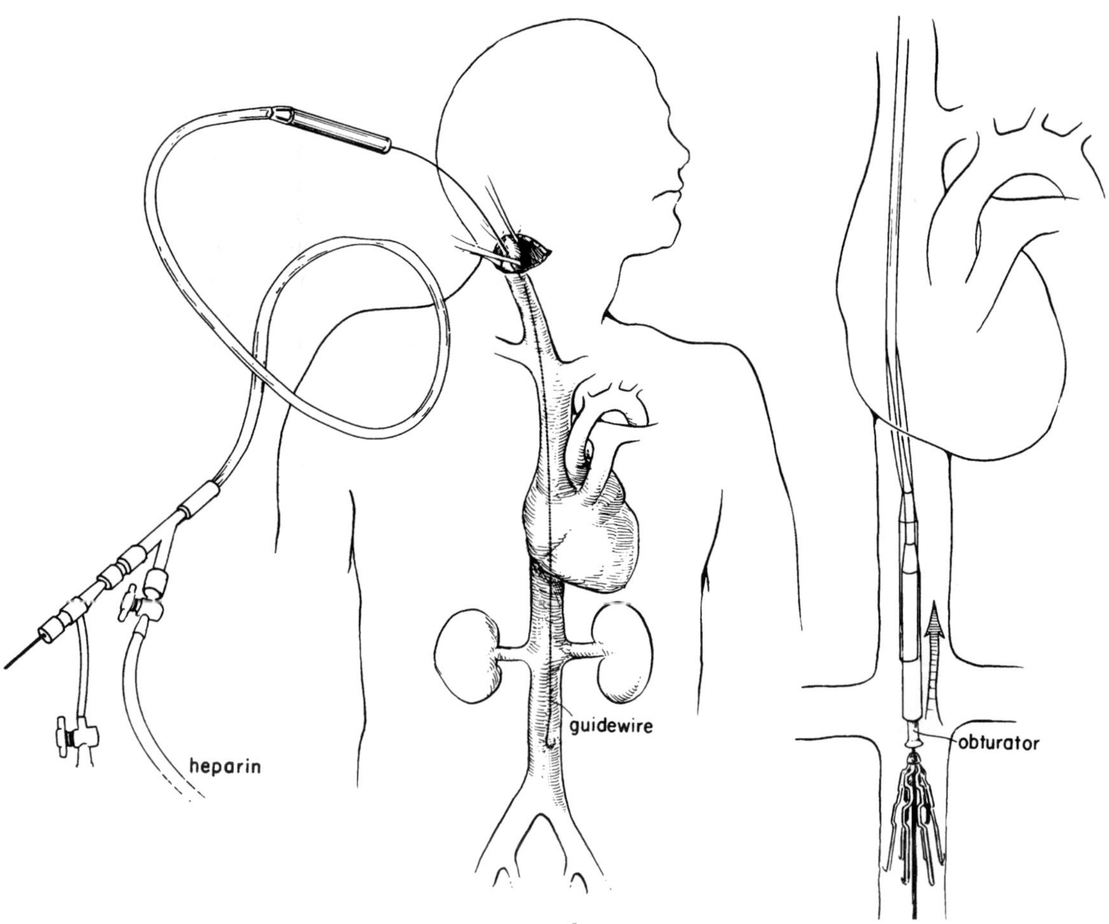

4

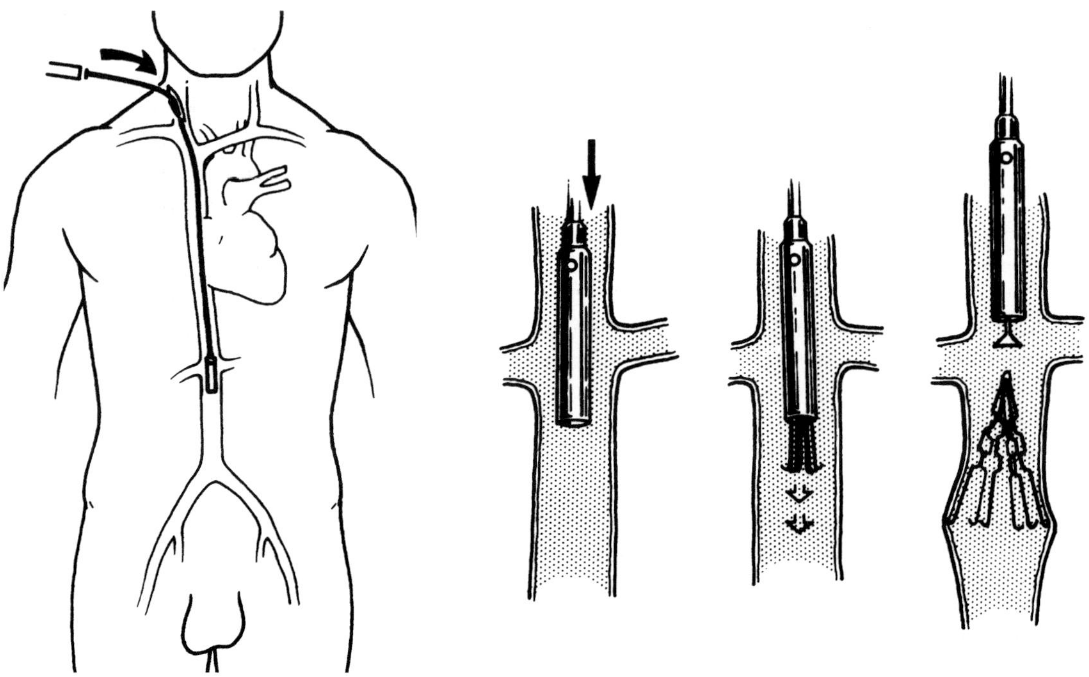

5

6

The carrier system and guidewire are withdrawn and the jugular venotomy is repaired using continuous polypropylene suture. Meticulous haemostasis is obtained and the wound is closed without drainage, usually with subcuticular closure. A compression dressing is applied with elastic adhesive tape.

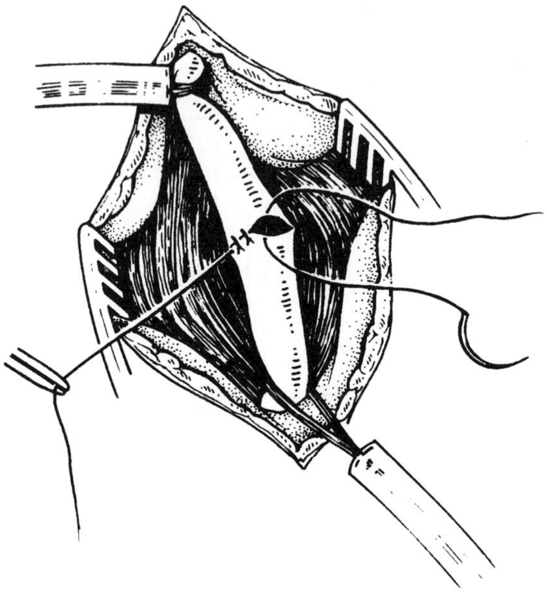

6

Percutaneous technique

7

Four percutaneous vena caval filters are currently approved for use by the FDA. These include the Bird's Nest filter (Cook, Bloomington IN), the Simon Nitinol filter (Nitinol Medical Technologies, Worburn, MA), the Vena Tech filter (Vena Tech, Evanston, IL) and the Greenfield Titanium Filter (Medi-Tech, Watertown, MA). Each device offers a low profile delivery system but they differ significantly in design and performance characteristics.

Placement is usually performed in the radiology suite, at the time of pulmonary angiography or venacavography. The presence of iliofemoral venous thrombosis is a contraindication to the use of that side for percutaneous filter insertion. Although the left common iliac vein is usually flattened by the crossover of the right common iliac artery, the smaller size of the TGF-MH carrier system allows it to be inserted from the left if no other route is available.

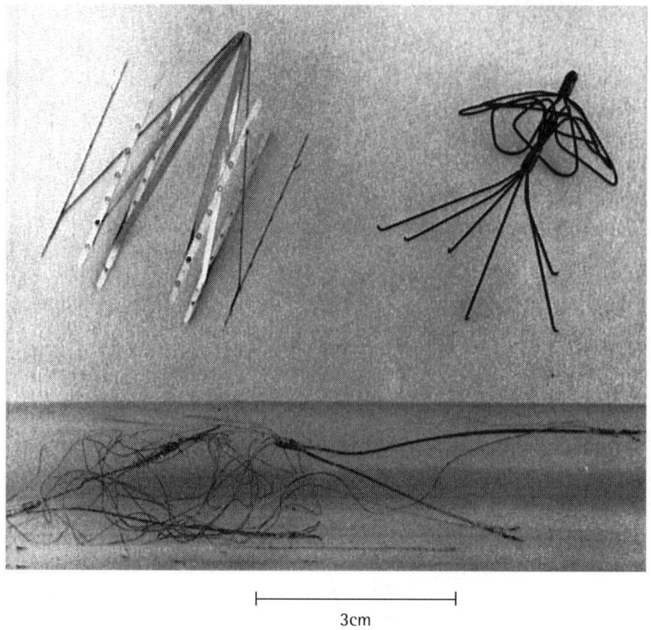

7

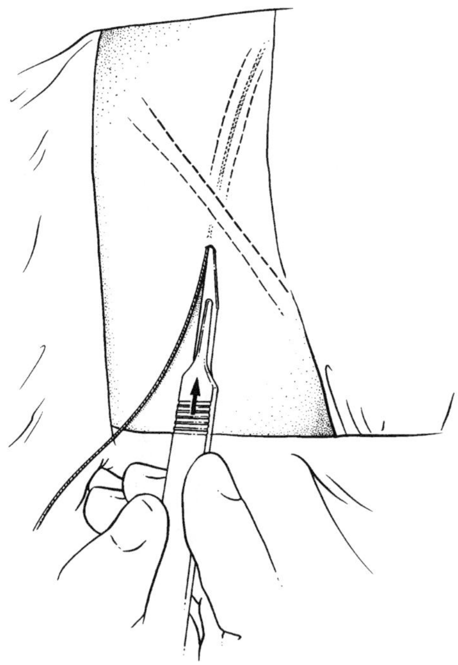

8

8

Under local anaesthesia, percutaneous needle aspiration of the common femoral vein is performed. A guidewire is passed through an attached plastic cannula once the needle is withdrawn. The cannula is removed and a small skin incision is made in order to allow passage of the dilator and sheath over the guidewire.

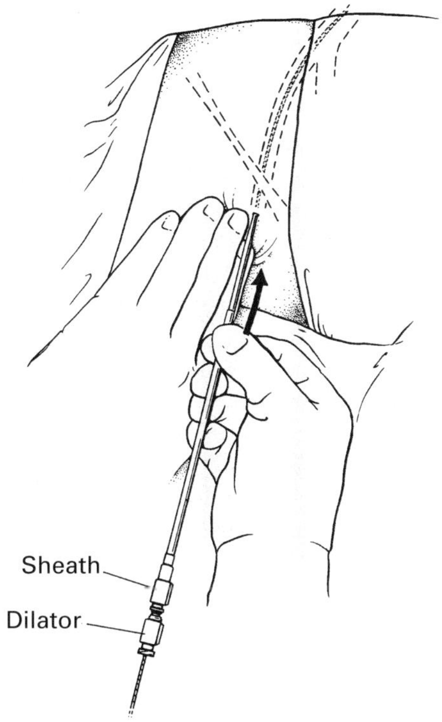

9

9

The dilator and sheath are passed under fluoroscopy over the guidewire into the inferior vena cava. Once the dilator and sheath are positioned in the vena cava, the dilator and guidewire are withdrawn, leaving the sheath in place.

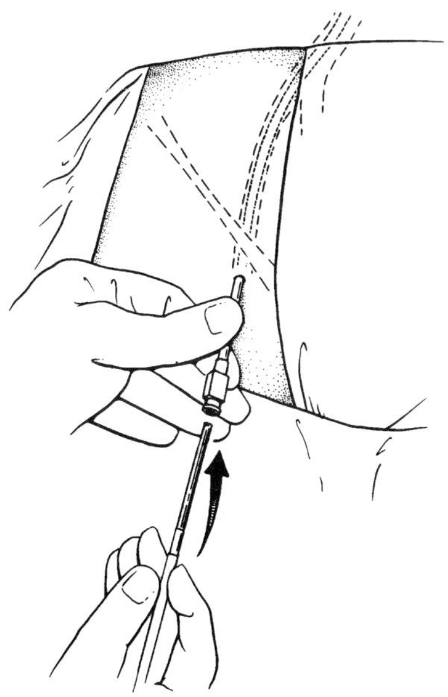

10

10

The filter carrier is then introduced into the sheath. Prior to insertion of the carrier system, the sheath should be flushed with heparinized saline to prevent air embolism and thrombus formation within the carrier system. Digital occlusion of the luerlock will avoid excessive blood loss.

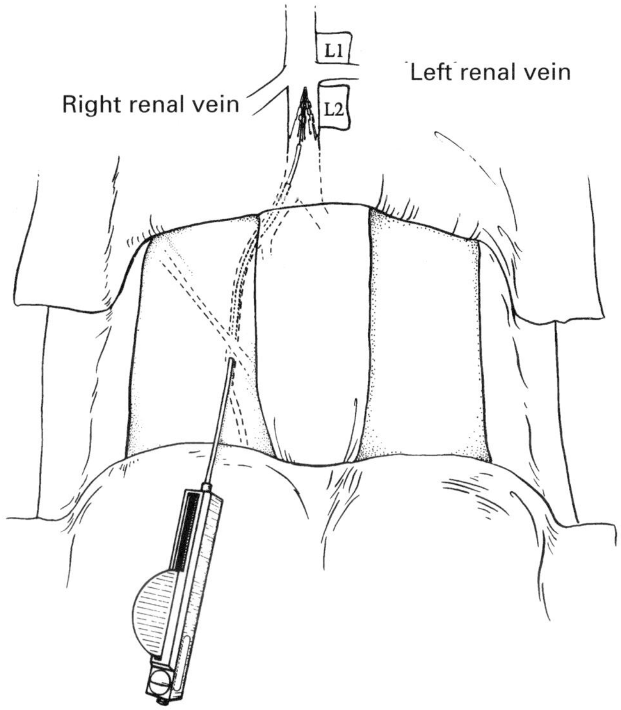

11

11

In order to prevent accidental release of the filter into the sheath, it is important to advance the carrier through the sheath until the sheath hub contacts the control handle. Using fluoroscopic guidance, the carrier should be positioned at the level of L3. The locking mechanism on the control handle is released by moving the control tab to the unlock position. The control tab is then slid backward which uncovers and discharges the filter. The carrier and sheath are withdrawn and pressure is applied to the puncture site to establish haemostasis. A pressure dressing may be applied.

Regardless of the method of delivery, a follow-up radiograph should be obtained to document filter position.

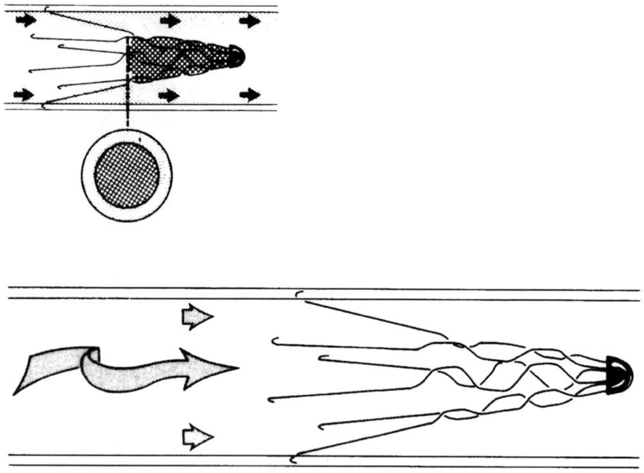

12

12

Long-term patency of the Greenfield filter is in excess of 95% due to its geometry (Greenfield, 1984; Greenfield *et al.*, 1981, 1982; Greenfield and Michna, 1988). The cone shape of the filter allows it to be filled to 70% of its depth by emboli without interfering with flow. Preservation of flow allows for spontaneous resolution of entrapped thrombi, with or without systemic anticoagulation. Anticoagulation should always be used to control the underlying thrombotic disorder, but is not necessary for long-term patency of the filter. The design also enhances entrapment of smaller thrombi, since axial flow is directed into the apex of the filter.

Complications

The use of Greenfield vena caval filters is associated with minimal morbidity. Reports of isolated limb penetration have been published but are rarely associated with clinical sequelae. The filter can be deformed and limbs extruded from the cava by external forces at the time of laparotomy or through the flaccid abdominal wall of the quadriplegic during a 'quad cough'. Misplacement of the filter at discharge is rare if the guidewire is used during surgical placement and is eliminated with the use of the sheath during percutaneous delivery. Apparent movement of the filter noted at follow-up is virtually without clinical significance and is often due to radiographic parallax or respiratory variation. Although a few cases of filter tilting have been noted, long-term follow-up studies fail to show a clinical relationship between tilt and the recurrence of PE (Messmer and Greenfield, 1985).

References

Brenner D, Brenner C, Scott J *et al.* (1992). Suprarenal Greenfield filter placement to prevent pulmonary embolus in patients with vena caval tumor thrombi. *J Urol* **147**: 19.

Greenfield L (1984). Current indications for and results of Greenfield filter placement. *J Vasc Surg* **1**: 502.

Greenfield L (1987). Vena caval filter placement for prevention of pulmonary embolism: Patient selection and results. *Pract Cardiol* **13**: 100.

Greenfield L, Michna B (1988). Twelve-year clinical experience with the Greenfield vena caval filter. *Surgery* **104**: 706.

Greenfield L, Peyton R, Crute S, Barnes R (1981). Greenfield vena caval filter experience: Late results in 156 patients. *Arch Surg* **116**: 11451.

Greenfield L, Cho KJ, Proctor M *et al.* (1982). Late results of suprarenal Greenfield vena cava filter placement. *Arch Surg* **127**: 969.

Hye R, Mitchell A, Dory C *et al.* (1990). Analysis of the transition to percutaneous placement of Greenfield filters. *Arch Surg* **125**: 1550.

Kantor A, Glanz S, Gordon DH, Sclafani SJ (1987). Percutaneous insertion of the Kimray-Greenfield filter: Incidence of femoral vein thrombosis. *Am J Roentgenol* **149**: 1065.

Messmer J, Greenfield L (1985). Greenfield caval filters: long-term radiographic follow-up study. *Radiology* **156**: 613.

Orsini R, Jarrell B (1984). Suprarenal placement of vena caval filters: Indications, techniques, and results. *J Vasc Surg* **1**: 125.

Owen E, Schoettle P, Harrington O (1992). Placement of a Greenfield filter in the superior vena cava. *Annl Thorac Surg* **53**: 896.

Pais O, Mirvis S, De Orchis D (1987). Percutaneous insertion of the Kimray-Greenfield filter: Technical considerations and problems. *Radiology* **165**: 377.

Rose B, Simon D, Hess M, Van Aman M (1987). Percutaneous transfemoral placement of the Kimray-Greenfield vena cava filter. *Radiology* **165**: 373.

Stewart J, Peyton W, Crute S, Greenfield L (1982). Clinical results of suprarenal placement of the Greenfield vena cava filter. *Surgery* **92**: 1.